MW01196841

Shoulder Arthroplasty
Principles and Practice

Shoulder Arthroplasty
Principles and Practice

LIBRARY OF CONGRESS SURPLUS DUPLICATE

EDITOR

Joseph D. Zuckerman, MD
Professor and Chair
Department of Orthopedic Surgery
NYU Grossman School of Medicine
Suregon-in-Chief
NYU Langone Orthopedic Hospital
NYU Langone Health
New York, New York

Illustrations by Bernie Kida

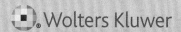
. Wolters Kluwer

Philadelphia • Baltimore • New York • London
Buenos Aires • Hong Kong • Sydney • Tokyo

Director, Medical Practice: Brian Brown
Senior Development Editor: Stacey Sebring
Editorial Coordinator: Lindsay Ries
Marketing Manager: Phyllis Hitner
Production Project Manager: Barton Dudlick
Design Coordinator: Stephen Druding
Manufacturing Coordinator: Beth Welsh
Prepress Vendor: TNQ Technologies

First edition

Copyright © 2022 Wolters Kluwer.

Copyright © 2022 Wolters Kluwer Health/Lippincott Williams & Wilkins. All rights reserved. This book is protected by copyright. No part of this book may be reproduced or transmitted in any form or by any means, including as photocopies or scanned-in or other electronic copies, or utilized by any information storage and retrieval system without written permission from the copyright owner, except for brief quotations embodied in critical articles and reviews. Materials appearing in this book prepared by individuals as part of their official duties as U.S. government employees are not covered by the above-mentioned copyright. To request permission, please contact Wolters Kluwer at Two Commerce Square, 2001 Market Street, Philadelphia, PA 19103, via email at permissions@lww.com, or via our website at shop.lww.com (products and services).

9 8 7 6 5 4 3 2 1

Printed in China

Library of Congress Cataloging-in-Publication Data

ISBN-13: 978-1-975157-66-1

Cataloging in Publication data available on request from publisher.

This work is provided "as is," and the publisher disclaims any and all warranties, express or implied, including any warranties as to accuracy, comprehensiveness, or currency of the content of this work.

This work is no substitute for individual patient assessment based upon healthcare professionals' examination of each patient and consideration of, among other things, age, weight, gender, current or prior medical conditions, medication history, laboratory data and other factors unique to the patient. The publisher does not provide medical advice or guidance and this work is merely a reference tool. Healthcare professionals, and not the publisher, are solely responsible for the use of this work including all medical judgments and for any resulting diagnosis and treatments.

Given continuous, rapid advances in medical science and health information, independent professional verification of medical diagnoses, indications, appropriate pharmaceutical selections and dosages, and treatment options should be made and healthcare professionals should consult a variety of sources. When prescribing medication, healthcare professionals are advised to consult the product information sheet (the manufacturer's package insert) accompanying each drug to verify, among other things, conditions of use, warnings and side effects and identify any changes in dosage schedule or contraindications, particularly if the medication to be administered is new, infrequently used or has a narrow therapeutic range. To the maximum extent permitted under applicable law, no responsibility is assumed by the publisher for any injury and/or damage to persons or property, as a matter of products liability, negligence law or otherwise, or from any reference to or use by any person of this work.

shop.lww.com

CCS0721

DEDICATION

My senior shoulder mentors, Robert H. Cofield, MD, and Frederick A. Matsen, MD, who developed my interest in shoulder arthroplasty and continued to provide their support throughout my career.

My colleague mentors, Pierre-Henri Flurin, MD, and Thomas W. Wright, MD, who for the past 18 years have greatly enhanced my knowledge and understanding of shoulder arthroplasty.

And of course, to my wonderful family, my wife, Janet Rivkin Zuckerman, and my children, Scott and Autumn Zuckerman and their sweet Avery, and Matthew Zuckerman and his partner Nicholas Pandolfi, you have made my life and career all it could possibly be.

JDZ

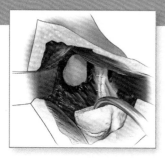

Contents

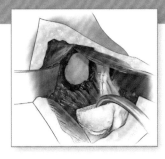

Contributors

Laurent Angibaud, Dipl. Ing.
Vice-President of Development
Exactech, Inc.
Gainesville, Florida

Samuel Antuña, MD, PhD
Director of Shoulder & Elbow Unit
Department of Orthopedic Surgery
Hospital Universitario La Paz
Madrid, Spain

Michael A. Boin, MD
Clinical Instructor
Department of Orthopaedic Surgery
NYU Langone Health
New York, New York

Joseph A. Bosco III, MD, FAAOS
Professor
Director of Quality and Patient Safety
Vice Chair for Clinical Affairs
Department of Orthopedic Surgery
NYU Langone Health
New York, New York

Stephen F. Brockmeier, MD
Associate Professor
Department of Orthopedic Surgery-Sports Medicine
University of Virginia
Charlottesville, Viginia

Daniel B. Buchalter, MD
Department of Orthopedic Surgery
NYU Langone Health
New York, New York

Geert Alexander Buijze, MD, PhD, FEBHS
Orthopedic Hand and Upper Extremity Surgeon
Department of Orthopaedic Surgery
Clinique Générale
Annecy, France
Department of Orthopaedic Surgery
Montpellier University
Lapeyronie Medical Center
Montpellier, France

Ian R. Byram, MD
Shoulder, Elbow and Sports Medicine
Bone and Joint Institute of Tennessee
Franklin, Tennessee

Jeffrey S. Chen, MD
Department of Orthopedic Surgery
NYU Langone Health
New York, New York

Chrissy J. Cherenfant, MD
Department of Anesthesiology
Weil Cornell Medicine
New York, New York

Ryan Colley, DO
Orthopedic Surgeon
Advanced Joint Replacement Center of Southern Oregon
Medford, Oregon

Cory G. Couch, MD
Department of Orthopedic Surgery
Mayo Clinic
Rochester, Minnesota

Bertrand Coulet, MD, PhD
Professor of Orthopaedic Surgery
Hand and Upper Extremity Surgery Unit
Montpellier University Medical Center
Montpellier, France

Lynn A. Crosby, MD
Clinical Professor
Department of Orthopaedic Surgery
University of Nebraska Medical Center
Omaha, Nebraska

Patrick Denard, MD
Oregon Shoulder Institute
Medford, Oregon

Matthew J. DiPaola, MD
Clinical Associate Professor
Department of Orthopaedics and Sports Medicine
University at Buffalo Jacobs School of Medicine
Buffalo, New York

Kenneth A. Egol, MD
Professor and Vice Chair
Department of Orthopedic Surgery
NYU Langone Orthopedic Hospital
NYU Langone Health
New York, New York

Josie Elwell, PhD
Product Design Engineer
Upper Extremities
Exactech, Inc.
Gainesville, Florida

Brandon J. Erickson, MD
Assistant Professor
Jefferson University School of Medicine
Zucker School of Medicine
Department of Orthopaedic Surgery
New York, New York

Kenneth J. Faber, MD, MHPE
Professor
Department of Surgery
Western University
London, Ontario

Kevin W. Farmer, MD
Peter Indelicato Professor in Orthopaedic Surgery and Sports
 Medicine
Department of Orthopaedic Surgery, Sports Medicine, and
 Shoulder Surgery
University of Florida
Gainesville, Florida

Pierre-Henri Flurin, MD
Shoulder Orthopedic Surgeon
C.E.O. Bordeaux Merignac Sport Clinic
Merignac, France

Mark A. Frankle, MD
Professor of Orthopedic Surgery
Department of Orthopaedics and Sports Medicine
University of South Florida Morsani College of Medicine
Florida Orthopaedic Institute, Shoulder Service
Tampa, Florida

Alex Friedman, DO
Department of Orthopaedic Surgery
Community Memorial Health System
Ventura, California

Richard J. Friedman, MD
Chief, Department of Shoulder and Elbow Surgery
Professor, Department of Orthopaedics
Medical University of South Carolina
Charleston, South Carolina

Christoph H. G. Fuchs, MD
Fellow, Department of Orthopaedic Surgery
The University of Texas Health Science Center at Houston
 - UT Orthopaedics
Houston, Texas

Robert K. Fullick, MD
Assistant Professor & Director of the Shoulder Service
Department of Orthopaedic Surgery
The University of Texas Health Science Center at Houston –
 UT Orthopaedics
Houston, Texas

Leesa M. Galatz, MD
Mount Sinai Professor and Chair
Leni & Peter May Department of Orthopedics
Icahn School of Medicine at Mount Sinai
Mount Sinai Health System
New York, New York

C. Parker Gibbs Jr, MD
Professor and Chief, Musuloskeletal Oncology
Department of Orthopaedic Surgery
University of Florida
Gainesville, Florida

Gregory J. Gilot, MD
Levitetz Department of Orthopaedic Surgery
Shoulder Service - Sports Health
Cleveland Clinic Florida
Weston, Florida

Alexander R. Graf, MD
Department of Orthopedic Surgery
Medical College of Wisconsin
Milwaukee, Wisconsin

Alexander T. Greene, BS
Field Clinical Engineer
Exactech, Inc.
Gainesville, Florida

Sean G. Grey, MD
Shoulder and Sports Medicine
Orthopedic and Spine Center of The Rockies
Fort Collins, Colorado

Steven I. Grindel, MD
Professor
Department of Orthopedic Surgery
Medical College of Wisconsin
Milwaukee, Wisconsin

Lawrence Gulotta, MD
Chief of Shoulder and Elbow Division
Sports Medicine Institute
Hospital for Special Surgery
Associate Professor
Department of Surgery (Orthopedics)
Weill Cornell School of Medicine
New York, New York

Georges Haidamous, MD
Department of Orthopaedics and Sports Medicine
University of South Florida Morsani College of Medicine
Florida Orthopaedic Institute, Shoulder Service
Tampa, Florida

Matthew L. Hansen, MD
OrthoArizona
Gilbert, Arizona

Joseph P. Iannotti, MD, PhD
Professor of Orthopaedic Surgery
Cleveland Clinic Lerner College of Medicine Case Western
  University
Chief of Staff
Chief Academic and Innovation Officer
Cleveland Clinic Florida
Weston, Florida

Reza Jazayeri, MD
Associate Professor
Department of Orthopaedic Surgery
Southern California Permanente Group
Woodlands Hills, California

Andrew R. Jensen, MD, MBE
Assistant Professor
Department of Orthopaedic Surgery
University of California
Los Angeles, California

Toufic R. Jildeh, MD
Department of Orthopaedic Surgery
Henry Ford Health System
Detroit, Michigan

Charles M. Jobin, MD
Louis U. Bigliani Associate Professor of Orthopedic Surgery
Residency Program Director
Associate Director, Shoulder and Elbow Fellowship
Center for Shoulder, Elbow and Sports Medicine
Columbia University Vagelos College of Physicians and
  Surgeons
NYP/Columbia University Medical Center
New York, New York

Richard B. Jones, MD
Southeastern Sports Medicine and Orthopedics
Asheville, North Carolina

Christopher M. Kilian, MD
Orthopaedic Associates of Wisconsin
Associate Professor
Department of Orthopaedic Surgery
Medical College of Wisconsin
Milwaukee, Wisconsin

Joseph J. King, MD
Associate Professor
Department of Orthopaedics and Rehabilitation
University of Florida
Gainesville, Florida

James Koo, PT, DPT
Outpatient Physical Therapy Department
Rusk Rehabilitation
NYU Langone Health
New York, New York

Young W. Kwon, MD, PhD
Associate Professor
Department of Orthopedic Surgery
NYU Langone Health
New York, New York

Joseph T. Labrum IV, MD
Department of Orthopaedic Surgery
Vanderbilt Medical Center
Nashville, Tennessee

G. Daniel Langohr, PhD
Assistant Professor
Department of Engineering
Western University
London, Ontario

William N. Levine, MD
Frank E. Stinchfield Professor and Chairman
Department of Orthopedic Surgery
Chief, Shoulder Service, Co-Director, Center for Shoulder,
  Elbow and Sports Medicine
Columbia University Vagelos College of Physicians and
  Surgeons
NYP/Columbia University Medical Center
New York, New York

Jonathan C. Levy, MD
Chief of Orthopedics
Department of Shoulder & Elbow Surgery
Program Director, Holy Cross Shoulder & Elbow Fellowship
Medical Director, Holy Cross Orthopedic Research Institute
Holy Cross Orthopedic Institute
Fort Lauderdale, Florida

Diego Lima, MD
Shoulder and Elbow / Sports Medicine Surgery
Adult Reconstruction Surgery
Department of Orthopaedics
Center for Bone and Joint Surgery
Wellington, Florida

Tyler A. Luthringer, MD
Department of Orthopedic Surgery
NYU Langone Health
New York, New York

Kevin M. Magone, MD
Shoulder and Elbow Surgery
CHI Saint Joseph Medical Group - Orthopedic Associates
London, United Kingdom

Jared M. Mahylis, MD
Department of Orthopedics
Midwestern University
Franciscan Health
Olympia Fields, Illinois

Peter D. McCann, MD
Professor
Department of Orthopedic Surgery
Zucker School of Medicine at Hofstra/Northwell
New York, New York

Brent Mollon, MD, MSc
Orthopaedic Surgeon, Simcoe-Muskoka Orthopaedics
Chief of Orthopaedics
Orillia Soldiers Memorial Hospital
Orillia, Ontario

Stephanie J. Muh, MD
Division Chief of Shoulder and Elbow Surgery
Deputy Chief, Orthopaedic Surgery Service - Henry Ford
    West Bloomfield Hospital
Associate Program Director - Sports Medicine Fellowship
Department of Orthopaedic Surgery
Henry Ford Health System
Detroit, Michigan

Surena Namdari, MD
Associate Professor
Department of Orthopaedic Surgery
The Sidney Kimmel Medical College at Thomas Jefferson
    University
Philadelphia, Pennsylvania

Curtis R. Noel, MD
Crystal Clinic Orthopaedic Center
Akron, Ohio

Rick F. Papandrea, MD
Orthopaedic Associates of Wisconsin
Associate Professor
Department of Orthopaedic Surgery
Medical College of Wisconsin
Milwaukee, Wisconsin

Stephen A. Parada, MD
Associate Professor, Director of Shoulder Surgery
Department of Orthopaedics
Medical College of Georgia at Augusta University
Augusta, Georgia

Brad Parsons, MD
Professor and Vice Chair of Education
Leni and Peter May Department of Orthopaedic Surgery
Icahn School of Medicine at Mount Sinai
New York, New York

Moby Parsons, MD
Attending Physician
The Knee Hip and Shoulder Center
Portsmouth, New Hampshire

Sri Pinnamaneni, MD
Shoulder and Elbow Division
Department of Orthopedics
Signature Orthopedics
St. Louis, Missouri

Eric T. Ricchetti, MD
Associate Professor
Cleveland Clinic Lerner College of Medicine of Case Western
    Reserve University
Staff, Department of Orthopaedic Surgery
Cleveland Clinic
Cleveland, Ohio

Christopher P. Roche, MSBE, MBA
Vice President, Extremities
Exactech, Inc.
Gainesville, Florida

Anthony A. Romeo, MD
Executive Vice President
Musculoskeletal Institute
Dupage Medical Group
Westmont, Illinois

Yoav Rosenthal, MD
Shoulder and Elbow Division
Department of Orthopaedic Surgery
Tel Aviv University
Petah Tikva, Israel

Howard D. Routman, DO
Assistant Professor
Department of Surgery
Nova Southeastern University
Davie, Florida

Kaveh R. Sajadi, MD
Kentucky Bone & Joint Surgeons
Assistant Professor
Department of Orthopaedics
University of Kentucky
Lexington, Kentucky

Joaquin Sanchez-Sotelo, MD, PhD
Consultant and Professor
Department of Orthopedic Surgery
Mayo Clinic and Mayo Clinic Alix School of Medicine
Rochester, Minnesota

Bradley S. Schoch, MD
Associate Professor
Department of Orthopedic Surgery
Mayo Clinic
Jacksonville, Florida

Blake J. Schultz, MD
Department of Orthopedic Surgery
NYU Langone Orthopedic Hospital
NYU Langone Health
New York, New York

Ryan W. Simovitch, MD
Director
Shoulder Division
Associate Medical Director Ambulatory Services
Hospital for Special Surgery
West Palm Beach, Florida

Jason B. Smoak, MD
Department of Orthopaedic Surgery
University at Buffalo
Buffalo, New York

John W. Sperling, MD, MBA
Professor
Department of Orthopedic Surgery
Mayo Clinic
Rochester, Minnesota

Jennifer Tangtiphaiboontana, MD
Assistant Professor
Department of Orthopaedic Surgery
University of California
San Francisco, California

Thomas (Quin) Throckmorton, MD
Professor and Vice Chief of Staff
Shoulder and Elbow Surgery
Department of Orthopaedic Surgery
University of Tennessee-Campbell Clinic
Memphis, Tennessee

Uchenna O. Umeh, MD
Assistant Professor
Associate Regional Fellowship Director
Co-Director, Ambulatory Anesthesia
Department of Anesthesiology, Perioperative Care and Pain
  Medicine
NYU Langone Health
NYU Langone Orthopedic Hospital
New York, New York

Thomas Vanasse, MS
Director of Engineering
Upper Extremities
Exactech, Inc.
Gainesville, Florida

Laura Vasquez-Welsh, MS, OT/L, CHT
Outpatient Hand Therapy Department
Rusk Rehabilitation
NYU Langone Health
New York, New York

Alexander J. Vervaecke, MD
Department of Orthopaedic Surgery
The Mount Sinai Hospital
New York, New York
University Hospital Antwerp
Antwerp, Belgium

Mandeep Singh Virk, MD
Assistant Professor
Department of Orthopedic Surgery
NYU Grossman School of Medicine
NYU Langone Orthopedic Hospital
NYU Langone Health
New York, New York

Jordan D. Walters, MD
Orthopedic Surgeon-Sports Medicine
Tallahassee Orthopedic Clinic
Tallahassee, Florida

Jessica Welter, DO
Staff Surgeon
Department of Orthopaedic Surgery
Mercy Clinic
Washington, Missouri

Jean-David Werthel, MD
Department of Orthopedic Surgery
Hopital Ambroise Pare
Boulogne-Billancourt, France

Gerald R. Williams Jr, MD
John M. Fenlin, Jr., MD Professor of Shoulder and Elbow
  Surgery
Department of Orthopaedic Surgery
The Sidney Kimmel Medical College at Thomas Jefferson
  University
Philadelphia, Pennsylvania

Thomas W. Wright, MD
Professor
Department of Orthopedic Surgery
University of Florida School of Medicine
Gainesville, Florida

Ari R. Youderian, MD
South County Orthopedic Specialists, a Division of
  Orthowest
Laguna Woods, California

Stephen Yu, MD
Department of Orthopedic Surgery
NYU Langone Health
New York, New York

Robert M. Zbeda, MD
Department of Orthopedic Surgery
Lenox Hill Hospital/Northwell Health
New York, New York

Joseph D. Zuckerman, MD
Professor and Chair
Department of Orthopedic Surgery
NYU Grossman School of Medicine
Surgeon-in-Chief
NYU Langone Orthopedic Hospital
NYU Langone Health
New York, New York

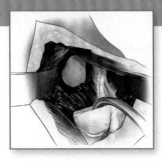

Foreword

It is indeed an honor to write a foreword for *Shoulder Arthroplasty: Principles and Practice* by Joseph D. Zuckerman and his colleagues. I have had the pleasure of knowing Joe since his first day as an orthopedic resident here at the University of Washington. From that point, it was apparent that he would become a major force in our field, subsequently exemplified by his presidencies of the American Shoulder and Elbow Surgeons and the American Academy of Orthopaedic Surgeons. His fellowship at the Brigham and Women's Hospital and his stay as a visiting clinician in shoulder surgery at the Mayo Clinic set the stage for his intense interest in investigating, performing, and teaching shoulder arthroplasty. That interest has now produced arguably the most comprehensive text on the subject, which, interestingly, begins with the evolution of shoulder arthroplasty and concludes with a view of the future of shoulder joint replacement. Along the way, we are treated to discussions and quality illustrations regarding biomechanics, glenohumeral pathology and pathoanatomy, surgical planning and technique, implant selection, complications, and outcomes for both anatomic and reverse shoulder arthroplasty. The concluding chapter considers the economics of shoulder arthroplasty in the context of our national healthcare budget—a topic that is exceedingly timely as we grapple with the realities of the COVID-19 pandemic. The readers of this text will be both informed and stimulated. Thank you, Joe and colleagues, for your comprehensive work.

FREDERICK A. MATSEN III, MD
Professor and Past Chair, Department of Orthopaedics and Sports Medicine
Inaugural Holder of the Douglas T. Harryman II
Endowed Chair for Shoulder Research
Founding Member and Past President, American Shoulder and Elbow Surgeons

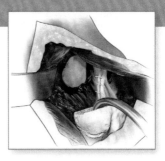

Foreword

It was approximately 25 years ago during the period between his residency with Dr. Matsen and beginning his practice in New York City our editor, Dr. Zuckerman, spent time with us at the Mayo Clinic in Minnesota. As promised by Dr. Matsen, he had unbounded energy, a mind organized for orthopedic surgery, skills, and drive. Time spent in Minnesota focused on reconstructive shoulder surgery, including publication of an article exposing poor pain relief in a segment of patients with osteoarthritis undergoing humeral head replacement. Since then, Dr. Zuckerman has remained focused on shoulder reconstruction: considered, studied, and reported on almost all questions posed about this subject. Luckily for all of us, he has pushed forward with his educational efforts—such as this book.

Both Dr. Zuckerman and I have had the opportunity to design a shoulder implant system and modify it over time, as science surrounding joint replacement has expanded. Fortunately, both he and I maintained active practices in hip and knee surgery so we could appreciate firsthand advances in those areas that could be translated to the shoulder. As a plus when being a part of an implant design team, one must understand anatomy, surgical pathology, biomechanics, and material characteristics.

This book is an outcome of the above experiences and acquisition of knowledge by our editor. Imagine what forming the structure of this text from understanding the past, recognizing what things a surgeon must know to perform these procedures, and defining future directions will do for the reader! Many thanks to Dr. Zuckerman and the more than 50 carefully selected authors for working so hard and effectively for our benefit.

ROBERT H. COFIELD, MD
Emeritus Chair, Department of Orthopedic Surgery
Mayo Clinic, Rochester, Minnesota
Founding Member and Past President, American Shoulder and Elbow Surgeons
Past Chair, International Board of Shoulder and Elbow Surgery

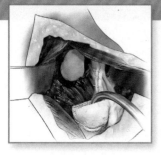

Video List

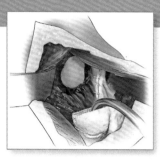

Preface

Embarking on a project to develop a comprehensive textbook on shoulder arthroplasty probably had its beginnings during my residency at the University of Washington. My earliest exposure to shoulder surgery and shoulder arthroplasty, specifically, occurred during residency working with Frederick Matsen, MD, one of the early leaders in shoulder surgery and a founding member of the American Shoulder and Elbow Surgeons. Dr. Matsen supported my interest in shoulder surgery during residency and has been an important and valuable mentor throughout my career. During my fellowship in adult reconstructive surgery under the direction of Clement B. Sledge, MD, at Brigham and Women's Hospital, I gained further experience in total shoulder arthroplasty as well as hip and knee replacement. When Victor Frankel, MD, PhD, recruited me to join the faculty of the Hospital for Joint Diseases (Dr. Frankel was the Chair of the Department of Orthopedic Surgery at the University of Washington during my first 3 years of residency), he encouraged me to pursue my interest in shoulder surgery and to develop a shoulder service. Dr. Matsen arranged an introduction to Robert H. Cofield, MD, at the Mayo Clinic who accepted me as a visiting clinician. During my time with Dr. Cofield, I was able to expand my knowledge and experience in shoulder surgery, especially shoulder arthroplasty. This was invaluable and Dr. Cofield, just like Dr. Matsen, became a source of tremendous mentorship and support throughout my career. My early growth and development as an academic orthopedic surgeon specializing in shoulder surgery was a product of my experiences with and the ongoing support provided by Drs. Matsen and Cofield and, of course, Dr. Frankel.

Dr. Frankel fully supported the development of a shoulder and elbow service at the Hospital for Joint Diseases. This included a research staff, the development of continuing education programs, and the initiation of a fellowship in shoulder and elbow surgery. Our shoulder and elbow service grew with additional faculty and increasing recognition as we were able to contribute to the orthopedic literature in this important and growing area. Becoming a member of the American Shoulder and Elbow Surgeons in 1986 allowed me to develop relationships with shoulder surgeons across the country. It was an opportunity to learn from the experience of others and further enhance my understanding and appreciation of shoulder surgery and, especially, shoulder arthroplasty.

My own clinical practice has also evolved through the years. When I started in practice, I focused on all types of shoulder and elbow surgery and also hip and knee arthroplasty. My training at the University of Washington in fracture care also resulted in an ongoing interest in the treatment of fractures, including hip fractures. As the years progressed, my practice became focused primarily on shoulder surgery and hip and knee arthroplasty. In the area of shoulder surgery, arthroplasty was always my main interest, and for the past 8 years, shoulder arthroplasty has been the only shoulder surgery I perform. I have continued to perform hip and knee arthroplasty, which I believe has given me an important perspective on arthroplasty that is somewhat unique compared to that of the vast majority of individuals who perform shoulder arthroplasty. It has enhanced my understanding of the surgical procedure, the techniques utilized, the design of the implants, and the materials used.

In 2003, I was approached by Darin Johnson from Exactech, Inc. inquiring as to whether I would be interested in joining a design team to develop a shoulder arthroplasty system. This was not something I had done before. In fact, I had generally been reluctant to be involved with industry in order to maintain my "academic" credibility. I met with Darin, who introduced me to Thomas W. Wright, MD, from the University of Florida and Pierre-Henri Flurin, MD, from the Merignac Clinic in Bordeaux, France. I immediately recognized that the value of joining this design team would be based upon the individuals I had the opportunity to work with. I agreed to join the team, and as they say, "the rest is history." My work with Tom Wright, Pierre-Henri Flurin along with Chris Roche, MS, and the team at Exactech, Inc. has further enhanced my understanding and appreciation of shoulder arthroplasty. It has allowed me to develop relationships with shoulder surgeons in the United States and around the world who have greatly enhanced my understanding of the procedure and have made me a better surgeon. It has also resulted in an extensive and growing compendium of shoulder arthroplasty research publications utilizing the clinical database we have developed over the past 15 plus years.

Throughout my career, I have been fortunate to serve as an editor of different textbooks related to shoulder surgery, fractures, orthopedic surgery techniques, shoulder fractures, and orthopedic residency training. I did not think my academic efforts would have been complete without a textbook devoted solely to shoulder arthroplasty, since this has been such an important area for my own clinical practice and academic pursuits. My early thoughts on the project led me to develop a table of contents and a description of the textbook. I am greatly appreciative of Brian Brown and his colleagues at Wolters Kluwer for accepting my proposal and their willingness to support the project. The next step was to select the contributors and seek their participation. Each and every colleague I asked agreed to participate. Not only did they agree to participate but they also provided outstanding contributions in every subject area including text, illustrative figures, and videos. This textbook could not have been possible without their efforts and I am tremendously appreciative of each and every contributor.

Moving a textbook through the production process requires the support of many, and this textbook is no different. The team at Wolters Kluwer has been outstanding, including Stacey Sebring, Senior Development Editor, Rajmohan Baskaran, Project Manager, and, of course, Bernie Kida, our expert and outstanding illustrator, who is responsible for all of the drawings in the textbook. Their efforts have allowed us to produce a finished product of which we can be very proud.

A project of this type could not have been possible without the support of all those around me. This includes my colleagues and friends on the faculty of the NYU Langone Health, Department of Orthopedic Surgery, and especially my colleagues in the Division of Shoulder and Elbow Surgery including Andrew Rokito, MD, Mandeep Singh Virk, MD, Young Kwon, MD, and Ramesh Gidumal, MD. Equally meaningful is the support provided by my office staff, including Lisa Lopez, Jim Madden, Naomi Perez, Migdalia Resto, and Robyn Smolen. They have helped to keep all of my other responsibilities on track while this project was being completed.

It is my hope that the readers of this textbook learn about the principles and practice of shoulder arthroplasty—that when they have a question about shoulder arthroplasty, they can open this textbook and find an answer to their question. If this textbook enhances each reader's knowledge and appreciation of shoulder arthroplasty and makes them a better clinician and surgeon, then my goals would have been fulfilled.

JOSEPH D. ZUCKERMAN, MD

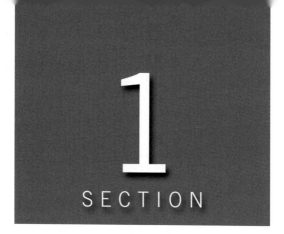
The Basics

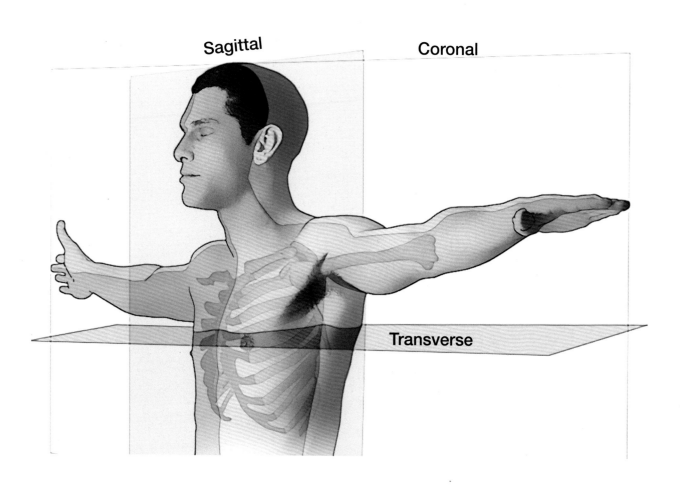

Sagittal

Coronal

Transverse

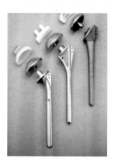

1 Evolution of Shoulder Arthroplasty

Reza Jazayeri, MD and Alex Friedman, DO

INTRODUCTION

Shoulder arthroplasty is now frequently performed to treat a variety of glenohumeral disorders. Its use has rapidly expanded over the past few decades as new innovations and designs have been developed and the indications have expanded. As we consider the role of shoulder arthroplasty today, it is both helpful and instructive to "start at the beginning" and understand the origins of the technology and recognize those individuals who have contributed to where we are today.

Historical Review of Early Implant Designs

Themistocles Gluck, a Romanian surgeon in the latter half of the 19th century, was the first to describe a prosthetic replacement as a potential treatment option in the shoulder.[1] His initial design was fabricated out of ivory and was anticipated to be used to treat tuberculosis infections in the shoulder. Unfortunately, there is no documentation that it was ever implanted in a patient.

The first recorded shoulder replacement was performed in 1893 by the French surgeon Jules Emile Péan for the treatment of tuberculosis in a 37-year-old baker at the Hôpital International in Paris.[2] The prosthesis design was originally inspired by Gluck, and it was fabricated by J. Porter Michaels, a dentist from Paris. The humeral stem was made of platinum that was connected by a wire to a rubber head coated with paraffin, creating a constrained implant (**FIGURE 1.1**). Although the patient initially had satisfactory results, the prosthesis eventually needed to be removed 2 years later because of a recurrent tuberculosis infection.

Nearly 60 years later, Frederick Krueger reported the use of a more anatomic shoulder prosthesis (**FIGURES 1.2** and **1.3**) constructed out of vitallium and molded from the proximal humeri of cadavers.[3] This was successfully used to treat a young patient with osteonecrosis of the humeral head. Despite the success of this implant, it did not appear to gain any significant traction until a few years later. The design and development of the early modern-day shoulder replacements was pioneered by Dr. Charles Neer. In 1953, in response to his dissatisfaction with the outcomes of the operative management of proximal humeral fractures, Neer developed the first

anatomic humeral prosthesis (**FIGURE 1.4**) for the treatment of a humeral head fracture.[4] This was followed by the development of a second design referred to as the Neer I prosthesis. This first-generation implant was a monoblock design made of vitallium, with a fixed inclination and a straight cylindrical stem that attempted to replicate the proximal humerus anatomy. In 1955, he reported his results in 12 patients who were treated for acute four-part proximal humeral fractures, fracture-dislocations, and in patients with osteonecrosis from prior fractures.[4] His results documented that 11 of 12 patients were pain free following this procedure. This led to an increased enthusiasm for the use of proximal humeral replacement to treat glenohumeral disorders. In 1964, Neer published a report describing the use of humeral head replacement for patients with a variety of glenohumeral disorders including acute fractures, fracture sequelae, and glenohumeral arthritis.[5] This initiated a period of significant expansion in the development of shoulder replacement designs.

The early designs by Neer and Kruger represented nonconstrained implants that recognized the underlying biomechanics of the glenohumeral joint. The humeral head replacement was eventually joined with a glenoid component to begin the era of total shoulder arthroplasty. At the same time, other implants were being developed by shoulder specialists around the world that represented more of a constrained design. For some period of time, constrained designs were being developed for use in all types of glenohumeral arthritis and not necessarily only for patients with underlying rotator cuff deficiency. Our discussion of the development of shoulder arthroplasty will follow two tracks: the development of unconstrained designs and the development of fixed-fulcrum or constrained designs.

UNCONSTRAINED DESIGNS

Early Designs

In the early 1970s, the design and implantation of glenoid components initiated the era of total shoulder arthroplasty. Neer designed a new humeral head replacement. The Neer II was characterized by a longer stem to dissipate the forces throughout the proximal humerus.[6]

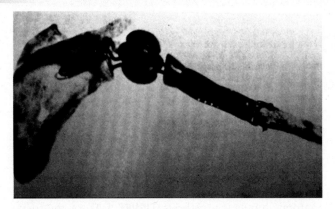

FIGURE 1.1 The first shoulder replacement created by Jules Emile Péan.

It consisted of a spherical head with a 22-mm radius that was available in two head heights of 15 and 22 mm **(FIGURE 1.5)**. The head had smooth rounded contours to accommodate the overlying rotator cuff tendons. This "monoblock" component is generally referred to as the "first-generation" shoulder arthroplasty. Neer also designed an all-polyethylene keeled cemented component that was rectangular in shape with a radius of curvature that matched the humeral component. In the 1970s and 1980s, the Neer II total shoulder arthroplasty was probably the nonconstrained shoulder arthroplasty system most commonly used for the treatment of traumatic, posttraumatic, and degenerative disorders of the glenohumeral joint.

The success of the Neer design led others to develop shoulder implant systems. The McNabb-English design **(FIGURE 1.6)** added more constraint to the articulation. The DANA design provided a nonconstrained option with a glenoid component that had a hood for increased constraint **(FIGURE 1.7)**.[7] Based upon the experiences with bipolar hip replacement, a bipolar shoulder design was also developed by Bateman. Nonconstrained implants had higher failure rates in the rotator cuff–deficient shoulder. This led Neer and others to develop more constrained designs, which will be discussed in the section on fixed-fulcrum designs.

Following the successful use of unconstrained designs, other implants were developed. The monoblock humeral component became a limiting factor because it did not address variations in humeral head size and dimension among different patients. The availability of one head radius (22 mm) and two head heights (15 and 22 mm) did not allow individual patient anatomy to be addressed. This occurred about the same time that modular components were being utilized for hip and knee replacement. Modularity then became part of total shoulder arthroplasty, which provided variable humeral head diameters and sizes that could be used to more closely match patient's individual anatomy and enhance the stability of the construct.[8] These modular components are generally referred to as "second-generation" implants **(FIGURE 1.8)**. These designs allowed for customization in sizing of the humeral head and the ability to combine humeral stems of different sizes with humeral heads of different

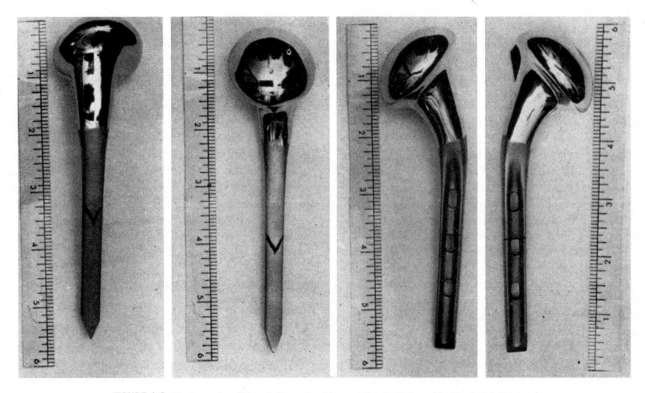

FIGURE 1.2 Photographs of the vitallium shoulder prosthesis designed by Frederick Krueger.

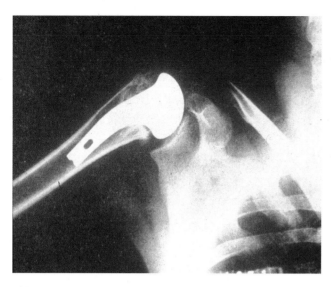

FIGURE 1.3 Radiograph of the vitallium stem designed by Frederick Krueger with fenestrations to allow for permeation with cancellous bone.

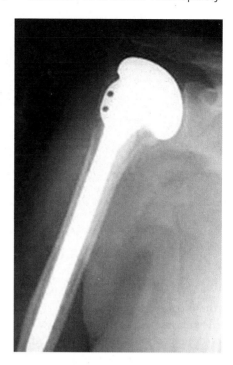

FIGURE 1.5 Radiograph of the Neer II shoulder prosthesis.

sizes.[8-10] Modularity improved the surgeon's ability to match certain aspects of the patient's individual anatomy, but it was soon recognized that it was not sufficient because the components did not account for the medial and posterior offset of the humeral head in relation to the shaft that characterizes proximal humeral anatomy.

In the 1980s, the anatomic studies by Boileau and Walch led to the development of "third-generation" implants.[10] Based upon their anatomic studies, they described the proximal humerus as a sphere and a cylinder. A portion of the sphere represents the articular surface of the proximal humerus, and the humeral shaft represents a cylinder. They found that the diameter

and thickness of the humeral head had a predictable relationship with each other but were highly variable between patients. In addition, they found that humeral neck inclination and retroversion were also highly variable. The humeral head (sphere) was offset posteriorly and medially from the humeral shaft (cylinder). These important findings led to the next phase of modularity,

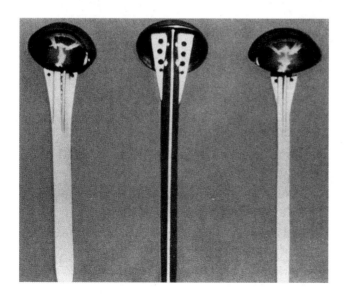

FIGURE 1.4 Photograph of Neer's early shoulder prosthesis designs from 1953.

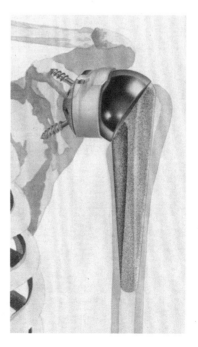

FIGURE 1.6 Illustration of the McNabb-English semiconstrained shoulder prosthesis design.

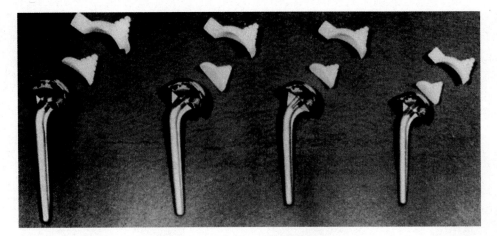

FIGURE 1.7 Photograph of the DANA nonconstrained shoulder prostheses.

with the design of eccentric humeral heads to provide a more anatomic restoration of the posterior and medial offset of the humeral head in relation to the shaft.[8,9] These "third-generation" modular designs provided variable options for head thickness, offset, and diameter, which were all designed to achieve a more anatomic restoration for each specific patient **(FIGURE 1.9)**. The principles behind the "third-generation" implants are for the prosthesis to be able to replicate the individual patient's anatomy rather than using an implant with limited options, which requires the patient's anatomy to adapt to the implant. This was a major step forward in implant design and resulted in improved patient outcomes.

Progression through second- and third-generation implants included a wide range of implant designs, including the Bateman bipolar prosthesis **(FIGURE 1.10)**, Global Advantage (DePuy, **FIGURE 1.11**), Cofield, which included a noncemented glenoid (Smith and Nephew, **FIGURE 1.12**), Solar (Stryker), Bigliani/Flatow (Zimmer), and Aequalis (Tornier, **FIGURE 1.13**).

Further design changes led to the "fourth generation" of nonconstrained total shoulder arthroplasty characterized by increased modularity that allowed for in situ adjustability of the humeral head offset as well

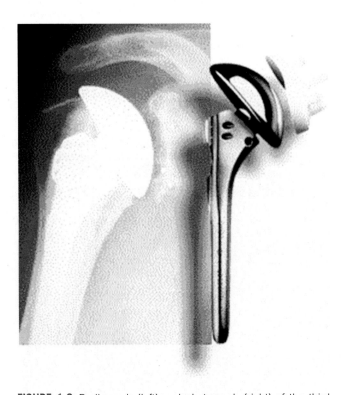

FIGURE 1.9 Radiograph (left) and photograph (right) of the third generation, modular prosthesis with a medial and posterior offset humeral head to better recreate the native anatomy of the proximal humerus.

FIGURE 1.8 Photograph of the second-generation, modular shoulder prostheses.

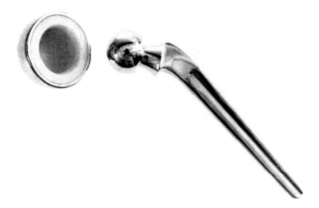

FIGURE 1.10 Photograph of the Bateman bipolar shoulder prosthesis.

as variation of inclination and version **(FIGURE 1.14)**. Progression of shoulder arthroplasty designs from the first generation to the fourth generation has been based upon the goal of reproducing individual patient anatomy, which has clearly been shown to correlate with improved functional outcomes.

Short-Stem and Stemless Implants

The successful use of press-fit standard length stems that relied primarily on metaphyseal fixation and some concerns about stress shielding and proximal humeral bone loss with longer stems led to the development of short humeral stems **(FIGURE 1.15)**.[11] These short-stem designs maintained metaphyseal fixation and also offered the same modularity and anatomic restoration as standard

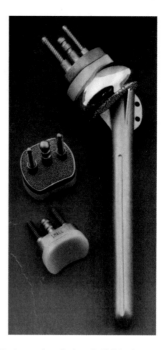

FIGURE 1.12 Photograph of the Cofield shoulder (second generation) prosthesis featuring a porous coating on the back of the humeral head. Also shown is the noncemented glenoid component. A cemented all-polyethylene keeled component was also available.

stems. Their use has become widespread and, for the most part, successful. Further shortening of the stem led to the development of stemless implants **(FIGURE 1.16)**. These were first introduced in Europe in 2004 and ultimately approved for use in the United States in 2015.[12] The benefits of short-stem and stemless implants include

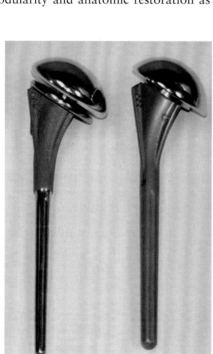

FIGURE 1.11 Photograph of the DePuy Global Advantage shoulder prostheses.

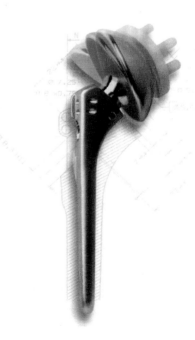

FIGURE 1.13 Photograph of the third-generation Aequalis shoulder prosthesis by Tornier.

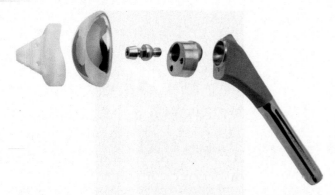

FIGURE 1.14 Photograph of the fourth-generation prosthesis with increased modularity for more anatomic recreation of the proximal humerus anatomy.

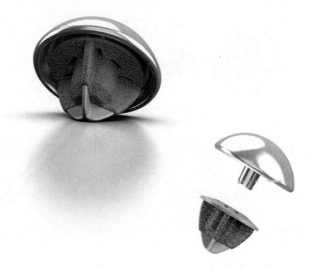

FIGURE 1.16 Photographs of a stemless humeral implant.

bone preservation and the ability to resurface the proximal humerus when a proximal humeral deformity is present.[13] Early results have certainly been encouraging, but longer term studies are needed to determine implant survival.[12,14,15]

Glenoid Implants

As total shoulder implants progressed through their development, the glenoid component also evolved through different development stages with design changes centered on preventing glenoid component loosening.[16] Neer's first glenoid design was a cemented all-polyethylene implant with a keel that was rectangular in shape with a radius of curvature that matched the humeral head component **(FIGURE 1.17)**.[6] Subsequent to this, different glenoid component designs that included cemented all-polyethylene keeled components with a convex back, cemented all-polyethylene keeled components with a flat back, cemented all-polyethylene pegged components with a convex back, and metal-backed designs were developed. The shape of the glenoid component also changed from rectangular to pear shaped to more closely replicate the anatomy of the glenoid in which the inferior width is greater than the superior width. Studies have generally shown that convex-back designs resist shear forces better than flat-back designs, which results in fewer radiolucent lines around the glenoid component and improved longevity, making it the preferred design. The question of whether a keeled or pegged design is preferred has not yet been answered. Successful outcomes have been reported with both designs. Nonetheless, at present, pegged designs are

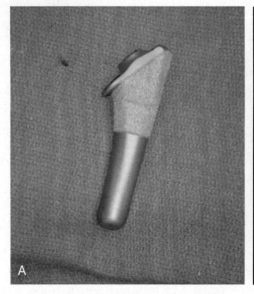
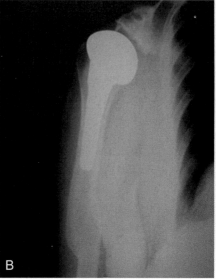

FIGURE 1.15 Photograph (**A**) and radiograph (**B**) of a short-stem shoulder prosthesis.

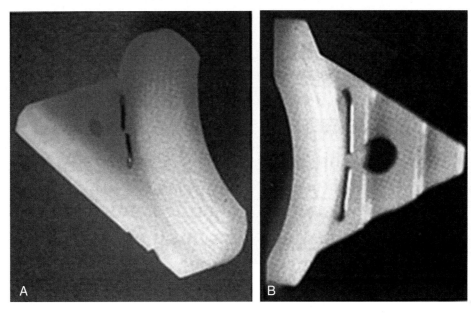

FIGURE 1.17 Photographs (**A** and **B**) of Neer's first glenoid design that was rectangular in shape with a radius of curvature that matched the humeral head component.

much more commonly utilized, in part, because of the need for less bone removal. Metal-backed implants were also designed based upon the early success of metal-backed acetabular components **(FIGURE 1.18)**. However, these designs were unsuccessful as a result of early loosening and polyethylene wear and dissociation.[17] Noncemented metal-backed designs with screw fixation were also developed. However, limitations on the thickness of the polyethylene led to increased polyethylene wear, dissociation, and an unacceptable rate

of failure. Most recently, design modifications have focused on hybrid glenoid components, which represent a combination of cemented and noncemented fixation. Some designs included an all-polyethylene component with a central bony ongrowth portion **(FIGURE 1.19)**, while others added bone ingrowth features including porous-coated metal backing combined with peripheral pegs **(FIGURE 1.20A and B)**.[17] Although all-polyethylene designs have been successful, the current state of the art is primarily based upon hybrid glenoids with a combination of noncemented

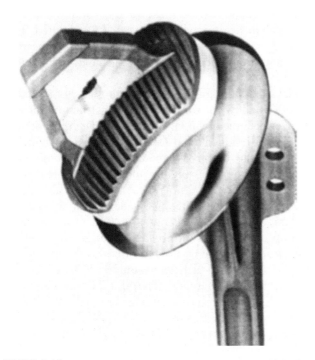

FIGURE 1.18 Photograph of an early metal-backed glenoid design.

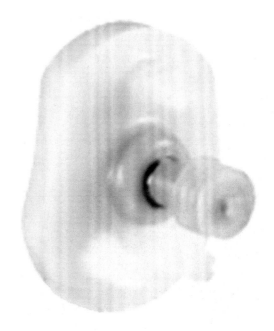

FIGURE 1.19 Photograph of an all-polyethylene glenoid implant with a central peg allowing for bony ongrowth.

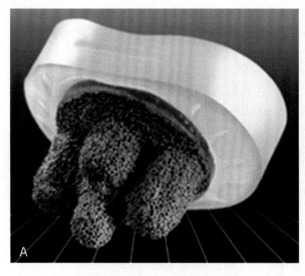
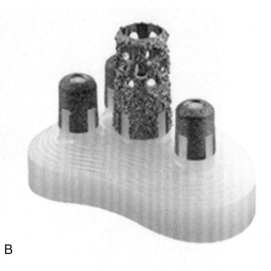

FIGURE 1.20 **A** and **B**, Photographs of hybrid glenoid implants with porous-coated metal backing combined with peripheral pegs.

and cemented fixation. The search for a successful entirely noncemented glenoid component continues but as yet has not been developed.

FIXED-FULCRUM DESIGNS

Early Designs

In their early experiences, it became evident to Neer and others that unconstrained prosthetic replacements were not successful in patients with rotator cuff deficiencies.[18] The early results of hemiarthroplasty and nonconstrained total shoulder arthroplasty for cuff tear arthropathy were unsuccessful in relieving pain and

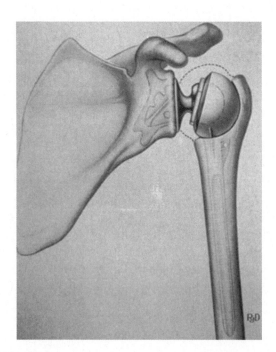

FIGURE 1.21 Illustration of the Mark I reverse total shoulder arthroplasty.

restoring function.[19] This led to the development of more constrained total shoulder arthroplasty designs based upon the principal that if the articulating surfaces had inherent stability, then the deltoid would be able to function in the role of the rotator cuff for the cuff-deficient shoulder.[20-22] This seemingly simple principle proved to be difficult to translate into a successful fixed-fulcrum prosthetic design.

Neer designed three constrained implant systems, each with modifications based upon the limitations of the previous design. The first of three designs, the Mark I (**FIGURE 1.21**), included a large glenoid implant that stabilized the prosthesis and prevented proximal humeral migration. The large glenoid component, however, prevented reattachment of the rotator cuff and presented difficulties when bone stock was limited. This resulted in early failures and poor outcomes from proximal migration, subacromial impingement, and glenoid loosening.[18,20]

The second design, the Mark II, consisted of a smaller glenoid to allow for rotator cuff reconstruction but was also characterized by poor outcomes.[18] The third design, the Mark III, added axial rotation between the humeral stem and the diaphysis in an attempt to limit constraint and improve range of motion.[23] Unfortunately, the results were also not successful, and ultimately, Neer abandoned his attempts to develop a constrained implant. During the same time, multiple other surgeons developed fixed-fulcrum prosthetic designs in an effort to achieve successful treatment for cuff tear arthropathy and the rotator cuff–deficient shoulder.[24] These included the Michael Reese shoulder (**FIGURE 1.22**), the Stanmore, which closely resembled a total hip replacement (**FIGURE 1.23**), Reeves (**FIGURE 1.24**), Kessel (**FIGURE 1.25**), Kölbel (**FIGURE 1.26**), Gristina (**FIGURE 1.27**), Bickel (**FIGURE 1.28**), and Fenlin (**FIGURE 1.29**) implants. These designs all had a common design flaw of a lateralized glenoid

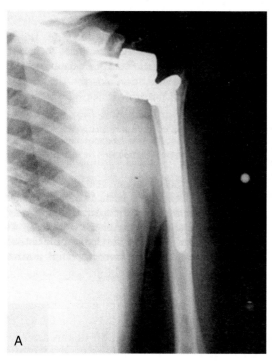
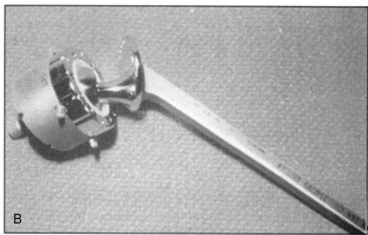

FIGURE 1.22 Radiograph (**A**) and photograph (**B**) of the constrained Michael Reese shoulder prosthesis designed by Mel Post, MD.

component (center of rotation) that produced excessive torque and stresses at the glenoid fixation site, resulting in a high rate of glenoid loosening, implant failure, and unsuccessful results.

Paul Grammont revolutionized shoulder arthroplasty in 1985 with his concept of medializing and lowering the center of rotation of the glenohumeral joint.[25] His prosthesis, termed the Delta reverse total shoulder arthroplasty (RTSA), used a semiconstrained ball-and-socket design, which eliminated the translational movement between the humeral head and the glenoid that occurs in a nonconstrained anatomic shoulder prosthesis. It was designed to compensate for an absent rotator cuff, improve stability, and decrease the risk of mechanical failure of the glenoid component. This improvement was primarily accomplished through removal of the

Stanmore
Total Shoulder
Replacement

FIGURE 1.23 Photograph of the Stanmore total shoulder replacement prosthesis, which closely resembles a total hip replacement prosthesis.

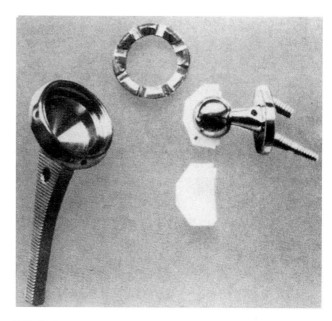

FIGURE 1.24 Photograph of the Reeves reverse shoulder prosthesis.

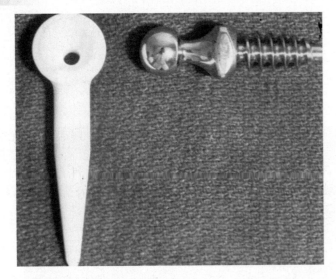

FIGURE 1.25 Photograph of the Kessel reverse prosthesis.

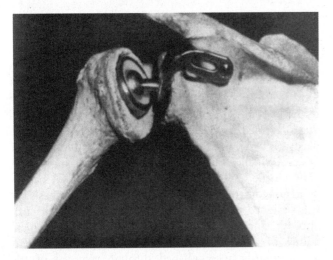

FIGURE 1.26 Photograph of the Kölbel reverse, fixed-fulcrum prosthesis.

glenoid neck, which medialized the center of rotation of the implant, thus transforming the previously shearing torque into compressive forces at the glenoid-bone interface.[25] Additionally, as the center of rotation of the prosthesis is medialized and lowered, the deltoid lever arm is increased. This places more tension on the deltoid muscle, making it more efficient and allowing it to perform shoulder abduction without relying on a functional rotator cuff.[26]

The first prototype of the Grammont RTSA consisted of a cemented glenosphere and an all-polyethylene humeral stem **(FIGURE 1.30)**.[27] In 1987, Grammont published his results in a series of eight patients and reported that although the center of rotation was medialized, it remained lateral to the native glenoid surface.[25] This placed more force at the implant-bone interface and resulted in loosening and failure of the glenoid component.

In 1991, Grammont designed the next generation of his RTSA, the Delta III **(FIGURE 1.31)**. This design further medialized the center of rotation of the prosthesis by changing the glenosphere from two-thirds of a sphere to one-half of a sphere. The baseplate (metaglene) was also changed to include a central press-fit peg and two divergent 3.5-mm screws. These design changes helped resist the unwanted shear forces at the bone-implant interface and resulted in stable fixation of the glenoid component, thereby solving the biggest challenge that had confronted all previous fixed-fulcrum designs.[23]

Grammont's third-generation design became available in 1994.[24] In this design, changes were focused on the humeral stem, which was changed from monoblock design to a modular design that consisted of a diaphyseal stem that was joined to a modular metaphyseal component. This implant design—referred to as the "Grammont

Trispherical total shoulder

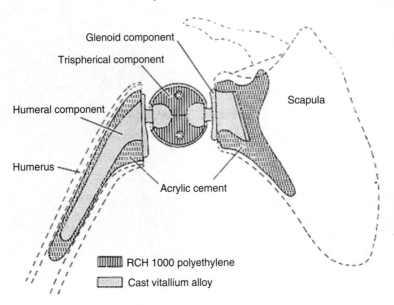

FIGURE 1.27 Illustration of the Gristina trispherical total shoulder replacement prosthesis.

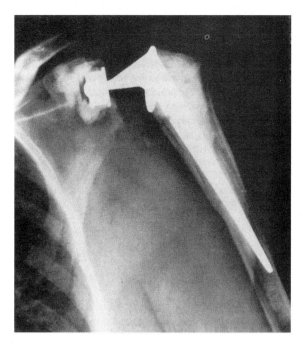

FIGURE 1.28 Radiograph of the Bickel shoulder prosthesis.

design"—has been the foundation for many of the current modern-day RTSA designs and has led to the development of many RTSAs that are currently available and being used.[27] Design modifications have included locking screws followed by variable angle locking screws with osseous-integrated baseplates to improve long-term glenoid fixation. The humeral side is also evolving, with variable neck-shaft angles and increased modularity to improve the ability to obtain correct deltoid tension and enhance the overall stability of the construct.

Subsequent to Grammont's work, Frankle introduced a RTSA design with a more lateralized center of rotation (**FIGURE 1.32**).[28] His early designs developed problems with failure of the glenoid baseplate because of screw breakage and loosening. However, subsequent design modifications have resolved this issue, and it has been used extensively and successfully. This lateralized design is commonly referred to as the "Frankel design" to differentiate it from the medialized "Grammont design."

Arthroplasty for Proximal Humeral Fractures

It is important to note that the reason Neer originally designed his humeral prosthesis was to treat proximal humeral fractures and their sequelae. His first report on its use was to treat patients with fractures, fracture-dislocations, and osteonecrosis following fracture.[4] For the next 50 years, the humeral implant used to treat glenohumeral arthritis was also used to treat proximal humerus fractures. The results of hemiarthroplasty for the treatment proximal fractures has generally been disappointing with respect to functional outcomes primarily because of problems with tuberosity fixation and healing. To address the problems related to the tuberosities, fracture-specific implants have been developed (**FIGURES 1.33** and **1.34**). The evolution of these implants has included design modifications that provide less proximal implant bulk with a fenestration to promote healing between the tuberosities for the placement of cancellous bone graft from the humeral head, easier and more secure reattachment of the tuberosities, and anatomic designs that differentiate the reattachment sites for the lesser and greater tuberosities. Although cemented fixation has been the standard for decades, more recently, emphasis

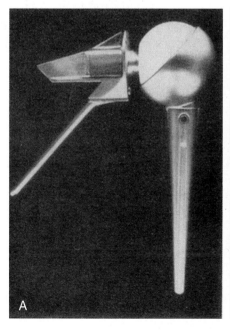
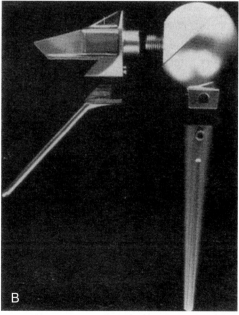

FIGURE 1.29 Photographs of the Fenlin constrained shoulder prosthesis with components articulated (**A**) and disarticulated (**B**).

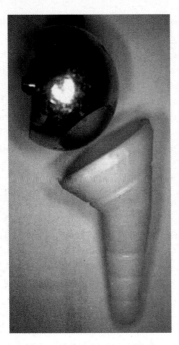

FIGURE 1.30 Photograph of the initial prototype of the Grammont reverse prosthesis.

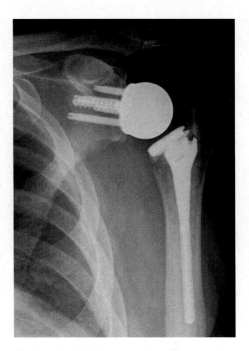

FIGURE 1.32 Radiograph of the Frankle design reverse total shoulder arthroplasty with a lateralized center of rotation.

has been placed on noncemented fixation designs. These design modifications, although thoughtful and creative, did not result in significant improvement in functional outcomes. The most significant change in treatment that has resulted in improvements compared to hemiarthroplasty has been the use of RTSA as the primary treatment for complex proximal humeral fractures.[29,30]

Conclusion

Since Pean's first shoulder implant in 1893, the work of shoulder specialists and engineers has led to the development of a variety of successful designs of anatomic total shoulder arthroplasty and RTSA that are used to

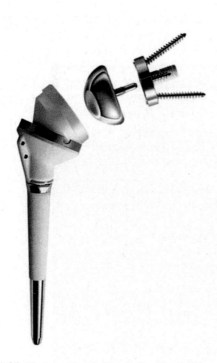

FIGURE 1.31 Photograph of the Delta III shoulder prosthesis designed by Grammont.

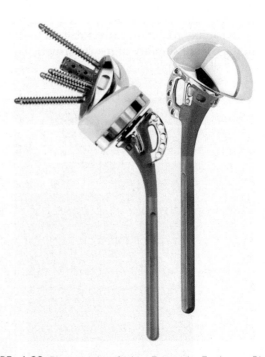

FIGURE 1.33 Photograph of the Exactech Equinoxe Platform Fracture Stem, with options for both reverse shoulder (left) and hemishoulder (right) arthroplasty. The stem has an anterior-lateral fin that allows for more anatomic reattachment of the greater and lesser tuberosities.

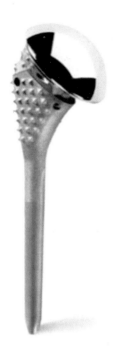

FIGURE 1.34 Photograph of the Biomet hemiarthroplasty fracture stem with fenestrations and roughened surfaces for tuberosity reattachment.

treat an expanding spectrum of glenohumeral disorders that affect hundreds of thousands of patients each year. The improvements in function and quality of life experienced by so many patients are a credit to those who have worked to develop these implants.

REFERENCES

1. Gluck T. Referat iJber die durch das moderne chirurgische Experfment gewonnenen positiven Resultate, betreffend die Naht und den Ersatz van Defecten hoherer Gewebe, sowie Jber die Verwerthung resorbirbarer und lebendiger Tampons in der Chirurgie. *Archiv für Klinische Chirurgie.* 1891;41:187-239.
2. Lugli T. Artificial shoulder joint by Péan (1893): the facts of an exceptional intervention and the prosthetic method. *Clin Orthop Relat Res.* 1978;133:215-218.
3. Krueger FJ. A vitallium replica arthroplasty on the shoulder: a case report of aseptic necrosis of the proximal end of the humerus. *Surgery.* 1951;30:1005-1011.
4. Neer CS II. Articular replacement for the humeral head. *J Bone Joint Surg Am.* 1955;37:215-228.
5. Neer CS II. Follow-up notes on articles previously published in the journal: articular replacement for the humeral head. *J Bone Joint Surg Am.* 1964;46:1607-1610.
6. Neer CS II. Replacement arthroplasty for glenohumeral osteoarthritis. *J Bone Joint Surg Am.* 1974;56:1-13.
7. Kölbel R, Friedebold G. Shoulder joint replacement. Article in German. *Arch Orthop Unfallchir.* 1973;76:31-39.
8. Flatow EL. Prosthetic design considerations in total shoulder arthroplasty. *Semin Arthroplasty.* 1995;6(4):233-244.
9. Pearl ML. Proximal humeral anatomy in shoulder arthroplasty: implications for prosthetic design and surgical technique. *J Shoulder Elbow Surg.* 2005;14:99S-104S.
10. Boileau P, Walch G. The three-dimensional geometry of the proximal humerus: implications for surgical technique and prosthetic design. *J Bone Joint Surg Br.* 1997;79(5):857-865.
11. Matsen FA III, Iannotti JP, Rockwood CA Jr. Humeral fixation by press-fitting of a tapered metaphyseal stem: a prospective radiographic study. *J Bone Joint Surg Am.* 2003;85(2):304-308.
12. Huguet D, DeClercq G, Rio B, Teissier J, Zipoli B; TESS Group. Results of a new stemless shoulder prosthesis: radiologic proof of maintained fixation and stability after a minimum of three years' follow-up. *J Shoulder Elbow Surg.* 2010;19:847-852.
13. Keener JD, Chalmers PN, Yamaguchi K. The humeral implant in shoulder arthroplasty. *J Am Acad Orthop Surg.* 2017;25:427-438.
14. Churchill RS, Chuinard C, Wiater JM, et al. Clinical and radiographic outcomes of the Simpliciti canal-sparing shoulder arthroplasty system: a prospective two-year multicenter study. *J Bone Joint Surg Am.* 2016;98:552-560.
15. Rasmussen JV, Harjula J, Arverud ED, etal. The short-term survival of total stemless shoulder arthroplasty for osteoarthritis is comparable to that of total stemmed shoulder arthroplasty: a Nordic Arthroplasty Register. *J Shoulder Elbow Surg.* 2019;28(8):1578-1586.
16. Gonzalez JF, Alami GB, Baque F, Walch G, Boileau P. Complications of unconstrained shoulder prostheses. *J Shoulder Elbow Surg.* 2011;20(4):666-682.
17. Pinkas D, Wiater B, Wiater JM. The Glenoid component in anatomic shoulder arthroplasty. *J Am Acad Orthop Surg.* 2015;23:317-326.
18. Neer CS II, Craig EV, Fukuda H. Cuff-tear arthropathy. *J Bone Joint Surg Am.* 1983;65:1232-1244.
19. Sanchez-Sotelo J, Cofield RH, Rowland CM. Shoulder hemiarthroplasty for glenohumeral arthritis associated with severe rotator cuff deficiency. *J Bone Joint Surg Am.* 2001;83A(12):1814-1822.
20. Franklin JL, Barrett WP, Jackins SE, Matsen FA III. Glenoid loosening in total shoulder arthroplasty. Association with rotator cuff deficiency. *J Arthroplasty.* 1988;3:39-46.
21. Reeves RB, Jobbins B, Flowers M. Biomechanical problems in the development of a total shoulder endoprosthesis. *J Bone Joint Surg Br.* 1972;54:193.
22. Coughlin MJ, Morris JM, West WF. The semiconstrained total shoulder arthroplasty. *J Bone Joint Surg Am.* 1979;61:574-581.
23. Neer CS II. *Shoulder Reconstruction.* WB Saunders Co; 1990:146-150.
24. Flatow El, Harrison AK. A history of reverse total shoulder arthroplasty. *Clin Orthop Relat Res.* 2011;469:2432-2439.
25. Grammont P, Trouilloud P, Laffay JP, Deries X. Concept study and realization of a new total shoulder prosthesis. Article in French. *Rhumatologie.* 1987;39:407-418.
26. De Wilde LF, Audenaert EA, Berghs BM. Shoulder prostheses treating cuff tear arthropathy: a comparative biomechanical study. *J Orthop Res.* 2004;22:1222-1230.
27. Boileau P, Watkinson DJ, Hatzidakis AM, Balg F. Grammont reverse prosthesis: design, rationale, and biomechanics. *J Shoulder Elbow Surg.* 2005;14(1 suppl):147S-161S.
28. Cuff D, Pupello D, Virani N, Levy J, Frankle M. Reverse shoulder arthroplasty for the treatment of rotator cuff deficiency. *J Bone Joint Surg Am.* 2008;90(6):1244-1251.
29. Martin TG, Iannotti JP. Reverse total shoulder arthroplasty for acute fractures and failed management after proximal humeral fractures. *Orthop Clin North Am.* 2008;39:451-457.
30. Jobin CM, Galdi B, Anakwenze OA, Ahmad CS, Levine WN. Reverse shoulder arthroplasty for the management of proximal humerus fractures. *J Am Acad Orthop Surg.* 2015;23(3):190-201.

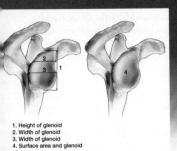

1. Height of glenoid
2. Width of glenoid
3. Width of glenoid
4. Surface area and glenoid shape

CHAPTER

2

Glenohumeral Anatomy and Implant Design

Kevin M. Magone, MD and Joseph D. Zuckerman, MD

INTRODUCTION

The glenohumeral joint is a complex, highly mobile joint that relies on the bony articulation between the humeral head and glenoid as well as the surrounding soft tissues for stability and balance.[1] The goal of shoulder arthroplasty is to re-create normal glenohumeral anatomy.[2] This can be a challenge not only because pathologic changes to the glenoid and humeral head can distort normal anatomy but also because of the inherent variation in "normal" anatomy that exists among patients.[1,3,4] When "normal" glenohumeral anatomy is more closely restored, shoulder arthroplasty results in better functional outcomes and longer implant survival.[1,5-7] This led to the development of glenoid and humeral implants that can accommodate the variations encountered. Furthermore, as our understanding of the anatomy and biomechanics of the glenohumeral joint has expanded, we have an opportunity to develop improved methods of preoperative planning and intraoperative navigation that could, ultimately, result in improved outcomes. In this chapter, we will review glenohumeral anatomy and its relationship to implant design.

GLENOID ANATOMY

The glenoid height, width, surface area, version, inclination, vault shape and size, and radius of curvature are all important anatomic parameters for prosthesis design. Multiple cadaveric and patient studies have reported the differences in these anatomic parameters among patients.

Glenoid height is the measurement from the most superior and to the most inferior portion of the glenoid (**FIGURE 2.1; TABLE 2.1**). Checroun et al evaluated 412 cadaver scapulae using direct measurement. These scapulae had an average age of 58 years (range, 24-87 years). The average glenoid height was 37.9 mm (range, 31.2-50.1 mm).[9] Kwon et al evaluated 12 cadaveric scapulae by CT imaging. The average glenoid height was 39.1 mm (range, 31-48 mm).[12] McPherson et al assessed 93 cadaveric shoulders radiographically using a custom computer software program. They reported an average glenoid height to be 33.9 mm.[19] Gender differences in glenoid height was assessed by Churchill et al in 344 scapulae

with an average age of 25 years (range, 20-30 years) using direct measurement. The average glenoid height for male and female specimens was 37.5 and 32.6 mm, respectively.[10] Lastly, Moineau et al assessed 41 arthritic glenoids using CT images. The average glenoid height was 41.33 mm (range, 31.5-55.1 mm), which supports the observation that glenohumeral arthritis results in glenoid enlargement primarily as a result of adaptive changes and osteophyte formation.[4]

Glenoid width is the measurement from the anterior rim to the posterior rim (**FIGURE 2.1; TABLE 2.1**). However, glenoid width varies depending on the level where the measurement is obtained because of the shape of the glenoid. Based upon anatomic studies, the glenoid shape or face is described as elliptical or pear shaped, with pear shaped being described in 71% of the specimens[9] (**FIGURE 2.1**). Checroun et al reported the average glenoid width at the midportion of the 412 cadaveric scapulae to be 29.3 mm (range, 22.6-41.5 mm).[9] Kwon et al reported the average width to be 25.2 mm (range, 21-34 mm), while McPherson et al described the average width to be 28.6 mm.[12,19] Churchill et al compared glenoid width between genders. From their review of 344 scapulae, the average glenoid width for male and female specimens was 27.8 and 23.6 mm, respectively.[10] Lastly, Moineau described the average glenoid width to be 29.35 mm (range, 19.6-44.8 mm) in 41 arthritic shoulders, again documenting the relative enlargement of the arthritic glenoid.

The glenoid surface area is the area of the entire articular surface (**FIGURE 2.1**). The variation in glenoid height and width results in a similar variation in glenoid surface area. Kwon reported the average glenoid surface area in 12 cadaveric scapulae based upon CT imaging to be 8.7 cm² (range, 7.0-14.2 cm²).[12]

Glenoid version is the angle of the glenoid face with respect to the transverse axis of the scapula (**FIGURE 2.2; TABLE 2.1**). Anteversion is present when the glenoid face is angled anteriorly with respect to the transverse axis, and retroversion is present when the glenoid face is angled posteriorly. Measuring glenoid version has been described by different methods. However, glenoid version is most often calculated using Friedman's method.[2,11,20-22] Based on aggregated studies reporting glenoid version in

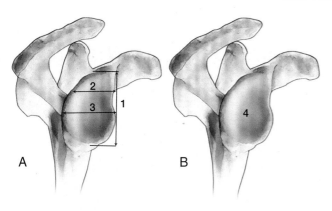

1. Height of glenoid
2. Width of glenoid
3. Width of glenoid
4. Surface area and glenoid shape

FIGURE 2.1 Sagittal view of the glenoid depicting the glenoid height, width, surface area, and shape. **A**, Glenoid height is the length of the glenoid from the superiormost aspect to the inferiormost aspect. The glenoid width is the measure from the anterior to the posterior glenoid rim. The glenoid width increases from superior to inferior. **B**, Surface area is the product of glenoid height and width. As these glenoid measurements vary, the surface area will also vary similarly. The glenoid shape is more consistently described as pear shaped.

1234 specimens, the average glenoid version was 6.3° of retroversion (range, 1°-12.1° retroversion).[2,4,9-11,20-24] Even though the range of the combined averages for these studies was 1° to 12.1° of glenoid retroversion, individual studies have reported glenoid version to be up to 23.2° of anteversion and up to 32° of retroversion, which clearly shows the wide variation of anatomic version in nonarthritic glenoids.[4,20]

Glenoid inclination is the slope of the articular surface from superior to inferior and is also based upon the transverse axis as a reference (**FIGURE 2.3**). Superior inclination is present when the glenoid articular surface is facing superiorly; conversely, with inferior inclination, the glenoid articular surface faces inferiorly. Ricchetti evaluated 57 shoulders with CT imaging and reported an average of 10° superior inclination.[2] Boileau assessed 47 shoulders with radiographs and CT images and reported glenoid inclination to be 15° superior based upon CT imaging and 10° superior based upon standard radiographs.[25] Gender differences were evaluated by Churchill who reported glenoid inclination to be 4° superior in men (range, 7° inferior to 15.8° superior) and 4.5° superior in women (range, 1.5° inferior to 15.3° superior).[10] Of note, this study emphasized the wide variability of inclination values encountered in the 344 cadaveric scapulae studied.

Various methods have been described to measure the glenoid inclination. At present, the beta angle is considered the most accurate method.[2,10,25,26] The beta angle is measured based upon the intersection of a line drawn on the floor of the supraspinatus fossa and a line drawn on the glenoid fossa that connects the superior and inferior margins[26] (**FIGURE 2.4**). Measuring glenoid inclination using the beta angle has been shown to be more accurate using CT coronal images than standard radiographs.[26] The beta angle has also been referred to as the total shoulder arthroplasty angle and the global glenoid inclination.[25] The beta angle is referred to as the global glenoid inclination as it incorporates the entire glenoid surface when measuring inclination. Typically, glenoid components for anatomic shoulder replacements are

Anatomic Parameter (mm Unless Noted)	Glenoid Height	Glenoid Width	Version Angle (°)	Glenoid Height/Lower Width Ratio
Bryce et al[8] (n = 40)	44.9	31.1	Not reported	Not reported
Checroun et al[9] (n = 412)	37.9 ± 2.7	29.3 ± 2.4	Not reported	1.3 ± 0.07
Churchill et al[10] (n = 344)	35.0	25.7	−1.2	Not reported
Iannotti et al[11] (n = 140)	39.0 ± 3.7	29.0 ± 3.1	Not reported	1.43 ± 0.02
Kwon et al[12] (n = 12)	39.1	25.2	−1.0	Not reported
Ljungquist et al[13] (n = 100)	35.2	25.3	Not reported	1.39
Mallon et al[14] (n = 28)	35.0	24.0	−2.0	Not reported
Merril et al[15] (n = 368,184 pairs)	35.4 ± 2.2	26.1 ± 3.5	Not reported	Not reported
Ohl et al[16] (n = 43)	35.3	25.9	−2.4	Not reported
Von Schroder et al[17] (n = 30)	36.4	28.6	Not reported	Not reported
Jacobson et al[18] (n = 74)	38.1 ± 4.5	29.6 ± 4.0	−6.2 ± 5.5	1.29 ± 0.10

TABLE 2.1 Summary of Published Data for Glenoid Dimensions

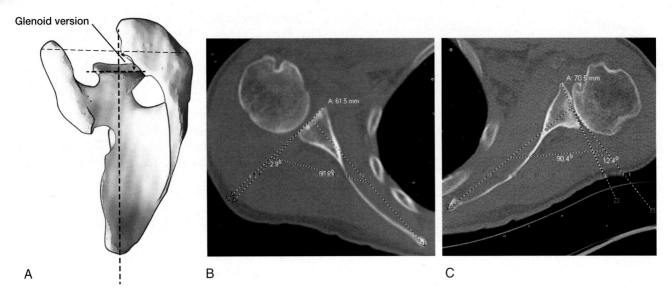

Glenoid version

A B C

FIGURE 2.2 A, Axial view of the glenoid to illustrate glenoid version. Glenoid version is the angle between the articular surface and the transverse plane of the scapular. **B**, Axial CT imaging of an intact glenohumeral joint with almost neutral version. **C**, Axial CT imaging of a glenohumeral joint with arthritis showing a biconcave glenoid and retroversion measuring approximately 12°.

implanted covering the entire glenoid; therefore, using a measurement that takes the entire glenoid into account is reasonable. In contrast, reverse shoulder arthroplasty baseplate designs utilize smaller baseplates that only

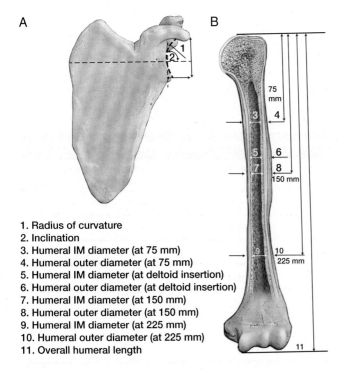

A B

1. Radius of curvature
2. Inclination
3. Humeral IM diameter (at 75 mm)
4. Humeral outer diameter (at 75 mm)
5. Humeral IM diameter (at deltoid insertion)
6. Humeral outer diameter (at deltoid insertion)
7. Humeral IM diameter (at 150 mm)
8. Humeral outer diameter (at 150 mm)
9. Humeral IM diameter (at 225 mm)
10. Humeral outer diameter (at 225 mm)
11. Overall humeral length

75 mm

150 mm

225 mm

FIGURE 2.3 A, Coronal view of the scapula illustrating the glenoid radius of curvature and glenoid inclination. The radius of curvatures is the radius of a circular arc that best approximates the curve of the articular surface. The glenoid inclination is the slope of the articular surface in the superior to inferior direction with reference to the transverse plane of the scapula. **B**, Coronal view of the humerus showing the variable intramedullary dimensions based upon the level of the humeral canal.

cover the inferior portion of the glenoid. Therefore, an inclination measurement focusing only on the inferior aspect of the glenoid has been proposed for inclination measurements for smaller baseplates that, when implanted, cover only the inferior aspect of the glenoid.[25] The reverse shoulder arthroplasty angle obtains an inclination measurement on the more inferior aspect of the glenoid surface for rotator cuff–deficient shoulders that will require a reverse shoulder prosthesis.[25]

The glenoid vault is best evaluated on axial CT imaging. The shape and size of the glenoid vault was described by Codsi et al. They evaluated 61 cadaveric scapulae with CT imaging and noted that from superior to inferior, the glenoid vault is triangular in shape[27] **(FIGURE 2.5)**. They used this information to propose five sizes of triangular-shaped implants that approximated all 61 glenoid vaults assessed.[27] These triangular-shaped implants closely resembled commonly used manufactured glenoid trials, but the study implants were never commercially produced.[27] Furthermore, it is important to understand the relationship between glenoid "vault anatomy" and "face anatomy." The glenoid triangular vault lies beneath the glenoid articular surface or "face" and between the anterior and posterior glenoid walls. However, the vault is not necessarily located centrally beneath the face **(FIGURE 2.6)**. Since the glenoid vault serves as the primary support for the glenoid component, understanding the relationship between glenoid "vault anatomy" and "face anatomy" will allow the surgeon to place the glenoid component centrally within the vault for optimal bony support.

The glenoid radius of curvature is the radius of the circular arc that best approximates the curve of

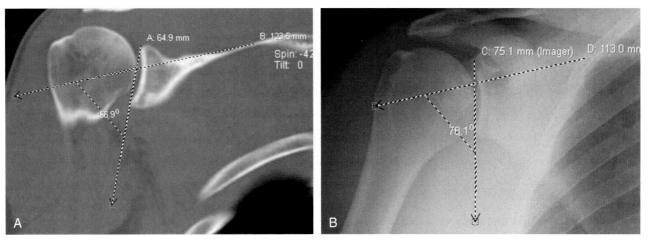

FIGURE 2.4 Coronal images of the glenohumeral joint illustrating the "beta angle" measurement of glenoid inclination. The beta angle is the angle between a line from the superior-inferior glenoid surface and a line through the floor of the supraspinatus fossa. The measurement is more accurate using coronal CT images (**A**) as opposed to AP radiographs (**B**).

the articular surface **(FIGURE 2.3)**. McPherson evaluated 93 shoulders with CT imaging using a custom computer software. They noted the mean radius of curvature to be 32.2 mm in the coronal plane and 40.6 mm in the axial plane, respectively.[19] Moineau also reported the radius of curvature for the glenoid in the coronal plane. They reported the average radius of curvature to be 34.9 mm (range, 21.7-65.5 mm) in 41 shoulders evaluated by CT imaging.[4] This is a particularly important anatomic parameter that is often compared to the humeral head radius of curvature. This comparison is referred to as the "radial mismatch"

and is replicated in the design of anatomic shoulder arthroplasty components in an effort to reproduce normal anatomy.

FLAT VERSUS CURVED COMPONENTS

Since the glenoid has a convex surface, the backside design of glenoid components has been a topic of study and discussion. Although replication of glenoid anatomy would appear to support a curved back design, both curved and flat designs have been used in an effort to limit rocking, micromotion, and displacement. Biomechanically, curved back components have performed better with respect to edge displacement during cyclic loading compared to flat glenoids.[28,29] Furthermore, curved glenoids require less reaming and preserve more bone.[19,30] Clinical outcomes and the incidence of radiolucent lines have been reported to be better with curved designs.[30,31]

HUMERAL ANATOMY

Proximal humeral anatomy has been studied extensively including humeral head diameter, height, shape, and radius of curvature; neck-shaft angle; humeral offset; and version. Metaphyseal and diaphyseal humeral anatomy has also been studied including the male and female differences. Understanding humeral anatomy has been instrumental in designing implants that provide the ability to reconstruct anatomy that reflects the individual variations often encountered.

Humeral head diameter is based at the anatomic neck level **(FIGURE 2.7; TABLE 2.2)**. This measurement is important since the goal of prosthetic replacement is to replicate the normal anatomy as closely as possible. McPherson et al evaluated 93 shoulders with radiographs and a custom computer software system. The

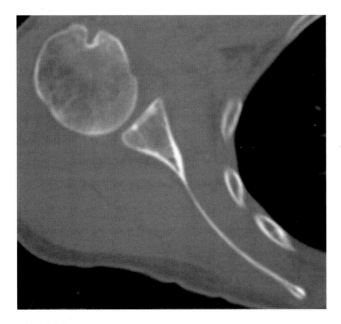

FIGURE 2.5 Axial CT image of the glenohumeral joint illustrating the triangular shape of the glenoid vault.

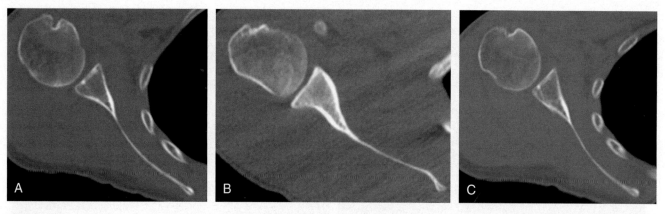

FIGURE 2.6 Axial CT images highlighting the glenoid "face" and "vault" relationship. **A,** In this image, the glenoid "vault" is neutral to the glenoid "face". **B,** In this image, the glenoid "vault" is anterior to the glenoid "face". **C,** In this image, the glenoid "vault" is posterior to the glenoid "face".

authors reported an average humeral head diameter to be 47.6 mm.[19] Boileau et al examined 65 cadaveric humeri with a digitized measuring device that allowed three-dimensional imaging with computer software. The average humeral head diameter was 46.2 mm, but the authors noted a significant variation with a range from 37.1 to 56.9 mm.[32] Lastly, Robertson et al evaluated 60 cadaveric humeri with CT imaging. The average humeral head diameter in their review was 46 mm (range, 34-56 mm).[6] All three of these studies documented similar findings.

The humeral head height is the measurement from the midportion of the anatomical neck to the superiormost portion of the articular surface **(FIGURE 2.7; TABLE 2.2).** This is often referred to as the humeral head thickness. Most shoulder arthroplasty systems have a variety of humeral head thicknesses to not only adapt to individual

anatomy but also allow tensioning of the periarticular soft tissues including the rotator cuff and posterior capsule during anatomic shoulder arthroplasty. Pearl et al examined 21 humeri with radiographs. The average humeral head height was 18.5 mm (range, 15-22 mm).[36] Jeong et al evaluated 36 cadaveric humeri and noted the average head height to be 18.24 mm (range, 15.3-21.5 mm).[37] Finally, Boileau et al and Robertson et al reported an average humeral head height to be 15.2 mm (range, 12.1-18.2 mm) and 19 mm (range, 15-24 mm), respectively.[6,32] These findings are interesting when considering the two head thicknesses—15 and 22 mm—offered by the original Neer humeral implant, which closely reflected this anatomic parameter.

The humeral head shape and offset are important anatomic parameters to understand since the goal of shoulder arthroplasty is, again, anatomic reconstruction.

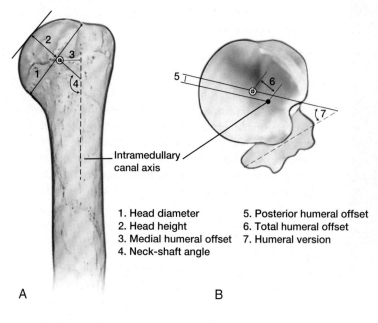

Intramedullary canal axis

1. Head diameter
2. Head height
3. Medial humeral offset
4. Neck-shaft angle

5. Posterior humeral offset
6. Total humeral offset
7. Humeral version

A   B

FIGURE 2.7 A, A coronal image of the proximal humerus illustrating head diameter, head height, medial offset, and neck-shaft angle. The diameter is measured by the length of the anatomical neck. The height is measured from the midportion of the anatomical neck to the superior most portion of the articular surface. The medial offset is measured by the center of rotation of the head in relation to the intramedullary canal of the humerus. The neck-shaft angle is the angle between the humeral medullary canal and a line bisecting the anatomical neck. **B,** Axial image of the humerus illustrating the posterior humeral offset, total humeral offset, and humeral version. The posterior offset is measured from the center of rotation of the humeral head to the central axis of the intramedullary canal. Total humeral offset is the sum of medial humeral offset and posterior humeral offset. The humeral version is the angle formed between the axis of the articular surface and the transepicondylar axis.

TABLE 2.2 Summary of Published Data of Humeral Dimensions							
Anatomic Parameter (mm unless noted)	HH Diameter	HH Thickness	HH Neck Angle (°)	HH Medial Offset	HH Posterior Offset	HH Retroversion	Humerus Length
Boileau et al[32] (n = 65)	46.2 ± 5.4	15.2 ± 1.6	129.6 ± 2.9	6.9 ± 2.0	2.6 ± 1.8	17.9 ± 13.7	Not reported
Hertel et al[33] (n = 200)	44.5 ± 4.0	17.0 ± 1.7	137.0 ± 3.6	6.0 ± 1.8	1.4 ± 1.4	23.3 ± 11.8	316.0 ± 23.0
Iannotti et al[11] (n = 140)	Not Reported	19 ± 2.4	135 ± 5	Not reported	Not reported	Not reported	Not reported
Roberts et al[34] (n = 39)	50.3 ± 1.01	Not reported	Not reported	Not reported	4.7 ± 1.1	21.4 ± 4.6	Not reported
Robertson et al[6] (n = 60)	46 ± 4	19 ± 2	131 ± 3	7 ± 2	2 ± 2	19 ± 6	330 ± 30
Takase et al[35] (n = 471)	54.3 ± 5.4	Not reported	140.4 ± 4.1	Not reported	Not reported	Not reported	Not reported
Jacobson et al[18] (n = 74)	46.8 ± 4.2	19.5 ± 2.5	134.5 ± 5.1	8.1 ± 3.3	3.2 ± 2.3	26.7 ± 12.1	321.1 ± 21.3

HH, humeral head.

The humeral head shape was noted to be elliptical rather than circular by McPherson et al.[19] This elliptical shape's major axis is superior-inferior, while the minor axis is anterior-posterior.[19] The humeral head offset is the measurement from the center of the humeral canal to the center of rotation of the humeral head. The humeral head is offset both medial and posterior to the axis of the humeral canal (**FIGURE 2.7; TABLE 2.2**). McPherson et al documented a mean medial offset of 7.6 mm and a posterior offset of 1.9 mm.[19] Pearl et al reported only a medial offset, which they documented to be 9.7 mm (range, 6-12 mm).[36] Boileau and Walch evaluated 65 cadaveric humeri and measured medial offset to be 6.9 mm (range, 2.9-10.8 mm) and posterior offset to be 2.6 mm (range, 0.8-6.1 mm).[32] Robertson et al also reported medial and posterior offset after evaluation of 60 cadaveric humeri. The authors reported the mean medial offset to be 7 mm (range, 4-12 mm) and the average posterior offset to be 2 mm (range, 1-8 mm).[6] Lastly, Jacobson et al evaluated 74 cadaveric shoulders with CT imaging. These authors reported a medial and posterior offset to be 8.1 and 3.2 mm, respectively.[18]

The humeral version has been described to represent the angle of the articular surface with respect to the long axis of the forearm, the transepicondylar axis of the distal humerus, and the trochlear axis of the distal humerus[38] (**FIGURE 2.7; TABLE 2.2**). Retroversion is present when the humeral head articular surface is facing posterior to these axes and anteversion is when the humeral head articular surface is facing anterior to these axes. Humeral head version has a wide variation reported in literature, in part, due to the multiple references utilized.[38] For example, the carrying angle of the elbow creates an angle between the forearm and trochlear axis, which represents an additional 10° to 15°.[38] The transepicondylar axis differs from the trochlear axis by 3° to 8°.[38] Although this may explain the range

of measurements reported for humeral version, there is an inherent individual variation that exists. By combining five anatomic studies that reported on a total of 592 shoulders, the mean humeral retroversion is 23.5° (range, 17.9°-29.8° of retroversion).[6,23,32,37,38] However, even though the range of the mean humeral retroversion was 17.9° to 29.8°, the individual studies have reported a much wider variation ranging from 2° of anteversion to 55° of retroversion.[23,38] This further supports the importance of identifying the individual variation that exists in achieving the goal of anatomic reconstruction. Just in one study, Jacobson et al measured the average humeral version to be 26.7° retroverted; however, the range encompassed 24.2° from 74 cadaveric specimens.[18]

The metaphyseal and diaphyseal diameters of the proximal humerus were reported by McPherson et al. Although the authors reported both periosteal and endosteal diameters, we will focus on the endosteal, intramedullary diameter since these dimensions are most relevant for humeral implant shape and press-fit fixation. The coronal endosteal diameters of the proximal humerus at the level of the surgical neck, 5 cm distal to the surgical neck, and 10 cm distal to the surgical neck are 2.7, 16, and 15.3 mm, respectively.[19] The sagittal endosteal diameters of the proximal humerus at the level of the surgical neck, 5 cm distal to the surgical neck, and 10 cm distal to the surgical neck are 16, 14.3, and 12.6 mm, respectively.[19] Furthermore, Pearl studied the diaphyseal diameter of the reamed humeral canal, which was found to be 12 mm (range, 10-14 mm).[36] Various humeral length measurements are listed in **FIGURE 2.3** and **TABLE 2.2**.

The neck-shaft angle is the angle between the anatomical neck of the humeral head and the long axis of the humeral diaphysis (**FIGURE 2.7; TABLE 2.2**). Using standard radiographs, McPherson et al evaluated 93 nonarthritic shoulders and noted a mean neck-shaft angle of 141° (range 132.4°-149.6°).[19] Using CT imaging to evaluate 2058 cadaveric humeri, Jeong et al reported the mean neck-shaft angle to be 134.7°.[37] More importantly, these authors noted the range of neck-shaft angles to be between 115° and 148°, with 78% of the measurements between 130° and 140°.[37]

Similar to the glenoid radius of curvature, the humeral head radius of curvature is the radius of a circular arc that best approximates the curve of the humeral head's articular surface. Pearl et al studied 21 cadaveric humeri and reported the radius of curvature to be 25.3 mm (range, 23-29 mm).[36] McPherson et al utilized radiographs of 93 cadaveric humeri to describe the radius of curvature of the humeral head in the true anteroposterior and axial-lateral projections. Both, the true anteroposterior and axial-lateral measurements were similar: the true anteroposterior radius of curvature was 23.1 mm and the axial-lateral radius of curvature was 22.9 mm.[19]

RADIAL MISMATCH

The difference in the radius of curvature of the glenoid and humeral head is referred to as the "radial mismatch."[3,39] This measurement describes the conformity of the articulation between the humeral head and the glenoid. In this context, a smaller radial mismatch represents increasing conformity (constraint), while a larger mismatch represents less conformity (constraint).[3,39] With a smaller radial mismatch, humeral head translation is more limited, which can create increased shear and edge loading on the glenoid implant.[3,39] With increased edge loading, the "rocking horse" phenomenon may occur, which is described as a cause of glenoid component loosening.[5,20,40] A larger radial mismatch creates less constraint, less shear, and less edge loading but is also a less stable configuration.[3,39] Furthermore, less constraint allows greater humeral head translation and thus, potentially, greater wear.[3,39] A radial mismatch of 4 mm has been reported to most accurately simulate the kinematics of a normal glenohumeral joint, although this amount of mismatch has been reported to be more variable in clinical outcome studies.[3,39,41,42] Since radial mismatch is an inherent part of glenohumeral anatomy, it should be replicated in shoulder arthroplasty component design and in the arthroplasty procedures performed.

CROSS-SECTIONAL PROXIMAL HUMERAL ANATOMY AND IMPLANT GEOMETRY

McPherson et al reported the axial shape of the proximal humeral canal to be oval or elliptical.[19] The anatomy of the humeral canal is reflected in the geometry of the different short humeral implant designs including circular (which is a more anatomic axial shape), semiangular, and angular.[43] These designs have been developed to decrease the potential for proximal stress shielding.[43] By varying the geometric design of the humeral stem,

physiologic stress can be transferred to the proximal humerus to limit stress shielding while still maintaining adequate torsional stability.[43]

CONCLUSION

Currently, the goal of shoulder arthroplasty is to re-create the native glenohumeral anatomy. This can be challenging when performing shoulder arthroplasty because of the variability of the individual glenohumeral anatomy, which is further altered by the arthritic processes. Glenoid anatomy that is pertinent to implant design includes height, width, surface area, version, vault shape and size, and radius of curvature. The concept of glenoid "face anatomy" and "vault anatomy" is also important to understand to accurately place the glenoid component into the central portion of the vault to optimize bony support of the implant. Proximal humeral anatomy that is pertinent to implant design includes humeral head diameter, height, shape, offset, version, humeral canal dimensions, neck-shaft angle, and radius of curvature. Additionally, the concept of radial mismatch allows a surgeon to reproduce normal kinematics of the glenohumeral joint to improve glenoid component longevity and survival. In general, glenoid and humeral implants have evolved to accommodate the variable anatomy to achieve an "anatomic reconstruction." Achieving this goal requires a clear understanding of glenohumeral anatomy and all of its variations. The increased success of shoulder arthroplasty has been attributed, in part, to a greater understanding of glenohumeral anatomy. The chapters that follow will address all facets of shoulder arthroplasty with the common thread of understanding the anatomy.

REFERENCES

1. Getz C, Ricchetti E, Verborgt O, Brolin T. Normal and pathoanatomy of the arthritic shoulder: considerations for shoulder arthroplasty. *J Am Acad Orthop Surg.* 2019;27:1068-1076.
2. Recchetti E, Hendel M, Collins D, Iannotti J. Is premorbid glenoid anatomy altered in patients with glenohumeral osteoarthritis? *Clin Orthop Relat Res.* 2013;471:2932-2939.
3. Strauss E, Roche C, florin PH, Wright T, Zuckerman J. The glenoid in shoulder arthroplasty. *J Shoulder Elbow Surg.* 2009;18:819-833.
4. Moineau G, Levigne C, Boileau P, Yaung A, Walch G. Three-dimensional measurement method of arthritic glenoid cavity morphology: feasibility and reproducibility. *Orthop Traumatol Surg Res.* 2012;98(6 suppl):139-145.
5. Shapiro T, McGarry M, Gupta R, Lee Y, Lee T. Biomechanical effects of glenoid retroversion in total shoulder arthroplasty. *J Shoulder Elbow Surg.* 2007;16:90-95.
6. Robertson D, Yuan J, Bigliani L, Flatow E, Yamaguchi K. Three-dimensional analysis of the proximal part of the humerus: relevance to arthroplasty. *J Bone Joint Surg Am.* 2000;82(11):1594-1602.
7. Flurin PH, Marczuk Y, Janout M, Wright T, Zuckerman J, Roche CP. Comparison of outcomes using anatomic and reverse total shoulder arthroplasty. *Bull Hosp Jt Dis (2013).* 2013;71(2):101-107.
8. Bryce CD, Pennypacker JL, Kulkarni N, Paul E, Hollenbeak C, Mosher T, Armstrong A. Validation of three-dimensional models of in situ scapulae. *J Shoulder Elbow Surg.* 2008;17(5):825-832.
9. Checroun A, Hawkins C, Kummer F, Zuckerman J. Fit of current glenoid component designs: an anatomic caver study. *J Shoulder Elbow Surg.* 2002;11:614-617.

10. Churchill R, Brems J, Kotschi H. Glenoid size, inclination, and version: an anatomic study. *J Shoulder Elbow Surg.* 2001;10: 327-332.

11. Iannotti J, Jun BJ, Patterson T, Ricchetti E. Quantitative measurement of osseous pathology in advanced glenohumeral osteoarthritis. *J Bone Joint Surg Am.* 2017;99:1460-1468.

12. Kwon Y, Powell K, Yum J, Brems J, Iannotti J. Use of three-dimensional computer tomography for the analysis of glenoid anatomy. *J Shoulder Elbow Surg.* 2005;14:85-90.

13. Ljungquist KL, Butler RB, Griesser MJ, Bishop JY. Prediction of coracoids thickness using a glenoid width-based model: implications for bone reconstruction procedures in chronic anterior shoulder instability. *J Shoulder Elbow Surg.* 2012;21(6):815-821.

14. Mallon WJ, Brown HR, Vogler JB, Martinez S. Radio-graphic and geometric anatomy of the scapula. *Clin Orthop Relat Res.* 1992;(277):142-154.

15. Merrill A, Guzman K, Miller SL. Gender differences in glenoid anatomy: an anatomic study. *Surg Radiol Anat.* 2009;31(3):183-189.

16. Ohl X, Billuart F, Lagacé P, Gagey O, Hagemeister N, Skalli W. 3D morphometric analysis of 43 scapulae. *Surg Radiol Anat.* 2012;34(5):447-453.

17. Von Schroeder HP, Kuiper SD, Botte MJ. Osseous anatomy of the scapula. *Clin Orthop Relat Res.* 2001;(383):131-139. Review.

18. Jacobson A, Gilot G, Hamilton M, et al. Glenohumeral anatomic study. A comparison of male and female shoulders with similar average age and BMI. *Bull Hosp Jt Dis (2013).* 2015;73(1):S68-S78.

19. McPherson EJ, Friedman RJ, An YH, Chokesi R, Dooley RL. Anthropometric study of normal glenohumeral relationships. *J Shoulder Elbow Surg.* 1997;6:105-112.

20. Friedman R, Hawthorne K, Genez B. The use of computerized tomography in the measurement of glenoid version. *J Bone Joint Surg Am.* 1992;74(7):1032-1037.

21. Bishop J, Kline S, Alderink K, Zauel R, Bey M. Glenoid inclination: in vivo measurements in rotator cuff tear patients and associations with superior glenohumeral joint translation. *J Shoulder Elbow Surg.* 2009;18:231-236.

22. Rouleau D, Kidder J, Pons-Villanueva J, Dynamidis S, Defranco M, Walch G. Glenoid version: how to measure it? Validity of different methods in two- and three- dimensional models. *J Shoulder Elbow Surg.* 2010;19:1230-1237.

23. Matsumura N, Ogawa K, Kobayashi S, et al. Morphologic features of humeral head and glenoid version in the normal glenohumeral joint. *J Shoulder Elbow Surg.* 2014;23:1724-1730.

24. Gannipathi A, McCarron J, Chen X, Iannotti J. Predicting normal glenoid version from pathologic scapula: a comparison of 4 methods in in 2- and 3- dimensional models. *J Shoulder Elbow Surg.* 2011;20:234-244.

25. Boileau P, Gauci M, Wagner E, et al. The reverse shoulder arthroplasty angle: a new measurement of glenoid inclination for reverse shoulder arthroplasty. *J Shoulder Elbow Surg.* 2019;28:1281-1290.

26. Dagget M, Werner B, Gauci M, Chaoui J, Walch G. Comparison of glenoid inclination angle using different imaging modalities. *J Shoulder Elbow Surg.* 2016;25(2):180-185.

27. Codsi M, Bennetts C, Gordiev K, et al. Normal glenoid vault anatomy and validation of a novel glenoid implant shape. *J Shoulder Elbow Surg.* 2008;17:471-478.

28. Anglin C, Wyss U, Pichora D. Mechanical testing of shoulder prostheses and recommendations for glenoid design. *J Shoulder Elbow Surg.* 2000;9:323-331.

29. Anglin C, Wyss U, Nyffeler R, Gerber C. Loosening performance of cemented glenoid prosthesis design pairs. *Clin Biomech (Bristol, Avon).* 2001;16:144-150.

30. Dauzere F, Arboucalot M, Lebon J, Elia F, Bonnevialle N, Mansat P. Evaluation of thirty-eight cemented pegged glenoid components with variable backside curvature: two-year minimum follow up. *Int Orthop.* 2017;41(11):2353-2360.

31. Szabo I, Buscayret F, Edwards B, Nemoz C, Boilaeu P, Walch G. Radiographic comparison of flat-back and convex-back glenoid components in total shoulder arthroplasty. *J Shoulder Elbow Surg.* 2005;14:636-642.

32. Boileau P, Walch G. The three-dimensional geometry of the proximal humerus. *J Bone Joint Surg Br.* 1997;79:857-865.

33. Hertel R, Knothe U, Ballmer FT. Geometry of the proximal humerus and implications for prosthetic design. *J Shoulder Elbow Surg.* 2002;11(4):331-338.

34. Roberts S, Foley A, Swallow H, Wallace W, Coughlan D. The geometry of the humeral head and the design of prostheses. *J Bone Joint Surg Br.* 1991;73(4):647-650.

35. Takase K, Yamamoto K, Imakiire A, Burkhead WZ. The radio-graphic study in the relationship of the glenohumeral joint. *J Orthop Res.* 2004;22(2):298-305.

36. Pearl M, Volk A. Coronal plane geometry of the proximal humerus relevant to prosthetic arthroplasty. *J Shoulder Elbow Surg.* 1996;5:320-326.

37. Jeong J, Bryan J, Iannotti J. Effect of variable prosthetic neck-shaft angle and the surgical technique on replication of normal humeral anatomy. *J Bone Joint Surg Am.* 2009;91:1932-1941.

38. Pearl M, Voil A. Retroversion of the proximal humerus in relationship to prosthetic replacement arthroplasty. *J Shoulder Elbow Surg.* 1995;4:286-289.

39. Karduna A, Williams G, Williams J, Iannotti J. Glenohumeral joint translations before and after total shoulder arthroplasty. *J Bone Joint Surg Am.* 1997;79(8):1166-1174.

40. Jacxsens M, Tangel A, Henninger H, Conick B, Mueller A, Wilde L. A three-dimensional comparative study in the scapulohumeral relationship in normal and osteoarthritic shoulders. *J Shoulder Elbow Surg.* 2016;25(10):1607-1615.

41. Walch G, Edwards T, boulahia A, Boileau P, Mole D, Adeleine P. The influence of glenohumeral prosthetic mismatch on glenoid radiolucent lines: results of a multicenter study. *J Bone Joint Surg Am.* 2002;84(10):2186-2191.

42. Schoch B, Wrigh T, Zuckerman J, et al. The effect of radial mismatch on radiographic glenoid loosening. *JSES Open Access.* 2019;3(4):287-291.

43. Barth J, Garret J, Geais L, Bothorel H, Saffarini M. Influence of uncemented humeral stem proximal geometry on stress distributions and torsional stability following total shoulder arthroplasty. *J Exp Orthop.* 2019;6:8.

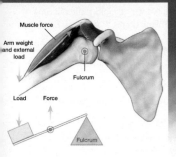

3

Biomechanics of Anatomic Total Shoulder Arthroplasty

Christopher P. Roche, MSE, MBA and Matthew L. Hansen, MD

MOTION OF THE SHOULDER

The motion of the shoulder is complex and created by the simultaneous action of three different joints and one articulation: the glenohumeral, sternoclavicular, and acromioclavicular joints and the scapulothoracic articulation **(FIGURE 3.1)**. To perform shoulder elevation, each is required to elevate and rotate the scapula while the humerus simultaneously rotates and lifts the arm in coordinated motion termed scapulohumeral rhythm **(FIGURE 3.2)**. As described by Codman et al and Inman, the approximate ratio of humeral to scapular rotation is 2:1, with scapulothoracic motion accounting for a maximum of 60° and humeral motion accounting for a maximum of 120° though most activities of daily living (ADLs) are completed with the scapula rotating no more than 30° and the humerus rotating no more than 60°.[1,2]

Inman et al described shoulder motion as being generated by three general muscle groupings: (1) scapulohumeral (muscles originating on the scapula and inserting on the humerus), (2) axiohumeral (muscles originating on the torso and inserting on the humerus), and (3) axioscapular muscles (muscles originating on the torso and inserting on the scapula).[2] The scapulohumeral muscles are the supraspinatus, infraspinatus, teres minor, subscapularis (collectively known as the rotator cuff), as well as the deltoid, and teres major. The scapulohumeral muscles work together to elevate and rotate the arm. The axiohumeral muscles are the latissimus dorsi and the pectoralis major (with a portion of the pectoralis originating on the clavicle), which act to internally rotate and elevate the arm. The axioscapular muscles are the trapezius, rhomboids, serratus anterior, levator scapulae, and the pectoralis minor, which all act to rotate the scapula (it should also be noted that the biceps brachii and the long head of the triceps originate from the scapula and cross the elbow joint to insert on the proximal radius and ulna, acting as shoulder stabilizers) **(FIGURE 3.3)**.

GLENOHUMERAL JOINT

Joint Form and Function

The form of each diarthrodial joint has evolved to carefully balance stability and motion for its particular function. Joints requiring more constraint to perform ADLs typically have more conforming and congruent articular geometries to ensure that the joint reaction force is directed toward the center of the articulation to maintain stability, even at the extremes of the range of motion (ROM). Conversely, joints that require greater mobility typically have less articular constraint to minimize bony impingement at the end points of motion. For these highly mobile joints, stability at the end points of motion is achieved by both static (ligamentous and capsular constraint) and by dynamic (coordinated contraction of the surrounding musculature) stabilizers.

The relationship between articular joint geometry and the surrounding musculature is highly refined, with the number, size, position, and orientation of muscles crossing a particular joint designed to both generate the torque necessary for a particular motion but also to constrain and control that motion. Agonist and antagonist muscle groupings are necessary for finely controlled motions, particularly in highly mobile joints like the shoulder complex. These muscle group pairs coordinate contraction to dynamically stabilize the joint at various positions in order to direct the joint reaction force toward the joint center despite large joint rotations and translations.[3,4]

The glenohumeral joint is the largest joint in the shoulder complex and is composed of the articulation of the proximal humerus (ie, the humeral head) and the scapula (ie, the glenoid) **(FIGURE 3.4)**. The concave humeral head articular geometry is large relative to the convex glenoid articular surface; and as the glenoid is approximately ¼ of the size of the humeral head, it provides little to no intrinsic osseous stability. Furthermore, since the bony joint curvatures are nonconforming, with the glenoid bone flatter than the relatively spherical humeral head, the glenohumeral joint osseous morphology has little intrinsic constraint or congruity. With these parameters, the analogy of a golf ball on a tee is often invoked to describe the humeral head and glenoid size relationship. However, glenohumeral joint conformity is increased by the presence of the glenoid labrum and variable thickness of the glenoid articular cartilage.[5-7] It should be noted that the glenoid is nonuniform and thicker on the periphery than in the glenoid center which increases joint congruency. Glenohumeral joint stability

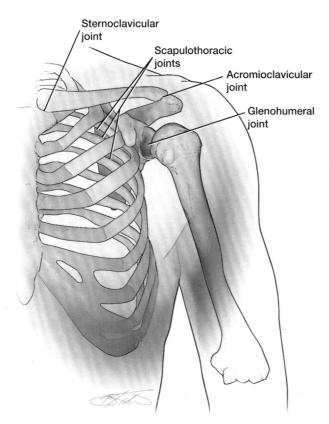

FIGURE 3.1 Components of the shoulder: glenohumeral, sterno-clavicular, and acromioclavicular joints and the scapulothoracic articulation.

changes with loading direction due to the varying glenoid morphology. As the glenoid is longer in the superior/inferior (S/I) direction than anterior/posterior (A/P) direction, the S/I glenoid is associated with additional depth as compared to the A/P glenoid.[8-12] As a result, the humeral head is more constrained in the S/I direction than in the A/P direction.

Glenohumeral Joint Motion

Due to this nonconforming geometry and lack of osseous constraint, the glenohumeral joint is the most mobile joint in the human body and requires dynamic and static soft-tissue action for both joint motion and stability. Specifically, glenohumeral joint motion and stability are assisted throughout the ROM by the coordinated action of muscle contractions, which vary according to joint position and the different types of motion.[3] The end points of motion are controlled by ligament and capsular tightening. Furthermore, due to both the minimal osseous constraint and the viscoelastic nature of the conforming articular cartilage and labrum, the glenohumeral joint center of rotation (CoR) can translate during motions. As such, glenohumeral joint motion has been described as (1) spinning (rotation only), (2) sliding (translation only), and (3) rolling (rotation + translation)[13,14] **(FIGURE 3.5)**.

There are three general types of arm motion enabled by these humeral head articulations against the glenoid, which are defined relative to the anatomic planes **(FIGURE 3.6)**. Abduction/adduction is defined as the motion of the humeral head that results in arm elevation/de-elevation in the scapular and/or coronal plane, and forward/backward in the transverse plane. Flexion/extension is defined as the motion of the humeral head that results in arm forward/backward elevation in the sagittal plane. Finally, internal/external rotation is defined as the motion of the humeral head around its longitudinal axis, with arm rotation toward the midline termed internal rotation and arm rotation away from the midline termed external rotation.

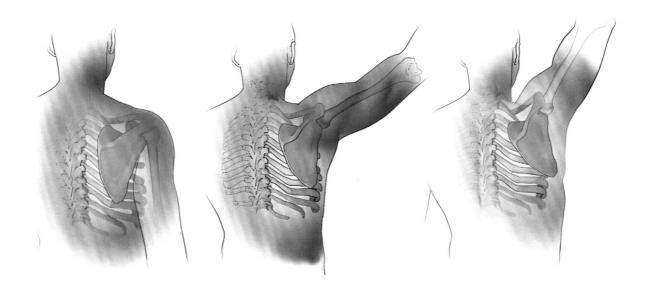

FIGURE 3.2 Scapulohumeral rhythm during arm elevation.

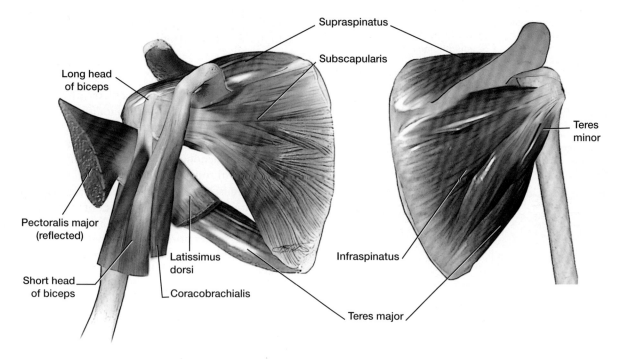

FIGURE 3.3 Anterior (left) and posterior (right) shoulder muscles.

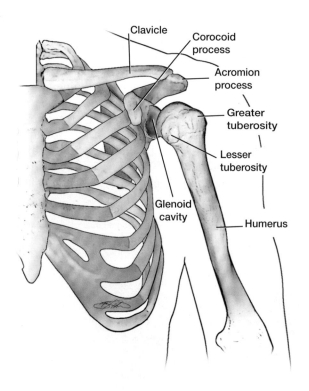

FIGURE 3.4 Shoulder joint anatomy.

GLENOHUMERAL MUSCLES

Muscles generate straight line forces that are converted to torques in proportion to their perpendicular distance between the joint CoR and the muscle's line of action.[3,4] This perpendicular distance is termed the muscle's moment arm. Muscle moment arms typically increase from deep to superficial. The torque generated by a particular muscle during contraction to either facilitate or stabilize a particular type of motion is determined by its moment arm position and orientation relative to the joint CoR. In general, shoulder muscles located anterior/posterior to the CoR internally/externally rotate the arm and muscles located superior/inferior to the CoR raise/lower the arm, respectively.

There are three types of muscle contraction. Concentric contractions generate submaximal tension during muscle shortening; eccentric contractions generate tension while the muscle elongates due to a larger opposing force; and isometric contractions generate muscle tension without a change in muscle length. Muscle contraction contributes to joint motion, typically in rotation, and may contribute to joint stability, depending on its line of action relative to the joint CoR. For finely controlled joint motions, muscles often function in groups as agonists (generating torque to cause joint rotation) or antagonists (contractions that oppose rotation). Agonists and antagonists typically mirror one another (A/P or S/I) for a particular type of motion and may work as force couples to increase the joint reaction force, thereby acting also to stabilize the joint. Individual muscles may also function in a biphasic manner, acting as agonists during one segment of motion and then acting as antagonists during another segment of motion because the muscle line of action crosses from one side of the CoR to the other as a result of joint motion.[3,4] The joint motion produced by a given shoulder muscle depends on the position of its origin and insertion relative to the CoR; thus, a shoulder

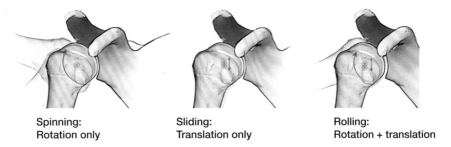

Spinning:
Rotation only

Sliding:
Translation only

Rolling:
Rotation + translation

FIGURE 3.5 Glenohumeral joint motion: spinning (left), sliding (middle), and rolling (right).

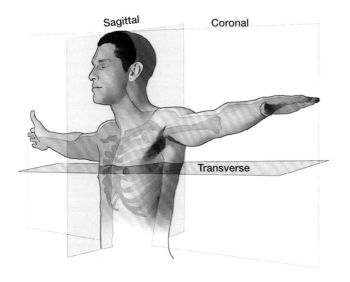

FIGURE 3.6 Anatomic planes.

muscle's function may change depending on arm position for each of the different motions.

The larger the muscle's moment arm, the greater its capacity to generate the torque required for motion and to support external loads. Thus, a larger moment arm may result in greater muscle efficiency, assuming the muscle mechanics inherent to a given muscle's architecture (eg, pennation angle, cross-sectional area, sarcomere structure) can accommodate greater excursion.[3] Muscles tend to specialize in varying degrees of force production or excursion. This is relevant for shoulder surgery and for shoulder prosthesis designs that alter the demands placed on shoulder muscles. Neurological status is also an important factor in muscle performance, as a poorly innervated muscle will not contract as well as a properly innervated muscle.

Most ADLs are performed with the arm internally rotated and elevated. As such, the largest muscles in the shoulder complex act to either elevate the arm and/or internally rotate the arm and to also stabilize the arm in those positions. External rotator muscles are also critical as they are necessary to resist internal rotation torque created by external loads as a result of elbow flexion. The deltoid is the largest muscle in the shoulder complex, and it is the primary elevator in the arm. The

deltoid consists of three distinct heads which originate on the scapula and clavicle and wrap around the lateral proximal humerus as it inserts midway down the humeral shaft. The three heads of the deltoid are as follows: (1) anterior deltoid (originating from the anterior acromion and clavicle); (2) middle deltoid (originating from the lateral margin of the acromion); and (3) the posterior deltoid (originating from the scapular spine). At low levels of abduction, the wrapping of the middle deltoid around the lateral proximal humerus generates a stabilizing compressive force **(FIGURE 3.7)**; however, this compressive force is small relative to that generated by the rotator cuff.[15-18]

The rotator cuff muscles generate the torque necessary for rotation of the humerus about the glenoid fossa while also compressing the humeral head into the glenoid concavity.[19] The rotator cuff muscles are aligned around the proximal humerus for effective joint compression at all glenohumeral joint positions, allowing it to balance the joint by creating a dynamic fulcrum. This enables arm elevation while inhibiting superior migration of the humeral head and acromial impingement. In doing so, the rotator cuff effectively compensates for the lack of osseous constraint in the glenohumeral joint.[20-22] Specifically, the anatomic arrangement of the anterior (subscapularis) and posterior (infraspinatus and teres minor) rotator cuff muscles creates a transverse force couple that centers the humeral head on the glenoid fossa in the A/P directions for all joint positions[23-25] **(FIGURE 3.8)**. The superior rotator cuff muscle (supraspinatus) is an abductor, which facilitates arm elevation, particularly at the initiation of motion. It also coordinates with the other rotator cuff muscles to generate a stabilizing compressive force to counteract the superiorly directed force generated by the deltoid, allowing for joint rotation as opposed to translation. This stabilizing mechanism of the rotator cuff interacting with the geometry of the glenohumeral joint has been termed concavity-compression.[19] Concavity-compression is the concept of stability achieved by pressing a convex surface into a concave surface, with additional resistance to shear forces achieved with greater compression. The stabilizing effect of concavity compression is illustrated by the difference in humeral head translation observed between active and

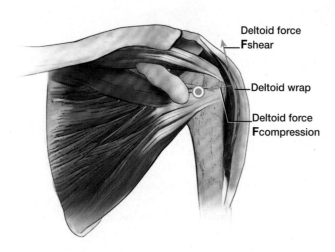

FIGURE 3.7 Deltoid wrapping around the greater tuberosity of the proximal humerus to generate a stabilizing compressive force.

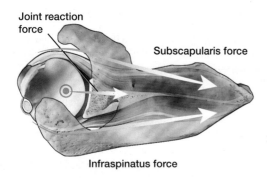

FIGURE 3.8 Transverse force couple of the anterior and posterior rotator cuff to create concavity compression of the humeral head into the glenoid.

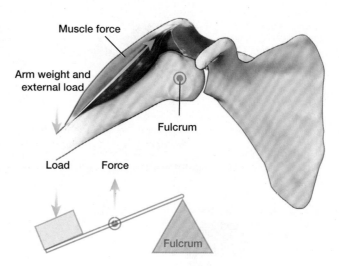

FIGURE 3.9 The shoulder joint represented as a class three lever.

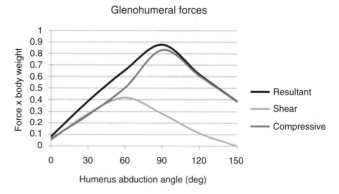

FIGURE 3.10 Compressive, shear, and joint reaction forces in the shoulder during unweighted abduction as a function of elevation angle. (Adapted from Poppen NK, Walker PS. Forces at the glenohumeral joint in abduction. *Clin Orthop Relat Res.* 1978;(135):165-170.)

passive motion, where humeral head translations during active motion are reported to be 1 to 4 mm in the S/I and A/P directions. During passive motion, humeral head translations can approach as much as 8 mm.[26-28]

Forces in the Shoulder

As shoulder muscle forces are applied between the CoR and the external load, the shoulder functions as a class three lever. While class one and class two levers amplify the input force at the expense of motion, class three levers place the input force at a mechanical disadvantage, requiring greater input force than the applied load. As such, the force exerted by the shoulder muscles must exceed that of the applied load **(FIGURE 3.9)**. Furthermore, as the shoulder muscles act to dynamically stabilize the joint by co-contraction and the aforementioned concavity-compression mechanism, the summation of these muscle forces further increases the overall joint reaction force. Assuming that the arm weighs 5% body weight (BW), Poppen and Walker demonstrated

that the maximum total joint reaction force in the shoulder occurs at 90° abduction and is approximately 0.89% BW, while the maximum shear force in the shoulder occurs at 60° abduction and is approximately 0.42% BW, based just upon the weight of the extremity[29] **(FIGURE 3.10)**. Poppen and Walker also reported that when 1 kg is held in the hand, the forces were increased by 60%.[29] Westerhoff et al reported joint reaction forces of up to 1700 N and 238% BW using an instrumented anatomic total shoulder arthroplasty (ATSA) prosthesis in patients performing common ADLs.[30-33] Thus, even though the shoulder joint is not "weight bearing," it can still experience significant loads.

The relative size and cross-sectional areas of the muscles in the shoulder can be indicative of their use and function. Basset et al reported that the three heads of the deltoid account for 24% of the total muscle volume in the shoulder, the pectoralis major accounts for 17%, the latissimus dorsi accounts for 13.5%, the subscapularis accounts for 10%, the combined infraspinatus and teres minor account for 9%, the biceps and triceps account for 7% each, the teres major accounts for 6.5%, the supraspinatus accounts for 3.5%, and finally the coracobrachialis accounts for 2% of the total muscle volume in the shoulder.[34] Basset et al also reported that the physiological cross-sectional area of the deltoid was 23 cm[2], the subscapularis was 16.3 cm[2], the combined infraspinatus and teres minor were 13.7 cm[2], the pectoralis major was 13.3 cm[2], the latissimus dorsi was 12 cm[2], the teres major was 8.8 cm[2], the supraspinatus was 5.7 cm[2], the biceps and triceps were 4 cm[2] each, and finally the coracobrachialis was 1.6 cm[2].[34] Similarly, Veeger et al reported that the physiological cross-sectional area of the deltoid was 26 cm[2], the pectoralis major was 13.7 cm[2], the subscapularis was 13.5 cm[2], the combined infraspinatus and teres minor were 12.4 cm[2], the teres major was 10.0 cm[2], the latissimus dorsi was 8.6 cm[2], and the supraspinatus was 5.2 cm[2].[35] The muscle volume, cross-sectional area, and moment arms all influence the magnitude of torque generated by each muscle for a given motion. As these muscles work together in agonist and antagonist groups, injury or impairment to just one muscle can reduce ROM and/or result in joint instability.

Glenohumeral Instability

Glenohumeral joint stability is achieved by the coordinated function of both the dynamic (muscles) and static (ligaments, capsule, and articular constraint) stabilizers to orient and position the joint reaction force toward the glenoid fossa at all joint positions. Specifically, in the shoulder, muscles can stabilize the glenohumeral joint by the following five mechanisms: (1) passive muscle tension, (2) contraction causing compression across the joint, (3) joint motion that secondarily tightens passive ligamentous constraints, (4) barrier effect of a contracted muscle, and (5) redirection of the joint reaction force to the center of the glenoid articular surface.[36]

In contrast, glenohumeral joint instability occurs when the joint reaction force is directed outside the glenoid fossa, which is typically associated with (1) muscle imbalance, (2) glenoid or humeral wear/deformity, and/or (3) soft-tissue injury caused by trauma, joint overloading, or congenital deficiencies. Due to the complexity of this static/dynamic interaction, injury to just one or more tissues can dramatically impact stability and result in humeral head subluxation, humeral head dislocations, and/or compromised ability to recenter the humeral head on the glenoid during active motion[19] **(FIGURE 3.11)**. The inability to dynamically recenter the humeral head can lead to eccentric glenoid loading, reduced surface contact area, and a joint load concentration that can induce degenerative changes in the glenoid and/or humeral head.[37-41]

One of the most common soft-tissue injuries in the shoulder is a rotator cuff tear. Disruption of rotator cuff

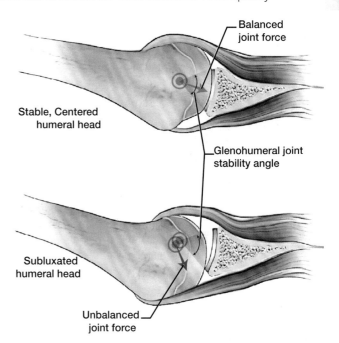

FIGURE 3.11 Instability resulting from the joint reaction force being directed outside of the glenoid articular surface. (Used with permission from Lippitt SB, Vanderhooft JE, Harris SL, Sidles JA, Harryman DT 2nd, Matsen FA 3rd. Glenohumeral stability from concavity-compression: A quantitative analysis. *J Shoulder Elbow Surg.* 1993;2(1):27-35. doi:10.1016/S1058-2746(09)80134-1.)

integrity, most commonly by a tear in one or more of the rotator cuff tendons, can have a significant impact on glenohumeral joint stability, with larger size and full-thickness tears resulting in greater loss of concavity-compression. As the rotator cuff fails to achieve concavity-compression and create a fulcrum that balances the superiorly directed deltoid force during arm elevation, the humeral head tends to migrate superiorly and impinge on the undersurface of the acromion **(FIGURE 3.12)**. This impingement can lead to further tearing of the rotator cuff, typically starting with the supraspinatus and propagating to the superior portions of the subscapularis and infraspinatus. An unrepaired rotator cuff tendon will have compromised blood flow and reduced function which eventually leads to irreversible fatty atrophy of the rotator cuff muscle. This further reduces its function and results in the onset of arthritic changes that are secondary to increased friction and a lack of nutrients supplied to the cartilage. Continued rotator cuff tearing propagates further impingement and results in humeral head collapse, biceps tendon dislocation, and erosion of the superior glenoid, acromion, and coracoid.[42,43] The resulting glenoid erosion can occur centrally or eccentrically; multiple classification systems[44-46] have been developed to define the location and magnitude of glenoid erosion.

Anatomic Total Shoulder Arthroplasty

The bony geometry of the glenohumeral joint is highly variable. As described in **TABLE 3.1**, numerous anatomic studies have demonstrated that the morphology of the

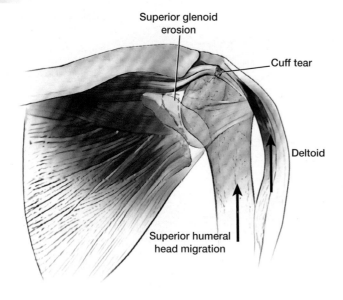

FIGURE 3.12 Superior humeral head migration resulting from loss of concavity compression by a rotator cuff tear.

humeral head in particular varies significantly relative to the intramedullary canal.[10,47-52] These anatomic findings are relevant to hemiarthroplasty and ATSA because the intramedullary axis is coincident with the axis of the humeral stem prosthesis, also known as the orthopedic axis. As such, the intramedullary canal establishes the position of the humeral head for the majority of first- and second-generation shoulder arthroplasty systems when attempting to reconstruct the joint for treatment of glenohumeral arthritis. Failure to restore the patient's

original anatomy and joint CoR is believed to result in poorer clinical outcomes.[53-58] Implanting too small a humeral head can result in excessive joint laxity and instability; whereas, implanting too large a humeral head can result in joint overstuffing and rotator cuff failure.

First-generation shoulder arthroplasty systems were defined by their monoblock nonmodular construction of the humeral head and humeral stem and were provided in too few sizes to account for anatomic variations. With the introduction of the glenoid prosthesis in the 1970s, ATSA was born.[59] Second-generation ATSA systems introduced in the 1980s incorporated a modular connection between the humeral head and humeral stem and provided additional humeral stem and humeral heads sizes for interchangeable configuration possibilities to facilitate a better anatomic reconstruction. This modular connection also permitted mixing of implant materials to improve wear (Co-28Cr-6Mo humeral heads) and fixation (Ti-6Al-4V humeral stems for press-fit usage and Co-28Cr-6Mo stems for cemented usage) when used for different indications. Later generation devices also incorporated an offset humeral head taper to fine tune the medial/posterior offset of the humeral head relative to the intramedullary canal and better tension the rotator cuff and balance the joint. However, even with offset humeral heads, these second-generation systems were unable to reproduce the native humeral head geometry for a large percentage of patients. An improved understanding of proximal humerus anatomy led to the development of third-generation shoulder arthroplasty systems in the early 1990s.[10,56,58] These shoulder arthroplasty systems permitted even better reconstruction of the medial/posterior offset of the humeral head relative

TABLE 3.1 Anatomy of the Proximal Humerus

Anatomic Parameter (mm Unless Noted)	HH Diameter	HH Thickness	HH Neck Angle (°)	HH Medial Offset	HH Posterior Offset	HH Retroversion	Humerus Length
Boileau et al[47] (n = 65)	46.2 ± 5.4	15.2 ± 1.6	129.6 ± 2.9	6.9 ± 2.0	2.6 ± 1.8	17.9 ± 13.7	Not reported
Hertel et al[48] (n = 200)	44.5 ± 4.0	17.0 ± 1.7	137.0 ± 3.6	6.0 ± 1.8	1.4 ± 1.4	23.3 ± 11.8	316.0 ± 23.0
Iannotti et al[10] (n = 140)	Not Reported	19 ± 2.4	135 ± 5	Not reported	Not reported	Not reported	Not reported
Roberts et al[49] (n = 39)	50.3 ± 1.01	Not reported	Not reported	Not reported	4.7 ± 1.1	21.4 ± 4.6	Not reported
Robertson et al[50] (n = 60)	46 ± 4	19 ± 2	131 ± 3	7 ± 2	2 ± 2	19 ± 6	330 ± 30
Takase et al[51] (n = 471)	54.3 ± 5.4	Not reported	140.4 ± 4.1	Not reported	Not reported	Not reported	Not reported
Jacobson et al[52] (n = 74)	46.8 ± 4.2	19.5 ± 2.5	134.5 ± 5.1	8.1 ± 3.3	3.2 ± 2.3	26.7 ± 12.1	321.1 ± 21.3

HH, humeral head.

to the intramedullary canal and also permitted selection of different humeral head neck angles by providing humeral stems at distinct angles, typically varying from 125° to 140° in 5° increments.

In the late 1990s and early 2000s, as usage of shoulder arthroplasty began to substantially increase, efforts were made to improve the precision of the anatomic reproduction, refine the stem geometry for different indications, and enhance their ease of use regardless of indication. These efforts led to the development of fourth-generation shoulder arthroplasty systems which utilize different humeral stem geometries for arthritis and fracture indications. These systems incorporate dual humeral offsets by use of an offset modular plate positioned between the humeral stem and offset humeral heads to decouple the medial and posterior humeral head offsets relative to the intramedullary canal. In some fourth-generation prosthesis designs, these offset modular plates also permit *in-situ* adjustability of humeral head neck angle and humeral head retroversion. With these adjustable features, fourth-generation shoulder systems permit reproduction of the patient's bony anatomy to best restore rotator cuff tension and balance the joint. Finally, some fourth-generation shoulder systems are defined by their platform humeral stems, which are used for both ATSA and reverse total shoulder arthroplasty (RTSA) applications; thereby, simplifying and reducing cost and time associated with revisions by permitting use of the same humeral stem during conversion from hemiarthroplasty or ATSA to RTSA[60-64] **(FIGURE 3.13)**.

Resurfacing humeral head arthroplasty offers a bone-conserving alternative to traditional humeral stemmed arthroplasty, as it does not require an anatomic humeral neck resection nor does it alter the humeral head position since it does not use the intramedullary canal as the reference for alignment. Instead, resurfacing humeral head arthroplasty simply requires spherical reaming to replace the humeral head articular surface. Despite this straightforward technique, Iannotti and colleagues reported that traditional stemmed arthroplasty may restore the joint CoR more accurately compared to resurfacing humeral head arthroplasty. Resurfacing humeral heads tend to overstuff the joint due to inaccuracies during humeral head reaming caused by the surgeon reaming too little bone and/or reaming in varus or valgus relative to the patient's actual humeral head neck angle.[65,66] Improvements in instrumentation and surgical technique can improve the accuracy and precision of anatomic reconstruction and better restore the joint CoR. Regarding this point, Chen et al reported that the joint CoR could be restored within 1 mm with resurfacing humeral head arthroplasty when a position 2 mm medial to the anatomic neck of the humeral head is used as a reference for reaming with a cannulated instrument technique.[67] Stemless humeral components **(FIGURE 3.14)** utilize an anatomic humeral neck resection that does not

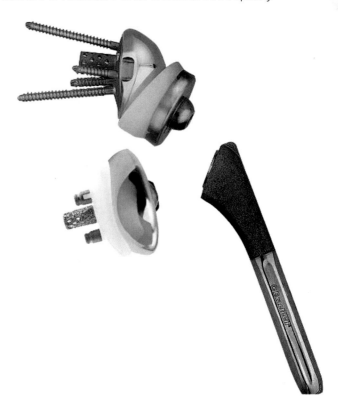

FIGURE 3.13 Equinoxe platform humeral stem system. (Used with permission from © Exactech, Inc.)

alter the humeral head position since it does not use the intramedullary canal as the reference for alignment. As such, stemless humeral components generally do not require different neck angles or offset humeral heads to reproduce the anatomy. As stemless humeral components are relatively new, additional clinical follow-up is necessary.

While aseptic humeral stem loosening is uncommon, other stem-related problems do exist in shoulder arthroplasty. In recent years, humeral stemmed components have shortened to a 70 mm minimum length permitted by the FDA via the 510k process to mitigate those concerns **(FIGURE 3.15)**. These "short stem" options have the potential to avoid some of the problems associated with standard length stems.[68,69] However, as clinical follow-up has evaluated these implants, numerous studies have reported high rates of stress shielding, bone remodeling, and "adaptations" with certain designs of short humeral stems.[70-72] Recent finite element analysis work by Langhor et al demonstrated that smaller diameter 70 mm length humeral stems are associated with more natural loading and stress profiles than larger diameter 70 mm length humeral stems, suggesting that observations of stress shielding with short humeral stems may be due to use of too large size stems for a given bone anatomy.[73] As humeral stem size selection with short-stem prostheses is no longer based upon the intramedullary canal diameter, new instrument and surgical technique refinement is necessary to provide intraoperative

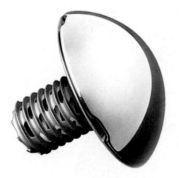 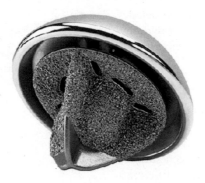 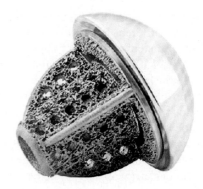

FIGURE 3.14 Arthrex eclipse (left), Wright Medical Simpliciti (right), and Exactech Equinoxe (right) stemless humeral components.

guidance on the appropriate short humeral stem size for given bony anatomy.

PATHOMECHANICS-INDUCED ATSA COMPLICATIONS

Anatomic reproduction of the CoR with ATSA should mitigate rotator cuff failures resulting from joint over-stuffing, while also mitigating instability that can result from an improperly balanced joint. However, rotator cuff tears can still occur and follow the same pathway as described for the native shoulder, which can result in loss of dynamic humeral head centering on the glenoid and instability. Secondarily, as the humeral head eccentrically loads the glenoid prosthesis, aseptic glenoid implant loosening can occur.

Aseptic glenoid loosening remains the unsolved and most common failure mode of ATSA and is the complication, which in most limits the long-term survival of the device. Glenoid loosening is caused by cyclic eccentric loading of the humeral head on the glenoid, inducing a torque on the bone-cement-implant fixation interface by a mechanism known as the rocking-horse phenomenon. Repetitive eccentric loading may also ultimately lead to glenoid failure by dissociation.[74-76]

Modern glenoid implants are designed to be uncon-strained and have a larger articular curvature than the humeral head. This permits humeral head translation and promotes more physiologic kinematics that minimize the shear forces on the fixation interfaces that occur from eccentric humeral head loading (relative to more con-forming and constrained designs). The difference between glenoid and humeral head articular surface curvatures is termed radial mismatch. There is no consensus regarding the ideal radial mismatch, though most implant systems are designed with a mismatch between 3 and 10 mm based upon results of different clinical and biomechani-cal studies.[27,75,77-81] Too small of a radial mismatch likely

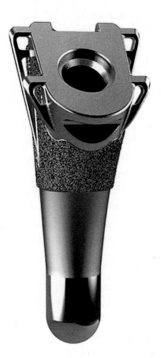 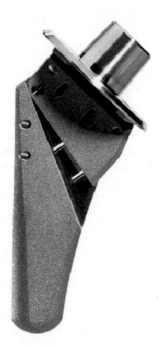 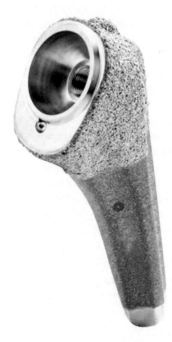

FIGURE 3.15 DJO AltiVate (left), Arthrex Univers Apex (middle), and Exactech Equinoxe preserve (right) short humeral stems.

constrains joint translation too much and increases shear on the fixation interfaces; too large of a radial mismatch may permit too much translation and decrease the surface contract area, potentially accelerating glenoid polyethylene wear. It is important to note that the ideal radial mismatch likely varies as a function of humeral head diameter as increasing humeral head diameter without also increasing radial mismatch results in a more conforming joint. For this reason, consideration of an ideal joint congruency ratio that permits sufficient joint translation across a size range may be more appropriate than a defined range of articular surface radial mismatches.

Significant glenoid implant design refinements have occurred since the first nonconstrained implants were introduced in the 1970s. Many of these design efforts have sought to improve fixation and reduce the occurrence of glenoid radiolucent lines. The incidence of radiolucent lines is reported in 22% to 95% of cemented keel or peg glenoid prostheses,[82-87] though clinical loosening is much less common, with 90% to 95% survivorship reported at 10 years.[88] Of note, Schoch et al demonstrated that the presence of radiolucent glenoid lines is associated with negative clinical outcomes.[89] Over the past decade, hybrid glenoid prostheses were developed, consisting of porous metal pegs or coatings attached to the polyethylene. Importantly, these new hybrid glenoid prostheses have no metal-backing, as metal-backed glenoids have had a high failure rate.[83,88,90-93] Clinical and biomechanical studies have demonstrated excellent bone ingrowth with these prostheses but have also reported problems with metal debris formation, fracture, and/or dissociation at the metal-polyethylene interface.[94-97] The initial clinical results of hybrid glenoids are now being reported.[98-104] Most significantly, Friedman et al conducted an age-, sex-, and follow-up–matched outcomes study of 632 patients comparing outcomes of a traditional cemented peg glenoid prosthesis compared with a hybrid glenoid prosthesis and reported improved clinical outcomes, less revisions, and most importantly, a 4.2× reduction in radiolucent glenoid lines (9% vs 38%) with the hybrid design at an average of 50 months follow-up.[100] However, Friedman et al also reported that four cage glenoids were revised due to a unique complication of polyethylene articular surface disassociation from the central fixation peg.[100] These results suggest that continued prosthesis, instrument, and surgical technique refinement is necessary to further reduce the occurrence of aseptic glenoid loosening.

Other important considerations that impact glenoid fixation include native glenoid retroversion and glenoid wear. Posterior glenoid wear is common in glenohumeral osteoarthritis and is normally quantified by measuring the amount of glenoid retroversion.[105] Tightening of the subscapularis and anterior musculature of the shoulder causes posterior humeral head subluxation and a posterior load concentration on the glenoid. This reduced contact area results in glenoid wear and eventually posterior humeral head subluxation. Farron et al demonstrated that glenoid prostheses implanted in scapula with posterior glenoid defects have a greater risk of aseptic loosening due to increased stresses in the bone, cement, and prosthesis, all of which increase implant micromotion—a precursor to loosening.[38] To correct a posterior glenoid defect, orthopedic surgeons typically eccentrically ream the anterior glenoid to correct the glenoid retroversion to an acceptable range and to allow recentering of the humeral head. Unfortunately, eccentric reaming undermines prosthesis support by removing the stronger (nonworn) anterior glenoid bone and medializes the joint line which has implications on both muscle tensioning and joint stability. Additionally, there is a functional limit of 10° to 15° of eccentric correction that can be performed prior to the bone being too small to support the implant and when cement fixation becomes compromised due to peg perforation.[37-41] As a result of these challenges, posterior augmented glenoid implants have been developed to conserve bone and better restore the joint line in patients with posterior glenoid defects undergoing ATSA.

Several posterior augmented glenoid designs have been developed, including step, wedge, and half-wedge prostheses. Some of these designs have been evaluated in computer analyses[41,106-111] and in mechanical bench tests.[112,113] The literature demonstrates that wedge-style posterior augmented glenoid designs remove less bone than step-style posterior augment glenoid designs and are also associated with better stress profiles and less muscle shortening.[41,106-108] Additionally, promising short- and midterm clinical results have recently been reported using these wedge style augmented glenoid implants, but longer-term studies are needed to determine the potential benefits of these implants.[114,115]

UNANSWERED ATSA BIOMECHANICS QUESTIONS

Despite substantial efforts to replicate anatomy and restore normal shoulder kinematics, the ATSA may not actually be governed by ball and socket joint mechanics.[116] Even in the setting of excellent clinical outcomes and the use of fourth-generation prosthesis designs, ATSA may not restore native shoulder function and achieve dynamic humeral head centering on the glenoid.[116] These findings suggest the need for continued refinement of prosthesis design, surgical technique, and rehabilitation in order to better restore postoperative biomechanics and optimize clinical outcomes.

As glenoid loosening remains the most common ATSA failure mode, perhaps the greatest need is to better understand the myriad of options available for glenoid fixation and better quantify the prosthesis performance requirements associated with each, to aid the orthopedic surgeon in selecting the appropriate prosthesis for a given patient. Increasingly, ATSA patients are younger and more active and desire to return to a higher level of daily activities and recreational sports after the procedure. As such, glenoid implant designs must adapt to accommodate these increased demands, and testing criteria must also evolve to be more rigorous and ensure safety at elevated loads and cycles relative to the current ASTM standard testing methodologies.[117] Performance characteristics should better define the limitations associated with each of the many options: metal-backed glenoids, hybrid glenoids, inlay glenoids, and the more traditional cemented keel and peg designs of various sizes and shapes, including augments.

Furthermore, ideal prosthesis selection for a given patient may not be obvious. Future biomechanical simulation, cadaveric studies, and clinical outcomes analyses combined with machine learning analytic techniques, as recently performed by Kumar et al, may elucidate previously unknown correlations related to prosthesis design, surgical technique, implant placement, and implant size/type selection that may predict better clinical outcomes.[118] The results and techniques could also be combined with three-dimensional (3D) image-based computer planning and navigation data to identify ideal implant and surgical technique recommendations for a specific patient that optimizes clinical outcomes following ATSA.

CONCLUSION

Since the first ATSA was introduced in the 1970s, ATSA has been demonstrated to be a reliable treatment option for patients with arthritis and other degenerative conditions of the glenohumeral joint. Advancements in ATSA prosthesis design and surgical technique development have continued in an effort to better restore native shoulder biomechanics and improve the reproducibility of the procedure. Given that the shoulder is the most mobile joint in the human body, significant effort has been made to develop devices that replicate the highly variable bony glenohumeral anatomy and also provide prosthetic solutions to accommodate for bony deformity in order to optimally balance an individual patient's soft-tissue envelope and provide stability while also maximizing ROM.

A greater understanding of ATSA biomechanics facilitates better surgeon decision-making for the multitude of options available to alleviate pain and restore function for their patients. While good clinical outcomes are often achieved by following biomechanical principles, failures and complications following ATSA can often be explained by pathomechanics. Biomechanical principles of the shoulder should guide future innovations in shoulder prosthesis design, patient selection algorithms, surgical technique development, and development of rehabilitation and recovery/strengthening programs, in an effort to further improve ATSA outcomes and reduce complication rates.

REFERENCES

1. Codman EA. *The Shoulder. Rupture of the Supraspinatus Tendon and Other Lesions in or About the Subacromial Bursa.* Classics of Medicine Library. 1934.
2. Inman VT, Saunders JB, Abbott LC. Observations of the function of the shoulder joint. *J Bone Joint Surg.* 1944;26-A:1-30.
3. Kuechle DK, Newman SR, Itoi E, Morrey BF, An KN. Shoulder muscle moment arms during horizontal flexion and elevation. *J Shoulder Elbow Surg.* 1997;6(5):429-439.
4. Otis JC, Jiang CC, Wickiewicz TL, Peterson MG, Warren RF, Santner TJ. Changes in the moment arms of the rotator cuff and deltoid muscles with abduction and rotation. *J Bone Joint Surg Am.* 1994;76(5):667-676.
5. Kelkar R, Wang VM, Flatow EL, et al. Glenohumeral mechanics: a study of articular geometry, contact, and kinematics. *J Shoulder Elbow Surg.* 2001;10(1):73-84.
6. Soslowsky LJ, Flatow EL, Bigliani LU, Mow VC. Articular geometry of the glenohumeral joint. *Clin Orthop Relat Res.* 1992;(285):181-190.
7. Soslowsky LJ, Flatow EL, Bigliani LU, Pawluk RJ, Ateshian GA, Mow VC. Quantitation of in situ contact areas at the glenohumeral joint: a biomechanical study. *J Orthop Res.* 1992;10(4):524-534.
8. Checroun AJ, Hawkins C, Kummer FJ, Zuckerman JD. Fit of current glenoid component designs: an anatomic cadaver study. *J Shoulder Elbow Surg.* 2002;11(6):614-617.
9. Churchill RS, Brems JJ, Kotschi H. Glenoid size, inclination, and version: an anatomic study. *J Shoulder Elbow Surg.* 2001;10(4):327-332.
10. Iannotti JP, Gabriel JP, Schneck SL, Evans BG, Misra S. The normal glenohumeral relationships. An anatomical study of one hundred and forty shoulders. *J Bone Joint Surg Am.* 1992;74(4):491-500.
11. Kwon YW, Powell KA, Yum JK, Brems JJ, Iannotti JP. Use of three-dimensional computed tomography for the analysis of the glenoid anatomy. *J Shoulder Elbow Surg.* 2005;14(1):85-90.
12. Mallon WJ, Brown HR, Vogler JB III, Martinez S. Radiographic and geometric anatomy of the scapula. *Clin Orthop Relat Res.* 1992;(277):142-154.
13. Morrey BF, Itoi E, An KN. Biomechanics of the shoulder. In: Rockwood CA, Matsen FA, ed. *The Shoulder.* Saunders; 1998:233-276.
14. Yu J, McGarry MH, Lee YS, Duong LV, Lee TQ. Biomechanical effects of supraspinatus repair on the glenohumeral joint. *J Shoulder Elbow Surg.* 2005;14(1 suppl S):65S-71S.
15. Billuart F, Gagey O, Skalli W, Mitton D. Biomechanics of the deltoideus. *Surg Radiol Anat.* 2006;28(1):76-81.
16. De Wilde L, Audenaert E, Barbaix E, Audenaert A, Soudan K. Consequences of deltoid muscle elongation on deltoid muscle performance: a computerised study. *Clin Biomech (Bristol, Avon).* 2002;17(7):499-505.
17. Gagey O, Hue E. Mechanics of the deltoid muscle. A new approach. *Clin Orthop Relat Res.* 2000;(375):250-257.
18. Lemieux PO, Hagemeister N, Tétreault P, Nuño N. Influence of the medial offset of the proximal humerus on the glenohumeral destabilising forces during arm elevation: a numerical sensitivity study. *Comput Methods Biomech Biomed Engin.* 2013;16(1):103-111. doi:10.1080/10255842.2011.607813
19. Lippitt SB, Vanderhooft JE, Harris SL, Sidles JA, Harryman DT II, Matsen FA III. Glenohumeral stability from concavity-compression: a quantitative analysis. *J Shoulder Elbow Surg.* 1993;2(1):27-35. doi:10.1016/S1058-2746(09)80134-1
20. Mura N, O'Driscoll SW, Zobitz ME, et al. The effect of infraspinatus disruption on glenohumeral torque and superior migration of the humeral head: a biomechanical study. *J Shoulder Elbow Surg.* 2003;12(2):179-184.
21. Parsons IM, Apreleva M, Fu FH, Woo SL. The effect of rotator cuff tears on reaction forces at the glenohumeral joint. *J Orthop Res.* 2002;20(3):439-446.
22. Sharkey NA, Marder RA. The rotator cuff opposes superior translation of the humeral head. *Am J Sports Med.* 1995;23(3):270-275.

23. Burkhart SS, Nottage WM, Ogilvie-Harris DJ, Kohn HS, Pachelli A. Partial repair of irreparable rotator cuff tears. *Arthroscopy.* 1994;10(4):363-370.

24. Halder AM, Zhao KD, Odriscoll SW, Morrey BF, An KN. Dynamic contributions to superior shoulder stability. *J Orthop Res.* 2001;19(2):206-212.

25. Labriola JE, Lee TQ, Debski RE, McMahon PJ. Stability and instability of the glenohumeral joint: the role of shoulder muscles. *J Shoulder Elbow Surg.* 2005;14(1 suppl S):32S-38S.

26. Harryman DT, Sidles JA, Harris SL, Lippitt SB, Matsen FA III. The effect of articular conformity and the size of the humeral head component on laxity and motion after glenohumeral arthroplasty. A study in cadavera. *J Bone Joint Surg Am.* 1995;77(4):555-563.

27. Karduna AR, Williams GR, Williams JL, Iannotti JP. Glenohumeral joint translations before and after total shoulder arthroplasty. A study in cadavera. *J Bone Joint Surg Am.* 1997;79(8):1166-1174.

28. Karduna AR, Williams GR, Williams JL, Iannotti JP. Kinematics of the glenohumeral joint: influences of muscle forces, ligamentous constraints, and articular geometry. *J Orthop Res.* 1996;14(6):986-993.

29. Poppen NK, Walker PS. Forces at the glenohumeral joint in abduction. *Clin Orthop Relat Res.* 1978;(135):165-170.

30. Bergmann G, Graichen F, Bender A, et al. In vivo gleno-humeral joint loads during forward flexion and abduction. *J Biomech.* 2011;44(8):1543-1552. doi:10.1016/j.jbiomech.2011.02.142

31. Westerhoff P, Graichen F, Bender A, et al. In vivo measurement of shoulder joint loads during activities of daily living. *J Biomech.* 2009;42(12):1840-1849. doi:10.1016/j.jbiomech.2009.05.035

32. Westerhoff P, Graichen F, Bender A, et al. In vivo measurement of shoulder joint loads during walking with crutches. *Clin Biomech (Bristol, Avon).* 2012;27(7):711-718. doi:10.1016/j.clinbiomech.2012.03.004

33. Westerhoff P, Graichen F, Bender A, et al. Measurement of shoulder joint loads during wheelchair propulsion measured in vivo. *Clin Biomech (Bristol, Avon).* 2011;26(10):982-989. doi:10.1016/j.clinbiomech.2011.05.017

34. Bassett RW, Browne AO, Morrey BF, An KN. Glenohumeral muscle force and moment mechanics in a position of shoulder instability. *J Biomech.* 1990;23(5):405-415.

35. Veeger HE, Van der Helm FC, Van der Woude LH, Pronk GM, Rozendal RH. Inertia and muscle contraction parameters for musculoskeletal modelling of the shoulder mechanism. *J Biomech.* 1991;24(7):615-629.

36. Halder AM, Itoi E, An KN. Anatomy and biomechanics of the shoulder. *Orthop Clin North Am.* 2000;31(2):159-176.

37. Clavert P, Millett PJ, Warner JJ. Glenoid resurfacing: what are the limits to asymmetric reaming for posterior erosion? *J Shoulder Elbow Surg.* 2007;16(6):843-848.

38. Farron A, Terrier A, Büchler P. Risks of loosening of a prosthetic glenoid implanted in retroversion. *J Shoulder Elbow Surg.* 2006;15(4):521-526.

39. Gillespie R, Lyons R, Lazarus M. Eccentric reaming in total shoulder arthroplasty: a cadaveric study. *Orthopedics.* 2009;32(1):21.

40. Nowak DD, Bahu MJ, Gardner TR, et al. Simulation of surgical glenoid resurfacing using three-dimensional computed tomography of the arthritic glenohumeral joint: the amount of glenoid retroversion that can be corrected. *J Shoulder Elbow Surg.* 2009;18(5):680-688. doi:10.1016/j.jse.2009.03.019

41. Roche CP, Diep P, Grey SG, Flurin PH. Biomechanical impact of posterior glenoid wear on anatomic total shoulder arthroplasty. *Bull Hosp Jt Dis (2013).* 2013;71(suppl 2):S5-S11.

42. Neer CS II, Craig EV, Fukuda H. Cuff-tear arthropathy. *J Bone Joint Surg Am.* 1983;65(9):1232-1244.

43. Visotsky JL, Basamania C, Seebauer L, Rockwood CA, Jensen KL. Cuff tear arthropathy: pathogenesis, classification, and algorithm for treatment. *J Bone Joint Surg Am.* 2004;86-A(suppl 2):35-40.

44. Bercik MJ, Kruse K II, Yalizis M, Gauci MO, Chaoui J, Walch G. A modification to the Walch classification of the glenoid in primary glenohumeral osteoarthritis using three dimensional imaging.

45. *J Shoulder Elbow Surg.* 2016;25(10):1601-1606. doi:10.1016/j.jse.2016.03.010

45. Walch G, Badet R, Boulahia A, Khoury A. Morphologic study of the glenoid in primary glenohumeral osteoarthritis. *J Arthroplasty.* 1999;14(6):756-760.

46. Huguet D, Favard L, Lautma S, et al. Epidemiology, imaging, and classification of glenohumeral osteoarthritis with massive and nonreparable rotator cuff tear. In: Walch G, Boileau P, Mole D, eds. *2000 Shoulder Prostheses: Two to Ten Year Follow-Up.* Sauramps Medical; 2001:233-240.

47. Boileau P, Walch G. The three-dimensional geometry of the proximal humerus. Implications for surgical technique and prosthetic design. *J Bone Joint Surg Br.* 1997;79(5):857-865.

48. Hertel R, Knothe U, Ballmer FT. Geometry of the proximal humerus and implications for prosthetic design. *J Shoulder Elbow Surg.* 2002;11(4):331-338.

49. Roberts SN, Foley AP, Swallow HM, Wallace WA, Coughlan DP. The geometry of the humeral head and the design of prostheses. *J Bone Joint Surg Br.* 1991;73(4):647-650.

50. Robertson DD, Yuan J, Bigliani LU, Flatow EL, Yamaguchi K. Three-dimensional analysis of the proximal part of the humerus: relevance to arthroplasty. *J Bone Joint Surg Am.* 2000;82-A(11):1594-1602.

51. Takase K, Yamamoto K, Imakiire A, Burkhead WZ Jr. The radiographic study in the relationship of the glenohumeral joint. *J Orthop Res.* 2004;22(2):298-305.

52. Jacobson A, Gilot GJ, Hamilton MA, et al. Glenohumeral anatomic study. A comparison of male and female shoulders with similar average age and bmi. *Bull Hosp Jt Dis (2013).* 2015;73(suppl 1):S68-S78.

53. Buchler P, Farron A. Benefits of an anatomical reconstruction of the humeral head during shoulder arthroplasty: a finite element analysis. *Clin Biomech (Bristol, Avon).* 2004;19:16-23.

54. Flurin PH, Roche CP, Wright TW, Zuckerman JD. Correlation between clinical outcomes and anatomic reconstruction with anatomic total shoulder arthroplasty. *Bull Hosp Jt Dis (2013).* 2015;73(suppl 1):S92-S98.

55. Nyffeler R, Sheikh R, Jacob HA, Gerber C. Influence of humeral prosthesis height on biomechanics of glenohumeral abduction. *J Bone Joint Surg Am.* 2004;86(3):575-580.

56. Pearl M, Kurutz S. Geometric analysis of commonly used prosthetic systems for proximal humeral replacement. *J Bone Joint Surg Am.* 1999;81(5):660-671.

57. Roche C, Angibaud L, Flurin PH, Wright TW, Fulkerson E, Zuckerman JD. Anatomic validation of an "Anatomical" shoulder system. *Bull Hosp Jt Dis (2013).* 2006;63(3-4):93-97.

58. Walch G, Boileau P. Prosthetic adaptability: a new concept for shoulder arthroplasty. *J Shoulder Elbow Surg.* 1999;8:443-451.

59. Neer CS II. Replacement arthroplasty for glenohumeral osteoarthritis. *J Bone Joint Surg Am.* 1974;56A:1-13.

60. Crosby LA, Wright TW, Yu S, Zuckerman JD. Conversion to reverse total shoulder arthroplasty with and without humeral stem retention: the role of a convertible-platform stem. *J Bone Joint Surg Am.* 2017;99(9):736-742. doi:10.2106/JBJS.16.00683

61. Flynn L, Patrick MR, Roche C, et al. Anatomical and reverse shoulder arthroplasty utilizing a single implant system with a platform stem: a prospective observational study with mid-term follow up. *Shoulder Elbow.* Forthcoming 2020;12(5):330-337.

62. Simovitch RW, Friedman RJ, Cheung EV, et al. Rate of improvement in clinical outcomes with anatomic and reverse total shoulder arthroplasty. *J Bone Joint Surg Am.* 2017;99(21):1801-1811. doi:10.2106/JBJS.16.01387

63. Simovitch R, Flurin PH, Wright T, Zuckerman JD, Roche CP. Quantifying success after total shoulder arthroplasty: the minimal clinically important difference. *J Shoulder Elbow Surg.* 2018;27(2):298-305. doi:10.1016/j.jse.2017.09.013

64. Simovitch R, Flurin PH, Wright T, Zuckerman JD, Roche CP. Quantifying success after total shoulder arthroplasty: the substantial clinical benefit. *J Shoulder Elbow Surg.* 2018;27(5):903-911. doi:10.1016/j.jse.2017.12.014

65. Alolabi B, Youderian AR, Napolitano L, et al. Radiographic assessment of prosthetic humeral head size after anatomic shoulder arthroplasty. *J Shoulder Elbow Surg.* 2014;23:1740-1746.

66. Youderian AR, Ricchetti ET, Drews M, Iannotti JP. Determination of humeral head size in anatomic shoulder replacement for glenohumeral osteoarthritis. *J Shoulder Elbow Surg.* 2014;23:955-963.

67. Chen EJ, Simovitch R, Savoie F, Noel CR. Assessment of the anatomic neck as an accurate landmark for humeral head resurfacing implant height placement. *Bull Hosp Jt Dis (2013).* 2015;73(suppl 1): S28-S32.

68. Berth A, Pap G. Stemless shoulder prosthesis versus conventional anatomic shoulder prosthesis in patients with osteoarthritis. *J Orthopaed Traumatol.* 2013;14:31-37.

69. Churchill RS. Stemless shoulder arthroplasty: current status. *J Shoulder Elbow Surg.* 2014;23:1409-1414.

70. Casagrande DJ, Parks DL, Torngren T, et al. Radiographic evaluation of short-stem press-fit total shoulder arthroplasty: short-term follow-up. *J Shoulder Elbow Surg.* 2016;25(7):1163-1169. doi:10.1016/j.jse.2015.11.067

71. Raiss P, Schnetzke M, Wittmann T, et al. Postoperative radiographic findings of an uncemented convertible short stem for anatomic and reverse shoulder arthroplasty. *J Shoulder Elbow Surg.* 2019;28(4):715-723. doi:10.1016/j.jse.2018.08.037

72. Schnetzke M, Coda S, Raiss P, Walch G, Loew M. Radiologic bone adaptations on a cementless short-stem shoulder prosthesis. *J Shoulder Elbow Surg.* 2016;25(4):650-657. doi:10.1016/j.jse.2015.08.044

73. Langohr GDG, Reeves J, Roche CP, Faber KJ, Johnson JA. The effect of short-stem humeral component sizing on humeral bone stress. *J Shoulder Elbow Surg.* 2020;29(4):761-767. doi:10.1016/j.jse.2019.08.018

74. Anglin C, Wyss UP, Nyffeler RW, Gerber C. Loosening performance of cemented glenoid prosthesis design pairs. *Clin Biomech (Bristol, Avon).* 2001;16(2):144-150.

75. Anglin C, Wyss UP, Pichora DR. Mechanical testing of shoulder prostheses and recommendations for glenoid design. *J Shoulder Elbow Surg.* 2000;9(4):323-331.

76. Anglin C, Wyss UP, Pichora DR. Shoulder prosthesis subluxation: theory and experiment. *J Shoulder Elbow Surg.* 2000;9(2):104-114.

77. Karduna AR, Williams GR, Williams JL, Iannotti JP. Joint stability after total shoulder arthroplasty in a cadaver model. *J Shoulder Elbow Surg.* 1997;6(6):506-511.

78. Diop A, Maurel N, Grimberg J, Gagey O. Influence of glenohumeral mismatch on bone strains and implant displacements in implanted glenoïds. An in vitro experimental study on cadaveric scapulae. *J Biomech.* 2006;39(16):3026-3035.

79. Sabesan VJ, Ackerman J, Sharma V, Baker KC, Kurdziel MD, Wiater JM. Glenohumeral mismatch affects micromotion of cemented glenoid components in total shoulder arthroplasty. *J Shoulder Elbow Surg.* 2015;24(5):814-822. doi:10.1016/j.jse.2014.10.004

80. Schoch BS, Wright TW, Zuckerman JD, et al. The effect of radial mismatch on radiographic glenoid loosening. *JSES Open Access.* 2019;3(4):287-291. doi:10.1016/j.jses.2019.09.007

81. Walch G, Edwards TB, Boulahia A, Boileau P, Mole D, Adeleine P. The influence of glenohumeral prosthetic mismatch on glenoid radiolucent lines: results of a multicenter study. *J Bone Joint Surg Am.* 2002;84(12):2186-2191.

82. Bohsali KI, Wirth MA, Rockwood CA Jr. Complications of total shoulder arthroplasty. *J Bone Joint Surg Am.* 2006;88(10):2279-2292.

83. Boileau P, Avidor C, Krishnan SG, Walch G, Kempf JF, Molé D. Cemented polyethylene versus uncemented metal-backed glenoid components in total shoulder arthroplasty: a prospective, double-blind, randomized study. *J Shoulder Elbow Surg.* 2002;11(4):351-359.

84. Boyd AD Jr, Thomas WH, Scott RD, Sledge CB, Thornhill TS. Total shoulder arthroplasty versus hemiarthroplasty. Indications for glenoid resurfacing. *J Arthroplasty.* 1990;5(4):329-336.

85. Brenner BC, Ferlic DC, Clayton ML, Dennis DA. Survivorship of unconstrained total shoulder arthroplasty. *J Bone Joint Surg Am.* 1989;71(9):1289-1296.

86. Norris BL, Lachiewicz PF. Modern cement technique and the survivorship of total shoulder arthroplasty. *Clin Orthop Relat Res.* 1996;(328):76-85.

87. Throckmorton TW, Zarkadas PC, Sperling JW, Cofield RH. Pegged versus keeled glenoid components in total shoulder arthroplasty. *J Shoulder Elbow Surg.* 2010;19(5):726-733. doi:10.1016/j.jse.2009.10.018

88. Fox TJ, Cil A, Sperling JW, Sanchez-Sotelo J, Schleck CD, Cofield RH. Survival of the glenoid component in shoulder arthroplasty. *J Shoulder Elbow Surg.* 2009;18(6):859-863. doi:10.1016/j.jse.2008.11.020

89. Schoch BS, Wright TW, Zuckerman JD, et al. Glenoid component lucencies are associated with poorer patient-reported outcomes following anatomic shoulder arthroplasty. *J Shoulder Elbow Surg.* 2019;28(10):1956-1963. doi:10.1016/j.jse.2019.03.011

90. Castagna A, Randelli M, Garofalo R, Maradei L, Giardella A, Borroni M. Mid-term results of a metal-backed glenoid component in total shoulder replacement. *J Bone Joint Surg Br.* 2010;92(10):1410-1415. doi:10.1302/0301-620X.92B10.23578

91. Fucentese SF, Costouros JG, Kühnel SP, Gerber C. Total shoulder arthroplasty with an uncemented soft-metal-backed glenoid component. *J Shoulder Elbow Surg.* 2010;19(4):624-631. doi:10.1016/j.jse.2009.12.021

92. Tammachote N, Sperling JW, Vathana T, Cofield RH, Harmsen WS, Schleck CD. Long-term results of cemented metal-backed glenoid components for osteoarthritis of the shoulder. *J Bone Joint Surg Am.* 2009;91(1):160-166. doi:10.2106/JBJS.F.01613

93. Wallace AL, Phillips RL, MacDougal GA, Walsh WR, Sonnabend DH. Resurfacing of the glenoid in total shoulder arthroplasty. A comparison, at a mean of five years, of prostheses inserted with and without cement. *J Bone Joint Surg Am.* 1999;81(4):510-518.

94. Budge MD, Kurdziel MD, Baker KC, Wiater JM. A biomechanical analysis of initial fixation options for porous-tantalum-backed glenoid components. *J Shoulder Elbow Surg.* 2013;22(5):709-715. doi:10.1016/j.jse.2012.07.001

95. Budge MD, Nolan EM, Heisey MH, Baker K, Wiater JM. Results of total shoulder arthroplasty with a monoblock porous tantalum glenoid component: a prospective minimum 2-year follow-up study. *J Shoulder Elbow Surg.* 2013;22(4):535-541. doi:10.1016/j.jse.2012.06.001

96. Endrizzi DP, Mackenzie JA, Henry PD. Early debris formation with a porous tantalum glenoid component: radiographic analysis with 2-year minimum follow-up. *J Bone Joint Surg Am.* 2016;98(12):1023-1029. doi:10.2106/JBJS.15.00410

97. Watson ST, Gudger GK Jr, Long CD, Tokish JM, Tolan SJ. Outcomes of Trabecular Metal-backed glenoid components in anatomic total shoulder arthroplasty. *J Shoulder Elbow Surg.* 2018;27(3):493-498. doi:10.1016/j.jse.2017.09.036

98. Churchill RS, Zellmer C, Zimmers HJ, Ruggero R. Clinical and radiographic analysis of a partially cemented glenoid implant: five-year minimum follow-up. *J Shoulder Elbow Surg.* 2010;19(7):1091-1097. doi:10.1016/j.jse.2009.12.022

99. Ford MC, Brolin TJ, Meehan EM, Smith R, Azar FM, Throckmorton TW. Two-year clinical and radiographic outcomes of total shoulder arthroplasty using a hybrid glenoid component with a central porous titanium post. *Tech Shoulder Elbow Surg.* 2017;18(2), 72-76. doi:10.1097/BTE.0000000000000094

100. Friedman RJ, Cheung E, Grey SG, et al. Clinical and radiographic comparison of a hybrid cage glenoid to a cemented polyethylene glenoid in anatomic total shoulder arthroplasty. *J Shoulder Elbow Surg.* 2019;28(12):2308-2316. doi:10.1016/j.jse.2019.04.049

101. Grey SG, Wright TW, Flurin PH, Zuckerman JD, Friedman R, Roche CP. Preliminary results of a novel hybrid cage glenoid compared to an all-polyethylene glenoid in total shoulder arthroplasty. *Bull Hosp Jt Dis (2013).* 2015;73(suppl 1):S86-S91.

102. Gulotta LV, Chambers KL, Warren RF, Dines DM, Craig EV. No differences in early results of a hybrid glenoid compared with a pegged implant. *Clin Orthop Relat Res.* 2015;473(12):3918-3924. doi:10.1007/s11999-015-4558-5

103. Nelson CG, Brolin TJ, Ford MC, Smith RA, Azar FM, Throckmorton TW. Five-year minimum clinical and radiographic outcomes of total shoulder arthroplasty using a hybrid glenoid component with a central

porous titanium post. *J Shoulder Elbow Surg.* 2018;27(8):1462-1467. doi:10.1016/j.jse.2018.01.012

104. Page RS, Pai V, Eng K, Bain G, Graves S, Lorimer M. Cementless versus cemented glenoid components in conventional total shoulder joint arthroplasty: analysis from the Australian Orthopaedic Association National Joint Replacement Registry. *J Shoulder Elbow Surg.* 2018;27(10):1859-1865. doi:10.1016/j.jse.2018.03.017

105. Friedman RJ, Hawthorne KB, Genez BM. The use of computerized tomography in the measurement of glenoid version. *J Bone Joint Surg Am.* 1992;74(7):1032-1037.

106. Allred JJ, Flores-Hernandez C, Hoenecke HR Jr, D'Lima DD. Posterior augmented glenoid implants require less bone removal and generate lower stresses: a finite element analysis. *J Shoulder Elbow Surg.* 2016;25(5):823-830. doi:10.1016/j.jse.2015.10.003

107. Hermida JC, Flores-Hernandez C, Hoenecke HR, D'Lima DD. Augmented wedge-shaped glenoid component for the correction of glenoid retroversion: a finite element analysis. *J Shoulder Elbow Surg.* 2014;23(3):347-354. doi:10.1016/j.jse.2013.06.008

108. Kersten AD, Flores-Hernandez C, Hoenecke HR, et al. Posterior augmented glenoid designs preserve more bone in biconcave glenoids. *J Shoulder Elbow Surg.* 2015;24(7):1135-1141.

109. Knowles NK, Ferreira LM, Athwal GS. Augmented glenoid component designs for type B2 erosions: a computational comparison by volume of bone removal and quality of remaining bone. *J Shoulder Elbow Surg.* 2015;24(8):1218-1226. doi:10.1016/j.jse.2014.12.018

110. Sabesan V, Callanan M, Sharma V, Iannotti JP. Correction of acquired glenoid bone loss in osteoarthritis with a standard versus an augmented glenoid component. *J Shoulder Elbow Surg.* 2014;23(7):964-973. doi:10.1016/j.jse.2013.09.019

111. Sabesan VJ, Lima DJL, Whaley JD, Pathak V, Zhang L. Biomechanical comparison of 2 augmented glenoid designs: an integrated kinematic finite element analysis. *J Shoulder Elbow Surg.* 2019;28(6):1166-1174. doi:10.1016/j.jse.2018.11.055

112. Iannotti JP, Lappin KE, Klotz CL, Reber EW, Swope SW. Liftoff resistance of augmented glenoid components during cyclic fatigue loading in the posterior-superior direction. *J Shoulder Elbow Surg.* 2013;22(11):1530-1536. doi:10.1016/j.jse.2013.01.018

113. Kirane YM, Lewis GS, Sharkey NA, Armstrong AD. Mechanical characteristics of a novel posterior-step prosthesis for biconcave glenoid defects. *J Shoulder Elbow Surg.* 2012;21(1):105-115. doi:10.1016/j.jse.2010.12.008

114. Grey SG, Wright TW, Flurin PH, Zuckerman JD, Roche CP, Friedman RJ. Clinical and radiographic outcomes with a posteriorly augmented glenoid for Walch B glenoids in anatomic total shoulder arthroplasty. *J Shoulder Elbow Surg.* 2020;29(5):e185-e195. doi:10.1016/j.jse.2019.10.008

115. Wright TW, Grey SG, Roche CP, Wright L, Flurin PH, Zuckerman JD. Preliminary results of a posterior augmented glenoid compared to an all polyethylene standard glenoid in anatomic total shoulder arthroplasty. *Bull Hosp Jt Di (2013).* 2015;73(suppl 1):S79-S85.

116. Massimini DF, Li G, Warner JP. Glenohumeral contact kinematics in patients after total shoulder arthroplasty. *J Bone Joint Surg Am.* 2010;92(4):916-926.doi:10.2106/JBJS.H.01610

117. Roche CP, Staunch C, Hahn W, et al. Analysis of glenoid fixation with anatomic total shoulder arthroplasty in an extreme cyclic loading scenario. *Bull Hosp Jt Dis (2013).* 2015;73(suppl 1):S57-S62.

118. Kumar V, Roche C, Overman S, et al. What is the accuracy of three different machine learning techniques to predict clinical outcomes after shoulder arthroplasty? *Clin Orthop Relat Res.* 2020;478(10):2351-2363. doi:10.1097/CORR.0000000000001263

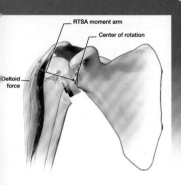

RTSA moment arm
Center of rotation
Deltoid force

4 Biomechanics of Reverse Total Shoulder Arthroplasty

Christopher P. Roche, MSE, MBA and Howard D. Routman, DO

HOW THE REVERSE SHOULDER WORKS

Reverse total shoulder arthroplasty (RTSA) inverts the native glenohumeral joint articulation to restore stability to an otherwise unstable glenohumeral joint. This is achieved by making the glenoid articulation convex and the humeral articulation concave to create a fixed fulcrum that geometrically prevents superior migration and acromial contact as the deltoid contracts to elevate the arm. Inverting the concavities inferiomedially translates both the center of rotation (CoR) and humeral position relative to that native shoulder (FIGURE 4.1). While RTSA prostheses vary in the degree of CoR and humeral translation, contemporary designs are associated with a 5 to 10 mm inferior[1-4] and 20 to 30 mm medial[2,3,5-8] translation of the CoR and a 25 to 40 mm inferior[2,3] and 5 to 20 mm medial[2,3] translation of the humerus relative to the native shoulder. Medially translating the CoR has the added benefit of increasing the length of the deltoid abductor moment arm from 10 to 30 mm[9-13] for the native shoulder with the arm at the side to 22 to 40 mm[13-16] for the RTSA construct (FIGURE 4.2). This increase in the length of the abductor moment arm improves the efficiency of the deltoid by requiring less muscle force to generate the same amount of torque.

Unlike the native shoulder, which has a nonconforming articulation that permits humeral head rotation, translation, and rolling on the glenoid, the RTSA articulation is conforming, so its motion is limited to humeral rotation without translation (FIGURE 4.3). In the native shoulder, the rotator cuff acts as a dynamic fulcrum that facilitates arm elevation by pivoting the humeral head against the glenoid as the deltoid contracts.[17] By comparison, in the RTSA shoulder, the inverted concavity converts the superiorly directed deltoid muscle vector into arm elevation and rotation. The magnitude of motion achieved with RTSA in each anatomic plane is dependent upon several factors including humeral liner constraint, humeral liner-scapular impingement, humeral neck angle, humeral retroversion, glenosphere inferior overhang, patient anatomy/morphology, and available musculature.[1-3,15,16,18-38]

Regarding the musculature required for active range of motion (ROM) with RTSA, a functioning deltoid is

necessary for arm abduction, forward flexion, and also for joint stability. A nonfunctioning deltoid is a contraindication of RTSA. Internal rotation is achieved by the action of the subscapularis, teres major, pectoralis major, latissimus dorsi, and/or anterior deltoid. A functioning teres minor, at a minimum, is necessary to achieve active external rotation, and while external rotation improvement after RTSA may be unpredictable, most patients will achieve more active external rotation if they also have a functioning infraspinatus. If neither the teres minor nor infraspinatus is functional, the posterior deltoid may contribute to external rotation, but a muscle transfer of one of the large internal rotator muscles, most commonly the latissimus dorsi, may also be necessary.

HISTORY OF THE REVERSE PROSTHESIS

The RTSA prosthesis was first designed in the 1970s; several prostheses were developed, including the Fenlin, Reeves-Leeds, Kessel, and Neer-Averill shoulders.[38-45] Each of these prostheses had a constrained and conforming articulation whose CoR was lateral to the glenoid fossa. These design features were associated with excessive torque on the glenoid bone-implant interface that compromised fixation and resulted in aseptic glenoid loosening and/or mechanical failure. Due to the high implant failure rates, the early RTSA designs were abandoned in the US market.[41,42]

Interest in RTSA reemerged when Dr. Paul Grammont introduced his Delta III reverse prosthesis in Europe in 1991 and in the United States in 2003. The Delta III RTSA prosthesis utilized a hemispherical glenosphere whose thickness was equal to its spherical radius to medially position the CoR directly on the glenoid fossa.[6,41,46-48] By medializing the CoR, the Grammont RTSA prosthesis minimized torque on the glenoid bone-implant interface to reduce the incidence of aseptic glenoid loosening, while also increasing the abductor moment arm length to improve deltoid efficiency and reduce the force required to elevate the arm. This medialized CoR concept is Dr. Grammont's great innovation that all contemporary RTSA designs generally share. These contemporary designs have been associated with predictable improvements in

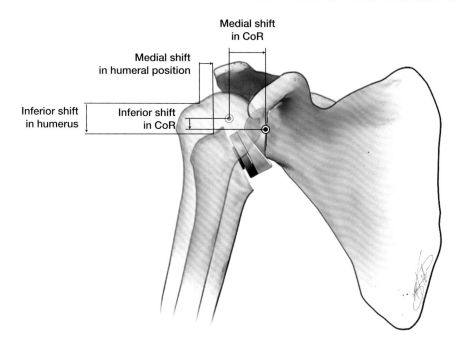

FIGURE 4.1 Inferiomedial translation of the center of rotation (CoR) and humeral position with RTSA, relative to the native shoulder.

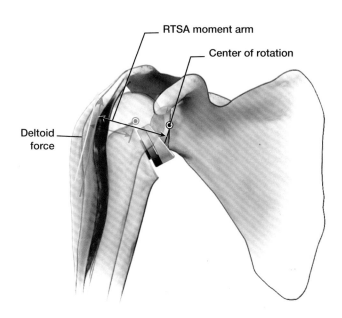

FIGURE 4.2 Increase in deltoid moment arm length with RTSA, relative to the native shoulder.

function and stability for a variety of difficult-to-treat degenerative conditions of the shoulder including cuff tear arthropathy, osteoarthritis with rotator cuff tears, proximal humeral fractures, arthroplasty with glenoid bone loss, arthroplasty with proximal humeral bone loss, and also revision arthroplasty.[48-61] Market response to these positive clinical experiences has dynamically altered the usage pattern of shoulder arthroplasty in the United States, as characterized by a sharp increase in RTSA since

its introduction, a significant decline in hemiarthroplasty, and a relative reduced growth of anatomic total shoulder arthroplasty (ATSA) **(FIGURE 4.4)**.

Medializing the CoR with the Grammont RTSA prosthesis inferiomedially translates the humerus and alters the native orientation of the humeral muscle insertions relative to the CoR. Doing so changes each muscle's moment arms and native lengths and modifies how each muscle influences motion relative to its native physiologic function. This inferiomedial humeral positioning has multiple negative biomechanical implications, including elongation of the deltoid by as much as 20%,[1-3,5,14-16,32,33,62,63] reduced deltoid wrapping around the greater tuberosity,[2,3,7,9,31,34,64,65] reduced ROM and impingement of the humeral liner with the scapular neck (leading to scapular notching),[18,20-24,29,32,33,35-37,58,66-70] and shortened rotator cuff muscle lengths, which impair their ability to generate internal/external rotation.[2,3,34,71-73] Shortening of the rotator cuff muscles[73] may be responsible for the modified scapulohumeral rhythm with RTSA, where additional scapular rotation occurs relative to the native shoulder, potentially as a compensatory mechanism for the lax scapulohumeral muscles during elevation[74] **(FIGURE 4.5)**.

IMPACT OF PROSTHESIS DESIGN ON RTSA BIOMECHANICS

RTSA biomechanics can be altered by prosthesis design parameters. Since the Delta III RTSA prosthesis was introduced in the United States in 2003, numerous RTSA prostheses have been developed, many of which

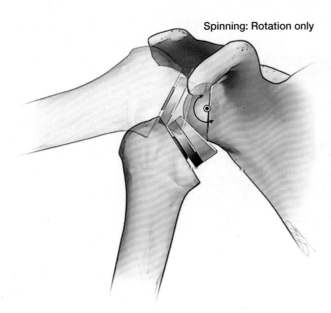

FIGURE 4.3 RTSA joint motion is limited to rotation due to the conforming articular geometry.

incorporate design improvements that address the aforementioned biomechanical limitations of the Grammont prosthesis. Specifically, RTSA prosthesis design changes sought to (1) preserve the amount of bone removed during implantation[75]; (2) enhance glenoid fixation and provide more options for glenoid bone loss in primary and revision procedures[75-83]; (3) improve ROM and reduce scapular notching[18,23,24,28,29,32,33,35,36,66,70]; and (4) lateralize the humerus to further increase abductor moment arms,[1,5,13-16,31,34,71] restore rotator cuff muscle length,[2,3,34,72,73] and restore deltoid wrapping.[2,3,34] These design modifications have largely resulted in positive clinical improvements by reducing the occurrence of certain complications such as instability,[34,84-86] acromial and scapular fractures,[87-91] and the incidence of scapular notching.[18,23,24,28,29,32,33,35,36,66,70] However, not all of these design changes have resulted in biomechanical improvements.

To mitigate scapular notching and improve ROM, several RTSA prostheses have attempted to lateralize the humerus by lateralizing the CoR through either use of thicker glenospheres[49,51] or by placing bone graft behind the glenoid baseplate.[53-55,92] Lateralizing the CoR has been demonstrated to reduce humeral liner impingement with the scapular neck.[1,32,33,49,51] However, lateralizing the CoR also increases the torque on the glenoid bone-implant interface (which can compromise fixation)[78,82,93] and decreases the length of the deltoid abductor moment arms (which reduces deltoid efficiency).[1,13,14,34,65,66,71] As the deltoid abductor moment arms are decreased, the deltoid becomes less effective as an abductor and requires a greater force to elevate the arm.[1,13,14,34,65,66,71] Additionally, these elevated muscle loads increase scapular bone stresses, thereby, increasing the risk of acromial and scapular insufficiency fractures, which occur at a higher rate in RTSA prostheses that lateralize the CoR relative to other design styles.[88,94-96]

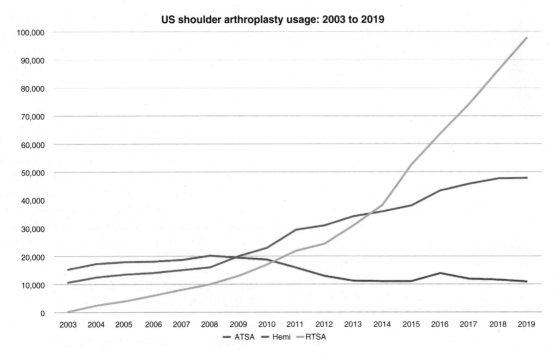

FIGURE 4.4 Shoulder arthroplasty usage in the United States from 2003 to 2019, based upon ICD-9 procedural codes, ICD-10 procedural codes, and all-payor data from the definitive database. ICD, International Classification of diseases.

humeral liner/stem design).[32,33] Onlay humeral tray designs also have the advantage of functioning as a platform humeral stem, modularly connecting to the same humeral stem that is used for both ATSA and RTSA applications, which potentially permits stem retention in revision procedures.[97] Numerous studies have demonstrated that lateralizing the humerus while maintaining Grammont medialized CoR is associated with multiple biomechanical advantages, including improved joint stability resulting from greater anatomic deltoid wrapping[2,3,34] **(FIGURE 4.6)**, improved deltoid efficiency resulting from larger deltoid moment arm lengths,[13,14,34,65,66,71] and improvement in active rotation resulting from more anatomic tensioning of the remaining rotator cuff muscles.[2,3,34,72,73] Furthermore, maintaining Grammont medialized CoR minimizes the torque on the glenoid bone-implant interface to reduce the risk of aseptic glenoid loosening.[78,82,93] While humeral lateralization offers numerous biomechanical advantages, it should be noted that overlateralizing the humerus may overtension these muscles in patients with small shoulders and also make concomitant repair of the subscapularis more difficult.

Given that prosthesis design parameters can impact RTSA biomechanics, surgical technique, and complication rates, an RTSA prosthesis classification system was developed to objectively categorize glenoid designs based upon how they position the CoR and separately categorize humeral designs based upon how they position the humerus, and then combine each together to account for the combined offset and interaction.[3,14,31,34] For the glenoid prosthesis classification, a glenosphere whose CoR is ≤5 mm lateral to the glenoid fossa is categorized as a medialized glenoid (MG) and a glenosphere whose CoR is >5 mm lateral is categorized as a lateralized glenoid (LG). The position of the CoR is determined by the difference between the glenosphere thickness and radius **(FIGURE 4.7)**. For the humeral prosthesis classification, a humeral component offset ≤15 mm is categorized as a medialized humerus (MH) and a humeral component offset >15 mm is categorized as a lateralized humerus (LH). Humeral offset is defined as the horizontal distance between the intramedullary canal/humeral stem axis to the center of the humeral liner and is influenced by humeral neck angle, humeral osteotomy, and use of an inlay liner/stem or an onlay humeral tray/stem design **(FIGURE 4.8)**. The combined interaction between these glenoid and humeral design categories defines the RTSA prosthesis classification system: MG/MH, LG/MH, MG/LH, and LG/LH[3,14,31,34] **(FIGURE 4.9)**. Recent work by Werthel et al further refined this classification system by adding one new humeral offset category, minimally lateralized humerus, and then grouping these implants into five different combined configurations by a measurement of global offset: medialized (M) RTSA, minimally lateralized (ML) RTSA, lateralized (L) RTSA, highly lateralized (HL) RTSA, and very highly

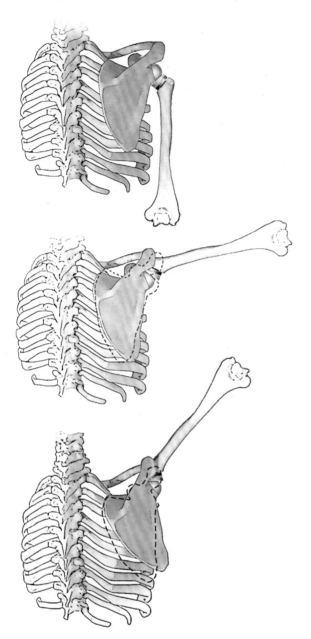

FIGURE 4.5 Modified scapulohumeral rhythm with RTSA, where additional scapular rotation occurs with RTSA relative to the scapulohumeral rhythm of the native shoulder (dotted line) during arm elevation.

Alternative methods to lateralize the humerus while maintaining a medialized CoR have been proposed. Roche et al demonstrated this can be accomplished by decreasing the humeral neck angle from the Delta III humeral neck angle of 155°, proportionally increasing the Grammont hemispherical glenosphere radius and thickness, decreasing the humeral liner constraint, and increasing the medial offset of the humeral liner relative to the humeral stem axis. Increasing humeral offset is most commonly performed by using an onlay humeral liner/tray design (as opposed to the Grammont inlay

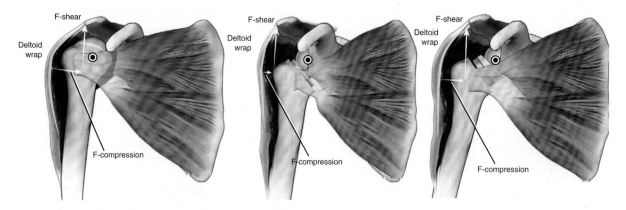

FIGURE 4.6 Wrapping of the middle deltoid around the lateral proximal humerus generates a stabilizing compressive force, where a greater amount of deltoid wrapping results in a larger compression vector that imparts greater joint stability: native shoulder (left), medial glenoid/medial humerus design (middle), and medial glenoid/lateral humerus design (right).

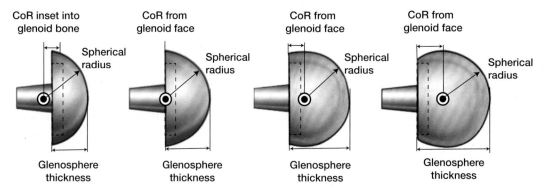

FIGURE 4.7 RTSA glenoid prosthesis design classification; representative images of four glenosphere designs having equivalent articular curvatures demonstrating that the relationship between glenoid thickness and articular radius, is directly related to the lateralization of the center of rotation (CoR) relative to the glenoid face.

lateralized (VHL) RTSA.[98] Werthel et al also quantified the offset of 24 different RTSA prostheses and sorted each into global offset configurations and reported 5 M RTSA, 5 ML RTSA, 7 L RTSA, 6 HL RTSA, and 1 VHL RTSA, demonstrating a wide range of design variability among these 24 different prosthesis available in the global marketplace.[98]

Liou et al utilized a computer muscle model to quantify the muscle and joint reaction forces associated with a native shoulder and three different RTSA prostheses (one MG/MH, one LG/MH, and one MG/LH) from the aforementioned design classification system.[65] They reported that all three RTSA prostheses demonstrated larger deltoid abductor moment arms, a decreased joint reaction force, and a decreased deltoid force during arm elevation relative to the native shoulder. Liou et al also reported the MG/LH RTSA prosthesis was associated with the lowest joint reaction force and lowest middle deltoid forces during both abduction and forward flexion as compared to the MG/MH and the LG/MH RTSA designs.[65] The biomechanical advantage created by humeral lateralization and the reduced advantage caused by CoR

lateralization of the glenoid was independently corroborated by Giles et al.[71] Biomechanical differences between prosthesis design configurations were also reported by Henninger et al who used a cadaveric shoulder controller study to investigate the impact of lateralizing the CoR by increasing glenoid thickness from 0 to 15 mm (in 5 mm increments) and reported the deltoid force during abduction increased with each 5 mm of CoR lateralization.[1] Similar to Liou et al,[65] Henninger et al reported lower deltoid forces during abduction with RTSA relative to the native shoulder, for the 0 and 5 mm lateral CoR configurations; however, they found that the deltoid force with the 10 and 15 mm lateral CoR configurations was not significantly different from the native shoulder.[1]

IMPACT OF SURGICAL TECHNIQUE ON RTSA BIOMECHANICS

RTSA biomechanics can be altered by different surgical techniques, as illustrated by the impact of concomitant subscapularis repair and also by muscle transfers in an external rotation deficient shoulder. Concomitant

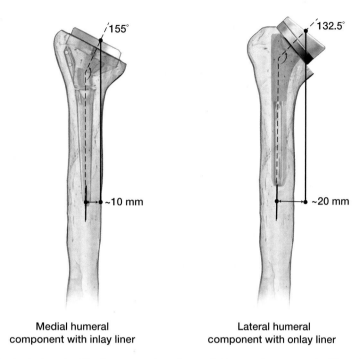

Medial humeral component with inlay liner

Lateral humeral component with onlay liner

FIGURE 4.8 RTSA humeral prosthesis design classification; examples of a medial humeral component with an inlay humeral liner (left) and a lateral humeral component with an onlay humeral liner (right).

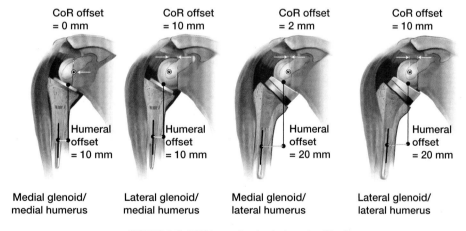

FIGURE 4.9 RTSA prosthesis design classification.

repair of the subscapularis with RTSA is controversial. Edwards et al reported a 5.1% dislocation rate with the Grammont prosthesis and concluded that the relative rate of dislocation with RTSA is doubled if the subscapularis is not repaired.[99] However, multiple other studies found no increased risk of instability or complications if the subscapularis is not repaired for RTSA that lateralize the humerus more than the Grammont design.[84,85,100] The subscapularis in the native shoulder functions predominately as an abductor and internal rotator. With RTSA, the inferiomedial humeral position causes the subscapularis to have a biphasic function, acting as an adductor at low/midelevations (ie, a line of action below the CoR) and as an abductor at high elevation

(ie, a line of action above the CoR) **(FIGURE 4.10)**. It should be noted that other surgical techniques, such as implanting the glenoid baseplate to achieve additional inferior glenosphere overhang, further distalizing the humerus through a smaller humeral osteotomy, or by using thicker humeral liners/trays, will further convert the subscapularis into an adductor at low elevation. The same is also true of the infraspinatus. The biomechanical consequence of this modified muscle function with RTSA has been investigated in a cadaveric shoulder controller by Hansen et al, who reported that subscapularis repair significantly increases the overall deltoid force, posterior rotator cuff force, and overall joint reaction force when elevating the arm with the elbow flexed as

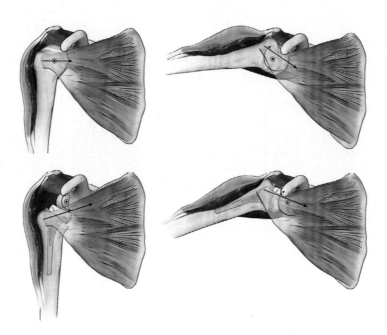

FIGURE 4.10 Subscapularis function with the native shoulder (top) and the RTSA (bottom). In the native shoulder at low elevation (top left image), the subscapularis line of action is in-line or above the center of rotation (CoR) to induce an abduction moment; however, with RTSA at both low elevation and midelevation (bottom left image), the subscapularis line of action is below the CoR to induce an adduction moment. At high elevations (right images), the subscapularis functions as an abductor in both the native shoulder and the RTSA.

compared to when the subscapularis is not repaired in RTSA.[101] Hansen postulated that because the posterior rotator cuff is often compromised in RTSA patients, subscapularis repair may lead to anterior/posterior imbalance in some patients since the infraspinatus and teres minor muscles may not be able to generate a sufficient countertorque if the infraspinatus and/or teres minor is impaired. Given these observations, it may be that subscapularis repair is necessary for RTSA prostheses that medialize the humerus but not required for RTSA prostheses that lateralize the humerus, as RTSA prostheses that lateralize the humerus achieve better tension on the rotator cuff muscles and have greater deltoid wrapping to improve stability.[3,85,100,101] Friedman et al quantified outcomes for patients with and without subscapularis repair using the same MG/LH RTSA prosthesis and reported no difference in complication or revision rates between cohorts. However, patients with subscapularis repair were associated with significantly better active internal rotation but significantly less active abduction than patients without subscapularis repair.[85]

Muscle transfers have been recommended when performing RTSA in patients with an impaired posterior rotator cuff that results in significant external rotation deficiency.[102-106] In the absence of a functioning posterior rotator cuff, the patient is unable to externally rotate their arm and also hold their arm in neutral during elevation, a condition commonly referred to as horn blower's sign.

This situation can be quite disabling. In general, internal rotator muscles (eg, muscles that attach anteriorly on the humerus) that have sufficient length (eg, the pectoralis or latissimus dorsi) can be transferred across the CoR to the posterior side of the humerus to convert their function to external rotation. The latissimus dorsi is the most common muscle transferred to remedy posterior rotator cuff insufficiency,[105] though additional muscles, like the teres major, can be transferred in combination with the latissimus as in the L'Episcopo procedure.[102,103] While muscle transfers have been demonstrated to successfully restore active external rotation, they may not be necessary if the teres minor is functional.[102,103,106]

IMPACT OF IMPLANT SIZE AND POSITIONING ON RTSA BIOMECHANICS

RTSA biomechanics can be altered by implant size and/or implant positioning. On the humeral side, implanting the RTSA humeral prosthesis in less humeral retroversion (eg, 0°) asymmetrically tensions the rotator cuff muscles by increasing tension of the posterior rotator cuff while further decreasing tension of the anterior rotator cuff.[2] Similarly, implanting the RTSA humeral prosthesis in more retroversion (eg, 40°) increases tension of the anterior rotator cuff but further decreases tension on the posterior rotator cuff.[2] Additionally, changing humeral retroversion also slightly alters the deltoid wrapping angle, with a few more degrees of wrapping occurring with less humeral retroversion.[2] While deltoid elongation occurs with all RTSA prostheses, taking a larger or smaller humeral osteotomy also influences deltoid tensioning and arm lengthening. Laaderman et al reported that arm lengthening up to 2 cm commonly occurs with RTSA and that more lengthening (at least up to an undefined point) correlates with improved active forward elevation.[62,63] De Wilde et al[7] reported that the Grammont and RSP (DJO, Inc) RTSA prostheses elongate the deltoid with the arm at 0° abduction by 16.4% and 13.0%, respectively, and Jobin et al[8] reported a 17% average deltoid elongation with three different RTSA prostheses with the arm at 0° abduction.[7,8] Similarly, in a computer muscle model comparing three different RTSA prostheses, Roche and colleagues[2,3] reported deltoid elongation between 12% and 22% relative to the native shoulder, where the magnitude of muscle elongation was influenced by humeral component type (inlay vs onlay), humeral implant retroversion, humeral implant position, and humeral tray/liner thickness.

On the glenoid side, Mollon et al compared the outcomes of 38 and 42 mm glenospheres and reported that patients with 42 mm glenospheres had significantly greater improvements in active forward elevation and active external rotation.[67] These clinical findings are supported by numerous computer analyses which conclude that larger glenosphere diameters are associated with improved ROM due to increased inferior overhang, more ROM, and less scapular impingement.[18,23,24,28,29,32,33,35,36,66,70] Various recommendations for glenoid baseplate positioning have been recommended to avoid scapular notching. Nyffeler et al[29] first recommended the glenoid baseplate be implanted with an inferior shift (with or without an inferior tilt). Implanting the baseplate with an inferior shift or tilt inferiorly shifts the joint CoR which also elongates the deltoid.[2,36] Implanting the baseplate with 15° inferior tilt also slightly medializes the humerus, decreases the

middle deltoid wrapping angle, and further decreases rotator cuff muscle tension because of this medialization.[2] Achieving inferior glenosphere tilt also requires reaming of the inferior glenoid, which has the advantage of removing bone that could impinge with the humeral liner, but the disadvantage of removing cortical bone which may compromise long-term fixation.[34,75] Boileau et al recommended placement of bone graft behind the baseplate in a nonworn glenoid (eg, bony increased-offset reverse total shoulder arthroplasty [BIO-RSA]) to lateralize the humerus and minimize humeral liner impingement.[92] While using bone graft behind the baseplate of a nonworn glenoid does improve muscle tensioning[72,92] and increases deltoid wrapping,[2] it also laterally shifts the CoR from the glenoid fossa which correspondingly decreases the deltoid abductor moment arm and reduces deltoid efficiency.[1,13,14,34] Lateralizing the CoR with bone graft also increases the torque at the implant-bone interface which increases the risk of loosening and introduces new potential complications.[82,92,107,108]

Building upon Dr. Grammont's fundamental concept of a medialized CoR to improve deltoid efficiency, Roche et al proposed a glenosphere design whose thickness is less than its radius; this 46 × 21 mm glenosphere medially insets the CoR within the glenoid bone to increase the deltoid abductor moment arms and further reduce the force necessary to elevate the arm.[13] In a computer muscle model measuring deltoid moment arms, this 46 × 21 mm glenosphere was evaluated against five different RTSA prostheses and was associated with a 4.8% to 40.7% increase in the average deltoid efficiency during abduction. This design conceptually illustrates the relationship between CoR and deltoid moment arm lengths and demonstrates that small changes in glenosphere thickness can result in biomechanically meaningful improvements[13] **(FIGURE 4.11)**. These results also suggest that many current RTSA prostheses have not yet been optimized from a biomechanical standpoint.

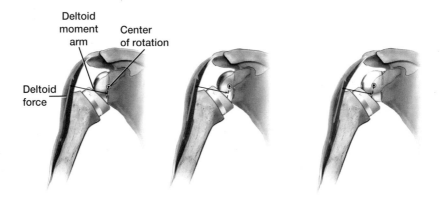

FIGURE 4.11 Increase in deltoid abductor moment arm length by medializing the center of rotation (CoR): inset CoR glenosphere (left), standard offset glenosphere (middle), and expanded glenosphere (right).

IMPACT OF PATIENT-SPECIFIC ANATOMY AND MORPHOLOGY ON RTSA BIOMECHANICS

RTSA biomechanics can be altered by patient-specific anatomic and morphological parameters. Just as proximal humeral anatomy is highly variable,[10,109-113] patient muscle size and muscle moment arms also vary. How muscles wrap around the proximal humeral anatomy alters the amount of deltoid wrapping, the deltoid's line of action at various joint positions, and, in turn, the amount of compression the deltoid can impart to the glenohumeral joint and the RTSA prosthesis. Jacobson et al demonstrated that middle deltoid moment arms change with gender and morphology: male shoulders had significantly larger deltoid moment arms than female shoulders. However, no gender differences were observed in the magnitude of deltoid wrapping.[10] Deltoid wrapping can vary as a function of greater tuberosity size, acromion size, acromial overhang, humeral head size, and humeral head offset (affecting the location of the CoR). Similarly, Jacobson et al reported that acromion size and width were significantly different between male and female scapulae.[10] As the middle and posterior heads of the deltoid originate on the acromion and scapular spine, acromion size can influence deltoid moment arm lengths, the amount of deltoid wrapping around the greater tuberosity, and the deltoid's line of action at various joint positions. Future work should investigate and identify the anatomic and morphological parameters that can further impact clinical outcomes and functional improvement after RTSA.

IMPACT OF GLENOID AND HUMERAL BONE LOSS ON RTSA BIOMECHANICS

RTSA biomechanics are altered when used in patients with glenoid wear. Glenoid wear further medializes the joint line which shortens the rotator cuff muscles and reduces deltoid wrapping around the greater tuberosity.[34,73] Norris et al demonstrated that with a sufficient amount of medial glenoid wear, the deltoid can actually generate a laterally directed distraction force that can result in instability.[55] Most commonly, surgeons address asymmetric glenoid wear with eccentric reaming to correct the defect. Unfortunately, reaming the glenoid further medializes the joint line and removes nonworn glenoid cortical bone which may compromise fixation.[76,80,81] Augmented glenoid baseplates were designed to conserve glenoid bone, increase prosthesis surface contact area with cortical bone, and better restore the native joint line when performing RTSA in eroded scapular morphologies.[34,61,73,114] Bench tests with these augmented baseplates have demonstrated adequate fixation can be achieved for various glenoid wear scenarios,[76,80] and promising short- and midterm clinical results using these augmented baseplates have recently been published.[61,114] Jones et al performed an outcomes analysis comparing the use of bone graft to augmented baseplates for patients with severe glenoid wear and reported equivalent outcome scores between RTSA cohorts but also observed significantly higher complication rates with bone grafting compared to augmented baseplates.[114]

RTSA biomechanics are altered when used in patients with proximal humeral bone loss. Edwards et al reported several cases of instability in patients with proximal humeral bone loss,[99] Simovitch et al reported that active external rotation was significantly less in three and four-part fracture patients who had greater tuberosity resorption as compared to those patients in whom the greater tuberosity healed,[57] and Sabesan et al reported that the loss of the greater tuberosity negatively affects shoulder biomechanics during external rotation.[115] This reduced external rotation is most likely due to compromised infraspinatus and teres minor function resulting from greater tuberosity resorption, and the findings of instability are presumably due, in part, to the loss of deltoid wrapping. By corollary, increasing humeral lateralization by use of an allograft or a metal augment can restore the proximal humeral morphology and increase deltoid wrapping to improve stability (**FIGURE 4.12**). Similarly, as RTSA are increasingly used in clinical situations with varying degrees of proximal humeral bone loss, humeral reconstruction prostheses have been utilized to provide greater lateralization to further enhance deltoid abductor moment arms and improve joint stability with increased deltoid wrapping (**FIGURE 4.13**).

MECHANICALLY INDUCED RTSA COMPLICATIONS

Scapular Notching

Scapular notching is the most commonly reported complication with RTSA. Scapular notching is caused by mechanical impingement of the humeral liner against the inferior scapular neck, resulting in scapular bone loss, humeral liner wear, and the generation of polyethylene debris. Scapular notching can be progressive and extend beyond the most inferior glenoid baseplate screw, suggesting an osteolytic response to the polyethylene debris. Previous studies have demonstrated that scapular notching is influenced by prosthesis design parameters, patient arm size and body habitus, and surgical technique, such as glenosphere inferior placement on the scapula.[18,23,24,28,29,32,33,35,36,66,70,116] The clinical consequences of scapular notching have been controversial, but it is now generally accepted that it negatively impacts clinical outcomes. Mollon et al first reported that the majority of clinical studies with sufficient statistical power demonstrated that scapular notching does, in fact, negatively impact clinical outcomes.[67] Mollon et al further demonstrated that the majority of studies which claimed scapular notching had no clinical effect were not sufficiently statistically powered to detect any difference.[67] Simovitch et al

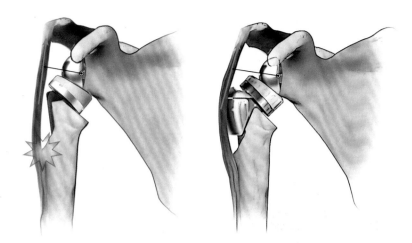

FIGURE 4.12 Use of an augmented humeral tray with RTSA in the case of proximal humeral bone loss to improve RTSA biomechanics by restoring the lateral tuberosity shape and increasing deltoid wrapping to improve stability while increasing the deltoid moment arm to improve deltoid efficiency.

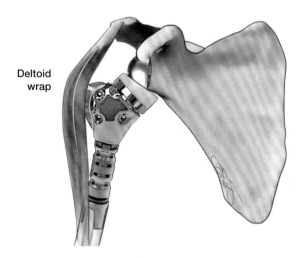

Deltoid wrap

FIGURE 4.13 Use of a humeral reconstruction prosthesis with variable sizes of modular proximal bodies to improve RTSA biomechanics by lateralizing the tuberosity and increasing deltoid wrapping to improve stability while increasing the deltoid moment arm to improve deltoid efficiency.

compared midterm outcomes of RTSA patients with and without scapular notching and demonstrated that patients with scapular notching had significantly lower postoperative patient-reported outcome measures, significantly less strength and ROM, and significantly higher complication and revision rates compared to patients without scapular notching.[68] Furthermore, one biomechanical study demonstrated that scapular notching can compromise baseplate fixation,[79] and another study raised concerns about the relationship between instability and implant failure due to notching.[117] In this context, scapular notching can be prevented by careful selection of implant design utilized, by close adherence to the technical aspects of glenoid component insertion and by integrating patient arm size and body habitus into both.

Instability

While the inverted concavities and fixed fulcrum of the RTSA articulation inherently provide joint stability, a net compressive joint reaction force acting on the glenosphere throughout the ROM is also required for RTSA stability. Instability is the most common cause for RTSA revisions. Instability/dislocation rates with RTSA have been reported between 1.5% and 31%.[118] Zumstein et al performed a meta-analysis of RTSA complications and reported an instability rate of 4.7%.[91] RTSA instability occurs when the joint reaction force is directed outside the humeral liner **(FIGURE 4.14)**, which is typically associated with (1) deltoid muscle laxity, weakness, or paralysis, (2) glenoid wear or humeral bone loss resulting in reduced muscle tensioning and reduced deltoid wrapping, (3) soft-tissue imbalance caused by lack of subscapularis repair, trauma, joint overloading, or congenital deformity, (4) humeral liner-scapular impingement induced dislocation of the humeral liner from the glenosphere, and/or (5) humeral liner or tray disassociation due to implant modular locking mechanism failure.

RTSA prosthesis geometry and implant size/type selection can influence the net joint compressive force. Liou et al utilized a computer muscle model to quantify joint reaction forces, including the resolved shear and compressive vectors for three different RTSA prosthesis designs during each of abduction, forward elevation, and internal/external rotation.[65] They reported that during forward elevation, the compression vector was the smallest component of the joint reaction force, and during abduction, the compression vector was the largest component of the joint reaction force for all three RTSA prosthesis designs.[65] Liou et al also reported a few differences in joint compression between prostheses for the different joint motions, where generally the MG/MH RTSA shoulder was associated with less joint compression as

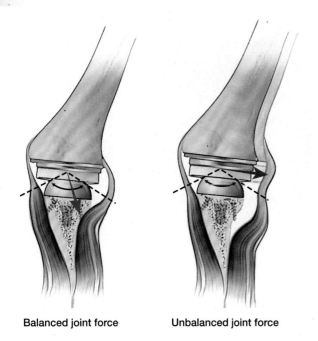

| Balanced joint force | Unbalanced joint force |

FIGURE 4.14 Instability resulting from the joint reaction force being directed outside of the humeral liner/glenosphere articulation (denoted by dotted lines) with RTSA.

compared to the LG/MH and MG/LH RTSA prostheses.[65] Two other computer muscle models demonstrated that prosthesis geometry and surgical technique can alter deltoid and rotator cuff muscle tensioning as well as the magnitude of deltoid wrapping,[2,3] all of which influence the magnitude and direction of the joint reaction force, including the relative contribution of the compressive vector. Clinically, several prosthetic options are available to treat the unstable RTSA to increase deltoid tensioning and joint stability. These options include use of a larger or thicker glenosphere, thicker/offset humeral trays, thicker/offset polyethylene liners, constrained humeral liners, or tuberosity augmentation to improve deltoid wrapping and stability in the cases of proximal humeral bone loss. Regarding constrained liners, they provide additional stability using a deeper concavity, and as result, they require a greater jump distance to dislocation.[19,33] However, this deeper concavity reduces motion[28] and may increase risk of scapular notching and impingement, which can induce dislocation. As a result, other measures should be considered first to improve stability before utilizing a constrained humeral liner.

Acromial and Scapular Insufficiency Fractures

Acromial and scapular fractures after RTSA are uncommon complications. The altered deltoid mechanics with RTSA can induce abnormal stresses in the scapula,[119] potentially leading to scapular fracture patterns unique to RTSA. These fractures can occur at various locations on the acromion and scapular spine and have been classified by Levy et al.[94] These fractures are discussed in

Chapter 38. From a biomechanical perspective, the magnitude of stress increase has been demonstrated to be influenced by RTSA prosthesis design. Wong et al conducted a finite element analysis and observed that lateralizing the CoR with RTSA was associated with a 17.2% increase in acromial stress whereas increasing humeral lateralization resulted in a nonsignificant change of only 1.7%.[119] Zumstein et al conducted a meta-analysis of RTSA between 1998 and 2008 and reported an acromion and scapular spine fracture rate of 1.5% (12 of 782 cases).[91] More recently, King et al conducted a meta-analysis between 2010 and 2018 and reported a fracture rate of 2.8% (253 of 9048 cases).[88] However, fracture rates of 10% have also been reported with RTSA prosthesis designs that lateralize the CoR.[94] Although there are several theories of the causes of these fractures after RTSA, the mechanical mechanism is unclear. One theory is that the inferiomedial shift of the humerus with RTSA elongates the deltoid and increases stress in the acromion and scapular spine.[94,120,121] Prosthesis design parameters likely have an influence on the rate of these fractures. King et al compared the acromion and scapular fracture rate associated with multiple RTSA prostheses and reported that the MG/LH RTSA prosthesis had a significantly lower fracture rate relative to other RTSA prosthesis design styles and that LG/MH prostheses had the highest fracture rate.[88] It is important to note that not all RTSA prostheses of the same design classification are associated with the same fracture rates. Ascione et al reported a 4.3% acromial and scapular fracture rate using one particular onlay MG/LH prosthesis,[120] which is nearly three times the 1.5% rate observed by Routman et al using a different onlay MG/LH prosthesis.[90] The most likely reason for these different fracture rates is that different onlay RTSA prostheses have different baseline offsets which result in different inferiomedial humeral translations.[3] These differences can presumably alter scapular stresses and fracture rates. Scapular fractures can also occur due to stress concentrations resulting from glenoid baseplate screw placement near the base of the acromion.[87,122,123] Another theory is that acromial and scapular fractures occur due to overactivity, increased activity following a period of inactivity, or by a traumatic event. Neyton et al reported that 15.8% of fractures were caused by trauma.[89]

UNANSWERED RTSA BIOMECHANICS QUESTIONS

The optimal RTSA joint tension at the time of intraoperative reduction is unknown and is highly variable based on physician experience, prosthesis design and sizing configuration, and patient factors. Overlengthening the arm has been implicated in complications such as acromial and scapular stress fractures, polyethylene wear, glenoid loosening, deltoid muscle strain, and brachial plexus injuries. Given the subjective and qualitative nature by which surgeons intraoperatively assess joint tensioning, Verstraete et al developed an instrumented load-sensing humeral trial to quantify joint loading and assess the point of contact during trial reduction and intraoperative ROM.[124] Verstraete et al reported use of this instrumented device in cadavers and measured RTSA joint forces between 1 and 70 lbs, though >98% of loads were <40 lbs. The largest joint loads were observed during forward elevation and at the extremes of rotation, and they observed ROM generally decreased with increasing joint tension.[124] The ability to quantify intraoperative RTSA joint loading is fundamental to our understanding of the normal load variability that occurs at different joint positions. In the near future, the data generated by such an instrumented tool can be used to standardize surgical decision-making relating to joint tensioning by characterizing how joint loads vary with different patient-specific factors, implant configurations, and surgical techniques. This joint loading data can then be combined with patient-specific factors, preoperative outcomes data, and implant size and position data using machine learning techniques[125] to predict patient-specific ROM, acromial and scapular stress fracture risk, and also instability risk.

The widespread adoption of three-dimensional computed tomography (3D CT) planning software has made questions of implant sizing and implant positioning an important focus for surgeons performing RTSA. Future work should utilize machine learning analytic techniques to characterize how implant positioning influences RTSA biomechanics and outcomes and, specifically, answer how much glenoid retroversion should be corrected for a posteriorly eroded glenoid, how much glenoid inclination should be corrected for a superiorly eroded glenoid, and provide guidance regarding when to eccentrically ream a glenoid, when to bone graft, and when to use augmented glenoid baseplates. These same predictive analytic techniques could potentially be used to identify the ideal implant size for a given patient's anatomy/morphology that will result in optimal ROM and/or outcomes. Identifying the implant and patient factors associated with active internal and external rotation is also necessary, as improvement in rotation remains unpredictable with RTSA.

The biomechanical causes of acromial and scapular insufficiency fractures after RTSA have not been fully explained. While patient risk factors[90,126] have been identified along with some prosthesis design configurations,[88,90,119] the mechanisms for failure are not fully understood, and most importantly, the appropriate mitigating actions to prevent occurrence have not been identified. Although it seems clear that using RTSA prostheses which lateralize the CoR concentrate stress at the base of the scapula,[119] there are certainly other factors that can contribute to their development. Coracoacromial ligament transection at the time of the RTSA procedure has been implicated as a potential contributor,[127] and an aggressive postoperative therapy program may also increase fracture risk. Future work should also seek to identify the optimal method of treatment of these complications.

Finally, recurrent instability after RTSA remains a perplexing clinical challenge. While traction on a reduced arm can clearly result in decoupling, there are mechanisms of instability that remain unclear, and some patients continue to dislocate despite revision arthroplasty in what appears to be a stable joint intraoperatively at the time of revision. The complex interactions between implant component size, implant position, the surrounding soft-tissue envelope, and patient activity are only beginning to be understood. With further analysis, the use of load-sensing tools, and clinical follow-up, we hope to identify why a particular RTSA becomes unstable and recommend patient-specific measures to restore stability and function.

CONCLUSION

The RTSA prosthesis can reliably restore stability and function to patients with a wide variety of degenerative conditions of the shoulder. Irrespective of the indications, the biomechanical mechanism for restored stability is the inverted articular concavities of the prosthesis, which creates a fixed fulcrum to minimize superior migration. The biomechanical mechanism for restored function is the medialized CoR of the prosthesis relative to the native shoulder, which increases the abductor moment arms and improves deltoid muscle efficiency to elevate the arm. RTSA biomechanics can be altered by prosthesis design parameters, surgical technique, implant size, implant position, and patient-specific anatomy and morphology, including different glenoid wear patterns and proximal humeral bone loss. While the risks associated with the RTSA prosthesis are well documented, the biomechanical mechanisms of these complications are not well understood and require future research.

REFERENCES

1. Henninger HB, Barg A, Anderson AE, Bachus KN, Burks RT, Tashjian RZ. Effect of lateral offset center of rotation in reverse total shoulder arthroplasty: a biomechanical study. *J Shoulder Elbow Surg.* 2012;21(9):1128-1135. doi:10.1016/j.jse.2011.07.034
2. Roche CP, Diep P, Hamilton M, et al. Impact of inferior glenoid tilt, humeral retroversion, bone grafting, and design parameters on muscle length and deltoid wrapping in reverse shoulder arthroplasty. *Bull Hosp Jt Dis (2013).* 2013;71(4):284-293.
3. Routman HD, Flurin PH, Wright T, Zuckerman J, Hamilton M, Roche C. Reverse shoulder arthroplasty prosthesis design classification system. *Bull Hosp Jt Dis (2013).* 2015;73(suppl 1):S5-S14.
4. Saltzman MD, Mercer DM, Warme WJ, Bertelsen AL, Matsen FA III. A method for documenting the change in center of rotation with reverse total shoulder arthroplasty and its application to a consecutive series of 68 shoulders having reconstruction with one of two different reverse prostheses. *J Shoulder Elbow Surg.* 2010;19(7):1028-1033. doi:10.1016/j.jse.2010.01.021

5. Ackland DC, Roshan-Zamir S, Richardson M, Pandy MG. Moment arms of the shoulder musculature after reverse total shoulder arthroplasty. *J Bone Joint Surg Am.* 2010;92(5):1221-1230. doi:10.2106/JBJS.I.00001

6. Boileau P, Watkinson DJ, Hatzidakis AM, Balg F. Grammont reverse prosthesis: design, rationale, and biomechanics. *J Shoulder Elbow Surg.* 2005;14(1 suppl S):147S-161S. doi:10.1016/j.jse.2004.10.006

7. De Wilde LF, Audenaert EA, Berghs BM. Shoulder prostheses treating cuff tear arthropathy: a comparative biomechanical study. *J Orthop Res.* 2004;22(6):1222-1230.

8. Jobin CM, Brown GD, Bahu MJ, et al. Reverse total shoulder arthroplasty for cuff tear arthropathy: the clinical effect of deltoid lengthening and center of rotation medialization. *J Shoulder Elbow Surg.* 2012;21(10):1269-1277. doi:10.1016/j.jse.2011.08.049

9. Elwell JA, Athwal GS, Willing R. Development and validation of a muscle wrapping model applied to intact and reverse total shoulder arthroplasty shoulders. *J Orthop Res.* 2018;36(12):3308-3317. doi:10.1002/jor.24131

10. Jacobson A, Gilot GJ, Hamilton MA, et al. Glenohumeral anatomic study. A comparison of male and female shoulders with similar average age and BMI. *Bull Hosp Jt Dis (2013).* 2015;73(suppl 1):S68-S78.

11. Otis JC, Jiang CC, Wickiewicz TL, Peterson MG, Warren RF, Santner TJ. Changes in the moment arms of the rotator cuff and deltoid muscles with abduction and rotation. *J Bone Joint Surg Am.* 1994;76(5):667-676.

12. Poppen NK, Walker PS. Forces at the glenohumeral joint in abduction. *Clin Orthop Relat Res.* 1978;(135):165-170.

13. Roche CP, Hamilton MA, Diep P, et al. Optimizing deltoid efficiency with reverse shoulder arthroplasty using a novel inset center of rotation glenosphere design. *Bull Hosp Jt Dis (2013).* 2015;73(suppl 1):S37-S41.

14. Hamilton MA, Diep P, Roche C, et al. Effect of reverse shoulder design philosophy on muscle moment arms. *J Orthop Res.* 2015;33(4):605-613. doi:10.1002/jor.22803

15. Kontaxis A, Johnson GR. The biomechanics of reverse anatomy shoulder replacement – A modeling study. *Clin Biomech (Bristol, Avon).* 2009;24(3):254-260.

16. Terrier A, Reist A, Merlini F, Farron A. Simulated joint and muscle forces in reversed and anatomic shoulder prostheses. *J Bone Joint Surg Br.* 2008;90(6):751-756. doi:10.1302/0301-620X.90B6.19708

17. Lippitt SB, Vanderhooft JE, Harris SL, Sidles JA, Harryman DT II, Matsen FA III. Glenohumeral stability from concavity-compression: a quantitative analysis. *J Shoulder Elbow Surg.* 1993;2(1):27-35. doi:10.1016/S1058-2746(09)80134-1

18. Chou J, Malak SF, Anderson IA, Astley T, Poon PC. Biomechanical evaluation of different designs of glenospheres in the SMR reverse total shoulder prosthesis: range of motion and risk of scapular notching. *J Shoulder Elbow Surg.* 2009;18(3):354-359. doi:10.1016/j.jse.2009.01.015

19. Clouthier AL, Hetzler MA, Fedorak G, Bryant JT, Deluzio KJ, Bicknell RT. Factors affecting the stability of reverse shoulder arthroplasty: a biomechanical study. *J Shoulder Elbow Surg.* 2013;22(4):439-444. doi:10.1016/j.jse.2012.05.032

20. De Wilde LF, Poncet D, Middernacht B, Ekelund A. Prosthetic overhang is the most effective way to prevent scapular conflict in a reverse total shoulder prosthesis. *Acta Orthop.* 2010;81(6):719-726. doi:10.3109/17453674.2010.538354

21. Elwell J, Choi J, Willing R. Quantifying the competing relationship between adduction range of motion and baseplate micromotion with lateralization of reverse total shoulder arthroplasty. *J Biomech.* 2017;52:24-30. doi:10.1016/j.jbiomech.2016.11.053

22. Elwell JA, Athwal GS, Willing R. Development and application of a novel metric to characterize comprehensive range of motion of reverse total shoulder arthroplasty. *J Orthop Res.* 2020;38(4):880-887. doi:10.1002/jor.24518

23. Kempton LB, Balasubramaniam M, Ankerson E, Wiater JM. A radiographic analysis of the effects of glenosphere position on scapular notching following reverse total shoulder arthroplasty. *J Shoulder Elbow Surg.* 2011;20(6):968-974. Doi: 10.1016/j.jse.2010.11.026.

24. Kempton LB, Balasubramaniam M, Ankerson E, Wiater JM. A radiographic analysis of the effects of prosthesis design on scapular notching following reverse total shoulder arthroplasty. *J Shoulder Elbow Surg.* 2011;20(4):571-576. doi:10.1016/j.jse.2010.08.024

25. Kolmodin J, Davidson IU, Jun BJ, et al. Scapular notching after reverse total shoulder arthroplasty: prediction using patient-specific osseous anatomy, implant location, and shoulder motion. *J Bone Joint Surg Am.* 2018;100(13):1095-1103. doi:10.2106/JBJS.17.00242

26. Li X, Knutson Z, Choi D, et al. Effects of glenosphere positioning on impingement-free internal and external rotation after reverse total shoulder arthroplasty. *J Shoulder Elbow Surg.* 2013;22(6):807-813. doi:10.1016/j.jse.2012.07.013

27. Middernacht B, De Roo PJ, Van Maele G, De Wilde LF. Consequences of scapular anatomy for reversed total shoulder arthroplasty. *Clin Orthop Relat Res.* 2008;466(6):1410-1418. doi:10.1007/s11999-008-0187-6

28. North LR, Hetzler MA, Pickell M, Bryant JT, Deluzio KJ, Bicknell RT. Effect of implant geometry on range of motion in reverse shoulder arthroplasty assessed using glenohumeral separation distance. *J Shoulder Elbow Surg.* 2015;24(9):1359-1366. doi:10.1016/j.jse.2014.12.031

29. Nyffeler RW, Werner CM, Gerber C. Biomechanical relevance of glenoid component positioning in the reverse Delta III total shoulder prosthesis. *J Shoulder Elbow Surg.* 2005;14(5):524-528. doi:10.1016/j.jse.2004.09.010

30. Paisley KC, Kraeutler MJ, Lazarus MD, Ramsey ML, Williams GR, Smith MJ. Relationship of scapular neck length to scapular notching after reverse total shoulder arthroplasty by use of plain radiographs. *J Shoulder Elbow Surg.* 2014;23(6):882-887. doi:10.1016/j.jse.2013.09.003

31. Roche C, Crosby L. *Kinematics and biomechanics of reverse total shoulder arthroplasty.* In: *AAOS Orthopaedic Knowledge Update.* 4th ed. 2013:45-54.

32. Roche C, Flurin PH, Wright T, Crosby LA, Mauldin M, Zuckerman JD. *Geometric analysis of the Grammont reverse shoulder prosthesis: an evaluation of the relationship between prosthetic design parameters and clinical failure modes.* In: *Proceedings of the 2006 ISTA Meeting.* New York, NY, October 6-9. 2006.

33. Roche C, Flurin PH, Wright T, Crosby LA, Mauldin M, Zuckerman JD. An evaluation of the relationships between reverse shoulder design parameters and range of motion, impingement, and stability. *J Shoulder Elbow Surg.* 2009;18(5):734-741. doi:10.1016/j.jse.2008.12.008

34. Roche C, Hansen M, Crosby L, et al. Biomechanical summary of reverse shoulder arthroplasty. Animation. AAOS Orthopaedic Video Theater. OVT-34. 2015.

35. Roche CP, Marczuk Y, Wright TW, et al. Scapular notching and osteophyte formation after reverse shoulder replacement: radiological analysis of implant position in male and female patients. *Bone Joint J.* 2013;95-B(4):530-535. doi:10.1302/0301-620X.95B4.30442

36. Roche CP, Marczuk Y, Wright TW, et al. Scapular notching in reverse shoulder arthroplasty: validation of a computer impingement model. *Bull Hosp Jt Dis (2013).* 2013;71(4):278-283.

37. Simovitch RW, Zumstein MA, Lohri E, et al. Predictors of scapular notching in patients managed with the Delta III reverse total shoulder replacement. *J Bone Joint Surg Am.* 2007;89(3):588-600.

38. Stephenson DR, Oh JH, McGarry MH, Rick Hatch GF III, Lee TQ. Effect of humeral component version on impingement in reverse total shoulder arthroplasty. *J Shoulder Elbow Surg.* 2011;20(4):652-658. doi:10.1016/j.jse.2010.08.020

39. Broström LA, Wallensten R, Olsson E, Anderson D. The Kessel prosthesis in total shoulder arthroplasty. A five-year experience. *Clin Orthop Relat Res.* 1992;(277):155-160.

40. Fenlin JM Jr. Semi-constrained prosthesis for the rotator cuff deficient patient. *Orthop Trans.* 1985;9:55.

41. Flatow EL, Harrison AK. A history of reverse total shoulder arthroplasty. *Clin Orthop Relat Res.* 2011;469(9):2432-2439. doi:10.1007/s11999-010-1733-6

42. Neer CS II. *Shoulder Reconstruction.* WB Saunders; 1990.

43. Redfern TR, Wallace WA. History of shoulder replacement surgery. In: Wallace WA, ed. *Joint Replacement in the Shoulder and Elbow.* Butterworth and Heinemann; 1998:6-16.

44. Reeves B, Jobbins B, Dowson D, Wright V. A total shoulder endoprosthesis. *Eng Med.* 1974;1:64-67.

45. Wretenberg PF, Wallensten R. The Kessel total shoulder arthroplasty. A 13- to 16-year retrospective followup. *Clin Orthop Relat Res.* 1999;(365):100-103.

46. Grammont PM, Trouilloud P, Laffay J, Deries X. Etude et realisation d'une novelle prosthese d'epaule. *Rhumatologie.* 1987;39:17-22.

47. Grammont PM, Baulot E. *Delta Shoulder Prosthesis: Biomechanical Principles.* 1991.

48. Boileau P, Watkinson D, Hatzidakis AM, Hovorka I. Neer Award 2005: the Grammont reverse shoulder prosthesis. Results in cuff tear arthritis, fracture sequelae, and revision arthroplasty. *J Shoulder Elbow Surg.* 2006;15(5):527-540. doi:10.1016/j.jse.2006.01.003

49. Cuff D, Pupello D, Virani N, Levy J, Frankle M. Reverse shoulder arthroplasty for the treatment of rotator cuff deficiency. *J Bone Joint Surg Am.* 2008;90:1244-1251.

50. De Wilde LF, Plasschaert FS, Audenaert EA, Verdonk RC. Functional recovery after a reverse prosthesis for reconstruction of the proximal humerus in tumor surgery. *Clin Orthop Relat Res.* 2005;(430):156-162.

51. Frankle M, Siegal S, Pupello D, Saleem A, Mighell M, Vasey M. The reverse shoulder prosthesis for glenohumeral arthritis associated with severe rotator cuff deficiency. A minimum two-year follow-up study of sixty patients. *J Bone Joint Surg Am.* 2005;87(8):1697-1705.

52. Guery J, Favard L, Sirveaux F, Oudet D, Mole D, Walch G. Reverse total shoulder arthroplasty. Survivorship analysis of eighty replacements followed for five to ten years. *J Bone Joint Surg Am.* 2006;88:1742-1747.

53. Neyton L, Boileau P, Nové-Josserand L, Edwards TB, Walch G. Glenoid bone grafting with a reverse design prosthesis. *J Shoulder Elbow Surg.* 2007;16(suppl 3):S71-S78. doi:10.1016/j.jse.2006.02.002

54. Neyton L, Walch G, Nové-Josserand L, Edwards TB. Glenoid corticocancellous bone grafting after glenoid component removal in the treatment of glenoid loosening. *J Shoulder Elbow Surg.* 2006;15(2):173-179. doi:10.1016/j.jse.2005.07.010

55. Norris TR, Kelly JD, Humphrey CS. Management of glenoid bone defects in revision shoulder arthroplasty: a new application of the reverse total shoulder prosthesis. *Tech Shoulder Elbow Surg* 2007;8(1):37-46. doi:10.1097/BTE.0b013e318030d3b7

56. Rittmeister M, Kerschbaumer F. Grammont reverse total shoulder arthroplasty in patients with rheumatoid arthritis and nonreconstructible rotator cuff lesions. *J Shoulder Elbow Surg.* 2001;10:17-22, doi:10.1067/mse.2001.110515

57. Simovitch RW, Roche CP, Jones RB, et al. Effect of tuberosity healing on clinical outcomes in elderly patients treated with a reverse shoulder arthroplasty for 3- and 4-part proximal humerus fractures. *J Orthop Trauma.* 2019;33(2):e39-e45. doi:10.1097/BOT.0000000000001348

58. Sirveaux F, Favard L, Oudet D, Huquet D, Walch G, Molé D. Grammont inverted total shoulder arthroplasty in the treatment of glenohumeral osteoarthritis with massive rupture of the cuff. Results of a multicentre study of 80 shoulders. *J Bone Joint Surg Br.* 2004;86(3):388-395.

59. Stechel A, Fuhrmann U, Irlenbusch L, Rott O, Irlenbusch U. Reversed shoulder arthroplasty in cuff tear arthritis, fracture sequelae, and revision arthroplasty. *Acta Orthop.* 2010;81:367-372. doi:10.3109/17453674.2010.487242

60. Werner CM, Steinmann PA, Gilbart M, Gerber C. Treatment of painful pseudoparesis due to irreparable rotator cuff dysfunction with the Delta III reverse-ball-and-socket total shoulder prosthesis. *J Bone Joint Surg Am.* 2005;87:1476-1486. doi:10.2106/JBJS.D.02342

61. Virk M, Yip M, Liuzza L, et al. Clinical and radiographic outcomes with a posteriorly augmented glenoid for Walch B2, B3, and C glenoids in reverse total shoulder arthroplasty. *J Shoulder Elbow Surg.* 2020;29(5):e196-e204. doi:10.1016/j.jse.2019.09.031

62. Lädermann A, Walch G, Lubbeke A, et al. Influence of arm lengthening in reverse shoulder arthroplasty. *J Shoulder Elbow Surg.* 2012;21(3):336-341. doi:10.1016/j.jse.2011.04.020

63. Lädermann A, Williams MD, Melis B, Hoffmeyer P, Walch G. Objective evaluation of lengthening in reverse shoulder arthroplasty.

64. Lemieux PO, Hagemeister N, Tétreault P, Nuño N. Influence of the medial offset of the proximal humerus on the glenohumeral destabilising forces during arm elevation: a numerical sensitivity study. *Comput Methods Biomech Biomed Engin.* 2013;16(1):103-111. doi:10.1080/10255842.2011.607813

65. Liou W, Yang Y, Petersen-Fitts GR, Lombardo DJ, Stine S, Sabesan VJ. Effect of lateralized design on muscle and joint reaction forces for reverse shoulder arthroplasty. *J Shoulder Elbow Surg.* 2017;26(4):564-572. doi:10.1016/j.jse.2016.09.045

66. Langohr GD, Giles JW, Athwal GS, Johnson JA. The effect of glenosphere diameter in reverse shoulder arthroplasty on muscle force, joint load, and range of motion. *J Shoulder Elbow Surg.* 2015;24(6):972-979. doi:10.1016/j.jse.2014.10.018

67. Mollon B, Mahure SA, Roche CP, Zuckerman JD. Impact of scapular notching on clinical outcomes after reverse total shoulder arthroplasty: an analysis of 476 shoulders. *J Shoulder Elbow Surg.* 2017;26:1253-1261. doi:10.1016/j.jse.2016.11.043

68. Simovitch R, Flurin PH, Wright TW, Zuckerman JD, Roche C. Impact of scapular notching on reverse total shoulder arthroplasty midterm outcomes: 5-year minimum follow-up. *J Shoulder Elbow Surg.* 2019;28(12):2301-2307. doi:10.1016/j.jse.2019.04.042

69. Torrens C, Corrales M, Gonzalez G, Solano A, Caceres E. Morphology of the scapula relative to the reverse shoulder prosthesis. *J Orthop Surg (Hong Kong).* 2009;17(2):146-150.

70. Valenti P, Sauzières P, Katz D, Kalouche I, Kilinc AS. Do less medialized reverse shoulder prostheses increase motion and reduce notching? *Clin Orthop Relat Res.* 2011;469(9):2550-2557. doi:10.1007/s11999-011-1844-8

71. Giles JW, Langohr GD, Johnson JA, Athwal GS. Implant design variations in reverse total shoulder arthroplasty influence the required deltoid force and resultant joint load. *Clin Orthop Relat Res.* 2015;473(11):3615-3626. doi:10.1007/s11999-015-4526-0

72. Herrmann S, König C, Heller M, Perka C, Greiner S. Reverse shoulder arthroplasty leads to significant biomechanical changes in the remaining rotator cuff. *J Orthop Surg Res.* 2011;6:42. doi:10.1186/1749-799X-6-42

73. Roche CP, Diep P, Hamilton MA, et al. Impact of posterior wear on muscle length with reverse total shoulder arthroplasty. *Bull Hosp Jt Dis (2013).* 2015;73(suppl 1):S63-S67.

74. Walker D, Matsuki K, Struk AM, Wright TW, Banks SA. Scapulohumeral rhythm in shoulders with reverse shoulder arthroplasty. *J Shoulder Elbow Surg.* 2015;24(7):1129-1134. doi:10.1016/j.jse.2014.11.043

75. Roche CP, Diep P, Hamilton MA, Flurin PH, Routman HD. Comparison of bone removed with reverse total shoulder arthroplasty. *Bull Hosp Jt Dis (2013).* 2013;71(suppl 2):S36-S40.

76. Friedman R, Stroud N, Glattke K, et al. The impact of posterior wear on reverse shoulder glenoid fixation. *Bull Hosp Jt Dis (2013).* 2015;73(suppl 1):S15-S20.

77. Roche C, DiGeorgio C, Yegres J, et al. Impact of screw length and screw quantity on reverse total shoulder arthroplasty glenoid fixation for 2 different sizes of glenoid baseplates. *JSES Open Access.* 2019;3(4):296-303. doi:10.1016/j.jses.2019.08.006

78. Roche CP, Stroud NJ, Flurin PH, Wright TW, Zuckerman JD, DiPaola MJ. Reverse shoulder glenoid baseplate fixation: a comparison of flat-back versus curved-back designs and oval versus circular designs with 2 different offset glenospheres. *J Shoulder Elbow Surg.* 2014;23(9):1388-1394. doi:10.1016/j.jse.2014.01.050

79. Roche CP, Stroud NJ, Martin BL, et al. The impact of scapular notching on reverse shoulder glenoid fixation. *J Shoulder Elbow Surg.* 2013;22(7):963-970. doi:10.1016/j.jse.2012.10.035

80. Roche CP, Stroud NJ, Martin BL, et al. Achieving fixation in glenoids with superior wear using reverse shoulder arthroplasty. *J Shoulder Elbow Surg.* 2013;22(12):1695-1701. doi:10.1016/j.jse.2013.03.008

81. Roche CP, Stroud NJ, Palomino P, et al. The impact of anterior glenoid defects on reverse shoulder glenoid fixation in a composite scapula model. *Bull Hosp Jt Dis (2013).* 2018;76(2):116-122.

82. Stroud N, DiPaola MJ, Flurin PH, Roche CP. Reverse shoulder glenoid loosening: an evaluation of the initial fixation associated

with six different reverse shoulder designs. *Bull Hosp Jt Dis (2013)*. 2013;71(suppl 2):S12-S17.

83. Stroud NJ, DiPaola MJ, Martin BL, et al. Initial glenoid fixation using two different reverse shoulder designs with an equivalent center of rotation in a low-density and high-density bone substitute. *J Shoulder Elbow Surg*. 2013;22(11):1573-1579. doi:10.1016/j.jse.2013.01.037

84. Clark JC, Ritchie J, Song FS, et al. Complication rates, dislocation, pain, and postoperative range of motion after reverse shoulder arthroplasty in patients with and without repair of the subscapularis. *J Shoulder Elbow Surg*. 2012;21(1):36-41. doi:10.1016/j.jse.2011.04.009

85. Friedman RJ, Flurin PH, Wright TW, Zuckerman JD, Roche CP. Comparison of reverse total shoulder arthroplasty outcomes with and without subscapularis repair. *J Shoulder Elbow Surg*. 2017;26(4):662-668. doi:10.1016/j.jse.2016.09.027

86. Gallo RA, Gamradt SC, Mattern CJ, et al. Instability after reverse total shoulder replacement. *J Shoulder Elbow Surg*. 2011;20(4):584-590. doi:10.1016/j.jse.2010.08.028

87. Kennon JC, Lu C, McGee-Lawrence ME, Crosby LA. Scapula fracture incidence in reverse total shoulder arthroplasty using screws above or below metaglene central cage: clinical and biomechanical outcomes. *J Shoulder Elbow Surg*. 2017;26(6):1023-1030. doi:10.1016/j.jse.2016.10.018

88. King JJ, Dalton SS, Gulotta LV, Wright TW, Schoch BS. How common are acromial and scapular spine fractures after reverse shoulder arthroplasty?: a systematic review. *Bone Joint J*. 2019;101-B(6):627-634. doi:10.1302/0301-620X.101B6.BJJ-2018-1187.R1

89. Neyton L, Erickson J, Ascione F, Bugelli G, Lunini E, Walch G. Grammont Award 2018: scapular fractures in reverse shoulder arthroplasty (Grammont style). Prevalence, functional, and radiographic results with minimum 5-year follow up. *J Shoulder Elbow Surg*. 2019;28(2):260-267. doi:10.1016/j.jse.2018.07.004

90. Routman HD, Simovitch RW, Wright TW, Flurin PH, Zuckerman JD, Roche CP. Acromial and scapular fractures after reverse total shoulder arthroplasty with a medialized glenoid and lateralized humeral implant: an analysis of outcomes and risk factors. *J Bone Joint Surg Am*. 2020;102(19):1724-1733. doi:10.2106/JBJS.19.00724.

91. Zumstein MA, Pinedo M, Old J, Boileau P. Problems, complications, reoperations, and revisions in reverse total shoulder arthroplasty: a systematic review. *J Shoulder Elbow Surg*. 2011;20(1):146-157. doi:10.1016/j.jse.2010.08.001

92. Boileau P, Moineau G, Roussanne Y, O'Shea K. Bony increased-offset reversed shoulder arthroplasty: minimizing scapular impingement while maximizing glenoid fixation. *Clin Orthop Relat Res*. 2011;469(9):2558-2567. doi:10.1007/s11999-011-1775-4

93. Harman M, Frankle M, Vasey M, Banks S. Initial glenoid component fixation in "reverse" total shoulder arthroplasty: a biomechanical evaluation. *J Shoulder Elbow Surg*. 2005;14(1 suppl S):162S-167S.

94. Levy JC, Anderson C, Samson A. Classification of postoperative acromial fractures following reverse shoulder arthroplasty. *J Bone Joint Surg Am*. 2013;95(15):e104. doi:10.2106/JBJS.K.01516

95. Levy JC, Blum S. Postoperative acromion base fracture resulting in subsequent instability of reverse shoulder replacement. *J Shoulder Elbow Surg*. 2012;21(4):e14-e18. doi:10.1016/j.jse.2011.09.018

96. Levy JC, Virani N, Pupello D, Frankle M. Use of the reverse shoulder prosthesis for the treatment of failed hemiarthroplasty in patients with glenohumeral arthritis and rotator cuff deficiency. *J Bone Joint Surg Br*. 2007;89(2):189-195.

97. Crosby LA, Wright TW, Yu S, Zuckerman JD. Conversion to reverse total shoulder arthroplasty with and without humeral stem retention: the role of a convertible-platform stem. *J Bone Joint Surg Am*. 2017;99(9):736-742. doi:10.2106/JBJS.16.00683

98. Werthel JD, Walch G, Vegehan E, Deransart P, Sanchez-Sotelo J, Valenti P. Lateralization in reverse shoulder arthroplasty: a descriptive analysis of different implants in current practice. *Int Orthop*. 2019;43(10):2349-2360.doi:10.1007/s00264-019-04365-3

99. Edwards TB, Williams MD, Labriola JE, Elkousy HA, Gartsman GM, O'Connor DP. Subscapularis insufficiency and the risk of shoulder dislocation after reverse shoulder arthroplasty. *J Shoulder Elbow Surg*. 2009;18(6):892-896. doi:10.1016/j.jse.2008.12.013

100. Routman HD. The role of subscapularis repair in reverse total shoulder arthroplasty. *Bull Hosp Jt Dis (2013)*. 2013;71(suppl 2):108-112.

101. Hansen ML, Nayak A, Narayanan MS, et al. Role of subscapularis repair on muscle force requirements with reverse shoulder arthroplasty. *Bull Hosp Jt Dis (2013)*. 2015;73(suppl 1):S21-S27.

102. Boileau P, Chuinard C, Roussanne Y, Bicknell RT, Rochet N, Trojani C. Reverse shoulder arthroplasty combined with a modified latissimus dorsi and teres major tendon transfer for shoulder pseudoparalysis associated with dropping arm. *Clin Orthop Relat Res*. 2008;466(3):584-593. doi:10.1007/s11999-008-0114-x

103. Boileau P, Rumian AP, Zumstein MA. Reversed shoulder arthroplasty with modified L'Episcopo for combined loss of active elevation and external rotation. *J Shoulder Elbow Surg*. 2010;19(2 suppl):20-30. doi:10.1016/j.jse.2009.12.011

104. Elhassan BT, Wagner ER, Werthel JD, Lehanneur M, Lee J. Outcome of reverse shoulder arthroplasty with pedicled pectoralis transfer in patients with deltoid paralysis. *J Shoulder Elbow Surg*. 2018;27(1):96-103. doi:10.1016/j.jse.2017.07.007

105. Gerber C, Pennington SD, Lingenfelter EJ, Sukthankar A. Reverse Delta-III total shoulder replacement combined with latissimus dorsi transfer. A preliminary report. *J Bone Joint Surg Am*. 2007;89(5):940-947.

106. Grey SG. Combined latissimus dorsi and teres major tendon transfers for external rotation deficiency in reverse shoulder arthroplasty. *Bull Hosp Jt Dis (2013)*. 2013;71(suppl 2):82-87.

107. Bateman E, Donald SM. Reconstruction of massive uncontained glenoid defects using a combined autograft-allograft construct with reverse shoulder arthroplasty: preliminary results. *J Shoulder Elbow Surg*. 2012;21(7):925-934. doi:10.1016/j.jse.2011.07.009

108. Melis B, Bonnevialle N, Neyton L, et al. Glenoid loosening and failure in anatomical total shoulder arthroplasty: is revision with a reverse shoulder arthroplasty a reliable option? *J Shoulder Elbow Surg*. 2012;21(3):342-349. doi:10.1016/j.jse.2011.05.021

109. Boileau P, Walch G. The three-dimensional geometry of the proximal humerus. Implications for surgical technique and prosthetic design. *J Bone Joint Surg Br*. 1997;79(5):857-865.

110. Hertel R, Knothe U, Ballmer FT. Geometry of the proximal humerus and implications for prosthetic design. *J Shoulder Elbow Surg*. 2002;11(4):331-338.

111. Iannotti JP, Gabriel JP, Schneck SL, Evans BG, Misra S. The normal glenohumeral relationships. An anatomical study of one hundred and forty shoulders. *J Bone Joint Surg Am*. 1992;74(4):491-500.

112. Pearl ML, Kurutz S. Geometric analysis of commonly used prosthetic systems for proximal humeral replacement. *J Bone Joint Surg Am*. 1999;81(5):660-671.

113. Pearl ML, Volk AG. Coronal plane geometry of the proximal humerus relevant to prosthetic arthroplasty. *J Shoulder Elbow Surg*. 1996;5(4):320-326.

114. Jones RB, Wright TW, Roche CP. Bone grafting the glenoid versus use of augmented glenoid baseplates with reverse shoulder arthroplasty. *Bull Hosp Jt Dis (2013)*. 2015;73(suppl 1):S129-S135.

115. Sabesan VJ, Lima DJL, Yang Y, Stankard MC, Drummond M, Liou WW. The role of greater tuberosity healing in reverse shoulder arthroplasty: a finite element analysis. *J Shoulder Elbow Surg*. 2020;29(2):347-354. doi:10.1016/j.jse.2019.07.022

116. Mau EM, Roche CP, Zuckerman JD. Effects of body mass index on outcomes in total shoulder arthroplasty. *Bull Hosp Jt Dis (2013)*. 2015;73(suppl 1):S99-S106.

117. Nam D, Kepler CK, Nho SJ, Craig EV, Warren RF, Wright TM. Observations on retrieved humeral polyethylene components from reverse total shoulder arthroplasty. *J Shoulder Elbow Surg*. 2010;19(7):1003-1012. doi:10.1016/j.jse.2010.05.014

118. Chae J, Siljander M, Wiater JM. Instability in reverse total shoulder arthroplasty. *J Am Acad Orthop Surg*. 2018;26(17):587-596. doi:10.5435/JAAOS-D-16-00408

119. Wong MT, Langohr GDG, Athwal GS, Johnson JA. Implant positioning in reverse shoulder arthroplasty has an impact on acromial stresses. *J Shoulder Elbow Surg*. 2016;25(11):1889-1895. doi:10.1016/j.jse.2016.04.011

120. Ascione F, Kilian CM, Laughlin MS, et al. Increased scapular spine fractures after reverse shoulder arthroplasty with a humeral onlay short stem: an analysis of 485 consecutive cases. *J Shoulder Elbow Surg.* 2018;27(12):2183-2190. doi:10.1016/j.jse.2018.06.007

121. Farshad M, Gerber C. Reverse total shoulder arthroplasty-from the most to the least common complication. *Int Orthop.* 2010;34(8):1075-1082. doi:10.1007/s00264-010-1125-2

122. Crosby LA, Hamilton A, Twiss T. Scapula fractures after reverse total shoulder arthroplasty: classification and treatment. *Clin Orthop Relat Res.* 2011;469:2544-2549.

123. Otto RJ, Virani NA, Levy JC, Nigro PT, Cuff DJ, Frankle MA. Scapular fractures after reverse shoulder arthroplasty: evaluation of risk factors and the reliability of a proposed classification. *J Shoulder Elbow Surg.* 2013;22(11):1514-1521. doi:10.1016/j.jse.2013.02.007

124. Verstraete M, Conditt MA, Parsons IM, et al. Assessment of intraoperative joint loads and mobility in reverse total shoulder arthroplasty through a humeral trial sensor. *Semin Arthroplasty: JSES.* 2020;30(1):2-12. doi:10.1053/j.sart.2020.03.001.

125. Kumar V, Roche C, Overman S, et al. What is the accuracy of three different machine learning techniques to predict clinical outcomes after shoulder arthroplasty? *Clin Orthop Relat Res.* 2020;478(10):2351-2363. doi:10.1097/CORR.0000000000001263

126. Werthel JD, Schoch BS, Van Veen SC, et al. Acromial fractures in reverse shoulder arthroplasty: a clinical and radiographic analysis. *J Shoulder Elbow Arthroplast.* 2018;2:1-9. doi:10.1177/2471549218777628

127. Taylor SA, Shah SS, Chen X, et al. Scapular ring preservation: coracoacromial ligament transection increases scapular spine strains following reverse total shoulder arthroplasty. *J Bone Joint Surg Am.* 2020;102(15):1358-1364. doi:10.2106/JBJS.19.01118

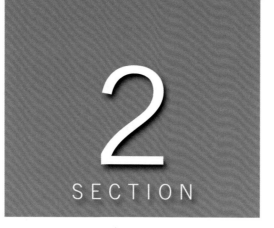

SECTION 2

Preoperative Considerations

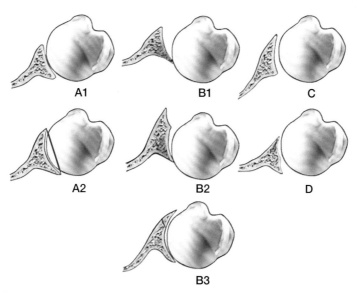

Modified Walch classification

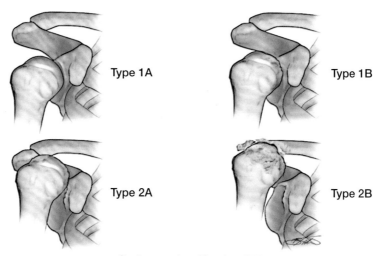

Seebauer classification CTA

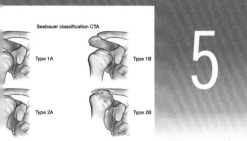

Seebauer classification CTA
Type 1A Type 1B
Type 2A Type 2B

5

The Spectrum of Glenohumeral Arthritis

Tyler A. Luthringer, MD and Joseph D. Zuckerman, MD

INTRODUCTION

The term "glenohumeral arthritis" encompasses a spectrum of degenerative conditions with a multitude of etiologies and characteristic presentations. Due to the variation in underlying pathology and patient functional demands, the management of glenohumeral arthritis requires an individualized approach. The use of shoulder arthroplasty for advanced glenohumeral arthritis has become commonplace in orthopedic surgery, and its evolution has paralleled our expanding appreciation for the range of presentations and contributing etiologies. For each type of glenohumeral arthritis, the orthopedic surgeon must consider the clinical, radiographic, and systemic manifestations when formulating a treatment approach in order to optimize patient function following shoulder arthroplasty.

The general indications for shoulder arthroplasty are similar to those for prosthetic replacement of other joints. Appropriate surgical candidates typically have severe shoulder pain and significant restrictions in range of motion that compromise their activities of daily living. Occasionally, individuals may present with minimal or no pain despite advanced radiographic disease and poor physical function. This often reflects a near-complete reliance on the opposite upper extremity for daily functioning. The history, physical examination, and initial radiographic assessment will generally be sufficient to determine the underlying etiology (or etiologies) of glenohumeral arthritis for the majority of patients. Advanced imaging and laboratory studies may infrequently be required to confirm a specific diagnosis in certain cases. Careful assessment of bony anatomy, quality of the surrounding soft tissues, and any systemic manifestations of disease are integral components of the clinical evaluation of all patients with glenohumeral arthritis.

In this chapter, we will review the different types of glenohumeral arthritis with respect to their clinical and radiographic characteristics and the general indications and contraindications for shoulder arthroplasty. Detailed discussion regarding the specific indications and contraindications for particular types of glenohumeral arthritis is provided in *Chapter 7*.

GENERAL CONSIDERATIONS

Bony Anatomy

Radiographs of the involved shoulder provide the basis for an evaluation of the bony anatomy. A complete radiographic assessment consists of four standard views: a true anteroposterior (AP) of the glenohumeral joint with internal and external rotation of the proximal humerus, scapular Y, and axillary view. The bony structures should be evaluated for "quantity, quality, and deformity." Bone *quantity* refers to the degree of bone loss that may be present as a result of inflammatory, degenerative, or traumatic processes. This most commonly applies to the humeral head and glenoid, but the acromion, distal clavicle, and coracoid may be affected as well. Bone *quality* refers to the structure of the available bone. The presence of both osteopenia and sclerosis should be noted, as each may present distinctly different challenges. Bone *deformity* is especially important in the posttraumatic patient and those with end-stage degenerative disease. In patients with a history of trauma, the greater and lesser tuberosities should be scrutinized for malunion, nonunion, and displacement. Similarly, any deformity of the humeral head and its relationship with the proximal humeral shaft must be considered when planning to insert a stemmed humeral prosthesis.

The added value of computed tomography (CT) for the evaluation of bone loss and deformity cannot be overstated. This is especially true for the glenoid. Both CT and three-dimensional (3D) CT reconstructions are particularly effective in understanding pathoanatomy, for the assessment of glenoid wear, scapular and glenoid vault morphology, as well as humeral head alignment and subluxation. This information is essential for preoperative planning and is discussed in detail in *Chapter 6*.

Soft Tissues

Assessment of the soft tissues is imperative when treating patients with glenohumeral arthritis. The degree of attainable motion and postoperative function following shoulder arthroplasty is largely dependent upon the integrity of the rotator cuff and deltoid muscles, as well as the overall balance of the shoulder's dynamic stabilizers. Muscle denervation and nerve injury must also be considered, as this too will influence surgical decision-making. History of trauma, prior surgery, and the type of glenohumeral arthritis each impact the status of the surrounding soft tissues, warranting preoperative attention and intraoperative preparedness for an array of technical challenges.

Magnetic resonance imaging (MRI) is particularly valuable for the assessment of concomitant rotator cuff pathology, which has implications for surgical planning, implant selection, and alignment of patient expectations regarding postoperative range of motion. In addition to evaluating for partial and complete rotator cuff tears, both MRI and CT can be used to determine the quality of remaining rotator cuff tissue.[1] The location and extent of rotator cuff fatty infiltration has been associated with specific patterns of glenoid wear, underscoring the interplay of bony and soft-tissue anatomy on the development of glenohumeral arthritis.[2]

Associated Conditions

Associated degenerative problems of the affected upper extremity require detailed assessment during the preoperative period. Foresight is particularly prudent in patients with polyarticular inflammatory arthritis who have ipsilateral elbow, wrist, and hand involvement; these issues may require staging of surgical procedures.[3] Intervening on hand and wrist pathology prior to shoulder reconstruction may optimize overall function and ease surgical recovery. Patients using antibiologic medications for inflammatory conditions are likely to require a regimen holiday during the perioperative window to minimize risks of infection and delayed wound healing.[4] Careful coordination among the patient, surgeon, rheumatologist, and all relevant medical providers is necessary to optimize the patient's biologic environment for surgery while continuing to mitigate the symptoms of ongoing systemic disease throughout the initial postoperative recovery.

Associated degenerative problems of the lower extremities, as well as the dependence on assistive devices for ambulation, must also be considered. Load bearing on assistive walking devices after shoulder arthroplasty may prematurely stress implant fixation or subscapularis repair, increasing the risk of early postoperative complications.[5,6] A patient with advanced glenohumeral arthritis who is also in need of a total hip or knee arthroplasty should completely recover from the lower extremity operation before shoulder arthroplasty is performed. It is our preference to wait at least 3 months and preferably closer to 6 months after shoulder arthroplasty before allowing the use of assistive devices for ambulation. Some individuals may require ambulatory aids for baseline function, independent of coexisting lower extremity conditions. The patient's care team should implement preventative measures such as preoperative rehabilitation for adaptive gait training with the goal of using the assistive device in the nonoperative extremity postoperatively until the patient has sufficiently recovered and can resume use of the operative extremity. Modifications to the home environment may also be necessary along with a plan for assistance at home.

PRIMARY OSTEOARTHRITIS

Primary osteoarthritis (OA) of the glenohumeral joint is degeneration of the humeral head and/or glenoid articular surfaces in the absence of an identifiable etiology or predisposing factor. It is characterized by the irreversible, progressive loss of articular cartilage with a hypertrophic reaction of subchondral bone. Though typically considered a monoarticular problem, it is not uncommon to have one or two major joints involved. Challenges in determining the early diagnosis, the timing of onset, and the absence of longitudinal data make estimates of the prevalence and incidence of OA imprecise. Nonetheless, primary OA has been the most common indication for shoulder arthroplasty in the United States for the past decade.[7,8] The cause of OA remains unknown but is classically attributed to "wear and tear." Age is considered the greatest risk factor for the development of primary glenohumeral OA.[9,10] Similar to other joints, additional contributors to OA development may include patient-specific factors (gender, nutrition, race, and ethnicity), intrinsic joint vulnerabilities, and the influence of environmental loading conditions.

Patients affected with primary glenohumeral OA tend to present older than 60 years. Women were initially thought to be more commonly affected than men, though recent data suggest the rate of primary glenohumeral OA is approximately equal between genders.[11-13] Pain with range of motion (as opposed to at rest), stiffness, and crepitus are common presenting complaints. Examination typically reveals equal loss of passive and active motion; anterior capsular contracture is commonly encountered and manifests as a significant loss of external rotation. Strength is usually maintained, as rotator cuff function is generally unaffected in primary glenohumeral OA. Although the rate of full-thickness rotator cuff tears associated with primary OA is considered to be less than 10%, the incidence of high-grade partial tears may be as high as 40%.[14-16]

Radiographically, the bone of the humeral head and glenoid appears sclerotic with extensive osteophyte formation **(FIGURE 5.1)**. Humeral head cartilage erosion predominates anteriorly, which eventually gives way to an aspherical (flattened) humeral head with an enlarged diameter.[17,18] Inferior osteophytes along the anatomic neck of the humerus give rise to the classic "goat's beard" appearance—the length of which may correlate

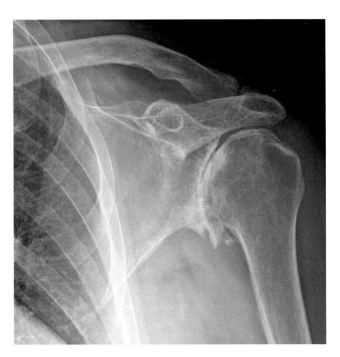

FIGURE 5.1 Anteroposterior (AP) radiograph of the left shoulder of a 64-year-old man with primary glenohumeral osteoarthritis showing humeral head flattening and osteophyte formation.

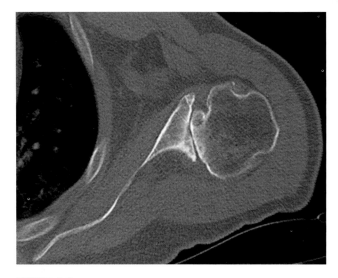

FIGURE 5.2 Axial computed tomographic (CT) image of the left shoulder demonstrating posterior glenoid erosion and humeral head subluxation in a 64-year-old man with primary glenohumeral osteoarthritis.

with the extent of humeral head deformity and glenoid erosion.[18] Generally, the osteoarthritic glenoid becomes flattened, enlarged, and increasingly retroverted due to asymmetric posterior wear **(FIGURE 5.2)**.[19-21] Walch et al originally classified glenoid morphology in glenohumeral OA on the basis of humeral head subluxation and glenoid retroversion.[22] The pathologic progression of glenoid deformity is complex and multifactorial and is discussed in *Chapter 6*.

INFLAMMATORY ARTHRITIS

Inflammatory arthritis describes a group of systemic conditions in which the body's joints and surrounding soft tissues are attacked by an overreactive immune system response. The etiology of the destructive inflammatory pathway can be spontaneous and autoimmune in nature as seen in rheumatoid arthritis (RA) and psoriatic arthritis. Alternatively, pathophysiologic processes such as crystalline deposition or recurrent hemarthrosis may cultivate a pernicious inflammatory response. Unlike the monoarticular presentation of primary OA that results from progressive joint "wear and tear," inflammatory arthropathies are generally characterized by symmetric polyarticular disease. Numerous forms of inflammatory arthritis can often be differentiated by their associated systemic manifestations, many of which require special perioperative attention and medical comanagement if shoulder arthroplasty is to be considered. The classic and most common form of inflammatory arthritis is RA.

Rheumatoid Arthritis

RA is a chronic systemic inflammatory disorder of unclear etiology characterized by a progressively debilitating, erosive, symmetrical polyarthritis. The estimated prevalence is 1% worldwide, with a female-to-male ratio of 3 to 5:1 that diminishes with age.[23] Prevalence increases starting in the third decade of life, and the disease affects more than 5% of the population older than 70 years.[24] Shoulder involvement remains a common finding in patients with long-standing RA (>5-year duration).[25] The incidence of end-stage shoulder RA has decreased considerably with the advent and improvement of antibiologic medication. The disease process is triggered by exposure of a genetically susceptible host to an arthritogenic antigen resulting in a breakdown of immunological self-tolerance and a chronic inflammatory reaction.[23] Acute arthritis is initiated in this manner. Ongoing autoimmune reaction, CD4+ helper T cell activation, and local release of inflammatory mediators and cytokines ultimately destroy the joint. Microvascular injury, synovial cell proliferation, and perivascular lymphocytosis result in the formation of an erosive, hyperplastic synovium (pannus) that grows over the articular surface. Immune complex deposition, complement activation, and production of cartilage matrix metalloproteinases cause proteoglycan and collagen degradation at the joint surface. The release of proinflammatory cytokines results in continued cartilage damage and increased osteoclast activity. This process yields bone erosion and soft-tissue degradation that frequently involves the insertion of the rotator cuff.[23]

The initial presentation of RA is highly variable; however, greater than 90% of patients report generalized symptoms of fatigue, musculoskeletal pain, variable fever, and weight loss.[24,25] During the initial phases of disease, the clinical course may be characterized by quiescence during periods of remission. Early involvement typically affects the small joints of the hand and foot, while larger joints are affected later. Rheumatoid involvement of the shoulder may present with an insidious onset of pain, swelling, and progressive loss of motion reflective of both articular and periarticular involvement. Unlike other joints involved, glenohumeral RA commonly contributes to nocturnal symptoms. All synovial joints around the shoulder may be affected, including the glenohumeral, acromioclavicular, and sternoclavicular articulations. Seventy-five percent of RA patients eventually develop rotator cuff pathology, with 20% to 50% developing full-thickness tears.[26,27] Findings on shoulder examination include those related to inflammation: tenderness, often diffuse but occasionally localized to the joint line; cutaneous warmth compared to surrounding areas; and variable swelling either due to glenohumeral effusion, or more often subacromial and subdeltoid fluid accumulation in the presence of a full-thickness rotator cuff tear. Erythema is not a typical symptom. Atrophy of the shoulder musculature due to rotator cuff pathology and/or disuse is usually present, though may be difficult to recognize due to generalized swelling or effusion. Active motion is typically compromised first, followed by both active and passive motion limitations. This can lead to fixed contractures in all three important planes of motion. Signs and symptoms of systemic involvement should also be noted in both the history and physical examination.

Laine has classified the progression of RA of the glenohumeral joint into three stages based on clinical and radiographic findings.[28] Stage I is characterized clinically by slight limitation of shoulder motion with mild to moderate pain, tenderness to palpation, and variable crepitation on range of motion; radiographs reveal only generalized osteopenia. Stage II describes moderate limitation of motion with crepitus and moderate to severe pain. Radiographic findings include osteopenia, erosive bony changes, and joint space narrowing. In stage III, severe functional deficits are present; range of motion is painful and limits activities of daily living. Radiographs show advanced erosive changes of both the humeral head and glenoid.[28]

The nature of radiographic lesions in glenohumeral RA vary considerably based on the duration and extent of disease, as well as the quality of medical management. Radiographic hallmarks of the disease include joint effusion, juxta-articular osteopenia with marginal erosions and cyst formation, concentric joint space narrowing with medialization of the glenohumeral joint line, and a lack of osteophyte formation (**FIGURE 5.3**). A decreased acromiohumeral interval is frequently present due to rotator cuff tear compromise, and acromioclavicular (synovial) joint destruction is also commonly present.

Numerous radiographic classifications of RA have been suggested in addition to that previously mentioned by Laine.[28] The most widely used system by Larsen et al describes six radiographic stages of RA (0-5) defined by the severity of the osteoarticular lesions and joint space narrowing; however, this method was not specifically designed for glenohumeral disease.[29] Specific to the shoulder, the four-stage classification by Walch et al describes earlier stages of rheumatoid involvement and provides prognostic information, where type C is the turning point beyond which destruction of the glenohumeral joint (type D) occurs inevitably within several months to 2 years.[30] The three-pattern scheme based on the sphericity of the humeral head and the upward migration of the humeral head in relation to the glenoid described by Lévigne and Franceschi (**FIGURE 5.4**) completes Walch's classification after the development of glenohumeral joint space loss.[31] The ascending form is the most common, which is encountered predominantly in older patients with rotator cuff lesions and leads to asymmetric wear of the superior portion of the glenoid with eventual pseudoarticulation between the humeral head and acromion (**FIGURE 5.5A**). In the centered form, rotator cuff tears are relatively rare and disease progression is slow; concentric glenoid erosion occurs medially (**FIGURE 5.5B**). In the destructive form, haphazardly distributed lesions of the joint surfaces lead to extensive erosions or "arthritis mutilans" (**FIGURE 5.5C**).

MRI is useful to determine the extent of joint effusion, synovial proliferation, pannus formation, bone and cartilage lesions, and rotator cuff pathology. It is particularly valuable for the evaluation of shoulder weakness and pain, not fully explained by bony changes visible on standard radiographs.[32] In addition to the assessment of glenoid erosion, CT allows for the characterization of humeral head defects that are not as easily detected on x-ray (**FIGURE 5.6**).[33]

Crystalline Arthropathy

Crystalline arthropathy may represent gout, pseudogout, or hydroxyapatite deposition disease ("Milwaukee shoulder syndrome") and is uncommon about the glenohumeral joint. Gout is characterized by hyperuricemia and resultant precipitation of monosodium urate crystals into joints and surrounding soft tissues. Lower temperatures facilitate monosodium urate crystal formation, causing gout to primarily manifest in small peripheral joints—shoulder involvement is only encountered with advanced, uncontrolled disease.[23] Gout has a strong predisposition toward men (20:1) and is the most common inflammatory arthropathy in males older than 40 years.[34] Pseudogout is also known as calcium pyrophosphate dihydrate (CPPD) deposition disease or chondrocalcinosis. Half as common as gout, it is characterized by CPPD crystal deposition into fibrocartilage

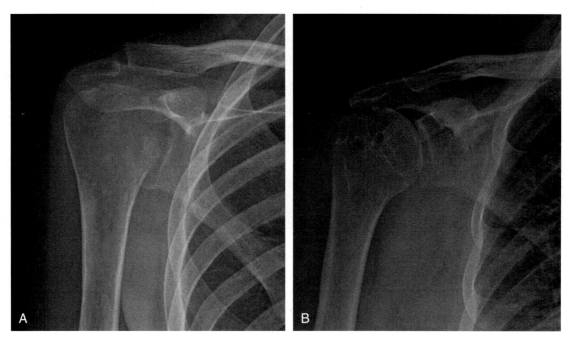

FIGURE 5.3 A, Anteroposterior (AP) radiograph of the right shoulder of a 39-year-old woman with rheumatoid arthritis showing generalized osteopenia, humeral head erosion, and superior migration. **B**, AP radiograph of the right shoulder of a 46-year-old woman with rheumatoid arthritis showing large areas of marginal erosions and humeral head cysts.

and hyaline cartilage via unclear mechanisms. There is no associated metabolic disturbance or gender predisposition.[23] The shoulder is the third most commonly involved joint after the knee and wrist.[23]

Intra-articular accumulation of both monosodium urate and CPPD crystals incite a common synovial inflammatory response in which chemotactic factors are released and propagated by polymorphonuclear phagocytosis.[23] Following repeated acute attacks, synovial hyperplasia and pannus formation can ensue—this perpetuates underlying cartilage damage, juxta-articular bone erosion, and joint destruction. Hydroxyapatite crystals do not incite the same degree of synovial response as seen in the other forms of crystalline arthropathy.[35] There has been some disagreement as to whether "Milwaukee shoulder syndrome" and rotator cuff arthropathy (RCA) represent the same or different disease entities. As Milwaukee shoulder and CTA have a unique clinical presentation that differs from gout and pseudogout, this entity will be discussed further in the subsequent section on CTA.

End-stage crystalline arthropathy is generally found in patients older than 70 years, with men more commonly affected than women. The degree of bony involvement as well as soft-tissue involvement is variable, ranging from the appearance of a mild inflammatory arthritis to one of extensive soft-tissue and bone destruction. Radiographically, late stages of disease may appear indistinguishable either from primary OA or RA. Chondrocalcinosis is often visible but is nonspecific, while gouty tophi are generally rare about the shoulder. Juxta-articular osteopenia and sharply outlined erosions, punched out with sclerotic margins, are classic x-ray findings **(FIGURE 5.7)**.

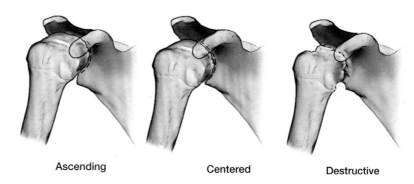

Ascending   Centered   Destructive

FIGURE 5.4 Three patterns of humeral head involvement in rheumatoid arthritis distinguished by Lévigne and Franceschi. (Adapted with permission from Levigne C, Franceschi J. Rheumatoid shoulder. Radiographic forms and results of shoulder arthroplasty. About 50 cases. In: Walch G, Boileau P, eds. *Shoulder Arthroplasty.* Springer; 1999:221-232.)

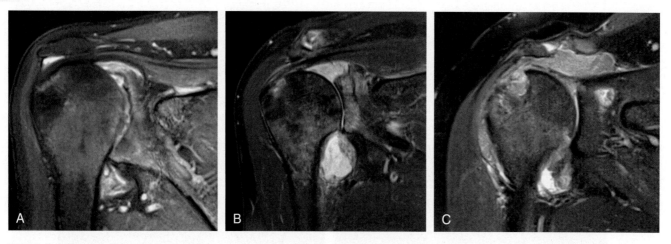

FIGURE 5.5 Coronal T2 magnetic resonance images (MRIs) demonstrating three patterns of erosion in glenohumeral rheumatoid arthritis described by Lévigne and Franceschi.[31] **A,** Upward migration in a 39-year-old woman. **B,** Concentric in a 53-year-old woman. **C,** Destructive in a 46-year-old woman. (Used with permission from Levigne C, Franceschi J. Rheumatoid shoulder. Radiographic forms and results of shoulder arthroplasty. About 50 cases. In: Walch G, Boileau P, eds. *Shoulder Arthroplasty.* Springer; 1999:221-232.)

Hemophiliac Arthropathy

Hemophiliac arthropathy is a rare form of inflammatory arthropathy that is primarily encountered in patients with hemophilia A (factor VIII deficiency) and hemophilia B (factor IX deficiency). von Willebrand disease and other factor deficiencies have also been implicated but are much less common. Hemophilia is classified as mild, moderate, or severe based on the clotting activity level. Spontaneous bleeding episodes are frequent in patients with severe disease, while those with mild deficiencies only experience bleeding episodes after trauma, surgery, or dental procedures. Greater than 60% of spontaneous bleeding events occur in joints, of which the shoulder is the fourth most common site.[36] The reported incidence of shoulder arthropathy among hemophiliacs ranges from 11% to 37% and increases with age and severity of the disease.[37-39] Men are much more commonly affected than women due to the sex-linked recessive nature of the disease. In hemophiliac arthropathy, hemosiderin deposition from recurrent hemarthroses leads to a chronic cycle of inflammatory synovitis and synovial hypertrophy.[40] Progressive cartilage destruction from synovial invasion and enzymatic degradation results in bony erosions, soft-tissue deterioration, and end-stage arthropathy over time.[40,41]

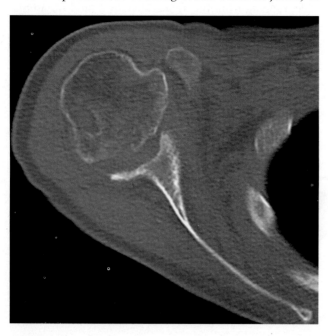

FIGURE 5.6 Axial computed tomographic (CT) image of the right shoulder demonstrating significant medial erosion and glenoid bone loss in a 39-year-old woman with rheumatoid arthritis.

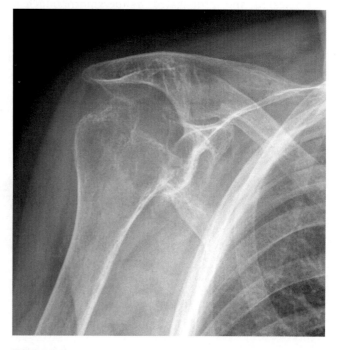

FIGURE 5.7 Anteroposterior (AP) radiograph of the right shoulder of a 79-year-old woman with crystalline arthropathy. The inflammatory component has resulted in significant humeral head erosion.

Contrary to the juvenile onset of lower extremity involvement (ie, ankle, knee), hemarthrosis and chronic synovitis of the shoulder typically occurs in adulthood. Nonetheless, hemophiliac arthropathy of the shoulder can result in intractable pain and severe functional impairment, with progression to end-stage disease by the fourth or fifth decade.[42] Age, lack of prophylactic therapy, and higher frequency of crutch use (typically from lower extremity involvement) are the most significant risk factors associated with recurrent shoulder bleeds.[39] Muscle atrophy and loss of motion occur early, often before the patient is aware of a significant problem. Impaired elbow motion can make the loss of shoulder function even more consequential. Oftentimes, early rehabilitation efforts may be thwarted by recurrent hemorrhage despite appropriate factor replacement therapy. Progression to end-stage arthropathy and arthrofibrosis requires many years but is the usual course, particularly in those with moderate to severe disease.[41] Concomitant soft-tissue pathology such as tendonitis of long head of the biceps and rotator cuff tears are common (up to 50% of patients with shoulder symptoms) but may be difficult to assess secondary to generalized pain on physical examination.[38,39] Clinical presentation correlates well with findings on imaging studies.[39]

Radiographically, hemophiliac arthropathy can appear similar to RA. A spectrum of changes may be seen beginning with mild subchondral irregularity and cyst formation progressing to osteopenia, joint space narrowing, marginal erosion, osseous deformity, and thinning of the glenoid **(FIGURE 5.8)**.[37] The Modified Arnold-Hilgartner arthropathy classification describes the general radiographic progression of hemophiliac arthropathy, though it is not specific to the shoulder.[43] Aside from rotator cuff assessment, MRI and ultrasonography are useful to gauge the extent of synovial hypertrophy and hyperemia, joint effusion, and articular cartilage change in the early phases of disease.[44] If arthroplasty is to be considered in this population, careful consideration must be given to intraoperative bleeding, transfusion requirements, and factor replacement.

ROTATOR CUFF TEAR ARTHROPATHY

Rotator cuff tear arthropathy (CTA) is best considered a pathologic endpoint characterized by progressive glenohumeral arthritis with clearly discernible morphological features resulting from a massive defect of the rotator cuff. While the concept of CTA has been acknowledged since the 17th century, the clinical entity was not defined until the description by Neer et al in 1977.[45] The cascade of events that precipitates CTA remains a topic of debate. Rheumatologists have supported an inflammatory-mediated degradation process and the pathogenic role of hydroxyapatite crystals, initially described in the CTA-like presentation of "Milwaukee shoulder syndrome" in

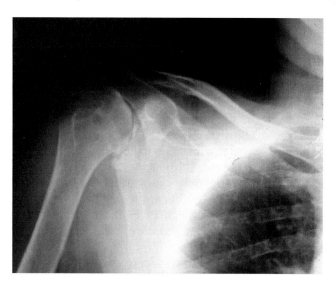

FIGURE 5.8 Anteroposterior (AP) radiograph of the right shoulder of a 46-year-old man with hemophiliac arthropathy.

1981.[46-48] In contrast, Neer postulated that both nutritional and mechanical factors play a role in its development.[45] He theorized that massive cuff tears lead to shoulder disuse, leakage of synovial fluid, and instability of the humeral head, resulting in articular cartilage attrition and osteoporosis of the subchondral bone.[45] It is likely that the cause of CTA is a combination of these theories.[49] While the incidence of CTA is difficult to determine, the natural history of nonoperatively treated, massive cuff tears has been shown to result in significant progression of glenohumeral arthritis, rotator cuff fatty infiltration, and tear size progression over the course of several years.[50,51]

Patients presenting with CTA are predominantly women in their seventh decade or older. The dominant upper extremity is more commonly affected, though bilateral shoulder involvement is sometimes seen.[52] Complaints frequently include a prolonged period of progressive pain with associated functional limitations (ie, inability to reach overhead or behind one's back). Night pain and a history of corticosteroid injections are also common, as in most patients with rotator cuff tears and arthritis. Systemic symptoms may be present in patients with CTA in association with RA or other inflammatory conditions. Weakness and loss of both active and passive motion worsen as the pathology progresses, becoming a hallmark finding of the physical examination attributable to the profound atrophy or loss of the rotator cuff.[45] Absence of the rotator cuff tendons yields significant instability via the compromised posterior mechanism, resulting in anterosuperior subluxation of the humeral head that is both palpable and visible. Fluid accumulation within the subacromial bursa may result in the classic "fluid sign," which yields blood-tinged fluid upon attempted aspiration. Synovial fluid analysis may reveal hemorrhagic stained fluid with calcium hydroxyapatite crystals that are only visible by electron microscopy or alizarin red S staining due to their size.[53] The loss of integrity of the glenohumeral joint also results in upward migration of the humerus, leading to secondary erosive changes of the underside of the acromion, the acromioclavicular joint, and the glenoid.

Standard radiographs are typically sufficient to confirm the diagnosis of CTA (**FIGURE 5.9**). Three prior radiographic classifications have graded the bony changes that develop throughout the progression of CTA. While overlapping characteristics are mutually considered, each highlights a different subset of associated findings. The Seebauer classification focuses on the degree of superior migration and the amount of instability from the center of rotation (**FIGURE 5.10**).[54] The Hamada classification system characterizes structural changes within the coracoacromial arch (**FIGURE 5.11**).[51,55] The Favard classification describes glenoid bone loss (**FIGURE 5.12**).[56] Generally, bone quality is osteopenic with variable osteophyte formation. An acromiohumeral interval of less than 7 mm is typically noted though is not considered diagnostic.[52,57] Sclerosis of the inferior acromion ("sourcil sign") may precede bony erosion. In severe presentations, acromial stress fractures have also been described.[57] Later stages of disease are also characterized by humeral head collapse, extensive subchondral cyst formation, and significant (often superior) glenoid erosion. In addition to the presence of a massive rotator cuff tear, Neer described the heralding characteristics of advanced CTA: superior migration and femoralization of the proximal humerus, collapse of the proximal aspect of the humeral articular surface, and undersurface erosion with eventual acetabularization of the acromion.[45] Advanced imaging may be beneficial in surgical planning, particularly to assess the extent of glenoid deformity and to delineate the extent of rotator cuff involvement (particularly that of the subscapularis) in patients who are difficult to examine due to disabling pain (**FIGURE 5.13**).

OSTEONECROSIS

Osteonecrosis (ON) is the in situ death of segment of bone—both osteocytes and marrow contents. Second to only the hip, the humeral head is the next most common site for ON to occur.[58,59] ON, also termed "avascular necrosis" or "aseptic necrosis," is best categorized as either posttraumatic or atraumatic. Both posttraumatic and atraumatic ON share the common pathway of disrupted vascular supply to the humeral head, resulting in subchondral bone death; however, underlying pathogenesis and patient presentation differentiate the two types. Posttraumatic ON is best considered a macrovascular disturbance to the main blood supply humeral head, 64% and 36% of which comes from the posterior and anterior humeral circumflex arteries, respectively.[60] The incidence of posttraumatic ON is mutually influenced by injury severity and management. In the setting of fracture sequelae, humeral head collapse from ON is often but a single component of the greater presentation of posttraumatic glenohumeral arthritis and will therefore be discussed in the next section. The remainder of section will focus atraumatic ON.

Atraumatic ON can occur in association with a number of predisposing conditions. Associated risk factors include corticosteroid therapy, alcoholism, smoking, hemoglobinopathies, lysosomal storage disorders, dysbarism, lipid metabolism disorders, connective tissue disorders—notably systemic lupus erythematosus, HIV, and cytotoxic drugs including chemotherapy and irradiation. Classically, corticosteroid therapy has been the most common reported cause of atraumatic ON; however, the incidence has decreased from approximately 25% to 5% secondary to increased awareness and adjustments in dosing.[61,62] Compared to the mechanical macrovasculature disruption that is associated with posttraumatic ON, the multifactorial pathogenesis of

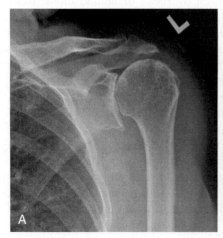
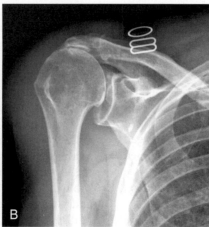
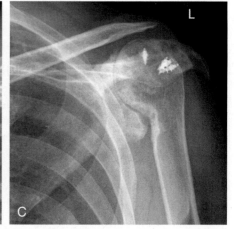

FIGURE 5.9 Series of anteroposterior (AP) radiographs demonstrating the progression of rotator cuff arthropathy in a (**A**) 76-year-old woman, (**B**) 68-year-old woman, and (**C**) 80-year-old man.

Seebauer classification CTA

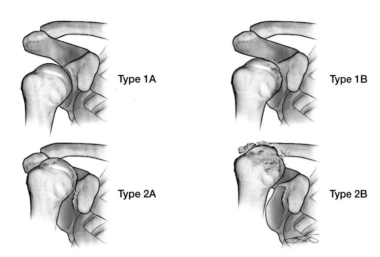

FIGURE 5.10 Seebauer classification of rotator cuff tear arthropathy (CTA). (Adapted with permission from Visotsky JL, Basamania C, Seebauer L, et al. Cuff tear arthropathy: pathogenesis, classification, and algorithm for treatment. *J Bone Joint Surg Am.* 2004;86-A(suppl 2):35-40.)

atraumatic ON occurs at the microvascular level due to thrombosis, embolic phenomena, increased intraosseous pressure, or some combination of the three.[61,63] There are presentations of atraumatic ON in which a predisposing condition cannot be identified. In these uncommon situations, the ON would be considered idiopathic.

Atraumatic ON of the humeral head is generally encountered in younger patients compared to those with primary OA.[64] Multiple joint involvement (frequently of the hips) may be present secondary to the possible systemic nature of the predisposing condition.[58]

Hamada classification CTA

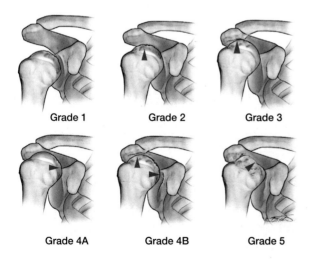

FIGURE 5.11 Hamada classification of rotator cuff tear arthropathy (CTA). Grade 1: AHI ≥ 6 mm. Grade 2: AHI ≤ 5 mm (arrow). Grade 3: AHI ≤ 5 mm with acetabularization (arrow). Grade 4A: glenohumeral arthritis (arrow) without acetabularization. Grade 4B: glenohumeral arthritis (arrow) with acetabularization (arrow). Grade 5: includes humeral head collapse (arrow). (Adapted with permission from Hamada K, Fukuda H, Mikasa M, Kobayashi Y. Roentgenographic findings in massive rotator cuff tears. A long-term observation. *Clin Orthop Relat Res.* 1990;254:92-96.)

Nonoperative management is often successful in limiting symptoms and maintaining function but is dependent on the adequate treatment of the associated condition or the feasibility of risk factor modification. Insidious shoulder pain with movement is the typical presentation. Mechanical symptoms, such as a painful click from joint incongruity, a cartilage flap, or a loose body, may also been described later in the process. Physical examination may reveal local tenderness, but active and passive motion is typically preserved until the later stages of disease. Active range of motion is compromised first secondary to pain. As secondary degenerative arthritis develops, capsular contracture becomes a common finding.

Radiographically, ON progresses through five stages as outlined by the Cruess classification system,[59] which is based on the Ficat-Arlet classification of ON of the femoral head.[65] In the first stage, ON is not visible on standard radiographs but can be detected on MRI as early subchondral edema with sensitivity approaching 100%.[66,67] Sclerosis on the superior middle portion of the humeral head that precedes collapse is usually the initial detectable sign on x-ray **(FIGURE 5.14A)**. Subchondral fracture follows and the appearance of the crescent sign heralds the onset of humeral head collapse. Initially, this may be limited to a relatively small area. Over time, progression to extensive humeral head collapse results in deformity, joint incongruity, and secondary arthritic change of both the humeral head and glenoid, often producing a picture more typical of OA **(FIGURE 5.14B)**.

POSTTRAUMATIC ARTHRITIS

In the broadest sense, posttraumatic arthritis (PTA) of the shoulder is the progressive degeneration of the glenohumeral articular surfaces incited by a significant traumatic event. Posttraumatic shoulder arthritis is most commonly encountered in association with fractures of

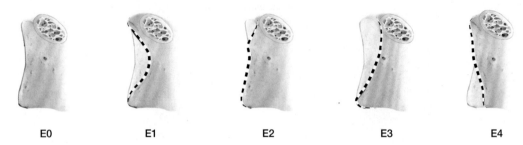

E0   E1   E2   E3   E4

FIGURE 5.12 Favard classification of glenoid bone loss in rotator cuff tear arthropathy (CTA). (Adapted with permission from Sirveaux F, Favard L, Oudet D, et al. Grammont inverted total shoulder arthroplasty in the treatment of glenohumeral osteoarthritis with massive rupture of the cuff. *J Bone Joint Surg Br.* 2004;86-B:388-395.)

the proximal humerus and can manifest following both nonoperative and operative initial management efforts. Fractures of the glenoid, proximal humerus fracture-dislocations, chronic glenohumeral dislocations, and recurrent instability may also lead to the development of PTA. The incidence of glenohumeral PTA varies widely depending on the nature and severity of the initial trauma, the time elapsed since the injury, and the efficacy and success of the index treatment. A 64% rate of PTA within 3 years has been reported among patients with displaced three- and four-part proximal humerus fractures treated nonoperatively or with internal fixation.[68] The pathology that contributes to the development of PTA is often multifactorial and constitutes its own spectrum. Potential factors include, but are not limited to, the extent of initial chondrocyte injury, joint incongruity from malunion, joint instability from surrounding soft-tissue injuries, disrupted vascular supply, intra-articular fibrosis, and the presence of malpositioned or migrated hardware. For surgical considerations and management guidelines, proximal humerus fracture sequelae may be grouped into two main categories according to the classification by Boileau et al: intracapsular, impacted fracture sequelae that require no tuberosity osteotomy and

extracapsular, disimpacted fracture sequelae that necessitate an osteotomy of the greater tuberosity.[69]

Patient presentation is often complex. Compared to primary OA, patients with PTA of the shoulder tend to be slightly younger with a mild predominance of females.[64,70] Physical examination should note the presence of prior incisions and assess for evidence of underlying infection and preexisting nerve injury. Strength and motion examination should specifically assess for internal and external rotation lag signs, which may be due to either rotator cuff attrition or tuberosity malunion/nonunion. The management of PTA presents unique challenges not encountered with primary OA. Many patients with mild disability may be managed nonoperatively with physical therapy, activity modification, and anti-inflammatory medications. Others, however, require significant surgical intervention to restore meaningful shoulder function. Whether the sequelae of the initial injury or prior surgery, numerous bone and soft-tissue abnormalities often need to be addressed to offer best chance of a satisfactory outcome following shoulder arthroplasty. Soft-tissue contracture, adhesions, obliteration of normal tissue planes, rotator cuff insufficiency, malunion, nonunion, heterotopic ossification, bone

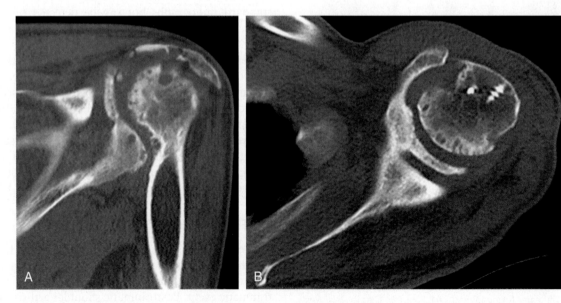

FIGURE 5.13 A, Coronal and (**B**) axial computed tomographic (CT) images of the left shoulder of an 80-year-old man with severe rotator cuff tear arthropathy.

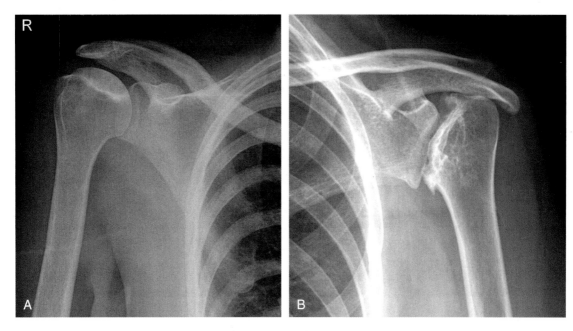

FIGURE 5.14 A, Anteroposterior (AP) radiograph of the right shoulder of a 57-year-old woman with sickle cell anemia demonstrating early (stage 2) osteonecrosis of the humeral head. B, AP radiograph of the left shoulder of a 41-year-old woman on long-term prednisone therapy for sarcoidosis demonstrating stage 4 osteonecrosis with complete humeral head collapse and secondary glenoid changes.

deficiency, nerve injury, and reflex sympathetic dystrophy are but some of the challenges that may be encountered. Active or indolent infection must also be ruled out in those who have previously undergone surgery.

Radiographs, CT, and MRI may all prove useful in the workup of PTA, each of which should be scrutinized for the potential associated pathology. Metal artifact reduction sequences may improve visualization on advanced imaging studies when hardware is present. Bone quality is usually sclerotic, and there may be significant collapse of the humeral head if there is associated ON (FIGURE 5.15).[59] Other common radiographic features include malunion of the greater and lesser tuberosities and articular segment, as well as malalignment of the proximal humerus and shaft. Glenoid morphology is variable based upon the degree of proximal humeral deformity and the duration of the problem. Fatty infiltration of the rotator cuff may be significant and should be considered an important factor in preoperative planning.

INSTABILITY-ASSOCIATED GLENOHUMERAL ARTHRITIS

Dislocation arthropathy describes the development of progressive degenerative changes of the glenohumeral articulation in the setting of shoulder instability (defined as at least one dislocation event, with or without surgical intervention). The term "dislocation arthropathy" was formally described by Samilson and Prieto in 1983, after Neer at al reported on a subset of patients with glenohumeral arthritis who had a history of shoulder instability or prior stabilization procedure.[26,71] Capsulorrhaphy arthropathy more specifically describes the development of glenohumeral arthritis as a complication of a prior

glenohumeral instability repair secondary to (1) overtightening the anterior capsule and/or (2) prominent suture anchors, staples, screws, or transferred coracoid bone that causes damage to the humeral head articular cartilage.[72] Associated trauma from a single dislocation,[73] repetitive injury from recurrent instability,[74] postsurgical alterations in shoulder biomechanics,[75-84] and complications of shoulder stabilization procedures have all been implicated in the development of dislocation arthropathy.[84-86] Thus, a specific etiology of joint degeneration and associated risk factors for its progression is

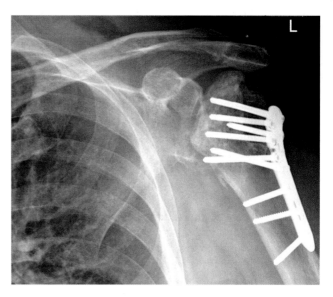

FIGURE 5.15 Anteroposterior (AP) radiograph of the left shoulder of a 64-year-old man with posttraumatic arthritis and osteonecrosis 32 months after open reduction and internal fixation of a proximal humerus fracture-dislocation.

difficult to define due to the heterogeneity of reported presentations. Older age at the time of initial dislocation and/or surgery is one of the most consistent risk factors for the development of dislocation arthropathy.[82,87] Bony injuries of the glenoid and humeral head impaction fractures can play a significant role in the development of future arthrosis,[87] though the contribution will depend on the size and location of the defect as well as the propensity to cause recurrent instability or a locked dislocation. While prior surgery has been considered the most important risk factor for the development of dislocation or capsulorrhaphy arthropathy, the associated risk is highly variable and dependent upon the appropriateness of the procedure performed.[75,76,78-83,87] By far, the most common etiology of dislocation or capsulorrhaphy arthropathy is when patients suffering from multidirectional instability undergo a "standard" operation for presumed unidirectional instability. The incidence of dislocation arthropathy, particularly in those who have not had stabilization procedures, is especially challenging to predict given the majority of shoulder dislocations occur in younger patients. Furthermore, the duration of time between the initial instability and presentation for arthropathy makes it difficult to control for interim events.

Instability-associated glenohumeral arthritis is generally encountered in a slightly younger, predominantly male population, representative of the group at highest risk of recurrent glenohumeral instability.[64,88] Presentation is highly variable. Individuals with capsulorrhaphy arthropathy due to a hardware complication (malpositioned or prominent) are more likely to present in an accelerated fashion than those with a fixed posterior subluxation from overtightened anterior structures. During the history and physical examination, particular attention should focus on the number of prior dislocations, direction of dislocation (if known), age at the time of initial dislocation, and any prior surgical interventions. Pain and restricted motion are the most common presenting complaints. Active and passive motion should be assessed with grading of rotator cuff strength, particularly of the subscapularis in patients who have previously undergone open surgery. Loss of motion may be due to a number of factors, including arthritic change and osteophyte formation, capsular contracture, posterior humeral head subluxation, and excessive tightening of the anterior capsule or subscapularis shortening.[86] Severe internal rotation contracture may indicate posterior glenoid wear, retroversion, and bone loss. In patients who have had previous surgery, careful attention should be paid to any evidence of infection, prior surgical incisions, neurologic status, and presence or absence of the coracoid. The anatomy encountered at the time of a secondary surgery may be significantly altered for a variety of reasons, necessitating careful dissection and attention to preoperative imaging.

Radiographically, dislocation arthropathy shares many features with primary OA; glenohumeral joint space narrowing, osteophyte and cyst formation, subchondral sclerosis, and posterior glenoid wear are all common findings in dislocation arthropathy. It should be noted that the presence of radiographic changes does not necessarily correlate with symptoms or assessment of function in many patients.[74] Samilson and Prieto described a radiographic classification of postdislocation glenohumeral arthropathy in 1983, which was later modified by Buscayret et al[71,87]; the progression of this classification is based on the diameter of the inferior humeral and glenoid osteophyte exostosis (stages 1-3) as well as joint space obliteration (stage 4). In addition, an AP internal rotation or Stryker notch view may reveal the presence of a Hill-Sachs impression fracture. Staples or screws from prior surgical procedures should be noted, and in some instances may be malpositioned or have migrated, contributing to secondary articular degradation (**FIGURE 5.16**). The axillary radiograph should be assessed for humeral head subluxation. In capsulorrhaphy arthropathy, tightening of the anterior capsule can result in posterior displacement of the humeral head, resulting in severe B2 or B3 glenoid wear patterns.[89-91] The anterior glenoid can simultaneously be worn from prior recurrent dislocations or posterior stabilization procedures, resulting in anterior humeral head subluxation.[92] Conversely, the anterior glenoid may have been previously reconstructed following a Latarjet, Bristow, or distal tibia allograft procedure. CT, particularly with 3D reconstruction, may be particularly helpful in detailing the osseous anatomy of the native glenoid and vault in these scenarios when arthroplasty is a consideration. In cases of mild to moderate arthropathy or earlier presentations, noncontrast MRI can be useful to assess the degree of cartilage loss in addition to evaluating for concurrent rotator cuff pathology.

POSTARTHROSCOPIC GLENOHUMERAL CHONDROLYSIS

Chondrolysis is the death of chondrocytes from apoptosis or the inability to produce and maintain cartilage matrix. It differs from primary OA in its rate of development (occurring over a period of months vs years) and the typical age of the affected population (young vs older). Postarthroscopic glenohumeral chondrolysis (PAGCL) is a rare complication in younger patients in which the articular cartilage undergoes rapid, irreversible degeneration after shoulder arthroscopy. Typically, PAGCL affects the entire cartilaginous surface of the glenohumeral joint rather than a localized area. The etiology of PAGCL is likely multifactorial, as numerous risk factors have been implicated in its development. The most frequently cited factors include direct surgical insults to cartilage, the use of thermal devices, prominence of anchor implants and knots on the articular surface, exposure

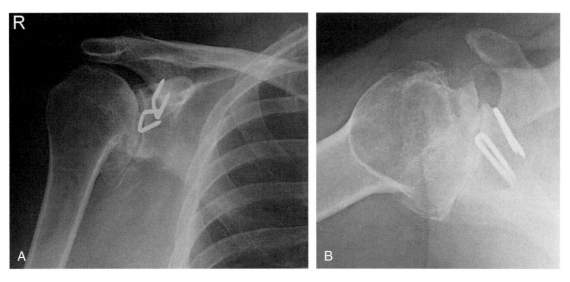

FIGURE 5.16 A, Anteroposterior (AP) and (**B**) axillary radiographs of the right shoulder of a 64-year-old man with dislocation arthropathy.

to harmful irrigation solutions, or high concentrations of local anesthetics (particularly intra-articular bupivacaine).[93-95] The incidence of PAGCL is rare, with only 91 shoulders identified as case reports in a 2009 systematic review. Awareness of the associated risk factors and appreciation of the disastrous effects of PAGCL in these younger patients should help to minimize this complication in the future.

For unclear reasons, PAGCL seems to occur most often in adolescents or those in their 20s, with a median age of 27 years (range 13-64) among reported cases.[93,96-99] The most frequent diagnoses for which the initial arthroscopy was performed are instability (32%) and superior labrum from anterior to posterior (SLAP) tears (23%),[93] though chondrolysis has also been seen following capsular release for adhesive capsulitis.[100] Relevant nonmodifiable risk factors that should be identified in the history include a family history of early arthritis, known arthritis conditions (particularly inflammatory), collagen disorders, or other synovial-based processes that may degrade hyaline cartilage.[93] Patients with PAGCL tend to present within weeks to 5 months after the offending procedure. Onset is characteristically marked by unexpected progressive pain both at rest and with activity, crepitus, and loss of active motion secondary to pain.[99] Often the pain is considered to be out of proportion to that expected in the normal postoperative period and is usually exacerbated at end range of motion. Immobilization may act to delay symptomatic manifestation.

Radiographic changes include joint-space narrowing on the true AP (Grashey) view, periarticular bone erosion, subchondral cysts, and a characteristic lack of osteophytosis (**FIGURE 5.17**). MRI is usually indicated and very helpful for confirmation of the diagnosis. Findings include diffuse loss of articular cartilage on both the humeral head and glenoid, cortical irregularity,

and patchy areas of altered signal intensity consistent with subchondral sclerosis and bone marrow edema.[97]

NEUROPATHIC ARTHROPATHY

Neuropathy arthropathy (NA) of the shoulder is a rare presentation defined as a chronic, progressive glenohumeral joint destruction that results from a neurosensory deficit due to an underlying neurologic condition.[101,102] Diabetes, syphilis (tabes dorsalis), and syringomyelia are the clinical entities most commonly associated with NA. Leprosy, spinal dysraphism, congenital insensitivity to pain, and numerous other disorders are also associated with the condition, although much less commonly. Syringomyelia is the most frequent cause of upper extremity presentations and accounts for almost 80% of all neuropathic shoulders.[103] Syringomyelia is a generic term for a condition in which a cyst or cavity (syrinx) forms within the spinal cord. It can be congenital (Arnold-Chiari malformation) or may arise as the result of malignancy, trauma, infection, vascular abnormalities, or degeneration.[104,105] With the condition, the decussating fibers of the lateral spinothalamic tract are the first structures damaged by the enlarging syrinx. This leads to abnormal innervation and *dissociative anesthesia* of the glenohumeral joint, in which motor function and proprioception are preserved in the absence of protective pain and temperature sensation.[106,107] Syrinx enlargement results in subsequent damage to the dorsal column and anterior horn cells, yielding a loss of proprioception, areflexia, muscle weakness, and atrophy.[106,108] Joint destruction ensues at a variable rate depending on a combination of patient and environmental factors.

The pathogenesis of NA has been a topic of debate since Charcot's first description in 1868. Currently, the most widely accepted etiology is that NA results from a combination of two prevailing theories: the

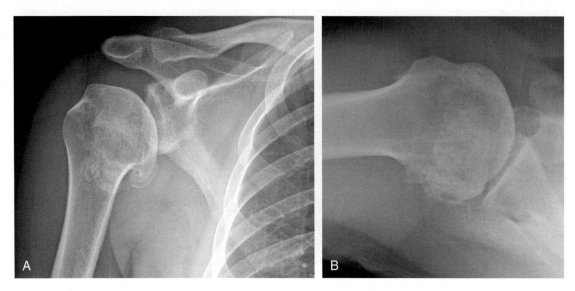

FIGURE 5.17 A, Anteroposterior (AP) and (**B**) axillary radiographs of a 28-year-old man with secondary glenohumeral arthritis due to postarthroscopic glenohumeral chondrolysis (PAGCL) following intra-articular pain pump use and laser capsulorrhaphy.

neurovascular and the neurotraumatic.[102,109] The neurovascular theory postulates that neurologic changes produced by an underlying medical disorder create a hypervascular region in the subchondral bone characterized by increased osteoclastic resorption and osteoporosis.[109] This leads to pathologic microfractures and eventual subchondral collapse, followed by joint destruction. The neurotraumatic theory postulates that a joint with abnormal sensory innervation, if unprotected, will undergo rapid destruction as a result of recurrent, unnoticed microtrauma secondary to the loss of somatic muscle reflexes and protective proprioception.[110] While the basis of the neurotraumatic theory has been supported both in an animal model and by clinical study,[111,112] the neurovascular theory has not been supported by histological evidence.[101,113] In all likelihood, NA is caused by some combination of these two mechanisms. Regardless of the etiology, the resultant inflammation is essential to the pathophysiology of NA, which can be simplified to a state of increased osteoclastogenesis with impaired mechanisms of bone remodeling and repair.[114-116] The neuropathic joint generally progresses through three distinct phases.[117] The first is the destructive phase, characterized by hyperemia, swelling, and osteoclastic resorption associated with repetitive trauma. The reparative phase follows with the formation of dense fibrous tissue within the joint, as well as osteophytosis, myositis ossifications, and the coalescence of bony and cartilaginous debris. The final, quiescent phase is characterized by decreased vascularity, stabilization of the periarticular reaction, and significant osseous sclerosis.

The average age of presentation for neuropathic arthropathy of the shoulder is 49 years.[103] It is nearly twice as common among men than it is in women.[103] A history of recognized trauma is only reported in

approximately 25% of cases; the remainder of patients tend to present later, often with more advanced disease.[103] Recognition of NA by the orthopedic surgeon is of utmost importance, as nearly 70% of cases present initially for shoulder-related complaints without a known underlying neurologic condition.[103] Bilateral shoulder involvement is rare, accounting for only 10% of reported presentations.[118-120] Patients typically complain of generalized discomfort and swelling about the shoulder region associated with gradual limitations of motion and progressive weakness. Neurosensory complaints in the ipsilateral upper extremity are also common. Findings on physical examination vary by the severity of joint degeneration at the time of presentation. Early in the course, a large joint effusion is usually present. In later stages, swelling may subside, but the joint maintains a boggy quality. Swelling is often associated with mild erythema and warmth, which may warrant aspiration and culture to rule out septic arthritis. If significant fragmentation has occurred, osseous debris may be palpable in the superficial soft tissues. Muscle atrophy is typically present but may be difficult to appreciate. Active range of motion is typically affected to a much greater degree than passive motion, and joint instability becomes evident as the destructive process progresses. Neurologic examination may reveal asymmetric deep tendon reflexes and abnormal pain and temperature sensation. While examination typically provokes pain to a certain extent, it is generally less than what might be expected on the basis of radiographic findings.

Radiographically, NA of the shoulder can be classified as atrophic or hypertrophic.[118,121] Atrophic NA is characterized by extensive osteolysis and bone resorption, while hypertrophic NA is associated with findings of sclerosis, debris, osseous fragmentation, and substantial osteophytes **(FIGURE 5.18)**. In either pattern, joint destruction can result in subluxation or frank dislocation of the joint. Bilateral shoulder x-rays should be obtained due to the rare incidence of bilateral disease and the indolent nature of presentation. MRI may be obtained to evaluate the extent of effusion, soft-tissue inflammation, articular destruction, as well as associated pathology (ie, rotator cuff tears). It should be stressed that the identification and management of the underlying neurological etiology is paramount if the disease process is to be positively impacted. A cervical MRI or CT myelogram should be obtained to assess for the presence of syringomyelia **(FIGURE 5.19)**. Neurology consultation and a series of laboratory studies to assess for possible contributing conditions are necessary in patients who primarily present for the shoulder. Nonoperative management is generally considered the first-line of treatment in patients with NA. Operative intervention by means of shoulder arthrodesis or arthroplasty should only be considered in patients after treatment of their primary condition, who demonstrate little or no changes in glenohumeral joint destruction over a minimum of 1 year, and have reasonable expectations regarding the goals of surgical management (mainly pain control).

SEPTIC ARTHRITIS

Septic arthritis is a degenerative joint disease incited by bacterial infection. It is considered an orthopedic emergency due to associated morbidity from rapid cartilage and bone destruction as well as the potential for systemic spread of infection. Native glenohumeral joint septic arthritis is a relatively rare occurrence, accounting for only 5% to 12% of all cases of native joint septic arthritis.[122-125] However, septic arthritis

of the shoulder has historically been associated with poor prognosis and frequent sequelae, including recurrent effusion, drainage, joint subluxation, dislocation, and osteomyelitis.[126] Prompt diagnosis and treatment is critical to minimize morbidity and achieve satisfactory outcomes. If not treated urgently and appropriately, the release of bacterial endotoxins as well as cytokines and destructive enzymes from the host immune system may result in degradation and erosion of the articular cartilage.[127] This cascade culminates in irreversible damage to the joint surfaces and may spread to adjacent bone (ie, osteomyelitis).[128] The presentation of septic arthritis is typically classified as acute or chronic. Modes of introduction include direct inoculation (traumatic or iatrogenic), or more commonly, hematogenous seeding from a confirmed primary source of infection.[129] In native glenohumeral joint infection, the most common offending organisms are *Staphylococcus* (>60%) and *Streptococcus* species (10%-20%).[125,129] Conversely, *Cutibacterium acnes* (formerly *Propionibacterium acnes*) is the most common infectious organism in the setting of prior shoulder surgery.[130-133] The topic of periprosthetic joint infection is discussed in *Chapter 32*.

Although all ages can be affected, septic arthritis is a disease that usually arises in elderly people or very young children. Preexisting joint pathology (ie, rheumatoid arthritis, crystalline arthropathy, osteoarthritis, and other inflammatory conditions) can predispose to the development of joint sepsis, though quantification of this increased risk is hard to establish.[134] Adult patients who present with glenohumeral septic arthritis are typically "susceptible" individuals with at least one of several medical comorbidities. Conditions associated with increased risk include diabetes mellitus, intravenous drug use, alcoholism, hemodialysis, cutaneous

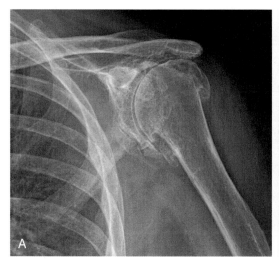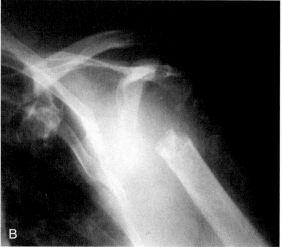

FIGURE 5.18 A, Anteroposterior (AP) radiograph of the left shoulder of a 65-year-old woman who developed bilateral hypertrophic neuropathic arthropathy secondary to syringomyelia. **B,** AP radiograph demonstrating atrophic neuropathic arthropathy.

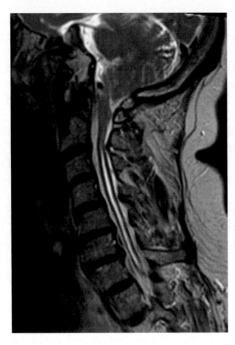

FIGURE 5.19 Sagittal T2 cervical magnetic resonance image (MRI) of a 65-year-old woman with syringomyelia and bilateral shoulder neuropathic arthropathy.

precede the manifestation of septic arthritis from hematogenous seeding.[136] Laboratory investigations should routinely include a complete blood count with differential, serum C-reactive protein, erythrocyte sedimentation rate, and blood cultures if systemic symptoms are present. Shoulder aspiration should be performed and synovial fluid sent for white blood cell count and differential, aerobic and anaerobic culture, and crystal examination.

Aside from evidence of an effusion and soft-tissue edema, radiographic findings in acute septic arthritis may be limited in the absence of preexisting degenerative joint disease. Late sequelae of septic arthritis include chronic progressive erosive changes that may resemble a late-stage inflammatory or a mixed pattern (inflammatory and primary osteoarthritis) of disease **(FIGURE 5.20)**. Advanced imaging modalities such as technetium bone scan, CT, and MRI can be used to assess the presence and extent of inflammation, destruction, and tissue response; however, they cannot accurately distinguish between infection and other causes of acute inflammatory arthritis.[134] MRI is helpful in evaluating for the presence of abscesses, sinus tracts, and coexisting osteomyelitis, the early stages of which can be recognized by increased signal intensity in the subchondral bone.[134,137]

Arthroplasty is strictly contraindicated in the setting of active infection. Initial management options for native shoulder septic arthritis include systemic antibiotics along with serial aspirations, arthroscopic irrigation and debridement (I&D), or arthrotomy I&D. Chronic sequelae of infection resulting in secondary joint degeneration may be considered for shoulder arthroplasty. In these cases, proper preoperative evaluation, intraoperative cultures, and pathology must confirm that infection has been eradicated prior to implantation of the prosthesis.

ulcerations or skin infections, and immunocompromised states.[125,129,134,135] Patients with septic arthritis of the glenohumeral joint usually present with warmth, effusion, cutaneous erythema, and painful restricted motion. Severity and duration of symptoms at the time of presentation may depend upon the virulence of the causative organism and the extent of preexisting degenerative joint disease. Symptoms related to systemic infection are less common than might be expected in the setting of primary septic arthritis from direct inoculation; conversely, fevers, chills, rigors, and sepsis may

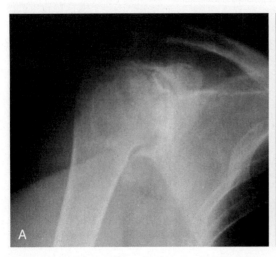
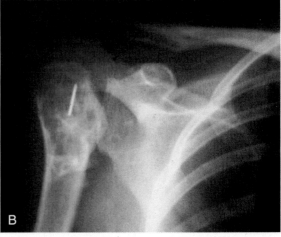

FIGURE 5.20 Anteroposterior (AP) radiographs of the right shoulder of two individuals demonstrating late sequelae of septic arthritis secondary to (**A**) tuberculosis and (**B**) failed open reduction and internal fixation (ORIF) requiring multiple procedures for debridement.

CONCLUSION

The goal of this chapter has been to provide a description of the many different types of degenerative conditions that can affect the glenohumeral joint. The vast majority can be considered indications for shoulder arthroplasty. In the chapters that follow, these conditions will be discussed in detail in conjunction with the specific shoulder arthroplasty techniques that can be used to provide effective treatment.

REFERENCES

1. Fuchs B, Weishaupt D, Zanetti M, Hodler J, Gerber C. Fatty degeneration of the muscles of the rotator cuff: assessment by computed tomography versus magnetic resonance imaging. *J Shoulder Elbow Surg.* 1999;8:599-605.
2. Donohue KW, Ricchetti ET, Ho JC, Iannotti JP. The association between rotator cuff muscle fatty infiltration and glenoid morphology in glenohumeral osteoarthritis. *J Bone Joint Surg Am.* 2018;100:381-387.
3. Friedman RJ, Ewald FC. Arthroplasty of the ipsilateral shoulder and elbow in patients who have rheumatoid arthritis. *J Bone Joint Surg Am.* 1987;69:661-666.
4. Goodman SM, Springer B, Guyatt G, et al. 2017 American College of Rheumatology/American Association of Hip and Knee Surgeons guideline for the perioperative management of antirheumatic medication in patients with rheumatic diseases undergoing elective total hip or total knee arthroplasty. *J Arthroplasty.* 2017;32:2628-2638.
5. Jordan RW, Sloan R, Saithna A. Should we avoid shoulder surgery in wheelchair users? A systematic review of outcomes and complications. *Orthop Traumatol Surg Res.* 2018;104:839-846.
6. Cuff DJ, Santoni BG. Reverse shoulder arthroplasty in the weight-bearing versus non–weight-bearing shoulder: mid-term outcomes with minimum 5-year follow-up. *Orthopedics.* 2018;41:e328-e333.
7. Kim SH, Wise BL, Zhang Y, Szabo RM. Increasing incidence of shoulder arthroplasty in the United States. *J Bone Joint Surg Am.* 2011;93:2249-2254.
8. Dillon MT, Ake CF, Burke MF, et al. The Kaiser Permanente shoulder arthroplasty registry. *Acta Orthop.* 2015;86:286-292.
9. Kobayashi T, Takagishi K, Shitara H, et al. Prevalence of and risk factors for shoulder osteoarthritis in Japanese middle-aged and elderly populations. *J Shoulder Elbow Surg.* 2014;23:613-619.
10. Oh JH, Chung SW, Oh CH, et al. The prevalence of shoulder osteoarthritis in the elderly Korean population: association with risk factors and function. *J Shoulder Elbow Surg.* 2011;20:756-763.
11. Schoenfeldt TL, Trenhaile S, Olson R. Glenohumeral osteoarthritis: frequency of underlying diagnoses and the role of arm dominance—a retrospective analysis in a community-based musculoskeletal practice. *Rheumatol Int.* 2018;38:1023-1029.
12. Harjula JNE, Paloneva J, Haapakoski J, et al. Increasing incidence of primary shoulder arthroplasty in Finland – A nationwide registry study. *BMC Muscoskel Disord.* 2018;19:245-252.
13. Yasuaki N, Hyakuna K, Otani S, Hashitani M, Nakamura T. Epidemiologic study of glenohumeral plain radiography. *J Shoulder Elbow Surg.* 1999;8:580-584.
14. Edwards TB, Boulahia A, Kempf JF, Boileau P, Nemoz C, Walch G. The influence of rotator cuff disease on the results of shoulder arthroplasty for primary osteoarthritis: results of a multicenter study. *J Bone Joint Surg Am.* 2002;84:2240-2248.
15. Norris TR, Iannotti JP. Functional outcome after shoulder arthroplasty for primary osteoarthritis: a multicenter study. *J Shoulder Elbow Surg.* 2002;11:130-135.
16. Choate WS, Shanley E, Washburn R, et al. The incidence and effect of fatty atrophy, positive tangent sign, and rotator cuff tears on outcomes after total shoulder arthroplasty. *J Shoulder Elbow Surg.* 2017;26:2110-2116.
17. Knowles NK, Carroll MJ, Keener JD, Ferreira LM, Athwal GS. A comparison of normal and osteoarthritic humeral head size and morphology. *J Shoulder Elbow Surg.* 2016;25:502-509.
18. Habermeyer P, Magosch P, Weiß C, et al. Classification of humeral head pathomorphology in primary osteoarthritis: a radiographic and in vivo photographic analysis. *J Shoulder Elbow Surg.* 2017;26:2193-2199.
19. Moineau G, Levigne C, Boileau P, Young A, Walch G; French Society for Shoulder & Elbow (SOFEC). Three-dimensional measurement method of arthritic glenoid cavity morphology: feasibility and reproducibility. *Orthop Traumatol Surg Res.* 2012;98:139-145.
20. Walch G, Mesiha M, Boileau P, et al. Three-dimensional assessment of the dimensions of the osteoarthritic glenoid. *Bone Joint J.* 2013;95-B:1377-1382.
21. Walker KE, Simcock XC, Jun BJ, Iannotti JP, Ricchetti ET. Progression of glenoid morphology in glenohumeral osteoarthritis. *J Bone Joint Surg Am.* 2018;100:49-56.
22. Walch G, Badet R, Boulahia A, Khoury A. Morphologic study of the glenoid in primary glenohumeral osteoarthritis. *J Arthroplasty.* 1999;14:756-760.
23. Rosenberg AE. Bones, joints, and soft-tissue tumors. In: Kumar V, Abbas AK, Fausto N, Aster JC, eds. *Robbins and Cotran Pathologic Basis of Disease.* 8th ed. Saunders; 2010:1205-1256.
24. Cuomo F, Greller MJ, Zuckerman JD. The rheumatoid shoulder. *Rheum Dis Clin North Am.* 1998;24:67-82.
25. Petersson CJ. Painful shoulders in patients with rheumatoid arthritis: prevalence, clinical and radiological features. *Scand J Rheumatol.* 1986;15:275-279.
26. Neer CS, Watson KC, Stanton FJ. Recent experience in total shoulder replacement. *J Bone Joint Surg Am.* 1982;64:319-337.
27. Thomas T, Noël E, Goupille P, Duquesnoy B, Combe B; GREP. The rheumatoid shoulder: current consensus on diagnosis and treatment. *Joint Bone Spine.* 2006;73:139-143.
28. Laine VAI, Vainio KJ, Pekanmaki K. Shoulder affections in rheumatoid arthritis. *Ann Rheum Dis.* 1954;13:157-160.
29. Larsen A, Dale K, Eek M. Radiographic evaluation of rheumatoid arthritis and related conditions by standard reference films. *Acta Radiol Diagn (Stockh).* 1977;18:481-491.
30. Walch G, Noel E, Guier C, et al. Rheumatoid arthritis of the shoulder: study of the clinical and radiographic evolution of 250 patients. In: Post M, Morey B, Hawkins R, eds. *Surgery of the Shoulder.* Mosby; 1990:267-269.
31. Levigne C, Franceschi J. Rheumatoid shoulder. Radiographic forms and results of shoulder arthroplasty. About 50 cases. In: Walch G, Boileau P, eds. *Shoulder Arthroplasty.* Springer; 1999:221-232.
32. Kieft GJ, Dijkmans BA, Bloem JL, Kroon HM. Magnetic resonance imaging of the shoulder in patients with rheumatoid arthritis. *Ann Rheum Dis.* 1990;49:7-11.
33. Albertsen M, Egund N, Jonsson E, Lidgren L. Assessment at CT of the rheumatoid shoulder with surgical correlation. *Acta Radiol.* 1994;35:164-168.
34. Roubenoff R. Gout and hyperuricemia. *Rheum Dis Clin North Am.* 1990;16:539-550.
35. Cawston TE, Dieppe PA, Mercer E, et al. Milwaukee shoulder—synovial fluid contains no active collagenase. *Rheumatology.* 1987;26:311-312.
36. Stephensen D, Tait R, Brodie N, et al. Changing patterns of bleeding in patients with severe haemophilia A. *Haemophilia.* 2009;15:1210-1214.
37. Cahlon O, Klepps S, Cleeman E, et al. A retrospective radiographic review of hemophilic shoulder arthropathy. *Clin Orthop Relat Res.* 2004;423:106-111.
38. MacDonald PB, Locht RC, Lindsay D, Levi C. Haemophilic arthropathy of the shoulder. *J Bone Joint Surg Br.* 1990;72:470-471.
39. Chen YC, Chen LC, Cheng SN, Pan RY, Chang ST, Li TY. Hemophilic arthropathy of shoulder joints. *J Bone Joint Surg Am.* 2013;95:e43-e48.
40. Stein H, Duthie R. The pathogenesis of chronic haemophilic arthropathy. *J Bone Joint Surg Br.* 1981;63B:601-609.

41. Luck JV, Silva M, Rodriguez-Merchan EC, Ghalambor N, Zahiri CA, Finn RS. Hemophilic arthropathy. *J Am Acad Orthop Surg.* 2004;12:234-245.

42. Wendt MC, Sperling JW, Cofield RH. Shoulder arthroplasty in hemophilic arthropathy. *J Shoulder Elbow Surg.* 2011;20:783-787.

43. Arnold W, Hilgartner M. Hemophilic arthropathy. Current concepts of pathogenesis and management. *J Bone Joint Surg Am.* 1977;59:287-305.

44. Hermann G, Gilbert MS, Abdelwahab IF. Hemophilia: evaluation of musculoskeletal involvement with CT, sonography, and MR imaging. *AJR Am J Roentgenol.* 1992;158:119.

45. Neer CS, Craig EV, Fukuda H. Cuff-tear arthropathy. *J Bone Joint Surg Am.* 1983;65:1232-1244.

46. Garancis JC, Cheung HS, Halverson PB, McCarty DJ. "Milwaukee shoulder"—association of microspheroids containing hydroxyapatite crystals, active collagenase, and neutral protease with rotator cuff defects. III. Morphologic and biochemical studies of an excised synovium showing chondromatosis. *Arthritis Rheum.* 1981;24:484-491.

47. McCarty DJ, Halverson PB, Carrera GF, Brewer BJ, Kozin F. "Milwaukee shoulder"—association of microspheroids containing hydroxyapatite crystals, active collagenase, and neutral protease with rotator cuff defects. I. Clinical aspects. *Arthritis Rheum.* 1981;24:464-473.

48. Halverson PB, Cheung HS, McCarty DJ, Garancis J, Mandel N. "Milwaukee shoulder"—association of microspheroids containing hydroxyapatite crystals, active collagenase, and neutral protease with rotator cuff defects. II. Synovial fluid studies. *Arthritis Rheum.* 1981;24:474-483.

49. Collins DN, Harryman DT. Arthroplasty for arthritis and rotator cuff deficiency. *Orthop Clin North Am.* 1997;28:225-239.

50. Zingg PO, Jost B, Sukthankar A, Buhler M, Pfirrmann CW, Gerber C. Clinical and structural outcomes of nonoperative management of massive rotator cuff tears. *J Bone Joint Surg Am.* 2007;89:1928-1934.

51. Hamada K, Fukuda H, Mikasa M, Kobayashi Y. Roentgenographic findings in massive rotator cuff tears. A long-term observation. *Clin Orthop Relat Res.* 1990;254:92-96.

52. Zeman CA, Arcand MA, Cantrell JS, Skedros JG, Burkhead WZ. The rotator cuff-deficient arthritic shoulder: diagnosis and surgical management. *J Am Acad Orthop Surg.* 1998;6:337-348.

53. Yamakawa K, Iwasaki H, Masuda I, et al. The utility of alizarin red s staining in calcium pyrophosphate dihydrate crystal deposition disease. *J Rheumatol.* 2003;30:1032-1035.

54. Visotsky JL, Basamania C, Seebauer L, et al. Cuff tear arthropathy: pathogenesis, classification, and algorithm for treatment. *J Bone Joint Surg Am.* 2004;86-A(suppl 2):35-40.

55. Hamada K, Yamanaka K, Uchiyama Y, Mikasa T, Mikasa M. A radiographic classification of massive rotator cuff tear arthritis. *Clin Orthop Relat Res.* 2011;469:2452-2460.

56. Sirveaux F, Favard L, Oudet D, Huquet D, Walch G, Molé D. Grammont inverted total shoulder arthroplasty in the treatment of glenohumeral osteoarthritis with massive rupture of the cuff. *J Bone Joint Surg Br.* 2004;86-B:388-395.

57. Frankle M, Siegal S, Pupello D, Saleem A, Mighell M, Vasey M. The reverse shoulder prosthesis for glenohumeral arthritis associated with severe rotator cuff deficiency: a minimum two-year follow-up study of sixty patients. *J Bone Joint Surg Am.* 2005;87:1697-1705.

58. Cruess RL. Corticosteroid-induced osteonecrosis of the humeral head. *Orthop Clin North Am.* 1985;16:789-796.

59. Cruess RL. Experience with steroid-induced avascular necrosis of the shoulder and etiologic considerations regarding osteonecrosis of the hip. *Clin Orthop Relat Res.* 1978;(130):86-93.

60. Hettrich CM, Boraiah S, Dyke JP, Neviaser A, Helfet DL, Lorich DG. Quantitative assessment of the vascularity of the proximal part of the humerus. *J Bone Joint Surg Am.* 2010;92:943-948.

61. Mankin HJ, Mankin HJ. Nontraumatic necrosis of bone (osteonecrosis). *N Engl J Med.* 1992;326:1473-1479.

62. Hattrup SJ, Cofield RH. Osteonecrosis of the humeral head: relationship of disease stage, extent, and cause to natural history. *J Shoulder Elbow Surg.* 1999;8:559-564.

63. Weinstein RS. Glucocorticoid-induced osteonecrosis. *Endocrine.* 2012;41:183-190.

64. Saltzman MD, Mercer DM, Warme WJ, Bertelsen AL, Matsen FA. Comparison of patients undergoing Primary shoulder arthroplasty before and after the age of fifty. *J Bone Joint Surg Am.* 2010;92:42-47.

65. Ficat R, Arlet T. Necrosis of the femoral head. In: Hungerford D, ed. *Ischemia Necrosis Bone.* Williams & Wilkins; 1980:171-182.

66. Coleman BG, Kressel HY, Dalinka MK, Scheibler ML, Burk DL, Cohen EK. Radiographically negative avascular necrosis: detection with MR imaging. *Radiology.* 1988;168:525-528.

67. Mitchell DG, Rao VM, Dalinka MK, et al. Femoral head avascular necrosis: correlation of MR imaging, radiographic staging, radionuclide imaging, and clinical findings. *Radiology.* 1987;162:709-715.

68. Zyto K, Kronberg M, Broström LA. Shoulder function after displaced fractures of the proximal humerus. *J Shoulder Elbow Surg.* 1995;4:331-336.

69. Boileau P, Trojani C, Walch G, Krishnan SG, Romeo A, Sinnerton R. Shoulder arthroplasty for the treatment of the sequelae of fractures of the proximal humerus. *J Shoulder Elbow Surg.* 2001;10:299-308.

70. Luthringer TA, Kester BS, Kolade O, et al. Shoulder arthroplasty for posttraumatic arthritis is associated with increased transfusions and longer operative times. *J Shoulder Elb Arthroplast.* 2019;3:1-8.

71. Samilson RL, Prieto V. Dislocation arthropathy of the shoulder. *J Bone Joint Surg Am.* 1983;65:456-460.

72. Matsen FI, Lippitt S, Rockwood CJ, Wirth M. Glenohumeral arthritis and its management. In: Rockwood CJ, Matsen FA, eds. *The Shoulder.* 5th ed. Elsevier; 2017:831-1042.

73. Norlin R. Intraarticular pathology in acute, first-time anterior shoulder dislocation: an arthroscopic study. *Arthroscopy.* 1993;9:546-549.

74. Hovelius L, Rahme H. Primary anterior dislocation of the shoulder: long-term prognosis at the age of 40 years or younger. *Knee Surg Sports Traumatol Arthrosc.* 2016;24:330-342.

75. Van Der Zwaag HM, Brand R, Obermann ER, Rozing PM. Glenohumeral osteoarthrosis after Putti-Platt repair. *J Shoulder Elbow Surg.* 1999;8:252-258.

76. Hawkins RJ, Angelo RL. Glenohumeral osteoarthrosis. A late complication of the Putti-Platt repair. *J Bone Joint Surg Am.* 1990;72:1193-1197.

77. Gill TJ, Zarins B. Open repairs for the treatment of anterior shoulder instability. *Am J Sports Med.* 2003;31:142-153.

78. Hovelius L, Sandström B, Saebö M. One hundred eighteen Bristow-Latarjet repairs for recurrent anterior dislocation of the shoulder prospectively followed for fifteen years: study II—the evolution of dislocation arthropathy. *J Shoulder Elbow Surg.* 2006;15:279-289.

79. Hovelius LK, Sandström B, Rösmark D, Saebö M, Sundgren KH, Malmqvist BG. Long-term results with the Bankart and Bristow-Latarjet procedures: recurrent shoulder instability and arthropathy. *J Shoulder Elbow Surg.* 2001;10:445-452.

80. Rachbauer F, Ogon M, Wimmer C, Sterzinger W, Huter B. Glenohumeral osteoarthrosis after the Eden-Hybbinette procedure. *Clin Orthop Relat Res.* 2000;373:135-140.

81. Elmlund AO, Ejerhed L, Sernert N, Rostgård LC, Kartus J. Dislocation arthropathy and drill hole appearance in a mid- to long-term follow-up study after arthroscopic Bankart repair. *Knee Surg Sports Traumatol Arthrosc.* 2012;20:2156-2162.

82. Plath JE, Aboalata M, Seppel G, et al. Prevalence of and risk factors for dislocation arthropathy radiological long-term outcome of arthroscopic Bankart repair in 100 shoulders at an average 13-year follow-up. *Am J Sports Med.* 2015;43:1084-1090.

83. Franceschi F, Papalia R, Buono AD, Vasta S, Maffulli N, Denaro V. Glenohumeral osteoarthritis after arthroscopic Bankart repair for anterior instability. *Am J Sports Med.* 2011;39:1653-1659.

84. Ahmad CS, Wang VM, Sugalski MT, Levine WN, Bigliani LU. Biomechanics of shoulder capsulorrhaphy procedures. *J Shoulder Elbow Surg.* 2005;14:12S-18S.

85. Zuckerman JD, Matsen FA. Complications about the glenohumeral joint related to the use of screws and staples. *J Bone Joint Surg Am.* 1984;66:175-180.

86. Wall MS, Warren RF. Complications of shoulder instability surgery. *Clin Sports Med.* 1995;14:973-1000.

87. Buscayret F, Edwards TB, Szabo I, et al. Glenohumeral arthrosis in anterior instability before and after surgical treatment: incidence and contributing factors. *Am J Sports Med.* 2004;32:1165-1172.

88. Robinson CM, Howes J, Murdoch H, Will E, Graham C. Functional outcome and risk of recurrent instability after primary traumatic anterior shoulder dislocation in young patients. *J Bone Joint Surg Am.* 2006;88:2326-2336.

89. Vezeridis PS, Ishmael CR, Jones KJ, Petrigliano FA. Glenohumeral dislocation arthropathy: etiology, diagnosis, and management. *J Am Acad Orthop Surg.* 2019;27:227-235.

90. Green A, Norris TR. Shoulder arthroplasty for advanced glenohumeral arthritis after anterior instability repair. *J Shoulder Elbow Surg.* 2001;10:539-545.

91. Bigliani LU, Weinstein DM, Glasgow MT, Pollock RG, Flatow EL. Glenohumeral arthroplasty for arthritis after instability surgery. *J Shoulder Elbow Surg.* 1995;4:87-94.

92. Brems JJ. Arthritis of dislocation. *Orthop Clin North Am.* 1998;29:453-466.

93. Solomon DJ, Navaie M, Stedje-Larsen ET, et al. Systematic review with video illustration glenohumeral chondrolysis after arthroscopy: a systematic review of potential contributors and causal pathways. *Arthroscopy.* 2009;25:1329-1342.

94. Yeh PC, Kharrazi DF. Postarthroscopic glenohumeral chondrolysis. *J Am Acad Orthop Surg.* 2012;20:102-112.

95. Busfield BT, Romero DM. Pain pump use after shoulder arthroscopy as a cause of glenohumeral chondrolysis. *Arthroscopy.* 2009;25:647-652.

96. Petty DH, Jazrawi LM, Estrada LS, Andrews JR. Glenohumeral chondrolysis after shoulder arthroscopy: case reports and review of the literature. *Am J Sports Med.* 2004;32:509-515.

97. Sanders TG, Zlatkin MB, Paruchuri NB, Higgins RW. Chondrolysis of the glenohumeral joint after arthroscopy: findings on radiography and low-field-strength MRI. *AJR Am J Roentgenol.* 2007;188:1094-1098.

98. Hardy JC, Hung M, Snow BJ, et al. Blood transfusion associated with shoulder arthroplasty. *J Shoulder Elbow Surg.* 2013;22:233-239.

99. Hansen BP, Beck CL, Beck EP, Townsley RW. Postarthroscopic glenohumeral chondrolysis. *Am J Sports Med.* 2007;35:1628-1634.

100. Jerosch J, Aldawoudy AM. Chondrolysis of the glenohumeral joint following arthroscopic capsular release for adhesive capsulitis: a case report. *Knee Surg Sports Traumatol Arthrosc.* 2007;15:292-294.

101. Alpert SW, Koval KJ, Zuckerman JD. Neuropathic arthropathy: review of current knowledge. *J Am Acad Orthop Surg.* 1996;4:100-108.

102. Yanik B, Tuncer S, Seçkin B. Neuropathic arthropathy caused by Arnold-Chiari malformation with syringomyelia. *Rheumatol Int.* 2004;24:238-241.

103. Rickert MM, Cannon JG, Kirkpatrick JS. Neuropathic arthropathy of the shoulder: a systemic review of classifications and treatments. *JBJS Rev.* 2019;7:e1.

104. Brodbelt A, Stoodley M. Post-traumatic syringomyelia: a review. *J Clin Neurosci.* 2003;10:401-408.

105. Klekamp J. The pathophysiology of syringomyelia – Historical overview and current concept. *Acta Neurochir (Wien).* 2002;144:649-664.

106. Cullen AB, Ofluoglu O, Donthineni R. Neuropathic arthropathy of the shoulder (Charcot shoulder). *MedGenMed.* 2005;7:29.

107. Jones J, Wolf S. Neuropathic shoulder arthropathy (Charcot joint) associated with syringomyelia. *Neurology.* 1998;50:825-827.

108. Tully JG, Latteri A. Paraplegia, syringomyelia tarda and neuropathic arthrosis of the shoulder: a triad. *Clin Orthop Relat Res.* 1978;134:244-248.

109. Brower AC, Allman RM. Pathogenesis of the neurotrophic joint: neurotraumatic vs. neurovascular. *Radiology.* 1981;139:349-354.

110. O'Connor BL, Visco DM, Brandt KD, Myers SL, Kalasinski LA. Neurogenic acceleration of osteoarthrosis. The effects of previous neurectomy of the articular nerves on the development of osteoarthrosis after transection of the anterior cruciate ligament in dogs. *J Bone Joint Surg Am.* 1992;74:367-376.

111. Eloesser L. On the nature of neuropathic affections of the joints. *Ann Surg.* 1917;66:201-207.

112. Johnson JT. Neuropathic fractures and joint injuries. Pathogenesis and rationale of prevention and treatment. *J Bone Joint Surg Am.* 1967;49:1-30.

113. Chantelau E, Onvlee GJ, Chantelaú E. Charcot foot in diabetes: farewell to the neurotrophic theory. *Horm Metab Res.* 2006;38:361-367.

114. Kaynak G, Birsel O, Güven MF, Oğüt T. An overview of the Charcot foot pathophysiology. *Diabet Foot Ankle.* 2013;4:21117.

115. Jeffcoate WJ, Game F, Cavanagh PR. The role of proinflammatory cytokines in the cause of neuropathic osteoarthropathy (acute Charcot foot) in diabetes. *Lancet.* 2005;366:2058-2061.

116. Irie K, Hara-Irie F, Ozawa H, Yajima T. Calcitonin gene-related peptide (CGRP)-containing nerve fibers in bone tissue and their involvement in bone remodeling. *Microsc Res Tech.* 2002;58:85-90.

117. Rosenbaum AJ, DiPreta JA. Classifications in brief: eichenholtz classification of Charcot arthropathy. *Clin Orthop Relat Res.* 2015;473:1168-1171.

118. Hatzis N, Kaar TK, Wirth MA, Toro F, Rockwood CA. Neuropathic arthropathy of the shoulder. *J Bone Joint Surg Am.* 1998;80:1314-1319.

119. Ueblacker P, Ansah P, Vogt S, Imhoff AB. Bilateral reverse shoulder prosthesis in a patient with severe syringomyelia. *J Shoulder Elbow Surg.* 2007;16:e48-e51.

120. Panagariya A, Sharma AK. Bilateral Charcot arthropathy of shoulder secondary to syringomyelia: an unusual case report. *Ann Indian Acad Neurol.* 2012;15:202-204.

121. Llanger J, Palmer J, Rosón N, Bagué S, Camins A, Cremades R. Nonseptic monoarthritis: imaging features with clinical and histopathologic correlation. *Radiographics.* 2000;20:S263-S278.

122. Kaandorp CJ, Dinant HJ, van de Laar MA, Moens HJ, Prins AP, Dijkmans BA. Incidence and sources of native and prosthetic joint infection: a community based prospective survey. *Ann Rheum Dis.* 1997;56:470-475.

123. Le Dantec L, Maury F, Flipo RM, et al. Peripheral pyogenic arthritis. A study of one hundred seventy-nine cases. *Rev Rhum Engl Ed.* 1996;63:103-110.

124. Weston VC, Jones AC, Bradbury N, Fawthrop F, Doherty M. Clinical features and outcome of septic arthritis in a single UK Health District 1982-1991. *Ann Rheum Dis.* 1999;58:214-219.

125. Jiang JJ, Piponov HI, Mass DP, Angeles JG, Shi LL. Septic arthritis of the shoulder: a comparison of treatment methods. *J Am Acad Orthop Surg.* 2017;25:e175-e184.

126. Gelberman RH, Menon J, Austerlitz MS, Weisman MH. Pyogenic arthritis of the shoulder in adults. *J Bone Joint Surg Am.* 1980;62:550-553.

127. Riegels-Nielson P, Frimodt-Möller N, Jensen JS. Rabbit model of septic arthritis. *Acta Orthop Scand.* 1987;58:14-19.

128. Bremell T, Abdelnour A, Tarkowski A. Histopathological and serological progression of experimental *Staphylococcus aureus* arthritis. *Infect Immun.* 1992;60:2976-2985.

129. Sweet MC, Sheena GJ, Liu S, et al. Clinical characteristics and long-term outcomes after septic arthritis of the native glenohumeral joint: a 20-year retrospective review. *Orthopedics.* 2019;42:e118-e123.

130. Settecerri JJ, Pitner MA, Rock MG, et al. Infection after rotator cuff repair. *J Shoulder Elbow Surg.* 1999;8:1-5.

131. Sperling JW, Kozak TK, Hanssen AD, Cofield RH. Infection after shoulder arthroplasty. *Clin Orthop Relat Res.* 2001;382:206-216.

132. Sperling JW, Cofield RH, Torchia ME, Hanssen AD. Infection after shoulder instability surgery. *Clin Orthop Relat Res.* 2003;414:61-64.

133. Khan U, Torrance E, Townsend R, et al. Low-grade infections in nonarthroplasty shoulder surgery. *J Shoulder Elbow Surg.* 2017;26:1553-1561.

134. Mathews CJ, Weston VC, Jones A, et al. Bacterial septic arthritis in adults. *Lancet.* 2010;375:846-855.

135. Assunção JH, Noffs GG, Malavolta EA, et al. Septic arthritis of the shoulder and elbow: one decade of epidemiological analysis at a tertiary referral hospital. *Rev Bras Ortop.* 2018;53:707-713.

136. Gupta MN, Sturrock RD, Field M. A prospective 2-year study of 75 patients with adult-onset septic arthritis. *Rheumatology.* 2001;40:24-30.

137. Kim SJ, Choi YR, Lee W, Jung WS, Chun YM. Arthroscopic debridement for septic arthritis of the shoulder joint: post-infectious arthritis is an inevitable consequence? *Arch Orthop Trauma Surg.* 2018;138:1257-1263.

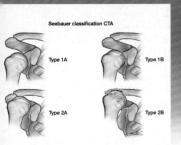

6

Assessment and Classification of Glenohumeral Deformity

Richard B. Jones, MD and Ari R. Youderian, MD

Shoulder arthroplasty has seen an enormous evolution in the last 2 decades. Subsequently, techniques to evaluate the glenohumeral joint and its related structures have evolved as well. In the past, surgeons relied heavily on physical examination and standard radiographs to evaluate disorders of the shoulder. This was followed by a progression to more advanced imaging modalities such as computed tomography (CT) and magnetic resonance imaging (MRI). Using these modalities, surgeons were able to identify more complex patterns of glenoid or humeral deformity, leading to classification systems and an enhanced ability to "quantify" deformities. Consequently, our understanding of how various glenohumeral deformities and anatomic parameters contribute to glenohumeral disorders and disease processes has improved. Similarly, our increased knowledge base has changed our approach to shoulder arthroplasty and allowed us to achieve better outcomes. Subsequent development of three-dimensional (3D) technology continues to advance the evaluation of bony deformity and has further progressed with preoperative planning software and navigation techniques.

Recognition of glenohumeral deformity or anatomic parameters that may impact patient outcomes after surgery is of paramount importance. Failure to do so may compromise the chances of successful surgical treatment of the patient's shoulder disorder. Hasan et al[1] evaluated characteristics of unsatisfactory shoulder arthroplasties and found that malposition of the components occurred in 28% of the cases. Others have shown that placement of an anatomic glenoid component in excessive retroversion leads to significantly decreased glenohumeral contact area, increased contact pressure, increased micromotion of the implant, and increased osteolysis around the pegs.[2-4]

Preoperative assessment of the extent and location of bony deformity, associated soft tissue pathology, and other scapular anatomic parameters is commonly performed with standard radiographs, axial CT scans through the glenohumeral joint, MRI, or 3D CT reconstructions.

IMAGING MODALITIES

Standard Radiographs

Despite the many advanced imaging techniques available for the shoulder, the initial evaluation usually includes standard radiographs. A shoulder radiographic series may vary among ordering physicians and can be tailored to address the various conditions being evaluated. A common shoulder series for glenohumeral arthritis includes a true scapular anteroposterior (AP) (Grashey) view, outlet view, and axillary view. Other common views include true AP views with the humerus in internal and external rotation.

While a standard AP view is a common component of a basic shoulder series, it may not be the best to evaluate the glenohumeral joint in arthritic conditions. Since the glenohumeral joint is often angled anteriorly 30° to 40°, this view results in overlap of the glenoid and humeral head. The Grashey view, on the other hand, is a true AP of the shoulder in the plane of the scapula (FIGURE 6.1). By rotating the patient posteriorly or angling the beam laterally, the overlap of the glenoid and humeral head is eliminated. This allows a more accurate view of the glenohumeral joint space and provides a better assessment of glenohumeral arthritis, humeral head subluxation, and joint congruity.[5] This view may be further modified to evaluate joint space narrowing by adding a weight and abduction, which applies an axial load to the joint.[6] The Grashey view allows an evaluation of glenoid inclination (GI), superior migration of the humeral head, as well as a general assessment of the acromioclavicular joint.

The axillary view is essential and provides an assessment of abnormal glenoid wear patterns, glenoid retroversion, and posterior subluxation of the humeral head. Since soft tissue can interfere with the appreciation of the glenohumeral joint line on an axillary view, a projection that shows a continuous line from the coracoid base and glenoid articular surface should be obtained.[7] (FIGURE 6.2)

The supraspinatus outlet view (FIGURE 6.3) is a modification of a standard scapular Y view with caudal tilt of the x-ray beam. It allows evaluation of the acromion and the subacromial space. An os acromiale, which may be of clinical importance during reverse shoulder

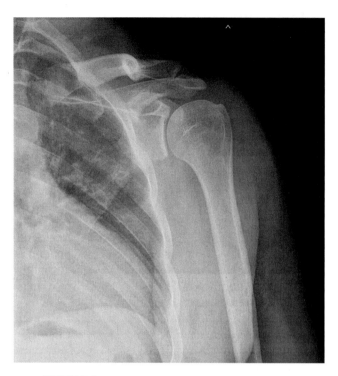

FIGURE 6.1 Anteroposterior (AP) Grashey radiograph.

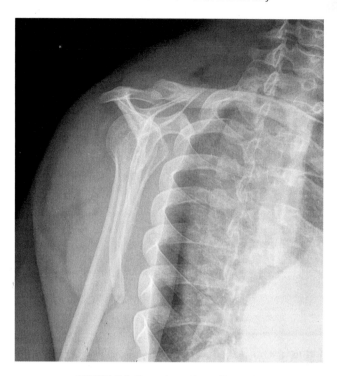

FIGURE 6.3 Scapular outlet radiograph.

arthroplasty (RSA), can also be visualized on this view as well as on the axillary view. Both the scapular Y and outlet views are also useful to detect humeral head subluxation or dislocation.

Characteristic radiographic changes occur as a result of the degenerative processes that impact the glenohumeral joint. Osteoarthritis (OA) leads to alterations in glenohumeral biomechanics, which can transform the anatomic features of the humerus and glenoid. Development of anterior contractures can lead to increased peripheral contact stresses on the glenoid

followed by increased glenoid posterior erosion and increased glenoid retroversion. This may lead to ultimate decentering and posterior subluxation of the humeral head.[8] Findings consistent with OA include marginal osteophytes around the anatomic neck of the humerus and glenoid, joint space narrowing, subchondral cysts, and subchondral sclerosis **(FIGURE 6.4)**. Post-traumatic arthritis may demonstrate more severe deformity of the humeral head or glenoid.

Rheumatoid arthritis (RA) may produce periarticular osteopenia, marginal erosions, and joint space narrowing with the absence of osteophytes **(FIGURE 6.5)**. Concentric erosion of the glenoid may occur causing medial migration of the humeral head. Concomitant rotator cuff disease is common in RA as well, which may lead to superior migration of the humeral head. This causes eventual erosion and thinning of the acromion and may lead to acetabularization of the glenohumeral joint and acromion.[5]

Rotator cuff tear arthropathy can demonstrate similar radiographic findings as OA or RA. Narrowing of the acromiohumeral interval in a nonrheumatoid patient indicates a large and chronic rotator cuff tear. The humeral head may articulate with the undersurface of the acromion, the superior portion of the glenoid, and the base of the coracoid process possibly leading to acetabularization of the glenohumeral joint and acromion. The head may eventually lose the contour of the greater tuberosity **(FIGURE 6.6)**.

While radiographs are routinely performed on patients considering shoulder arthroplasty, they do

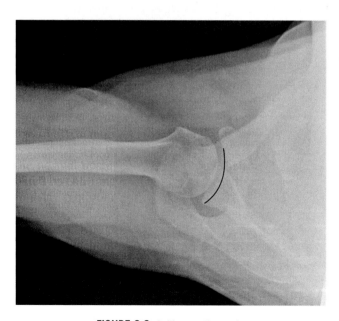

FIGURE 6.2 Axillary radiograph.

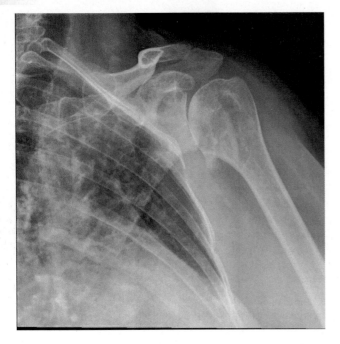

FIGURE 6.4 AP Grashey view demonstrating findings consistent with osteoarthritis including marginal osteophytes around the anatomic neck of the humerus and glenoid, joint space narrowing, subchondral cysts, and subchondral sclerosis.

contain limitations. Nyffeler et al[9] showed that glenoid retroversion was overestimated on axillary radiographs 86% of the time with a maximum difference of 21°. The authors noted three factors that may contribute to this: (1) Most axillary radiographs are not aligned properly with the superior and inferior margins of the glenoid superimposed; (2) Often, on axillary views, the medial border of the scapula is not visualized due to the patient's neck preventing sufficient medial placement of

the cassette; and (3) The quality of the images depends on the orientation of the beam relative to the patient's scapula. Small changes in this relationship can alter the version measurement. The authors concluded that glenoid version could not be accurately determined on standard radiographs and recommended a more reproducible imaging modality such as CT scans.

Computed Tomography

It is now common for shoulder surgeons to employ more advanced imaging modalities such as CT or MRI in the evaluation of the glenohumeral joint. CT scans have been used in standard two-dimensional (2D) format, 3D reformatted 2D scans in the plane of the scapula, and more recently, 3D CT imaging often combined with preoperative surgical planning software. This has prompted abundant investigation as to which modality is most accurate to assess the glenoid.

Friedman[10] first introduced the technique of using 2D CT scans to measure glenoid version. However, the accuracy of traditional 2D clinical CT scans has been questioned. 2D clinical CT scans are axial cuts traditionally aligned to the patient's torso. Because of the natural tilt of the scapula, which is typically oriented in 20° to 30° of anteversion with respect to the coronal plane of the body, these axial slices are rarely aligned perpendicular to the scapula body. The mean angle between the direction of axial scans and the scapular body is approximately 35°, which may lead to inaccurate measurement of glenoid version.[11] **(FIGURE 6.7)** The average error in version measurement using this technique has been demonstrated to be ±5°; however, the maximum error is even higher at 16°.[11] Subsequent research has shown that obtaining accurate and reproducible glenoid measurements, at least

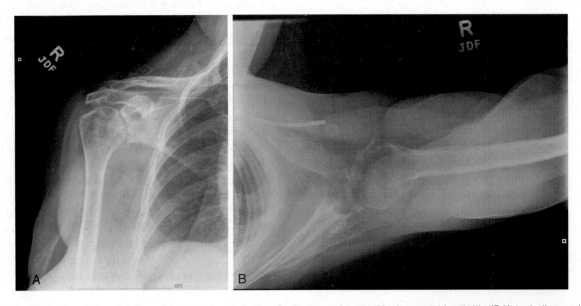

FIGURE 6.5 AP Grashey (**A**) and axillary (**B**) views demonstrating findings consistent with rheumatoid arthritis (RA) including periarticular osteopenia, marginal erosions, and joint space narrowing with the absence of osteophytes.

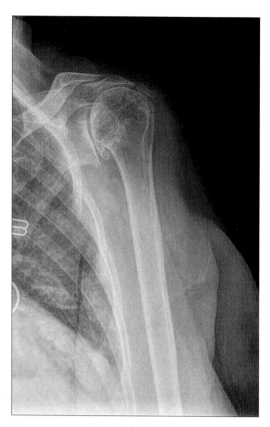

FIGURE 6.6 This Grashey view shows, in rotator cuff tear arthropathy, the humeral head may articulate with the undersurface of the acromion, the superior portion of the glenoid, and the base of the coracoid process possibly leading to acetabularization of the glenohumeral joint and acromion.

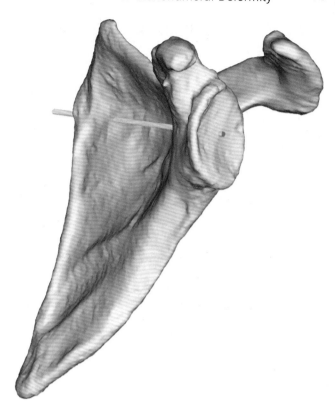

FIGURE 6.8 Three-dimensional reconstruction of computed tomography (CT) scan showing Friedman line.

of version, requires CT scans using axial slices that have been reoriented in the plane of the scapula.[11-16] CT scans that are not reoriented have shown significant overestimation of version and inclination.[11-13,15]

Rotation of the scapula in relation to the CT orientation can also affect measured version. Minor rotation of the scapula can alter the accuracy of glenoid version measurement by up to 10°. It is recommended that the glenoid articular surface should be perpendicular to plane of CT cut.[14]

More recently, much investigation has focused on 3D reconstructed CT scans in the evaluation of the

glenohumeral joint. 3D reconstruction of CT scan images offers the potential to evaluate the bony erosion without positional errors. 3D reconstructed CT scans have shown improved assessment of glenoid bone loss in patients with instability[17,18] as well as glenohumeral arthritis.[19,20] **(FIGURE 6.8)** 3D CT images also have shown better interrater reliability[19] and more accurate measurements of version and inclination[21] compared to 2D measurements. 3D CT reconstruction techniques have furthermore led to preoperative planning techniques allowing for templating of implant size and positioning and has been shown to be reproducible and beneficial for surgical decision-making.[19,21,22]

Magnetic Resonance Imaging

While CT scans remain the gold standard for advanced imaging of the glenohumeral joint, MRI can be useful and has certain advantages. MRI allows superior imaging of the soft tissues resulting in better assessment of the rotator cuff, deltoid, and other soft tissue structures around the shoulder, which can assist decision-making in shoulder arthroplasty **(FIGURE 6.9)**. While CT scans are still the standard, the capacity of MRI to visualize bone morphology has improved with advancing technology. Compared to radiographs, MRI has been shown to provide a more accurate and reproducible assessment of glenoid version[23] with better inter- and intrarater reliability in identifying glenoid morphology and classification.[23,24]

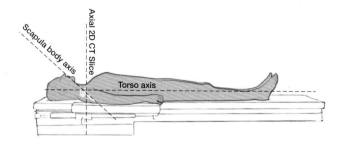

FIGURE 6.7 The mean angle between the direction of axial scans and the scapular body is approximately 35°, which may lead to inaccuracy in version measurement.

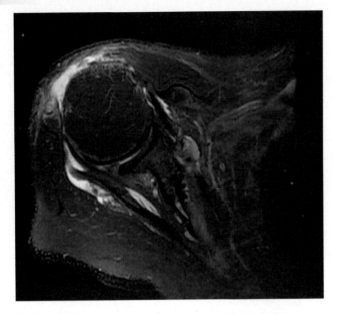

FIGURE 6.9 Axial magnetic resonance image (MRI).

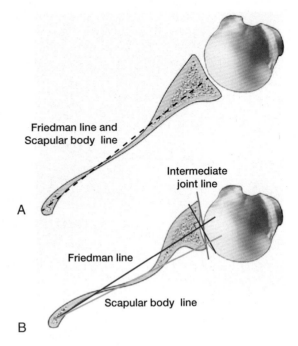

FIGURE 6.10 A, In a scapula with no deformity, Friedmans line and the scapular body line will be the same. **B**, In a more deformed scapula, Friedmans line and the scapular body line may differ causing variability in version calculation between the two methods. (A and B, Redrawn with permission from Friedman RJ, Hawthorne KB, Genez BM. The use of computerized tomography in the measurement of glenoid version. *J Bone Joint Surg Am.* 1992;74(7):1032-1037, and Randelli M, Gambrioli PL. Glenohumeral osteometry by computed tomography in normal and unstable shoulders. *Clin Orthop Relat Res.* 1986;(208):151-156.)

MRI has also been shown to be comparable to CT in the assessment of glenoid bone loss[25,26] and version.[27] Lowe et al,[27] in their study comparing MRI to CT scan in the evaluation of the glenoid, found that MRI is largely comparable to CT scan for evaluation of the glenoid, with similar measurements of version and identification of less severe glenoid deformity. However, MRI is less accurate at distinguishing between Walch type B2 and C glenoids.

SCAPULAR ANATOMIC PARAMETERS AND THEIR IMPLICATIONS

Much work has been done evaluating various scapular anatomic parameters and their influence on shoulder disorders, most commonly glenohumeral OA and rotator cuff tears (RCT). Version and inclination of the glenoid, size and shape of the glenoid vault, and acromial morphology including lateral extension, size, tilt, and rotation have been investigated. Identifying anatomic parameters and their causal relationship to shoulder disorders may allow the surgeon to identify patients at risk for particular problems or modify these factors at surgery to improve outcomes.

Glenoid Version

Abnormal glenoid version can have adverse consequences in shoulder arthroplasty. In anatomic total shoulder arthroplasty (ATSA), numerous studies have demonstrated increased forces in the cement mantle, glenoid implant, and glenoid bone as well as increased micromotion with implantation in excessive retroversion, all of which contribute to early glenoid loosening.[2,4,28,29] During reverse total shoulder arthroplasty (RTSA), abnormal placement of the glenoid component can adversely affect

ROM, stability, and scapular notching.[30-33] Therefore, proper determination of the patient's preoperative version can be crucial to a successful arthroplasty.

Axillary radiographs have been demonstrated to be inaccurate in the measurement of glenoid version.[9] Friedman et al[10] were among the first to use CT scans to characterize the relationship between glenoid retroversion and OA. They described a technique to calculate glenoid version using the transverse axis of the scapula, defined as a line drawn from the tip of the medial border of the scapula to the midpoint of the glenoid fossa. The first slice distal to the coracoid is usually chosen for measurement. Randelli and Gambrioli[34] also proposed a technique that uses the scapular body line to calculate glenoid version (scapular body method). In both of these methods, a line drawn perpendicular to the axis along the glenoid surface was defined as neutral version, and the angle from either the posterior margin or the anterior margin of the glenoid defined the native version **(FIGURE 6.10)**. Rouleau et al[35] compared the validity of both of these measurement methods for determining glenoid version. The authors showed that both methods demonstrated excellent reliability but suggested the use of the Friedman method citing it as more user-friendly in the presence of a curved scapula for all glenoid types.

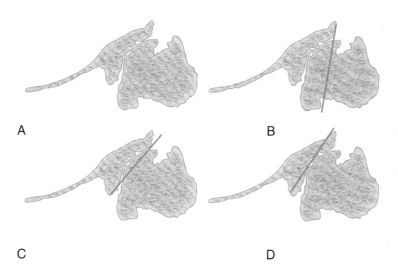

A

B

C

D

FIGURE 6.11 A, Arthritic shoulder showing glenoid with posterior wear and eccentric erosion. **B**, Paleoglenoid (original glenoid surface), (**C**) intermediate glenoid (line from anterior and posterior edge), (**D**) neoglenoid (posterior erosion surface). (Redrawn with permission from Rouleau DM, Kidder JF, Pons-Villanueva J, Dynamidis S, Defranco M, Walch G. Glenoid version: how to measure it? Validity of different methods in two-dimensional computed tomography scans. *J Shoulder Elbow Surg.* 2010;19(8):1230-1237.)

The authors also introduced new reference lines to characterize a glenoid surface with posterior wear and eccentric erosion. These included the paleoglenoid (original glenoid surface), intermediate glenoid (line from anterior and posterior edge), and neoglenoid (posterior erosion surface) **(FIGURE 6.11)**. They indicated that in the presence of a B2 glenoid and posterior erosion, the choice of an intermediate glenoid line is more reliable for measurement. This line also represents the surface that could be obtained with minimal bone loss after limited reaming of the glenoid surface during total shoulder arthroplasty

(TSA). Poon et al[36] introduced a third method of version measurement using a 2D CT slice focusing solely on the glenoid vault. The authors felt their technique was more relevant to glenoid implant placement and was generally more simple and accessible to everyone **(FIGURE 6.12)**. However, the vault method has been shown to have less reliability and more variability according to CT slice height or angulation than the Friedman method in glenoid version measurement.[37]

3D CT reconstructions are quickly becoming the standard for assessing the glenohumeral joint, often in

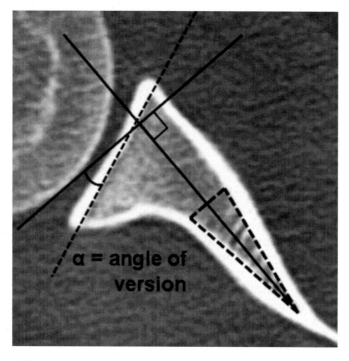

FIGURE 6.12 Poon two-dimensional (2D) glenoid vault method. (Reproduced with permission from Poon PC, Ting FS. A 2-dimensional glenoid vault method for measuring glenoid version on computed tomography. *J Shoulder Elbow Surg.* 2012;21(3):329-335.)

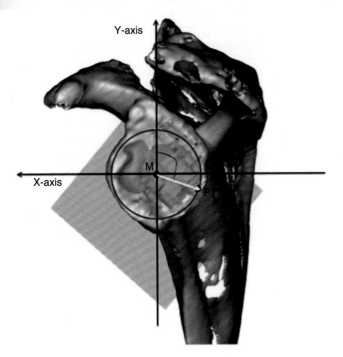

FIGURE 6.13 Three-dimensional (3D) measurement technique showing maximum erosion in type B1 glenoids is situated more posteroinferiorly. (Reproduced with permission from Beuckelaers E, Jacxsens M, Van Tongel A, De Wilde LF. Three-dimensional computed tomography scan evaluation of the pattern of erosion in type B glenoids. *J Shoulder Elbow Surg.* 2014;23(1):109-116.)

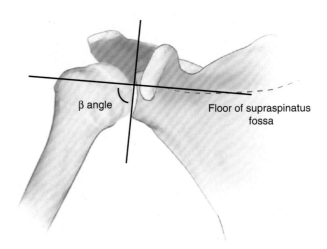

FIGURE 6.14 The beta angle is defined as the angle formed between the floor of the supraspinatus fossa and the glenoid fossa measured on an anteroposterior (AP) Grashey view.

concert with preoperative planning software. Kwon et al[38] used 3D CT imaging of cadaveric specimens and showed that on average, the glenoid version angles measured from the 3D CT images were within 1.0° ± 0.7° of those from the actual specimen. The measurements from the 3D CT images also showed high interobserver and intraobserver reliability. Beuckelaers et al[39] described a 3D technique to quantify glenoid erosion and measure version in a population with primary glenohumeral arthritis and posterior subluxation of the humeral head. They concluded that the amount of erosion in glenoids with a Walch type B1 morphology can be underestimated using 2D CT evaluation because the orientation of the maximum erosion in type B1 glenoids is situated more posteroinferiorly **(FIGURE 6.13).**

Inclination of the Glenoid

The inclination of the glenohumeral joint is an important variable. Increased GI has been associated with RCT[40-42] and superior migration of the humeral head.[43,44] Inclination of the glenoid can also play an important role in TSA. Proper positioning of the glenoid component is the most important factor for implant longevity and avoiding clinical failure.[45] Excessive superior or inferior placement of the glenoid component has been shown to create the highest stress on the cement mantle.[46] Downward tilting of

the glenoid component has been shown to decrease superior migration of the humeral head,[47] subluxation of the humeral head and implant tilting,[48] as well as balance supraspinatus insufficiency.[49] In RTSA, excessive superior inclination can lead to increased risks of baseplate loosening, whereas excessive inferior tilt may increase impingement on the neck of the scapula leading to scapular notching.[50]

Maurer et al[51] described the most commonly accepted technique for accurate and reproducible measurement of GI on standardized AP radiographs and CT images. The authors described the beta angle as being the most reproducible measurement for GI on conventional AP radiographs, providing a resistance to positional variability of the scapula and good interrater reliability. Radiographically, the beta angle is defined as the angle formed between the floor of the supraspinatus fossa and the glenoid fossa measured on an AP Grashey view **(FIGURE 6.14).** On CT images, the coronal section at the deepest point of the supraspinatus fossa is used. The measurement line is placed along the cortical margin of the floor of the supraspinatus fossa. As with glenoid version, measurements of GI have been shown to be most accurate using 3D reformatted scans in the plane of the scapula. Nonreformatted CT scans as well as standard radiographs are less accurate.[52] More recently, MRI has shown to be comparable to CT scan in accurately measuring GI using the beta angle.[42]

Boileau et al[53] drew our attention to problems using the beta angle technique to measure inclination prior to RTSA. Baseplates are routinely placed on the inferior portion of the glenoid with slight overhang to reduce scapular notching. The authors point out that

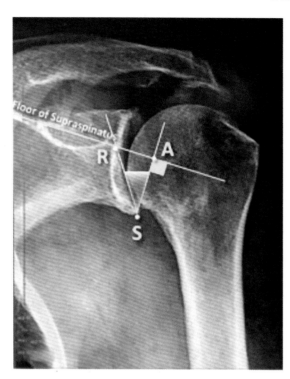

FIGURE 6.15 The reverse shoulder arthroplasty angle. (Reproduced with permission from Boileau P, Gauci MO, Wagner ER, et al. The reverse shoulder arthroplasty angle: a new measurement of glenoid inclination for reverse shoulder arthroplasty. *J Shoulder Elbow Surg.* 2019;28(7):1281-1290.)

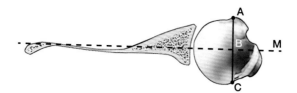

FIGURE 6.16 Shoulder subluxation index: Using a mid-axial computed tomography (CT) slice, Friedman line is drawn from medial scapula across mid-point on glenoid (M) and extended across humeral head. Line AC is drawn from anterior to posterior humeral head intersecting Friedman line at point B. The subluxation index is calculated by the ratio BC/AC × 100.

in patients with central erosion of the glenoid (Favard E1), there is risk for placing the baseplate in superior tilt if this is not taken into account. The beta angle will underestimate the superior orientation of the baseplate by using the entire glenoid fossa in the measurement. They introduce a new measurement for inclination called the RSA angle (**FIGURE 6.15**). The RSA angle was defined as the angle between the inferior part of the glenoid fossa and the perpendicular to the floor of the supraspinatus fossa. In their investigation, the RSA angle averaged 20° ± 5° versus the TSA (or beta) angle, which was on average 10° ± 5° lower. This difference needs to be corrected to achieve neutral inclination of the baseplate.

Humeral Head Subluxation

The early descriptions of glenohumeral arthritis described the combined attributes of posterior subluxation and glenoid retroversion.[54] Since then, several techniques to assess subluxation along with theories regarding the pathogenesis have been proposed. Recommendations for surgical techniques and the ability to restore normal glenohumeral stability have followed.

The glenohumeral joint is dynamically stabilized by the soft tissue constraints of its ligaments and the medially directed pull of the rotator cuff tendons. To a lesser degree, the bony anatomy also plays a role.

Traditionally, subluxation has been defined as the percentage of translation of the humeral head in reference to the scapular plane using Friedman line.[55,56] The first methods used a 2D mid-axial CT slice, Friedman line, and the midpoint of a line drawn across the humeral head (**FIGURE 6.16**). Improvements in this measurement have included the use of 3D imaging, defining the various glenoid version indices such as the glenoid pathologic plane (humeral-glenoid alignment)[57] or the glenoid native plane[58] and using the actual humeral head center of rotation.

The normal shoulder joint typically exhibits some degree of dynamic translation.[55] It is commonly accepted that beyond 45% anterior and 55% posterior subluxation is pathologic. In OA, pathologic subluxation is present in almost half of cases.[56] However, these values do vary based on imaging modality and arm position with radiographs underestimating subluxation compared to CT and, to a greater degree, 3D CT imaging.[59]

The correlation between subluxation and glenoid retroversion has also been assessed with varying results.[56,57,59,60] Significant correlations are seen when measuring subluxation via the scapular plane method versus using the pathologic glenoid plane[57,61] or the native glenoid plane.[59]

It's been speculated that the pathogenesis of humeral retroversion in glenohumeral arthritis is related to abnormal force generation on the posterior glenoid due to pathologic subluxation.[56] The Walch B0 glenoid has also been proposed as a finding in younger patients with a preosteoarthritic posterior subluxation of the humeral head (PPSHH) prior to the development of other signs and symptoms. These patients exhibited early dynamic instability that may later develop into a static decentering.[62-65]

Ultimately, the use of a subluxation index in combination with understanding the bony and soft tissue presentation may be helpful in defining which surgical cases

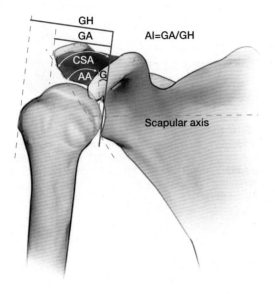

FIGURE 6.17 The acromial index (AI) is the ratio of the distance between a line from the superior to inferior border of the glenoid to the lateral border of the acromion (GA) and the same glenoid line to the lateral border of the greater tuberosity (GH).

should or can be corrected and by which means.[60,66,67] Corrective reaming, posterior bone grafting, and posterior glenoid augments have been shown to correct posterior subluxation in a majority of shoulders undergoing ATSA.[60,68-70] The use of primary RTSA may also play a significant role in restoring stability and protecting the longevity of implants.[71]

Acromion Index/Critical Shoulder Angle

The amount of lateral extension of the acromion and its combination with GI has been postulated to have an effect on the development of glenohumeral arthritis as well as RCT.[40,41,72,73] Nyffeler et al[72] were the first to describe a measurement of the amount of lateral acromial extension. The acromial index(AI) was defined as the ratio of the distance between a line from the superior to inferior border of the glenoid to the lateral border of the acromion and the same glenoid line to the lateral border of the greater tuberosity on an AP Grashey view **(FIGURE 6.17)**. The authors theorized that an increased lateral extension of the acromion caused a more vertically oriented force vector on the deltoid, leading to increased strain in the supraspinatus due to the horizontal force needed to stabilize the humeral head. They subsequently showed that the AI was higher in patients with RCT.

The AI, however, did not take into consideration the inclination of the glenoid, which has also been shown to play a potential role in RCT.[40-42] Moor et al[74] introduced a measurement which combined the two anatomic parameters of GI and the AI, the critical shoulder angle(CSA). Unlike the AI, the CSA does not involve the shape or orientation of the humeral head in the measurement, which in OA may become deformed and flattened leading to inaccuracies. The CSA is defined as the angle between a line connecting the superior and inferior margins of the glenoid and a second from the inferior edge of the glenoid to the lateral border of the acromion on an AP Grashey view **(FIGURE 6.18)**. In their investigation, with almost 300 patients consisting of asymptomatic controls

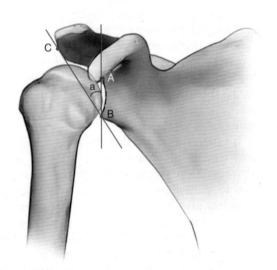

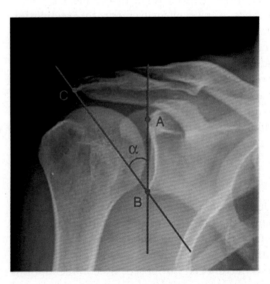

FIGURE 6.18 The critical shoulder angle (CSA) is the angle between a line connecting the superior and inferior margins of the glenoid (AB) and a second from the inferior edge of the glenoid to the lateral border of the acromion (BC). (Right image used with permission from Moor BK, Bouaicha S, Rothenfluh DA, Sukthankar A, Gerber C. Is there an association between the individual anatomy of the scapula and the development of rotator cuff tears or osteoarthritis of the glenohumeral joint? A radiological study of the critical shoulder angle. *Bone Joint J.* 2013;95-B(7):935-941.)

and those with RCT and glenohumeral arthritis, Moor et al[74] demonstrated a mean CSA of 33.1°. Decreased CSA (<30°) has been shown to correlate with the development of glenohumeral OA, whereas increased CSA (>35°) has been associated with increased incidence of RCT.[74-78] It is believed that as the CSA decreases, forces on the deltoid shift becoming more horizontal, causing the forces on the glenohumeral joint to become more compressive, thereby resulting in greater loading of the cartilage and subsequent OA. Conversely, as the CSA increases the vertical shear forces and instability across the joint increase, leading to higher stresses and force in the supraspinatus required to stabilize the joint. This potentially leads to increased impingement and RCT.[74,79,82] Because AI and GI may have opposite effects on the measurement, CSA may be a better indicator for the risk of tendon tear, but AI may be more efficient to predict the risk of OA.[80]

The CSA has recently been correlated with surgical outcomes in terms of retear rates after rotator cuff repair and glenoid implant loosening after ATSA. Increase in CSA of 10° or more has been associated with a 6.2-fold increased odds of having an at-risk glenoid for loosening on radiographs.[81] The CSA may be a modifiable factor to improve outcomes and implant longevity after TSA.

Other Scapular Parameters

Further investigations evaluating the influence of acromial and scapular morphology on shoulder disease processes have focused on acromial shape, rotation, and inclination in the sagittal plane. Beeler et al[83] analyzed the 3D orientation and shape of the lateral acromion in patients with concentric OA and RCT using CT scans. They found that a more externally rotated (axial plane), more downward tilted (coronal plane), and wider posterior covering acromion was more frequent in patients with massive RCT. A following investigation also using CT scans to evaluate acromial and glenoid relationships demonstrated that the combination of a flat posterior acromial slope and an increased posterior glenoid version are risk factors strongly associated with posterior glenoid wear and posterior static subluxation of the humeral head.[84] **(FIGURE 6.19)**

THE GLENOID VAULT MODEL

Iannoti and colleagues described and validated a standardized 3D model of the glenoid vault. Using 61 specimens of varying sizes and custom software, they described a common 3D shape of the endosteal surface of the glenoid vault.[85] It has since been shown to be a powerful tool in predicting the amount of glenoid bone loss[86] and the native, or premorbid, glenoid version and inclination.[87-89] 2D versions using the glenoid vault have also been described.[36] The glenoid vault model not only complements other methods that predict the native

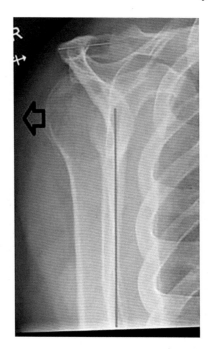

FIGURE 6.19 Flat posterior acromial slope and an increased posterior glenoid version are risk factors strongly associated with posterior glenoid wear and posterior static subluxation of the humeral head. (With permission from Meyer DC, Riedo S, Eckers F, Carpeggiani G, Jentzsch T, Gerber C. Small anteroposterior inclination of the acromion is a predictor for posterior glenohumeral erosion (B2 or C). *J Shoulder Elbow Surg.* 2019;28(1):22-27.)

glenoid morphology[35,90] but also useful information in cases of severe glenoid wear without notable bony surface landmarks. Unfortunately, the lack of commercial availability within current preoperative planning software applications does limit the use and further investigation of this technique **(FIGURE 6.20)**.

CLASSIFICATION SYSTEMS FOR GLENOHUMERAL ARTHRITIS

Numerous classification systems have been proposed to describe the pathoanatomy of different types of glenohumeral arthritis. These have been used in the shoulder arthroplasty literature in an attempt to both quantify and qualify factors involved in the pathology including bone morphology, soft tissue changes, and relative positioning of the humeral head in relation to the glenoid. The most often referenced classification systems will be described along with their validity and a discussion of their impact on treatment regimens, surgical decision-making, and outcome measures.

PRIMARY GLENOHUMERAL OA

Original Walch Classification (1999)

The most referenced classification for glenohumeral OA was proposed by Walch et al in 1999.[91] Prior to this, assessment was based upon a qualitative description of

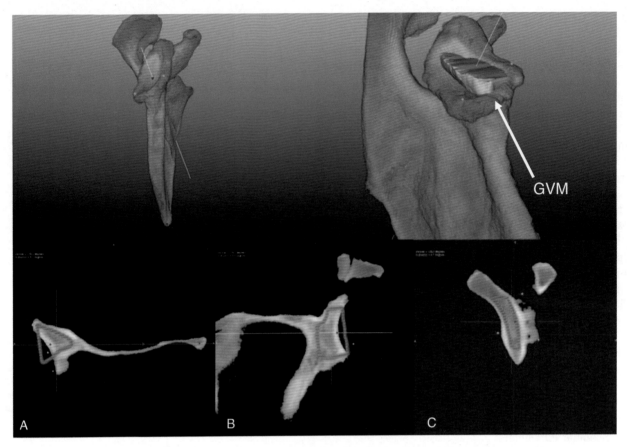

FIGURE 6.20 Example of the glenoid vault model (GVM) in a patient with severe glenoid retroversion. The model is sized and aligned to the endosteal border of the anterior glenoid on axial (**A**), the suprascapular notch on coronal (**B**), and the anterior glenoid rim on sagittal (**C**) and can be used to predict the native glenoid version and native joint line.

the findings that focused on posterior glenoid wear and posterior subluxation of the humeral head.[54] Walch et al proposed a descriptive anatomic system using a mid-axial cut on 2D CT scans to describe and categorize the features of glenoid wear and subluxation together. They proposed three main classes based on a review of 113 CT scans of osteoarthritic shoulders. Type A described a centered humeral head without (A1) and with (A2) centralized wear. Type B described posterior subluxation of the humeral head without (B1) and with (B2) obvious posterior glenoid erosion. The authors further distinguished the congenitally dysplastic glenoid from typical arthritis wear patterns as type C with over 25° retroversion regardless of humeral head location.

Despite its widespread use, the utility and reliability of the original Walch classification has been variable and inconsistent. The original article reported good inter- and intraobserver reliability scores, but they did not include all subtypes. Subsequently, others have published independent reviews including Scalise et al.[92] Their findings showed only fair inter- and intraobserver reliability scores when all five subtypes were used. Nowak et al[93] similarly found only moderate interobserver reliability

with substantial intrarater scores. The trend for better intraobserver reliability was further confirmed by Kiddler et al[94] who also found only moderate interobserver reliability.

The utility of the classification system based upon an axillary radiograph[95] and MRI[27] has also been reported. In comparison between radiographs and CT scans, radiographs had a higher intra- and interobserver agreement. Lowe et al[27] evaluated MRI compared to CT scan using the Walch classification. MRI was found to be similar in agreement overall, but MRI lacked the sensitivity of CT imaging to help distinguish between B2 and C glenoids. Based upon these inconsistent results, a modified Walch classification was proposed.

Modified Walch Classification (2016)

With advances in 3D imaging technology and an enhanced understanding of glenoid pathoanatomy,[39] Bercik et al[96] proposed a modification to the original classification (**FIGURE 6.21**). The first clarification was to describe the type C glenoid as one with over 25° of retroversion not caused by pathologic erosion. A subtype B3 glenoid was described as consisting of

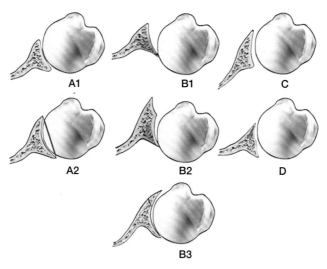

Modified Walch classification

FIGURE 6.21 The modified Walch classification: Additions include the B3 glenoid with retroversion and recentering of the humeral head, D with anterior subluxation, and clarifications of the A2 and C. (Redrawn with permission from Bercik MJ, Kruse K II, Yalizis M, Gauci MO, Chaoui J, Walch G. A modification to the Walch classification of the glenoid in primary glenohumeral osteoarthritis using three-dimensional imaging. *J Shoulder Elbow Surg.* 2016;25(10):1601-1606. doi:10.1016/j.jse.2016.03.010. PMID: 27282738.)

a monoconcavity with posterior wear and at least 15° of retroversion and/or at least 70% posterior humeral head subluxation. The B3 is distinguished from the B1 glenoid by the presence of posterior wear. The B3 glenoid was speculated to develop as either a direct monoconcavity with posterior erosion or as a conversion from a B2 biconcave glenoid secondary to additional erosion. A new type D glenoid was added and described as any glenoid with anteversion and/or anterior subluxation. Lastly, the A2 glenoid was better defined as one in which a line drawn from the anterior to posterior native glenoid transects the humeral head. The authors used 3D-aligned CT scans for their reevaluation of reliability. They reported a significant improvement in both intra- and interobserver agreement when compared to the original Walch classification.

Shukla et al[97] were the first to independently evaluate the modified Walch classification using both radiographs and CT scans. Intraobserver agreement was found to be substantial for both imaging techniques. The interobserver agreement was reported as fair for both radiographs and CT scans. Although these results are not as strong as reported by the original authors, it does represent an improvement over the original classification.[95]

Despite its criticisms, the now "modified" Walch classification has provided a platform for preoperative assessment of glenohumeral OA as well as a common language to discuss the pathoanatomy,[63] surgical techniques to address deformity (bone grafting, augmented glenoids, primary RTSA),[3,67] and clinical outcome.[3,60,67,98]

Clinical patterns have emerged including findings that osteoarthritic B2 glenoids have significantly higher retroversion measurements (−14° ± 6°) compared to normal, age-matched controls (−5° ± 5°).[99] In a large sample of prearthroplasty patients, Matsen et al[100] found that men had a higher frequency of B2 glenoids, and type A1 and C glenoids were found more commonly in younger patients. OA patients were more likely to have B2 morphology, but they did not report any worse preoperative self-assessment scores. Further assessments of the B3 glenoid have concluded that it is an acquired monoconcavity with an absent paleoglenoid and further characterized by medialization, retroversion, and subluxation. The subluxation significantly increases with increased retroversion, as referenced in the scapular plane.[101]

REVISION SHOULDER ARTHROPLASTY

Antuna Classification

Failure of the glenoid component in TSA is a leading cause of revision surgery. Implant loosening and glenoid bone loss in revision situations are common from both pathologic bone resorption and mechanical bone loss during removal of implants. The *Antuna classification*[102] has been used since 2001 as a means to classify glenoid bone loss in revision arthroplasty **(FIGURE 6.22)**. This will be discussed extensively in Chapter 42.

CUFF TEAR ARTHROPATHY CLASSIFICATIONS

Following the original description of cuff tear arthropathy (CTA) in 1983,[103] the patterns of bony changes have since been described and classified.

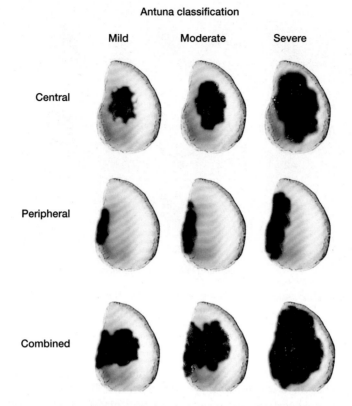

FIGURE 6.22 The Antuna classification of glenoid bone loss for revision arthroplasty specifying the location and degree of bone loss on the glenoid face. (Redrawn with permission from Antuna SA, Sperling JW, Cofield RH, Rowland CM. Glenoid revision surgery after total shoulder arthroplasty. *J Shoulder Elbow Surg.* 2001;10:217-224.)

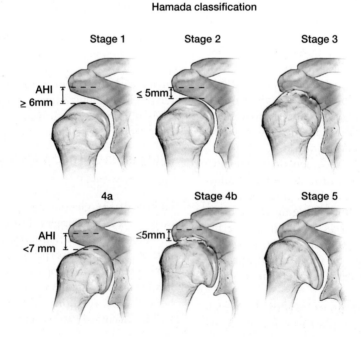

FIGURE 6.23 The Hamada classification of rotator cuff arthropathy showing progressive changes between the humerus and acromion as well as the humerus and glenoid. (Redrawn with permission from Hamada K, Fukuda H, Mikasa M, Kobayashi Y. Roentgenographic findings in massive rotator cuff tears. A long-term observation. *Clin Orthop Relat Res.* 1990;92-96.)

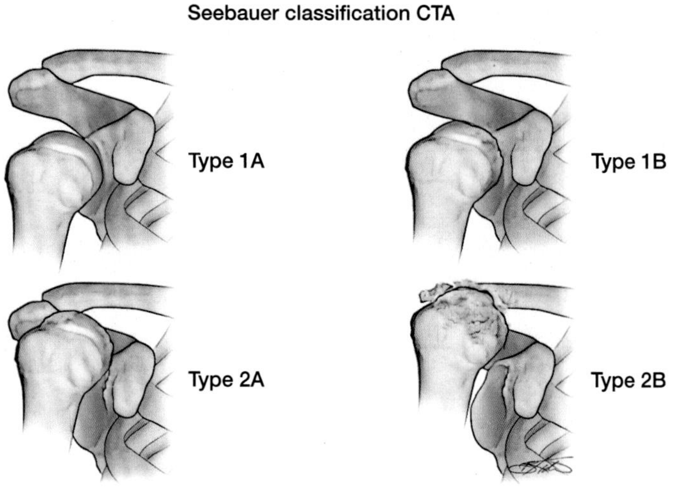

Seebauer classification CTA

Type 1A

Type 1B

Type 2A

Type 2B

FIGURE 6.24 The Seebauer classification depicting rotator cuff arthropathy cases with progressive destabilization of the glenohumeral joint. (Redrawn from VisotskyJL, Basamania C, Seebauer L, Rockwood CA, Jensen KL. Cuff tear arthropathy: pathogenesis, classification, and algorithm for treatment. *J Bone Joint Surg Am.* 2004;86-A(suppl 2):35-40.)

Hamada Classification

The *Hamada classification* **(FIGURE 6.23)** was based upon an analysis of standard radiographs in patients with massive RCT.[104] The authors proposed five categories based on the degree of narrowing of the acromiohumeral interval and the associated degenerative changes of the glenohumeral and acromioclavicular joints Reliability studies have indicated interrater reliability as assess both the early and late stages of the disease.[106]

Seebauer Classification

The *Seebauer classification*[107] **(FIGURE 6.24)** focuses on the progressive destabilization of the glenohumeral joint that occurs in CTA. The two main types are centered (type 1) and decentered (type 2). With progression, the subtypes define the progressive loss of dynamic joint stabilization and subsequent erosions either medially (IB), superiorly (IIA), or complete loss of stabilization with anterosuperior escape (IIB). This classification references advanced stages of the disease and has been found to have fair to moderate interrater reliability.[107]

Favard Classification

The *Favard classification*[108-110] **(FIGURE 6.25)** is recognized as being the most reliable overall[106] and distinguishes the glenoid patterns of erosion in CTA. The E2 erosion patterns have been further reported as having maximum erosion in the posterior superior quadrant of the glenoid and are most progressive in higher grade subscapularis tears.[111] Understanding these wear patterns may make surgical decisions easier for both the placement of[109] and choice of implants such as superior, posterior-superior, or custom-augmented baseplates.[111,112]

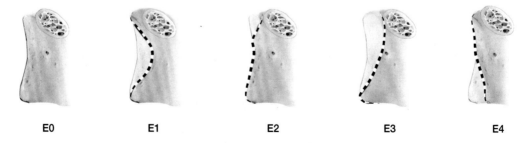

E0   E1   E2   E3   E4

FIGURE 6.25 The Sirveaux classification depicting patterns of glenoid erosion in cuff tear arthropathy. E0 superior migration without erosion, E1 concentric erosion, E2 superior erosion, and E3 erosion with extension inferiorly. (Redrawn with permission from Sirveaux F, Favard L, Oudet D, Huquet D, Walch G, Mole D. Grammont inverted total shoulder arthroplasty in the treatment of glenohumeral osteoarthritis with massive rupture of the cuff. Results of a multicentre study of 80 shoulders. *J Bone Joint Surg Br.* 2004;86:388-395.)

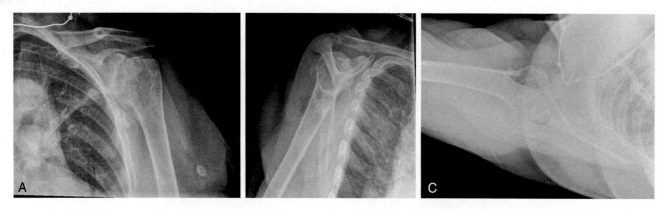

FIGURE 6.26 Standard shoulder x-ray series. **A**, Anteroposterior (AP) Grashey view, (**B**) outlet view, and (**C**) axillary view.

In reviewing the reliability of these classification schemes for CTA, Iannotti et al[105] noted radiographic criteria to be most important relative to superior humeral head migration and escape. Inclusion of clinical data such as patient age, degree of active elevation, and presence of pseudoparalysis improved the utilization of the radiographic-based classification schemes. Importantly, these classifications are based on a continuous spectrum of disease pathology, so classification of discrete grades within the spectrum makes it difficult for agreement among evaluators. Quality radiographs and advanced imaging may help improve the reliabilities.

AUTHOR'S PREFERRED APPROACH

The case example shown is a 75-year-old female presenting with OA and consideration for reverse TSA. Our preferred preoperative evaluation for shoulder arthroplasty patients always begins with plain x-rays. The standard shoulder series includes an AP Grashey view, outlet view, and axillary view (**FIGURE 6.26**). The AP Grashey view allows us to assess for narrowing of the glenohumeral joint space and acromiohumeral space. Acromiohumeral space of less than 7 mm may indicate rotator cuff tearing, which in some cases may need to be worked up with an MRI prior to surgery. We also use this view to assess the beta angle indicating the amount of inclination of the glenoid, which may need to be addressed at the time of surgery (**FIGURE 6.27**). In cases of RCT arthropathy, the shoulder is graded using the Hamada and Sirveaux classification from this view as well. The outlet view allows us to assess the angulation and slope of the acromion and may show an os acromiale. The axillary view is used to further assess glenohumeral joint space narrowing and get a feel for posterior humeral subluxation and the Walch type. We usually use this view to measure posterior subluxation of the humeral head (**FIGURE 6.28**) but do not make an

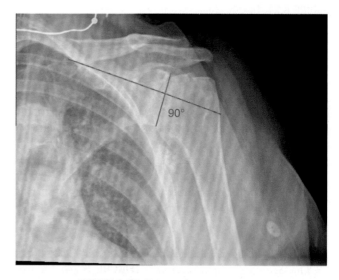

FIGURE 6.27 Beta angle measurement.

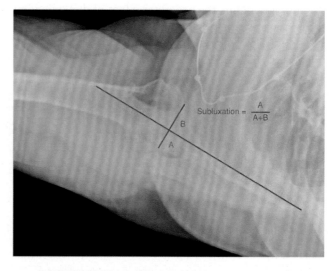

FIGURE 6.28 Humeral head subluxation measurement.

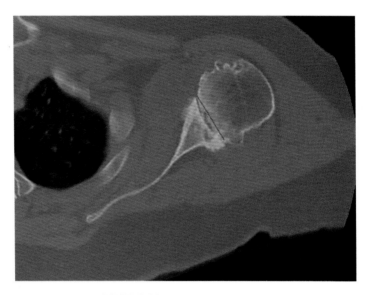

FIGURE 6.29 Walch type A2 glenoid.

official version measurement as it has been shown to be less accurate than CT measurements.

Secondary evaluation routinely includes a CT scan using a protocol with 1 mm cuts in the plane of the scapula. This allows us to later incorporate the CT data into preoperative planning software, which is the final measurement and planning stage. From the 2D axial CT image, a final grade of the glenoid using the modified Walch classification is determined. In this case, the glenoid is a Walch type A2, as a line drawn from the anterior to posterior edge of the glenoid intersects the humeral head. The head is also centered within the glenoid **(FIGURE 6.29)**. We then use the Friedman method to calculate glenoid version **(FIGURE 6.30)**. Evaluation of rotator muscle atrophy can be evaluated on the CT as well.

Finally, we move to the preoperative planning software, which allows us to evaluate 3D as well as 2D images. Here, a final assessment of version and inclination is made based on Friedman line during the CT segmentation process **(FIGURE 6.31)**. Notice the version measurement of 10° is slightly higher than the measurement on the 2D CT which was 6°. We also assess vault depth and determine the best fit for implants **(FIGURE 6.32)**. Finally, reaming depth and bone loss can be determined in cases where eccentric reaming or augmented implants are being considered.

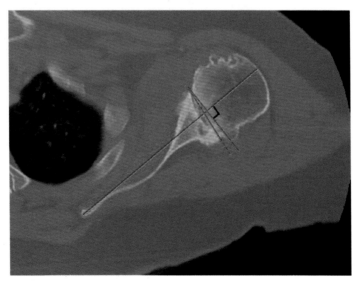

FIGURE 6.30 Glenoid version measurement using Friedman method.

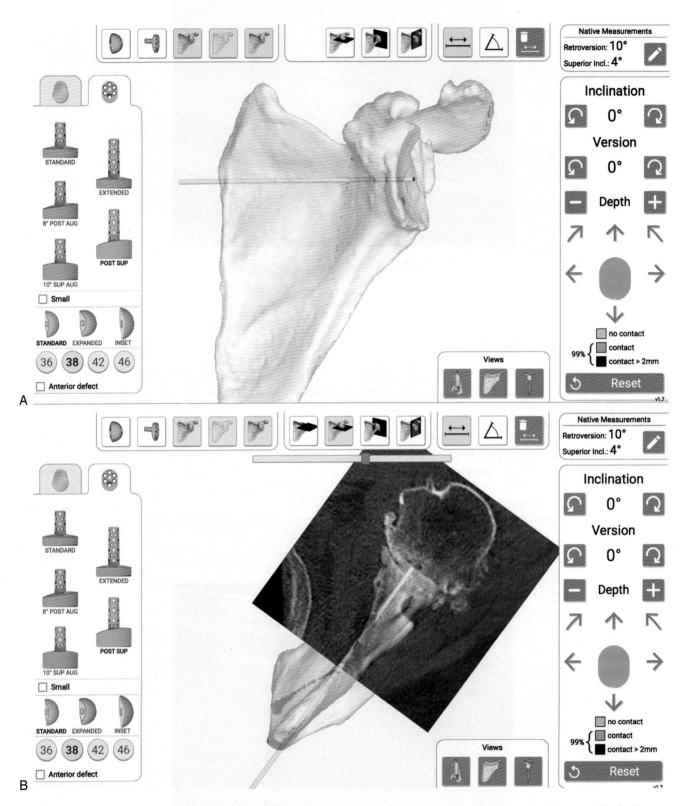

FIGURE 6.31 A and B, Three-dimensional (3D) image from preoperative planning software showing Friedman line. Version and inclination are shown in the top right corner.

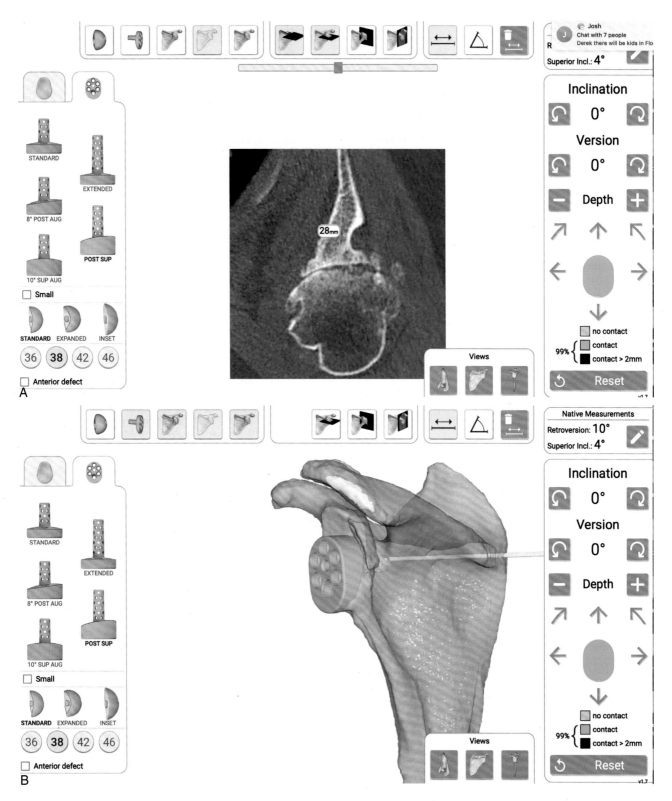

FIGURE 6.32 A, Vault depth measurement. **B**, Final implant placement.

REFERENCES

1. Hasan SS, Leith JM, Campbell B, Kapil R, Smith KL, Matsen FA III. Characteristics of unsatisfactory shoulder arthroplasties. *J Shoulder Elbow Surg.* 2002;11(5):431-441. doi:10.1067/mse.2002.125806

2. Farron A, Terrier A, Büchler P. Risks of loosening of a prosthetic glenoid implanted in retroversion. *J Shoulder Elbow Surg.* 2006;15(4):521-526. doi:10.1016/j.jse.2005.10.003

3. Ho JC, Sabesan VJ, Iannotti JP. Glenoid component retroversion is associated with osteolysis. *J Bone Joint Surg Am.* 2013;95(12):e82. doi:10.2106/JBJS.L.00336

4. Shapiro TA, McGarry MH, Gupta R, Lee YS, Lee TQ. Biomechanical effects of glenoid retroversion in total shoulder arthroplasty. *J Shoulder Elbow Surg.* 2007;16(3 suppl):S90-S95. doi:10.1016/j.jse.2006.07.010

5. Goud A, Segal D, Hedayati P, Pan JJ, Weissman BN. Radiographic evaluation of the shoulder. *Eur J Radiol.* 2008;68(1):2-15. doi:10.1016/j.ejrad.2008.02.023

6. Apple AS, Pedowitz RA, Speer KP. The weighted abduction Grashey shoulder method. *Radiol Technol.* 1997;69(2):151-156.

7. Ebraheim NA, Mekhail AO, Haman SP. Axillary view of the glenoid articular surface. *J Shoulder Elbow Surg.* 2000;9(2):115-119.

8. Sears BW, Johnston PS, Ramsey ML, Williams GR. Glenoid bone loss in primary total shoulder arthroplasty: evaluation and management. *J Am Acad Orthop Surg.* 2012;20(9):604-613. doi:10.5435/JAAOS-20-09-604

9. Nyffeler RW, Jost B, Pfirrmann CW, Gerber C. Measurement of glenoid version: conventional radiographs versus computed tomography scans. *J Shoulder Elbow Surg.* 2003;12(5):493-496. doi:10.1016/s1058-2746(03)00181-2

10. Friedman RJ, Hawthorne KB, Genez BM. The use of computerized tomography in the measurement of glenoid version. *J Bone Joint Surg Am.* 1992;74(7):1032-1037.

11. Hoenecke HR Jr, Hermida JC, Flores-Hernandez C, D'Lima DD. Accuracy of CT-based measurements of glenoid version for total shoulder arthroplasty. *J Shoulder Elbow Surg.* 2010;19(2):166-171. doi:10.1016/j.jse.2009.08.009

12. Zale CL, Pace GI, Lewis GS, Chan J, Kim HM. Interdepartmental imaging protocol for clinically based three-dimensional computed tomography can provide accurate measurement of glenoid version. *J Shoulder Elbow Surg.* 2018;27(7):1297-1305. doi:10.1016/j.jse.2017.11.020

13. Budge MD, Lewis GS, Schaefer E, Coquia S, Flemming DJ, Armstrong AD. Comparison of standard two-dimensional and three-dimensional corrected glenoid version measurements. *J Shoulder Elbow Surg.* 2011;20(4):577-583. doi:10.1016/j.jse.2010.11.003

14. Bokor DJ, O'Sullivan MD, Hazan GJ. Variability of measurement of glenoid version on computed tomography scan. *J Shoulder Elbow Surg.* 1999;8(6):595-598. doi:10.1016/s1058-2746(99)90096-4

15. Chalmers PN, Salazar D, Chamberlain A, Keener JD. Radiographic characterization of the B2 glenoid: the effect of computed tomographic axis orientation. *J Shoulder Elbow Surg.* 2017;26(2):258-264. doi:10.1016/j.jse.2016.07.021

16. van de Bunt F, Pearl ML, Lee EK, Peng L, Didomenico P. Glenoid version by CT scan: an analysis of clinical measurement error and introduction of a protocol to reduce variability. *Skeletal Radiol.* 2015;44(11):1627-1635. doi:10.1007/s00256-015-2207-4

17. Kubicka AM, Stefaniak J, Lubiatowski P, et al. Reliability of measurements performed on two dimensional and three dimensional computed tomography in glenoid assessment for instability. *Int Orthop.* 2016;40(12):2581-2588. doi:10.1007/s00264-016-3253-9

18. Magarelli N, Milano G, Baudi P, et al. Comparison between 2D and 3D computed tomography evaluation of glenoid bone defect in unilateral anterior gleno-humeral instability. *Radiol Med.* 2012;117(1):102-111. doi:10.1007/s11547-011-0712-7

19. Scalise JJ, Codsi MJ, Bryan J, Brems JJ, Iannotti JP. The influence of three-dimensional computed tomography images of the shoulder in preoperative planning for total shoulder arthroplasty. *J Bone Joint Surg Am.* 2008;90(11):2438-2445. doi:10.2106/JBJS.G.01341

20. Lombardo DJ, Khan J, Prey B, Zhang L, Petersen-Fitts GR, Sabesan VJ. Quantitative assessment and characterization of glenoid bone loss in a spectrum of patients with glenohumeral osteoarthritis. *Musculoskelet Surg.* 2016;100(3):179-185. doi:10.1007/s12306-016-0406-3

21. Werner BS, Hudek R, Burkhart KJ, Gohlke F. The influence of three-dimensional planning on decision-making in total shoulder arthroplasty. *J Shoulder Elbow Surg.* 2017;26(8):1477-1483. doi:10.1016/j.jse.2017.01.006

22. Moineau G, Levigne C, Boileau P, Young A, Walch G; French Society for Shoulder & Elbow (SOFEC). Three-dimensional measurement method of arthritic glenoid cavity morphology: feasibility and reproducibility. *Orthop Traumatol Surg Res.* 2012;98(6 suppl):S139-S145. doi:10.1016/j.otsr.2012.06.007

23. Raymond AC, McCann PA, Sarangi PP. Magnetic resonance scanning vs axillary radiography in the assessment of glenoid version for osteoarthritis. *J Shoulder Elbow Surg.* 2013;22(8):1078-1083. doi:10.1016/j.jse.2012.10.036

24. Kopka M, Fourman M, Soni A, Cordle AC, Lin A. Can glenoid wear be accurately assessed using x-ray imaging? Evaluating agreement of x-ray and magnetic resonance imaging (MRI) Walch classification. *J Shoulder Elbow Surg.* 2017;26(9):1527-1532. doi:10.1016/j.jse.2017.03.014

25. Gyftopoulos S, Hasan S, Bencardino J, et al. Diagnostic accuracy of MRI in the measurement of glenoid bone loss. *AJR Am J Roentgenol.* 2012;199(4):873-878. doi:10.2214/AJR.11.7639

26. Lee RK, Griffith JF, Tong MM, Sharma N, Yung P. Glenoid bone loss: assessment with MR imaging. *Radiology.* 2013;267(2):496-502. doi:10.1148/radiol.12121681

27. Lowe JT, Testa EJ, Li X, Miller S, DeAngelis JP, Jawa A. Magnetic resonance imaging is comparable to computed tomography for determination of glenoid version but does not accurately distinguish between Walch B2 and C classifications. *J Shoulder Elbow Surg.* 2017;26(4):669-673. doi:10.1016/j.jse.2016.09.024

28. Nowak DD, Bahu MJ, Gardner TR, et al. Simulation of surgical glenoid resurfacing using three-dimensional computed tomography of the arthritic glenohumeral joint: the amount of glenoid retroversion that can be corrected. *J Shoulder Elbow Surg.* 2009;18(5):680-688. doi:10.1016/j.jse.2009.03.019

29. Allred JJ, Flores-Hernandez C, Hoenecke HR Jr, D'Lima DD. Posterior augmented glenoid implants require less bone removal and generate lower stresses: a finite element analysis. *J Shoulder Elbow Surg.* 2016;25(5):823-830. doi:10.1016/j.jse.2015.10.003

30. Simovitch RW, Zumstein MA, Lohri E, Helmy N, Gerber C. Predictors of scapular notching in patients managed with the Delta III reverse total shoulder replacement. *J Bone Joint Surg Am.* 2007;89(3):588-600. doi:10.2106/JBJS.F.00226

31. Roche CP, Marczuk Y, Wright TW, et al. Scapular notching and osteophyte formation after reverse shoulder replacement: radiological analysis of implant position in male and female patients. *Bone Joint J.* 2013;95-B(4):530-535. doi:10.1302/0301-620X.95B4.30442

32. Nyffeler RW, Werner CM, Gerber C. Biomechanical relevance of glenoid component positioning in the reverse Delta III total shoulder prosthesis. *J Shoulder Elbow Surg.* 2005;14(5):524-528. doi:10.1016/j.jse.2004.09.010

33. Friedman R, Stroud N, Glattke K, et al. The impact of posterior wear on reverse shoulder glenoid fixation. *Bull Hosp Jt Dis (2013).* 2015;73(suppl 1):S15-S20.

34. Randelli M, Gambrioli PL. Glenohumeral osteometry by computed tomography in normal and unstable shoulders. *Clin Orthop Relat Res.* 1986;(208):151-156.

35. Rouleau DM, Kidder JF, Pons-Villanueva J, Dynamidis S, Defranco M, Walch G. Glenoid version: how to measure it? Validity of different methods in two-dimensional computed tomography scans. *J Shoulder Elbow Surg.* 2010;19(8):1230-1237. doi:10.1016/j.jse.2010.01.027

36. Poon PC, Ting FS. A 2-dimensional glenoid vault method for measuring glenoid version on computed tomography. *J Shoulder Elbow Surg.* 2012;21(3):329-335. doi:10.1016/j.jse.2011.04.006

37. Cunningham G, Freebody J, Smith MM, et al. Comparative analysis of 2 glenoid version measurement methods in variable axial slices on 3-dimensionally reconstructed computed tomography scans. *J Shoulder Elbow Surg.* 2018;27(10):1809-1815. doi:10.1016/j.jse.2018.03.016

38. Kwon YW, Powell KA, Yum JK, Brems JJ, Iannotti JP. Use of three-dimensional computed tomography for the analysis of the glenoid anatomy. *J Shoulder Elbow Surg.* 2005;14(1):85-90. doi:10.1016/j.jse.2004.04.011

39. Beuckelaers E, Jacxsens M, Van Tongel A, De Wilde LF. Three-dimensional computed tomography scan evaluation of the pattern of erosion in type B glenoids. *J Shoulder Elbow Surg.* 2014;23(1):109-116. doi:10.1016/j.jse.2013.04.009

40. Hughes RE, Bryant CR, Hall JM, et al. Glenoid inclination is associated with full-thickness rotator cuff tears. *Clin Orthop Relat Res.* 2003;(407):86-91. doi:10.1097/00003086-200302000-00016

41. Kandemir U, Allaire RB, Jolly JT, Debski RE, McMahon PJ. The relationship between the orientation of the glenoid and tears of the rotator cuff. *J Bone Joint Surg Br.* 2006;88(8):1105-1109. doi:10.1302/0301-620X.88B8.17732

42. Chalmers PN, Beck L, Granger E, Henninger H, Tashjian RZ. Superior glenoid inclination and rotator cuff tears. *J Shoulder Elbow Surg.* 2018;27(8):1444-1450. doi:10.1016/j.jse.2018.02.043

43. Wong AS, Gallo L, Kuhn JE, Carpenter JE, Hughes RE. The effect of glenoid inclination on superior humeral head migration. *J Shoulder Elbow Surg.* 2003;12(4):360-364. doi:10.1016/s1058-2746(03)00026-0

44. Bishop JL, Kline SK, Aalderink KJ, Zauel R, Bey MJ. Glenoid inclination: in vivo measures in rotator cuff tear patients and associations with superior glenohumeral joint translation. *J Shoulder Elbow Surg.* 2009;18(2):231-236. doi:10.1016/j.jse.2008.08.002

45. Strauss EJ, Roche C, Flurin PH, Wright T, Zuckerman JD. The glenoid in shoulder arthroplasty. *J Shoulder Elbow Surg.* 2009;18(5):819-833. doi:10.1016/j.jse.2009.05.008

46. Hopkins AR, Hansen UN, Amis AA, Emery R. The effects of glenoid component alignment variations on cement mantle stresses in total shoulder arthroplasty. *J Shoulder Elbow Surg.* 2004;13(6):668-675. doi:10.1016/S1058274604001399

47. Konrad GG, Markmiller M, Jolly JT, et al. Decreasing glenoid inclination improves function in shoulders with simulated massive rotator cuff tears. *Clin Biomech.* 2006;21(9):942-949. doi:10.1016/j.clinbiomech.2006.04.013

48. Oosterom R, Rozing PM, Bersee HE. Effect of glenoid component inclination on its fixation and humeral head subluxation in total shoulder arthroplasty. *Clin Biomech.* 2004;19(10):1000-1008. doi:10.1016/j.clinbiomech.2004.07.001

49. Terrier A, Merlini F, Pioletti DP, Farron A. Total shoulder arthroplasty: downward inclination of the glenoid component to balance supraspinatus deficiency. *J Shoulder Elbow Surg.* 2009;18(3):360-365. doi:10.1016/j.jse.2008.11.002

50. Gerber C, Pennington SD, Nyffeler RW. Reverse total shoulder arthroplasty. *J Am Acad Orthop Surg.* 2009;17(5):284-295. doi:10.5435/00124635-200905000-00003

51. Maurer A, Fucentese SF, Pfirrmann CW, et al. Assessment of glenoid inclination on routine clinical radiographs and computed tomography examinations of the shoulder. *J Shoulder Elbow Surg.* 2012;21(8):1096-1103. doi:10.1016/j.jse.2011.07.010

52. Daggett M, Werner B, Gauci MO, Chaoui J, Walch G. Comparison of glenoid inclination angle using different clinical imaging modalities. *J Shoulder Elbow Surg.* 2016;25(2):180-185. doi:10.1016/j.jse.2015.07.001

53. Boileau P, Gauci MO, Wagner ER, et al. The reverse shoulder arthroplasty angle: a new measurement of glenoid inclination for reverse shoulder arthroplasty. *J Shoulder Elbow Surg.* 2019;28(7):1281-1290. doi:10.1016/j.jse.2018.11.074

54. Neer CS II, Watson KC, Stanton FJ. Recent experience in total shoulder replacement. *J Bone Joint Surg Am.* 1982;64(3):319-337.

55. Papilion JA, Shall LM. Fluoroscopic evaluation for subtle shoulder instability. *Am J Sports Med.* 1992;20(5):548-552. doi:10.1177/036354659202000511

56. Walch G, Boulahia A, Boileau P, Kempf JF. Primary glenohumeral osteoarthritis: clinical and radiographic classification. The Aequalis Group. *Acta Orthop Belg.* 1998;64(suppl 2):46-52.

57. Sabesan VJ, Callanan M, Youderian A, Iannotti JP. 3D CT assessment of the relationship between humeral head alignment and glenoid retroversion in glenohumeral osteoarthritis. *J Bone Joint Surg Am.* 2014;96(8):e64. doi:10.2106/JBJS.L.00856

58. Jacxsens M, Van Tongel A, Henninger HB, Tashjian RZ, De Wilde L. The three-dimensional glenohumeral subluxation index in primary osteoarthritis of the shoulder. *J Shoulder Elbow Surg.* 2017;26(5):878-887. doi:10.1016/j.jse.2016.09.049

59. Jacxsens M, Karns MR, Henninger HB, Drew AJ, Van Tongel A, De Wilde L. Guidelines for humeral subluxation cutoff values: a comparative study between conventional, reoriented, and three-dimensional computed tomography scans of healthy shoulders. *J Shoulder Elbow Surg.* 2018;27(1):36-43. doi:10.1016/j.jse.2017.06.005

60. Gerber C, Costouros JG, Sukthankar A, Fucentese SF. Static posterior humeral head subluxation and total shoulder arthroplasty. *J Shoulder Elbow Surg.* 2009;18(4):505-510. doi:10.1016/j.jse.2009.03.003

61. Terrier A, Ston J, Farron A. Importance of a three-dimensional measure of humeral head subluxation in osteoarthritic shoulders. *J Shoulder Elbow Surg.* 2015;24(2):295-301. doi:10.1016/j.jse.2014.05.027

62. Walch G, Ascani C, Boulahia A, Nové-Josserand L, Edwards TB. Static posterior subluxation of the humeral head: an unrecognized entity responsible for glenohumeral osteoarthritis in the young adult. *J Shoulder Elbow Surg.* 2002;11(4):309-314. doi:10.1067/mse.2002.124547

63. Domos P, Checchia CS, Walch G. Walch B0 glenoid: preosteoarthritic posterior subluxation of the humeral head. *J Shoulder Elbow Surg.* 2018;27(1):181-188. doi:10.1016/j.jse.2017.08.014

64. von Eisenhart-Rothe RM, Jäger A, Englmeier KH, Vogl TJ, Graichen H. Relevance of arm position and muscle activity on three-dimensional glenohumeral translation in patients with traumatic and atraumatic shoulder instability. *Am J Sports Med.* 2002;30(4):514-522. doi:10.1177/03635465020300041101

65. von Eisenhart-Rothe R, Müller-Gerbl M, Wiedemann E, Englmeier KH, Graichen H. Functional malcentering of the humeral head and asymmetric long-term stress on the glenoid: potential reasons for glenoid loosening in total shoulder arthroplasty. *J Shoulder Elbow Surg.* 2008;17(5):695-702. doi:10.1016/j.jse.2008.02.00

66. Iannotti JP, Norris TR. Influence of preoperative factors on outcome of shoulder arthroplasty for glenohumeral osteoarthritis. *J Bone Joint Surg Am.* 2003;85(2):251-258. doi:10.2106/00004623-200302000-00011

67. Walch G, Moraga C, Young A, Castellanos-Rosas J. Results of anatomic nonconstrained prosthesis in primary osteoarthritis with biconcave glenoid. *J Shoulder Elbow Surg.* 2012;21(11):1526-1533. doi:10.1016/j.jse.2011.11.030

68. Habermeyer P, Magosch P, Lichtenberg S. Recentering the humeral head for glenoid deficiency in total shoulder arthroplasty. *Clin Orthop Relat Res.* 2007;457:124-132. doi:10.1097/BLO.0b013e31802ff03c

69. Ho JC, Amini MH, Entezari V, et al. Clinical and radiographic outcomes of a posteriorly augmented glenoid component in anatomic total shoulder arthroplasty for primary osteoarthritis with posterior glenoid bone loss. *J Bone Joint Surg Am.* 2018;100(22):1934-1948. doi:10.2106/JBJS.17.01282

70. Grey SG, Wright TW, Flurin PH, Zuckerman JD, Roche CP, Friedman RJ. Clinical and radiographic outcomes with a posteriorly augmented glenoid for Walch B glenoids in anatomic total shoulder arthroplasty. *J Shoulder Elbow Surg.* 2020;29:e185-e195. doi:10.1016/j.jse.2019.10.008

71. Mizuno N, Denard PJ, Raiss P, Walch G. Reverse total shoulder arthroplasty for primary glenohumeral osteoarthritis in patients with a biconcave glenoid. *J Bone Joint Surg Am.* 2013;95(14):1297-1304. doi:10.2106/JBJS.L.00820

72. Nyffeler RW, Werner CM, Sukthankar A, Schmid MR, Gerber C. Association of a large lateral extension of the acromion with rotator cuff tears. *J Bone Joint Surg Am.* 2006;88(4):800-805. doi:10.2106/JBJS.D.03042

73. Moor BK, Wieser K, Slankamenac K, Gerber C, Bouaicha S. Relationship of individual scapular anatomy and degenerative rotator cuff tears. *J Shoulder Elbow Surg.* 2014;23(4):536-541. doi:10.1016/j.jse.2013.11.008

74. Moor BK, Bouaicha S, Rothenfluh DA, Sukthankar A, Gerber C. Is there an association between the individual anatomy of the scapula and the development of rotator cuff tears or osteoarthritis of the glenohumeral joint? A radiological study of the critical shoulder angle. *Bone Joint Lett J.* 2013;95-B(7):935-941. doi:10.1302/0301-620X.95B7.31028

75. Heuberer PR, Plachel F, Willinger L, et al. Critical shoulder angle combined with age predict five shoulder pathologies: a retrospective analysis of 1000 cases. *BMC Musculoskelet Disord.* 2017;18(1):259. doi:10.1186/s12891-017-1559-4

76. Mantell MT, Nelson R, Lowe JT, Endrizzi DP, Jawa A. Critical shoulder angle is associated with full-thickness rotator cuff tears in patients with glenohumeral osteoarthritis. *J Shoulder Elbow Surg.* 2017;26(12):e376-e381. doi:10.1016/j.jse.2017.05.020

77. Blonna D, Giani A, Bellato E, et al. Predominance of the critical shoulder angle in the pathogenesis of degenerative diseases of the shoulder. *J Shoulder Elbow Surg.* 2016;25(8):1328-1336. doi:10.1016/j.jse.2015.11.059

78. Daggett M, Werner B, Collin P, Gauci MO, Chaoui J, Walch G. Correlation between glenoid inclination and critical shoulder angle: a radiographic and computed tomography study. *J Shoulder Elbow Surg.* 2015;24(12):1948-1953. doi:10.1016/j.jse.2015.07.013

79. Li X, Olszewski N, Abdul-Rassoul H, Curry EJ, Galvin JW, Eichinger JK. Relationship between the critical shoulder angle and shoulder disease. *JBJS Rev.* 2018;6(8):e1. doi:10.2106/JBJS.RVW.17.00161

80. Engelhardt C, Farron A, Becce F, Place N, Pioletti DP, Terrier A. Effects of glenoid inclination and acromion index on humeral head translation and glenoid articular cartilage strain. *J Shoulder Elbow Surg.* 2017;26(1):157-164. doi:10.1016/j.jse.2016.05.031

81. Watling JP, Sanchez JE, Heilbroner SP, Levine WN, Bigliani LU, Jobin CM. Glenoid component loosening associated with increased critical shoulder angle at midterm follow-up. *J Shoulder Elbow Surg.* 2018;27(3):449-454. doi:10.1016/j.jse.2017.10.002

82. Garcia GH, Liu JN, Degen RM, et al. Higher critical shoulder angle increases the risk of retear after rotator cuff repair. *J Shoulder Elbow Surg.* 2017;26(2):241-245. doi:10.1016/j.jse.2016.07.009. Published correction appears in *J Shoulder Elbow Surg.* 2017;26(4):732.

83. Beeler S, Hasler A, Getzmann J, Weigelt L, Meyer DC, Gerber C. Acromial roof in patients with concentric osteoarthritis and massive rotator cuff tears: multiplanar analysis of 115 computed tomography scans. *J Shoulder Elbow Surg.* 2018;27(10):1866-1876. doi:10.1016/j.jse.2018.03.014

84. Meyer DC, Riedo S, Eckers F, Carpeggiani G, Jentzsch T, Gerber C. Small anteroposterior inclination of the acromion is a predictor for posterior glenohumeral erosion (B2 or C). *J Shoulder Elbow Surg.* 2019;28(1):22-27. doi:10.1016/j.jse.2018.05.041

85. Codsi MJ, Bennetts C, Gordiev K, et al. Normal glenoid vault anatomy and validation of a novel glenoid implant shape. *J Shoulder Elbow Surg.* 2008;17(3):471-478. doi:10.1016/j.jse.2007.08.010

86. Scalise JJ, Bryan J, Polster J, Brems JJ, Iannotti JP. Quantitative analysis of glenoid bone loss in osteoarthritis using three-dimensional computed tomography scans. *J Shoulder Elbow Surg.* 2008; 17: 328-335. doi:10.1016/j.jse.2007.07.013

87. Scalise JJ, Codsi MJ, Bryan J, Iannotti JP. The three-dimensional glenoid vault model can estimate normal glenoid version in osteoarthritis. *J Shoulder Elbow Surg.* 2008;17(3):487-491. doi:10.1016/j.jse.2007.09.006

88. Ganapathi A, McCarron JA, Chen X, Iannotti JP. Predicting normal glenoid version from the pathologic scapula: a comparison of 4 methods in 2- and 3-dimensional models. *J Shoulder Elbow Surg.* 2011;20(2):234-244. doi:10.1016/j.jse.2010.05.024

89. Ricchetti ET, Hendel MD, Collins DN, Iannotti JP. Is premorbid glenoid anatomy altered in patients with glenohumeral osteoarthritis? *Clin Orthop Relat Res.* 2013;471(9):2932-2939. doi:10.1007/s11999-013-3069-5

90. Verstraeten TR, Deschepper E, Jacxsens M, Walravens S, De Coninck B, De Wilde LF. Operative guidelines for the reconstruction of the native glenoid plane: an anatomic three-dimensional computed tomography-scan reconstruction study. *J Shoulder Elbow Surg.* 2012;21(11):1565-1572. doi:10.1016/j.jse.2011.10.030

91. Walch G, Badet R, Boulahia A, Khoury A. Morphologic study of the glenoid in primary glenohumeral osteoarthritis. *J Arthroplasty.* 1999;13:756-760.

92. Scalise JJ, Codsi MJ, Brems JJ, Iannotti JP. Inter-rater reliability of an arthritic glenoid morphology classification system. *J Shoulder Elbow Surg.* 2008;17:575-577. doi:10.1016/j.jse.2007.12.006

93. Nowak DD, Gardner TR, Bigliani LU, Levine WN, Ahmad CS. Interobserver and intraobserver reliability of the Walch classification in primary glenohumeral arthritis. *J Shoulder Elbow Surg.* 2010;19:180-183. doi:10.1016/j.jse.2009.08.003

94. Kidder JF, Rouleau DM, DeFranco MJ, Pons-Villanueva J, Dynamidis S. Revisited: Walch classification of the glenoid in glenohumeral osteoarthritis. *Shoulder Elbow.* 2012;4:11-15. doi:10.1111/j.1758-5740.2011.00151.x

95. Aronowitz JG, Harmsen WS, Schleck CD, Sperling JW, Cofield RH, Sánchez-Sotelo J. Radiographs and computed tomography scans show similar observer agreement when classifying glenoid morphology in glenohumeral arthritis. *J Shoulder Elbow Surg.* 2017;26(9):1533-1538. doi:10.1016/j.jse.2017.02.015

96. Bercik MJ, Kruse K II, Yalizis M, Gauci MO, Chaoui J, Walch G. A modification to the Walch classification of the glenoid in primary glenohumeral osteoarthritis using three-dimensional imaging. *J Shoulder Elbow Surg.* 2016;25(10):1601-1606. doi:10.1016/j.jse.2016.03.010. PMID: 27282738.

97. Shukla DR, McLaughlin RJ, Lee J, Cofield RH, Sperling JW, Sánchez-Sotelo J. Intraobserver and interobserver reliability of the modified Walch classification using radiographs and computed tomography. *J Shoulder Elbow Surg.* 2019;28(4):625-630. doi:10.1016/j.jse.2018.09.021. PMID: 30528438.

98. Iannotti JP, Greeson C, Downing D, Sabesan V, Bryan JA. Effect of glenoid deformity on glenoid component placement in primary shoulder arthroplasty. *J Shoulder Elbow Surg.* 2012;21(1):48-55. doi:10.1016/j.jse.2011.02.011

99. Knowles NK, Ferreira LM, Athwal GS. Premorbid retroversion is significantly greater in type B2 glenoids. *J Shoulder Elbow Surg.* 2016;25(7):1064-1068. doi:10.1016/j.jse.2015.11.002

100. Matsen FA II, Whitson A, Hsu JE, Stankovic NK, Neradilek MB, Somerson JS. Prearthroplasty glenohumeral pathoanatomy and its relationship to patient's sex, age, diagnosis, and self-assessed shoulder comfort and function. *J Shoulder Elbow Surg.* 2019;28(12):2290-2300. doi:10.1016/j.jse.2019.04.043

101. Chan K, Knowles NK, Chaoui J, et al. Characterization of the Walch B3 glenoid in primary osteoarthritis. *J Shoulder Elbow Surg.* 2017;26(5):909-914. doi:10.1016/j.jse.2016.10.003

102. Antuna SA, Sperling JW, Cofield RH, Rowland CM. Glenoid revision surgery after total shoulder arthroplasty. *J Shoulder Elbow Surg.* 2001;10:217-224.

103. Neer CS II, Craig EV, Fukuda H. Cuff-tear arthropathy. *J Bone Joint Surg Am.* 1983;65(9):1232-1244.

104. Hamada K, Fukuda H, Mikasa M, Kobayashi Y. Roentgenographic findings in massive rotator cuff tears. A long-term observation. *Clin Orthop Relat Res.* 1990;(254):92-96.

105. Kappe T, Cakir B, Reichel H, Elsharkawi M. Reliability of radiologic classification for cuff tear arthropathy. *J Shoulder Elbow Surg.* 2011;20(4):543-547. doi:10.1016/j.jse.2011.01.012

106. Iannotti JP, McCarron J, Raymond CJ, et al. Agreement study of radiographic classification of rotator cuff tear arthropathy. *J Shoulder Elbow Surg.* 2010;19(8):1243-1249. doi:10.1016/j.jse.2010.02.010

107. Visotsky JL, Basamania C, Seebauer L, Rockwood CA, Jensen KL. Cuff tear arthropathy: pathogenesis, classification, and algorithm for treatment. *J Bone Joint Surg Am.* 2004;86-A(suppl 2):35-40.

108. Favard L, Lautmann S, Sirveaux F, Oudet D, Kerjean Y, Huguet D. Hemiarthroplasty versus reverse arthroplasty in the treatment of osteoarthritis with massive rotator cuff tear. In: Walch G, Boileau

P, Molé D, eds. *2000 Shoulder Prostheses. Two to Ten Years Follow-up*. Sauramps Médical; 2001:261-268.

109. Sirveaux F, Favard L, Oudet D, Huquet D, Walch G, Mole D. Grammont inverted total shoulder arthroplasty in the treatment of glenohumeral osteoarthritis with massive rupture of the cuff. Results of a multicentre study of 80 shoulders. *J Bone Joint Surg Br.* 2004;86:388-395. doi:10.1302/0301-620X.86B3.14024

110. Lévigne C, Garret J, Boileau P, Alami G, Favard L, Walch G. Scapular notching in reverse shoulder arthroplasty: is it important to avoid it and how? *Clin Orthop Relat Res.* 2011;469(9):2512-2520

111. Abdic S, Knowles NK, Walch G, Johnson JA, Athwal GS. Type E2 glenoid bone loss orientation and management with augmented implants. *J Shoulder Elbow Surg.* 2020;29:1460-1469. doi:10.1016/j.jse.2019.11.009

112. Liuzza L. Roche C. Virk M. Zuckerman J. Outcomes using superior and posterior-superior augmented baseplates in reverse total shoulder arthroplasty for glenoid wear: short term follow up compared to match control. *J Shoulder Elbow Surg.* 2019;28(6):E214-E215. doi:10.1016/j.jse.2018.11.030

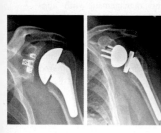

7 Decision-Making:
Anatomic or Reverse Shoulder Arthroplasty

Kevin M. Magone, MD and Joseph D. Zuckerman, MD

INTRODUCTION

In 2003, the first reverse shoulder prosthesis was approved in the United States. Prior to its approval, shoulder arthroplasty surgeons in the United States utilized hemiarthroplasty, resurfacing, and anatomic total shoulder arthroplasty (ATSA) for various etiologies. The classic indication for ATSA has been osteoarthritis. However, degenerative conditions with a deficient rotator cuff were typically treated with hemiarthroplasty because of the increased concern that abnormal glenohumeral motion and eccentric glenoid loading would result in subsequent component loosening.[1] Initially, the reverse shoulder prosthesis was approved for cuff tear arthropathy (CTA) in elderly, low-demand patients.[1-3] Since 2003, the use of shoulder arthroplasty, and in particular, reverse total shoulder arthroplasty (RTSA), has expanded considerably.[1-3] The initial narrow indications for RTSA were expanded based upon the initial successful results, evolving technology, and an increasing level of comfort with the procedure such that, currently, the majority of shoulder arthroplasties performed are of the reverse design.[1-3] The expanded indications for RTSA include massive irreparable rotator cuff tear without arthritis, rheumatoid and other inflammatory glenohumeral arthritis, tumor, acute fractures, posttraumatic arthritis, osteoarthritis with significant bone loss or deformity, and chronic glenohumeral dislocation.[1-3] In this chapter we will focus on clinical situations in which both ATSA and RTSA are treatment options and the factors to consider when determining the preferred approach.

OSTEOARTHRITIS WITH AN INTACT ROTATOR CUFF: ATSA

Osteoarthritis is the most common indication for an ATSA.[4,5] In the United States, one-third of the population have osteoarthritis, and the glenohumeral joint is the third most common joint to be replaced.[5,6] Outcome studies consistently report good and excellent outcomes following ATSA, and it is considered a successful treatment for end-stage glenohumeral arthritis.[5-12] The average age for a patient undergoing ATSA has decreased over the past decade and has been reported to be as low

as 64 years.[1,6] ATSA decreases pain, improves range of motion and function, and achieves high rates of patient satisfaction.[4-7,10,12] For patients with glenohumeral osteoarthritis and an intact rotator cuff, it is evident that ATSA is the preferred treatment (**FIGURE 7.1**).

The importance of an intact rotator cuff for a successful ATSA cannot be overemphasized, and identifying patients with rotator cuff tears or dysfunction is important in deciding whether ATSA is the best option. Of note, up to 10% of patients undergoing ATSA have rotator cuff tears.[5,7,9] If a patient has rotator cuff pathology, the supraspinatus tendon is typically involved with half of the tears partial thickness and half of the tears full thickness.[7-9] Simone et al reported on 33 ATSAs with simultaneous rotator cuff repair with an average follow-up of 5 years. Of the 33 shoulder replacements, 10 had small tears, 14 had medium tears, 9 had large tears, and none had massive tears.[9] While all patients reported improved pain, function, and satisfaction, those patients with small tears had greater improvement of forward elevation.[9] Six of the medium- and large-sized tears exhibited postoperative instability indicating that the rotator cuff repair did not heal.[9] Postoperative instability was not identified in the small tear group.[9] Therefore, smaller, isolated tears of the supraspinatus should not be considered a contraindication for ATSA.[7,9] However, in older patients with larger rotator cuff tears, RTSA would be the preferred option.[9] Livesey et al also retrospectively reviewed patients who underwent ATSA with concurrent rotator cuff repair. These authors reported on 45 procedures with a minimum follow-up of 2 years.[8] From this cohort, 31% had a poor result, while 18% required another operation.[8] This study provided further support for the use of RTSA in patients with glenohumeral arthritis and a larger concurrent rotator cuff tear even if the tear is repairable.

OSTEOARTHRITIS WITH INCREASING AGE: ATSA AND RTSA

As shoulder arthroplasty surgeons have become increasingly confident about the outcomes of RTSA, there has been a trend toward considering RTSA as the preferred option in patients with osteoarthritis and an intact

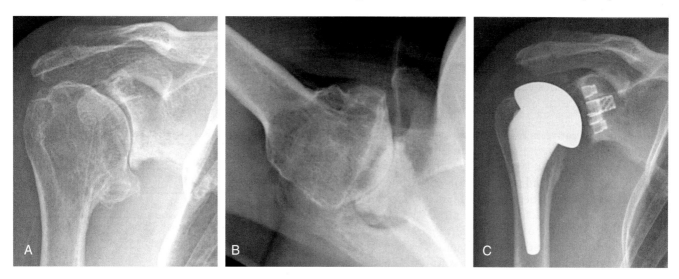

FIGURE 7.1 A and **B**, A 71-year-old woman with primary osteoarthritis of the right shoulder. Primary osteoarthritis is characterized by inferior humeral head and glenoid osteophytes, glenohumeral joint space narrowing, slight medial and posterior glenoid erosion (10° retroversion on axial CT scan), and the absence of humeral head superior migration. **C**, Anatomic shoulder replacement performed with metaphyseal fitting stem and hybrid all-polyethylene glenoid.

rotator cuff based primarily on increasing age. There is a general agreement that an ATSA requires an intact and functioning rotator cuff for a successful outcome. There is also a general agreement that as patients age, there is concurrent rotator cuff degeneration. There are situations in which a "structurally" intact rotator cuff may not be "functionally" intact, particularly after the manipulation that occurs during a shoulder arthroplasty. We have certainly encountered patients with ATSA, who at the time of surgery clearly had a structurally intact rotator cuff. However, postoperatively, these patients are unable to regain active range of motion and present with the clinical appearance of rotator cuff deficiency. This generally occurs in older patients in their 70s and 80s, and this situation has led to the question of whether RTSA is preferred for patients with osteoarthritis with an intact rotator cuff based solely on advancing age **(FIGURE 7.2)**.

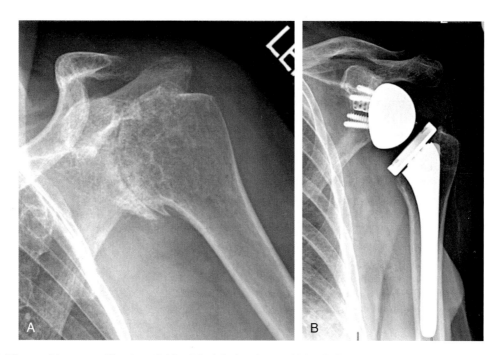

FIGURE 7.2 A, A 92-year-old woman with osteoarthritis of the left glenohumeral joint. **B**, Reverse total shoulder arthroplasty performed based primarily on patient age and potential for associated rotator cuff compromise.

Currently, there is no age-specific indication for RTSA in patients with glenohumeral arthritis and an intact rotator cuff. However, there is some literature that provides important information. Wright et al specifically compared ATSA and RTSA for the treatment of glenohumeral osteoarthritis with an intact cuff. In this series of 135 patients, all patients were older than 70 years and had preoperative active forward elevation of less than 90° despite imaging showing an intact cuff.[13] Of the 135 patients, 33 underwent RTSA and 102 underwent ATSA.[13] They found no differences in complication rates, revision rates, patient-reported outcomes, patient satisfaction, and pain scores.[13] Both groups reported a high level of satisfaction with a final range of motion that allowed performance of overhead activities.[13] The authors recommended an expanded role for RTSA in older patients with glenohumeral arthritis and an intact rotator cuff.[13] Furthermore, Brewley et al reported a retrospective cohort study of 1250 shoulder replacements, which included 518 ATSAs and 732 RTSAs.[14] With an average follow-up of 50 months, all shoulder replacements improved pain, function, and range of motion.[14] However, patients younger than 65 years with ATSAs and those younger than 60 years with RTSAs were noted to have higher revision rates.[14] ATSA had a three times higher and RTSA had a five times higher revision rate.[14] This study adds support that there may be an age indication for specific shoulder arthroplasty procedures.

To gain a more global perspective on the impact of age and the use of RTSA in patients with osteoarthritis and an intact rotator cuff, a multicenter international database was analyzed (Exactech, Gainesville, Florida). Specifically, this database included 2940 shoulder replacements performed between 2007 and 2018 in patients with glenohumeral arthritis and an intact rotator cuff **(TABLE 7.1)**. For ATSA, the mean age of the first 200 patients was 67.5 years; the mean age for the last 200 ATSA patients decreased to 65.5 years. For RTSA, the mean age of the first 200 patients was 74.6 years; the mean age for the last 200 RTSA patients decreased to 72.6 years. These data indicate that for patients with glenohumeral osteoarthritis and an intact rotator cuff, as experience with RTSA has increased, there is a trend toward reserving ATSA for younger patients and also performing RTSA in younger patients. Using this same database, patients undergoing ATSA and RTSA were subdivided based upon age. ATSA was more commonly performed in all age groups up to age 76 to 79 years, at which point the trend changed to RTSA. Based upon this database, in patients with glenohumeral osteoarthritis with an intact rotator cuff, RTSA is now being performed at a younger age and has become the preferred procedure in patients in the 76- to 79-year age group. Although there is no definitive age-specific indication currently, it is certainly an option in this patient population based upon surgeon assessment and preference.

TABLE 7.1 Age Distribution of 2940 ATSAs and RTSAs for Glenohumeral Osteoarthritis With an Intact Rotator Cuff in 3-Year Increments. RTSA Becomes More Commonly Utilized Beginning in the 76- to 79-Year Age Group

Age	RTSA	ATSA	ATSA and RTSA
<40	0	19	19
40-43	0	12	12
43-46	2	14	16
46-49	2	26	28
49-52	3	59	62
52-55	11	114	125
55-58	24	136	160
58-61	36	194	230
61-64	37	230	267
64-67	92	288	380
67-70	123	284	407
70-73	136	242	378
73-76	135	187	322
76-79	115	115	230
79-82	92	68	160
82-85	65	26	91
85-88	31	6	37
>88	13	3	16

ATSA, anatomic total shoulder arthroplasty; RTSA, reverse total shoulder arthroplasty.

CUFF TEAR ARTHROPATHY: RTSA

Approximately 4% of complete rotator cuff tears progress to CTA, which is characterized by superior migration of the humeral head leading to progressive degenerative changes of the glenoid, acromion, and humeral head.[15-17] The superior migration of the humeral head is caused by an unopposed pull of the deltoid due to an unbalanced force couple.[16] CTA is more common in elderly women and may present with the classically described "pseudoparalysis."[15,16] Prior to RTSA, hemiarthroplasty was utilized for CTA.[17] The initial indication for RTSA in the United States was CTA, and it is now the preferred treatment of choice.[15-21] The reverse prosthesis design creates a more distal and medial center of rotation, which allows the deltoid to restore arm elevation and abduction.[17,18,20] The outcomes of RTSA for CTA have been consistently successful and much improved compared with earlier results using hemiarthroplasty.[16,17,19-21]

These results with RTSA are sustained over long-term follow-up as Gerber et al recently reported. For 22 CTA patients treated with RTSA and a minimum 15 year follow-up, forward elevation improved from 53° to 101° and abduction improved from 55° to 86°.[19] Furthermore, RTSA for CTA has been noted to have greater improvement compared to RTSA performed for other glenohumeral pathologies.[16,17,20] For CTA, RTSA is clearly the preferred arthroplasty option (**FIGURE 7.3**).

MASSIVE IRREPARABLE ROTATOR CUFF TEAR WITHOUT ARTHRITIS: RTSA

Rotator cuff tears are commonly diagnosed with increasing patient age and often occur in the absence of glenohumeral arthritis.[22] Treatment options for patients with irreparable rotator cuff tears without arthritis have included débridement with or without subacromial decompression, tuberoplasty, biceps tenotomy or tenodesis, partial rotator cuff repair, and superior capsular reconstruction with varying levels of success.[22-26] Based upon the success of RTSA in patients with rotator cuff deficiency and glenohumeral arthritis, the indications for RTSA have been expanded to include massive, irreparable rotator cuff tears in the absence of arthritis. In this patient population, RTSA has proven to be very successful with implant survival greater than 90% at 10 years[22,24-26] (**FIGURE 7.4**).

Mulieri et al reported on 58 RTSAs for the treatment of irreparable rotator cuff tears without arthritis, of which 26 RTSAs had undergone previous rotator cuff repair.[26] At an average follow-up of 52 months, pain and function improved, even though some residual discomfort persisted.[26] Forward elevation improved from 53° to 134°, abduction improved from 49° to 125°, and external rotation improved from 27° to 51°.[26] However, there was a 20% complication rate.[26] Ernstbrunner et al also reported their experience with RTSA for the treatment of irreparable rotator cuff tears without arthritis. These authors retrospectively evaluated 23 RTSAs in 20 patients who were all younger than 60 years.[25] With an average follow-up of 12 years, forward elevation improved from 64° to 117° and abduction improved from 58° to 111°.[25] Additionally, strength, pain, and functional scores all improved, but the complication rate in this series was 39%.[25] Although most studies report good long-term outcomes, not all patients have shown clinical improvement.[22,23] Patients younger than 60 years, those with concurrent upper extremity neurologic dysfunction, and those with increased preoperative function have not gained as much clinical improvement.[22,23] This is particularly concerning with patients who have irreparable rotator cuff tears and also maintain very good active range of motion. In this challenging patient population, the indication for RTSA is pain relief. Before proceeding with surgery, it is important to discuss that the range of motion postoperatively may be less than the preoperative range and that the procedure is being done for pain relief. Although range of motion will be functional, it may be less than anticipated.

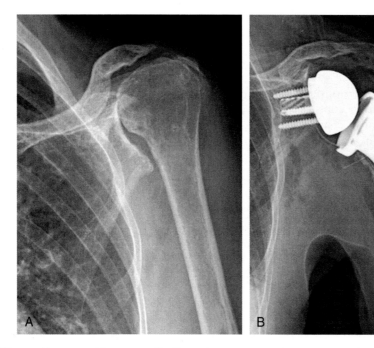

FIGURE 7.3 A, A 78-year-old woman with rotator cuff arthropathy characterized by superior migration of the humeral head, asymmetric superior erosion of the glenoid, acetabularization of the acromion, and femoralization of the humeral head. **B**, Reverse total shoulder arthroplasty performed with a diaphyseal fitting stem and a 10° superiorly augmented baseplate to address asymmetric superior glenoid erosion.

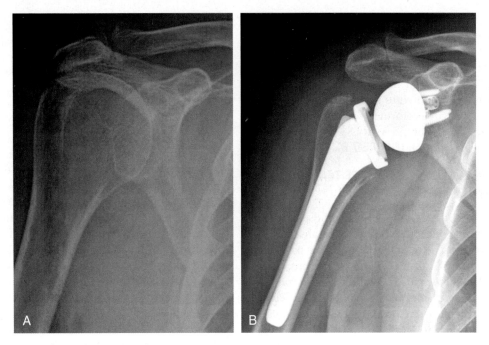

FIGURE 7.4 A, A 70-year-old woman with a massive irreparable rotator cuff tear following initial anterior dislocation followed by multiple recurrent episodes of instability. Superior migration of the humeral head is noted without significant arthritic changes. **B**, Treatment with reverse total shoulder arthroplasty addresses the massive rotator cuff tear and restores stability.

RHEUMATOID ARTHRITIS AND OTHER INFLAMMATORY CONDITIONS: ATSA AND RTSA

Early in the progression of rheumatoid arthritis (RA), the glenohumeral joint is typically spared. However, as the disease process progresses, the shoulder will become involved in most patients.[27] RA and other inflammatory conditions release proinflammatory mediators that not only destroy the articular surface but also impact the surrounding connective tissues including the rotator cuff.[27-31] Patients with RA and other inflammatory glenohumeral conditions typically have radiographs characterized by osteopenia, erosive changes of the humeral head and glenoid, superior migration consistent with rotator cuff compromise, and similar changes of the acromioclavicular joint.[28,30,32-34] These changes occur on a spectrum from mild to advanced. With the development of disease-modifying medications, the natural history of this disease can be altered. In patients with an intact rotator cuff and adequate bone stock, ATSA has been utilized with significant success, although outcomes are not as consistent as in patients with osteoarthritis **(FIGURE 7.5)**. Good to excellent outcomes are reported at 2-, 5-, and 10-year follow-up, while implant survivorship is reported to be 96.1% and 92.9% at 5 and 10 years.[27,28,32,35]

Most of the outcomes of ATSA in patients with RA were reported prior to the more extensive use of RTSA. With inflammatory conditions, ATSA is recognized to have an increased risk of soft-tissue complications including progressive subscapularis and rotator cuff dysfunction.[29,33] In patients with more advanced bone and soft-tissue changes, RTSA becomes a more important reconstructive option, which has shown similar good to excellent outcomes at short- and mid-term follow-up.[30,34,36] **(FIGURE 7.6)**. In patients with RA, RTSA revision-free survivorship has been reported to be 99% at both 2 and 5 years.[34,36]

For patients with RA and other inflammatory conditions that impact the glenohumeral joint, the degree of soft tissue and bony changes will be the primary factors determining whether ATSA or RTSA is the preferred option. However, other important factors such as patient age, activity level, expectations, and response to medical management will also influence treatment decisions. Fortunately, the availability of RTSA has expanded our ability to successfully treat shoulders compromised by RA and other inflammatory conditions.

OSTEOARTHRITIS WITH GLENOID DEFORMITY: ATSA AND RTSA

Glenohumeral osteoarthritis is associated with varying degrees of asymmetric posterior glenoid wear.[37-41] As the degenerative process progresses, the degree of posterior glenoid erosion and posterior humeral head subluxation increases along with a progressive loss of glenoid bone stock.[37-41] The combination of increasing glenoid retroversion and posterior humeral head subluxation makes it more challenging to achieve a stable construct with ATSA. In addition, the long-term survival of ATSA performed for osteoarthritis with significant posterior

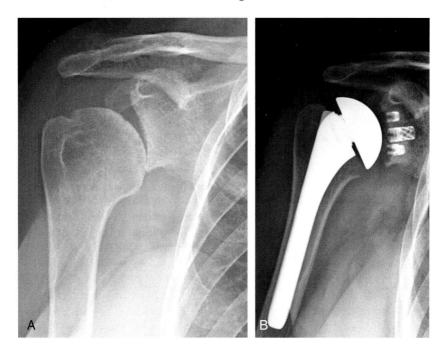

FIGURE 7.5 A, A 60-year-old woman with polyarticular rheumatoid arthritis. Shoulder radiographs characterized by the marginal erosions about the humeral head and glenoid, subchondral cyst, absence of osteophytes, and generalized osteopenia. **B**, Anatomic total shoulder arthroplasty with a diaphyseal fitting stem and all-polyethylene glenoid was performed due to limited bony erosion and an intact and well-functioning rotator cuff.

glenoid erosion has been shown to be less reliable because of glenoid component loosening and residual posterior subluxation.[38,40,41] Correcting glenoid retroversion to less than 10° will decrease the stress at the implant-cement-bone interfaces.[42,43] Correction of posterior subluxation is also essential to avoid eccentric loading of the implant as residual posterior subluxation has been noted to have inferior postoperative outcomes.[38,40-43]

ATSA can be successfully utilized in patients with posterior glenoid erosion and posterior humeral head

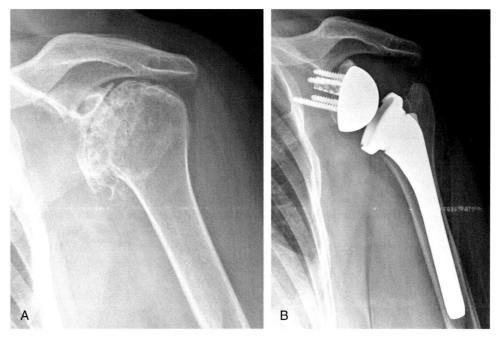

FIGURE 7.6 A, A 70-year-old woman with rheumatoid arthritis of the left shoulder. Rheumatoid arthritis is characterized by the glenoid and humeral erosions, glenoid medialization, and limited osteophyte formation. **B**, Reverse total shoulder arthroplasty performed based upon glenoid erosion and associated rotator cuff compromise.

subluxation. However, the ability to adequately correct the deformity will be important to achieve a successful outcome. Correcting excessive glenoid retroversion may be accomplished by eccentric reaming, bone grafting, use of posteriorly augmented implants, or by using a combination of these techniques.[43-46] Eccentric reaming has been used to correct version up to 15°. However, when greater correction is needed, more eccentric reaming is required, which ultimately leaves less glenoid bone stock remaining. The remaining glenoid bone may be compromised with respect to component contact, support, and coverage that may not be ideal for long-term implant survival.[47-49] There has been limited experience and success with the use of bone grafts in ATSA, which has led to the development and more extensive use of augmented components. Wright et al recently retrospectively reviewed 24 patients treated with ATSA and posteriorly augmented all-polyethylene glenoids. These authors compared their outcomes to a matched cohort without augmented glenoid components.[12] With a minimum 2-year follow-up, all patients improved with range of motion, pain, and functional outcome measures.[12] Furthermore, even though the augmented glenoid component group had greater retroversion preoperatively, there were no revisions necessary, and in 17 of 20 shoulders, the humeral head remained concentrically reduced on final follow-up radiographs.[12] Other early results with augmented components to correct deformity have been promising, but longer term follow-up is still needed.[43-46]

Posterior subluxation of the humeral head can also be challenging to correct with ATSA. Techniques utilized with varying degrees of success have included rotator interval closure, posterior capsular plication, and anterior eccentric head placement.[37,38,40,41,50] The Mayo Clinic reported their experience with posterior capsular plications in ATSA. From their retrospective review of 28 ATSAs, soft-tissue balancing as evidenced by concentric alignment was restored in 71% of shoulders, while 8 % required revision to address residual posterior instability.[40] The Mayo Clinic also reported a matched cohort study comparing ATSA and posterior capsular plication with RTSA for biconcave, osteoarthritic glenoids with an intact rotator cuff.[41] There were 15 ATSAs and 16 RTSAs with an average follow-up of 43 and 73 months, respectively.[41] Both cohorts reported comparable excellent outcomes. However, the ATSA group experienced more complications.[41]

Furthermore, Mizuno et al reported a retrospective review of 27 RTSAs used to treat biconcave, arthritic glenoids with an intact rotator cuff. The glenoids in this series had an average retroversion of 27° and an average humeral head subluxation of 87%.[38] At an average follow-up of 54 months, they reported excellent clinical outcomes, no residual posterior instability, but a 15% complication rate.[38] Based upon the experiences reported, there is a role for ATSA with increasing

glenoid deformity and posterior humeral head subluxation as long as adequate correction can be achieved (**FIGURE 7.7**). However, with increasing glenoid retroversion, erosion, and posterior humeral head subluxation, there is an important role for RTSA even in patients with an intact rotator cuff. Individualizing each case by integrating clinical factors with a clear understanding of the pathoanatomy is essential to determine the preferred procedure (**FIGURE 7.8**).

POSTTRAUMATIC ARTHRITIS: ATSA AND RTSA

Posttraumatic glenohumeral arthritis encompasses a wide spectrum of clinical and radiographic characteristics ranging from isolated articular incongruity with intact soft tissues to extensive proximal humeral deformity with extensive soft-tissue compromise, scarring, and adhesions. The evaluation of the patient with posttraumatic arthritis must combine a careful assessment of the clinical findings with a complete understanding of the deformity based upon appropriate imaging studies. Integration of this information will determine whether ATSA or RTSA is the most appropriate treatment.

Beredjiklian et al retrospectively reviewed 39 patients with a range of posttraumatic disorders of the glenohumeral joint. Injury sequelae included greater and lesser tuberosity malunions, incongruity of the articular surface, malunion of the articular surface, and soft-tissue injuries including contracture, rotator cuff tears, and impingement.[51] They concluded that proximal humeral malunions and posttraumatic arthritis are osseous and soft tissue-injuries, and both require correction to have a successful outcome. At an average 44-month follow-up, satisfactory results were only obtained with 69% (27/39) of the patients treated operatively.[51] Of those 27 patients who obtained satisfactory results, 96% had complete correction of the osseous and soft-tissue deformity.[51] However, this series was reported before the availability of RTSA. Arthroplasty options in this series included only hemiarthroplasty or ATSA. Similarly, the Mayo Clinic recently reported on 37 hemiarthroplasties and 45 ATSAs used for the treatment of posttraumatic arthritis.[52] The authors found that both options improved pain, forward elevation, and external rotation.[52] However, ATSA had less pain and greater patient satisfaction at final follow-up.[52] This is most likely due to the progressive glenoid erosion that can occur after hemiarthroplasty.[52] Long-term survivorship was also better following ATSA. At 15 years, survivorship was 79.5% after hemiarthroplasty and 83% after ATSA.

Traditionally, hemiarthroplasty and ATSA have been utilized for the sequelae of proximal humerus fractures.[53-55] More recently, RTSA has been used more extensively to treat complications following proximal humerus fractures. While the need for a greater tuberosity osteotomy has been reported to be a significant factor

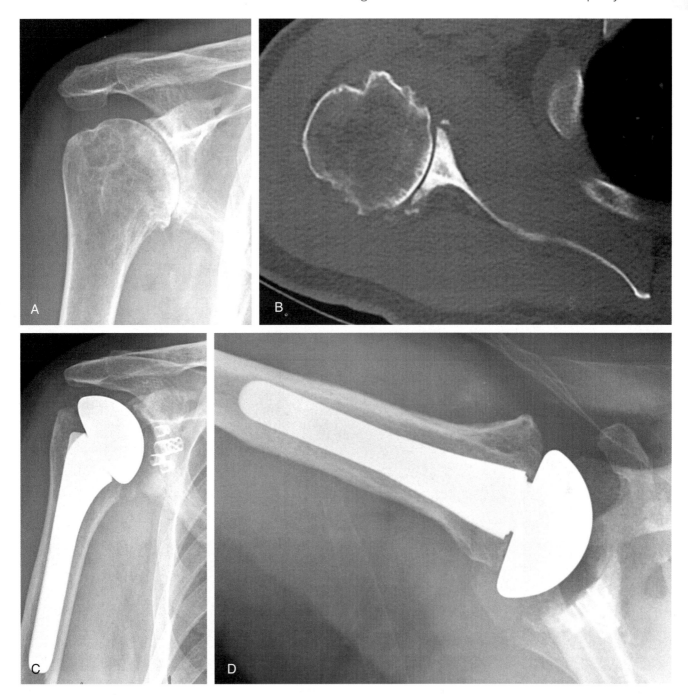

FIGURE 7.7 A, A 75-year-old man with osteoarthritis of the right glenohumeral joint with well-functioning rotator cuff. **B**, Axial CT imaging shows medial wear and reduced glenoid vault. **C** and **D**, Anatomic total shoulder arthroplasty performed utilizing preoperative planning and intraoperative navigation for placement and positioning of a posteriorly augmented glenoid component.

affecting outcomes following shoulder arthroplasty for posttraumatic arthritis, this was reported before the use of RTSA in the United States.[54] Alentorn-Geli et al prospectively evaluated 32 patients, in which 20 patients were treated with RTSA for proximal humerus osteonecrosis with head collapse, humeral neck nonunion, greater tuberosity malunion, and chronic dislocations. The average age of these patients was 80 years with an average follow-up of 4 years.[53] All patients had improved

pain, function, and range of motion scores.[53] Willis et al also reviewed RTSA for the treatment of proximal humerus fracture malunions in 16 patients with a minimum follow-up of 2 years.[55] All patients had improved range of motion, function, and pain scores.[55] With these newer reports confirming the successful use of RTSA for proximal humerus fracture sequelae, it is now a valuable treatment option for these patients who require arthroplasty. The associated soft-tissue changes and bony

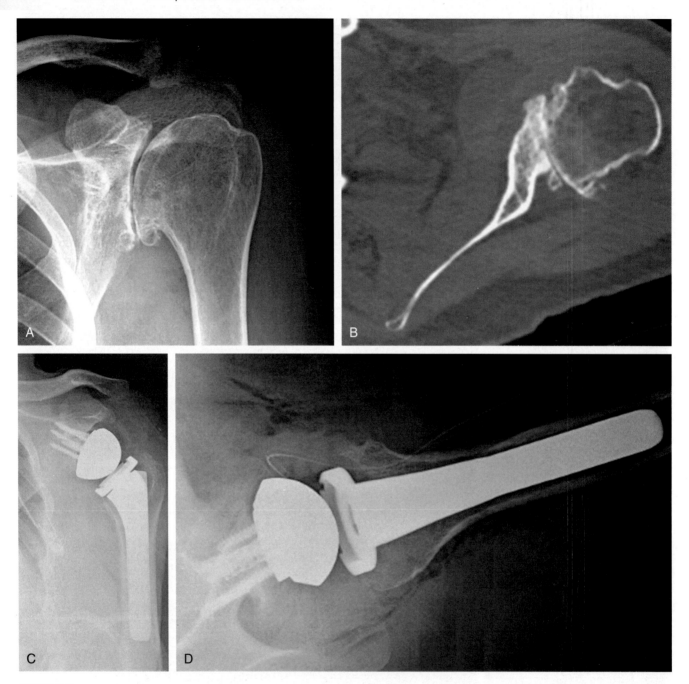

FIGURE 7.8 A, A 67-year-old man with osteoarthritis of the left glenohumeral joint. **B,** Axial CT image of the left shoulder shows significant posterior wear, biconcave glenoid, and medial erosion resulting in a narrowed vault. **C** and **D,** Reverse total shoulder arthroplasty with augmented baseplate performed based upon the extensive glenoid wear pattern and bone loss.

deformity that characterizes posttraumatic arthritis have made RTSA the preferred procedure in the majority of situations **(FIGURE 7.9).**

GLENOHUMERAL ARTHRITIS IN YOUNGER PATIENTS: ATSA

Glenohumeral arthritis in a young patient can present in the absence of an underlying etiology. When pain and associated disability can no longer be managed by nonoperative measures, shoulder arthroplasty has been shown to be an effective treatment. The use of total shoulder arthroplasty in young patients has been a concern because of the perceived increased risk of glenoid component loosening.[56-58] As a result, multiple surgical options have been utilized, including hemiarthroplasty, hemiarthroplasty with concentric glenoid reaming, humeral resurfacing, and hemiarthroplasty with biologic glenoid resurfacing.[56] Although hemiarthroplasty provides good pain relief, the outcomes with respect to pain relief, patient satisfaction, and range of motion have been inferior to ATSA.[56] This

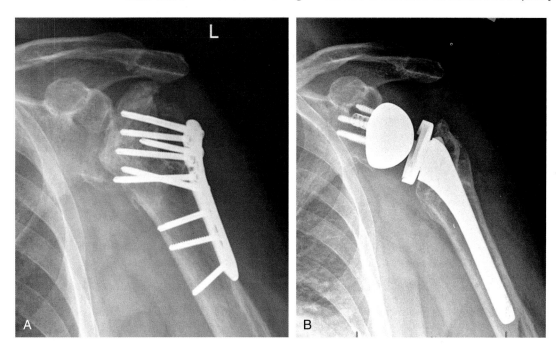

FIGURE 7.9 A, A 64-year-old man 3 years following open reduction and internal fixation of left proximal humerus fracture with posttraumatic arthritis and osteonecrosis. Greater tuberosity resorption is also noted. **B**, Reverse total shoulder arthroplasty performed with removal of plate and screws and extensive lysis of adhesions.

has also been the experience when compared with hemi-arthroplasty with biologic glenoid resurfacing, which has had high failure and reoperations rates.[56,58-62] As a result, there is general agreement that in the presence of humeral head and glenoid degenerative changes, ATSA is the preferred surgical treatment[56,63,64] **(FIGURE 7.10)**.

With technological advances, ATSA implant survival is reported to be greater than 90% at 15 to 20 years; thereby, making it a more attractive option in younger patients.[56] Levy et al specifically reviewed 42 noncemented shoulder arthroplasties in patients younger than 50 years of age for a variety of diagnoses. The average

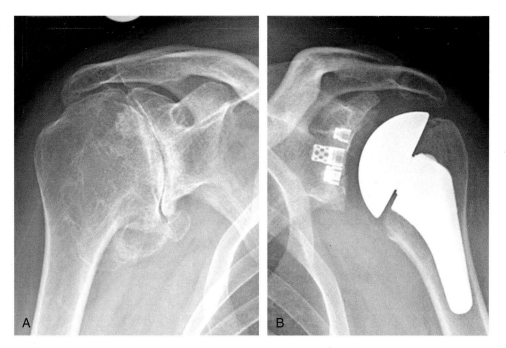

FIGURE 7.10 A, A 47-year-old man with primary osteoarthritis of the left shoulder. Osteoarthritis is characterized by inferior humeral head osteophyte and joint space narrowing of the glenohumeral joint. **B**, Anatomic shoulder arthroplasty was performed with a metaphyseal fitting humeral component and an all-polyethylene glenoid.

age of the patients was 39 years, and the average follow-up was 15 years.[65] Of the 42 shoulder arthroplasties, 17 were ATSA and 37 were hemiarthroplasties.[65] All patients improved with functional, pain, and satisfaction scores.[65] However, the revision rate was 18.5% raising understandable concerns about the longevity of shoulder arthroplasty in a younger patient population. Gauci et al also retrospectively reviewed younger patients who underwent ATSA for osteoarthritis. This series included 69 ATSAs, of which 46 ATSAs were cemented all-polyethylene glenoids and 23 were noncemented metal-backed glenoids.[66] The average age was 54 years, with all patients younger than 60 years. With a 12-year follow-up, there was 74% implant survival and a 20% revision rate for the patients with an all-polyethylene glenoid.[66] These results emphasize the challenge of treating glenohumeral arthritis in young patients. However, on balance, in the presence of both humeral and glenoid involvement, ATSA is the preferred option.

OSTEOARTHRITIS WITH PARKINSON DISEASE: RTSA

In the United States, Parkinson disease affects 1% to 2% of the population older than 65 years.[67] Musculoskeletal manifestations of this disease include rigidity, bradykinesia, postural instability, impaired balance and coordination which result in frequent falls, resting tremor, dyskinesia, and choreiform movements.[67-69] The associated conditions make this a very challenging patent population to treat. Treatment of glenohumeral arthritis with hemiarthroplasty and ATSA in patients with Parkinson disease has been associated with high rates

of unsatisfactory results including an increase in periprosthetic fractures and implant loosening.[67] The Mayo Clinic reported on 36 patients with Parkinson disease who underwent 43 ATSAs with an average 8-year follow-up. Overall, patients reported decreased pain and improved function. However, there were 47% unsatisfactory results primarily related to postoperative instability. Cusick et al, in a matched cohort study, compared RTSA in 10 patients with Parkinson disease with 40 patients without Parkinson disease. Compared to patients without Parkinson disease, patients with Parkinson disease had a similar improvement in pain but reported inferior functional results and an unpredictable range of motion improvement. This would certainly be anticipated based upon the underlying condition. Furthermore, the complication rate in the Parkinson patients was reported to be 40% compared to 15% in the comparison cohort.[70] As the risk of postoperative complications and compromised outcomes is higher in patients with Parkinson disease, shoulder arthroplasty should be considered carefully. However, in patients who are identified as reasonable candidates for surgery, RTSA is the preferred treatment **(FIGURE 7.11)**.

CONCLUSION

The original indication for an ATSA was osteoarthritis. However, as the procedure developed, the indications were expanded to a much wider range of degenerative and traumatic conditions of the glenohumeral joint. The initial indication for RTSA was rotator cuff arthropathy. Similarly, with experience and technological

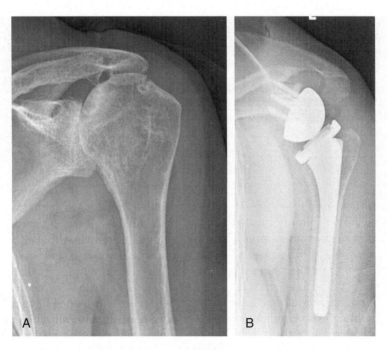

A

B

FIGURE 7.11 A, A 82-year-old woman with Parkinson disease. Radiograph shows advanced glenohumeral arthritis with superior humeral head migration. **B**, Reverse total shoulder arthroplasty performed based upon underlying Parkinson disease, patient age, and rotator cuff compromise.

improvements, the indications have expanded significantly. Patients who present with glenohumeral arthritis of different etiologies may be candidates for shoulder arthroplasty. The decision of whether to consider an ATSA or RTSA should always be based upon a comprehensive evaluation of clinical factors, patient factors, and imaging studies. There are clinical situations in which an ATSA is clearly indicated and others in which an RTSA is clearly indicated. However, there are also situations in which the indication for one procedure or the other is not as evident. Understanding the advantages and disadvantages of each procedure as well as the specific patient being evaluated will allow the surgeon to determine the best course of treatment. In this chapter, the goal was to establish guidelines for ATSA and RTSA. Ultimately, the goal is to provide the patients with the most successful outcome, which will always be a combination of patient selection, technical skills, and the implant utilized. Furthermore, it is important to recognize that as techniques and technology advance, these indications can be expected to change going forward just as they have previously.

REFERENCES

1. Chalmers P, Salazar D, Romeo A, Keener J, Yamaguchi K, Chamberlain A. Comparative utilization of reverse and anatomic total shoulder arthroplasty: a comparison analysis of a high-volume center. *J Am Acad Orthop Surg.* 2018;26(24):e504-e510.
2. Smith C, Guyver P, Bunker T. Indications for reverse shoulder replacement. *J Bone Joint Surg Br.* 2012;94-B(5):577-583.
3. Hyun Y, Huri G, Garbis N, McFarland E. Uncommon indications for reverse total shoulder arthroplasty. *Clin Orthop Surg.* 2013;5(4):243-255.
4. Rasmussen J, Amundsen A, Sorensen A, et al. Increased use of total shoulder arthroplasty for osteoarthritis and improved patient-reported outcomes in Denmark, 2006-2015: a nationwide cohort study from the Danish Shoulder Arthroplasty Registry. *Acta Orthop.* 2019;90(5):489-494.
5. Norris T, Iannotti J. Functional outcome after shoulder arthroplasty for primary osteoarthritis: a multicenter study. *J Shoulder Elbow Surg.* 2002;11(2):130-135.
6. Pandya J, Johnson T, Low A. Shoulder replacement for osteoarthritis: a review of surgical management. *Maturitas.* 2018;108:71-76.
7. Iannotti J, Norris T. Influence of preoperative factors on outcome of shoulder arthroplasty for glenohumeral osteoarthritis. *J Bone Joint Surg Am.* 2003;85(2):251-258.
8. Liversey M, Horneff J, Sholder D, Lazarus M, Williams G, Namdari S. Functional outcomes and predictors of failure after rotator cuff repair during total shoulder arthroplasty. *Orthopedics.* 2018;4(3):e334-e339.
9. Simone J, Struebel P, Sperling J, Schleck C, Cofield R, Athwal G. Anatomical total shoulder replacement with rotator cuff repair for osteoarthritis of the shoulder. *Bone Joint J.* 2014;96-B(2):224-228.
10. Bulhoff M, Spranz D, Maier M, Raiss P, Bruckner T, Zeifang F. Mid-term results with an anatomic stemless shoulder prosthesis in patients with primary osteoarthritis. *Acta Orthop Traumatol Turc.* 2019;53(3):170-174.
11. Rasmussen J, Hole R, Metlie T, et al. Anatomical total shoulder arthroplasty used for glenohumeral osteoarthritis has higher survival rates than hemiarthroplasty: a Nordic registry based study. *Osteoarthritis Cartilage.* 2018;26(5):659-665.
12. Wright T, Flurin P, Crosby C, Struk A, Zuckerman J. Total shoulder arthroplasty outcome for treatment of osteoarthritis: a multicenter study using a contemporary implant. *Am J Orthop (Belle Mead NJ).* 2015;44(11):523-526.
13. Wright M, Keener J, Chamberlain A. Comparison of clinical outcomes after anatomic total shoulder arthroplasty and reverse shoulder arthroplasty in patients 70 years and older with glenohumeral osteoarthritis and an intact rotator cuff. *J Am Acad Orthop Surg.* 2020;28(5):e222-e229.
14. Brewley E, Christmas K, Gorman R, Downes K, Mighell M, Frankle M. Defining the younger patient: age as a predictor factor for outcomes in shoulder arthroplasty. *J Shoulder Elbow Surg.* 2020;29(suppl 7):S1-S8.
15. MaCaulay A, Greiwe M, Bigliani L. Rotator cuff deficient arthritis of the glenohumeral joint. *Clin Orthop Surg.* 2010;2:197-202.
16. Wellman M, Struck M, Pastor M, Gettmann A, Weadhagen H, Smith T. Short and midterm results of reverse shoulder arthroplasty according to the preoperative etiology. *Arch Orthop Trauma Surg.* 2013;133:463-471.
17. Rugg C, Gallo R, Craig E, Feeley B. The pathogenesis and management of cuff tear arthropathy. *J Shoulder Elbow Surg.* 2018;27(12):2271-2283.
18. Ortmaier R, Hitzl W, Matis N, Mattiassich G, Hochreiter J, Resch H. Reverse shoulder arthoplasty combined with latissimus dorsi transfer: a systematic review. *Orthop Traumatol Surg Res.* 2017;103(6):853-859.
19. Gerber C, Canonica S, Catanzaro S, Erustbrunner L. Longitudinal observational study of reverse total shoulder arthroplasty for irreparable rotator cuff dysfunction: results after 15 years. *J Shoulder Elbow Surg.* 2018;27(5):831-838.
20. Petrillo S, Longo V, Papalia R, Denaro V. Reverse shoulder arthroplasty for massive irreparable rotator cuff tears and cuff tear arthropathy: a systematic review. *Musculoskelet Surg.* 2017;101(2):105-112.
21. Seebauer L, Walter W, Keyl W. Reverse total shoulder arthroplasty for the treatment of defect arthropathy. Article in German. *Oper Orthop Traumatol.* 2005;17(1):1-24.
22. Sellers T, Abdelfattah A, Frankle M. Massive rotator cuff tear: when to consider reverse shoulder arthroplasty. *Curr Rev Musculoskelet Med.* 2018;11:131-140.
23. Hartzler R, Steen B, Hussey M, et al. Reverse shoulder arthroplasty for massive rotator cuff tear: risk factors for poor functional improvement. *J Shoulder Elbow Surg.* 2015;24(11):1698-1706.
24. Allert J, Sellers T, Simon P, Christmas K, Patel S, Frankle M. Massive rotator cuff tears in patients older than sixty-five: indications for cuff repair versus reverse total shoulder arthroplasty. *Am J Orthop (Belle Mead NJ).* 2018;47(12).
25. Ernstbrunner L, Suter A, Catanzaro S, Rahm S, Gerber C. Reverse total shoulder arthroplasty for massive, irreparable rotator cuff tears before the age of 60 years. *J Bone Joint Surg Am.* 2017;99(20):1721-1729.
26. Mulieri P, Dunning P, Klein S, Pupello D, Frankle M. Reverse shoulder arthoplasty for the treatment of irreparable rotator cuff tear without glenohumeral arthritis. *J Bone Joint Surg Am.* 2010;92(15):2544-2556.
27. Waldman B, Figgie M. Indications, technique and results of total shoulder arthroplasty in rheumatoid arthritis. *Orthop Clin North Am.* 1998;29(3):435-444.
28. Barlow J, Yuan B, Schleck C, Harmsen W, Cofield R, Sperling J. Shoulder arthroplasty for rheumatoid arthritis: 303 consecutive cases with minimum 5 year follow up. *J Shoulder Elbow Surg.* 2014;23:791-799.
29. Lim S, Sun J, Kekatpure A, Chun J, Jeon I. Rotator cuff surgery in patients with rheumatoid arthritis: clinical outcome comparable to age, sex and tear size matched non-rheumatoid patients. *Ann R Coll Surg Engl.* 2017;99(7):579-583.
30. Choi W, Lee K, Park J, Lee B. Bilateral bony increased-offset reverse shoulder arthroplasty in rheumatoid arthritis shoulder with sever glenoid bone defect: a case report. *Acta Orthop Traumatol Turc.* 2017;51(3):262-265.
31. Tiusanen H, Sarantsin P, Stenholm M, Mattie R, Saltycher M. Ranges of motion after reverse shoulder arthroplasty improve significantly the frist year after surgery in patients with rheumatoid arthritis. *Eur J Orthop Surg Traumatol.* 2016;26(5):447-452.
32. Collins D, Harryman D, Wirth M. Shoulder arthroplasty for the treatment of inflammatory arthritis. *J Bone Joint Surg Am.* 2004;86:2489-2496.

33. Lee Y, Jeong J, Park C, Kang S, Yoo J. Evaluation of the risk factors for a rotator cuff retear after repair surgery. *Am J Sports Med.* 2017;45(8):1755-1761.

34. Hattrup S, Sanchez-Sotelo J, Sperling J, Cofield R. Reverse shoulder replacement for patients with inflammatory arthritis. *J Hand Surg Am.* 2012;37(9):1888-1894.

35. Schwyzer H, Loehr J, Simmen B. Indications for shoulder prosthesis in degenerative and inflammatory diseases. Article in German. *Ther Umsch.* 1998;55(3):203-209.

36. Mangold D, Wagner E, Cofield R, Sanchez-Sotelo J, Sperling J. Reverse shoulder arthroplasty for rheumatoid arthritis since the introduction of disease-modifying drugs. *Int Orthop.* 2019;43(11):2593-2600.

37. Collin P, Herve A, Walch G, Boileau P, Manuandy M, Chelli M. Midterm results of reverse shoulder arthroplasty for glenohumeral osteoarthritis with posterior glenoid deficiency and humeral subluxation. *J Shoulder Elbow Surg.* 2019;28(10):2023-2030.

38. Mizuno N, Denard P, Raiss P, Walch G. Reverse total shoulder arthroplasty for primary glenohumeral osteoarthritis in patients with a biconcave glenoid. *J Bone Joint Surg Am.* 2013;95:1297-304.

39. Paul R, Knowles N, Chaoui J, et al. Characterization of the dysplastic Walch type C glenoids. *Bone Joint J.* 2018;100-B(8):1074-1079.

40. Alentorn-Geli E, Assenmacher A, Sperling J, Cofield R, Sanchez-Sotelo J. Plication of the posterior capsule for intraoperative posterior instability during anatomic total shoulder arthroplasty. *J Shoulder Elbow Surg.* 2017;26(6):982-989.

41. Alentorn-Geli E, Wanderman N, Assenmacker A, Sperling J, Cofield R, Sanchez-Sotelo J. Anatomic total shoulder arthroplasty with posterior capsular plication versus reverse shoulder arthroplasty in patients with biconcave glenoids: a matched cohort study. *J Orthop Surg (Hong Kong).* 2018;26(2):1-8.

42. Farron A, Terrier A, Buchler P. Risks of loosening of a prosthetic glenoid implanted in retroversion. *J Shoulder Elbow Surg.* 2006;15:521-526.

43. Sowa B, Bochenek M, Braun S, et al. Replacement options for the B2 glenoid in osteoarthritis of the shoulder: a biomechanical study. *Arch Orthop Trauma Surg.* 2018;138(7):891-899.

44. Priddy M, Zare Zadeh A, Farmer K, et al. Early results of augmented anatomic glenoid components. *J Shoulder Elbow Surg.* 2019;28:138-145.

45. Sandow M, Schutz C. Total shoulder arthroplasty using trabecular metal augments to address glenoid retroversion: the preliminary result of 10 patients with minimum 2-year follow-up. *J Shoulder Elbow Surg.* 2016;25(4):598-607.

46. Rice R, Sperling J, Miletti J, Schleck C, Cofield R. Augmented glenoid compnents for bone deficiency in shoulder arthroplasty. *Clin Orthop Relat Res.* 2008;466:579-583.

47. Gillespie R, Lyons R, Lazarus M. Eccentric reaming in total shoulder arthroplasty: a cadaver study. *Orthopedics.* 2009;32(1):21.

48. Nowak D, Bahu M, Gardner T, et al. Simulation of surgical glenoid resurfacing using three-dimensional computed tomography of the arthritic glenohumeral joint: the amount of glenoid retroversion that can be corrected. *J Shoulder Elbow Surg.* 2009;18:680-688.

49. Olszewski A, Ramne A, Maerz T, Freehill M, Warner J, Bedi A. Vault perforation after eccentric glenoid reaming for deformity correction in anatomic total shoulder arthroplasty. *J Shoulder Elbow Surg.* 2020;29(7):1450-1459.

50. Hsu J, Gee A, Lucas R, Somerson J, Warme W, Matsen F. Management of intraoperative posterior decentering in shoulder arthroplasty using anteriorly eccentric humeral head components. *J Shoulder Elbow Surg.* 2016;25(12):1980-1988.

51. Beredjiklian P, Iannotti J, Norris T, Williams G. Operative treatment of malunion of A fracture of the proximal aspect of the humerus. *J Bone Joint Surg Am.* 1998;80(10):1484-1497.

52. Schoch B, Barlow J, Schleck C. Cofield R, Sperling J. Shoulder arthroplasty for post-traumatic osteonecrosis of the humeral head. *J Shoulder Elbow Surg.* 2016;25:406-412.

53. Alentorn-Geli E, Guirro P, Santana F, Torreas C. Treatment of fracture sequelea of the proximal huemrus: comparison of hemiarthroplasty and reverse total shoulder arthroplasty. *Arch Orthop Trauma Surg.* 2014;134:1545-1550.

54. Boileau P, Trojani C, Walch G, Krishnan S, Romeo A, Sinnerton R. Shoulder arthroplasty for the treatment of the sequelae of fractures of the proximal humerus. *J Shoulder Elbow Surg.* 2001;10(4):299-308.

55. Willis M, Min W, Brooks J, et al. Proximal humeral malunion treated with reverse shoulder arthroplasty. *J Shoulder Elbow Surg.* 2012;21:507-513.

56. Keller J, Vadaski K, Biliani L. Arthroplasty in the young patient. *Br J Hosp Med (Lond).* 2009;70(5):266-270.

57. Saltzman B, Leroux T, Verma N, Romeo A. Glenohumeral osteoarthritis in the young patient. *J Am Acad Orthop Surg.* 2018;26:361-370.

58. Muh S, Streit J, Shishani Y, Dubrow S, Nowinski R, Bogezie R. Biologic resurfacing of the glenoid with humeral head resurfacing for glenohumeral arthritis in the young patient. *J Shoulder Elbow Surg.* 2014;23(8):e185-e190.

59. Hammond J, Lin EC, Harwood D, et al. Clinical outcomes of hemiarthroplasty and biological resurfacing in patients aged younger than 50 years. *J Shoulder Elbow Surg.* 2013;22:1345-1351.

60. Puskas G, Meyer D, Lebschi J, Gerber C. Unacceptable failure of hemiarthroplasty combined with biological glenoid resurfacing in the treatment of glenohumeral arthritis in the young. *J Shoulder Elbow.* 2015;24(12):1900-1907.

61. Strauss E, Verma N, Salata M, et al. The high failure rate of biologic resurfacing of the glenoid in young patients with glenohumeral arthritis. *J Shoulder Elbow Surg.* 2014;23:409-419.

62. Nicholson G, Goldstein J, Romeo A, et al. Lateral meniscus allograft biologic glenoid arthroplasty in total shoulder arthroplasty for young shoulders with degenerative joint disease. *J Shoulder Elbow Surg.* 2007;16(suppl 5):S261-S266.

63. Padegimas E, Maltenfort M, Lazarus M, Ramsey M, Williams G, Namdari S. Future patient demand for shoulder arthroplasty by younger patients: national projections. *Clin Orthop Relat Res.* 2015;473:1860-1867.

64. Davis D, Acevedo D, Williams A, Williams G. Total shoulder arthroplasty using an inlay mini-glenoid component for glenoid deficiency: a 2 year follow up of 9 patients. *J Shoulder Elbow Surg.* 2016;25(8):1354-1361.

65. Levy O, Tsvieli O, Merchant J, et al. Surgace replacement arthroplasty for glenohumeral arthropathy in patients aged younger than fifty years: results after a minimum ten-year follow up. *J Shoulder Elbow Surg.* 2015;24(7):1049-1060.

66. Gauci M, Bonnevialle N, Moineau G, Baba M, Walch G, Boileau P. Anatomical total shoulder arthroplasty in young patients with osteoarthritis. *Bone Joint J.* 2018;100-B:485-92.

67. Burrus M, Werner B, Cancienne J, Gwathmey F, Brochmeier S. Shoulder arthroplasty in patients with Parkinson's disease is associated with increased complications. *J Shoulder Elbow Surg.* 2015;24(12):1881-1887.

68. Skedros J, Smith J, Langston T, Adondakis M. Reverse total shoulder arthroplasty as treatment for rotator cuff-tear arthropathy and shoulder dislocations in an elderly male with Parkinson's disease. *Case Rep Orthop.* 2017;2017:5051987.

69. Giannotti S, Bottai V, Dell'Osso G, Bugelli G, Guido G. Stemles humeral component in reverse shoulder prosthesis in patient with Parkinson's disease: a case report. *Clin Cases Miner Bone Metab.* 2015;12(1):56-59.

70. Cusick M, Otto R, Clark R, Frankle M. Outcome of reverse shoulder arthroplasty for patients with Parkinson's disease: a matched cohort study. *Orthopedics.* 2017;40(4);e675-e680.

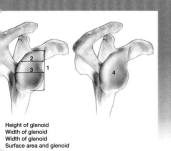

Height of glenoid
Width of glenoid
Width of glenoid
Surface area and glenoid
...ape

CHAPTER

8

Preoperative Planning:
Patient-Specific Instrumentation

Brandon J. Erickson, MD, Patrick Denard, MD, and Anthony A. Romeo, MD

INTRODUCTION

Anatomic total shoulder arthroplasty (ATSA) is an effective treatment option for the management of glenohumeral osteoarthritis and aims to provide patients with pain relief and improvement in function.[1,2] Similarly, reverse total shoulder arthroplasty (RTSA) has emerged as an excellent treatment option for older patients with cuff tear arthropathy, proximal humerus fractures, patients with glenohumeral osteoarthritis and a poorly functioning or nonfunctional rotator cuff, patients with severe glenoid deformity in the setting of osteoarthritis, and other evolving indications.[3-5] Given the success of ATSA and RTSA, the number of these procedures performed continues to rise each year, and there is every indication this trend will continue.[6]

While the outcomes following ATSA and RTSA are encouraging, there are still complications that occur. One of the most common complications and/or reason for a poor outcome following ATSA and RTSA is a problem with the glenoid component.[7,8] Obtaining optimal exposure of the glenoid can be challenging in certain cases, and, once the glenoid is exposed, placing the component in the ideal position can also be difficult. As such, glenoid component problems can occur in the early or later postoperative setting and include loosening, migration, polyethylene dissociation, malposition leading to shoulder instability, and notching.[9-11] Studies have cited the rate of glenoid loosening at 1.2% per year following ATSA with a recorded revision rate of 0.8% per year.[8] Similarly, the rate of glenoid loosening following RTSA has been cited at 1.7% to 13% and is often attributed to malposition of the glenoid baseplate (most commonly superiorly inclined).[12] Therefore, if glenoid position could be improved such that the glenoid was placed in the "optimal" position reproducibly and reliably from case to case, complications following ATSA and RTSA may decrease.

One potential method for improving glenoid component position in every case is the use of preoperative three-dimensional (3D) planning and patient-specific instrumentation (PSI).[13] 3D planning allows the surgeon to understand patient-specific glenoid inclination and version. PSI can then be created for each specific patient based upon preoperative advanced imaging that, in turn, will allow the surgeon to reproducibly place the glenoid in the ideal position in each case by positioning the glenoid pin in an optimal position. This chapter will discuss the evolution of PSI, its role in both ATSA and RTSA, and the results following use of 3D planning and PSI for glenoid placement in shoulder arthroplasty.

EVOLUTION OF PATIENT-SPECIFIC INSTRUMENTATION

The idea of using technology to improve glenoid component position in shoulder arthroplasty began with intraoperative computer-assisted navigation.[14,15] This technology was first attempted in cadaveric shoulders where pre- and postoperative computed tomography (CT) scans were obtained to help plan the glenoid placement and then to check the version and inclination of the implanted glenoid component.[15] Nguyen et al compared traditional with computer-assisted glenoid placement in 16 paired cadaveric shoulders.[15] The authors found the computer-assisted technique was more accurate in achieving the correct version of the glenoid component as measured on postoperative CT scans. The authors also noted that the largest errors with traditional glenoid implantation occurred during drilling and reaming and that the common error with the traditional method was to overly retrovert the glenoid. This technique was evaluated in patients by Kircher et al who performed a prospective randomized controlled trial, where 26 patients with shoulder osteoarthritis were randomized to traditional glenoid placement or intraoperative navigation glenoid placement.[14] The authors measured glenoid version on preoperative CT scans for baseline values and then assessed the glenoid component position on postoperative CT scans at 6 weeks. The authors found that average change of retroversion was significantly better in the navigation group where the glenoid version of the navigation group improved from 15.4° preoperatively to 3.7° postoperatively compared to 14.4° preoperatively to 10.9° postoperatively in the traditional, nonnavigation group. However, the navigation process was aborted for six patients because of technical issues, and the authors noted operating time was significantly longer in the navigation group (170 vs

111

138 minutes). Unfortunately, the purpose of this study was simply to gauge the accuracy of the navigation and not to determine if placement of the components in an improved position led to improved patient outcomes. While the navigation seemed to improve placement of the components, it was not a feasible long-term solution given the technical complications and added time in the operating room (OR). A new technique that would similarly improve glenoid position but not at a great monetary or time consumption expense had to be developed.

This improvement became known as 3D planning and PSI and was first described by Hendel et al in 2012.[13] Hendel et al performed a randomized prospective clinical trial in which 31 patients were randomized for glenoid component placement to either the novel 3D CT scan planning software combined with PSI or a conventional two-dimensional (2D) CT scan, with standard instrumentation. The study was appropriately powered to detect differences in glenoid position based on CT scans between groups. The authors found that PSI significantly decreased the average deviation of the glenoid component position in inclination and medial/lateral offset compared to the non-PSI group and also decreased the frequency of malpositioned implants. This study demonstrated that PSI was not only reproducible but it also improved the accuracy of glenoid component position, both of which were critical factors when evaluating the effectiveness of new technology.

IDEAL PLACEMENT OF THE GLENOID IN ANATOMIC AND REVERSE TOTAL SHOULDER ARTHROPLASTY

Proper placement of the glenoid in ATSA and RTSA is one of the most controversial topics in shoulder arthroplasty. While PSI can allow precise and accurate glenoid placement based on a preoperative plan, this is irrelevant if the preoperative plan has the glenoid placed in a poor position. Unfortunately, there is significant debate as to the ideal placement of the glenoid in ATSA and RTSA. Some advocate for restoring normal anatomy, while others will use the patient's current anatomy to place the glenoid component. In the author's opinion, the ideal position of the glenoid component would be to recreate of the patient's native version, inclination, and center of rotation. Native position can either be based on of estimates of the "normal" population or by using computer modeling of the premorbid state such as the glenoid vault model.[16] Churchill et al used 172 matched pairs of cadaver glenoids in an attempt to determine average native glenoid version, inclination, and size in the general population as a baseline.[17] They used 50 black male, 50 white male, 50 black female, and 22 white female cadavers aged between 20 and 30 years. The authors reported that glenoid version for all cadavers averaged 1.23° of retroversion. Interestingly, there

was a statistically significant difference in average glenoid version between black and white patients (0.20° vs 2.65° of retroversion, respectively), between black and white males (0.11° vs 2.87° of retroversion, respectively), and between black and white females (0.30° vs 2.16° of retroversion, respectively). However, there was no statistical difference in glenoid version between men and women of the same race and no statistical difference in glenoid inclination based on race or sex. The obvious issues with using such estimates are that these means do not take into consideration individual anatomy and, perhaps more importantly, were based on nonpathologic specimens. An alternative to using mean values is to estimate the premorbid anatomy of the individual based on the glenoid vault method described by Iannotti and Scalise.[16] Iannotti, Codsi, Scalise, and others described and validated a 3D glenoid vault model as a template to predict a normal glenoid version in patients undergoing shoulder arthroplasty.[16,18,19] This method allows for determination of what the patient's native glenoid version and inclination was prior to onset of their arthritis, thereby allowing the surgeon to recreate the patients normal anatomy at the time of surgery.

To obtain an "ideal" position, the glenoid component must be placed in proper version and inclination without removing too much bone. Chen et al performed a computational study on 25 CT-reconstructed B2 glenoids and demonstrated that version correction as low as 10° reduced glenoid bone density for glenoid fixation.[20] They noted that as version correction increased, there was a gradual depletion of high-quality bone from the anterior portion of B2 glenoids. Hence, while correction of deformity may be necessary to achieve success in ATSA, removing too much subchondral bone during glenoid preparation can compromise fixation of the glenoid component. Decreasing the amount of reaming and accepting some deformity or using an augmented glenoid design are options to maintain glenoid bone stock.

Some authors have found that placing the glenoid component without correcting any deformity has led to excellent short-term outcomes. Service et al reported the 2-year results of 71 ATSAs and compared the results of those patients (n = 21) in whom the glenoid component was implanted in 15° or greater retroversion (mean ± standard deviation [SD], 20.7° ± 5.3°) with those patients (n = 50) in whom the glenoid was implanted in less than 15° retroversion (mean ± SD, 5.7° ± 6.9°).[21] The authors found no difference in clinical outcomes scores between the retroverted and nonretroverted group. Furthermore, no patient in either group complained of posterior shoulder instability, and there was no difference in revision rates between the groups. While these results are interesting and worthy of discussion, the results are short term, and there is concern that posterior instability can occur over time leading to glenoid loosening.

There are differences in implant design and biomechanics between ATSA and RTSA and, in the authors' opinion, ideal placement of the glenoid is different for each procedure. Furthermore, there are patient-specific considerations that should be incorporated into glenoid placement as no two glenoids are exactly the same. Placement of a glenoid in a patient with neutral version and inclination is very different than placement of a glenoid in patients with 15° of superior inclination and 30° of retroversion with 85% posterior humeral head subluxation.

Anatomic Total Shoulder Arthroplasty

The goal of glenoid placement in ATSA is to maximize contact between the glenoid component and the native bone while avoiding violation of the subchondral bone, to avoid overstuffing the joint, and to minimize the potential for postoperative glenoid failure from loosening through version/inclination malpositioning. Several studies have evaluated glenoid placement, and unfortunately, no consensus on placement has been reached. Karelse et al used CT scans of 152 patients undergoing ATSA to place virtual glenoid components and determine forces on these components, which could lead to the rocking horse phenomenon.[22] The authors found that by using a best-fit circle based on the inferior glenoid rim rather than a best-fit circle based on the superior glenoid rim, there was a significant reduction in shear forces on the glenoid component. Hence, when preoperatively planning a case for the use of PSI, ensuring the glenoid component fits the inferior portion of the native glenoid may reduce shear forces on the implanted glenoid component.

Some studies surrounding PSI in total shoulder arthroplasty (TSA) have templated the cases to 0° of version and 0° of inclination, while many studies do not mention the templated inclination and version but rather report the difference between the preoperative plan and the postoperative outcome.[13,23,24] In the authors' opinion, if the glenoid vault method is not available to determine the patient's premorbid anatomy, ideal positioning of the glenoid component should include retroversion of 10° or less, correcting any asymmetry in inclination (the native glenoid averages approximately 10° of superior tilt) and centering where the glenoid is positioned on the scapula.

Reverse Total Shoulder Arthroplasty

Similar to ATSA, ideal placement of the glenoid in RTSA remains a matter of debate among experienced shoulder arthroplasty surgeons. The goals of glenoid placement in RTSA are to obtain adequate contact/seating of the baseplate with the native glenoid, appropriately tension the deltoid, minimize excessive abutment (impingement) of the humeral component against the scapula (that could lead to scapular notching), achieve stability of the glenohumeral articulation, prevent undue stress on the baseplate through inclination/version correction, and maximize shoulder range of motion (ROM). This is done through adjustments in version, inclination, and lateralization of the glenoid component. Minimizing scapular notching is imperative as excessive notching can lead to osteolysis, potentially compromising the stability of the glenoid component.[25] Keener et al attempted to determine the optimal glenoid and humeral RTSA component design and position by utilizing advanced software and ROM analysis on 10 CT scans.[26] The authors concluded that optimal ROM was achieved with 10-mm lateralization of the baseplate and neutral to 5° of retroversion paired with a 135° humeral implant. Werner et al performed a study that used virtual computer simulation to evaluate the influence of humeral neck shaft angle and glenoid lateralization on ROM in onlay design RTSA.[27] The authors concluded that the 135° humeral neck shaft angle implant with 5 mm of glenoid lateralization provided the best results in impingement-free ROM with the exception of abduction. However, they did not evaluate >5 mm of lateralization in this study, so it is unclear what role greater lateralization would have had. Hence, it appears that glenoid lateralization with a lower neck shaft angle of the humerus is ideal.

In the authors' opinion, ideal glenoid baseplate placement based on normative population data is 10° or less of retroversion, neutral or less inclination (inferior tilt of up to 10°), and placement of the glenoid baseplate lower on the glenoid face, so that the glenosphere covers or is slightly extended beyond the inferior glenoid rim. As far as the lateral position, it is unknown what the ideal lateralization position is; however, there is growing evidence that 5 to 10 mm of lateralization from the glenoid face provides a position that allows for stability, appropriate soft tissue tension, and improved internal and external rotation.

PLANNING A CASE

When using PSI, the surgeon must plan the case before proceeding to the OR. This occurs a few days to several weeks in advance depending on whether the PSI device is reusable (days) or must be manufactured (weeks). Each patient is asked to obtain a CT scan, typically with 1-mm slices that include the medial border of the scapula to allow the preoperative planning software to properly report the glenoid version and inclination (**FIGURES 8.1** and **8.2**), which are then uploaded to the planning software program. For systems based on measurements of anatomic landmarks, it is imperative that the entire scapula be included in the CT scan as several studies have demonstrated improved accuracy of glenoid version and inclination measurements when the medial border of the scapula is included.[28,29] Some software programs also measure humeral head subluxation, while others do not.

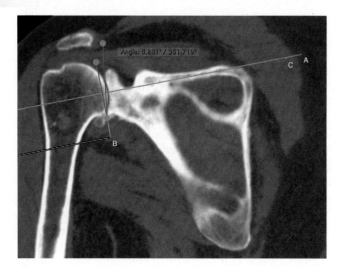

FIGURE 8.1 Preoperative coronal computed tomography scan oriented in the plane of the scapula demonstrating glenoid inclination. Line A is the line drawn along the supraspinatus fossa and line B is perpendicular to this line. A line is drawn connecting the superior and inferior border of the scapula. The measurement is derived from the line connecting the superior and inferior glenoid and the line perpendicular to the supraspinatus fossa line.

This will be provided as a percent, indicating what percentage of the humeral head is translated relative to the midpoint of the glenoid.

Once the CT scan is uploaded, the software uses one of the two primary measuring techniques (anatomic landmarks to determine the plane of the scapula or an average scapula plane and best-fit sphere) to report the glenoid inclination and version and, in some cases, the

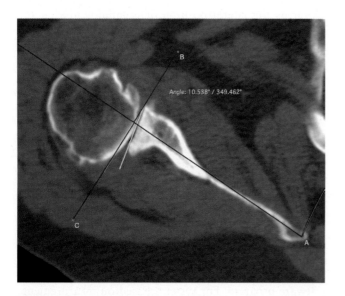

FIGURE 8.2 Preoperative axial computed tomography scan oriented in the plane of the scapula demonstrating glenoid version. Line A is drawn from the medial border of the scapula through the center of the glenoid on the axial slice just distal to the inferior aspect of the coracoid. This is known as the scapular axis (Friedman line). Line BC is perpendicular to line A. The angle measurement is derived from the glenoid version and the line perpendicular to Friedman line.

humeral head subluxation. The software also creates a tentative plan of where the placement of the glenoid pin should be, explains the amount of version and inclination correction the pin position will achieve, and provides the estimated final version and inclination once the final glenoid component is in place (**FIGURE 8.3A** and **B**). Some systems also allow planning of the humeral component. This initial plan is then modified by the surgeon to his or her liking. In systems that have augmented glenoid components, these can be added and subtracted from the preoperative plan to determine if the patient would benefit from an augment to correct version and or inclination as opposed to eccentric reaming or placement of a bone graft. Once the plan is complete, the PSI can be created if desired (**FIGURE 8.4**). If a reusable PSI guide is to be used, a paper plan will be produced, and it will allow for adjustment of the reusable PSI guide based on coordinates to mirror the preoperative plan (**FIGURE 8.5A-D**). Other systems print a single-use 3D-printed guide that can be used at the time of surgery and is machined to fit the patient's bony anatomy. These single-time use guides can be machined with a glenoid/scapular component to allow the surgeon to visualize where on the native glenoid the guide should sit to replicate the preoperative plan. Once the center pin is drilled, the guide is removed and the glenoid is reamed to the appropriate depth. This will vary based on the system utilized and whether an augmented component is selected. Once this is completed, the glenoid component is placed and secured. In the case of RTSA, screw lengths may be templated beforehand on the planning software. Ensuring that the screw length measurements obtained at the time of surgery match the preoperative plan is a good way to verify that the position of the glenoid component mirrors that of the plan.

HOW REPRODUCIBLE IS PATIENT-SPECIFIC INSTRUMENTATION?

Several studies have evaluated the reproducibility of PSI for glenoid component position.[30-33] Gauci et al reported the results of 17 patients who underwent ATSA with the use of PSI.[31] The mean error in the orientation of the glenoid component was 3.4° (SD of 5.1°) for version and 1.8° (SD of 5.3°) for inclination. Heylen et al compared the β-angle (angle between the glenoid baseplate and the floor of the supraspinatus fossa) of 36 patients who underwent shoulder arthroplasty (18 with the use of PSI and 18 with standard instrumentation).[32] The PSI group had lower β-angle for both ATSA and RTSA and had smaller variability in implant positioning compared to the standard instrumentation group. These studies indicate a decreased amount of variability with the use of PSI, indicating that the instrumentation is achieving its goal.

In a cadaveric model, Iannotti et al compared the use of 2D CT versus 3D CT for preoperative planning

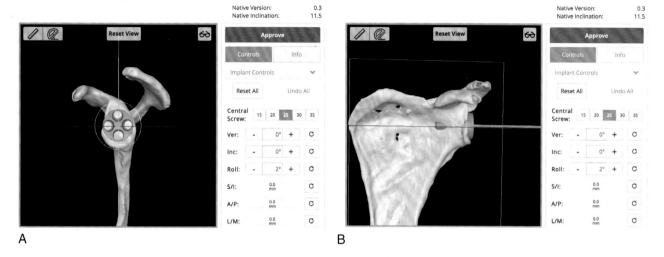

FIGURE 8.3 A and **B**, Initial plan provided by the preoperative planning software with proposed glenoid placement. Native version and inclination are provided on the top right of the images, and the adjusted version and inclination are seen on the control panel.

as well as the use of PSI versus standard instrumentation for glenoid pin placement in nine bone models.[23] The results demonstrated that standard instrumentation combined with 3D preoperative planning software improved guide pin positioning compared with standard instrumentation and preoperative planning using 2D imaging. Furthermore, the use of PSI and preoperative 3D planning improved the pin position when compared with standard instrumentation and the 3D software. Hence, this study demonstrated the use of 3D preoperative planning software had a significant positive impact

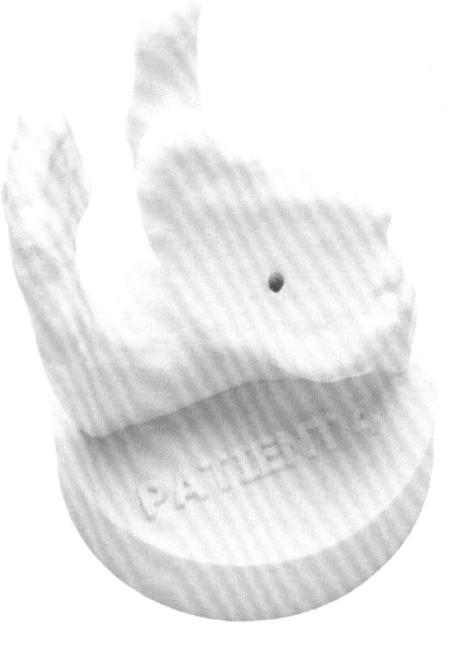

FIGURE 8.4 Three-dimensional model created from the preoperative plan that can be used in the surgery for glenoid pin placement.

on pin position both with the use of PSI and with standard instrumentation.

In clinical studies, the differences between preoperative 3D planning and PSI have not been as substantial. Iannotti et al evaluated 173 patients who underwent primary TSA to determine if PSI improved implant positioning compared to standard instrumentation.[24] All patients in this study underwent a preoperative 3D CT that was used to plan the case. The authors divided the patients into five groups: (1) standard instrumentation, (2) standard instrumentation combined with use of a 3D glenoid bone model containing the guide pin, (3) use of the 3D glenoid bone model combined with single-use PSI, (4) use of the 3D glenoid bone model combined with reusable PSI, and (5) use of reusable PSI with an adjustable, reusable base. Groups 1 and 2 were similar as they used standard instrumentation, group 3 utilized a single-use PSI, and groups 4 and 5 utilized reusable PSI. The authors found no significant differences in deviation from the preoperative plan among groups in regard to glenoid implant location or orientation. Lau et al reported on 11 patients in whom PSI was used to place the glenoid component (seven ATSA and four RTSA).[34] The authors found a mean retroversion of 8° ± 10° and mean inclination of 1° ± 4° for the ATSA group compared to a mean retroversion of 10° ± 10° and mean inclination of −1° ± 5° for the RTSA group. They noted five cases of outliers where the postoperative version was >10° of anteversion or retroversion. Thus, while the numbers were small, in the clinical setting, 3D planning alone improves component placement compared to 2D planning, but the differences between 3D planning and PSI are not as substantial as demonstrated in cadaveric models.

Finally, several systematic reviews have evaluated PSI in shoulder arthroplasty.[30,35,36] Burns et al performed a systematic review and meta-analysis of nine studies

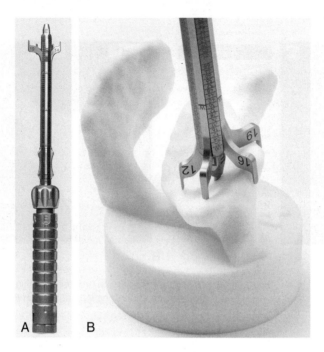

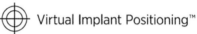

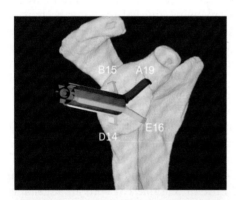

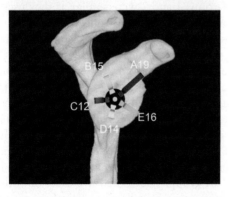

Preoperative Plan and 5-D Glenoid Targeter Instructions	
Patient	Arthrex VIP
MRN	1
Surgeon	Dr. VIP
Customer Order Number	1
Procedure / Side	RSA / Right
Date of Surgery	2020-May-17
Native Version (deg)	**-1.4**
Native Inclination (deg)	**5.2**
Implant	Arthrex MGS BP
Implant Size	24mm ø, 25mm Screw
Glenosphere or Inlay	36mm ø Standard
Implant Version (deg)	**0**
Implant Inclination (deg)	**0**
Implant Roll (deg)	12
Humeral Head Size (mm)	47.6
Planning Engineer	plannervip@arthrex.com
Expiration Date	2020-Oct-10
Comments	

Slot	Targeter Leg Length (mm)	5D Glenoid Calibrator Height Settings
A	19 mm	Z 31 Anterior Overhang
B	15 mm	X 41 On Surface
C	12 mm	Y 30 On Surface
D	14 mm	X 33 On Surface
E	16 mm	Y 30 Anterior Overhang

Glenoid
Targeter

FIGURE 8.5 A, Reusable guide for glenoid pin placement. The legs of the guide are set based on the preoperative plan to allow for proper pin placement. **B**, Image of the targeting guide placed on the three-dimensional model to illustrate how this sits intraoperatively. This model can be used by the surgeon to get a feel for how the guide should sit on the patient's glenoid. **C** and **D**, Example of a preoperative plan that can be used as a reference for the surgeon intraoperatively. This allows the surgeon to check the length of each leg on the targeter that is set up on the back table and allows the surgeon to understand how to properly position the targeter on the patient's glenoid.

with 258 patients to compare radiographic positioning outcomes using standard instrumentation, surgical navigation, and PSI for glenoid component positioning in ATSA and RTSA.[30] The authors concluded that both navigation and PSI had a statistically significant effect on improving glenoid implant position, while standard instrumentation resulted in a high rate of glenoid component malposition. Villatte et al found similar results in a systematic review and meta-analysis of 12 studies compromising 227 patients, in which the authors concluded that deviations from the preoperative plan in regard to version and inclination as well as the number of outliers (>10° of deviation) was lower when using PSI compared to standard instruments.[36] Cabarcas et al also performed a systematic review that included 22 studies with 518 patients (352 ATSAs and 166 RTSAs) to determine whether PSI significantly improved the accuracy of component positioning during shoulder arthroplasty.[35] The analysis demonstrated postoperative errors in both version and inclination angles were 5° or less in 20 of the 22 studies (90.9%). They noted that the effect of PSI on cost and operative time was not evaluated in these studies. Interestingly, many reviews included results in both cadavers and patients. Hence, based on the available evidence, it appears that 3D planning and PSI reduce the variability in glenoid placement in ATSA and RTSA, but there may be no difference between the technologies in the clinical (noncadaveric) setting.

While PSI in general has often been shown to allow the surgeon to reproduce the preoperative plan, little research has been done to evaluate how accurate the preoperative planning software is at generating version and inclination measurements. Furthermore, as there are several preoperative planning software programs available, it is possible that different programs could provide different measurements on the same patient for preoperative glenoid version and inclination. Denard et al used preoperative 3D CT scans of 63 consecutive patients undergoing primary shoulder arthroplasty to compare glenoid version and inclination values obtained by two different planning software systems.[37] These two systems used two different methods for measuring glenoid version and inclination; one used an average scapular plane and an automated best-fit sphere system (Blueprint; Wright Medical , Memphis, TN, USA), while the other used manual landmark-based software system (VIP; Arthrex Corporation, Naples, FL, USA). The authors found that glenoid version based on Blueprint was −10.9° compared with −9.3° for VIP (P = 0.04), while inclination was 9.0° with Blueprint compared with 9.7° for VIP (P = 0.463). The mean differences were thus small. However, in many cases, there was considerable variability between the systems. For inclination, the difference between VIP and Blueprint was 5° to 10° in 17 cases (27.0%) and greater than 10° in 12 cases (19.0%). For version, the difference

between VIP and Blueprint was 5° to 10° in 12 cases (19.0%) and greater than 10° in 7 cases (11.1%). This study highlights the variability with preoperative planning software systems. It also highlights the differences in measuring glenoid version and inclination based on the measurement tool used. Unfortunately, it is unclear from the study which measurement method is more accurate.

In order to address this question, we performed a study to compare version and inclination measurements between five fellowship-trained sports medicine and shoulder and elbow surgeons and then compared the average measurements among the surgeons to four commercially available preoperative planning software programs. We used 81 consecutive shoulder CT scans obtained for preoperative planning purposes for shoulder arthroplasty and analyzed these using commercially available software from Blueprint (Wright Medical, Memphis, TN), GPS (Exactech, Gainesville, FL), Materialise (DJO, Vista, CA), and VIP (Arthrex, Naples, FL). The first program uses a 3D mean to determine the scapular plane and best-fit sphere for the glenoid, while all other systems use an anatomic landmark-based approach. Inclination, version, and subluxation of the humerus were measured in a blinded fashion by the five surgeons on axial and coronal sequences at the midglenoid. Surgeon measurements were analyzed for agreement and were compared to the four commercial programs. We found surgeon reliability was acceptable for version (intraclass correlation coefficient [ICC]: 0.876), inclination (ICC: 0.84), and subluxation (ICC: 0.523), indicating the five surgeons were in agreement in all measured parameters. However, significant differences were found between surgeon and commercial software measurements in version (P = 0.03), inclination (P = 0.023), and subluxation (P < 0.001). The results revealed that software measurements tended to be more superiorly inclined (average: −2°-2° greater), more retroverted (average: 2°-5° greater) and more posteriorly subluxed (average: 7°-10° greater) than surgeon measurements. Interestingly, in comparing imaging software measurements between preoperative planning programs, only Blueprint produced significantly different version measurements than surgeon measurements (P = 0.02). Further work is needed to determine the ideal measurement method for glenoid version and inclination to allow precision and accuracy across all software planning systems.

OUTCOMES FOLLOWING THE USE OF PATIENT-SPECIFIC INSTRUMENTATION

The clinical results following ATSA and RTSA using PSI have been excellent, with the vast majority of patients achieving a reduction in pain, improvement in function, and improvement in sleep quality (**FIGURE 8.6A-E**).[38-40]

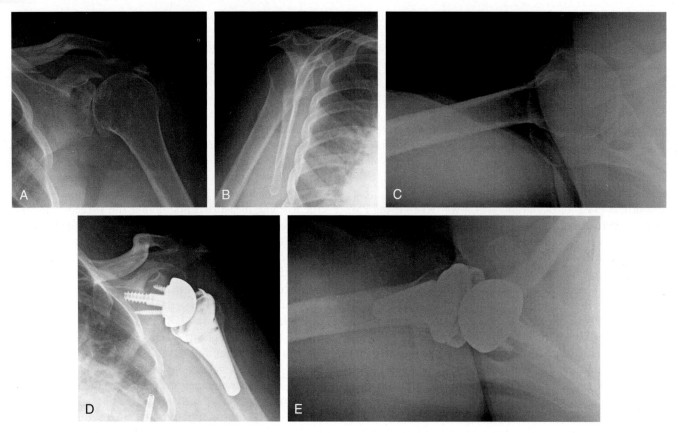

FIGURE 8.6 A-E, Preoperative anteroposterior (**A**), scapular Y (**B**), and axillary (**C**) radiographic views from a 79-year-old woman with rotator cuff tear arthropathy. Postoperative anteroposterior (**D**) and axial (**E**) radiographs following left reverse total shoulder arthroplasty demonstrating proper glenoid placement in which a reusable patient-specific instrumentation guide was used.

Patel et al recently reported the results of 1135 patients who underwent ATSA at a mean follow-up of 4 years and found excellent clinical outcomes with significant improvements in ROM and pain scores.[39] Most studies of PSI have focused on implant position in the acute postoperative setting and not on patient-reported outcome scores or postoperative complications. Lau et al reported on 11 patients who underwent ATSA (n = 7) and RTSA (n = 4) with the use of preoperative planning software and PSI.[34] The authors noted two postoperative complications, both in the RTSA group that included one case of scapular notching and one case of a soft-tissue infection. The study did not comment on patient-reported outcome scores at the 1-year follow-up. This highlights the limited clinical evidence regarding success of PSI with respect to improved patient outcomes. Furthermore, no study to date has directly compared patient-reported outcomes and future revision surgery rates between patients who underwent ATSA/RTSA with PSI versus standard instrumentation.[41] Hence, it is currently unclear if the use of PSI translates to improved clinical outcomes as no direct comparison in a randomized study has been made.

CONCLUSION

3D planning and PSI have the potential to improve glenoid component position in shoulder arthroplasty. While the technology is not perfect, most studies agree that the use of PSI improves glenoid position when compared to freehand guides in the cadaveric setting. In the clinical setting, it appears both 3D planning and PSI show improvements in glenoid position, but there may not be a significant difference between the two. However, despite improved glenoid position, it is still unclear if this had resulted in an improvement in patient-reported outcomes and a decrease in complication rates following shoulder arthroplasty. Now that the accuracy, reproducibility, and radiographic benefit have been clearly demonstrated, further work is needed to determine the clinical benefit of PSI.

REFERENCES

1. Basques BA, Erickson BJ, Leroux T, et al. Comparative outcomes of outpatient and inpatient total shoulder arthroplasty: an analysis of the Medicare dataset. *Bone Joint J*. 2017;99-B(7):934-938.
2. Boileau P, Cheval D, Gauci MO, Holzer N, Chaoui J, Walch G. Automated three-dimensional measurement of glenoid version and inclination in arthritic shoulders. *J Bone Joint Surg Am*. 2018;100(1):57-65.

3. Boileau P, Alta TD, Decroocq L, et al. Reverse shoulder arthroplasty for acute fractures in the elderly: is it worth reattaching the tuberosities? *J Shoulder Elbow Surg.* 2019;28(3):437-444.

4. Erickson BJ, Bohl DD, Cole BJ, et al. Reverse total shoulder arthroplasty: indications and techniques across the world. *Am J Orthop (Belle Mead NJ).* 2018;47(9). doi:10.12788/ajo.2018.0079.

5. Erickson BJ, Ling D, Wong A, et al. Does having a rotator cuff repair prior to reverse total shoulder arthroplasty influence the outcome? *Bone Joint J.* 2019;101-B(1):63-67.

6. Kim SH, Wise BL, Zhang Y, Szabo RM. Increasing incidence of shoulder arthroplasty in the United States. *J Bone Joint Surg Am.* 2011;93(24):2249-2254.

7. Ladermann A, Schwitzguebel AJ, Edwards TB, et al. Glenoid loosening and migration in reverse shoulder arthroplasty. *Bone Joint J.* 2019;101-B(4):461-469.

8. Papadonikolakis A, Neradilek MB, Matsen FA III. Failure of the glenoid component in anatomic total shoulder arthroplasty: a systematic review of the English-language literature between 2006 and 2012. *J Bone Joint Surg Am.* 2013;95(24):2205-2212.

9. Erickson BJ, Frank RM, Harris JD, Mall N, Romeo AA. The influence of humeral head inclination in reverse total shoulder arthroplasty: a systematic review. *J Shoulder Elbow Surg.* 2015;24(6):988-993.

10. Erickson BJ, Harris JD, Romeo AA. The effect of humeral inclination on range of motion in reverse total shoulder arthroplasty: a systematic review. *Am J Orthop (Belle Mead NJ).* 2016;45(4):E174-E179.

11. Singh JA, Sperling JW, Cofield RH. Revision surgery following total shoulder arthroplasty: analysis of 2588 shoulders over three decades (1976 to 2008). *J Bone Joint Surg Br.* 2011;93(11):1513-1517.

12. Boileau P. Complications and revision of reverse total shoulder arthroplasty. *Orthop Traumatol Surg Res.* 2016;102(1 suppl):S33-S43.

13. Hendel MD, Bryan JA, Barsoum WK, et al. Comparison of patient-specific instruments with standard surgical instruments in determining glenoid component position: a randomized prospective clinical trial. *J Bone Joint Surg Am.* 2012;94(23):2167-2175.

14. Kircher J, Wiedemann M, Magosch P, Lichtenberg S, Habermeyer P. Improved accuracy of glenoid positioning in total shoulder arthroplasty with intraoperative navigation: a prospective-randomized clinical study. *J Shoulder Elbow Surg.* 2009;18(4):515-520.

15. Nguyen D, Ferreira LM, Brownhill JR, et al. Improved accuracy of computer assisted glenoid implantation in total shoulder arthroplasty: an in-vitro randomized controlled trial. *J Shoulder Elbow Surg.* 2009;18(6):907-914.

16. Scalise JJ, Codsi MJ, Bryan J, Iannotti JP. The three-dimensional glenoid vault model can estimate normal glenoid version in osteoarthritis. *J Shoulder Elbow Surg.* 2008;17(3):487-491.

17. Churchill RS, Brems JJ, Kotschi H. Glenoid size, inclination, and version: an anatomic study. *J Shoulder Elbow Surg.* 2001;10(4):327-332.

18. Codsi MJ, Bennetts C, Gordiev K, et al. Normal glenoid vault anatomy and validation of a novel glenoid implant shape. *J Shoulder Elbow Surg.* 2008;17(3):471-478.

19. Scalise JJ, Bryan J, Polster J, Brems JJ, Iannotti JP. Quantitative analysis of glenoid bone loss in osteoarthritis using three-dimensional computed tomography scans. *J Shoulder Elbow Surg.* 2008;17(2):328-335.

20. Chen X, Reddy AS, Kontaxis A, et al. Version correction via eccentric reaming compromises remaining bone quality in B2 glenoids: a computational study. *Clin Orthop Relat Res.* 2017;475(12):3090-3099.

21. Service BC, Hsu JE, Somerson JS, Russ SM, Matsen FA III. Does postoperative glenoid retroversion affect the 2-year clinical and radiographic outcomes for total shoulder arthroplasty? *Clin Orthop Relat Res.* 2017;475(11):2726-2739.

22. Karelse A, Van Tongel A, Verstraeten T, Poncet D, De Wilde LF. Rocking-horse phenomenon of the glenoid component: the importance of inclination. *J Shoulder Elbow Surg.* 2015;24(7):1142-1148.

23. Iannotti J, Baker J, Rodriguez E, et al. Three-dimensional preoperative planning software and a novel information transfer technology improve glenoid component positioning. *J Bone Joint Surg Am.* 2014;96(9):e71.

24. Iannotti JP, Walker K, Rodriguez E, Patterson TE, Jun BJ, Ricchetti ET. Accuracy of 3-dimensional planning, implant templating, and patient-specific instrumentation in anatomic total shoulder arthroplasty. *J Bone Joint Surg Am.* 2019;101(5):446-457.

25. Levigne C, Garret J, Boileau P, Alami G, Favard L, Walch G. Scapular notching in reverse shoulder arthroplasty: is it important to avoid it and how? *Clin Orthop Relat Res.* 2011;469(9):2512-2520.

26. Keener JD, Patterson BM, Orvets N, Aleem AW, Chamberlain AM. Optimizing reverse shoulder arthroplasty component position in the setting of advanced arthritis with posterior glenoid erosion: a computer-enhanced range of motion analysis. *J Shoulder Elbow Surg.* 2018;27(2):339-349.

27. Werner BS, Chaoui J, Walch G. The influence of humeral neck shaft angle and glenoid lateralization on range of motion in reverse shoulder arthroplasty. *J Shoulder Elbow Surg.* 2017;26(10):1726-1731.

28. Berhouet J, Gulotta LV, Dines DM, et al. Preoperative planning for accurate glenoid component positioning in reverse shoulder arthroplasty. *Orthop Traumatol Surg Res.* 2017;103(3):407-413.

29. Chalmers PN, Salazar D, Chamberlain A, Keener JD. Radiographic characterization of the B2 glenoid: is inclusion of the entirety of the scapula necessary? *J Shoulder Elbow Surg.* 2017;26(5):855-860.

30. Burns DM, Frank T, Whyne CM, Henry PD. Glenoid component positioning and guidance techniques in anatomic and reverse total shoulder arthroplasty: a systematic review and meta-analysis. *Shoulder Elbow.* 2019;11(2 suppl):16-28.

31. Gauci MO, Boileau P, Baba M, Chaoui J, Walch G. Patient-specific glenoid guides provide accuracy and reproducibility in total shoulder arthroplasty. *Bone Joint J.* 2016;98-B(8):1080-1085.

32. Heylen S, Van Haver A, Vuylsteke K, Declercq G, Verborgt O. Patient-specific instrument guidance of glenoid component implantation reduces inclination variability in total and reverse shoulder arthroplasty. *J Shoulder Elbow Surg.* 2016;25(2):186-192.

33. Throckmorton TW, Gulotta LV, Bonnarens FO, et al. Patient-specific targeting guides compared with traditional instrumentation for glenoid component placement in shoulder arthroplasty: a multi-surgeon study in 70 arthritic cadaver specimens. *J Shoulder Elbow Surg.* 2015;24(6):965-971.

34. Lau SC, Keith PPA. Patient-specific instrumentation for total shoulder arthroplasty: not as accurate as it would seem. *J Shoulder Elbow Surg.* 2018;27(1):90-95.

35. Cabarcas BC, Cvetanovich GL, Gowd AK, Liu JN, Manderle BJ, Verma NN. Accuracy of patient-specific instrumentation in shoulder arthroplasty: a systematic review and meta-analysis. *JSES Open Access.* 2019;3(3):117-129.

36. Villatte G, Muller AS, Pereira B, Mulliez A, Reilly P, Emery R. Use of Patient-Specific Instrumentation (PSI) for glenoid component positioning in shoulder arthroplasty. A systematic review and meta-analysis. *PLoS One.* 2018;13(8):e0201759.

37. Denard PJ, Provencher MT, Ladermann A, Romeo AA, Parsons BO, Dines JS. Version and inclination obtained with 3-dimensional planning in total shoulder arthroplasty: do different programs produce the same results? *JSES Open Access.* 2018;2(4):200-204.

38. Grey SG, Wright TW, Flurin PH, Zuckerman JD, Roche CP, Friedman RJ. Clinical and radiographic outcomes with a posteriorly augmented glenoid for Walch B glenoids in anatomic total shoulder arthroplasty. *J Shoulder Elbow Surg.* 2020;29(5):e185-e195.

39. Patel RB, Muh S, Okoroha KR, et al. Results of total shoulder arthroplasty in patients aged 55 years or younger versus those older than 55 years: an analysis of 1135 patients with over 2 years of follow-up. *J Shoulder Elbow Surg.* 2019;28(5):861-868.

40. Weinberg M, Mollon B, Kaplan D, Zuckerman J, Strauss E. Improvement in sleep quality after total shoulder arthroplasty. *Phys Sportsmed.* 2020;48(2):194-198.

41. Virk MS, Steinmann SP, Romeo AA, Zuckerman JD. Managing glenoid deformity in shoulder arthroplasty: role of new technology (computer-assisted navigation and patient-specific instrumentation). *Instr Course Lect.* 2020;69:583-594.

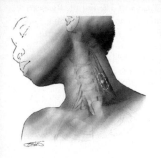

9 Anesthesia for Shoulder Arthroplasty

Uchenna O. Umeh, MD and Chrissy J. Cherenfant, MD

INTRODUCTION

Each year, the number of both in-hospital and ambulatory shoulder surgeries continues to increase in the United States. Examples of some common shoulder procedures include anatomic and reverse total shoulder arthroplasty, hemiarthroplasty, and shoulder arthroscopy. Surgery is indicated for management for many conditions such as rotator cuff repair, fractures, impingement syndrome, instability, and degenerative arthritis. As the elderly population undergoes many of these procedures and our population continues to age and live longer, more patients undergo elective shoulder replacement surgery to improve their quality of life by alleviating pain and restoring function.[1-5]

A vital aspect of shoulder surgery is the anesthesia provided, as it may often impact a patient's postoperative pain, opioid utilization, and clinical outcome. The anesthetic plan for each patient is individualized and determined by factors such as the medical history, duration of surgery, positioning, and body habitus.[6,7] With the emergence of many anesthetic techniques, it is essential to evaluate the anesthetic options for shoulder surgery and the elements that influence the anesthesiologist's decision on the preferred plan (VIDEO 9.1).

TYPES OF ANESTHESIA FOR SHOULDER SURGERY

Depending on the nature of the shoulder surgery, a patient may be awake, be sedated, or undergo general anesthesia (GA) with appropriate airway management. Often, the anesthesiologist's initial decision is determining whether general or regional anesthesia will be the primary mode of anesthesia.[7]

GA encompasses amnesia, unconsciousness, analgesia, autonomic and sensory blockade of responses to noxious surgical stimulation, and immobilization or muscle relaxation. As a result, patients have decreased awareness and recall with simultaneously controlled autonomic reflexes such as breathing.[8-11] Despite these advantages and its common use, GA has drawbacks. Some disadvantages include necessary airway management, greater effect on cardiac and pulmonary function, possible increased morbidity and mortality risk in patients with multiple medical comorbidities, and inadequate postoperative pain control. With the sole use of GA, without regional anesthesia, patients will likely require more opioids intraoperatively and postoperatively. They may also be subject to a variety of side effects such as nausea, vomiting, pruritus, and drowsiness.[7] In addition, compared to regional anesthesia for shoulder surgeries, GA is associated with an increased likelihood of pulmonary complications, blood transfusions, intensive care unit transfers, longer stays in the postanesthesia care unit, and more readmissions for pain, sedation, nausea/vomiting, and other complications.[7,12-16] GA for shoulder surgery in the beach chair position is associated with reductions in cerebral oxygenation and consequential higher risk of neurological damage.[6,15] Due to the many benefits of regional anesthesia, many patients undergoing GA will also receive a peripheral nerve block, such as an interscalene block (ISB). Compared to GA alone, this combination of care has been associated with shorter extubation time, faster recovery, less analgesic consumption, and lower pain scores, heart rate, systolic blood pressure, and incidence of adverse events.[7,17,18]

Although regional anesthesia has many advantages, it is important to note that it may not be 100% successful, and conversion to GA may occur in the setting of inadequate analgesia.[7] Nevertheless, regional anesthesia promotes postoperative recovery and allows for shoulder surgery with less or without the need for GA and less opioid use intraoperatively and postoperatively, which also decreases the potential for the associated risks. Regional anesthesia can also be used in conjunction with other forms of anesthesia for sedation, with the outcome of patients achieving optimal postoperative pain management, care, comfort, and satisfaction.[6,7,19-21] Regional anesthesia suitable for shoulder arthroplasty encompasses peripheral nerve blocks such as interscalene nerve blocks, supraclavicular nerve blocks, suprascapular nerve blocks (SSNBs), and axillary nerve blocks. Anesthesia for shoulder surgeries may also include intraarticular local anesthesia injections.

PERIPHERAL NERVE BLOCKS

Interscalene Block

An interscalene nerve block or ISB covers most of the brachial plexus (C5-T1), upper and middle trunks, which supplies the upper extremity while sparing the ulnar nerve (C8-T1) **(FIGURES 9.1** and **9.2)**. An ISB is composed of a local injection of 15 to 25 mL of a long-acting anesthetic such as bupivacaine or ropivacaine. The block may last for about 12 to 24 hours and results in anesthesia of the shoulder, distal clavicle, and proximal humerus. The interscalene groove is often identified with ultrasound visualization of the needle and vital structures such as the subclavian artery, first rib, anterior and middle scalene muscles, and nerve roots of the brachial plexus. The positioning of this block entails the patients with their head turned away from the side of the block while in a supine position. Palpation and identification of the sternal notch, clavicle, and heads of the sternocleidomastoid muscle are often used to discern the interscalene space. Although less utilized compared to ultrasound, nerve stimulation is another method used to locate a peripheral nerve or nerve plexus and facilitate the performance of a nerve block.[6,7,19,22]

Complications of an ISB are often due to needle or local anesthetic placement, including pneumothorax with an incidence of 0.2%, and blockade of the phrenic nerve that can cause transient ipsilateral hemiparesis of the diaphragm (78.75%-100%), which may lead to a 25% reduction in pulmonary function.[6,22-29] Hoarseness may occur with an incidence of 3% to 31% as a result of recurrent laryngeal nerve blockade.[24,27,30] Horner syndrome may result from blockage of the sympathetic trunk at an incidence of 1% to 59.6%, which is most likely an underestimation.[23,25,27,29,31,32] Other rare complications include bleeding or hematoma formation, infection, vascular structure puncture, nerve damage, local anesthetic toxicity, or epidural or subarachnoid injection. Allergic reactions to local anesthesia are uncommon but also possible.[6,22-24]

ISBs can be done as a single-shot interscalene block (SSISB) with an injection of a local anesthetic or as a continuous interscalene block (CISB) by percutaneous insertion of a catheter adjacent to the brachial plexus. SSISB provides better analgesia, less nausea, and improved satisfaction than single-shot intra-articular injections or SSNBs.[33] SSISB is also associated with less risk of neurological injury compared to CISB.[34] However, some patients may benefit from greater analgesic coverage after surgery since SSISB has a limited duration. A CISB consists of an infusion of local anesthetic that allows prolonged analgesia and decreases opioid requirements.[35-38] Compared to SSISB, CISB has been associated with a shorter length of stay; however, some studies have shown the contrary, with increased length of stay and increased barriers to discharge.[39,40] Overall, an ISB is an effective anesthetic and analgesic technique that is commonly used for shoulder arthroplasty.

Supraclavicular Block

A supraclavicular block **(FIGURE 9.3)** is another anesthetic technique used for analgesia for shoulder arthroplasty. It rapidly blocks the brachial plexus at the nerve trunk level, which affects the distal two-thirds of the upper extremity such as the elbow, forearm, wrist, and hand. It can also block proximal nerves that supply the shoulder. However, there is concern that the nerves supplying the shoulder may be missed, depending on the anesthetic placement in the interscalene groove.[7,23] The positioning for a supraclavicular block is similar to an ISB, with the addition of some preferring a 30° elevation of the head of the bed.[41]

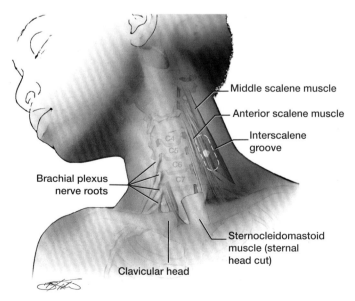

Middle scalene muscle

Anterior scalene muscle

Interscalene groove

Brachial plexus nerve roots

Sternocleidomastoid muscle (sternal head cut)

Clavicular head

FIGURE 9.1 Anatomic relationship of the brachial plexus in relation to the head and neck.

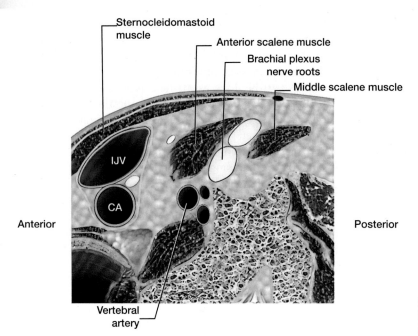

Sternocleidomastoid muscle

Anterior scalene muscle

Brachial plexus nerve roots

Middle scalene muscle

IJV

CA

Anterior

Posterior

Vertebral artery

FIGURE 9.2 Cross-sectional anatomy of the interscalene brachial plexus block. The brachial plexus is seen between the anterior and middle scalene muscles.

In the past, prior to widespread ultrasound use, there was reluctant utilization of the supraclavicular block due to the high incidence of pneumothorax. With ultrasound guidance, it is now known as a safe alternative to ISB that provides pain relief, with fewer potential side effects or complications like pneumothorax with an incidence of 0% to 6.1%.[7,23-27,29,31,42,43] The possible complications of a supraclavicular block are similar to those of an ISB, including nerve injury, pneumothorax, vascular puncture, intravascular injection causing anesthetic toxicity, recurrent laryngeal nerve blockade, phrenic nerve blockade, and Horner syndrome.[23,24,43,44] However, when compared to an ISB, studies have found supraclavicular blocks to have a greater motor blockade and reduced incidence of hoarseness (4.3%-22%),

hemidiaphragmatic paresis (1%-65.2%), and Horner syndrome (1%-19.6%).[23-27,29,31,43] Yet, it has not been found to be more efficacious than ISB for sensory blockade and pain control, where supraclavicular blocks compared to ISBs have not had any statistically significant difference in postoperative analgesia duration. Thus, a supraclavicular block is an effective option for anesthesia for shoulder arthroplasty.[7,23-27,31,42]

Suprascapular and Axillary (Circumflex) Nerve Block

The suprascapular nerve (SSN) originates from C5 and C6 nerve roots **(FIGURE 9.4)**. It innervates the posterior shoulder capsule, acromioclavicular joint, subacromial bursa, and coracoclavicular ligament. The SSN supplies the majority of the shoulder, at about 70%, with the

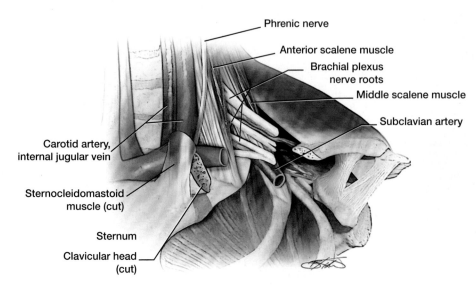

Phrenic nerve

Anterior scalene muscle

Brachial plexus nerve roots

Middle scalene muscle

Subclavian artery

Carotid artery, internal jugular vein

Sternocleidomastoid muscle (cut)

Sternum

Clavicular head (cut)

FIGURE 9.3 The brachial plexus can be seen emerging between the anterior and middle scalene muscles and traveling above the subclavian artery.

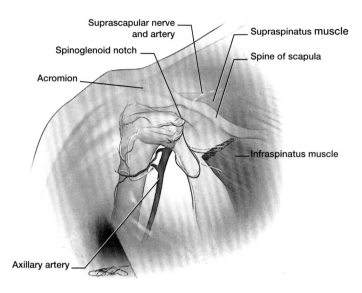

FIGURE 9.4 The suprascapular nerve originates from the upper trunk of the brachial plexus. It travels through the upper part of the scapula providing sensory branches to the shoulder joint and capsule. It travels under the suprascapular ligament to the suprascapular fossa providing motor innervation to the supraspinatus and infraspinatus muscles.

axillary nerve providing the remaining innervation, followed by the lateral pectoral nerve. Thus, an SSNB is a suitable form of pain relief for shoulder arthroplasty. An SSNB and axillary nerve block combined is another alternative to an ISB for shoulder surgery anesthesia. The positioning for SSNB can vary depending on whether the approach is posterior or anterior. For the posterior approach of a combined axillary and SSN block, the patient is in a sitting position, with their ipsilateral hand over the contralateral shoulder to move the scapula and provide more space for ultrasound visualization. In contrast, the patient is positioned supine with their head turned away for the anterior approach.[7,23,26,45]

The SSN and axillary combination nerve block does not block the phrenic nerve and is therefore especially useful for shoulder anesthesia among patients with risk factors such as severe chronic obstructive pulmonary disease and contralateral hemidiaphragmatic paresis.[23] However, this combination has the disadvantage that the patient must undergo two, separate injections and a possibility of incomplete analgesia due to proximal branches to the injection not being blocked. As a result, supplementation with GA, local anesthesia infiltration, and intravenous analgesics is often needed. Similar to other peripheral nerve blocks, possible complications include nerve damage, vascular structure damage, intravascular injection, and a small risk of pneumothorax.[23,46] Aside from ISBs providing better pain control in the recovery room and SSNB having fewer side effects, studies have found no other clinically meaningful analgesic differences between suprascapular and ISBs, especially in the first 24 hours. The suprascapular and axillary combination nerve block has prospects of providing effective to nonequivalent postoperative relief for shoulder surgeries compared to ISB and with fewer complications.[7,23,46-48] Although SSNB and axillary nerve blocks have no superior analgesic effect compared to ISB, these

diaphragm-sparing nerve blocks are a feasible and effective alternative for patients who are not candidates for an ISB.[7,23,49-51]

ADJUVANTS

A drawback to peripheral nerve blocks is that the duration of their effect is limited, commonly lasting to the patient's first postoperative evening or night.[7,52] A strategy to alleviate this shortcoming is to use adjuvant drugs that prolong analgesia after nerve blockade and can consequently reduce postoperative pain and rescue analgesic use. Drugs that have been studied for this purpose include epinephrine, clonidine, fentanyl, buprenorphine, morphine, ketamine, midazolam, tramadol, magnesium, neostigmine, dexmedetomidine, and dexamethasone. However, epinephrine, buprenorphine, clonidine, magnesium, dexmedetomidine, and dexamethasone have been found to be more consistent in prolonging peripheral nerve blockade.[7,52-57] Tramadol as an adjuvant to ropivacaine in ISBs also has prospects in improving time of onset and duration of analgesia.[58] Notably, dexamethasone is commonly incorporated into clinical practice because many studies have shown its prolonging analgesic effect.[7,59-62] However, there is a concern for the side effects of these adjuvant drugs, such as neurotoxicity, neurological complications, and intravascular injection, all of which require further investigation through research.[53-56]

More recent advancements include using charged molecules like tonicaine and n-butyl tetracaine and using liposomal microspheres and cyclodextrin formulations as encapsulating delivery mechanisms for anesthetics. All of these approaches provide the main benefit of having a longer duration of block action and pain control.[56,63,64] For instance, liposomal bupivacaine may have a duration of up to 72 hours, reducing pain and opioid consumption.[65,66] These formulations may be delivered as blocks or local infiltrations intraoperatively. Studies comparing intraoperative infiltration of liposomal bupivacaine versus ISB of ropivacaine or bupivacaine found comparable pain control, with no increase in complications or length of stay.[67-70] Yet, formulations may be more effectively used as blocks rather than local infiltration, where the value and success in adding an infiltration of liposomal bupivacaine to ISB are dependent on technique.[71-73] Studies have found liposomal bupivacaine to lower pain, increase patient satisfaction, and decrease opioid use when added to an ISB of standard bupivacaine.[74,75] Liposomal bupivacaine also has comparable pain relief and fewer major complications and costs than CISB for shoulder arthroplasty.[76,77] Prior to these formulations, especially liposomal bupivacaine, being consistently integrated into clinical practice for the optimal pain regimen of shoulder surgeries, more research is needed.[54,63,67,78]

AUTHOR'S PREFERRED APPROACH

All interscalene or supraclavicular nerve blocks for shoulder surgery are performed under ultrasound guidance. The patient is positioned supine with the head facing away from the surgical site (**FIGURE 9.5**). The area above the clavicle on the operative side is cleaned with an alcohol-based prep solution. A linear ultrasound transducer (3-12 MHz) is placed right above the patient's clavicle on the operative side. The transducer should be pointing slightly caudad toward the lung and should be midclavicle. The optimal image at this point is that of a pulsating subclavian artery with the supraclavicular plexus directly lateral to the vessel (**FIGURE 9.6**). Two hyperechoic lines will be prominent below the subclavian artery. The superior line represents the first rib. The second hyperechoic line is the pleura of the lung, note the pleural sliding movement during respiration.

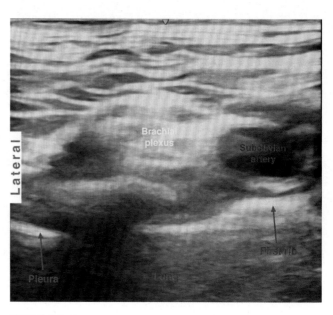

FIGURE 9.6 The supraclavicular brachial plexus is located superficial and posterolateral to the subclavian artery. The brachial plexus is covered by a connective tissue sheath. The first rib, pleura, and lung can be seen below the brachial plexus.

To image the interscalene space, obtain the image of the supraclavicular brachial plexus as described above. Keeping the plexus at the center of the image screen, move the ultrasound transducer slowly cephalad toward the patient's head. Follow the brachial plexus and watch as the hyper- and hypoechoic bundle of nerves typically described as a "bunch of grapes" transitions to three distinct hypoechoic nerve roots lined up next to each other. This is usually referred to as the "traffic light" (**FIGURE 9.7**). At this point, your transducer should be transverse on the neck, about 3 to 4 cm above the clavicle and over the external jugular vein.

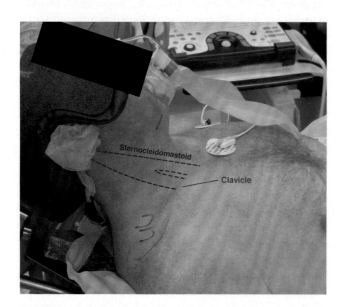

FIGURE 9.5 For ultrasound-guided brachial plexus block, appropriate patient positioning is important and facilitates block placement. The patient is in the semisitting position with the head turned to the opposite side.

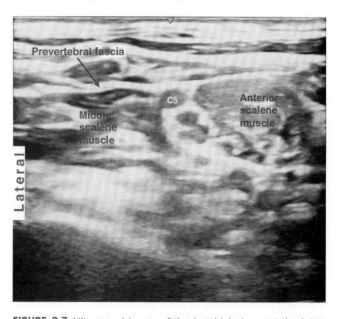

FIGURE 9.7 Ultrasound image of the brachial plexus at the interscalene level. C5 nerve root is highlighted between the anterior and middle scalene muscles.

To perform a supraclavicular block, identify the supraclavicular plexus lateral to the subclavian artery. This is the ideal image for needle placement. Make a needle puncture about 1 cm lateral to the transducer and identify the needle in the ultrasound image. Move the needle in a lateral to medial direction and approach the supraclavicular plexus. Pierce through the fascia surrounding the plexus and inject the local anesthetic solution. The supraclavicular plexus comprises three trunks (upper, middle, and lower) bundled together. It is important to ensure that the lower trunk of the brachial plexus is not missed while performing your supraclavicular block. Inject a few milliliters of local anesthetic in the "corner pocket" immediately lateral to the subclavian artery and above the first rib.

To perform an ISB, obtain the image of the "traffic light" as described above. This "green" and the "yellow" traffic lights represent the C5 and C6 nerve roots. For a safe and effective ISB, the needle entry point is posterior, in-plane, and in a lateral to medial direction. The needle will pierce and travel through the middle scalene muscle. The needle should always be aimed in between the nerve roots so as to decrease the risk of nerve injury. Once the needle has punctured the fascia surrounding the nerves, inject the local anesthetic. Observe the spread around the nerve roots, behind the anterior scalene muscle, and in front of the middle scalene. The block may not be effective if good spread of local anesthetic is not noted.

Once the patient has been successfully blocked, the anesthetic plan is typically intravenous sedation with propofol, plus or minus dexmedetomidine and ketamine with supplementary oxygen via nonrebreather face mask.

Depending on the patient's body habitus, history of obstructive sleep apnea, abnormal anatomy, or anticipated difficult airway, the decision may be made to place an oral airway or nasal trumpet to prevent airway obstruction and ensure that the patient is adequately ventilating throughout the procedure. If the patient continues to obstruct the airway despite the assistive device, the next step would be to convert to GA and place a laryngeal mask airway or an endotracheal tube.

CONCLUSION

There are a variety of anesthetic techniques suitable for shoulder arthroplasty surgery. The chosen anesthetic plan is determined by the patient's physical examination and medical history. Compared to solely using GA, utilizing regional anesthesia is advantageous for patients by minimizing or excluding the need for GA, decreasing postoperative pain and opioid consumption, and reducing readmissions. Thus, regional anesthesia, in the form of peripheral nerve blocks, is frequently employed as anesthesia for shoulder surgeries, either in conjunction

with sedation or GA. An interscalene nerve block is commonly used as a safe, effective form of regional anesthesia for shoulder surgeries. However, alternative anesthetic techniques such as blockades of the supraclavicular nerve, SSN, and axillary nerve are effective options of analgesia for shoulder arthroplasty, especially when an ISB may be unfavorable such as in patients with poor pulmonary function. Anesthesia for shoulder arthroplasty requires a solid understanding of anatomy and utilization of ultrasound plus or minus nerve stimulation. Ultrasound allows for better visualization of the nerve, vascular structures, needle, and anesthetic delivery. Although the safety of regional anesthesia has increased with ultrasound guidance, it is important to be aware of the complications that may occur. Lastly, with a continued focus on patient safety and comfort, there remains a need for further research on anesthesia for shoulder arthroplasty, especially in terms of advancements such as liposomal formulations that can augment the efficacy of anesthesia.

REFERENCES

1. Landy DC, Boyadjian H, Shi LL, Lee MJ. General health measures in shoulder surgery: are we powered for success? *J Shoulder Elbow Surg.* 2019;28(7):1341-1346.
2. Jain NB, Higgins LD, Losina E, Collins J, Blazar PE, Katz JN. Epidemiology of musculoskeletal upper extremity ambulatory surgery in the United States. *BMC Musculoskelet Disord.* 2014;15:4.
3. Palsis JA, Simpson KN, Matthews JH, Traven S, Eichinger JK, Friedman RJ. Current trends in the use of shoulder arthroplasty in the United States. *Orthopedics.* 2018;41(3):e416-e423.
4. Cancienne JM, Brockmeier SF, Gulotta LV, Dines DM, Werner BC. Ambulatory total shoulder arthroplasty: a comprehensive analysis of current trends, complications, readmissions, and costs. *J Bone Joint Surg Am.* 2017;99(8):629-637.
5. Kim SH, Wise BL, Zhang Y, Szabo RM. Increasing incidence of shoulder arthroplasty in the United States. *J Bone Joint Surg Am.* 2011;93(24):2249-2254.
6. Santoprete S, Chierichini A, Micci DM. Anesthesia in shoulder arthroscopy. In: Milano G, Grasso A, eds. *Shoulder Arthroscopy.* Springer; 2014.
7. Sulaiman L, Macfarlane RJ, Waseem M. Current concepts in anaesthesia for shoulder surgery. *Open Orthop J.* 2013;7:323-328.
8. Grasshoff C, Rudolph U, Antkowiak B. Molecular and systemic mechanisms of general anaesthesia: the 'multi-site and multiple mechanisms' concept. *Curr Opin Anaesthesiol.* 2005;18(4):386-391.
9. Mashour GA, Forman SA, Campagna JA. Mechanisms of general anesthesia: from molecules to mind. *Best Pract Res Clin Anaesthesiol.* 2005;19(3):349-364.
10. Smith G, Goldman J. *General anesthesia for surgeons.* In: *StatPearls.* StatPearls Publishing; 2019.
11. Ding DY, Mahure SA, Mollon B, Shamah SD, Zuckerman JD, Kwon YW. Comparison of general versus isolated regional anesthesia in total shoulder arthroplasty: a retrospective propensity-matched cohort analysis. *J Orthop.* 2017;14(4):417-424.
12. Eroglu A, Apan A, Erturk E, Ben-shlomo I. Comparison of the anesthetic techniques. *ScientificWorldJournal.* 2015;2015:650684.
13. Brown AR, Weiss R, Greenberg C, Flatow EL, Bigliani LU. Interscalene block for shoulder arthroscopy: comparison with general anesthesia. *Arthroscopy.* 1993;9(3):295-300.
14. D'alessio JG, Rosenblum M, Shea KP, Freitas DG. A retrospective comparison of interscalene block and general anesthesia for ambulatory surgery shoulder arthroscopy. *Reg Anesth.* 1995;20(1):62-68.

15. Pohl A, Cullen DJ. Cerebral ischemia during shoulder surgery in the upright position: a case series. *J Clin Anesth.* 2005;17(6):463-469.

16. Herrick MD, Liu H, Davis M, Bell JE, Sites BD. Regional anesthesia decreases complications and resource utilization in shoulder arthroplasty patients. *Acta Anaesthesiol Scand.* 2018;62(4):540-547.

17. Yan S, Zhao Y, Zhang H. Efficacy and safety of interscalene block combined with general anesthesia for arthroscopic shoulder surgery: a meta-analysis. *J Clin Anesth.* 2018;47:74-79.

18. Lehmann LJ, Loosen G, Weiss C, Schmittner MD. Interscalene plexus block versus general anaesthesia for shoulder surgery: a randomized controlled study. *Eur J Orthop Surg Traumatol.* 2015;25(2):255-261.

19. Edwards TB, Morris BJ, Gartsman GM. *Anesthesia, patient positioning, and patient preparation.* In: *Shoulder Arthroplasty.* 2nd ed. Elsevier; 2019:29-34.

20. Wu CL, Rouse LM, Chen JM, Miller RJ. Comparison of postoperative pain in patients receiving interscalene block or general anesthesia for shoulder surgery. *Orthopedics.* 2002;25(1):45-48.

21. Hughes MS, Matava MJ, Wright RW, Brophy RH, Smith MV. Interscalene brachial plexus block for arthroscopic shoulder surgery: a systematic review. *J Bone Joint Surg Am.* 2013;95(14):1318-1324.

22. Zisquit J, Nedeff N. *Interscalene block.* In: *StatPearls.* StatPearls Publishing; 2019.

23. Bowens C, Sripada R. Regional blockade of the shoulder: approaches and outcomes. *Anesthesiol Res Pract.* 2012;2012:971963.

24. Liu SS, Gordon MA, Shaw PM, Wilfred S, Shetty T, Yadeau JT. A prospective clinical registry of ultrasound-guided regional anesthesia for ambulatory shoulder surgery. *Anesth Analg.* 2010;111(3):617-623.

25. Guo CW, Ma JX, Ma XL, et al. Supraclavicular block versus interscalene brachial plexus block for shoulder surgery: a meta-analysis of clinical control trials. *Int J Surg.* 2017;45:85-91.

26. Kim BG, Han JU, Song JH, Yang C, Lee BW, Baek JS. A comparison of ultrasound-guided interscalene and supraclavicular blocks for postoperative analgesia after shoulder surgery. *Acta Anaesthesiol Scand.* 2017;61(4):427-435.

27. Schubert AK, Dinges HC, Wulf H, Wiesmann T. Interscalene versus supraclavicular plexus block for the prevention of postoperative pain after shoulder surgery: a systematic review and meta-analysis. *Eur J Anaesthesiol.* 2019;36(6):427-435.

28. Long TR, Wass CT, Burkle CM. Perioperative interscalene blockade: an overview of its history and current clinical use. *J Clin Anesth.* 2002;14(7):546-556.

29. Horloker TT, Kopp SL, Wedel DJ. *Peripheral nerve blocks.* In: *Miller's Anesthesia.* vol 1. 8th ed. Elsevier/Saunders; 2015:1726-1728.

30. Kim H, Jang H, He H, et al. Ipsilateral vocal cord paralysis after interscalene brachial plexus block for clavicle surgery: anatomical considerations and technical recommendations – a case report. *Int J Clin Exp Med.* 2019;12.10132-10138.

31. Ryu T, Kil BT, Kim JH. Comparison between ultrasound-guided supraclavicular and interscalene brachial plexus blocks in patients undergoing arthroscopic shoulder surgery: a prospective, randomized, parallel study. *Medicine (Baltimore).* 2015;94(40):e1726.

32. Al-Khafaji JM, Ellias MA. Incidence of horner syndrome with interscalene brachial plexus block and its importance in the management of head injury. *Anesthesiology.* 1986;64(1):127.

33. Singelyn FJ, Lhotel L, Fabre B. Pain relief after arthroscopic shoulder surgery: a comparison of intraarticular analgesia, suprascapular nerve block, and interscalene brachial plexus block. *Anesth Analg.* 2004;99(2):589-592.

34. Holbrook HS, Parker BR. Peripheral nerve injury following interscalene blocks: a systematic review to guide orthopedic surgeons. *Orthopedics.* 2018;41(5):e598-e606.

35. Shah A, Nielsen KC, Braga L, Pietrobon R, Klein SM, Steele SM. Interscalene brachial plexus block for outpatient shoulder arthroplasty: postoperative analgesia, patient satisfaction, and complications. *Indian J Orthop.* 2007;41(3):230-236.

36. Lehtipalo S, Koskinen LO, Johansson G, Kolmodin J, Biber B. Continuous interscalene brachial plexus block for postoperative analgesia following shoulder surgery. *Acta Anaesthesiol Scand.* 1999;43(3):258-264.

37. Klein SM, Nielsen KC, Martin A, et al. Interscalene brachial plexus block with continuous intraarticular infusion of ropivacaine. *Anesth Analg.* 2001;93(3):601-605.

38. Nielsen KC, Greengrass RA, Pietrobon R, Klein SM, Steele SM. Continuous interscalene brachial plexus blockade provides good analgesia at home after major shoulder surgery-report of four cases. *Can J Anaesth.* 2003;50(1):57-61.

39. Chalmers PN, Salazar D, Fingerman ME, Keener JD, Chamberlain A. Continuous interscalene brachial plexus blockade is associated with reduced length of stay after shoulder arthroplasty. *Orthop Traumatol Surg Res.* 2017;103(6):847-852.

40. Thompson M, Simonds R, Clinger B, et al. Continuous versus single shot brachial plexus block and their relationship to discharge barriers and length of stay. *J Shoulder Elbow Surg.* 2017;26(4):656-661.

41. *Ultrasound-Guided Supraclavicular Brachial Plexus Block.* NYSORA; 2019. Accessed January 13, 2020. https://www.nysora.com/regional-anesthesia-for-specific-surgical-procedures/upper-extremity-regional-anesthesia-for-specific-surgical-procedures/anesthesia-and-analgesia-for-elbow-and-forearm-procedures/ultrasound-guided-supraclavicular-brachial-plexus-block/

42. Karaman T, Karaman S, Aşçı M, et al. Comparison of ultrasound-guided supraclavicular and interscalene brachial plexus blocks in postoperative pain management after arthroscopic shoulder surgery. *Pain Pract.* 2019;19(2):196-203.

43. Perlas A, Lobo G, Lo N, Brull R, Chan VW, Karkhanis R. Ultrasound-guided supraclavicular block: outcome of 510 consecutive cases. *Reg Anesth Pain Med.* 2009;34(2):171-176.

44. Chan VW, Perlas A, Rawson R, Odukoya O. Ultrasound-guided supraclavicular brachial plexus block. *Anesth Analg.* 2003;97(5):1514-1517.

45. Barber FA. Suprascapular nerve block for shoulder arthroscopy. *Arthroscopy.* 2005;21(8):1015.

46. Pani N, Routray SS, Pani S, Mallik S, Pattnaik S, Pradhan A. Postoperative analgesia for shoulder arthroscopic surgeries: a comparison between inter-scalene block and shoulder block. *Indian J Anaesth.* 2019;63(5):382-387.

47. Lee SM, Park SE, Nam YS, et al. Analgesic effectiveness of nerve block in shoulder arthroscopy: comparison between interscalene, suprascapular and axillary nerve blocks. *Knee Surg Sports Traumatol Arthrosc.* 2012;20(12):2573-2578.

48. Dhir S, Sondekoppam RV, Sharma R, Ganapathy S, Athwal GS. A comparison of combined suprascapular and axillary nerve blocks to interscalene nerve block for analgesia in arthroscopic shoulder surgery: an equivalence study. *Reg Anesth Pain Med.* 2016;41(5):564-571.

49. Hussain N, Goldar G, Ragina N, Banfield L, Laffey JG, Abdallah FW. Suprascapular and interscalene nerve block for shoulder surgery: a systematic review and meta-analysis. *Anesthesiology.* 2017;127(6):998-1013.

50. Desroches A, Klouche S, Schlur C, Bauer T, Waitzenegger T, Hardy P. Suprascapular nerve block versus interscalene block as analgesia after arthroscopic rotator cuff repair: a randomized controlled noninferiority trial. *Arthroscopy.* 2016;32(11):2203-2209.

51. Kay J, Memon M, Hu T, et al. Suprascapular nerve blockade for postoperative pain control after arthroscopic shoulder surgery: a systematic review and meta-analysis. *Orthop J Sports Med.* 2018;6(12):2325967118815859.

52. Brattwall M, Jildenstål P, Warrén stomberg M, Jakobsson JG. Upper extremity nerve block: how can benefit, duration, and safety be improved? An update. *F1000Res.* 2016;5:907. doi:10.12688/f1000research.7292.1.

53. Kirksey MA, Haskins SC, Cheng J, Liu SS. Local anesthetic peripheral nerve block Adjuvants for prolongation of analgesia: a systematic qualitative review. *PLoS One.* 2015;10(9):e0137312.

54. Swain A, Nag DS, Sahu S, Samaddar DP. Adjuvants to local anesthetics: current understanding and future trends. *World J Clin Cases.* 2017;5(8):307-323.

55. Jeon YH. The use of adjuvants to local anesthetics: benefit and risk. *Korean J Pain.* 2018;31(4):233-234.

56. Brummett CM, Williams BA. Additives to local anesthetics for peripheral nerve blockade. *Int Anesthesiol Clin.* 2011;49(4):104-116.

57. Yadeau JT, Dines DM, Liu SS, et al. What pain levels do TSA patients experience when given a long-acting nerve block and multimodal analgesia? *Clin Orthop Relat Res.* 2019;477(3):622-632.

58. Soulioti E, Tsaroucha A, Makris A, et al. Addition of 100 mg of tramadol to 40 mL of 0.5% ropivacaine for interscalene brachial plexus block improves postoperative analgesia in patients undergoing shoulder surgeries as compared to ropivacaine alone-A randomized controlled study. *Medicina (Kaunas).* 2019;55(7):399.

59. Hewson D, Bedforth N, Mccartney C, Hardman J. Dexamethasone and peripheral nerve blocks: back to basic (science). *Br J Anaesth.* 2019;122(4):411-412.

60. Cummings KC, Napierkowski DE, Parra-sanchez I, et al. Effect of dexamethasone on the duration of interscalene nerve blocks with ropivacaine or bupivacaine. *Br J Anaesth.* 2011;107(3):446-453.

61. Pehora C, Pearson AM, Kaushal A, Crawford MW, Johnston B. Dexamethasone as an adjuvant to peripheral nerve block. *Cochrane Database Syst Rev.* 2017;11:CD011770.

62. Webb BG, Sallay PI, Mcmurray SD, Misamore GW. Comparison of interscalene brachial plexus block performed with and without steroids. *Orthopedics.* 2016;39(6):e1100-e1103.

63. Park SK, Choi YS, Choi SW, Song SW. A comparison of three methods for postoperative pain control in patients undergoing arthroscopic shoulder surgery. *Korean J Pain.* 2015;28(1):45-51.

64. Patel MA, Gadsden JC, Nedeljkovic SS, et al. Brachial plexus block with liposomal bupivacaine for shoulder surgery improves analgesia and reduces opioid consumption: results from a multicenter, randomized, double-blind, controlled trial. *Pain Med.* 2020;21(2):387-400.

65. Malik O, Kaye AD, Kaye A, Belani K, Urman RD. Emerging roles of liposomal bupivacaine in anesthesia practice. *J Anaesthesiol Clin Pharmacol.* 2017;33(2):151-156.

66. Sethi PM, Brameier DT, Mandava NK, Miller SR. Liposomal bupivacaine reduces opiate consumption after rotator cuff repair in a randomized controlled trial. *J Shoulder Elbow Surg.* 2019;28(5):819-827.

67. Okoroha KR, Lynch JR, Keller RA, et al. Liposomal bupivacaine versus interscalene nerve block for pain control after shoulder arthroplasty: a prospective randomized trial. *J Shoulder Elbow Surg.* 2016;25(11):1742-1748.

68. Namdari S, Nicholson T, Abboud J, Lazarus M, Steinberg D, Williams G. Randomized controlled trial of interscalene block compared with injectable liposomal bupivacaine in shoulder arthroplasty. *J Bone Joint Surg Am.* 2017;99(7):550-556.

69. Cao X, Pan F. Comparison of liposomal bupivacaine infiltration versus interscalene nerve block for pain control in total shoulder arthroplasty: a meta-analysis of randomized control trails. *Medicine (Baltimore).* 2017;96(39):e8079.

70. Sun H, Li S, Wang K, et al. Do liposomal bupivacaine infiltration and interscalene nerve block provide similar pain relief after total shoulder arthroplasty: a systematic review and meta-analysis. *J Pain Res.* 2018;11:1889-1900.

71. Namdari S, Nicholson T, Abboud J, Lazarus M, Steinberg D, Williams G. Interscalene block with and without intraoperative local infiltration with liposomal bupivacaine in shoulder arthroplasty: a randomized controlled trial. *J Bone Joint Surg Am.* 2018;100(16):1373-1378.

72. Joshi GP, Hawkins RJ, Frankle MA, Abrams JS. Best practices for periarticular infiltration with liposomal bupivacaine for the management of pain after shoulder surgery: consensus recommendation. *J Surg Orthop Adv.* 2016;25(4):204-208.

73. Angerame MR, Ruder JA, Odum SM, Hamid N. Pain and opioid use after total shoulder arthroplasty with injectable liposomal bupivacaine versus interscalene block. *Orthopedics.* 2017;40(5):e806-e811.

74. Vandepitte C, Kuroda M, Witvrouw R, et al. Addition of liposome bupivacaine to bupivacaine HCl versus bupivacaine HCl alone for interscalene brachial plexus block in patients having major shoulder surgery. *Reg Anesth Pain Med.* 2017;42(3):334-341.

75. Ford E, Saini S, Szukics P, Assiamah AA, Mcmillan S. Patient-reported outcomes after arthroscopic shoulder surgery with interscalene brachial plexus nerve block using liposomal bupivacaine: a prospective observational study. *Surg Technol Int.* 2019;35:319-322.

76. Weller WJ, Azzam MG, Smith RA, Azar FM, Throckmorton TW. Liposomal bupivacaine mixture has similar pain relief and significantly fewer complications at less cost compared to indwelling interscalene catheter in total shoulder arthroplasty. *J Arthroplasty.* 2017;32(11):3557-3562.

77. Sabesan VJ, Shahriar R, Petersen-fitts GR, et al. A prospective randomized controlled trial to identify the optimal postoperative pain management in shoulder arthroplasty: liposomal bupivacaine versus continuous interscalene catheter. *J Shoulder Elbow Surg.* 2017;26(10):1810-1817.

78. Wang K, Zhang HX. Liposomal bupivacaine versus interscalene nerve block for pain control after total shoulder arthroplasty: a systematic review and meta-analysis. *Int J Surg.* 2017;46:61-70.

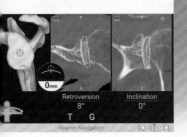

10 Intraoperative Navigation

Pierre-Henri Flurin, MD and Laurent Angibaud, Dipl. Ing.

INTRODUCTION

Computer-assisted orthopedic surgery (CAOS) systems, such as navigation platforms, have been developed for various applications since the 1990s as an opportunity to improve the accuracy of the alignment of implants.[1-5] CAOS application dedicated to the field of total shoulder arthroplasty (TSA) has been more difficult to achieve, hampered by technical difficulties related to the reliability of the equipment[6] and the challenges of reduced visibility due to the shoulder's limited exposure.

However, the clinical result of a TSA highly depends on the quality of anatomical and biomechanical restitution of the glenohumeral joint.[7-9] The difficulties of proper appreciation of the anatomical landmarks combined with the narrowness of the surgical field tend to challenge the accuracy of the bone cut and preparation, resulting in a crucial need for TSA-dedicated guidance solutions such as personalized surgical instrumentation (PSI) and CAOS systems.[10-16]

Combined advances in computed tomography (CT) medical imaging and technical improvements in computer and tracking systems have enabled the development of a new generation of image-based CAOS system for shoulder prosthetic application.[17-21]

There is currently only one widely used computer-aided navigation system on the market for TSA application, whose technical and clinical evaluations are encouraging.[22-27] This initial system is expected to be joined by other technological platforms over the upcoming years, all further enhanced by the development of augmented and/or virtual reality, robotic, sensor, and machine learning. In this chapter, we will describe the history as well as the general principles of CAOS in the field of orthopedics. Then, we will describe, more precisely, the globally launched computer-aided navigation dedicated to TSA. Finally, we will present the results of validation studies and the current clinical evaluation of this technology.

HISTORY OF NAVIGATION

The initial concepts of CAOS emerged almost 30 years ago, with the first clinical applications[1-4] being reported in the mid-1990s. From these early days, numerous technologies in the field of CAOS were developed for a large range of clinical applications such as total hip arthroplasty, total knee arthroplasty (TKA), spine, and a variety of other procedures. The overachieving goal behind each of these technologies was to provide guidance to the surgeon to improve the accuracy of implant positioning and reproducibility as an attempt to ultimately improve clinical outcomes.

Over the years, CAOS has morphed into different types of technology. The initial development related to active robotic systems intended to perform the machining of the envelope of the expected femoral stem based on preoperative CT-based plan.[5] The inherent complexity and cost of these active robots limited their adoption in the operating room.

In parallel, semiactive systems were developed, where the robot prepositions a cutting instrument according to a preoperative CT-based plan, but the bone cut/preparation is ultimately performed by the surgeon.[28]

The most widely used family of CAOS systems relates to the passive systems such as computer-aided navigation, where the surgeon follows guidance and/or information displayed on a screen at the time of surgery.[29-34] These navigation systems rely on surgical plans that, in turn, may be based on intraoperative measurements (aka imageless system) or on preoperative three-dimensional (3D) models derived from CT (aka image-based system).

Image-based navigation systems are based on two key technologies: 3D model reconstruction from a CT scan and a real-time surgical guidance tracking system, used at the preoperative and intraoperative stage, respectively.

At the preoperative stage, a CT of the patient is performed, and a reconstructed 3D model is established. A planning application allows the surgeon to establish a surgical plan by selecting the proper size and type of implant and then planning the position and orientation of the selected implant relative to the reconstructed 3D model.

At the time of surgery, key anatomical landmarks are acquired in order to establish the relationship between the patient's anatomy and the reconstructed 3D model. Once the verification of the registration is completed, the surgeon follows the displayed information to guide the orientation and position of the cutting tools to prepare the bone according to the preestablished surgical plan.

In their current form, navigation systems have demonstrated superior results in terms of alignment by substantially reducing the occurrence of outliers.[29-34] Also, because of their real-time guidance, these systems represent an effective educational tool to upskill the most junior surgeons.[35,36] However, usual navigation systems tend to be perceived as compromising the efficiency in the operating room by adding operative time.[30,33,34,37] In addition, some of these systems may appear as being too complex, which directly impacts the user experience. Finally, the most active debate relates to the benefit of using CAOS in terms of clinical outcomes, which may explain its somewhat limited adoption over the years. A recent study using data from the Australian Orthopaedic Association National Joint Replacement Registry showed that the revision rate for TKA patients less than 65 years old was reduced by ~20% if computer-assisted navigation was used.[38] Notably, the authors found that its usage led to a significant reduction in the rate of revision due to loosening/lysis ($P = 0.001$), which is the leading reason for revision TKA. Along the same lines, another study demonstrated that CAOS produced better clinical outcomes compared to traditional surgery in TKA after 1 year.[39] Such evidence tends to demonstrate that greater accuracy of implantation results in an improved survival rate. Finally, it can be hypothesized that navigation systems provide added value for difficult indications such as those associated with reduced exposure or bone defects and deformity when visual landmarks are limited, such as in TSA.

DESCRIPTION OF A CONTEMPORARY CAOS PLATFORM FOR TSA

The presented CAOS system (ExactechGPS [eGPS], Blue Ortho, Gières, France) has been developed with a particular focus on enriching the user experience through added efficiency and efficacy. The first clinical application for TKA was released in 2010 and then seconded by an application dedicated to TSA in 2016. Since then, the application has been used in almost 30,000 surgeries. The eGPS is considered as a closed platform, being only compatible with the Equinoxe shoulder implant from the same manufacturer.

The eGPS includes (1) a display unit composed of a proprietary infrared charge-coupled device camera and a touchscreen tablet intended to be located in the sterile field and directly accessible by the surgeon during the surgery and (2) a set of wireless active trackers. The camera is intended to define the 3D position and orientation within 6° of freedom of the trackers rigidly attached to patient bone and surgical instruments as well as the system-specific probe used to acquire the anatomical landmarks during the registration phase. The infrared camera provides an extra-large field of vision (>135°) for maintaining the line of sight during the surgery.[40] Based on the limited distance between the localizer and the camera, the high frequency of the camera, and other proprietary attributes (eg, algorithms), this hardware has been proven to offer both accurate and precise surgical resection measurements during simulated TKA.[41]

The eGPS for TSA includes two dedicated software applications. The preoperative planning application (Equinoxe Planning App, Blue Ortho, Gières, France) allows surgeons to establish a surgical plan regarding the preparation of the glenoid based on a reconstructed 3D model of the scapula referencing the Friedman axis connecting the center of the glenoid to the trigonum.[42] The intraoperative application (ExactechGPS Shoulder Application, Blue Ortho, Gières, France) is intended to provide real-time visual guidance and alignment in order to execute the surgical plan at the time of the surgery.

Finally, the last aspect of the eGPS relates to the navigated mechanical instrument, which includes a navigated modular driver for a series of drills as well as side-specific blocks intended to rigidly attach the reference tracker to the scapula at the level of the coracoid.

SURGICAL NAVIGATION

Preoperative Navigation Steps

A preoperative CT scan is performed for each patient requiring a TSA according to a precise protocol with 1-mm-thick sections of the entire scapula.

Subsequently, the CT is uploaded to the preoperative application with the objective of performing surgical planning according to two distinct options:

- If the planning is only intended for visualization, then the immediate reconstruction feature of the application is used to establish an automated 3D-reconstructed scapula on which selected implants can be assessed in terms of position and/or orientation relative to a referential based on the Friedman axis connecting the center of the glenoid to the trigonum established by the user.
- If the planning is intended to be used for surgical navigation, then a manual 3D reconstruction performed by Blue Ortho specialists is required.

After completion of the manual reconstruction, a detailed 3D rendering of the scapula featuring the Friedman axis is available for planning purposes using the dedicated application. In this application, the surgeon plans the glenoid portion of an anatomical TSA (ATSA) or a reverse TSA (RTSA) in order to optimize the choice and position of the implant.

The inclination of the selected glenoid implant is calculated relative to the frontal plane of the scapula. This plane is defined by Friedman axis and the most inferior point of the scapula.

The version of the selected glenoid implant is calculated relative to a plane passing through Friedman axis, orthogonal to the frontal plane of the scapula.

Preoperative planning allows the user to visualize the deformity and/or bone defect in 3D and to select the most suitable implant (eg, size, length of the central peg, posterior or superior augment, standard or expanded glenosphere for RTSA). The possibility of adjusting the position and orientation of the glenoid implant in terms of inclination, version, and depth is even more useful in cases of substantial deformity or a small glenoid, which allows the user to anticipate eccentric reaming or the use of augmented implants.

In addition to the usual solid 3D body rendering, the application offers a transparent 3D body as well as the possibility of adding CT-based slices in order to enrich the visualization. This will further limit the risk of perforation. Planning allows for an optimized correction with minimal reaming in order to respect the native bone stock **(FIGURE 10.1)**.

This preoperative planning can be changed at any time before being uploaded onto the navigation system and can also be changed intraoperatively using the eGPS touchscreen. The planning can be leveraged by the team from the operating room to gain efficiency by proactively checking the availability of the implants and preparing the selected implants and instrumentation for the surgery. Looking forward, the planning could play an even more important role for the management of implant inventory.

Intraoperative Navigation Steps

Patient and Station Positioning

The system has been designed so as not to modify either the usual operating technique or patient positioning. The surgery is performed with the patient in a beach chair position, and the display unit of the eGPS is fixed on the contralateral side of the patient at approximately 1 m from the operated shoulder and away from patient's head in order to limit interposition between sensors.

The touchscreen of the display unit remains accessible during surgery, thanks to a dedicated transparent

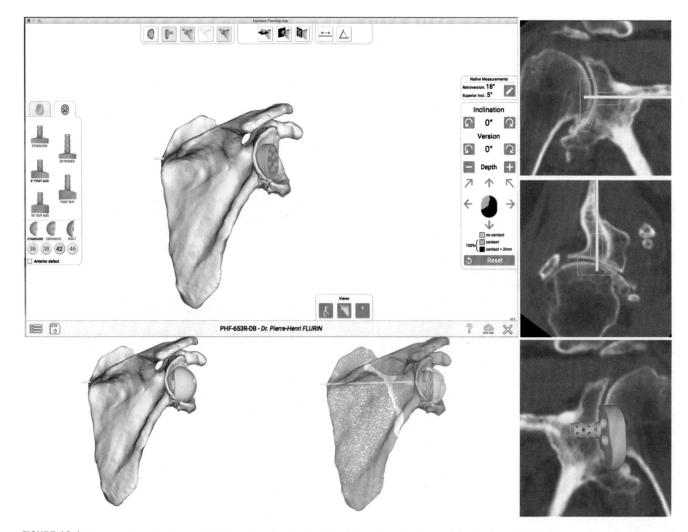

FIGURE 10.1 Preoperative planning application allows to visualize the deformity and or bone defect in three dimensions and to select the most suitable implant.

sterile drape covering the display unit. The rest of the draping is usual, but it is essential to ensure a line of sight between the tracker to be fixed onto the coracoid process and the camera. In this regard, it is necessary to be particularly attentive to the position of the patient's head, the airway probe, and breathing tubes as they may obstruct the view of the expected trackers **(FIGURE 10.2)**.

Particularity of the Surgical Exposure

The system was designed to be used preferably through a deltopectoral approach, which allows the user to set up for either ATSA or RTSA. An incision of standard length (11-13 cm) starts at the lower edge of the clavicle and follows the deltopectoral interval passing above the coracoid process and moving toward the deltoid insertion.

The only adaption of the approach relates to a slight superior translation of the incision to expose the coracoid process for placement of the tracker's block.

Once the humeral head resection is completed, the glenoid is approached and the soft tissues around the glenoid are released, as well as the upper surface and the base of the coracoid, so as to be able to integrate a number of anatomical landmarks with the patient's preoperative CT data.

Trackers

A total of three trackers are needed to complete the surgery: the glenoid (G) tracker references the glenoid/scapula, the tool (T) tracker references the navigated instruments, and the probe tracker is intended to acquire the anatomical landmarks. These three trackers are wirelessly paired with the camera. The G tracker's block is then affixed to the upper portion of the coracoid process using two self-tapping screws **(VIDEO 10.1)**.

Registration of the Anatomical Landmarks

At this point, the surgeon performs the acquisitions of the anatomical landmarks, by placing the tip of the probe on specific points and surfaces of interest according to the steps sequentially announced on the screen. After completion of the acquisitions, the system displays the result of the registration between the patient's anatomy and the reconstructed 3D model from the CT images. Green points indicate proper accuracy and yellow or red points indicate lower accuracy. To complete the assessment of the accuracy, the probe tip can be used to touch different surfaces on the scapula and visualize the probe tip on the screen.

Instruments Guidance

Once the registration is completed, the preparation of the glenoid according to the surgical plan is performed by following the detailed on-screen guidance steps. First, the modular driver is assembled by attaching a T tracker for its guidance as well as the proper drill bit. The screen of the station displays the spatial orientation and position of the navigated instruments synchronized with the CT scan slices and provides real-time feedback to the surgeon **(FIGURE 10.3)**. Based on this valuable information, the surgeon is able to prepare the glenoid based upon the preoperative plan. The learning curve is thus shortened by simplifying the operative technique.

Each navigation step is very clearly represented on the screen and also displays the proper instrument construct to be used.

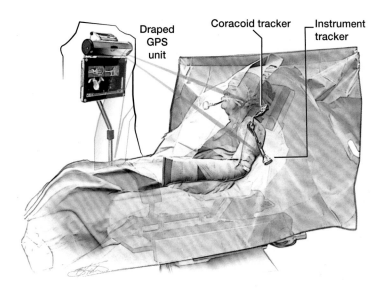

Draped GPS unit   Coracoid tracker   Instrument tracker

FIGURE 10.2 The touchscreen remains accessible during the surgery through a transparent sterile drape. The airway probe and breathing tubes should not obstruct the view of the expected trackers.

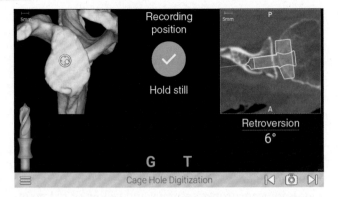

FIGURE 10.3 The numbers shown for version and inclination are displayed according to the preoperative plan.

For the drilling stages, the tip of the instrument is displayed in yellow on the screen and must be superimposed on a blue dot corresponding to the preoperative planning in order to achieve the proper position. The final orientation is achieved by aligning the simulated axis of the instrument (displayed as a target) with the yellow dot **(VIDEO 10.2)**. CT scan slices are displayed simultaneously on the screen to control the correct positioning of the drilling. The version and tilt axes are accurately indicated in real time **(FIGURE 10.3)**.

The reaming of the glenoid is controlled in the same way, first by aligning the target on the yellow dot and second by representation of the reamer on the CT slices **(FIGURE 10.4; VIDEO 10.3)**. It is thus possible to visually control both the orientation and depth of reaming. The version, tilt, and depth axes data are displayed on the screen in real time.

After reaming, the central cage hole is then drilled precisely to where the glenoid component was positioned preoperatively.

The surgeon can then use the on-screen prompts to place and impact the implant properly according to the plan **(FIGURE 10.5; VIDEO 10.4)**.

For the implantation of an RTSA, the glenoid fixation screws can be navigated **(FIGURE 10.6)**, as the system allows the user to visualize the orientation and the length of the screws on the CT scan slices.

Each step of the operating technique is sequentially displayed on the navigation screen, but the surgeon remains in control and therefore free to skip a step or to go back at any time by interacting directly on the touchscreen **(VIDEO 10.5)**. The interactive 3D model and section views continuously inform the orientation of the implant relative to Friedman "ideal" axis.

Management of Technical Issues

The confidence that the surgeon gradually invests in the navigation system imposes a rigorous control of the specific patient being treated, on the CT scan, on the planning software, and on the navigation system. Nonetheless, confirming selection of the correct case in the navigation system must therefore be added to the preoperative check list.

When the navigation system is started at the beginning of surgery, the trackers must be recognized by the station. After a certain number of sterilizations, a tracker may no longer function properly. In this situation, it is then necessary to check the battery and have a backup tracker available in order to continue the procedure under guidance.

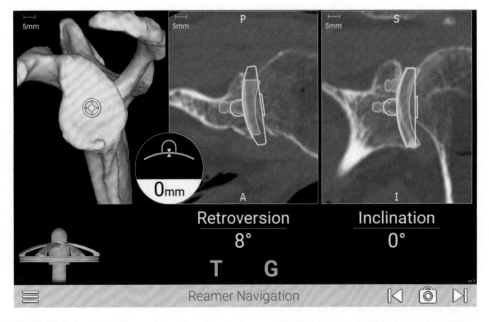

FIGURE 10.4 During drilling and reaming, the version and tilt axis are accurately indicated in real time.

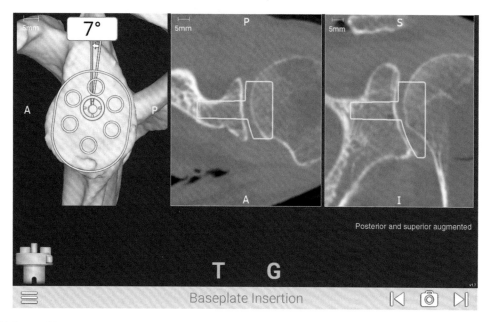

FIGURE 10.5 Yellow and blue dots are aligned while referencing the angular measurements, to impact the implant based on the plan.

The fixation of the G tracker onto the coracoid process is a new step for the surgeon who has not yet utilized navigation, and it is therefore necessary to obtain proper good exposure of the horizontal portion of the coracoid process and to make certain that the bicortical screw fixation is secure. This type of fixation is, in our experience, sufficient, even in elderly patients with osteoporosis. In patients who have undergone a previous Latarjet procedure, fixation of the tracker may be more challenging. However, in our experience, fixation of the tracker can be achieved on the remaining part of the coracoid. When this is not feasible, then the surgeon should be prepared to proceed without the use of the navigation system.

When the glenoid exposure is limited and specifically in cases of severe posterior glenoid erosion and deformity, it can be difficult to work in line with the axis imposed by the navigation system, which, according to planning, is close to Friedman axis. In this situation, additional soft-tissue releases and modified retractor placement may provide the needed exposure. If adequate exposure is not achieved, then we have utilized a transdeltoid approach for passage of the drill using the navigation screen to direct position and placement.

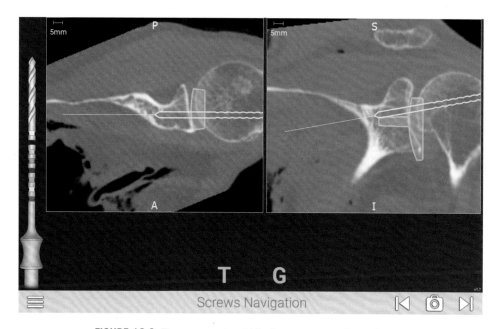

FIGURE 10.6 The reverse glenoid fixation screws can be navigated.

Navigation is a sophisticated digital tool that represents an additional cost compared to a nonnavigated shoulder arthroplasty. In addition, the fact that this technology is still relatively new has not yet made it the standard of care, and, as such, it is not available in all operating rooms. Going forward, issues related to cost and availability will be gradually resolved when outcomes confirm the superiority of navigation compared to the traditional approach, in terms of patient satisfaction, anatomic reconstruction, reduction in complications, and implant survival.

Benefits in Challenging Cases

The navigation system will be particularly useful when a metal screw or other implant that is technically difficult to remove may interfere with the glenoid implantation. During planning, this system allows the surgeon to select a location that avoids the obstacle and achieves proper placement (**FIGURE 10.7**).

In cases of significant glenoid wear and deformity, the planning system allows the surgeon to choose the most suitable augmented implant and to define more precisely the need for and the size and shape of a graft. The navigation system allows the user to plan and make decisions about the details of the surgery before the procedure, rather than making all of these decisions intraoperatively (**VIDEO 10.6**).

During revision surgery, the system allows the user to plan the case but does not allow navigation due to interference related to prosthetic metal artifacts on the preoperative CT scan. Indeed, the extraction of metal parts during modeling makes the mapping of bone surfaces insufficiently precise to guide the navigation system and does not offer the same reliability as in a primary reconstruction.

VALIDATION

In Vitro Accuracy Validation

The overall accuracy of the eGPS has been validated by a cadaveric study involving five surgeons who planned and operated on two shoulders each (ATSA, $n = 1$; and RTSA, $n = 1$). The implants used for this study were impregnated with Barium in order to assess their position and orientation on a postoperative CT scan, which was then used to compare final implantation to the targeted plan. The average implantation error was less than 2 mm and less than 2° for position and orientation, respectively.[22,23] These results were below the margins of error described as acceptable in the published studies[43-47] on implantation accuracy (**FIGURE 10.8**).

In Vivo Accuracy Validation

A first validation of a shoulder navigation system accuracy was performed by Habermeyer in 2009, but the validity of the study was limited by the small number of cases and the relatively high percentage of technical issues during the surgeries.[6]

Therefore, it was deemed necessary to conduct a prospective study with postoperative CT scan control of navigated TSA to assess the in vivo accuracy provided by the eGPS to achieve the targeted implantation parameters.

A total of 31 cases (ATSA, $n = 9$ and RTSA, $n = 22$) performed using the CAOS system were reviewed with a CT scan between 6 and 12 months after the surgery. Postoperative CT scans were performed according to the same protocol as the preoperative stage in order to verify the orientation of the implant.

The accuracy was evaluated by comparing the version and inclination of the implant relative to Friedman axis between the preoperative surgical plan level (targeted)

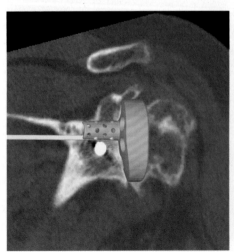
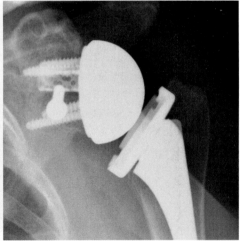

FIGURE 10.7 The navigation system will be particularly useful when a metal screw of foreign body that is technically difficult to remove may interfere with the glenoid implantation.

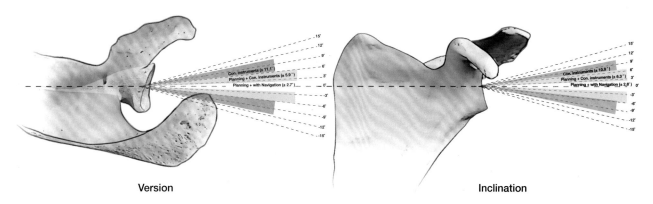

Version   Inclination

FIGURE 10.8 In vitro validation of navigation compared with conventional instruments and personalized surgical instrumentation (PSI).

and the postoperative CT scan (measured). Positive values were assigned to superior inclination and retroversion, and negative values were assigned to inferior inclination and anteversion.

The accuracy error of the navigation system is described as the average of these angular deviations with the corresponding standard deviation.

For inclination, the accuracy error was 1.11° ± 1.62° and 1.77° ± 0.77° for ATSA and RTSA, respectively.

For version, the accuracy error was 1.33° ± 1.22° and 0.77° ± 0.92° for ATSA and RTSA, respectively.

Finally, the mean accuracy error was 1.58° ± 1.75° and 1.13° ± 0.81° for inclination and for version, respectively, and was less than or equal to 2° in 97% of the cases for version and in 80% of cases for inclination **(FIGURE 10.9)**.

The measured differences were positive, meaning there was a bias toward superior inclination and retroversion, as if the surgical technique, and in particular the reaming stage, pushed the surgeon's hand to a slight accentuation of the initial glenoid wear superiorly and posteriorly.

Other recent studies using the same CAOS system reported similar positive results regarding the ability to deliver high levels of accuracy and precision to achieve the targeted surgical plan.[24-26]

Also, based on the postoperative CT scan, it was found that central peg penetration was 13% (less than 1 mm in 3/4 of these cases). Similarly, a recent study reported that the same navigation system was associated with a significantly reduced incidence of perforation of the central cage compared to traditional technique (17.7% vs 52.4%, $P = 0.04$).[27]

In conclusion, these in vivo studies demonstrate the ability of the eGPS system to accurately execute the preoperative surgical plan with an angular error less than or equal to 2° in more than 80% of the cases.

Clinical Results

It was hypothesized that the usage of the CAOS system would result in an improvement of clinical and radiographic results.

We have then studied the clinical results in 49 patients (ATSA, $n = 14$; and RTSA, $n = 35$) operated upon by the same surgeon using the eGPS with a minimum follow-up of 2 years.

The 2-year postoperative visit results were compared with those of a homogeneous comparison group in terms of sex, age, and postoperative follow-up from a multicentric database using the same implant system.

The navigated ATSA group was composed of 57% men versus 54% in the comparison group ($P = 0.91$); mean age was 67.3 and 66.9 years, respectively ($P = 0.88$), and average follow-up was 25 and 24.8 months, respectively ($P = 0.75$).

Postoperatively, slightly better range of motion was observed for the navigated ATSAs for forward flexion, external rotation, and internal rotation, although only the improvement in external rotation was statistically significant. Clinical scores were similar between the two groups.

The radiographic analysis did not detect any difference in terms of radiolucent lines at 2-year follow-up, but there were two cases of symptomatic glenoid loosening requiring revision surgery in the group of nonnavigated ATSAs.

The navigated and nonnavigated groups of RTSA were also homogeneous with respect to sex (49% men vs 40% in the control group; $P = 0.34$), mean age (72.5 vs 72.9 years; $P = 0.77$), and follow-up (24.15 vs 24.3 months; $P = 0.26$).

Postoperatively, significantly better range of motion was observed in the navigated group in forward flexion ($P = 0.01$) and internal rotation ($P = 0.0001$) as well as a greater strength ($P = 0.003$) **(TABLE 10.1)**.

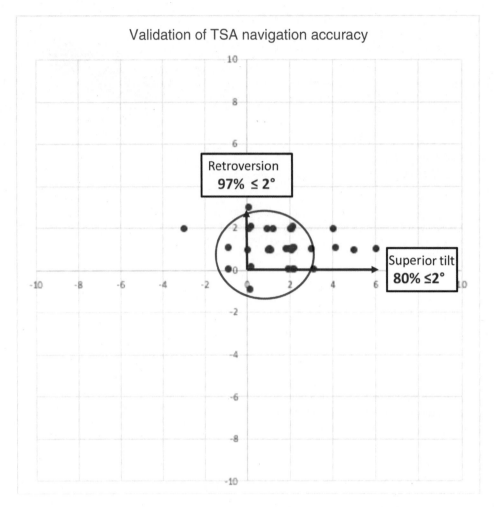

FIGURE 10.9 In vivo validation of navigation accuracy: the average error is 1.58° in inclination and 1.13° in version, with less than 2° for 97% of cases in version and 80% of cases for inclination. TSA, total shoulder arthroplasty.

The postoperative clinical scores were equivalent between the two groups, except for the Constant score that was greater in the navigated group ($P = 0.0012$).

The radiographic analysis found no difference in terms of radiolucent lines at 2 years ($P = 0.75$). The incidence of scapular notching was higher for the nonnavigated RTSA, but the difference was not statistically significant probably as a result of the low overall incidence of scapular notching.

SURGICAL TIME AND LEARNING CURVE

An analysis of surgical time was performed by one of the early adopters of this technology (P.H.F) based upon a comparison of the first navigated cases compared with the last navigated cases in an overall cohort of 150 navigated cases. This was also compared with surgical time for nonnavigated cases.

For ATSA, the average time was 70 minutes for conventional surgery. The average operating time of the first

TABLE 10.1 Comparison of Clinical Results Between Navigated and Nonnavigated RTSA

Postoperative, Average	FF	IR	ER	Strength (lbs)
Navigated RTSA	157°	5.5	40°	11
Nonnavigated RTSA	144°	4.2	39°	8
P-value	0.01	0.00016	0.76	0.003

ER, external rotation; FF, forward flexion; IR, external rotation; RTSA, reverse total shoulder arthroplasty.

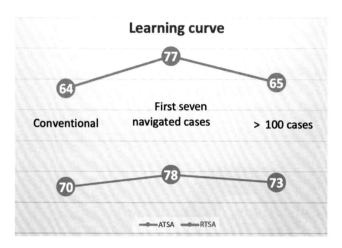

FIGURE 10.10 Surgical time and learning curve. ATSA, anatomical total shoulder arthroplasty; RTSA, reverse total shoulder arthroplasty.

seven navigated cases was 78 minutes and the last five navigated cases was 73 minutes. The average additional surgical time for ATSA after the initial learning curve was 3 minutes for navigation.

For RTSA, the average time was 64 minutes for conventional surgery. The average operating time of the first seven navigated cases was 77 minutes and the last five navigated cases was 65 minutes. The average additional surgical time for RTSA after the initial learning curve was 1 minute for navigation (**FIGURE 10.10**).

A cumulative control chart analysis study using five surgeons was performed to examine the learning curve for RTSA and found that the observed learning duration for all five surgeons was approximately seven cases. In this analysis, one surgeon demonstrated statistically significant lower surgical time after learning and lower average surgical time than without navigation.[48] Similarly, Wang, in 2020, showed the learning curve to be approximately eight cases for an experienced shoulder surgeon with an overall surgical time almost identical to nonnavigated cases.[26]

One of the purposes of using navigation is to improve the reproducibility and accuracy of implant placement. Although its use by experienced shoulder arthroplasty surgeons has been shown to be beneficial, one can imagine that this system would be of even greater interest in guiding lower volume shoulder arthroplasty surgeons and as a tool in training orthopedic residents and fellows. In this context, this tool could be easily used in the spirit of an "edutrainment" or a "serious game" during sawbone workshops or even cadaver laboratories.

FUTURE DEVELOPMENTS

Despite its clearly established advantages, such CAOS system still has numerous opportunities to further expand its added value and gain greater adoption among the TSA surgeons.

Potential improvements relate to the increase of the scope of the functionalities offered by the CAOS with the development of the humeral side navigation. In addition, in an attempt to implement a more personalized approach as part of the planning, patient-reported outcome measures and other patient-specific data can be leveraged as inputs to customize the plan to the patient.

Some improvements are intrinsically linked to the continuous development of the technology, notably in terms of connectivity, which can be leveraged for basic functions (eg, upload a preoperative planning from the cloud-based application to the eGPS before a case) as well as more advanced functions (eg, real-time support).

Similarly, there are opportunities for the eGPS to become more integrated with the operating room environment. For example, the camera can be embedded into the surgical light in order to optimize the line of sight. Another possibility relates to the connection of the system with the management of the operating rooms in order to provide accurate updates regarding the progress of the surgery based on the specific step being navigated.

Similar integration can be envisioned between the CAOS system and other technologies intended to augment it. This type of integration is particularly relevant in the field of sensors, where sensor-based technology can provide intraoperative information (eg, soft-tissue tension), thereby allowing the surgeon to modify the surgical plan based on this additional information.

Another area of development relates to the addition of augmented and virtual reality, in which the surgeon would be able to visualize the guidance looking directly at the site instead of the screen or to superpose guidance/information (eg, 3D model) on top of the operative site.

With respect to the hardware, there is the potential to challenge the passive method of bone preparation by considering robotic applications with a lower footprint and higher flexibility than the system described in terms of active and/or semiactive systems.

Finally, and certainly most importantly, the CAOS system should not be perceived as a sole intraoperative solution, but rather as a major component of the overall ecosystem (**FIGURE 10.11**); in which detailed preoperative patient-specific data obtained from wearables as well as imaging are combined to establish a personalized surgical plan for the patient. At the time of the surgery, based upon intraoperative information obtained from sensors integrated to the system, the surgeon is able to gain an additional layer of information and then to potentially fine-tune the surgical plan. Once the surgery is completed, the surgical log including quantified information is uploaded to the clinical record of the patient as well as to the active clinical research database (assuming the patient is enrolled). The addition of postoperative follow-up of the patient provides the ultimate set of information. Using machine learning, all the longitudinal data collected can then be used to provide predictive modeling and therefore provide the patient with a proactive appreciation of the expected outcomes.[49]

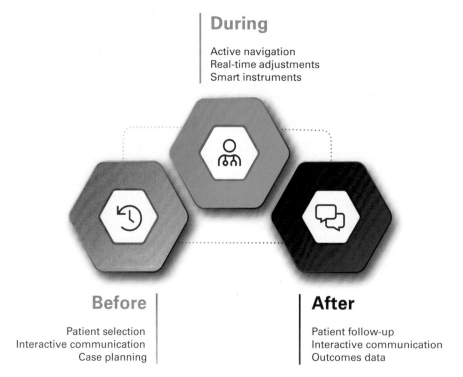

During

Active navigation
Real-time adjustments
Smart instruments

Before

Patient selection
Interactive communication
Case planning

After

Patient follow-up
Interactive communication
Outcomes data

FIGURE 10.11 Illustration of a comprehensive ecosystem based on the active synergy between the technologies along the continuum of care.

CONCLUSION

The precise placement of a TSA is particularly important for the quality of the clinical result, the reduction of complications, and the longevity of the implant fixation.

Navigation provides enhanced precision that can improve current clinical practice, especially since the learning curve is short and the operating time is not significantly lengthened compared to nonnavigated technique. It allows for better reproducibility of the procedure, for the experienced arthroplasty surgeon, and for the lower volume arthroplasty surgeon and offers the surgeon in training a security and an acceleration of their learning curve.

The clinical results are encouraging but require longer term follow-up to confirm improved survival of the implants. Today, intraoperative navigation is primarily limited to a single system deployed commercially and only for glenoid navigation. However, with further development, it can be generalized to all shoulder arthroplasty systems, include navigation of the humeral implant, enhance soft-tissue balancing, and integrate virtual reality and progressive robotization of the surgical technique.

The planning tool coupled with the precision of the system will allow more statistical correlations between pathology, patients, technical choices, selected implants, and clinical results. In the near future, machine learning predictive models will guide the surgeon starting with the indications and preoperative planning. It could also provide better patient information with a more precise risk-benefit balance and probably a much better alignment between the expectations of the patient and the surgeon and the anticipated postoperative functional result.

REFERENCES

1. Nolte LP, Visarius H, Arm E, Langlotz F, Schwarzenbach O, Zamorano L. Computer-aided fixation of spinal implants. *J Image Guid Surg.* 1995;1(2):88-93.
2. Dessenne V, Lavallée S, Julliard R, Orti R, Martelli S, Cinquin P. Computer-assisted knee anterior cruciate ligament reconstruction: first clinical tests. *J Image Guid Surg.* 1995;1(1):59-64.
3. Nolte LP, Zamorano LJ, Jiang Z, Wang Q, Langlotz F, Berlemann U. Image-guided insertion of transpedicular screws. A laboratory set-up. *Spine.* 1995;20(4):497-500.
4. Lavallée S, Sautot P, Troccaz J, Cinquin P, Merloz P. Computer-assisted spine surgery: a technique for accurate transpedicular screw fixation using CT data and a 3-D optical localizer. *J Image Guid Surg.* 1995;1(1):65-73.
5. Spencer EH. The ROBODOC clinical trial: a robotic assistant for total hip arthroplasty. *Orthop Nurs.* 1996;15(1):9-14.
6. Kircher J, Wiedemann M, Magosh P, Lichtenberg S, Habermeyer P. Improved accuracy of glenoid positioning in total shoulder arthroplasty with intraoperative navigation: a prospective randomized clinical study. *J Shoulder Elbow Surg.* 2009;18(4):515-520.
7. Flurin PH, Roche C, Wright T, Zuckerman J. Correlation between clinical outcomes and anatomic reconstruction with anatomic total shoulder arthroplasty. *Bull Hosp Jt Dis (2013).* 2015;73:S92-S98.
8. Iannoti JP, Spenser EE, Winter U, Deffenbaugh D, Williams G. Prosthetic positioning in total shoulder arthroplasty. *J Shoulder Elbow Surg.* 2005;14(1 suppl):111S-121S.
9. Papadonikolakis A, Neradilek MB, Matsen FA III. Failure of the glenoid component in anatomic total shoulder arthroplasty: a systematic review of the English-language literature between 2006 and 2012. *J Bone Joint Surg Am.* 2013;95(24):2205-2212.
10. Berhouet J, Gulotta LV, Dines DM, et al. Pre-operative planning for accurate glenoid component positioning in reverse shoulder arthroplasty. *Orthop Traumatol Surg Res.* 2017;103:407-413.
11. Hendel MD, Bryan JA, Barsoum WK, et al. Comparison of patient-specific instruments with standard surgical instruments in determining glenoid component position: a randomized prospective clinical trial. *J Bone Joint Surg Am.* 2012;94:2167-2175.
12. Gauci MO, Boileau P, Baba M, Chaoui J, Walch G. Patient-specific-glenoid guides provide accuracy and reproducibility in total shoulder arthroplasty. *Bone Joint J.* 2016;98:1080-1085.

13. Jacquot A, Gauci MO, Chaoui J, et al. Proper benefit of a three-dimensional preoperative planning software for glenoid component positioning in total shoulder arthroplasty. *Int Orthop.* 2018;42:2897-2906.

14. Iannoti JP, Weiner S, Rodriguez E, et al. Three-dimensional imaging and templating improve glenoid implant positioning. *J Bone Joint Surg Am.* 2015;97:651-658.

15. Throckmorton TW, Gulotta LV, Bonnarens FO, et al. Patient-specific targeting guides compared with traditional instrumentation for glenoid component placement in shoulder arthroplasty: a multi-surgeon study in 70 arthritic cadaver specimens. *J Shoulder Elbow Surg.* 2015;24:965-971.

16. Verborgt O, Hachem AI, Eid K, Vuylsteke K, Ferrand M, Hardy P. Accuracy of patient-specific guided implantation of the glenoid component in reverse shoulder arthroplasty. *Orthop Traumatol Surg Res.* 2018;104:767-772.

17. Flurin PH, Sirveaux F. Is CT indispensable in shoulder arthroplasty in 2019? *Orthop Traumatol Surg Res.* 2019;105(2):199-201.

18. Nguyen D, Ferreira LM, Brownhill JR, Faber KJ, Johnson JA. Design and development of a computer assisted glenoid implantation technique for shoulder replacement surgery. *Comput Aided Surg.* 2007;12:152-159.

19. Bicknell RT, Delude JA, Kedgley AR, et al. Early experience with computer assisted shoulder hemiarthroplasty for fractures of the proximal humerus: development of a novel technique and an in vitro comparison with traditional methods. *J Shoulder Elbow Surg.* 2007;16:117S-125S.

20. Gregory TM, Sankey A, Augereau B, et al. Accuracy of glenoid component placement in total shoulder arthroplasty and its effect on clinical and radiological outcome in a retrospective longitudinal open study. *PLoS One.* 2013;8(10):e75791.

21. Werner BS, Hudek R, Burkhart KJ, Gohlke F. The influence of three-dimensional planning on decision-making in total shoulder arthroplasty. *J Shoulder Elbow Surg.* 2017;26:1477-1483.

22. Greene A, Jones RB, Wright TW, et al. Distribution of glenoid implant options for correcting deformities using a preoperative planning tool. *Bull Hosp Jt Dis (2013).* 2015;73(suppl 1):S52-S56.

23. Hamilton MA, Polakovic S, Saadi P, Jones RB, Parsons IM, Cheung EV. Evaluation of pre-operative implant placement in total shoulder arthroplasty. *Bull Hosp Jt Dis (2013).* 2015;73(suppl 1):S47-S51.

24. Barrett I, Ramakrishnan A, Cheung E. Safety and efficacy of intraoperative computer-navigated versus non-navigated shoulder arthroplasty at a tertiary referral. *Orthop Clin North Am.* 2019;50(1):95-101. doi:10.1016/j.ocl.2018.08.004

25. Nashikkar PS, Scholes CJ, Haber MD. Computer navigation re-creates planned glenoid placement and reduces correction variability in total shoulder arthroplasty: an in vivo case-control study. *J Shoulder Elbow Surg.* 2019;28(12):e398-e409. doi:10.1016/J.JSE.2019.04.037

26. Wang AW, Hayes A, Gibbons R, Mackie KE. Computer navigation of the glenoid component in reverse total shoulder arthroplasty: a clinical trial to evaluate the learning curve. *J Shoulder Elbow Surg.* 2020;29:617-623.

27. Nashikkar PS, Scholes CJ, Haber MD. Role of intraoperative navigation in the fixation of the glenoid component in reverse total shoulder arthroplasty: a clinical case-control study. *J Shoulder Elbow Surg.* 2019;28(9):1685-1691.

28. Barrett AR, Davies BL, Gomes MP, et al. Computer-assisted hip resurfacing surgery using the acrobot navigation system. *Proc Inst Mech Eng H.* 2007;221(7):773-785.

29. Rosenberger RE, Hoser C, Quirbach S, Attal R, Hennerbichler A, Fink C. Improved accuracy of component alignment with the implementation of image-free navigation in total knee arthroplasty. *Knee Surg Sports Traumatol Arthrosc.* 2008;16(3):249-257.

30. Zhang GQ, Chen JY, Chai W, Liu M, Wang Y. Comparison between computer-assisted-navigation and conventional total knee arthroplasties in patients undergoing simultaneous bilateral procedures: a randomized clinical trial. *J Bone Joint Surg Am.* 2011;93(13):1190-1196.

31. Leenders T, Vandevelde D, Mahieu G, Nuyts R. Reduction in variability of acetabular cup abduction using computer assisted surgery: a prospective and randomized study. *Comput Aided Surg.* 2002;7(2):99-106.

32. Sparmann M, Wolke B, Czupalla H, Banzer D, Zink A. Positioning of total knee arthroplasty with and without navigation support. A prospective, randomised study. *J Bone Joint Surg Br.* 2003;85(6):830-835.

33. Jenny JY, Clemens U, Kohler S, Kiefer H, Konermann W, Miehlke RK. Consistency of implantation of a total knee arthroplasty with a non-image-based navigation system: a case-control study of 235 cases compared with 235 conventionally implanted prostheses. *J Arthroplasty.* 2005;20(7):832-839.

34. Haaker RG, Stockheim M, Kamp M, roof G, Breitenfelder J, Ottersbach A. Computer-assisted navigation increases precision of component placement in total knee arthroplasty. *Clin Orthop Relat Res.* 2005;(433):152-159.

35. Iorio R, Mazza D, Bolle G, et al. Computer-assisted surgery: a teacher of TKAs. *Knee.* 2013;20(4):232-235.

36. Love GJ, Kinninmonth AW. Training benefits of computer navigated total knee arthroplasty. *Knee.* 2013;20(4):236-241.

37. Bauwens K, Matthes G, Wich M, et al. Navigated total knee replacement. A meta-analysis. *J Bone Joint Surg Am.* 2007;89(2):261-269.

38. de Steiger RN, Liu YL, Graves SE. Computer navigation for total knee arthroplasty reduces revision rate for patients less than sixty-five years of age. *J Bone Joint Surg Am.* 2015;97(8):635-642.

39. Lehnen K, Giesinger K, Warschkow R, Porter M, Koch E, Kuster MS. Clinical outcome using a ligament referencing technique in CAS versus conventional technique. *Knee Surg Sports Traumatol Arthrosc.* 2011;19(6):887-892.

40. Dai Y, Angibaud L, Harris B, Hamad C. Evaluation of tracker visibility during computer-assisted total knee arthroplasty. *Orthop Proc.* 2016;98-B(suppl 8):20.

41. Angibaud LD, Dai Y, Liebelt RA, Gao B, Gulbransen SW, Silver XS. Evaluation of the accuracy and precision of a next generation computer-assisted surgical system. *Clin Orthop Surg.* 2015;7(2):225-233.

42. Friedman RJ, Hawthorne KB, Genez BM. The use of computerized tomography in the measurement of glenoid version. *J Bone Joint Surg Am.* 1992;74:1032-1037.

43. Stübig T, Petri M, Zeckey C, et al. 3D navigated implantation of the glenoid component in reversed shoulder arthroplasty. Feasibility and results in an anatomic study. *Int J Med Robot.* 2013;9:480-485.

44. Edwards TB, Gartsman GM, O'Conner DP, Sarin VK. Safety and utility of computer-aided shoulder arthroplasty. *J Shoulder Elbow Surg.* 2008;17:503-508.

45. Nguyen D, Ferreira LM, Brownhill JR, et al. Improved accuracy of computer assisted glenoid implantation in total shoulder arthroplasty: an in-vitro randomized controlled trial. *J Shoulder Elbow Surg.* 2009;18(6):907-914.

46. Verborgt O, De Smet T, Vanhees M, Clockaerts S, Parizel PM, Van Glabbeek F. Accuracy of placement of the glenoid component in reversed shoulder arthroplasty with and without navigation. *J Shoulder Elbow Surg.* 2011;20(1):21-26.

47. Sadoghi P, Vavken J, Leithner A, Vavken P. Benefit of intraoperative navigation on glenoid component positioning during total shoulder arthroplasty. *Arch Orthop Trauma Surg.* 2015;135:41-47.

48. Parsons IM, Greene AT, Harris AB, et al. *Assessing the Learning Curve of a Shoulder Arthroplasty Navigation System Using Advanced CUSUM Analysis.* AAOS; 2019.

49. Kumar V, Roche C, Overman S, et al. What is the accuracy of three different machine learning techniques to predict clinical outcomes after shoulder arthroplasty? *Clin Orthop Relat Res.* 2020;478(10):2351-2363. doi:10.1097/CORR.0000000000001263

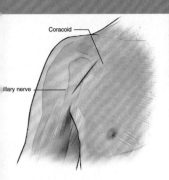

11 Operative Approach:
Deltopectoral and Anterosuperior

Yoav Rosenthal, MD and Young W. Kwon, MD, PhD

INTRODUCTION

Shoulder arthroplasty has been performed with high rates of patient satisfaction, decreased pain levels, and improved function to treat a variety of pathologies about the shoulder.[1-5] Due to its efficacy, the prevalence of shoulder arthroplasty has almost doubled in the United States in less than 10 years.[6]

The deltopectoral approach and the anterosuperior approach have been the most commonly utilized approaches for shoulder arthroplasty. Both approaches may yield comparable clinical outcomes with a different complication profile. This chapter describes the two approaches from patient positioning to deep exposure, emphasizing on the surgical technique, advantages, and potential complications. Further information regarding the capsular release, subscapularis management, humerus and glenoid exposure can be found in the corresponding surgical technique chapters.

DELTOPECTORAL APPROACH

Historically, shoulder arthroplasty is performed through an anterior approach. The first shoulder arthroplasty was performed by Jules Emile Péan in 1893, using an anterior incision passing down vertically from the acromion, between the deltoid and the biceps.[7] Subsequently, Arnold K. Henry described the extensile anterior approach in 1945.[8] To the best of our knowledge, however, the first full description of the use of the anterior deltopectoral approach for shoulder arthroplasty was published by Charles S. Neer in 1963.[9]

The deltopectoral approach for the shoulder, which is considered as the "work-horse" of all shoulder approaches, is useful for various surgical indications **(VIDEO 11.1)**. This approach utilizes an internervous plane between the axillary nerve on the lateral side and the medial and lateral pectoral nerves on the superficial medial side and the musculocutaneous nerve on the deep medial side. In addition, it provides wide exposure and excellent access to the glenohumeral joint.

Indications for Deltopectoral Approach

- Shoulder arthroplasty
- Revision shoulder arthroplasty

- Anterior glenohumeral stabilization
- Proximal humerus fracture open reduction and fixation
- Septic joint irrigation and debridement
- Tumor biopsy and excision

Advantages

The deltopectoral approach utilizes a true anatomic plane that is internervous, intermuscular, and atraumatic. Preservation of deltoid muscle integrity is paramount for successful outcome after the surgery. This is especially crucial for reverse shoulder arthroplasty, which is powered primarily by the deltoid muscle for active motion. The deltopectoral approach provides initial wide exposure and allows an extensile approach to the entire humerus, if necessary, for revision arthroplasty, fracture management, and tumor resection with subsequent reconstruction. Furthermore, this approach provides excellent exposure, especially to the superior, anterior, and inferior structures, eg, the inferior glenoid pole and humeral neck osteophytes. The versatile deltopectoral approach is suitable for all types of arthroplasty, regardless of the etiology or the presence of an intact rotator cuff. If indicated, it even provides access for a latissimus dorsi tendon transfer.[10-12]

Disadvantages

Despite its merits and popularity, the deltopectoral approach has several limitations. Since glenoid exposure depends on posterior retraction of the deltoid muscle, adequate glenoid exposure may be limited in muscular patients with a hypertrophied deltoid. Furthermore, the deltopectoral approach may offer limited access to posterior structures about the glenohumeral joint. For example, imbrication of posterior capsule during arthroplasty cases or isolation of the displaced greater tuberosity fragment in fracture cases can be challenging through the deltopectoral interval.[10-12]

Surprisingly, despite having the theoretical advantage of being an internervous approach, the deltopectoral was found to have a higher incidence of neurologic complications than the anterosuperior approach for anatomic shoulder arthroplasty.[13] Comparing the two approaches,

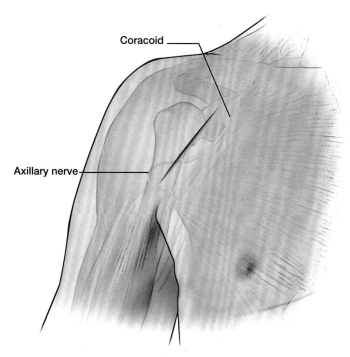

Coracoid

Axillary nerve

FIGURE 11.1 While performing the deltopectoral approach, the surgeon should be aware of the proximity of several neurovascular structures, eg, the cephalic vein, the axillary nerve, the musculocutaneous nerve, and the brachial plexus.

Lynch and colleagues found neurologic complications involving the brachial plexus in 4.7% of the deltopectoral approach patients and 0% in the anterosuperior approach patients, none of which involved the axillary nerve.[13]

Dangers

Despite being relatively safe, several neurovascular structures are in close proximity and can be injured during the deltopectoral approach, either by a direct insult or indirectly by excessive traction. These include the cephalic vein, ascending branches of the anterior circumflex artery, axillary artery and vein, the musculocutaneous nerve, axillary nerve, and the brachial plexus **(FIGURE 11.1)**.

Surgical Technique (Table 11.1)

Patient Positioning and Draping

The patient is placed in a "beach chair" position with the torso flexed in about 30° to 45°. At this angle, the venous pressure is reduced, and the arm may be comfortably manipulated for the humeral preparation. The head and neck should be secured in a designated headrest, and the trunk should be stabilized in order to accurately estimate the glenoid version during the procedure. In addition, the arm must be allowed to fully extend in order to provide complete humeral head and canal exposure. Prior to surgical preparation, the final positioning of the patient should be rechecked and secured as adjustments will be quite difficult after draping. For the majority of the procedure, the arm must be secured

TABLE 11.1 Deltopectoral Approach Steps
• Patient positioning in a beach chair and draping
• Skin incision and subcutaneous tissue dissection
• Cephalic vein exposure
• Deltopectoral interval division
• Mobilization of the subdeltoid and subacromial spaces
• Division of the clavipectoral fascia and coracohumeral ligament release
• Retraction of the deltoid and cephalic vein laterally and the pectoralis major and conjoint tendon medially
• Long head of biceps soft tissue tenotomy/tenodesis

in various positions. This can be accomplished by a surgical assistant with or without the use of a padded surgical stand or with a commercially available arm holder **(FIGURE 11.2)**.

Initial Incision Marking

The bony landmarks are palpated and marked. They include the acromion, clavicle, tip of the coracoid process, and the deltoid tuberosity of the humerus. The line for proposed surgical incision starts at the level of the clavicle and is extended distally through the tip of the coracoid process, aiming toward the deltoid tuberosity (or midhumeral line) to the level of the axilla. This line should measure approximately 12 to 14 cm **(FIGURE 11.3)**.

Superficial Dissection

While keeping tension on both sides of the line, the incision is carried out through the skin and the subcutaneous

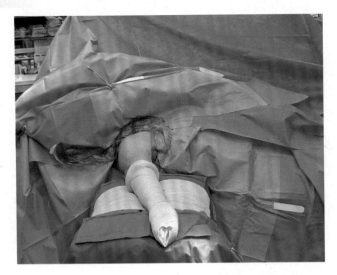

FIGURE 11.2 The patient is positioned in a "beach chair" position with the torso flexed in 30° to 45°. The arm may be fully extended when necessary.

may provide fewer alterations to the natural blood blow. Alternatively, as the vein is more likely to be damaged during deltoid retraction for glenoid exposure, it may be better protected if it is retracted medially with the pectoralis. Clinically, there is no evidence to suggest that retraction of the vessel to either direction is superior.

At this stage, the directions of muscle fibers of the pectoralis and the deltoid should be clearly visible such that the intermuscular interval can be easily identified. If the deltopectoral interval is not immediately obvious, the coracoid process can be palpated as it typically marks the superior most portion of the interval. The interval is gently dissected to avoid damage to the muscle tissue, while small vascular branches (usually in the proximal and distal part of the interval) are cauterized to prevent bleeding. The subdeltoid and the subacromial spaces are mobilized to allow continuity between the two spaces. With any previous surgical procedures including shoulder arthroscopy, there may be significant residual scar tissue in this region. In such instances, it is generally more effective to identify the subacromial space and then extend the exposure distally to include the subdeltoid space. While mobilizing this space, it is also helpful to place the shoulder in slight flexion, abduction, and internal rotation to improve access. Subsequently, the mobilized deltoid is retracted laterally and the pectoralis major is retracted medially to expose the clavipectoral facia (**FIGURE 11.5**).

Deep Layer Exposure

The clavipectoral fascia is divided longitudinally up to the coracoacromial ligament. For additional exposure,

tissue down to the deltopectoral fascia. After achieving hemostasis, lateral and medial skin flaps are developed, and appropriate retractors are placed. At this stage, the fat stripe, which envelops the cephalic vein, should be visible. The cephalic vein is exposed in its entirety about the deltopectoral interval (**FIGURE 11.4**). Caution should be taken while dissecting the vein as several branches drain into the main vessel both proximally and distally. Pending surgeon preference, the cephalic vein can be mobilized and retracted medially with the pectoralis or laterally with the deltoid. Since the cephalic vein drains more branches from the deltoid muscle, lateral retraction

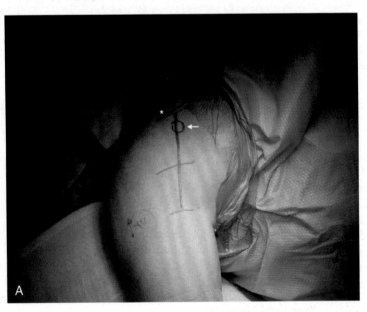

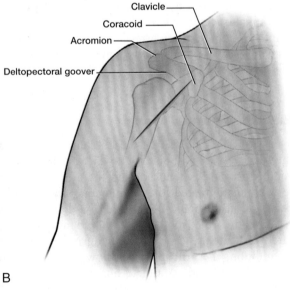

FIGURE 11.3 A and B, Prior to skin incision marking, the bony landmarks are identified. The incision starts at the tip of the coracoid process (arrow), aiming toward the deltoid tuberosity and extends approximately 12 to 14 cm. The acromion, clavicle, and acromioclavicular joint (asterisk) are identified as well.

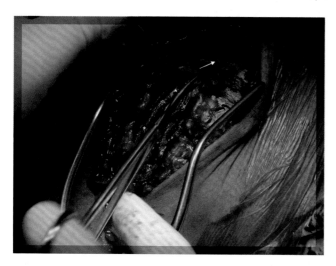

FIGURE 11.4 The cephalic vein (asterisks) is exposed and dissected in its entirety about the deltopectoral approach from distal to proximal, toward the coracoid process (white arrow).

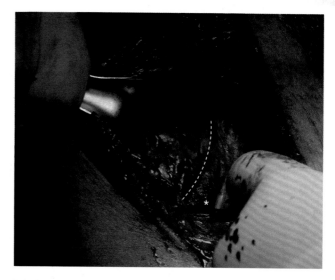

FIGURE 11.6 The fascia of the conjoint tendon is divided (dashed line) and must be mobilized with its associated muscle fibers (asterisk), which are just lateral to the tendon (black arrow).

the coracoacromial ligament can be either partially or completely released. For anatomic shoulder arthroplasty, however, to maintain the integrity of the coracoacromial arch and prevent anterior superior escape of the humeral head, the ligament may need to be maintained.

The conjoint tendon (brachioradialis and short head of biceps) is identified, and its fascia is divided to allow mobilization. It should be noted, however, that the tendon must be mobilized with its associated muscle fibers, which are often just lateral to the tendon (**FIGURE 11.6**). By retracting the deltoid muscle laterally and the conjoint tendon (with the pectoralis major) medially, the entire glenohumeral joint can be exposed. The musculo-cutaneous nerve lies on the deep surface of the conjoint tendon about 5.6 cm (range 3.1-8.2 cm) distal to the tip of the coracoid process.[14] However, its most proximal

branch penetrates the coracobrachialis muscle at about 3.4 cm (range 2.38-4.3 cm) distal to the tip of the coracoid proces[15] (**FIGURE 11.7**). Therefore, the retractor should be placed and secured proximally underneath the conjoint tendon in order to avoid injuring the nerve.

For additional inferior exposure and to allow greater rotation of the humerus during joint manipulation, many surgeons will release the superior 1 cm of the pectoralis major insertion. As the tendon is quite broad (7-9 cm in diameter[16]), releasing the proximal 1 cm or so, does not appear to compromise pectoralis major function. Immediately deep to the pectoralis major insertion is the long head of the biceps tendon. If there is substantial pathology about the biceps tendon, the proximal portion of the tendon can be excised while the distal portion of the tendon is fixed to the pectoralis major tendon insertion using heavy nonabsorbable suture (**FIGURE 11.8**). The biceps tendon is then traced proximally to identify the rotator interval and the lesser tuberosity with the subscapularis tendon insertion (**FIGURE 11.9**).

Complications of the Deltopectoral Approach

Since the deltopectoral approach is an internervous plane, injuries to major blood vessels or nerves are unlikely. However, blood vessels and nerves can still be iatrogenically injured.

For example, the cephalic vein can be injured at any point throughout the procedure, but it is most prone to injury during initial vein dissection with deltoid retraction for glenoid preparation and during deltopectoral interval closure. In the case of cephalic vein puncture, meticulous ligation of the vein is recommended to prevent postoperative hematoma. Similarly, the posterior circumflex arterial branches to the humerus can also

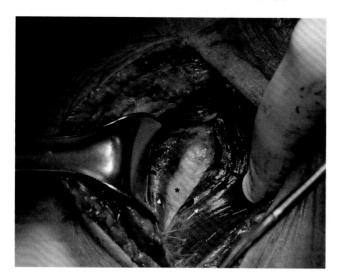

FIGURE 11.5 While dividing the deltopectoral interval, the deltoid (arrowhead) is retracted laterally and the pectoralis major (arrows) is retracted medially to expose the clavipectoral fascia (black asterisk).

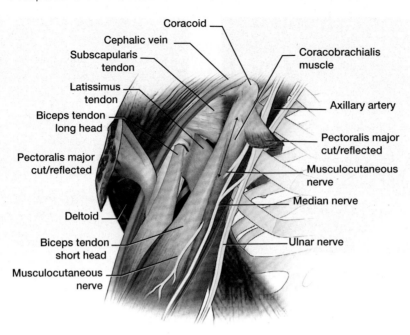

FIGURE 11.7 The most proximal branch of the musculocutaneous nerve penetrates the coracobrachialis muscle at about 3.4 cm distal to the tip of the coracoid process (bidirectional arrowhead).

be injured during mobilization of the subdeltoid space just distal to the surgical neck of the proximal humerus. The prevalence of neurological complications through the deltopectoral approach has been reported to be 1% to 4.7%.[17] Specifically, the prevalence of axillary nerve and musculocutaneous impairment after deltopectoral approach is approximately 1.8% and 3.8%, respectively, for all types of shoulder arthroplasty.[18] Although the majority of these injuries are transient neuropraxic

injuries with spontaneous recovery, on rare occasions, these neurologic deficits may remain persistent.[17,18]

Finally, excessive retraction even with blunt instruments may damage the conjoint tendon and the deltoid muscle. This is especially concerning for the deltoid as any significant damage to the muscle may lead to an inferior clinical outcome after shoulder arthroplasty. Therefore, continued vigilance during surgery is required in order to avoid significant and permanent damage to the muscles.

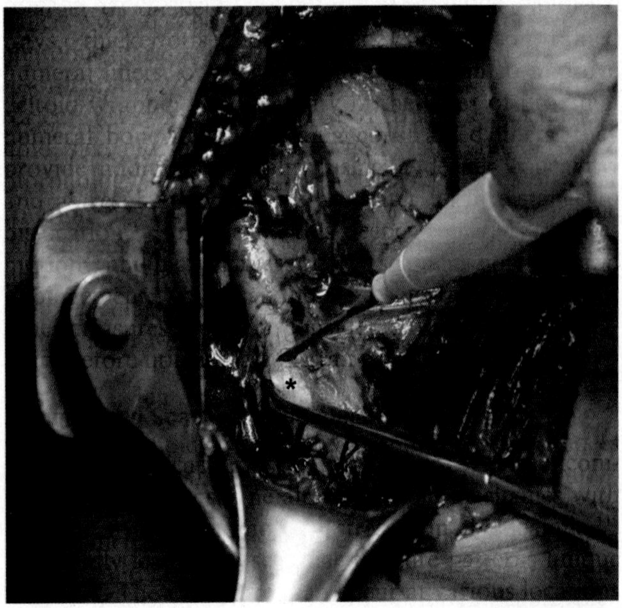

Tips and Hazards

Anatomic Orientation

The coracoid process is the "lighthouse" of the shoulder. It guides the surgeon through the incision, the superficial and deep dissection, and glenoid implant positioning. It is the anatomic border of the "safe zone" (lateral to the coracoid) and the "danger zone" (medial to the coracoid). Furthermore, the coracoid process can often serve as an anchor for intraoperative navigation and patient-specific instrumentation. Therefore, the relative position of the surgical field to the coracoid process should always be noted during the procedure.

Another useful anatomic landmark is the bicipital groove. At the level of the humeral head, the bicipital groove divides the lesser tuberosity from the greater tuberosity with insertion of the subscapularis and the supraspinatus tendons, respectively. In addition, it also marks the rotator interval that can be opened to inspect the joint and estimate physiological humeral head retroversion.

FIGURE 11.8 The long head of biceps tendon (asterisk) is fixed to pectoralis major insertion (sutures) and released.

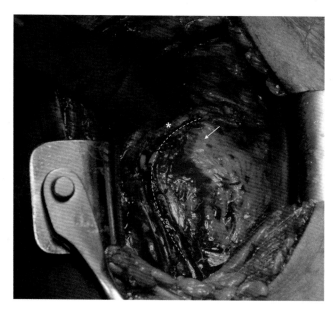

FIGURE 11.9 The long head of the biceps tendon is traced proximally (dashed line) to identify the rotator interval, supraspinatus (asterisk), and subscapularis (arrow).

Positioning and Draping

In order to position the patient in 30° to 45° of torso flexion, it is recommended to place the table in 20° to 30° of Trendelenburg and 60° to 75° of torso flexion. This "true" beach chair position will prevent the patient from sliding down toward the foot of the bed during surgery. Adding 10° to 15° of tilt to the contralateral side is also helpful in preventing the patient from sliding toward the surgical side when the arm is externally rotated during the surgery. For positioning of the arm during the procedure, the authors' preferred method is to use a separate sterile surgical stand. During the initial surgical approach, the arm is rested on the surgical stand (see **FIGURE 11.2**). Then, during various portions of the surgery, the shoulder can be extended or flexed slightly to enhance the surgical exposure by adjusting the height of the surgical stand.

Skin Incision

Standard surgical incision should be adequate for majority of the patients. However, for some very muscular patients with a hypertrophic anterior deltoid muscle, it is advantageous to establish the incision slightly more laterally. After the skin incision, a larger skin flap will need to be established medially to identify and develop the deltopectoral interval. However, after this initial dissection, by lateralizing the skin incision, it will be easier to retract the muscle and the associated soft tissues more laterally to allow improved exposure of the joint, especially the glenoid.

ANTEROSUPERIOR APPROACH

The anterosuperior approach for shoulder replacement was first introduced by Donald B. Mackenzie in 1993 (**VIDEO 11.2**).[19] By using this approach, he aimed to optimize the glenoid surface exposure. Unlike the deltopectoral approach, however, it does not utilize an internervous plane. Rather, the approach requires detachment of the anterior deltoid from the acromion.

Indications

- Shoulder arthroplasty
- Open rotator cuff repair
- Proximal humerus fracture (limited distal exposure due to axillary nerve)

Absolute Contraindications

The anterosuperior approach is contraindicated in osteoarthritis associated with dwarfism since branches of the axillary nerve may be encountered as close as 1 cm from the acromioclavicular joint.[19]

Relative Contraindications

If one of the following criteria is met, the risk of improper placement of the prosthesis and perioperative complications may increase[11]:

- Irreducible proximally migrated humeral head under anesthesia
- Inadequate passive external rotation of the arm (<25°)
- Presence of significant inferior humeral osteophytes
- Revision arthroplasty that may require osteotomy of the humerus

Advantages

The anterosuperior approach is simple to perform and can be completed quickly. It provides excellent glenoid surface exposure, as direct visualization perpendicular to the glenoid surface can be obtained. This exposure is especially useful in cases with significant glenoid retroversion that must be surgically corrected. Moreover, it is also superior in mobilizing posterior structures such as the posterior capsule and the infraspinatus tendon.

The anterosuperior approach for reverse total shoulder replacement may allow preservation of the subscapularis tendon, and therefore may be associated with a lower incidence of postoperative anterior instability. Unlike the deltopectoral approach, it also avoids the cephalic vein. Finally, although controversial, the anterosuperior approach may lead to a decreased incidence of acromial stress fractures following reverse shoulder arthroplasty.[10,11,20]

Disadvantages

Due to difficulty in distracting the humeral head and adequately exposing the inferior glenoid rim, the risk of inaccurate glenoid component positioning (superior translation or superior tilt) is increased. In order to improve the inferior glenoid exposure, a lower humeral neck cut may be necessary which, in turn, can result in loss of bone stock and possibly inferior

TABLE 11.2 Anterosuperior Approach Steps

- Patient positioning in beach chair and draping
- Skin incision and subcutaneous tissue dissection
- Deltoid split
- Mobilization of the subdeltoid space and coracoacromial ligament division
- Long head of biceps soft tissue tenotomy/tenodesis

humeral component fixation.[21] The difficulty in inferior exposure also limits the ability to remove inferior humeral neck osteophytes. Furthermore, especially for obese patients, due to difficulty in completely adducting the arm for canal preparation, there is a tendency of the humeral prosthesis to be placed in a slight valgus position.

After releasing the anterior deltoid from the acromion, this approach also requires separation of the anterior and the middle deltoid muscles. Excessively splitting of this interval may, in turn, lead to iatrogenic injury to the anterior branches of the axillary nerve. In fact, compared to the deltopectoral approach, the proximity to the axillary nerve limits the distal exposure and prevents this approach from being more versatile.[10,11,20]

Surgical Technique (Table 11.2)

Patient Positioning and Draping

The patient is positioned in a beach chair position in a manner similar to the deltopectoral approach. However, the torso is more vertical and recommended to be positioned at approximately 70° (**FIGURE 11.10**).

Similar to the deltopectoral approach, the bony landmarks, including the lateral and anterior edges of the acromion, coracoid process, acromioclavicular joint, and the anterior and posterior margins of the humerus, should be identified and marked. The line for proposed surgical incision starts about 1 cm posterior to the acromioclavicular joint, runs parallel to the anterior edge of the acromion to the mid-humeral

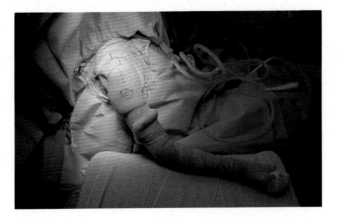

FIGURE 11.10 The patient is positioned in a beach chair position with the torso flexed at approximately 70°.

line about 6 to 8 cm distal to the lateral border of the acromion (**FIGURE 11.11**).

Superficial Dissection

The incision is carried down through the skin and the subcutaneous tissue until the overlying fascia of the deltoid muscle. After hemostasis, full-thickness anterior and posterior skin flaps are developed. Then, from the acromioclavicular joint, the anterior deltoid is peeled off the anterior acromion and reflected in a subperiosteal manner. This release is carried distally through the raphe between the anterior and middle deltoid muscles (**FIGURE 11.12**). According to one anatomic study, the axillary nerve horizontally crosses this area about 4.3 to 6.4 cm from the anterolateral corner of the acromion. Other studies have measured this distance to be as high as 7.2 cm. Likely, the actual distance depends on the size of the patient and may be calculated using the formula: *Axillary nerve distance* (cm) = $(0.155 \times humeral\ length$ [cm]) + 0.628.[22-24] Alternatively, the axillary nerve may be palpated on individual patients to establish the inferior border of the split (**FIGURE 11.13**). Many surgeons will then put a "stay" suture on the distal-most portion of the split raphe, reattaching the anterior and middle deltoid muscles in order to prevent further splitting of the raphe that can potentially damage the axillary nerve (**FIGURE 11.14**).

After releasing the deltoid, the coracoacromial ligament can be resected from the undersurface of the acromion. The acromial branch to the thoracoacromial artery is identified and ligated. At this stage, if required, acromial spurs can be resected using a Rongeur, but an official acromioplasty is generally not required.

Deep Layer Exposure

The subdeltoid space is mobilized both anteriorly and posteriorly, and the subdeltoid bursa is excised. Then, the biceps tendon is located and used to identify the rotator interval and the greater and lesser tuberosities. Again, if there is sufficient pathology, the proximal biceps tendon can be resected while the distal portion is fixed to the local soft tissues using heavy nonabsorbable sutures. If there is a preexisting large defect of the rotator cuff tendons (eg, rotator cuff arthropathy), the glenohumeral joint should be visible, and the humeral head may be resected without violating the subscapularis tendon insertion at the lesser tuberosity (**FIGURE 11.15**), and the glenoid is exposed (**FIGURE 11.16**).

Complications of the Anterosuperior Approach

The most significant complication related to the anterosuperior approach is loss of the deltoid function, which may result from axillary nerve injury or postoperative deltoid dehiscence.

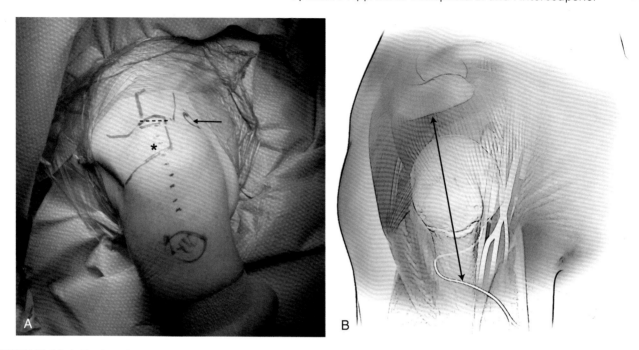

FIGURE 11.11 A, The bony landmarks, including the acromion (asterisk), coracoid process (arrow), and acromioclavicular joint (dashed line), are identified and marked. **B**, The line for proposed surgical incision for the anterosuperior approach starts about 1 cm posterior to the acromioclavicular joint, runs parallel to the anterior edge of the acromion to the mid-humeral line about 6 to 8 cm distal to the lateral border of the acromion.

Fortunately, the incidence of iatrogenic damage to the anterior branches of the axillary nerve has been reported to be quite low at 0% to 0.8%.[11,13,18] However, since no adequate alternative shoulder flexor muscle can compensate for the loss of the powerful anterior deltoid,[25] functional outcome may be notably diminished with significant morbidity.[26]

Deltoid dehiscence (or detachment) has an unknown incidence. Limited studies report an incidence of up to

5% in patients undergoing shoulder arthroplasty via the anterosuperior approach.[11] Extrapolated literature taken from rotator cuff repair surgery performed through a similar approach reveals an incidence of up to 9%.[27] Patient with deltoid dehiscence report a poor functional outcome, pain, and deformity, with the majority require revision surgery to reattach the deltoid. Even with the surgical reattachment, however, the resulting outcome may still be compromised.[11,26,27]

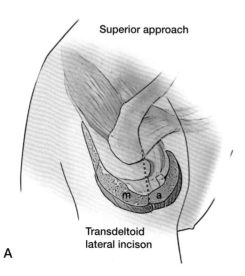

Superior approach

m   a

Transdeltoid
lateral incison

A

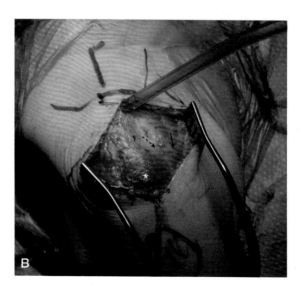

FIGURE 11.12 A, The skin incision is superficial to the raphe between the anterior (a) and middle (m) deltoid muscles. **B**, The raphe (dashed arrow) between the anterior (arrow) and middle deltoid (asterisk) muscles is identified and split.

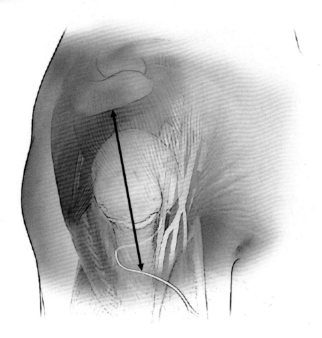

FIGURE 11.13 The axillary nerve horizontally crosses vertically at about 4.3 to 6.4 cm distal from the anterolateral corner of the acromion (bidirectional arrowhead).

Tips and Hazards

Patient Selection

The ideal patient for this approach is thin, with smaller deltoid muscles, thick humeral cortices to resist the force required for retraction, and a reduceable proximally migrated humeral head. While this approach has been used for anatomic shoulder arthroplasty,[28,29] it is optimally suited for reverse total shoulder arthroplasty in

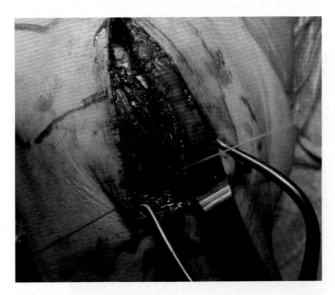

FIGURE 11.14 A "stay" suture on the distal-most portion of the split raphe is placed, reattaching the anterior and middle deltoid muscles in order to prevent further splitting of the raphe that can potentially damage the axillary nerve.

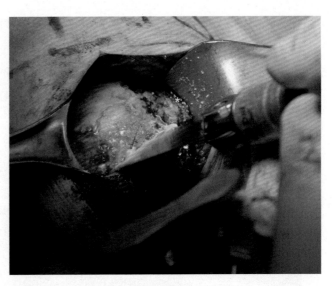

FIGURE 11.15 The humeral head is resected without violating the subscapularis tendon insertion at the lesser tuberosity (yellow asterisk).

patients with preexisting massive rotator cuff tears. In addition, revision arthroplasty cases where extensive manipulation of the humerus may be required would be quite challenging with this surgical approach and should be avoided.

Closure

Significant care and effort should be taken to optimally reattach the anterior deltoid muscle back to the acromion to minimize the likelihood of deltoid dehiscence. Generally, this requires multiple heavy nonabsorbable sutures that are passed through bone tunnels in the anterior acromion.[26] In addition, the split raphe between the anterior and middle deltoid muscle should also be reapproximated. Even with sufficient repair, most

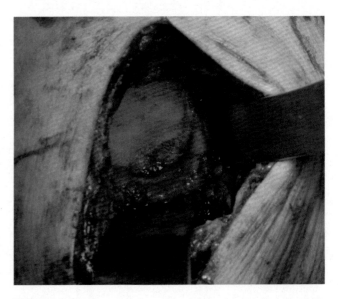

FIGURE 11.16 After resection of the humeral head, the glenoid is visible "en face."

surgeons favor postoperative restrictions to protect the repair. Therefore, active forward elevation is generally restricted for the first 4 to 6 weeks after surgery.

CONCLUSION

Both the deltopectoral and anterosuperior approaches provide adequate exposure for shoulder arthroplasty. Each approach has its distinct advantages and disadvantages. Despite several studies that have compared the two approaches, long-term comparative prospective data on clinical outcome after shoulder arthroplasty is lacking. Therefore, the specific surgical approach should be selected according to the surgeon's experience and individual patient's needs.

REFERENCES

1. Patel RB, Muh S, Okoroha KR, et al. Results of total shoulder arthroplasty in patients aged 55 years or younger versus those older than 55 years: an analysis of 1135 patients with over 2 years of follow-up. *J Shoulder Elbow Surg.* 2019;28:861-868.
2. Flurin PH, Marczuk Y, Janout M, Wright TW, Zuckerman J, Roche CP. Comparison of outcomes using anatomic and reverse total shoulder arthroplasty. *Bull Hosp Jt Dis (2013).* 2013;71(suppl 2):101-107.
3. Dillon MT, Chan PH, Inacio MCS, Singh A, Yian EH, Navarro RA. Yearly trends in elective shoulder arthroplasty, 2005-2013. *Arthritis Care Res (Hoboken).* 2017;69:1574-1581.
4. Simovitch R, Flurin PH, Wright T, Zuckerman JD, Roche CP. Quantifying success after total shoulder arthroplasty: the substantial clinical benefit. *J Shoulder Elbow Surg.* 2018;27:903-911.
5. Jeong J, Bryan J, Iannotti JP. Effect of a variable prosthetic neck-shaft angle and the surgical technique on replication of normal humeral anatomy. *J Bone Joint Surg Am.* 2009;91:1932-1941.
6. Sadoghi P, Vavken J, Leithner A, Vavken P. Benefit of intraoperative navigation on glenoid component positioning during total shoulder arthroplasty. *Arch Orthop Trauma Surg.* 2015;135:41-47.
7. Lugli T. Artificial shoulder joint by Pean (1893): the facts of an exceptional intervention and the prosthetic method. *Clin Orthop Relat Res.* 1978;(133):215-218.
8. Henry AK. Extensile to shoulder joint and to elbow joint. In: Henry AK, ed. *Extensile Exposure,* 2nd ed. Edinburgh and London, Great Britain. E. & S. Livingstone; 1970:25-37.
9. Neer CS II. Prosthetic replacement of the humeral head: indications and operative technique. *Surg Clin North Am.* 1963;43:1581-1597.
10. Mole D, Wein F, Dezaly C, Valenti P, Sirveaux F. Surgical technique: the anterosuperior approach for reverse shoulder arthroplasty. *Clin Orthop Relat Res.* 2011;469:2461-2468.
11. Gillespie RJ, Garrigues GE, Chang ES, Namdari S, Williams GR Jr. Surgical exposure for reverse total shoulder arthroplasty: differences in approaches and outcomes. *Orthop Clin North Am.* 2015;46:49-56.
12. Nove-Josserand L, Clavert P. Glenoid exposure in total shoulder arthroplasty. *Orthop Traumatol Surg Res.* 2018;104:S129-S135.
13. Lynch NM, Cofield RH, Silbert PL, Hermann RC. Neurologic complications after total shoulder arthroplasty. *J Shoulder Elbow Surg.* 1996;5:53-61.
14. Flatow EL, Bigliani LU, April EW. An anatomic study of the musculocutaneous nerve and its relationship to the coracoid process. *Clin Orthop Relat Res.* 1989;(244):166-171.
15. Reboucas F, Filho RB, Filardis C, Pereira RR, Cardoso AA. Anatomical study of the musculocutaneous nerve in relation to the coracoid process. *Rev Bras Ortop.* 2010;45:400-403.
16. de Figueiredo EA, Terra BB, Cohen C, et al. The pectoralis major footprint: an anatomical study. *Rev Bras Ortop.* 2013;48:519-523.
17. Ladermann A, Lubbeke A, Melis B, et al. Prevalence of neurologic lesions after total shoulder arthroplasty. *J Bone Joint Surg Am.* 2011;93:1288-1293.
18. Ball CM. Neurologic complications of shoulder joint replacement. *J Shoulder Elbow Surg.* 2017;26:2125-2132.
19. Mole D. The antero-superior exposure for total shoulder replacement. *Orthop Traumatol.* 1993;7:71-77.
20. Sager BW, Khazzam M. Surgical approaches in shoulder arthroplasty. In: Sonar SB, ed. *Advances in Shoulder Surgery.* IntechOpen; 2018.
21. Ladermann A, Lubbeke A, Collin P, Edwards TB, Sirveaux F, Walch G. Influence of surgical approach on functional outcome in reverse shoulder arthroplasty. *Orthop Traumatol Surg Res.* 2011;97:579-582.
22. Ikemoto RY, Nascimento LG, Bueno RS, Almeida LH, Strose E, Murachovsky J. Axillary nerve position in the anterosuperior approach of the shoulder: a cadaveric study. *Acta Ortop Bras.* 2015;23:26-28.
23. Traver JL, Guzman MA, Cannada LK, Kaar SG. Is the axillary nerve at risk during a deltoid-splitting approach for proximal humerus fractures? *J Orthop Trauma.* 2016;30:240-244.
24. Leechavengvongs S, Teerawutthichaikit T, Witoonchart K, et al. Surgical anatomy of the axillary nerve branches to the deltoid muscle. *Clin Anat.* 2015;28:118-122.
25. Burkhead WZ Jr, Scheinberg RR, Box G. Surgical anatomy of the axillary nerve. *J Shoulder Elbow Surg.* 1992;1:31-36.
26. Groh GI, Simoni M, Rolla P, Rockwood CA. Loss of the deltoid after shoulder operations: an operative disaster. *J Shoulder Elbow Surg.* 1994;3:243-253.
27. Gumina S, Di Giorgio G, Perugia D, Postacchini F. Deltoid detachment consequent to open surgical repair of massive rotator cuff tears. *Int Orthop.* 2008;32:81-84.
28. Levy O, Copeland SA. Cementless surface replacement arthroplasty of the shoulder. 5- to 10-year results with the Copeland mark-2 prosthesis. *J Bone Joint Surg Br.* 2001;83:213-221.
29. Mullett H, Levy O, Raj D, Even T, Abraham R, Copeland SA. Copeland surface replacement of the shoulder. Results of an hydroxyapatite-coated cementless implant in patients over 80 years of age. *J Bone Joint Surg Br.* 2007;89:1466-1469.

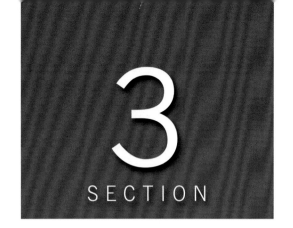

SECTION 3

Anatomic Total Shoulder Arthroplasty

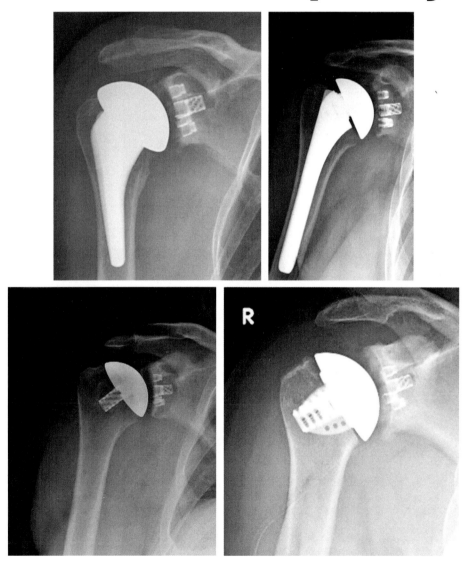

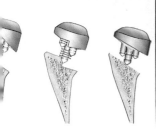

12 Implant Options

Kenneth J. Faber, MD, MHPE and G. Daniel Langohr, PhD

HISTORY

Shoulder arthroplasty has undergone considerable change since the early contemporaneous attempts by Pean[1] and Gluck[2] to treat tuberculous arthritis with a prosthesis. The initial shoulder arthroplasties were understandably failures, and the procedure was essentially abandoned until the 1950s when Neer revisited arthroplasty as a treatment for proximal humerus fractures.[3,4] The early successes of this treatment resulted in an expansion of the indications of shoulder arthroplasty for the treatment of end-stage glenohumeral arthritis.[5] Over the past 4 decades, clinical, anatomical, and biomechanical studies have improved our understanding of anatomic total shoulder arthroplasty (TSA) and led to advances in implant materials, design, and fixation methods.

HUMERAL STEM OPTIONS

Humeral components have undergone profound changes over the past 4 decades. Stem fixation techniques have improved, and implant size has steadily diminished to reduce bone resection, preserve host bone, simplify the treatment of proximal humeral deformity, and minimize stress shielding.

Humeral Implant Materials

Titanium is the most commonly used material for the humeral stem. This material is relatively inert, has excellent biocompatibility, and a modulus of elasticity resembling normal bone that can promote ingrowth to create a stable bone-implant interface. Cobalt chrome (CoCr) has a modulus of elasticity that is considerably greater than titanium and is a material that is infrequently used for humeral stems.[6]

Fixation Options: Cemented

Shoulder cementing techniques have benefitted from improvements and advances in hip and knee arthroplasty cementation **(FIGURE 12.1)**. Current cementing techniques include the use of cement restrictors, canal cleansing, and cement pressurization.

There are several advantages to cement fixation. Cement provides immediate early stem fixation and avoids the risks of stem subsidence. The stem size can be reduced to facilitate accurate positioning within the canal that optimizes head coverage of the humerus resection. Cemented stems have an excellent performance record with low rates of aseptic stem loosening.[7-10]

There are several disadvantages to cement fixation. Cement can extrude from the intramedullary canal through nutrient artery fenestrations and compromise the radial nerve.[11] Well-fixed cemented stems are often challenging to remove, and complications such as iatrogenic fracture and thermal injury to bone and neurological structures have been reported.[12] Occasionally, an intentional humeral osteotomy is required for stem removal, and the subsequent reconstruction may require bone grafting and supplemental fixation that can delay postoperative rehabilitation.[13-15]

Fixation Options: Cementless

The transition to cementless (or uncemented) stem fixation has been motivated by the technical challenges associated with the extraction and revision of cemented stems and the increasing ease and familiarity with the use of cementless devices.[16,17] Cementless humeral stems can be broadly categorized as metaphyseal or diaphyseal filling implants **(FIGURE 12.2)**. Metaphyseal filling stems rely on proximal bone ingrowth/ongrowth to a textured surface. Initial proximal stability can be enhanced by the addition of cancellous autograft harvested from the resected humeral head.[18] Diaphyseal filling stems are dependent on endosteal fixation adjacent to the metaphysis.

Uncemented stems have several advantages. Humerus preparation and prosthesis implantation are simplified and less time-consuming than implantation of cemented stems. Shortened case times and the avoidance of disposable canal preparation equipment such as pulse lavage, restrictors, and cement may provide increased value.

The disadvantages of cementless fixation include iatrogenic fracture, incomplete implant seating, implant migration, and stress shielding. Iatrogenic fracture can occur during canal reaming, broaching,

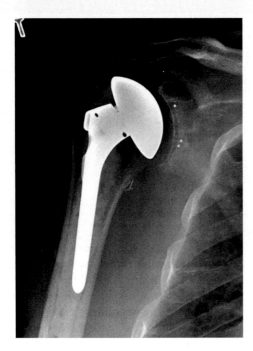

FIGURE 12.1 Cemented humeral stem. A 75-year-old man with a well-functioning shoulder replacement 13 years following surgery for primary osteoarthritis.

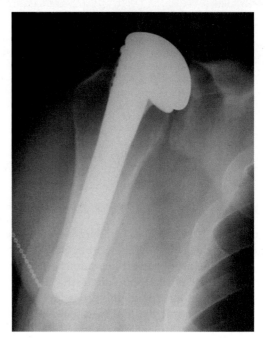

FIGURE 12.3 A 58-year-old man who is painful 2 years following total shoulder arthroplasty for osteoarthritis. The implant is well-fixed, diaphyseal filling, and incompletely seated.

or implantation. Stable fractures can be treated with a modified rehabilitation program or cerclage wire fixation. Unstable fractures can be converted to a smaller cemented stem with cerclage wire fixation. Incomplete

implant seating can alter joint loading, rotator cuff tensioning and cause persistent postoperative pain requiring revision **(FIGURE 12.3)**.[19]

Similarly, implant migration can alter normal glenohumeral alignment resulting in pain or instability **(FIGURE 12.4)**.

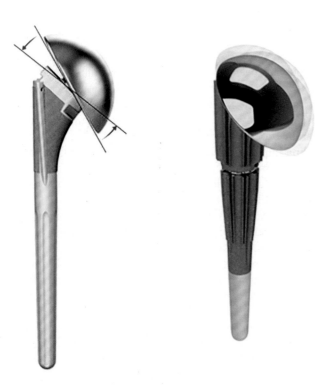

FIGURE 12.2 Examples of metaphyseal (left) and diaphyseal fixation (right) cementless humeral stems. (Courtesy of DePuy Synthes. Image of the product used under license of Limacorporate S.p.A. – Italy.)

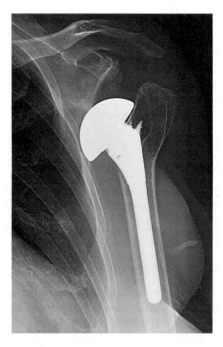

FIGURE 12.4 A 72-year-old woman 1-year postop hemiarthroplasty for arthritis with severe implant subsidence.

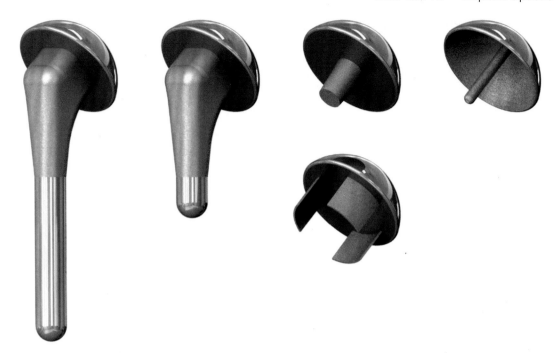

FIGURE 12.5 From left to right; standard stem, short stem, central stemless (top) and peripheral stemless (bottom), and humeral resurfacing implants.

CONVERTIBLE STEMS

Common reasons for clinical failure of anatomic TSA include progressive rotator cuff disease, glenoid component loosening, and shoulder instability. In each of these instances, the humeral stem may be well fixed and well aligned. The development of convertible platform systems specifically addresses this clinical scenario and permits revision to a reverse prosthesis without removal of the stem. Clinical studies of platform systems indicate that fewer complications occur and blood loss is diminished when compared to revisions requiring stem removal, but there may be a risk of excessive humeral lengthening.[20,21]

Humeral Stem Options: Length, Geometry, and Surface Characteristics

Humeral stem vary in length **(FIGURE 12.5)**, ranging from standard-length stems having an overall length between 100 to 150 mm, short stems having overall lengths between 50 to 100 mm, to stemless designs which have lengths of less than 50 mm.[22]

Stem width also varies and is commonly classified in terms of filling ratio **(FIGURE 12.6)**, which is the size of the stem relative to the diameter of the humeral bone.[23] Generally, a larger filling ratio is associated with more bone removal and may contribute to humerus stress shielding. The presence (or absence) of a proximal collar that provides initial stability and transfers implant loading to the proximal cortex is also a common variant in humeral stem design.

Humeral stem geometry and design are both major factors in determining the type of humeral fixation achieved, which can be metaphyseal (proximal), diaphyseal (distal), or some combination of both.

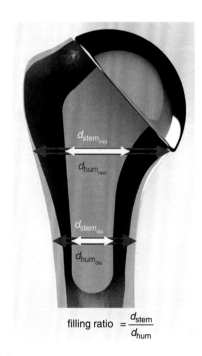

$$\text{filling ratio} = \frac{d_{stem}}{d_{hum}}$$

FIGURE 12.6 Metaphyseal (top) and diaphyseal (bottom) filling ratios.

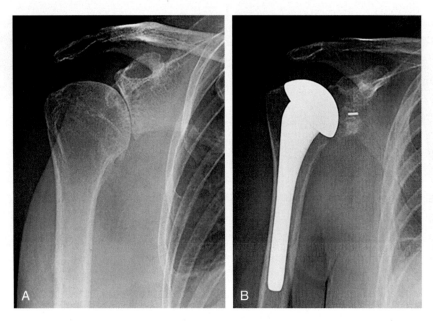

FIGURE 12.7 A 67 year old woman with primary osteoarthritis (**A**) that was treated with a standard-length stem shoulder arthroplasty (**B**).

Standard Stem

Standard-length stems include a fixation structure that extends distally from the humeral resection plane into the humeral canal (**FIGURES 12.5** and **12.7**). The surface characteristics of the standard stem are dependent on whether it is cemented or uncemented. Cemented variants typically have a constant polished or slightly roughened surface finish that provides an interface for adhesion between the stem and cement. Uncemented stems have a metaphyseal surface that is treated to create a rough and/or porous surface to promote proximal bony ingrowth, while the distal aspect of the stem is commonly polished to prevent distal fixation. Some manufacturers have dedicated stems for cemented and uncemented applications,

while others have a universal stem with uncemented surface characteristics that is intended for both fixation techniques. The filling ratio is typically larger proximally and smaller distally for metaphyseal fixation stems, while the opposite occurs with diaphyseal fixation stems.

As a result of the high prevalence of stress shielding with standard uncemented stems, shorter humeral stems have been introduced.

Short Stem

Short-stem humeral components maintain the proximal metaphyseal contact surfaces, but the distal stem is either absent or greatly reduced (**FIGURES 12.5** and **12.8**). Short-stem humeral components are also available

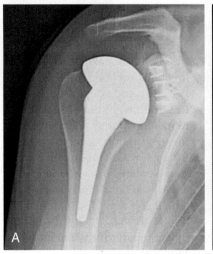
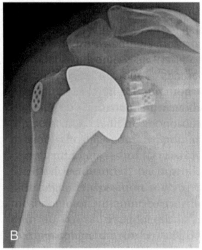

FIGURE 12.8 Examples of short stem uncemented shoulder arthroplasties for osteoarthritis (**A** and **B**). (Courtesy Dr. R. Simovitch.)

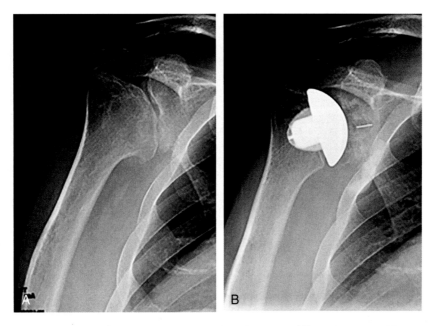

FIGURE 12.9 Glenohumeral arthritis in a 50-year-old with multiple epiphyseal dysplasia (**A**) causing proximal humerus offset and shaft-bowing deformity treated with a stemless total shoulder arthroplasty (**B**).

for cemented and uncemented fixation, with the former typically exhibiting constant smooth polished or roughened contact surfaces, and the latter employing various forms of spatially varying rough and/or porous surfaces to promote bone ingrowth for fixation. Like standard stems, the filling ratio of short stems typically decreases moving distally.

To further address the concern of humeral stress shielding, as well as to increase bone preservation, stemless humeral fixation components have most recently been developed.

Stemless

Stemless humeral fixation components incorporate fixation structures, which interface only with the most proximal humeral bone (**FIGURES 12.5** and **12.9**) and include two classifications of fixation; central and peripheral fixation. Central fixation engages the central aspect of the humeral trabecular bone beneath the humeral resection plane, whereas peripheral fixation involves the interaction of the peripheral region of humeral trabecular bone closer to the cortex. The amount of load transfer at the proximal cortex of the humeral resection plane also plays a role in determining the load transfer from the implant to the surrounding bone.

Stemless humeral reconstruction allows accurate positioning of the humeral head on the resection surface without referencing the distal canal. This is particularly helpful when treating arthritis that is associated with proximal humeral deformity (**FIGURE 12.9**). In addition, failed stemless components can often be removed without damaging the proximal humerus and revised to conventional components (**FIGURE 12.10**). Early clinical

results with stemless devices are encouraging, and this may be partially due to the more anatomic positioning of the humeral head, although the long-term clinical outcomes are still not known.[22]

Resurfacing

Humeral resurfacing prostheses are implanted after removal of the remaining articular cartilage and subchondral bone. The humeral head cancellous bone is preserved, and fixation is achieved with cancellous bone ingrowth to the hydroxyapatite or plasma sprayed back surface of the component and the central alignment post (**FIGURES 12.5** and **12.11**). Conservation of the cancellous bone makes glenoid exposure more difficult, and resurfacing devices are being gradually displaced by stemless devices.[7]

HUMERAL STRESS SHIELDING

Stress shielding, which manifests itself as a reduction in proximal bone following humeral reconstruction, occurs as a result of bone remodeling in response to applied stress according to Wolff Law. In the case of humeral reconstruction, this occurs due to the reduction in loading of the proximal humerus as a result of the insertion of the humeral stem, which now carries a proportion of the joint load distally. The first clinical reports of stress shielding were based on observations of extensively coated implants that were intended to achieve metaphyseal and diaphyseal fixation[23,24] (**FIGURE 12.12**). In some cases, the stress shielding was profound and mimicked observations of extensively coated uncemented hip arthroplasty stems.[25,26]

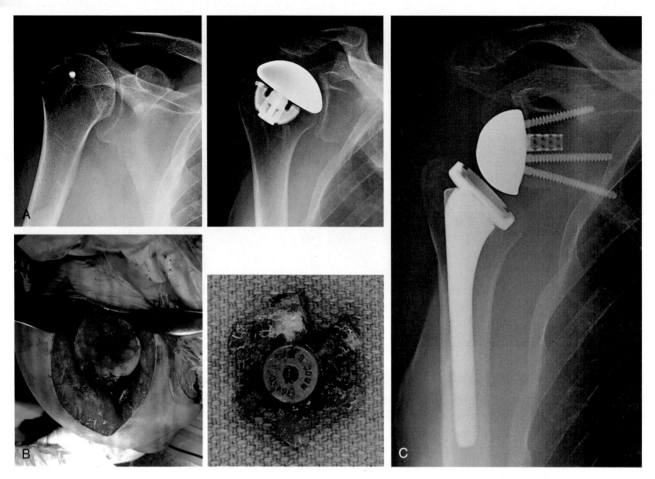

FIGURE 12.10 A 62-year-old man 7 years following stemless hemiarthroplasty (**A**) for rotator cuff arthropathy with preserved active motion. Symptoms progressed, and the prosthesis was removed (**B**) and revised to a standard length uncemented reverse arthroplasty (**C**).

Standard stems are at risk of facilitating stress shielding if the distal portion of the stem is well-fixed in the diaphysis. Clinical reports of a variety of standard stem humeral implants have found the prevalence of stress shielding in uncemented stems to range from 5% to 63% of patients.[23,27,28] Larger filling ratios have also been correlated with increased remodeling and proximal bone resorption.[23,29]

In the case of short stems, the elimination of the distal stem theoretically reduces the risk of distal fixation and stress shielding. Computational studies have shown that as humeral stem length is reduced, so does the

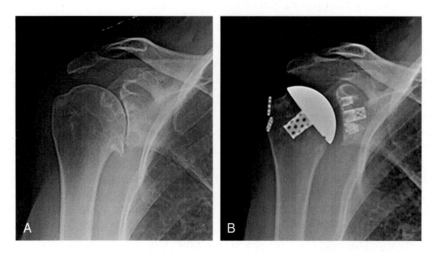

FIGURE 12.11 Resurfacing total shoulder arthroplasty for primary osteoarthritis (**A** and **B**). (Courtesy Dr M Parsons.)

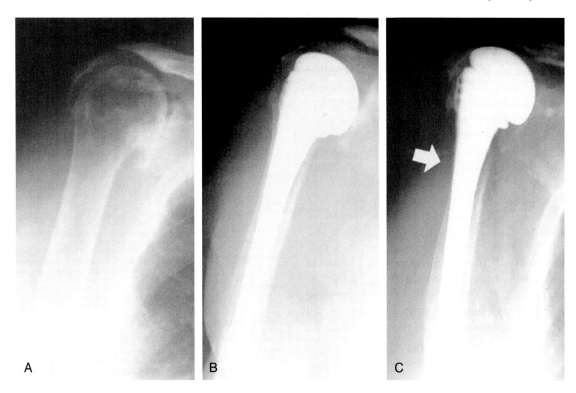

FIGURE 12.12 Humeral stress shielding showing progression from the preoperative state (**A**), immediately postoperative (**B**), and after 7 years of follow-up (**C**). (Reproduced with permission from Nagels J, Stokdijk M, Rozing PM. Stress shielding and bone resorption in shoulder arthroplasty. *J Shoulder Elbow Surg.* 2003;12:35-39.)

corresponding change in humeral bone stress compared to native bone, meaning that shorter stems have the potential to reduce the risk of proximal humeral stress shielding.[30] However, clinical reports have shown stress shielding still occurs with short stem humeral components ranging in prevalence from 14% to 52%[31,32] and radiolucencies or bony adaptations present in 71% to 80% of patients[33,34] (**FIGURE 12.13**).

It has also been reported that up to 9% to 17% have been found to be either loose or at risk of loosening,[33,35] although the presence of proximal ingrowth coating has been shown to reduce the risk of loosening significantly.[36] Although short stems still can result in humeral stress shielding, they are better than standard stems, with comparative clinical results showing less prevalence of cortical thinning (50% vs 74%) and partial calcar osteolysis (23% vs 31%).[37]

Short humeral stems are also sensitive to filling ratio. For example, short stem humeral components with smaller filling ratios were found to be less likely to exhibit cortical thinning,[22] which agrees with a finite element study that showed that the use of smaller-sized implants resulted in less changes in bone stress compared to the intact state, as well as a smaller proportion of bone that was expected to resorb immediately following reconstruction.[38] A second-factor contributing to stress shielding, that is unique to short stems, is varus or valgus component misalignment. In this instance, the tip of

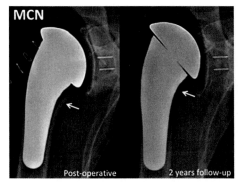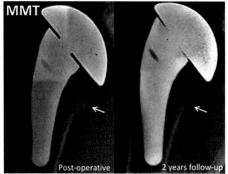

FIGURE 12.13 Examples of bone remodeling following implantation of a short stem uncemented humeral component. MCN, medial cortical narrowing; MMT, medial metaphyseal thinning. (Reproduced with permission from Peduzzi L, Goetzmann T, Wein F, et al. Proximal humeral bony adaptations with a short uncemented stem for shoulder arthroplasty: a quantitative analysis. *JSES Open Access.* 2019;3:278-286.)

the stem deviates from the canal's central axis and abuts against the endosteum effectively locking the stem distally. Clinically, filling ratios greater than 0.7, as well as distal cortical contact are both associated with a higher risk of stress shielding.[34,39,40] There are many short-stem humeral designs currently available, all of which vary significantly in geometry and design, and existing clinical reports may not be representative of all short stems.

Clinical reports of humeral stress shielding in stemless implants are favorable, with many reporting no radiolucencies with follow-ups ranging from 2 to 9 years.[41-43] Another study reported radiolucencies in 1%, osteolysis in 4%, and decreased bone density in 35% to 54% of short stem recipients,[44] although this finding may have been a result of imaging artifacts.[45] Bone stresses following reconstruction with a stemless implant seem to be dependent on the shape of the fixation feature, with computational studies suggesting that central fixation designs may produce less expected bone resorption when compared to peripheral fixation designs.[46]

HUMERAL HEAD OPTIONS

Humeral Head Implant Materials

Most humeral head components are manufactured from CoCr. The articulating surface is highly polished to minimize generation of particulate wear debris. Titanium heads are available and intended for patients with nickel allergy. However, the surface polishing and hardness is inferior to CoCr, and accelerated polyethylene wear that is described in hip arthroplasty may occur.[47,48]

Alternate bearing surfaces, such as pyrolytic carbon and ceramic, have excellent biocompatibility and can have superior wear characteristics when compared to their metal counterparts. Bell reported fewer radiolucent lines around the glenoid component and less humeral osteolysis in patients treated with a ceramic bearing surface and a stemless humeral component when compared to a standard stem and CoCr bearing surface. It is unclear whether the observed differences were solely due to the bearing surface or due to the stem geometry, and further investigation is warranted.[49,50] At the present time, there is little clinical information that supports or refutes the use of these materials.[51]

Humeral Head Shape

Most humeral head resections are effectively covered with a hemispherical component. This is achieved with head modularity options including offset heads and modular variable angle necks (**FIGURE 12.14**). In some instances, the resection plane is incompletely covered despite existing modularity options. This may be a result of normal variations in anatomy[52,53] or departures from

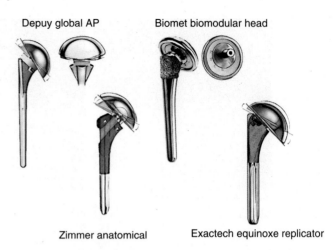

FIGURE 12.14 Modular neck devices. (Courtesy of DePuy Synthes. Used with permission from © Zimmer Biomet. Used with permission from © Exactech, Inc.)

the intended anatomic humeral resection plane. Several anatomic studies have identified variation in humeral head geometry, and the anatomic resection plane may be more accurately described as an ellipse rather than a circle. There are in vitro advantages of a nonspherical design with respect to improved motion and joint kinematics that more closely approximate the normal joint, but this design concept remains unproven in clinical studies.[54]

The effect of backside surface treatments is poorly understood. For example, the difference between flat back and hollow back devices on stem stability and the long-term effect on stress shielding is unknown. In addition, the impact of various surface characteristics of the head backside is also unknown.

GLENOID OPTIONS

Neer's first anatomic total shoulder replacement had an all polyethylene glenoid component with a radius of curvature (ROC) that matched the ROC of the humeral head.[5] The rationale for matching the ROC was to prevent joint translation to minimize strain on the rotator cuff and the joint capsule and to prevent edge loading on the component that would result in premature loosening. Second-generation implants included humeral component modularity and a ROC mismatch between the humeral head and glenoid components. The glenoid modifications were intended to more precisely reconstruct the anatomy, improve soft-tissue tensioning, and permit some joint translation. Interestingly, the translation permitted with ROC mismatch may have introduced a new mechanism of implant failure: Franklin and colleagues introduced the term "rocking horse" (**FIGURE 12.15**) to describe premature glenoid loosening that was attributed to excessive superior translation observed in rotator cuff deficient shoulders.[55]

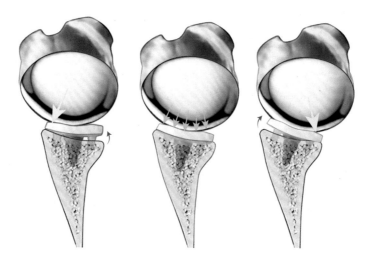

FIGURE 12.15 Rocking Horse Lift off occurs when an eccentric load is applied to the glenoid component. (Redrawn with permission from Matsen FA, Iannotti JP, Rockwood CA. Humeral fixation by press-fitting of a tapered metaphyseal stem. A prospective radiographic study. *J Bone Joint Surg Am.* 2003;85:304-308. doi:10.2106/00004623-200302000-00018.)

Glenoid Implant Materials

Polyethylene Types

Ultra-high-molecular-weight polyethylene (UHMWPE) has material properties including a low coefficient of friction, abrasion resistance, and impact strength that make it suitable as a bearing surface in shoulder arthroplasty.[56] Molded UHMWPE has better wear characteristics than machined UHMWPE, but both are susceptible to scratching, pitting, and delamination.[57,58] Although UHMWPE is the gold standard glenoid-bearing surface, there are concerns about the induction of osteolysis, bone resorption, and component failure by polyethylene wear particles. Alternatives such as highly cross-linked UHMWPE with and without vitamin E enrichment[50,59] have been investigated in vitro and have promising wear characteristics, but clinical outcome data to support the use of alternate bearing surfaces is lacking.

Glenoid Implant Options

Onlay

The most common type of implant used is an onlay keeled or pegged component that is secured to the glenoid with bone cement. Onlay components have excellent early clinical outcomes, but implant failures with loosening have been attributed to malpositioning, progressive rotator cuff disease resulting in component edge loading, infection, cement fracture, and osteolysis induced by particulate debris. Implant toggling and perimeter "lift-off" **(FIGURE 12.15)** may enable synovial fluid ingress/egress beneath the component, promote cement mantle fracture, and accelerate implant loosening.[60,61] Keeled convex-backed implant longevity has been investigated by Walch and colleagues who reported satisfactory clinical outcomes and low revision rates

with cemented keeled implants but noted frequent and progressive radiolucent lines that were associated with excessive removal of the subchondral plate during bone preparation.[62] They advised against striving to achieve neutral implant alignment with excessive reaming and recommended preservation of the subchondral plate. In a similar study examining outcomes of pegged cemented components, McLendon[63] not only noted satisfactory clinical outcomes and low revision rates but also noted concerning radiographic findings of implant loosening in 40% of glenoids.

Biomechanical studies suggest that pegged glenoid components have superior stability when compared to keel or inverted "Y" components.[64,65] Radiostereometric analysis (RSA) has also demonstrated that less implant migration occurs with existing pegged glenoids when compared to keeled glenoids.[66] In prospective comparative studies of keeled and pegged glenoids, radiolucent lines are more commonly seen with keeled glenoids, but clinical outcomes and revision rates are similar with both implants.[67,68] Several risk factors associated with progressive radiolucent line formation and loosening include younger age, dominant limb, bone erosion, and surgeon experience.[63,69] Glenoid component loosening remains a challenge in anatomic total shoulder replacement.

Augmented

Glenoid deformities commonly encountered in osteoarthritis can be managed with eccentric anterior reaming, corrective bone grafting, or augmented glenoid components **(FIGURES 12.16–12.18)**. Eccentric reaming is not technically demanding but results in joint line medialization, further loss of glenoid bone, and risks peg perforation through the glenoid vault.[70,71] Corrective bone

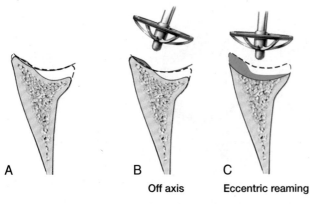

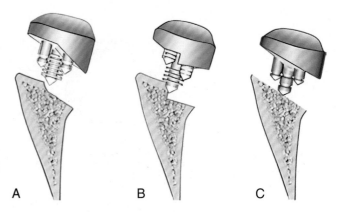

FIGURE 12.16 Reaming techniques to reconstruct posterior glenoid bone defects: (**A**) representative posterior bone defect, (**B**) concentric reaming used with augmented wedge-shaped glenoids, (**C**) eccentric (high side) reaming used with standard glenoid components or shoulder hemiarthroplasty. (Used with permission from © Exactech, Inc.)

FIGURE 12.18 Examples of augmented glenoids: (**A**) partial wedge, (**B**) step augment, (**C**) full wedge.

grafting using the humeral head autograft is more technically challenging and is associated with satisfactory clinical outcomes particularly if the graft incorporates.[72-75]

An alternative to eccentric reaming is implanting an augmented glenoid (see **FIGURE 12.18**). There are two differing conceptual strategies in augmented glenoid component design. The first concept involves resecting additional posterior bone to create prepared surfaces that are parallel to the backside of the stepped glenoid component. This is meant to minimize shear stresses at

the component-cement-bone interfaces but requires further posterior bone resection.[76] The second design concept uses hemi or full wedge augments that preserve host bone.[77-79] The glenoid is prepared with concentric "off-axis" reaming using a single or double convexity reamer. Augmented glenoids require less bone resection than eccentric anterior reaming, reduce joint line medialization, and may minimize the risk of peg perforation.[79-81] A potential disadvantage of wedged designs is that joint compressive forces can be converted to shear forces at the component-cement-bone interfaces.[82] Early clinical results with augmented glenoids are promising, and additional long-term outcome data is required to determine if the newer augmented implants are more durable than standard implants.[83,84]

Metal Back Glenoids

Interest in metal back uncemented glenoids (**FIGURE 12.19**) has been present for several decades primarily to reduce rates of aseptic loosening that have been attributed to the use of bone cement.[24] Several different design configurations have been studied including press-fit glenoids secured with screws and press-fit porous metal structures.

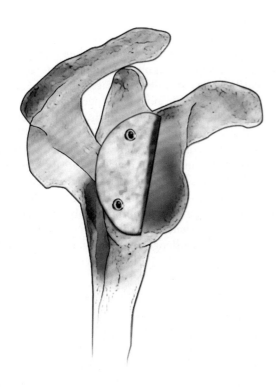

FIGURE 12.17 Bone grafting to reconstruct an asymmetric posterior glenoid erosion.

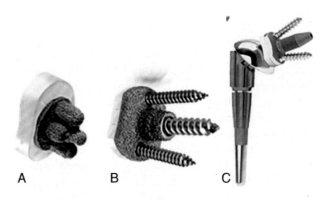

FIGURE 12.19 Examples of metal back glenoids: Zimmer Biomet (**A** and **B**) and Lima Corporate (**C**). (A and B, Used with permission from © Zimmer Biomet. C, Image of the product used under license of Limacorporate S.p.A.–Italy.)

Although early clinical results have been favorable, longer term follow-up has been less rewarding, and failure rates are high.[85-91] Failures are due to excessive polyethylene wear, component disassembly, and aseptic loosening. Many of the failures can be attributed to engineering and manufacturing challenges associated with the design of a modular metal back component. Current materials mandate a nominal polyethylene thickness to reduce the risk of delamination. When this is applied to a metal glenoid component, the joint line is lateralized, compressive forces on the polyethylene increase, and accelerated polyethylene wear occurs.[92,93] Improvements in implant longevity are unlikely to develop until there are advances in tribology and material science that result in implants with durable fixation and superior wear characteristics and that can provide reconstructions that more accurately approximate normal kinematics than existing devices.

Hybrid

Hybrid glenoids are a recent innovation intended to reduce glenoid radiolucent lines and component loosening and incorporate metallic fixation structures without a metal backing. The conceptual framework includes minimal cementation of peripheral pegs and bony ingrowth of a central titanium peg **(FIGURE 12.20)**. Hybrid glenoids are currently available from two manufacturers, but limited clinical data exists. Early clinical results show equivalent outcomes to UHMWPE-pegged glenoids with significantly less frequent radiolucent lines.[94] Potential long-term concerns include dissociation of metal pegs from molded polyethylene due to repeated loading.

Inset

Inset glenoids attempt to address glenoid component loosening by altering the net displacement of the implant during loading with the preservation of a circumferential rim of glenoid bone. The perimeter of an onlay glenoid behaves like an umbrella when loaded, and the margins of the implant deflect away from the supporting bone while the central portion of the implant subsides medially into the vault.[60,61] This behavior may be altered with an inset glenoid that has peripheral support from the host bone. Biomechanical testing of an inset glenoid has shown that this deflection is reduced and may theoretically reduce loosening rates.[95,96] An inset glenoid requires removal of the subchondral bone to fully seat the implant when native cartilage is absent **(FIGURE 12.21)**. Although this avoids joint line lateralization, the long-term effect of subchondral bone removal on implant stability and subsidence is not known. Results reported in small cases series are favorable, and additional study of larger comparative cohorts with greater follow-up is necessary.[97,98]

CONCLUSION

Shoulder arthroplasty implants have undergone tremendous change over the past 4 decades. Humeral stems have steadily diminished in size to preserve bone and, more accurately, recreate normal anatomy. Designs have changed to optimize cementless fixation and simplify implantation and revision. The development of convertible platform stems is an innovation that permits retention of stable and well-aligned humeral components during revision to reverse (TSA). All-polyethylene glenoid component loosening remains problematic, and alternate bearing surfaces and fixation methods are being investigated and developed to improve survivorship and simplify revision of failed glenoid components.

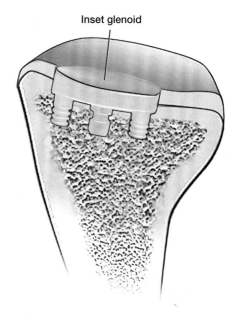

Inset glenoid

FIGURE 12.21 Inset glenoid example. A circumferential rim of cortical bone is preserved at the perimeter of the implant. Shoulder innovations.

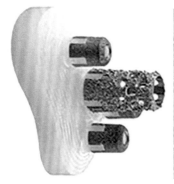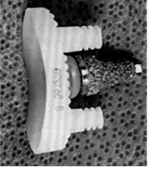

FIGURE 12.20 Hybrid glenoid examples. (Used with permission from © Exactech, Inc. Used with permission from © Zimmer Biomet.)

REFERENCES

1. Lugli T. Artificial shoulder joint by Péan (1893): the facts of an exceptional intervention and the prosthetic method. *Clin Orthop Relat Res.* 1978;(133):215-218. doi:10.1097/00003086-197806000-00025:215-8

2. Bankes MJK, Emery RJH. Pioneers of shoulder replacement: Themistocles Gluck and Jules Emile Péan. *J Shoulder Elbow Surg.* 1995;4:259-262.

3. Brand RA, Bigliani LU. Biographical sketch Charles S. Neer, II, MD (1917-2011). *Clin Orthop Relat Res.* 2011;469:2407-2408.

4. Neer CS. Articular replacement for the humeral head. *J Bone Joint Surg Am.* 1955;37:215-228.

5. Neer CS. Replacement arthroplasty for glenohumeral osteoarthritis. *J Bone Joint Surg Am.* 1974;56:1-13.

6. Hahn H, Palich W. Preliminary evaluation of porous metal surfaced titanium for orthopedic implants. *J Biomed Mater Res.* 1970;4:571-577. doi:10.1002/jbm.820040407

7. Australian Orthopaedic Association. *Australian Orthopaedic Association National Joint Replacement Registry (AOANJRR). Hip, knee & shoulder arthroplasty Annual report 2019, Adelaide; 2017: 1-17.* 2019:366.

8. Litchfield RB, McKee MD, Balyk R, et al. Cemented versus uncemented fixation of humeral components in total shoulder arthroplasty for osteoarthritis of the shoulder: a prospective, randomized, double-blind clinical trial—a JOINTs Canada Project. *J Shoulder Elbow Surg.* 2011;20:529-536.

9. Torchia ME, Cofield RH, Settergren CR. Total shoulder arthroplasty with the Neer prosthesis: long-term results. *J Shoulder Elbow Surg.* 1997;6:495-505.

10. Sanchez-Sotelo J, O'Driscoll SW, Torchia ME, et al. Radiographic assessment of cemented humeral components in shoulder arthroplasty. *J Shoulder Elbow Surg.* 2001;10:526-531.

11. Sherfey MC, Edwards TB. Cement extrusion causing radial nerve palsy after shoulder arthroplasty: a case report. *J Shoulder Elbow Surg.* 2009;18:e21-e24.

12. Goldberg SH, Cohen MS, Young M, et al. Thermal tissue damage caused by ultrasonic cement removal from the humerus. *J Bone Joint Surg.* 2005;87:583-591.

13. Sperling JW, Cofield RH. Humeral windows in revision shoulder arthroplasty. *J Shoulder Elbow Surg.* 2005;14:258-263.

14. Johnston PS, Creighton RA, Romeo AA. Humeral component revision arthroplasty: outcomes of a split osteotomy technique. *J Shoulder Elbow Surg.* 2012;21:502-506.

15. Petersen SA, Hawkins RJ. Revision of failed total shoulder arthroplasty. *Orthop Clin North Am.* 1998;29:519-533.

16. Levy JC, Berglund D, Vakharia R, et al. Midterm results of anatomic total shoulder arthroplasty with a third-generation implant. *J Shoulder Elbow Surg.* 2019;28:698-705.

17. Sperling JW, Cofield RH, O'Driscoll SW, et al. Radiographic assessment of ingrowth total shoulder arthroplasty. *J Shoulder Elbow Surg.* 2000;9:507-513.

18. Lucas RM, Hsu JE, Gee AO, et al. Impaction autografting: bone-preserving, secure fixation of a standard humeral component. *J Shoulder Elbow Surg.* 2016;25:1787-1794.

19. Franta AK, Lenters TR, Mounce D, et al. The complex characteristics of 282 unsatisfactory shoulder arthroplasties. *J Shoulder Elbow Surg.* 2007;16:555-562.

20. Crosby LA, Wright TW, Yu S, et al. Conversion to reverse total shoulder arthroplasty with and without humeral stem retention: the role of a convertible-platform stem. *J Bone Joint Surg Am.* 2017;99:736-742. doi:10.2106/JBJS.16.00683

21. Werner BS, Boehm D, Gohlke F. Revision to reverse shoulder arthroplasty with retention of the humeral component. *Acta Orthop.* 2013;84:473-478.

22. Denard PJ, Raiss P, Gobezie R, et al. Stress shielding of the humerus in press-fit anatomic shoulder arthroplasty: review and recommendations for evaluation. *J Shoulder Elbow Surg.* 2018;27:1139-1147.

23. Nagels J, Stokdijk M, Rozing PM. Stress shielding and bone resorption in shoulder arthroplasty. *J Shoulder Elbow Surg.* 2003;12:35-39.

24. McElwain JP, English E. The early results of porous-coated total shoulder arthroplasty. *Clin Orthop Relat Res.* 1987;218:217-224.

25. Engh CA, Bobyn JD, Glassman AH. Porous-coated hip replacement. The factors governing bone ingrowth, stress shielding, and clinical results. *J Bone Joint Surg.* 1987;69:45-55.

26. Engh CA, Young AM, Engh CA, et al. Clinical consequences of stress shielding after porous-coated total hip arthroplasty. *Clin Orthop Relat Res.* Lippincott Williams and Wilkins. 2003;(417):157-163.

27. Verborgt O, El-Abiad R, Gazielly DF. Long-term results of uncemented humeral components in shoulder arthroplasty. *J Shoulder Elbow Surg.* 2007;16:S13-S18. doi:10.1016/j.jse.2006.02.003

28. Raiss P, Edwards TB, Deutsch A, et al. Radiographic changes around humeral components in shoulder arthroplasty. *J Bone Joint Surg.* 2014;96:e54.

29. Matsen FA, Iannotti JP, Rockwood CA. Humeral fixation by press-fitting of a tapered metaphyseal stem. A prospective radiographic study. *J Bone Joint Surg.* 2003;85:304-308. doi:10.2106/00004623-200302000-00018

30. Razfar N, Reeves JM, Langohr DG, et al. Comparison of proximal humeral bone stresses between stemless, short stem, and standard stem length: a finite element analysis. *J Shoulder Elbow Surg.* 2016;25:1076-1083.

31. Schnetzke M, Coda S, Raiss P, et al. Radiologic bone adaptations on a cementless short-stem shoulder prosthesis. *J Shoulder Elbow Surg.* 2016;25:650-657.

32. Jost PW, Dines JS, Griffith MH, et al. Total shoulder arthroplasty utilizing mini-stem humeral components: technique and short-term results. *HSS J.* 2011;7:213-217. doi:10.1007/s11420-011-9221-4

33. Casagrande DJ, Parks DL, Torngren T, et al. Radiographic evaluation of short-stem press-fit total shoulder arthroplasty: short-term follow-up. *J Shoulder Elbow Surg.* 2016;25:1163-1169.

34. Peduzzi L, Goetzmann T, Wein F, et al. Proximal humeral bony adaptations with a short uncemented stem for shoulder arthroplasty: a quantitative analysis. *JSES Open Access.* 2019;3:278-286.

35. Romeo AA, Thorsness RJ, Sumner SA, et al. Short-term clinical outcome of an anatomic short-stem humeral component in total shoulder arthroplasty. *J Shoulder Elbow Surg.* 2018;27:70-74.

36. Morwood MP, Johnston PS, Garrigues GE. Proximal ingrowth coating decreases risk of loosening following uncemented shoulder arthroplasty using mini-stem humeral components and lesser tuberosity osteotomy. *J Shoulder Elbow Surg.* 2017;26:1246-1252.

37. Denard PJ, Noyes MP, Walker JB, et al. Proximal stress shielding is decreased with a short stem compared with a traditional-length stem in total shoulder arthroplasty. *J Shoulder Elbow Surg.* 2018;27:53-58. doi:10.1016/j.jse.2017.06.042. http://elinks.library.upenn.edu/sfx_local?sid=EMBASE&issn=15326500&id=doi:10.1016%2Fj.jse.2017.06.042&atitle=Proximal+stress+shielding+is+decreased+with+a+short+stem+compared+with+a+traditional-length+stem+in+total+shoulder+arthroplasty&stitle=J.+Shoulder+Elbow+Surg.&title=Journal+of+Shoulder+and+Elbow+Surgery&volume=27&issue=1&spage=53&epage=58&aulast=Denard&aufirst=Patrick+J.&auinit=P.J.&aufull=Denard+P.J.&coden=JSESB&isbn=&pages=53-58&date=2018&auinit1=P&auinit

38. Langohr GDG, Reeves J, Roche CP, et al. The effect of short-stem humeral component sizing on humeral bone stress. *J Shoulder Elbow Surg.* 2020;29:761-767.

39. Raiss P, Schnetzke M, Wittmann T, et al. Postoperative radiographic findings of an uncemented convertible short stem for anatomic and reverse shoulder arthroplasty. *J Shoulder Elbow Surg.* 2019;28:715-723.

40. Denard PJ, Noyes MP, Walker JB, et al. Radiographic changes differ between two different short press-fit humeral stem designs in total shoulder arthroplasty. *J Shoulder Elbow Surg.* 2018;27:217-223.

41. Churchill RS, Chuinard C, Wiater JM, et al. Clinical and radiographic outcomes of the simpliciti canal-sparing shoulder arthroplasty system: a prospective two-year multicenter study. *J Bone Joint Surg Am.* 2016;98:552-560. doi:10.2106/JBJS.15.00181

42. Huguet D, DeClercq G, Rio B, et al. Results of a new stemless shoulder prosthesis: radiologic proof of maintained fixation and stability after a minimum of three years' follow-up. *J Shoulder Elbow Surg.* 2010;19:847-852.

43. Hawi N, Magosch P, Tauber M, et al. Nine-year outcome after anatomic stemless shoulder prosthesis: clinical and radiologic results. *J Shoulder Elbow Surg*. 2017;26:1609-1615. doi:10.1016/j.jse.2017.02.017. http://vu.on.worldcat.org/atoztitles/link?sid=EMBASE&issn=15326500&id=doi:10.1016%2Fj.jse.2017.02.017&atitle=Nine-year+outcome+after+anatomic+stemless+shoulder+prosthesis%3A+clinical+and+radiologic+results&stitle=J.+Shoulder+Elbow+Surg.&title=Journal+of+Shoulder+and+Elbow+Surgery&volume=26&issue=9&spage=1609&epage=1615&aulast=Hawi&aufirst=Nael&auinit=N.&aufull=Hawi+N.&coden=JSESB&isbn=&pages=1609-1615&date=2017&auinit1=N&auinitm=

44. Habermeyer P, Lichtenberg S, Tauber M, et al. Midterm results of stemless shoulder arthroplasty: a prospective study. *J Shoulder Elbow Surg*. 2015;24:1463-1472. doi:10.1016/j.jse.2015.02.023

45. Hudek R, Werner B, Abdelkawi AF, et al. Radiolucency in stemless shoulder arthroplasty is associated with an imaging phenomenon. *J Orthop Res*. 2017;35:2040-2050. doi:10.1002/jor.23478

46. Reeves JM, Langohr GDG, Athwal GS, et al. The effect of stemless humeral component fixation feature design on bone stress and strain response: a finite element analysis. *J Shoulder Elbow Surg*. 2018;27:2232-2241. doi:10.1016/j.jse.2018.06.002

47. Philippot R, Boyer B, Farizon F. *Study of a Titanium Dual-Mobility Socket With a Mean Follow-up of 18 Years: Total Hip Arthroplast. Wear Behaviour of Different Articulations*. Springer-Verlag Berlin Heidelberg; 2013:161-168.

48. Hernandez JR, Keating EM, Faris PM, et al. Polyethylene wear in uncemented acetabular components. *J Bone Joint Surg*. 1994;76:263-266.

49. Bell S, Coghlan J, Edwards G. Medium term outcomes of stemless, ceramic head, anatomic shoulder replacement in patients with type B and C glenoids. Results better than expected. *JSES Open Access*. 2019;3:258.

50. Peers S, Moravek JE Jr, Budge MD, et al. Wear rates of highly cross-linked polyethylene humeral liners subjected to alternating cycles of glenohumeral flexion and abduction. *J Shoulder Elbow Surg*. 2015;24:143-149.

51. Mueller U, Braun S, Schroeder S, et al. Influence of humeral head material on wear performance in anatomic shoulder joint arthroplasty. *J Shoulder Elbow Surg*. 2017;26:1756-1764.

52. Hertel R, Knothe U, Ballmer FT. Geometry of the proximal humerus and implications for prosthetic design. *J Shoulder Elbow Surg*. 2002;11:331-338.

53. Iannotti JP, Gabriel JP, Schneck SL, et al. The normal glenohumeral relationships. An anatomical study of one hundred and forty shoulders. *J Bone Joint Surg Am*. 1992;74:491-500.

54. Jun BJ, Iannotti JP, McGarry MH, et al. The effects of prosthetic humeral head shape onglenohumeral joint kinematics: a comparison of non-spherical and spherical prosthetic heads to the native humeral head. *J Shoulder Elbow Surg*. 2013;22:1423-1432.

55. Franklin JL, Barrett WP, Jackins SE, et al. Glenoid loosening in total shoulder arthroplasty: association with rotator cuff deficiency. *J Arthroplasty*. 1988;3:39-46.

56. McGeough JA. *The Engineering of Human Joint Replacements*. John Wiley & Sons, Incorporated; 2013.

57. Benson EC, Faber KJ, Athwal GS. *Glenoid fixation in total shoulder arthroplasty: what type of glenoid component should we use?* In: *Evidence-Based Orthopedics*. Wiley; 2011.

58. Benson LC, Desjardins JD, Laberge M. Effects of in vitro wear of machined and molded UHMWPE tibial inserts on TKR kinematics. *J Biomed Mater Res*. 2001;58:496-504.

59. Alexander JJ, Bell SN, Coghlan J, et al. The effect of vitamin E–enhanced cross-linked polyethylene on wear in shoulder arthroplasty—a wear simulator study. *J Shoulder Elbow Surg*. 2019;28:1771-1778.

60. Glennie RAA, Giles JWJW, Johnson JAJA, et al. An in vitro study comparing limited to full cementation of polyethylene glenoid components. *J Orthop Surg Res*. 2015;10:142.

61. Anglin C, Wyss UP, Pichora DR. Mechanical testing of shoulder prostheses and recommendations for glenoid design. *J Shoulder Elbow Surg*. 2000;9:323-331.

62. Walch G, Young AA, Melis B, et al. Results of a convex-back cemented keeled glenoid component in primary osteoarthritis: multicenter study with a follow-up greater than 5 years. *J Shoulder Elbow Surg*. 2010;20:385-394.

63. McLendon PB, Schoch BS, Sperling JW, et al. Survival of the pegged glenoid component in shoulder arthroplasty: part II. *J Shoulder Elbow Surg*. 2017;26:1469-1476.

64. Knowles NK, Langohr GDG, Athwal GS, et al. Polyethylene glenoid component fixation geometry influences stability in total shoulder arthroplasty. *Comput Methods Biomech Biomed Engin*. 2018;0:1-9.

65. Geraldes DM, Hansen U, Amis AA. Parametric analysis of glenoid implant design and fixation type. *J Orthop Res*. 2017;35:775-784.

66. Nuttall D, Haines JF, Trail IA. The early migration of a partially cemented fluted pegged glenoid component using radiostereometric analysis. *J Shoulder Elbow Surg*. 2012;21:1191-1196.

67. Collin P, Tay AKL, Melis B, et al. A ten-year radiologic comparison of two-all polyethylene glenoid component designs: a prospective trial. *J Shoulder Elbow Surg*. 2011;20:1217-1223.

68. Edwards TB, Labriola JE, Stanley RJ, et al. Radiographic comparison of pegged and keeled glenoid components using modern cementing techniques: a prospective randomized study. *J Shoulder Elbow Surg*. 2010;19:251-257.

69. Lazarus MD, Jensen KL, Southworth C, et al. The radiographic evaluation of keeled and pegged glenoid component insertion. *J Bone Joint Surg*. 2002;84:1174-1182.

70. Hsu JE, Ricchetti ET, Huffman GR, et al. Addressing glenoid bone deficiency and asymmetric posterior erosion in shoulder arthroplasty. *J Shoulder Elbow Surg*. 2013;22:1298-1308.

71. Chen X, Reddy AS, Kontaxis A, et al. Version correction via eccentric reaming compromises remaining bone quality in B2 glenoids: a computational study. *Clin Orthop Relat Res*. 2017;475:3090-3099.

72. Klika BJ, Wooten CW, Sperling JW, et al. Structural bone grafting for glenoid deficiency in primary total shoulder arthroplasty. *J Shoulder Elbow Surg*. 2014;23:1066-1072.

73. Nicholson GP, Cvetanovich GL, Rao AJ, et al. Posterior glenoid bone grafting in total shoulder arthroplasty for osteoarthritis with severe posterior glenoid wear. *J Shoulder Elbow Surg*. 2017;26:1844-1853.

74. Hill JM, Norris TR. Long-term results of total shoulder arthroplasty following bone-grafting of the glenoid. *J Bone Joint Surg*. 2001;83:877-883.

75. Steinmann SP, Cofield RH. Bone grafting for glenoid deficiency in total shoulder replacement. *J Shoulder Elbow Surg*. 2000;9:361-367.

76. Iannotti JP, Lappin KE, Klotz CL, et al. Liftoff resistance of augmented glenoid components during cyclic fatigue loading in the posterior-superior direction. *J Shoulder Elbow Surg*. 2013;22:1530-1536.

77. Allred JJ, Flores-Hernandez C, Hoenecke HR, et al. Posterior augmented glenoid implants require less bone removal and generate lower stresses: a finite element analysis. *J Shoulder Elbow Surg*. 2016;25:823-830.

78. Roche CP, Diep P, Grey SG, et al. Biomechanical impact of posterior glenoid wear on anatomic total shoulder arthroplasty. *Bull Hosp Jt Dis (2013)*. 2013;71:S5.

79. Kersten AD, Flores-Hernandez C, Hoenecke HR, et al. Posterior augmented glenoid designs preserve more bone in biconcave glenoids. *J Shoulder Elbow Surg*. 2015;24:1135-1141.

80. Olszewski A, Ramme AJ, Maerz T, et al. Vault perforation after eccentric glenoid reaming for deformity correction in anatomic total shoulder arthroplasty. *J Shoulder Elbow Surg*. 2020;29:1450-1459. doi:10.1016/j.jse.2019.11.011

81. Knowles NK, Ferreira LM, Athwal GS. Augmented glenoid component designs for type B2 erosions: a computational comparison by volume of bone removal and quality of remaining bone. *J Shoulder Elbow Surg*. 2015;24:1218-1226.

82. Wang T, Abrams GD, Behn AW, et al. Posterior glenoid wear in total shoulder arthroplasty: eccentric anterior reaming is superior to posterior augment. *Clin Orthop Relat Res*. 2015;473:3928-3936.

83. Wright TW, Grey SG, Roche CP, et al. Preliminary results of a posterior augmented glenoid compared to an all polyethylene standard glenoid in anatomic total shoulder arthroplasty. *Bull Hosp Jt Dis (2013)*. 2015;73:S79.

84. Grey SG, Wright TW, Flurin P-H, et al. Clinical and radiographic outcomes with a posteriorly augmented glenoid for Walch B glenoids in anatomic total shoulder arthroplasty. *J Shoulder Elbow Surg.* 2020;29:e185-e195.

85. Tammachote N, Sperling JW, Vathana T, et al. Long-term results of cemented metal-backed glenoid components for osteoarthritis of the shoulder. *J Bone Joint Surg.* 2009;91:160-166.

86. Watson ST, Gudger GK, Long CD, et al. Outcomes of Trabecular Metal–backed glenoid components in anatomic total shoulder arthroplasty. *J Shoulder Elbow Surg.* 2018;27:493-498.

87. Boileau P, Avidor C, Krishnan SG, et al. Cemented polyethylene versus uncemented metal-backed glenoid components in total shoulder arthroplasty: a prospective, double-blind, randomized study. *J Shoulder Elbow Surg.* 2002;11:351-359.

88. Budge MD, Nolan EM, Heisey MH, et al. Results of total shoulder arthroplasty with a monoblock porous tantalum glenoid component: a prospective minimum 2-year follow-up study. *J Shoulder Elbow Surg.* 2013;22:535-541.

89. Castagna A, Randelli M, Garofalo R, et al. Mid-term results of a metal-backed glenoid component in total shoulder replacement. *J Bone Joint Surg.* 2010;92:1410-1415.

90. Fox TJ, Cil A, Sperling JW, et al. Survival of the glenoid component in shoulder arthroplasty. *J Shoulder Elbow Surg.* 2009;18:859-863.

91. Wallace AL, Phillips RL, MacDougal GA, et al. Resurfacing of the glenoid in total shoulder arthroplasty: a comparison, at a mean of five years, of prostheses inserted with and without cement. *J Bone Joint Surg Am.* 1999;81:510-518.

92. Kocsis G, Payne CJ, Wallace A, et al. Wear analysis of explanted conventional metal back polyethylene glenoid liners. *Med Eng Phys.* 2018;59:1-7.

93. Budge MD, Kurdziel MD, Baker KC, et al. A biomechanical analysis of initial fixation options for porous-tantalum-backed glenoid components. *J Shoulder Elbow Surg.* 2013;22:709-715.

94. Grey SG, Wright TW, Flurin PH, et al. Preliminary results of a novel hybrid cage glenoid compared to an all-polyethylene glenoid in total shoulder arthroplasty. *Bull Hosp Joint Dis (2013).* 2015;73:S86-S91.

95. Gunther SB, Lynch TL, O'Farrell D, et al. Finite element analysis and physiologic testing of a novel, inset glenoid fixation technique. *J Shoulder Elbow Surg.* 2012;21:795-803.

96. Gagliano JR, Helms SM, Colbath GP, et al. A comparison of onlay versus inlay glenoid component loosening in total shoulder arthroplasty. *J Shoulder Elbow Surg.* 2017;26:1113-1120.

97. Gunther SB, Tran SK. Long-term follow-up of total shoulder replacement surgery with inset glenoid implants for arthritis with deficient bone. *J Shoulder Elbow Surg.* 2019;28:1728-1736.

98. Gunther SB, Lynch TL. Total shoulder replacement surgery with custom glenoid implants for severe bone deficiency. *J Shoulder Elbow Surg.* 2012;21:675-684.

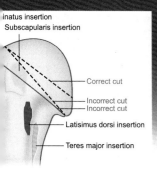

inatus insertion
Subscapularis insertion
Correct cut
Incorrect cut
Incorrect cut
Latisimus dorsi insertion
Teres major insertion

13 Operative Technique Anatomic Total Shoulder Arthroplasty

Sean G. Grey, MD

Anatomic total shoulder arthroplasty is a reliable and reproducible procedure to treat multiple degenerative conditions about the shoulder. Successful total shoulder arthroplasty requires several critical technical steps, including adequate humeral and glenoid exposure, appropriate management of the subscapularis tendon, meticulous glenoid and humeral preparation, anatomic implant selection, and precise soft tissue balancing (VIDEO 13.1).

PATIENT POSITIONING

The patient is positioned in a modified or lazy beach chair position (FIGURE 13.1). Care is taken not to elevate the head higher than 30° to 40°. Less flexion helps facilitate the visualization of the assistant on the superior side of the shoulder. The patient should be placed far enough on the lateral side of the table to allow free motion of the arm, including free extension of the arm to 90° for visualization and preparation of the humeral canal. All bony prominences should be padded appropriately, and the head should be securely stabilized. After positioning, the range of motion of the shoulder is assessed to guarantee adequate ability to manipulate the arm as needed during the surgery. During the surgical procedure, the arm may be placed in one of many commercially available arm holders. My preference is to place the arm free on a padded Mayo stand. The Mayo stand allows the surgeon to shift the arm position freely during the procedure, as well as removing and replacing the stand throughout the surgery.

Retractor selection is critical in obtaining adequate exposure. Multiple combinations of retractors can be used effectively. Each surgeon may identify a combination of retractors that works well for their specific needs. As a general rule, smaller and fewer retractors may be helpful when working in the shoulder where space is limited. Particularly with glenoid exposure, it is helpful to have not only an initial set of retractors but also alternative retractors, which may be useful in patients with unique anatomic challenges. Each surgeon is encouraged to experiment with multiple retractor combinations in various anatomic situations. Our standard retractors include the following (FIGURE 13.2): a Darrach for sweeping the subacromial and subdeltoid spaces, as well

as levering the humeral head; a Browne deltoid retractor; a posterior humeral head retractor; various Richardson retractors; multiple 2-point retractors; a bent spiked Hohmann; various posterior glenoid retractors; and a self-retaining deltoid retractor with multiple blades.

APPROACH

For primary anatomic arthroplasty, I use a standard deltopectoral approach. The deltopectoral approach is familiar to most surgeons and allows for an extensile approach as needed in revision cases. This approach provides excellent exposure of both the humeral and glenoid side of the joint while preserving the deltoid and protecting the surrounding neurovascular structures. Landmarks for the skin incision include the coracoid, distal one-third of the clavicle, and the distal deltoid insertion. A straight skin incision is made directly over the coracoid following the predictable path of the deltopectoral interval (FIGURE 13.3). Small subcutaneous flaps are raised on either side of the incision as well as proximally and distally. The cephalic vein is identified and used as a landmark for the deltopectoral interval. If the cephalic vein is absent, then the interval can be identified by palpating just proximal to the coracoid and identifying a small triangle devoid of muscle tissue between the pectoralis major and the deltoid.[1] This step can be facilitated by externally rotating the arm and putting the pectoralis major fibers on stretch. When present, the cephalic vein may be taken either medially or laterally. My preference is to mobilize the vein laterally with the deltoid. Lateral mobilization of the vein prevents the need for coagulation of multiple branches that enter laterally from the deltoid. However, this places the vein under more tension throughout the procedure. To prevent injury in cases where the vein has been taken laterally, it is helpful to mobilize the vein proximally toward the clavicle and distally well past the pectoralis major muscle insertion. After the development of the deltopectoral interval, the deltoid is retracted laterally with a Richardson retractor, and the deep landmarks are identified, including the coracoid, conjoined tendon, coracoacromial ligament, rotator interval, biceps tendon, and pectoralis major tendon insertion (FIGURE 13.4).

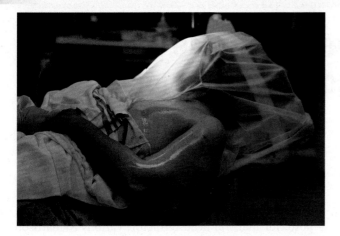

FIGURE 13.1 Patient placed in the beach chair position for anatomic shoulder arthroplasty. The head should not be elevated more than 30° to 40°.

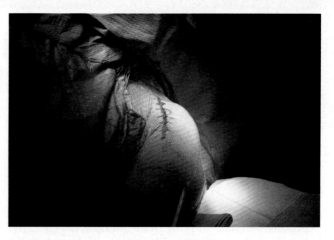

FIGURE 13.3 Skin marking for standard deltopectoral incision.

A Darrach retractor or the surgeon's index finger is used to mobilize and connect the subacromial and subdeltoid spaces. A Browne deltoid retractor is placed beneath the deltoid in the subacromial and subdeltoid spaces. At this point, the surgeon sweeps the subcoracoid space between the conjoined tendon and the subscapularis for placement of the blades of a self-retaining deltoid retractor. During this step, it is helpful to identify the axillary nerve with the tip of the surgeon's index finger. "Tug test" **(FIGURE 13.5)** can be helpful here in identifying the location of the axillary nerve, which is at some risk during the remainder of the procedure. Familiarity with the location of the nerve can help minimize the risk of injury throughout the case.[2]

The humeral insertion of the pectoralis major tendon is located. The release of the upper portion of the pectoralis tendon facilitates exposure of the lower one-third of the subscapularis tendon **(FIGURE 13.6)**. In unusually

large or excessively stiff patients, further release of the pectoralis tendon improves exposure. In rare cases of difficult exposure, if necessary, the entire tendon may be released, greatly enhancing the posterior displacement of the humerus and thereby improving glenoid exposure. It is helpful to leave as much of the identifiable tendon on the insertion of the humeral side for later repair. The dorsal side of the pectoralis major tendon has additional tendon fibers not visible from the ventral approach. A tag suture placed on the superior border of the muscular side of the tendon aids with retraction and helps align repair during the closure. After the removal of any excessive clavipectoral fascia, the border of the subscapularis should be visible. Superiorly, the rotator interval is identified by finding the soft spot just below the confluence of the conjoined tendon and the coracoacromial ligament. External rotation of the arm can assist in locating the interval. Opening the interval allows for visualization of the biceps tendon. Tracing the biceps tendon distal to the upper border of the pectoralis

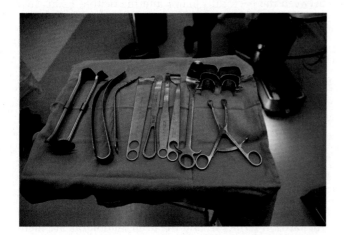

FIGURE 13.2 Standard retractors for shoulder arthroplasty include (left to right): Richardson retractors, multiple 2-point retractors, Darrach elevators, posterior humeral head retractor, Browne deltoid retractor, and self-retaining deltoid retractor with multiple blades.

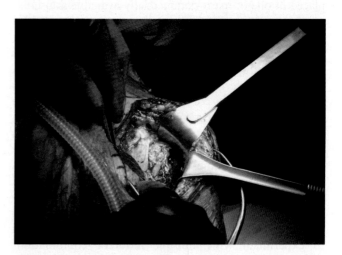

FIGURE 13.4 After development of the deltopectoral interval, the deeper structures are identified including the coracoid process, conjoined tendon, coracoacromial ligament, rotator interval, biceps tendon, and pectoralis major tendon insertion.

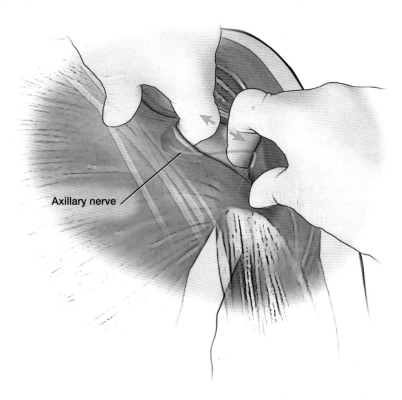

Axillary nerve

FIGURE 13.5 The "tug test" can be helpful in identifying the location of the axillary nerve and preventing injury.

major tendon locates the lateral border of the subscapularis. The anterior humeral circumflex vessels denote the inferior border. Once the anterior humeral circumflex vessels are identified, they should be ligated or cauterized at the level of the humeral neck.

Attention is then turned toward the management of the long head of the biceps tendon. The tendon should be released, and the intra-articular portion is removed in all cases, as it may serve as a source of pain and stiffness postoperatively. After release, a biceps tenodesis is

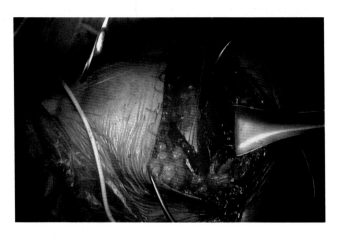

FIGURE 13.6 The upper one-third of the pectoralis major tendon insertion should be released to expose the lower portion of the subscapularis tendon.

carried out in the majority of arthroplasty cases. Several acceptable alternatives exist for tenodesis management. I prefer to secure the biceps into the pectoralis major tendon near the conclusion of the case during wound closure. Tenodesis to the pectoralis major tendon directly after release is also acceptable but may limit the ease of releasing further pectoralis major tendon later in the case if that becomes necessary. Despite the method chosen, the anatomic tension of the biceps tendon is restored during tenodesis to prevent postoperative pain or deformity. If the surgeon elects to perform tenodesis of the long head of the biceps tendon at the conclusion of the case, this is accomplished with the repair of the pectoralis major tendon using two high-tensile sutures and incorporating the long head of the biceps tendon within the repair of the pectoralis major tendon. The borders of the subscapularis tendon are now clearly defined, including the open rotator interval superiorly, the released biceps tendon laterally, and the anterior humeral circumflex vessels inferiorly. With the subscapularis borders clearly defined, attention is turned toward the release of the subscapularis tendon.

SUBSCAPULARIS MANAGEMENT

Subscapularis management is critical for a successful outcome following an anatomic total shoulder replacement. Failure of subscapularis repair represents one of the most common causes of early failure after anatomic arthroplasty.[3] Subscapularis management should not solely be considered the method of tendon release, but also the management of the tendon during the surgical procedure as well as the meticulous nature of repair during the closure. For example, overaggressive mobilization during glenoid-sided releases can result in denervation by disruption of the upper and lower subscapular nerves as they enter the dorsal surface of the subscapularis medially. Additionally, the method of repair may be at least as important as the type of release performed.

Three primary options are available for the release of the tendon. In the "peel" techniques, the subscapularis is removed subperiosteally and repaired back to the lesser tuberosity with drill holes through bone. In the "tenotomy" technique, the tendon is split vertically, approximately 1 cm medial to the lesser tuberosity attachment, leaving adequate tendon laterally for tendon-to-tendon repair. In the "osteotomy" techniques, the tendon is removed by performing an osteotomy with a small portion of the lesser tuberosity still attached to the subscapularis tendon, which is then reattached to the humerus using one of a variety of techniques. Controversy exists as to which method is superior, and all three methods have shown good outcomes in the literature.[3,4] None of the methods have shown conclusive superiority, and selection of the approach is based primarily on surgeon preference. The following text focuses on my preferred method of subperiosteal peeling of the tendon from the lesser tuberosity; however, we have included specific techniques of the tenotomy and the osteotomy in the video library.

The subperiosteal subscapularis peel provides several advantages. In patients with severe internal rotation contracture, the tendon is released laterally and repaired along the humeral neck, in a slightly more medial position. Each 1 cm of medialization provides approximately 15° of increased external rotation.[1] The peel, unlike the osteotomy, does not disrupt the existing proximal humeral osseous anatomy. Furthermore, repair of the peel is performed with multiple transosseous sutures, which provide a reliable postoperative construct. Performing the subscapularis release with the arm in an adducted and slightly externally rotated position provides protection of the axillary nerve. Increasing the abduction of the arm moves the axillary nerve progressively more laterally, increasing its risk for injury. The rotator interval is released medially to the anterosuperior glenoid. From the window of the rotator interval, the superior subscapularis attachment to the lesser tuberosity is identified and released with a #10 blade (**FIGURE 13.7**). Care is taken not to leave any tendon attachment laterally, which allows for maximum tendon excursion when later repaired. The upper two-thirds, or tendinous portion, of the tendon is released with a knife. The lower one-third, or muscular portion, is released with a needle tip electrocautery, directing the needle tip

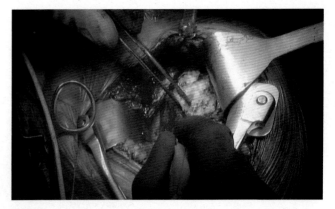

FIGURE 13.7 The subscapularis tendon is released subperiosteally from the lesser tuberosity.

between the previously ligated anterior humeral circumflex vessels. The dissection is continued distally in a subperiosteal fashion until encountering the upper borders of the latissimus dorsi tendon (**FIGURE 13.8**). The latissimus dorsi tendon serves as an excellent landmark for the inferior extent of the dissection, particularly in patients with extensive glenohumeral joint contracture. Multiple #2 Ethibond stay sutures are placed in the released subscapularis tendon to facilitate retraction throughout the case and assist in later repair of the tendon. Attention is now turned toward the remaining humeral releases and exposure.

HUMERAL RELEASE

The humeral release is continued from the inferior extent of the subscapularis release. The arm should remain in a fully adducted position. Progressive external rotation of the arm combined with gentle flexion allows for the release of the humeral attachments of the inferior glenohumeral ligaments.[5] Subperiosteal dissection using a needle tip electrocautery combined with adduction, external rotation, and gentle flexion significantly facilitates the protection of the axillary nerve. The inferior

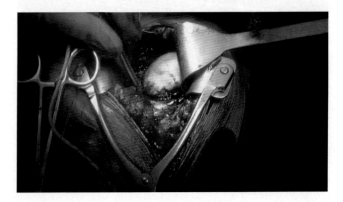

FIGURE 13.8 The inferior glenohumeral joint capsule is released in an anterior to posterior direction up to the border of the latissimus dorsi tendon attachment.

glenohumeral ligaments are released posteriorly beyond the 6 o'clock position to about the 7 o'clock position.

The humeral head is now dislocated using a Darrach retractor to lever the head while externally rotating and extending the arm. If present, a self-retaining deltoid retractor should be removed to prevent traction injury to the musculocutaneous nerve. A posterior humeral head retractor is placed. Removal of all humeral head osteophytes facilitates exposure of the true anatomic humeral neck. Completely dislocate the humeral head by levering forward with the posterior humeral head retractor as the arm is placed into full extension with adduction and external rotation. If a Mayo stand is being used to support the arm, lowering the Mayo stand allows the arm to come into full extension and adduction. In this position, the margins of the articular surface should be entirely visualized **(FIGURE 13.9)**. Visualization of the articular margin is critical for performing humeral osteotomy and avoiding complications.[6] Landmarks to recognize should include the following: the superolateral margin of the articular surface adjacent to the greater tuberosity and rotator cuff insertion, the posterior rotator cuff attachment, the bare area of the humerus, and the inferomedial margin where the articular surface exits at the medial calcar. The above landmarks are essential for the humeral osteotomy, and if not fully visualized, the surgeon should retrace the humeral releases until achieving adequate visualization.

HUMERAL OSTEOTOMY AND PREPARATION

The specifics of the humeral osteotomy and preparation are dependent on the surgeon's selected system. However, in all cases of anatomic arthroplasty, general principles of humeral osteotomy are followed. Included in these principles are the height, retroversion, and inclination angle of the osteotomy.[7] Despite being often overlooked, these factors are critical in the short-term and long-term success of the prosthesis.[6] For example, humeral osteotomies, which do not remove the entire articular surface, result in overstuffing of the joint, subsequently reduced motion, potential rotator cuff failure, and increased risk of early glenoid loosening. Alternatively, overaggressive humeral osteotomy may result in the disruption of the superior or posterior rotator cuff. Osteotomy inclination should follow the path of the native articular surface and not be misguided by residual osteophytes **(FIGURE 13.10)**. A vertical osteotomy resulting in a varus cut disrupts the medial calcar and stability of the humeral component. Likewise, an excessively valgus cut may result in disruption of the rotator cuff insertion or overstuffing. Principles of the given system determine the exact humeral retroversion. Typically, these systems follow the patient's anatomic retroversion or are predetermined somewhere between 20° and 40°. The majority of available systems have either intramedullary or extramedullary guides that align with the patient's forearm and assist in the determination of desired retroversion and inclination angle.

After the osteotomy, attention is turned toward the preparation of the humeral canal. Humeral stem options include short and standard stems, as well as stemless prosthesis, and are covered in more specific detail in other chapters. The majority of standard- and short-stem systems follow a preparation template combining serial reaming and broaching of the humeral canal. With the humerus placed in the extended and adducted

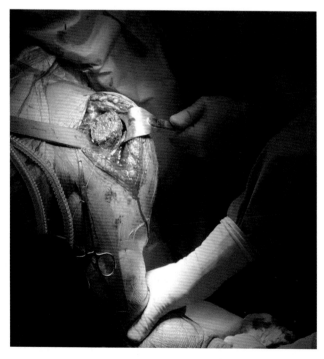

FIGURE 13.9 With the humerus in extension and external rotation, it can be placed on a Mayo stand for support with excellent visualization of the humeral head.

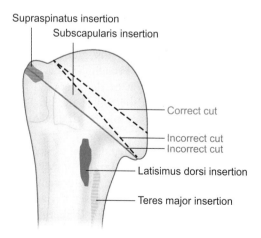

FIGURE 13.10 The location and angle of the humeral head osteotomy is determined after proper exposure and removal of osteophytes.

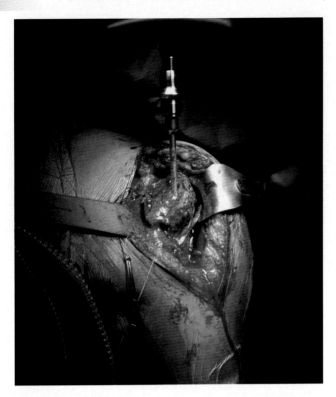

FIGURE 13.11 With the arm in extension and external rotation, sequential reaming is performed.

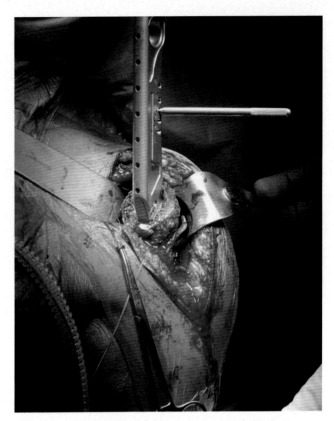

FIGURE 13.12 Following reaming, sequential broaching is performed to the selected size.

position, a starting hole is made in the superolateral aspect of the humeral osteotomy. The bicipital groove serves as a landmark to establish the starting location for the reamer. Sequential hand reaming is carried out until encountering cortical chatter (**FIGURE 13.11**). Depending on bone density, minimal cortical contact distally will most likely result in adequate fixation. Excessive cortical reaming, particularly using power, should be avoided. Once encountering cortical chatter, the reamer size used serves as a reference for the corresponding broaching and final implant. Sequential broaching should follow the reaming with a broach one to two sizes smaller than the last used reamer. Sequential broaching is carried out to the broach size that corresponds with the last used reamer (**FIGURE 13.12**). A version guide, which aligns with the forearm, on the broach handle, helps confirm the appropriate version of the prepared humerus. Additionally, the plate on the top of the broach assists in determining the accuracy of the desired osteotomy inclination.

Once broaching is completed, the surgeon decides about the humeral fixation and stability. My preference in the vast majority of cases is to use uncemented fixation. Standard-length stem prostheses derive their stability from distal cortical fixation. If there appears to be poor proximal fill of the prosthesis, cancellous bone from the resected head can be impacted into the prepared proximal humeral metaphysis. If this provides inadequate fixation, the surgeon may consider upsizing the

humeral preparation to the next available stem size. In rare cases, with significant osteopenic bone, cement fixation may be selected. As humeral loosening is an uncommon complication, it is my preference to avoid cement fixation when possible due to difficulty in cemented stem revisions. In those cases where I determine cement fixation necessary, my preferred method is to use a limited cement technique around only the proximal 3 to 4 cm of metaphyseal bone, as distal diaphyseal cement mantles often present the most significant challenge in revision cases. Upon completion of proximal humeral preparation, the surgeon decides whether to place a trial humeral stem or the definitive implant before turning attention to the glenoid side exposure. My choice in anatomic arthroplasty is to seat the definitive humeral stem as the need to change the stem in anatomic arthroplasty is unlikely.

GLENOID EXPOSURE

Focus now turns toward adequate glenoid exposure. Many of the critical steps in successful glenoid exposure have been accomplished with the humeral-sided preparation. Adequate humeral-sided releases allow for relaxation and posterior displacement of the humerus relative to the glenoid. Accomplishing posterior humeral displacement requires mobilization of the subacromial and subdeltoid spaces, the release of the pectoralis major tendon, adequate humeral head osteotomy, removal of osteophytes, and release of the inferior glenohumeral ligaments on the humeral side. If, with the placement of the first posterior glenoid retractor, the humeral head will not freely sublux behind the posterior inferior glenoid, the surgeon should consider retracing these steps.

I tilt the bed approximately 20° away from the operative side to help with the visualization of the glenoid. Utilization of the Mayo stand for arm placement is advantageous during this step. Adjusting the Mayo stand height and the position of the arm as it lays free on the padded Mayo stand allows the operating surgeon to find a position in which the soft tissues are maximally relaxed. Preferably, the arm is in approximately 30° of abduction with slight external rotation. Progressively increasing amounts of abduction brings the axillary nerve closer to the inferior capsule and increases the risk of injury during the subsequent releases. A posterior glenoid retractor is placed at the posterior inferior corner of the glenoid. As discussed earlier, our preference is to use as small and few glenoid retractors as possible, allowing for the minimal intrusion of the retractors on the limited working space available. My primary choice for the posterior glenoid retractor is a modified curved Darrach-type retractor.

Attention is turned toward further mobilization of the subscapularis tendon. The releases are started superiorly by completing the release of the rotator interval medial to the level of the glenoid, including the release of the superior glenohumeral ligament **(FIGURE 13.13)**. Traction is applied to the stay sutures previously placed on the released end of the subscapularis tendon, allowing visualization of the middle glenohumeral ligament. The middle glenohumeral ligaments and anterior capsule are subsequently released with a needle tip electrocautery just lateral to the labral attachment **(FIGURE 13.14)**. Performing the release medially on the glenoid side of the subscapularis allows for the capsular tissue laterally to remain with the subscapularis tendon, improving structural integrity for later repair. The release of the inferior glenohumeral ligaments is continued inferiorly

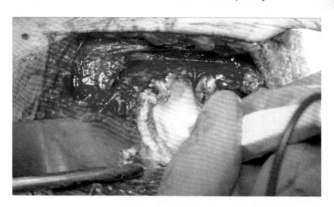

FIGURE 13.14 The anterior capsule is released which also allows mobilization of the subscapularis tendon.

approximately to the 6 o'clock position. The axillary nerve is at the most significant risk of injury during this portion of the releases.[2] The following techniques mitigate risk to the axillary nerve: (1) The surgeon should remain aware of the location of the axillary nerve at all times despite the inability of direct visualization of the nerve. (2) The use of the needle tip electrocautery acts as a nerve stimulator, alerting the surgeon to the proximity of the nerve. (3) The inferior muscular portion of the subscapularis isolates the releases from the path of the nerve.

After completion of the inferior capsular releases, a spiked two-pronged retractor is placed on the anterior neck of the glenoid, improving anterior exposure. My preference is to then place a spiked bent Hohmann at the posterior superior corner of the glenoid just behind the biceps tendon attachment **(FIGURE 13.15)**. By palpating the subscapularis recess, remaining osteocartilaginous loose bodies are identified and removed. The anterior labrum and remaining capsule are removed with a needle tip electrocautery. The released medial portion of the long head of the biceps tendon is used as a tether to remove the superior and posterior labral tissue. Extreme care should be taken in anatomic arthroplasties not to release the posterior glenohumeral ligaments, which may result in posterior glenohumeral instability.

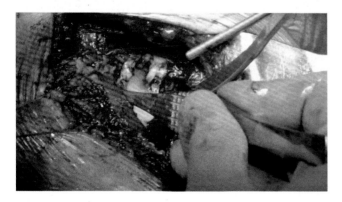

FIGURE 13.13 Capsular releases are essential for proper glenoid exposure including release of the superior glenohumeral ligament.

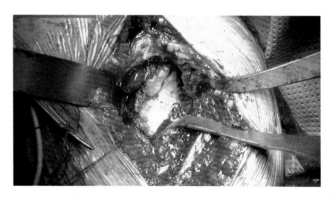

FIGURE 13.15 Placement of glenoid retractors is essential for proper glenoid exposure.

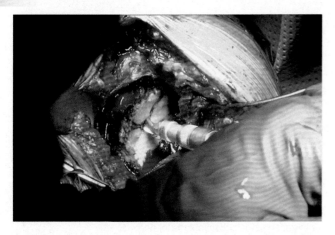

FIGURE 13.16 Glenoid exposure should provide direct perpendicular access to the face of the glenoid.

The final step is to release the inferior capsular attachments from the inferior glenoid subperiosteally. The release is carried 1 cm medial on the inferior neck of the glenoid to the location of the long head of the triceps insertion. The retractor position may now be optimized, and adequacy of the glenoid exposure evaluated.

Before proceeding with the preparation of the glenoid component, the surgeon should critically evaluate exposure to the glenoid face. The humeral head should be relaxed and be posteriorly subluxed behind the glenoid. Exposure should allow for perpendicular access onto the face of the glenoid for preparation instruments (**FIGURE 13.16**). If these parameters are not achieved, the surgeon should retrace the steps of humeral releases, glenoid releases, and retractor placement until these goals met. For example, if the humeral head is not fully posteriorly subluxed, further release of the pectoralis major tendon or humeral-sided inferior capsule may significantly improve overall exposure. Additionally, various retractor substitutions may aid exposure in patients with unique anatomic variations. After obtaining sufficient exposure, the focus shifts toward the preparation of the glenoid component.

GLENOID PREPARATION

The goal of glenoid preparation is to have the final appropriate size prosthesis centered and symmetrically supported on native subchondral bone. Several significant improvements in glenoid implant technology, including augmentation, hybrid fixation, and inset glenoids, have resulted in multiple options to deal with significant glenoid-sided challenges. Implant options, dealing with deformity, and inset glenoids are covered in more detail elsewhere in this textbook. This chapter focuses on the use of a pegged hybrid glenoid implant in patients with moderate to no significant posterior glenoid deformity.

Aseptic glenoid loosening remains one of the primary modes of intermediate and late failure for anatomic total shoulder arthroplasty. Appropriate positioning and preservation of subchondral bony support are critical for glenoid implant longevity.[8] Preoperative planning, including high-quality true AP and axillary lateral radiographs, as well as computed tomography (CT) imaging, in many cases, are strongly recommended. CT imaging allows the operating surgeon a more accurate representation of bone deformity, as well as being necessary for use in preoperative planning software, patient-specific instrumentation, and use of guided intraoperative navigation. Based on the CT findings, preoperative assessment of the glenoid size, osteophyte location, deformity, and glenoid center can be determined. Determination of the actual center of the glenoid is vital to reaching our goals, as mentioned earlier, for glenoid preparation. A central hole that is not in the actual center results in excessive reaming of subchondral bone, undersizing of the implant, or likely both. I use electrocautery to mark the center point of the glenoid with hash marks superior to inferior and anterior to posterior (see **FIGURE 13.16**). In patients with minimal or no deformity, the exact center lies at this point. In patients with more significant posterior wear, the center point lies just anterior to this point, typically on the ridge between the native and neo glenoid (**FIGURE 13.17**). Guided navigation and patient-specific instrumentation can be particularly helpful in these cases. After identifying the actual glenoid center, a pilot-tipped drill hole is placed perpendicular to the face of the native glenoid in preparation for reaming. In patients with minimal deformity and adequate glenoid exposure, the reamer should be easily placed perpendicular to the face of the glenoid. In excessively stiff and progressively more deformed patients, perpendicular insertion may be more difficult. In these cases, the surgeon should again check that adequate humeral and glenoid releases have been performed as well as consider modification of retractor placement. Sometimes it is helpful to have the assistant give extra traction on the posterior glenoid retractor to place the reamer within the joint and then fully relax on the retractor during the

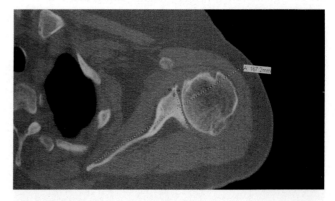

FIGURE 13.17 Computed tomography (CT) scans show significant posterior glenoid wear in which the center point of the glenoid is located more anteriorly on the face of the glenoid.

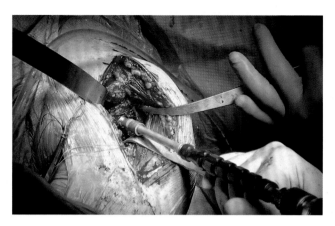

FIGURE 13.18 Perpendicular access to the glenoid allows sequential reaming to be performed.

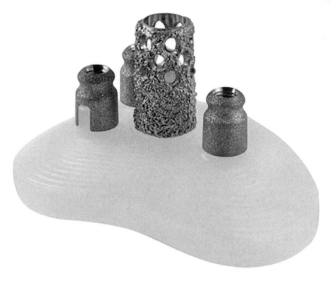

FIGURE 13.19 Anatomic total shoulder arthroplasty utilizing a hybrid glenoid implant which allows for central bone ingrowth and peripheral cement fixation.

actual reaming. The tip of the reamer is inserted into the pilot hole, and reaming is initiated before the reamer fully contacts bone. Sequential reaming is carried up from the smallest reamer until identifying the appropriate size **(FIGURE 13.18)**. The selection of the appropriate glenoid size is based on coverage of the glenoid surface and glenohumeral prosthetic radial mismatch.[5] Variability in glenohumeral radial mismatch is dependent on the implant system used, and the surgeon should be aware of the specific recommendations of the manufacturer of their chosen system. Most modern shoulder prosthetic implant systems allow for a significant mismatch between the humeral head and glenoid component size by providing various radius of curvatures at given sizes. As stated earlier, a primary goal of reaming is for the final implant to have complete or near-complete concentric support. In patients with excessive posterior wear, the posterior portion of the glenoid may fail to be fully supported. In my experience, if greater than 15% of the glenoid remains unsupported posteriorly, the patient may be better served with a more stable glenoid-sided fixation provided by a reverse shoulder arthroplasty. Avoid cement placed on the backside of the implant to compensate for unsupported areas.

Further preparation of the glenoid depends on the type of implant selected, keeled versus pegged. In general, both implants have obtained excellent results, and selection is based on surgeon preference.[9] My preference in the majority of cases is to use a hybrid pegged implant **(FIGURE 13.19)**. The central cage on this implant allows for initial interference fit as well as long-term bone through growth.[10] The initial interference fit allows for stable implant positioning during cement polymerization.

Preparation for a pegged implant begins with the placement of the central hole. By placing the central hole in the same location as the pilot reaming hole and perpendicular to the face of the glenoid, the surgeon ensures the central hole is in the actual glenoid center. As previously stated, central hole placement is vital for the remainder of glenoid preparation as well as appropriate implant sizing. The assistance of navigation or patient-specific instrumentation significantly enhances central hole accuracy. In the absence of navigation, a guide provided by the specific system identifies the location of the central hole. The specific guide to be used may require selection of final implant size, or sizing of the implant can occur after preparation of the peg holes. The central drill guide should be placed flush on the prepared, reamed surface of the glenoid **(FIGURE 13.20)**. The central guide facilitates the placement of the central hole perpendicular to the glenoid face, which is critical when using an interference fit hybrid central cage glenoid component. Care should be taken that soft tissues and retractors do not displace the drill anteriorly, resulting in a central hole placed in a posteriorly angled direction. Central hole perforation should be unlikely with careful

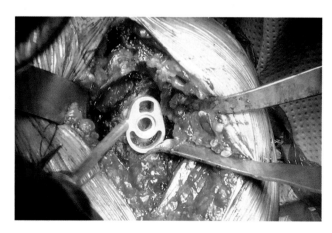

FIGURE 13.20 Placement of the drill guide allows preparation of the central hole for the hybrid glenoid implant.

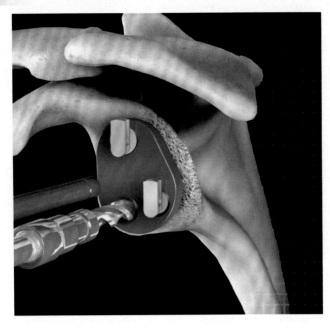

FIGURE 13.21 A second guide is used to prepare the peripheral peg holes.

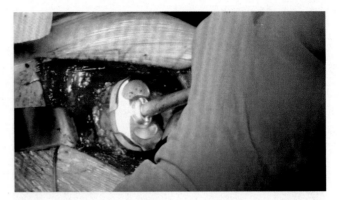

FIGURE 13.22 Insertion of the glenoid component requires direct perpendicular access to the glenoid.

preoperative planning, glenoid preparation, and precise central hole placement. A peripheral hole guide is placed in the just-completed central hole. When fully seated, the body of the guide should be circumferentially flush with the reamed glenoid surface, allowing for perpendicular preparation of the peripheral peg holes **(FIGURE 13.21)**. Antirotation pins are placed as subsequent peripheral peg holes are drilled. After glenoid preparation, check each peg hole to confirm perforation has not occurred, and the trial implant is placed. If the trial implant fails to sit flush on the prepared glenoid, consider further preparation or conversion to reverse arthroplasty.

CEMENTATION

Attention is turned toward cementation. With a hybrid-style implant, only the peripheral holes are cemented. In the unlikely event of peripheral hole perforation, it is my preference to bone graft and press-fit the perforated hole or holes. A cement restriction peg is placed in the central hole and any bone grafted peripheral holes to prevent the migration of cement from the cemented peripheral holes during pressurization. A pulse lavage irrigates and removes all blood and debris from the peripheral holes. In my experience, rapid setting polymethyl methacrylate inserted with a commercially available disposable pressurizing syringe results in minimal postoperative radiolucent lines. After appropriate pressurization of the cement, the hybrid cage pegged implant is inserted. It is imperative with this type of implant that insertion, just as the preparation, occurs precisely perpendicular to the glenoid face **(FIGURE 13.22)**. The stability of the

implant during polymethyl methacrylate polymerization is achieved with an interference fit of the central cage.[10] When cementing an all-polyethylene implant, whether pegged or keeled, the prosthesis must be held stable in a position to prevent micromotion. When using an instrument to stabilize the prosthesis during polymerization, prevent posterior soft tissues and retractors from tipping the implant. After assessing the position and stability of the implant, remove all excess cement.

ASSESSING AND ACHIEVING STABILITY

Once the final glenoid implant is secured, attention is returned to humeral sizing and assessing stability. Modern shoulder arthroplasty systems effectively adapt to individual patient anatomy and significantly help soft tissue balancing. However, proper soft tissue balancing is still essential to the active function and long-term survival of the prosthesis. Both overstuffing and undersizing the prosthesis can lead to postoperative complications. Given that the majority of anatomic arthroplasties are performed for osteoarthritis, overstuffing and stiffness are of primary concern. At this point in the surgical procedure, options for soft tissue balancing include the selection of the humeral head size and thickness, as well as soft tissue releases and capsulorrhaphy.[5,11]

Humeral head trialing should begin with the size that provides coverage to the resected humerus and correlates with the prosthetic glenohumeral mismatch of the selected glenoid component. The majority of prosthetic systems allow for significant variability between humeral head size and glenoid size while continuing to ensure an appropriate radius of curvature mismatch. Eccentric or dual eccentricity implants aid coverage of the resected humerus. Base the thickness of the selected trial on preoperative templating and the amount of resected bone. With these parameters as a starting point, a trial reduction can be performed.

There are four parameters the surgeon can use for assessment of soft tissue balancing. First, with the shoulder reduced in approximately 20° to 30° of external rotation, the humeral head should sublux 30% to 50% of the humeral head diameter posteriorly with a posteriorly directed force on the arm. The humeral head should reduce spontaneously when the posterior force is relieved. Second, the humeral head should translate 30% to 50% inferiorly when applying a traction force to the arm and spontaneously reduce when the force is relieved. Third, with the arm in 30° of external rotation, the subscapularis should return to the lesser tuberosity without significant tension. Fourth, no dislocation of the shoulder should occur with either cross-arm adduction or external rotation with the arm in an adducted position. Fortunately, with adequate soft tissue releases during exposure and anatomic arthroplasty systems, the majority of cases meet these criteria.

In cases where excessive posterior translation occurs, and the prosthesis will not spontaneously reduce, the instability can be addressed in three ways. First, repair of the subscapularis with rotator interval closure can restore stability in the majority of these cases. Second, consideration should be given to increasing humeral head thickness and, potentially, the diameter. Third, if these fail to control instability, a posterior capsulorrhaphy is likely necessary. My preferred method of posterior capsulorrhaphy is to use a lamina spreader between the humeral head and glenoid **(FIGURE 13.23)** and place multiple Ethibond capsulorrhaphy sutures from medial to lateral in the posterior capsular tissue.[12] Reassess stability and add capsulorrhaphy stitches as needed. In patients requiring added capsulorrhaphy sutures, it is my preference to immobilize them postoperatively in a neutral rotation sling.

Alternatively, in patients who do not achieve the desired posterior to inferior humeral head subluxation (ie, too tight), decreasing humeral head thickness and size should be considered first. Second, reevaluate the competence of the humeral and glenoid releases. Third, the surgeon should confirm adequate humeral head resection with the initial osteotomy. Only in rare cases and with caution, will I perform additional posterior capsular releases.

In cases where the subscapularis fails to return to the lesser tuberosity, retrace the initial steps of subscapularis releases. Often subscapularis excursion is limited by inadequate releases of the inferior glenohumeral joint capsule or the rotator interval. Care should be taken to avoid overaggressive releases on the medial aspect of the dorsal subscapularis that can result in denervation of the muscle. After completion of final soft tissue balancing, the definitive humeral component is seated, the shoulder reduced, one last check of soft tissue balancing is evaluated, and attention is turned toward closure.

CLOSURE

Closure begins with the meticulous repair of the subscapularis. As noted earlier, failure of the subscapularis repair remains one of the most common early postoperative complications of anatomic arthroplasty. Meticulous and structurally rigid repair is vital to prevent postoperative dehiscence. Repair of the subscapularis after subperiosteal takedown consists of the following four principles. First, the use of multiple transosseous high-tensile nonabsorbable sutures for tendon repair. Second, the use of a rip-stop suture technique through the subscapularis tendon to prevent longitudinal failure of the repair sutures. Third, at least two of the transosseous sutures should also be fixed to the humeral prosthesis to prevent the failure of the bone tunnels. Fourth, closure of the rotator interval, which may result in some loss of external rotation, but significantly improves the load to failure of the repaired tendon.

My preferred technique is to pass five #2 FiberWire sutures through small drill holes 1 to 2 cm distal to the humeral osteotomy, beginning superolaterally in the dense bone of the bicipital groove and extending inferomedially to the anterior humeral calcar **(FIGURE 13.24)**. The central three sutures are at the highest risk of pulling through their transosseous tunnels; therefore, pass at least two of these sutures around the humeral component. Pass each of the transosseous sutures exiting from the medullary canal through the subscapularis in a modified Mason-Allen pattern **(FIGURE 13.25)**. Only after the passing of all five sutures are the sutures tied.

Adequately pretensioning the sutures to relieve any laxity improves the structural integrity of the repair. This is particularly true for the sutures passed around the prosthesis. Finally, the rotator interval is closed laterally to medially. In the majority of cases, my rotator interval closure involves the lateral 50% of the interval or less. In cases with significant posterior subluxation, more aggressive medial rotator interval closure may be helpful but will result in some loss of external rotation. After the closure of the interval, assess the integrity of the subscapularis repair with passive external rotation. These numbers are documented and used to help guide postoperative rehabilitation parameters. The pectoralis major tendon, if previously released, is now repaired with #2 FiberWire. If the long head of the biceps tendon was not previously tenodesed, then the tendon can be incorporated into the repair suture for the pectoralis major tendon providing for tenodesis. In cases where the pectoralis major tendon is not released throughout the surgical procedure, the biceps tendon is tenodesed into the upper one-third of the intact pectoralis major tendon.

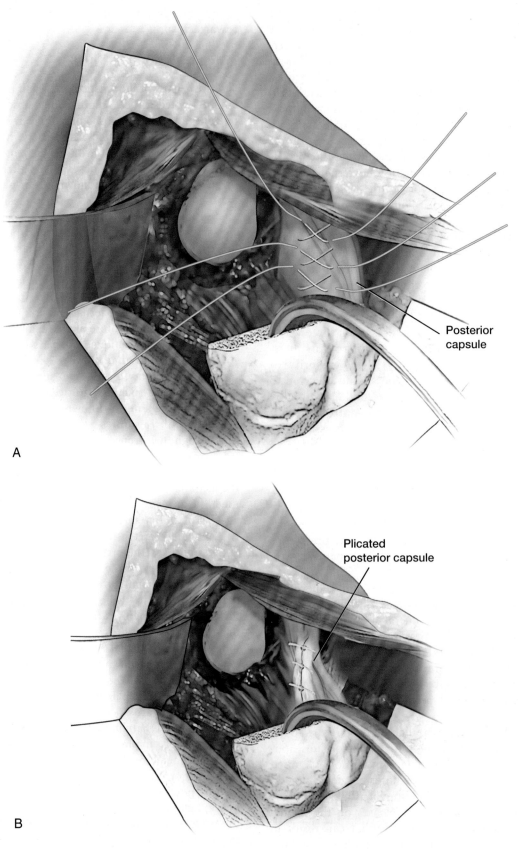

FIGURE 13.23 A and **B**, Posterior capsulorrhaphy may be necessary if there is residual posterior laxity or instability. A lamina spreader is placed between the humeral head and the glenoid, and multiple nonabsorbable sutures are placed in the posterior capsular tissue from a medial to lateral direction to imbricate and shorten the capsule.

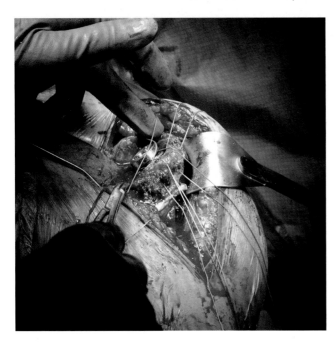

FIGURE 13.24 Technique for reattachment of the subscapularis with sutures passed through drill holes in the area of the lesser tuberosity.

Attention is then turned toward the superficial wound closure. I prefer not to use drains in the majority of anatomic shoulder arthroplasty cases. However, in patients on bridging anticoagulation medication, and patients with greater than usual intraoperative blood loss, a suction Hemovac drain is placed in the subacromial and subdeltoid spaces. The cephalic vein is examined for intraoperative damage and is ligated if necessary. The

deltopectoral interval is left unclosed. The subcutaneous tissue is closed with interrupted absorbable vicral sutures, and I close the skin with a commercially available noninvasive *zip tie* closure system.

Technical nuances exist between differing implant systems, specific techniques dealing with deformity, and for resurfacing-type implants. However, the principles outlined in this chapter serve as a foundation for successful anatomic arthroplasties of all types. Optimal exposure, anatomic reconstruction, and precise soft tissue balancing are the fundamental framework of clinical outcomes and implant longevity.

REFERENCES

1. Zuckerman JD. *Advanced Reconstruction Shoulder*. American Academy of Orthopaedic Surgeons; 2007.
2. LiBrizzi CL, Rojas J, Joseph J, Bitzer A, McFarland EG. Incidence of clinically evident isolated axillary nerve injury in 869 primary anatomic and reverse total shoulder arthroplasties without routine identification of the axillary nerve. *JSES open access*. 2019;3(1):48-53. doi:10.1016/j.jses.2018.12.002
3. Choate WS, Kwapisz A, Momaya AM, Hawkins RJ, Tokish JM. Outcomes for subscapularis management techniques in shoulder arthroplasty: a systematic review. *J Shoulder Elbow Surg*. 2018;27(2):363-370. doi:10.1016/j.jse.2017.08.003
4. Aibinder WR, Bicknell RT, Bartsch S, Scheibel M, Athwal GS. Subscapularis management in stemless total shoulder arthroplasty: tenotomy versus peel versus lesser tuberosity osteotomy. *J Shoulder Elbow Surg*. 2019;28(10):1942-1947. doi:10.1016/j.jse.2019.02.022
5. Edwards TB, Morris BJ, Gartsman GM. *Shoulder Arthroplasty*. Elsevier; 2019.
6. Keener JD, Chalmers PN, Yamaguchi K. The humeral implant in shoulder arthroplasty. *J Am Acad Orthop Surg*. 2017;25(6):427-438. doi:10.5435/JAAOS-D-15-00682
7. Craig EV. Total shoulder replacement with intact bone and soft tissue. In: Craig EV, ed. *Master Techniques in Orthopaedic Surgery: The Shoulder*. Lippincott Williams & Wilkins; 2004.
8. Hsu JE, Hackett DJ Jr, Vo KV, Matsen FA III. What can be learned from an analysis of 215 glenoid component failures? *J Shoulder Elbow Surg*. 2018;27(3):478-486. doi:10.1016/j.jse.2017.09.029
9. Kilian CM, Press CM, Smith KM, et al. Radiographic and clinical comparison of pegged and keeled glenoid components using modern cementing techniques: midterm results of a prospective randomized study. *J Shoulder Elbow Surg*. 2017;26(12):2078-2085. doi:10.1016/j.jse.2017.07.016
10. Friedman RJ, Cheung E, Grey SG, et al. Clinical and radiographic comparison of a hybrid cage glenoid to a cemented polyethylene glenoid in anatomic total shoulder arthroplasty. *J Shoulder Elbow Surg*. 2019;28(12):2308-2316. doi:10.1016/j.jse.2019.04.049
11. Ibarra C, Craig EV. Soft-tissue balancing in total shoulder arthroplasty. *Orthop Clin North Am*. 1998;29(3):415-422. doi:10.1016/s0030-5898(05)70017-1
12. Alentorn-Geli E, Assenmacher AT, Sperling JW, Cofield RH, Sánchez-Sotelo J. Plication of the posterior capsule for intraoperative posterior instability during anatomic total shoulder arthroplasty. *J Shoulder Elbow Surg*. 2017;26(6):982-989. doi:10.1016/j.jse.2016.10.008

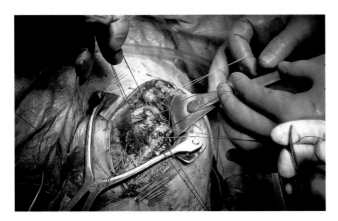

FIGURE 13.25 The transosseous sutures are then placed through the subscapularis tendon in a modified Mason-Allen pattern.

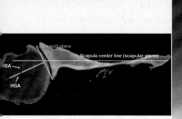

14 Addressing Glenoid Deformity in Anatomic Total Shoulder Arthroplasty

Jared M. Mahylis, MD, Eric T. Ricchetti, MD, and Joseph P. Iannotti, MD, PhD

INTRODUCTION

Surgical treatment of the glenoid remains the most challenging portion of anatomic total shoulder arthroplasty (ATSA). A spectrum of glenoid deformity can be encountered, and each morphologic pattern presents its own surgical obstacles. This chapter will highlight the surgical treatment options for glenoid deformity in the setting of ATSA.

DEFINING GLENOID PATHOLOGY IN GLENOHUMERAL OSTEOARTHRITIS

Classification

Glenohumeral (GH) osteoarthritis (OA) exhibits unique eccentric wear patterns in contrast to OA in other large joints.[1-3] Walch et al were the first to formally classify these patterns in GH OA. This classification did have notable weaknesses due to poor reproducibility[4,5] and has since undergone modifications.[6,7] Bercik et al expanded the classification system to include new types of B3 glenoid and D glenoids (FIGURE 14.1). Using three-dimensional computed tomography (3D-CT), they described the B3 glenoid as a progression from a B2 glenoid with continued posterior glenoid wear but loss of biconcavity (monoconcave) with at least 15° of retroversion and/or at least 70% posterior humeral head subluxation relative to the scapula. The C glenoid was further defined as having at least 25° of retroversion not caused by posterior erosion to prevent incorrect classification as a more severe B glenoid.[6] Subsequently, Iannotti et al further defined the B3 glenoid and added a new subtype, the C2 glenoid. Utilizing 3D-CT with the previously validated 3D glenoid vault model, the B3 glenoid definition was expanded to having minimal or no paleoglenoid, high retroversion due to posterior wear, and more medialization than B2 glenoids (FIGURE 14.2A). The C2 glenoid was introduced as a biconcave variant similar to a B2 glenoid, but with underlying glenoid dysplasia and thus a greater premorbid glenoid retroversion. The new C2 glenoid also exhibited greater posterior humeral head subluxation compared with C1 glenoids resulting from the "acquired" biconcavity (FIGURE 14.2B).[7]

Imaging Assessment of the Glenoid

Assessment of GH pathology is important to surgically addressing deformity. However, radiographs have shown poor reproducibility and frequently overestimate glenoid retroversion.[8] Studies have shown that x-rays demonstrate fair to good assessment of glenoid morphology and Walch classification when compared to CT.[9,10] However, intra- and interreader reliability remains only fair to moderate when comparing standard radiographs to more advanced imaging such as CT and magnetic resonance imaging (MRI).[10,11]

CT remains the standard for assessment of glenoid pathology.[12-14] Two-dimensional CT has shown fair reproducibility in assessing retroversion and classifying morphology,[2,4,5] but with development of 3D-CT reconstruction and surgical planning software, multiple studies have shown superiority of 3D-CT in assessing glenoid morphology.[13,15,16] MRI studies assessing glenoid architecture remain mixed.[17,18] Raymond et al showed superiority of MRI to axillary radiographs in assessment of retroversion.[17] However, Lowe et al found MRI had poor accuracy in assessing the advanced glenoid bone loss and retroversion of B2 and C glenoids.[18] Overall, 3D-CT provides a more detailed evaluation of the glenoid in OA.[12]

Humeral Head Relationship to Glenoid and Scapula in OA

Neer first noted posterior humeral head subluxation with asymmetric GH OA,[19] which Walch et al later detailed.[2] Walch described a humeral head subluxation index, relative to the center of the glenoid, between 45% and 55% to be a centered humeral head, while 0% was considered an anterior dislocation and 100% a posterior dislocation.[2] This study, however, did not compare subluxation to normal controls.

Recently, Sabesan et al utilized 3D-CT comparing 60 patients with advanced OA to 15 non-OA controls to define the baseline relationship between the center of the humeral head to the glenoid fossa plane and to the plane of the scapula (FIGURE 14.3).[20] Humeral-scapular alignment (HSA) averaged −8.43 ± 5.58 mm or −17.1% ± 11.3% relative to humeral head diameter in OA patients, compared to −0.998 ± 1.85 mm or −2.27% ± 4.18% in

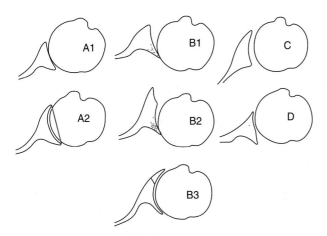

FIGURE 14.1 Modified Walch classification. Note that a line drawn from the anterior to posterior native glenoid rim transects the humeral head in A2 glenoid but not in the A1 glenoid. (Redrawn with permission from Bercik MJ, Kruse K II, Yalizis M, Gauci MO, Chaoui J, Walch G. A modification to the Walch classification of the glenoid in primary glenohumeral osteoarthritis using three-dimensional imaging. *J Shoulder Elbow Surg.* 2016;25(10):1601-1606.)

controls. A near-perfect linear relationship between glenoid retroversion and HSA ($P < 0.001$) was seen, as well as a significant relationship between glenoid bone loss and HSA ($P < 0.001$). Humeral-glenoid alignment (HGA) averaged -1.16 ± 3.81 mm or $-2.48\% \pm 7.3\%$ relative to humeral head diameter in OA patients, compared to 0.48 ± 1.33 mm or $0.87\% \pm 2.6\%$ in controls. The relationship between glenoid retroversion and HGA was not significant, but the relationship between glenoid bone loss and HGA was ($P < 0.001$). The authors concluded that the two methods of defining humeral head subluxation are different and independent of one another. While HSA is highly correlated with glenoid retroversion, HGA is more variable and related to factors other than bony glenoid anatomy that may include soft-tissue contracture or humeral head deformity.[20]

Chan et al. showed similar findings when assessing the B3 glenoid. They found a mean posterior humeral head subluxation of $80\% \pm 8\%$ for HSA, while HGA showed a mean posterior humeral head subluxation of $54\% \pm 6\%$. The authors suggested a centering of the humeral head with respect to the neoglenoid articulation. They found a significant correlation between glenoid version and degree of posterior humeral head subluxation related to HSA, with every 1° increase in glenoid retroversion resulting in a 1% increase in posterior humeral head subluxation ($P < 0.001$), but no significant correlation with HGA and glenoid retroversion ($P = 0.409$).[21]

Gender Specifics in OA

Epidemiologic studies show high prevalence of OA,[22-24] with men and women having different rates of OA,[25,26] which does include the shoulder. Nakagawa et al found significantly greater proportion of primary GH OA in female patients compared to males with shoulder disease ($P = 0.0178$).[26] The differences in prevalence and onset between men and women also appear to be different with women having greater prevalence and later onset.[26,27] Schoenfeldt et al found women to be affected in 54% of cases of primary GH OA, with an older age at time of presentation for treatment compared to men (72.9 ± 11.2 vs 66.1 ± 12.4; $P = 0.0005$).[27] Lastly, multiple studies have shown asymmetric glenoid wear to be far more prevalent in males, with four to five times greater incidence of B2 and B3 glenoid morphology in males.[28-30]

Natural History and Progression of Disease

The pathogenesis and pathophysiology of GH OA remains poorly understood.[1] Historically, primary GH OA was thought to begin on the glenoid.[1,2] Yet, few studies have assessed pathologic progression of disease looking at bony and soft-tissue changes in primary OA.[31] Walker et al recently performed a retrospective CT assessment of 65 shoulders with GH OA analyzing the amount and location of glenoid bone loss on at least two CT scans performed 24 months apart. Rotator cuff fatty infiltration was calculated and assignment of modified Walch classification was performed on all scans. Of the 65 shoulders assessed, 42 were A-type glenoids and 23 B-type glenoids. Successive CT scans showed 8 of 42 A1 glenoids had evidence of pathologic progression compared to 17 of 19 B1 glenoids (15 to B2 and 2 to B3) ($P < 0.001$) (**FIGURE 14.4A-C**). The odds of progressive joint-line medialization were 8.1 times higher for B-type glenoids. B-type glenoids showed a higher association with percentage of infraspinatus muscle fatty infiltration compared with A-type glenoids both initially (14% vs 7%; $P < 0.001$) and at final CT follow-up (16% vs 10%; $P = 0.003$). The authors concluded progressive asymmetric bone loss seldomly develops in A1 glenoids, whereas initial posterior humeral head translation (B1 glenoids) is associated with subsequent development and progression of posterior glenoid bone loss.[28]

Donohue et al further examined the relationship of glenoid morphology and rotator cuff fatty infiltration in 175 patients who underwent TSA for GH OA. Using 3D-CT analysis, glenoid pathologic version, and joint line, modified Walch classification and Goutallier classification were determined. High-grade posterior rotator cuff fatty infiltration (combined infraspinatus and teres minor) was seen in 16% B2 and 55% of B3 glenoids compared to 8% and 12% for A1 and A2 glenoids, respectively ($P < 0.001$). Higher fatty infiltration of the infraspinatus, teres minor, and combined posterior rotator cuff muscles was associated with increasing glenoid retroversion ($P < 0.05$), while higher fatty infiltration of all four rotator cuff muscles and combined posterior rotator cuff muscles was associated with increasing joint-line medialization ($P < 0.05$).[29]

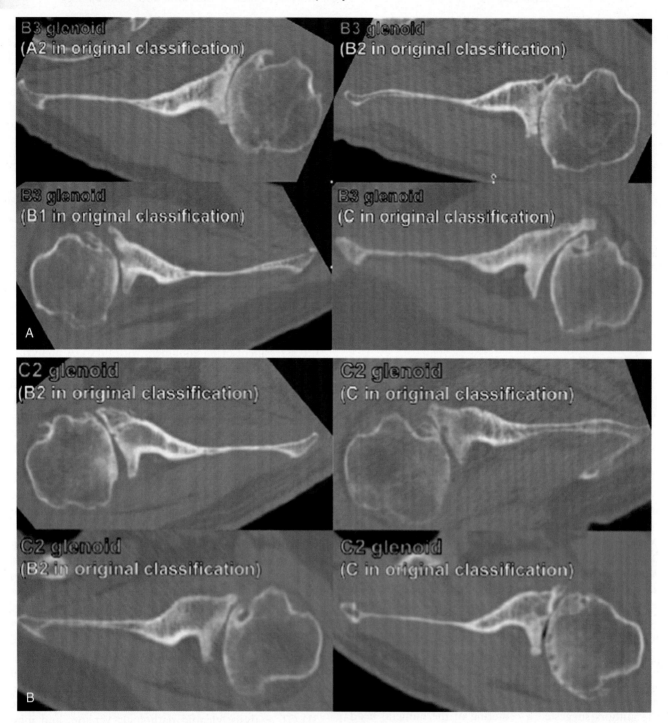

FIGURE 14.2 A, Computed tomography (CT) scan examples of four B3 glenoids and classification according to the original Walch classification. Note the B3 glenoid has both central and asymmetric posterior bone loss, increased medialization, and little to no paleoglenoid unlike the B2. **B,** CT scan examples of four C2 glenoids and classification according to the original Walch classification. In similarity to the B2 glenoid, the C2 glenoid has a biconcave surface with associated posterior humeral head subluxation; however, pathologic glenoid retroversion and the premorbid glenoid version are both greater in the C2 glenoid. (Reprinted with permission from Lippincott Williams & Wilkins from Iannotti JP, Jun BJ, Patterson TE, Ricchetti ET. Quantitative measurement of osseous pathology in advanced glenohumeral osteoarthritis. *J Bone Joint Surg Am.* 2017;99(17):1460-1468.)

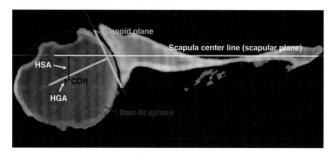

FIGURE 14.3 Preoperative humeral alignment. In relation to the scapular plane, the humeral-scapular alignment (HSA) is measured between the center of rotation (COR) of a best-fit sphere and the scapular center line. In relation to the pathologic glenoid fossa, the humeral-glenoid alignment (HGA) is measured from the COR to a line perpendicular to the glenoid plane from the center of the glenoid. The measurements are normalized to the humeral head diameter. (Reprinted with permission from Lippincott Williams & Wilkins from Sabesan VJ, Callanan M, Youderian A, Iannotti JP. 3D CT assessment of the relationship between humeral head alignment and glenoid retroversion in glenohumeral osteoarthritis. *J Bone Joint Surg Am.* 2014;96(8):e64.)

SURGICAL TREATMENT OPTIONS FOR GLENOID DEFORMITY

Correction of Anatomy: Eccentric Reaming and Use of a Standard Glenoid Component

Eccentric or asymmetric reaming (AR) with use of a standard glenoid component currently remains the most common method of addressing glenoid asymmetry (eg, B2 glenoid) in ATSA (**FIGURE 14.5A**). Glenoid asymmetry such as biconcavity is corrected by reaming the paleoglenoid. Using this technique, surgeons are able to treat approximately 5 to 8 mm of posterior bone loss while also being able to correct version between 10° and 15°.[32] This does lead to joint-line medialization (**FIGURE 14.5B**), which requires greater implant thickness to make up for this bone loss.[33] Good clinical outcomes have been reported with this method,[34-36] although they are limited by study design and duration of follow-up.

The technique does have limitations. Correcting retroversion greater than 15° to 20° results in excessive

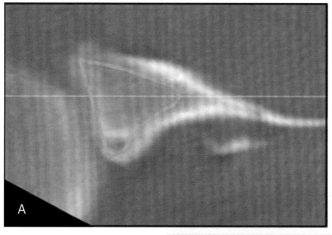

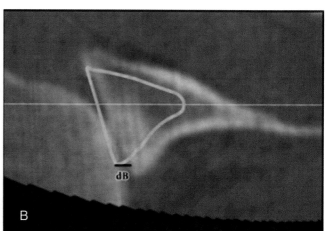

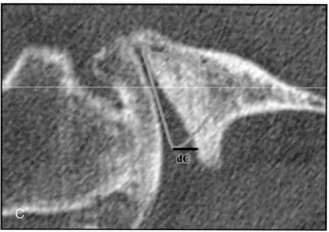

FIGURE 14.4 A-C, Images depicting B-type glenoid progression. A B1 glenoid with subluxation of the humeral head is seen on the initial computed tomography (CT) scan (**A**), with progression to a B2 glenoid on a 4-year interim CT scan (**B**) and further progression of posterior glenoid bone loss seen at 10 years (**C**). The vault model (blue) and the glenoid center axis (white line) are depicted. In B-type glenoids, the joint-line medialization was measured in reference to the vault model at the posterior aspect of the glenoid. On the initial CT scan, there is no measurable difference between the vault model and the glenoid surface. Line dB (4.22 mm) and line dC (7.96 mm) show the joint-line medialization measurements at 4 and 10 years, respectively. (Reprinted with permission from Lippincott Williams & Wilkins from Walker KE, Simcock XC, Jun BJ, Iannotti JP, Ricchetti ET. Progression of glenoid morphology in glenohumeral osteoarthritis. *J Bone Joint Surg Am.* 2018;100(1):49-56.)

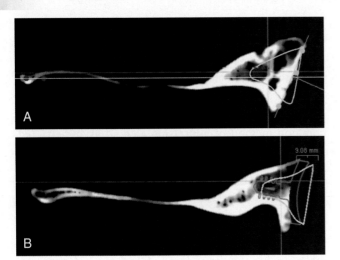

FIGURE 14.5 A, A 58-year-old man with B2 glenoid with superimposed vault model, with retroversion of 23.6° and inclination of 3.9°. **B**, B2 glenoid after simulated asymmetric reaming to accommodate an Anchor Peg Glenoid (Depuy, Warsaw, IN, USA). Reamed volume measures 9.1 mL with correction of version to −8°. Significant medialized location of the glenoid component (blue) relative to the vault model (orange).

joint-line medialization that is associated with glenoid implant perforation,[33,37] loss of cortical bone support, and narrowed glenoid dimension that may impact implant stability.[38,39] Sabesan et al suggested correcting glenoid retroversion to 6° rather than 0° in order to minimize joint-line medialization and best restore normal anatomy.[40]

Correction of Anatomy: Augmented Glenoid Component

Current Available Implants

Augmented glenoid components allow for better bone preservation, restoration of the joint line, and better soft-tissue tensioning compared to asymmetric glenoid reaming. These implants also eliminate the need for

bone grafting. An early metal-backed wedged design (Smith & Nephew; London, UK) was plagued by similar failure rates as other metal-backed implants. Cil et al reported a 31% 10-year revision-free survival rate of this implant.[41] Three posteriorly augmented glenoid components are currently available in the United States, a stepped design (StepTech; Depuy Synthes, Warsaw, Indiana; **FIGURE 14.6A**), a full-wedge design (Equinoxe Posterior Augment; Exactech, Gainesville, Florida; **FIGURE 14.6B**), and a posterior wedge design (Aequalis Perform+, Wright Medical Group N.V., Memphis, Tennessee; **FIGURE 14.6C**).[42]

Surgical Technique Differences Between Implants

All currently available implants attempt to limit the bone loss associated with AR while correcting or maintaining the native joint line. Each implant manufacturer's surgical technique should be utilized for detailed steps on correct sizing and insertion of the implant. The following description highlights differences between implants and should not be used in lieu of the manufacturers recommended technique. The shape of the implant augment may be important in determining its best use between a biconcave (B2) glenoid and a glenoid with more symmetric posterior glenoid bone loss (B3). All three manufacturers utilize preoperative planning 3D-CT software to assist with determining the optimal implant position at the time of surgery (TrueMatch, Depuy Synthes, Warsaw, Indiana; GPS, Exactech, Gainesville, Florida; and BluePrint, Wright Medical Group N.V., Memphis, Tennessee).[42-44]

For the DePuy StepTech implant, the paleoglenoid is first reamed over a central guide pin to create an even, concave surface from the 12-o'clock to 6-o'clock position. A posterior glenoid guide corresponding to the desired size step (3, 5, 7 mm) is then used to ream the neoglenoid with an oscillating rasp and create the posterior step surface.[43]

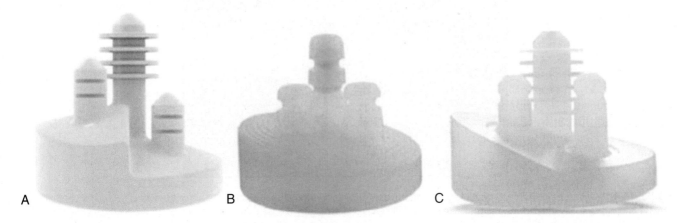

FIGURE 14.6 A, StepTech from Depuy Synthes available in +3, +5, and +7 mm augmented stepped glenoids. **B**, Equinoxe posterior augment wedge glenoid from Exactech (Gainesville, FL) available in 8° and 16° full wedge. Also available with hybrid metal-coated pegs (not pictured). **C**, Aequalis Perform+ posterior wedged augmented glenoid from Wright Medical Group N.V. (Memphis, TN) available in 15°, 25°, and 35° posterior wedge.

The Exactech Equinoxe implant allows for both a freehand and cannulated technique. For brevity, the cannulated technique is outlined. A 0° Kirschner wire (K-wire) is inserted into the glenoid relative to the central scapular axis. A second K-wire is inserted through a guide 8° or 16° relative to the first guide pin. The glenoid is then reamed on the second wire to create the desired posterior wedge surface (8° or 16°).[44]

The Aequalis Perform+ implant technique is also performed in a cannulated fashion. The paleoglenoid is first reamed to form an even, concave surface from the 12-o'clock to 6-o'clock position. A specialized, adjustable Neoreamer (**FIGURE 14.7D**) is then used to ream the neoglenoid according to the desired posterior half-wedge size (15°, 25°, 35°) to create the posterior half-wedge surface (**FIGURE 14.7A-C**).[45]

In Vitro and In Vivo Data for Correction by Augmented Implant Type

Correcting glenoid retroversion with minimal bone removal is the goal with utilization of an augmented component, regardless of implant design. Clinical (in vivo) and simulated (in vitro) studies have shown the ability to achieve this goal.[30,40,46-49]

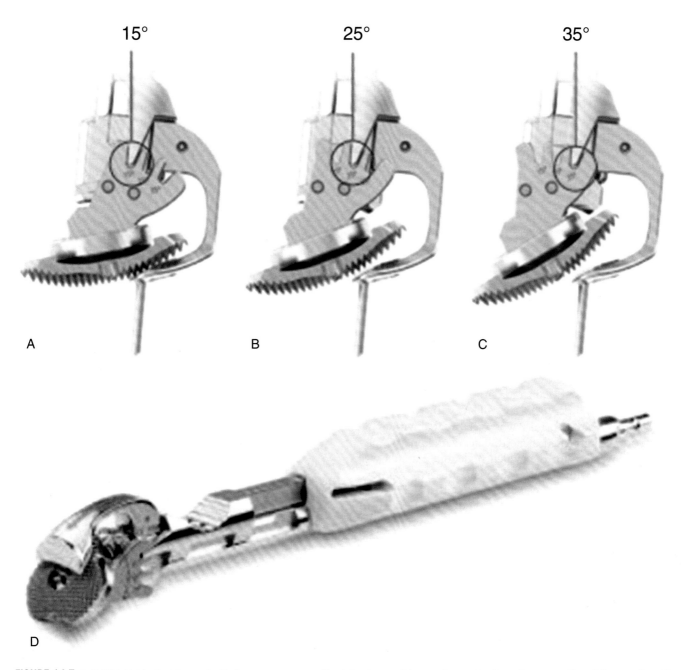

FIGURE 14.7 **A-D**, Wright Medical Aequalis Perform+ neoreamer. The interchangeable reaming angle allows for preparation of the neoglenoid corresponding to the desired posterior half-wedge: (**A**) 15°, (**B**) 25°, and (**C**) 35°. **D**, Neoreamer.[44]

Posterior Stepped Glenoid

Sabesan et al performed a simulation analysis of correction obtained with a posterior augmented stepped component. Thirty patients who underwent ATSA with an augmented glenoid component had preoperative 3D-CT planning to compare correction with augmented and standard components to 0° (perpendicular) and 6° retroversion relative to the scapular plane. The augmented component corrected version with significantly less joint-line medialization than the standard component. The average medialization when retroversion was corrected to 0° was 8.3 ± 4.1 mm with use of the standard glenoid versus 3.8 ± 3.3 mm with the augmented glenoid component ($P < 0.001$). The average medialization with correction to 6° retroversion was 7.2 ± 4.2 mm for the standard glenoid versus 3.36 ± 2.9 mm with the augmented glenoid component ($P < 0.05$).[40] In a clinical study using standard radiographs, Ko et al compared the ability to correct version by AR with standard glenoid and posterior stepped augmented glenoid (PAG) components. In their assessment of 48 AR and 49 PAG patients, they found that mean version improved 6.8° in the AR group and mean version improved 8.8°, 13.4°, and 12.8° with 3, 5, and 7 mm augments, respectively, in the PAG group.[46] Stephens et al assessed 21 patients with a PAG using standard radiographs and found preoperative retroversion averaged 20.8° (range, 12°-37°), with mean postoperative version correction of 9° (range, 0°-32°).[47] Finally, in clinical and radiographic assessment of 71 patients with Walch B2 and B3 glenoids, Ho et al showed mean improvement in glenoid version from −24° ± 7° to −11° ± 6° ($P < 0.0001$), with 52 (73%) of the 71 shoulders having less than 15° of glenoid retroversion postoperatively.[30]

Full-Wedged Glenoid

Grey et al assessed plain radiographic outcomes of 68 patients undergoing primary ATSA with OA and a Walch B glenoid deformity who were treated with an 8° posteriorly augmented glenoid. The average native glenoid retroversion for the Walch B glenoid patients was 17.3° ± 5.9°, with B3 glenoids being observed to have significantly more retroversion than both B1 (21.3° vs 13.7°, $P < 0.0005$) and B2 (21.3° vs 17.0°, $P < 0.0300$) glenoid types. At latest follow-up, the average glenoid retroversion for the augmented glenoid patients was 4.8° ± 7.3°, with no difference in glenoid version observed between Walch B glenoid types.[48]

Posterior Wedged Glenoid

Das et al. assessed a noncommercial posterior half-wedged component in 11 TSAs in 10 patients and found a mean preoperative retroversion of 16° (13°-23°) corrected to a mean of 0° postoperatively with 63% having radiological correction (0°-5°) of retroversion.[49]

Biomechanical Assessment and Finite Element Analysis of Augmented Glenoids

Posterior Stepped and Full-Wedged Glenoid

Multiple studies have assessed augmented glenoid designs biomechanically in the setting of asymmetric posterior glenoid wear. A recent study compared a wedged posterior component to stepped component using finite element analysis (FEA). Both implants were tested with a simulated 20° retroverted glenoid model, and implant designs were fit to simulate desired retroversion correction using a +7 mm stepped design and 16° wedged design. The step design showed greater micromotion than the wedge design during simulated abduction; however, the wedge design provided less joint stability (36% less) than the step design as measured by force ratio.[50] Another FEA study compared a wedge augmented glenoid to a stepped augmented glenoid and standard glenoid placed in 0° version after reaming the high side.[51] The investigators found the wedge design had more backside contact and less volume of bone at risk for strain damage compared with the standard glenoid after reaming the high side, but no differences were seen between the wedge design and stepped design.[51] Another FEA study compared the wedged augment with a standard component in retroversion and found that the wedged augment required a smaller cement mantle and had greater bone fatigue life.[52] Finally, Iannotti et al assessed early and late fixation states in a biomechanical study of stepped augmented components compared with spherical asymmetric, spherical symmetric, flat angled, and standard pegged implants. Implants were assessed for resistance to anterior liftoff when posteriorly loaded. The stepped augmented component had decreased anterior glenoid liftoff compared with the other designs, and the authors concluded the design may lead to improved long-term durability.[53]

Posterior Wedged Glenoid Compared to Other Designs

In looking at all three designs, Knowles et al performed a modeling study comparing the commercially available augmented glenoids (full wedge, stepped, and posterior wedge). Components were placed in B2 glenoids corrected to 0° version, and the amount of bone removal and bone quality remaining was assessed. They demonstrated the posterior wedge design resulted in less bone removal compared with the full-wedge and stepped designs. Remaining posterior bone density was noted to be higher with the stepped design.[54,55] In a more recent FEA study of a full-wedge, stepped, and posterior wedge glenoid, this group showed the posterior wedge implant resulted in the lowest amount of reactive posterior glenoid bony displacement. With anterior directed loads, anterior liftoff was decreased and neoglenoid bone displacements were reduced in all implants.[56]

Correction of Anatomy: Bone Graft With Glenoid Component Placement

Posterior glenoid bone grafting is a technically demanding method to correct deformity too severe to treat with AR and is an alternative to use of augmented glenoid components in ATSA. The glenoid is exposed and the needed size bone graft measured (**FIGURE 14.8A-C**). A portion of bone autograft from the resected humeral head is measured, cut, and contoured to fit the glenoid defect (**FIGURE 14.8D** and **E**). The graft is secured to the glenoid with cannulated screws (**FIGURE 14.8F** and **G**) superiorly and inferiorly passed in a posterior to anterior direction. The grafted glenoid is gently reamed and prepared, and a standard glenoid component is placed (**FIGURE 14.8H-J**). Correcting glenoid retroversion and bone loss is dependent upon graft union.[32] Five case series have evaluated the use of posterior bone graft in ATSA and have shown good clinical results at short- to midterm follow-up, but complications of incomplete graft incorporation, graft resorption, and high glenoid radiolucencies persist.[57-61] We will discuss additional details on outcomes later in this chapter.

Treatment Without Correction of Glenoid Anatomy: Inset Glenoid Prosthesis

In cases with severe retroversion from dysplasia or bone loss, correction with AR may further reduce bone stock, and use of an augmented glenoid may lead to vault perforation of multiple pegs.[62] Newer inlay glenoid components have been proposed as an alternative, showing less edge loading force compared to onlay implants and less loosening with cyclic loading ($P < 0.0001$).[63] Good clinical outcomes for both symmetric and asymmetric glenoid OA have been seen in short case series.[64,65] This concept is detailed in Chapter 18.

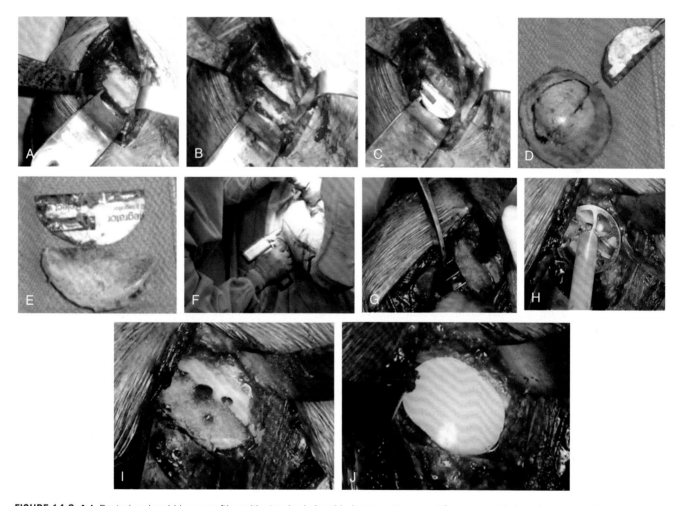

FIGURE 14.8 A-J, Posterior glenoid bone grafting with standard glenoid placement to correct for asymmetric bone loss and pathologic retroversion. **A,** Glenoid exposure and identification of neoglenoid bone loss. **B,** Step cut prepared neoglenoid. **C,** Sterile paper utilized for measurement of bone graft dimensions. **D,** Native humeral head used as donor site for glenoid bone autograft with measured template. **E,** Comparison of template and prepared donor autograft for glenoid. **F,** Percutaneous technique for cannulated screw fixation of glenoid bone graft. **G,** Glenoid bone graft following cannulate wire placement. **H,** Reaming of native glenoid and graft to create uniform bony backside support for glenoid implant. **I,** Glenoid following bone grafting and drilling of central peg and peripheral pegs. **J,** Final glenoid implant after cementation to bone grafted glenoid.

OUTCOMES FOR EACH TREATMENT METHOD (ASYMMETRIC REAMING, AUGMENTED GLENOID IMPLANT, AND BONE GRAFTING)

Asymmetric Reaming With Standard Glenoid Implant

Walch et al assessed 92 ATSAs in 75 patients with B2 glenoids treated with AR at a mean of 77 months (range, 14-180 months). The mean Constant score improved significantly (32.4-68.8) at final follow-up (P = 0.0001), but 15 revisions (16.3%) were performed for glenoid loosening (6.5%), posterior instability (5.5%), or soft-tissue problems (4.3%). Glenoid loosening was observed in 20.6% and was significantly associated with posterior bone erosion in depth (P = 0.005), humeral head subluxation (P = 0.01), and glenoid retroversion (P = 0.001).[34] Recently, Orvets et al evaluated 92 patients with B2 glenoids treated with ATSA and high-side corrective reaming at average 50-month follow-up (range, 24-97 months). Goals of surgery were final retroversion of 10° to 15° or less and minimum 80% backside glenoid component support. Fifty-two patients showed mean improvement in American Shoulder and Elbow Surgeon (ASES) scores from 35.4 to 84.3, and Simple Shoulder Test (SST) score improved from 4.5 to 9.1. No difference was found in the rate of progression of glenoid radiolucencies on radiographs between shoulders with a preoperative glenoid retroversion of less than or equal to 20° (27.8%) compared to those with greater than 20° (22.7%, P = 0.670). No shoulders were revised for glenoid loosening or instability.[35] Chin et al assessed 104 type B (B1 and B2) glenoids with use of corrective reaming and standard glenoid implants. Glenoids were asymmetrically reamed to achieve retroversion of 0° to 10° with removal of less than 5 mm of bone. At mean 60-month follow-up (range, 23-120 months), significant improvement in pre- and postoperative QuickDASH scores was seen, with no difference when comparing B1 to B2 morphology. However, 51.5% of the B1 glenoids and 47.9% of the B2 glenoids demonstrated glenoid loosening with incomplete radiolucent lines on plain radiographs.[36]

Augmented Glenoids

In an assessment of 21 patients (19 B2 glenoids, 2 C glenoids), Stephens et al showed significant improvements in ASES scores, SST, range of motion (ROM), pain, glenoid version, humeral head alignment, and no glenoid failures at a mean of 35 months of follow-up with a stepped augment glenoid in ATSA.[47] Similarly, Favorito et al reported on 22 shoulders (20 B2 glenoids, 2 C glenoids) using stepped augmented glenoids. At a mean of 36 months of follow-up, patients showed significant improvements in visual analog scale, Western Ontario Osteoarthritis of the Shoulder (WOOS) index, 36-Item Short Form, and ROM. This series showed low glenoid lucency rates and two reported cases of implant instability.[66]

Two studies assessed the use of full-wedge augmented glenoids for correction in ATSA. Grey et al showed average preoperative-to-postoperative glenoid retroversion correction of 12.6° ± 8.4° at mean 50-month follow-up.[48] The second study showed improvement in Constant scores from 47.6 ± 15.0 to 82.7 ± 12.9 (P = 0.016) and ASES scores from 45.3 ± 12.3 to 86.8 ± 14.7 (P = 0.04) at average follow-up of 38 months.[67]

In the largest study to date, Ho et al assessed 71 patients with median 2.4-year follow-up (range, 1.9-5.7 years), with B2 and B3 glenoids treated with ATSA using a posterior augmented step glenoid. The Penn Shoulder Score (PSS) improved from a median of 30 (interquartile range [IQR], 16-43) to 94 (IQR = 88-98) (P < 0.0001). Glenoid version measured on plain radiographs improved from −24° ± 7° (range, −42° to −9°) to −11° ± 6° (range, −28° to 1°). Posterior humeral head subluxation was present in 60 of 71 shoulders (85%) preoperatively, with prosthetic humeral head centering seen in 60 of 71 shoulders (85%) postoperatively (P < 0.0001). Of 71 shoulders, 64 shoulders (90%) had a PSS of 80 or higher, 52 shoulders (73%) had postoperative glenoid retroversion less than 15°, and only 11 shoulders (15%) had center peg osteolysis. ROM improved from a median forward elevation of 110° preoperatively (IQR, 90°-140°; range, 60°-170°) to 160° postoperatively (IQR, 150°-170°; range, 90°-180°) and from median external rotation of 20° (IQR, 10°-30°; range, 0°-60°) to 50° (IQR, 40°-60°; range, 10°-80°; P < 0.0001).[47] Patients with center peg osteolysis of the glenoid component had a greater amount of preoperative joint-line medialization (5.5 ± 2.7 mm vs 3.2 ± 2.5 mm; P = 0.024) and posterior glenoid bone loss (7.0 ± 2.0 mm vs 5.5 ± 2.3 mm; P = 0.032) compared to cases without center peg osteolysis. This study was the first to define the limitations of the step glenoid augmented implant relative to the severity of bone loss in OA.[30] We have subsequently evaluated a patient cohort undergoing postoperative 3D-CT analysis and demonstrated a higher rate of central peg osteolysis at minimum 2-year follow-up in B3 glenoids with a posterior augmented step component, with greater postoperative joint-line medialization in the B3 glenoids with augmented components compared to B2 glenoids with augmented components. The shape of the posterior augmented step component can better match the biconcave deformity of the B2 glenoid when compared to the monoconcave deformity of the B3 glenoid, making it more difficult to restore the native joint line in a B3 glenoid with this implant in the setting of moderate to severe posterior glenoid bone loss[68-70] (**FIGURE 14.9A-E**).

Glenoid Bone Grafting With Standard Implant

Five case series have reported on posterior glenoid bone grafting in ATSA.[57-61] The earliest studies reported good results in 82% to 84% of patients with complete graft integration. However, incomplete glenoid component

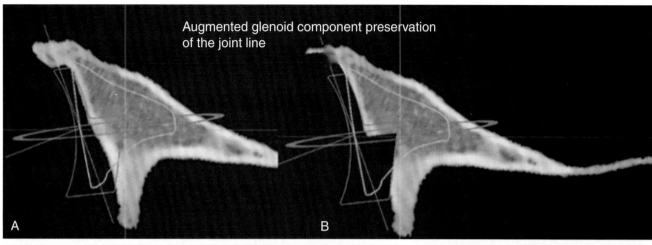

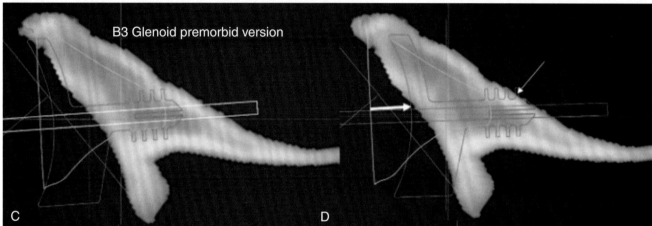

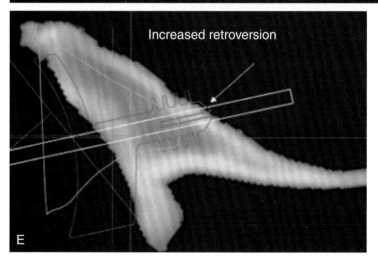

FIGURE 14.9 A, B2 glenoid after simulated placement of +5 mm posterior augmented stepped glenoid (StepTech APG, Depuy, Warsaw, IN, USA) prior to reaming of neoglenoid. **B**, B2 glenoid after simulated placement of +5 mm posterior augmented stepped glenoid with simulated neoglenoid reaming. Note full seating and backside support of glenoid component (pink) with restoration of native joint line and version represented by the vault model (blue). **C**, B3 glenoid with simulated +7 mm posterior augmented stepped glenoid with attempts to restore native joint line and version represented by vault model. Note incomplete seating of implant. **D**, Same B3 glenoid with simulated +7 mm posterior augmented stepped glenoid prior to reaming showing corrected retroversion but significant medialization to obtain complete seating resulting in central peg perforation (white arrow) and inability to restore native joint line. **E**, Same B3 glenoid with simulated +7 mm posterior augmented glenoid prior to simulated reaming placed with increased retroversion to obtain bony seating. Note medialization and central peg perforation (white arrow) in addition to increased retroversion.

lucent lines and glenoid component displacement were noted complications.[57,58] Sabesan et al reported good clinical results in 12 patients (9 B2 glenoids) with mean follow-up of 53 months. The mean preoperative glenoid retroversion improved from 44° to 21.3° postoperatively, mean PSS improved from 38.7 to 79.4, and mean forward flexion improved to 156°. Ten of 12 (83%) shoulders had graft incorporation without resorption and two had minor resorption. Failed graft fixation in two cases was attributed to early postoperative trauma and *Cutibacterium acnes* infection.[59] Klika et al reported favorable clinical outcomes in 23 of 25 shoulders (92%) at average follow-up of 8.7 years, despite 13 cases of postoperative GH subluxation, 20 cases of glenoid radiolucency, 6 cases of glenoid component shift, and 6 cases of bone graft resorption. The authors determined 10 glenoids (40%) were at risk for failure, 5 of which had metal-backed components.[60] Finally, Nicholson et al assessed 28 of 34 patients at minimum 2-year follow-up. Mean ASES improved from 39 ± 18 to 90 ± 10 ($P < 0.001$), forward elevation improved from 89° ± 24° to 149° ± 19°, and retroversion improved from a mean of 28° ± 4° to 4° ± 2° postoperatively. All bone grafts were noted to have integration despite five patients with broken screws.

AUTHORS PREFERRED SURGICAL TECHNIQUE

In cases of GH OA with moderate to severe asymmetric glenoid bone loss and retroversion, as seen in B2 glenoids, our preferred treatment technique is utilization of a posterior augmented component to restore the native version and joint line. Below we detail use of ATSA with a stepped augmented glenoid component. The clinical outcomes of this technique have been described above in the study by Ho et al.[30]

Preoperative 3D-CT Planning

We routinely use 3D-CT imaging for preoperative planning in cases of moderate to severe posterior glenoid bone loss. Multiple prior studies utilizing 3D-CT have shown more accurate assessment of glenoid anatomy and improved surgeon ability to place the planned glenoid implant in the desired location.[71-73] We believe this surgical tool allows optimal implant choice based on the degree of pathologic correction and a detailed assessment of the proposed implant to restore the premorbid version and joint line with the use of an augmented or standard glenoid (**FIGURE 14.9A-E**).

Operative Technique

A standard deltopectoral approach is utilized. The subscapularis is mobilized via lesser tuberosity osteotomy (LTO), allowing release of the underlying capsule from the muscle and tendon of the subscapularis and bone-to-bone healing at the time of repair. The capsule is carefully released along the anatomic neck of the humeral head as posterior as possible to allow for maximal glenoid exposure via increased posterior humeral retraction. The humeral head is dislocated, osteophytes are removed from the anatomic neck, and the native humeral head is marked. The humeral head is osteotomized at approximately 20° to 30° of retroversion, exiting approximately 2 to 3 mm above the superior and posterior rotator cuff reflection (ie, bare spot of posterior humeral head). The humeral cut protector is applied and attention turned to the glenoid.

Appropriate glenoid exposure is vital to attaining optimal glenoid preparation and placement of an augmented glenoid component. A glenoid retractor is placed along the posterior inferior border of the glenoid to displace the humerus posteriorly out of the surgical field. Another glenoid retractor is placed along the anterior glenoid rim for exposure and to protect the axillary nerve. We regularly perform a resection of the anterior and inferior joint capsule to maximize glenoid exposure (**FIGURE 14.10A**). The plane between the subscapularis and anterior capsule is developed with care to protect the axillary nerve during dissection. The anterior and inferior capsule and entire labrum are excised (**FIGURE 14.10B**). The posterior capsule is released as needed for visualization. A superior glenoid retractor is placed to fully visualize the glenoid face. Residual soft tissue is removed to precisely inspect the neo- and paleoglenoid (**FIGURE 14.10B**). The central glenoid guide pin is placed using standard or patient-specific instrumentation (PSI) as determined by the 3D-CT preoperative plan (**FIGURE 14.10C**). Use of a posterior step augmented glenoid (StepTech, DePuy Synthes, Warsaw, IN) is performed in a cannulated fashion, and the anterior paleoglenoid is reamed to a level defined by the planning software and the shape of the augmented glenoid component (**FIGURE 14.10D**). The centering hole for the central anchor peg is then drilled over the guide pin, and the guide pin is removed.

A posterior reaming guide for the neoglenoid is next placed into the center hole and secured with antirotation pins (**FIGURE 14.10E**). The neoglenoid is prepared with a high-speed burr/rasp for the appropriate posterior step augmented glenoid (3, 5, or 7 mm). The high-speed burr is useful to remove bone centrally initially, where the majority of bone is removed to create the posterior step cut, with the guided rasp reamer (**FIGURE 14.10F**) used to finish the step cut. Peripheral holes for the anchor peg glenoid are drilled (**FIGURE 14.10G**) with a guide, and the glenoid trial is placed to ensure appropriate seating of the component. Peg holes are irrigated and dried, then peripheral holes are filled with pressurized cement, and the grooves of the center anchor peg are filled with cancellous autograft bone prior to final impaction (**FIGURE 14.10H**). After the glenoid component is placed (**FIGURE 14.10I**), we complete the humeral preparation. The trial humeral implant should be reduced to assess for proper soft-tissue tensioning prior to placement of the final implant. Subscapularis repair of the LTO is done through bone tunnels and use of multiple nonabsorbable sutures passed around the implant with closure of the rotator interval.

Expert Pearls

Glenoid exposure, including capsular release and retractor positioning, is crucial to precise placement of augmented glenoids. Glenoid exposure can be more difficult depending on the amount of posterior humeral head subluxation and patient size. In large muscular males, exposure can be difficult due to the deltoid muscle belly or a tight posterior capsule. Posterior capsular release should be dependent on the amount of humeral head subluxation and soft-tissue laxity and may be needed for adequate glenoid visualization. Full anterior and inferior capsulectomy (**FIGURE 14.10A**) and circumferential removal of the labrum are important for maximal glenoid exposure and preparation (**FIGURE 14.10B**).

Appropriate reaming of the paleoglenoid is important to allow for complete seating of the implant while allowing for preservation of as much of the cortical bone as possible. With a stepped augmented glenoid, using a high-speed burr can aid with initial shaping of the posterior step, followed by use of the manufacturer's reamer to finish the step cut. The high-speed burr can also be used to correct any bony imperfections in the step cut to ensure full backside implant seating. Selecting the optimal sized posterior augment is important to allow for correction of retroversion, preservation of posterior bone, and minimization of joint-line medialization. This can all be achieved by 3D-CT preoperative planning and implant templating. Use of PSI or computer navigation intraoperatively can also improve the ability of the surgery to accurately execute the preoperative plan.

Pitfalls and Bailouts/Salvage

Release of the posterior capsule should not be performed with use of a standard glenoid when residual glenoid retroversion or significant joint-line medialization remains. This can result in postoperative humeral head instability or residual posterior humeral head translation. Posterior release of the capsule should be reserved for cases where use of augmented glenoid components will result in correction of retroversion without significant joint-line medialization. For a stepped augmented glenoid, care should be taken to prevent disruptions of the posterior glenoid rim with preservation of the better cortical bone to ensure good implant backside support. With a stepped glenoid, neoglenoid preparation should focus on central bone removal to create the posterior step (**FIGURE 14.10F**). Selecting the correct augment size is imperative. Too small a posterior augment may lead to incomplete

version correction, while too large an augment can result in excessive posterior bone removal causing peg perforation and inadequate bone support.

If posterior instability is present when trialing the humeral component, the first step is to perform a posterior capsulorrhaphy with three purse-string sutures placed and tied in the midportion of the posterior capsule. These sutures should be placed 1 cm apart from superior to inferior, thereby shortening the anteroposterior dimension of the posterior capsule. Following this salvage, use of an external rotation brace is commonly needed for 4 weeks postoperatively. Use of a larger or "soft-tissue balancing" humeral head is a less desirable option to gain stability, as this can lead to tightening of the anterior soft tissues and overstuffing of the joint but can be a secondary bailout option. Increasing humeral anteversion has been advocated as another salvage option, but it is the least effective given the very short lateral humeral offset in all anatomic stems. The need for these bailout options can be avoided by selecting the optimal augmented implant to avoid undercorrection of version and/or medialization of the joint line.

Postoperative Care and Rehabilitation

Standard rehabilitation for ATSA is instituted after surgery. Passive supine forward flexion up to 120°, protected passive external rotation limited to 30°, and pendulum exercises are initiated on postoperative day 1. Six weeks after surgery, ROM exercises are advanced and a gentle strengthening regimen is initiated. Strengthening is advanced at 3 months, and typically patients are released to activity as tolerated by 6 months postoperatively. Routine clinical and radiographic follow-up is continued at 1, 2, and 5 years postoperatively, and every 5 years afterward to monitor for component loosening or clinical status. Obtaining a high-quality axillary view in the early postoperative period (within 4 weeks) is important to evaluate the location and healing of the LTO.

Clinical and Radiographic Outcomes of the Technique

The clinical and radiographic outcomes of our surgical technique have been described above in Section 3, including the study by Ho et al and our postoperative CT analysis.[37]

CONCLUSION

Asymmetric glenoid deformity in GH OA remains a treatment challenge for surgeons. Multiple options are available for addressing deformity with ATSA, particularly in the setting of increased retroversion and posterior bone loss as encountered in patterns such as the B2 glenoid. In cases with mild posterior glenoid bone loss and retroversion, eccentric reaming with use of a standard glenoid component can address the glenoid pathology without significant bone removal and medialization

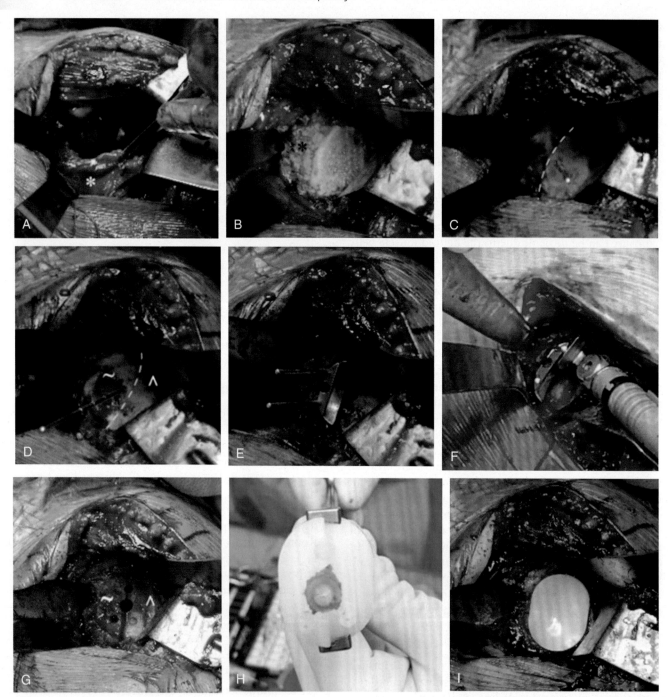

FIGURE 14.10 A, Isolation of the anterior inferior capsule (white *) prior to resection to aid in glenoid exposure. **B,** Exposed glenoid prior to reaming with seen with posterior bone loss of neoglenoid and paleoglenoid anteriorly (black *). **C,** Demonstration of biconcavity of B2 glenoid (white dashed line demarcating transition of paleoglenoid to neoglenoid with typical posterior inferior bone loss). **D,** Glenoid after anterior paleo-glenoid reaming (white ~) to position corresponding to three-dimensional computed tomography (3D-CT) plan (yellow dashed line) and prior to reaming of the posterior neoglenoid (white ^). **E,** Glenoid with step reaming guide sitting flush on reamed anterior glenoid surface. **F,** Reaming of neoglenoid using posterior reaming guide and manufacture's oscillating rasp. **G,** Final glenoid preparation with peripheral peg holes drilled, reamed paleoglenoid (white ~), and posterior step cut of paleoglenoid (white ^). **H,** En face view of the glenoid component with reamings in the central anchor peg. **I,** Implanted glenoid component.

of the joint line. However, we believe that correction of pathology to restore both premorbid joint line and version is best accomplished with use of a posterior augmented glenoid component when moderate to severe posterior glenoid bone loss and retroversion are present in the B2 glenoid. The goal for all surgeons should be to minimize bone loss and restore function at the time of surgery.

REFERENCES

1. Collins DN. Pathophysiology, classification, and pathoanatomy of glenohumeral arthritis and related disorders. In: Iannotti JP, ed. *Disorders of the Shoulder: Diagnosis & Management Volume 1-Shoulder Reconstruction.* 3rd ed. Lippincott Williams & Wilkins; 2014:222-285.
2. Walch G, Badet R, Boulahia A, Khoury A. Morphologic study of the glenoid in primary glenohumeral osteoarthritis. *J Arthroplasty.* 1999;14(6):756-760.
3. Beuckelaers E, Jacxsens M, Van Tongel A, De Wilde LF. Three-dimensional computed tomography scan evaluation of the pattern of erosion in type B glenoids. *J Shoulder Elbow Surg.* 2014;23(1):109-116.
4. Scalise JJ, Codsi MJ, Brems JJ, Iannotti JP. Inter-rater reliability of an arthritic glenoid morphology classification system. *J Shoulder Elbow Surg.* 2008;17(4):575-577.
5. Nowak DD, Gardner TR, Bigliani LU, Levine WN, Ahmad CS. Interobserver and Intraobserver reliability of the Walch classification in primary glenohumeral arthritis. *J Shoulder Elbow Surg.* 2010;19(2):180-183.
6. Bercik MJ, Kruse K II, Yalizis M, Gauci MO, Chaoui J, Walch G. A modification to the Walch classification of the glenoid in primary glenohumeral osteoarthritis using three-dimensional imaging. *J Shoulder Elbow Surg.* 2016;25(10):1601-1606.
7. Iannotti JP, Jun BJ, Patterson TE, Ricchetti ET. Quantitative measurement of osseous pathology in advanced glenohumeral osteoarthritis. *J Bone Joint Surg Am.* 2017;99(17):1460-1468.
8. Nyffeler RW, Jost B, Pfirrmann CW, Gerber C. Measurement of glenoid version: conventional radiographs versus computed tomography scans. *J Shoulder Elbow Surg.* 2003;12(5):493-496.
9. Aronowitz JG, Harmsen WS, Schleck CD, Sperling JW, Cofield RH, Sanchez-Sotelo J. Radiographs and computed tomography scans show similar observer agreement when classifying glenoid morphology in glenohumeral arthritis. *J Shoulder Elbow Surg.* 2017;26(9):1533-1538.
10. Shukla DR, McLaughlin RJ, Lee J, Cofield RH, Sperling JW, Sanchez-Sotelo J. Intraobserver and interobserver reliability of the modified Walch classification using radiographs and computed tomography. *J Shoulder Elbow Surg.* 2019;28(4):625-630.
11. Kopka M, Fourman M, Soni A, Cordle AC, Lin A. Can glenoid wear be accurately assessed using x-ray imaging? Evaluating agreement of x-ray and magnetic resonance imaging (MRI) Walch classification. *J Shoulder Elbow Surg.* 2017;26(9):1527-1532.
12. Mahylis JM, Entezari V, Jun BJ, Iannotti JP, Ricchetti ET. Imaging of the B2 Glenoid: an assessment of glenoid wear. *J Shoulder Elbow Arthroplast.* 2019;3(1):1-9.
13. Budge MD, Lewis GS, Schaefer E, Coquia S, Flemming DJ, Armstrong AD. Comparison of standard two dimensional and three-dimensional corrected glenoid version measurements. *J Shoulder Elbow Surg.* 2011;20(4):577-583.
14. Chalmers PN, Salazar D, Chamberlain A, Keener JD. Radiographic characterization of the B2 glenoid: the effect of computed tomographic axis orientation. *J Shoulder Elbow Surg.* 2017;26(2):258-264.
15. Ganapathi A, McCarron JA, Chen X, Iannotti JP. Predicting normal glenoid version from the pathologic scapula: a comparison of 4 methods in 2- and 3-dimensional models. *J Shoulder Elbow Surg.* 2011;20(2):234-244.
16. Kwon YW, Powell KA, Yum JK, Brems JJ, Iannotti JP. Use of three-dimensional computed tomography for the analysis of the glenoid anatomy. *Shoulder Elbow Surg.* 2005;14(1):85-90.
17. Raymond AC, McCann PA, Sarangi PP. Magnetic resonance scanning vs axillary radiography in the assessment of glenoid version for osteoarthritis. *J Shoulder Elbow Surg.* 2013;22(8):1078-1083.
18. Lowe JT, Testa EJ, Li X, Miller S, DeAngelis JP, Jawa A. Magnetic resonance imaging is comparable to computed tomography for determination of glenoid version but does not accurately distinguish between Walch B2 and C classifications. *J Shoulder Elbow Surg.* 2017;26(4):669-673.
19. Neer CS II, Watson KC, Stanton FJ. Recent experience in total shoulder replacement. *J Bone Joint Surg Am.* 1982;64:319-337.
20. Sabesan VJ, Callanan M, Youderian A, Iannotti JP. 3D CT assessment of the relationship between humeral head alignment and glenoid retroversion in glenohumeral osteoarthritis. *J Bone Joint Surg Am.* 2014;96(8):e64.
21. Chan K, Knowles NK, Chaoui J, et al. Characterization of the Walch B3 glenoid in primary osteoarthritis. *J Shoulder Elbow Surg.* 2017;26(5):909-914.
22. Kerr R, Resnick D, Pineda C, Haghighi P. Osteoarthritis of the glenohumeral joint: a radiologic-pathologic study. *AJR Am J Roentgenol.* 1985;144(5):967-972.
23. Petersson CJ. Degeneration of the glenohumeral joint. An anatomical study. *Acta Orthop Scand.* 1983;54(2):277-283.
24. Oh JH, Chung SW, Oh CH, et al. The prevalence of shoulder osteoarthritis in the elderly Korean population: association with risk factors and function. *J Shoulder Elbow Surg.* 2011;20(5):756-763.
25. Cushnaghan J, Dieppe P. Study of 500 patients with limb joint osteoarthritis. I. Analysis by age, sex, and distribution of symptomatic joint sites. *Ann Rheum Dis.* 1991;50(1):8-13.
26. Nakagawa Y, Hyakuna K, Otani S, Hashitani M, Nakamura T. Epidemiologic study of glenohumeral osteoarthritis with plain radiography. *J Shoulder Elbow Surg.* 1999;8(6):580-584.
27. Schoenfeldt TL, Trenhaile S, Olson R. Glenohumeral osteoarthritis: frequency of underlying diagnoses and the role of arm dominance-a retrospective analysis in a community-based musculoskeletal practice. *Rheumatol Int.* 2018;38(6):1023-1029.
28. Walker KE, Simcock XC, Jun BJ, Iannotti JP, Ricchetti ET. Progression of glenoid morphology in glenohumeral osteoarthritis. *J Bone Joint Surg Am.* 2018;100(1):49-56.
29. Donohue KW, Ricchetti ET, Ho JC, Iannotti JP. The association between rotator cuff muscle fatty infiltration and glenoid morphology in glenohumeral osteoarthritis. *J Bone Joint Surg Am.* 2018;100(5):381-387.
30. Ho JC, Amini MH, Entezari V, et al. Clinical and radiographic outcomes of a posteriorly augmented glenoid component in anatomic total shoulder arthroplasty for primary osteoarthritis with posterior glenoid bone loss. *J Bone Joint Surg Am.* 2018;100(22):1934-1948.
31. Ansok CB, Muh SJ. Optimal management of glenohumeral osteoarthritis. *Orthop Res Rev.* 2018;10:9-18.
32. Donohue KW, Ricchetti ET, Iannotti JP. Surgical management of the biconcave (B2) glenoid. *Curr Rev Musculoskelet Med.* 2016;9(1):30-39.
33. Nowak DD, Bahu MJ, Gardner TR, et al. Simulation of surgical glenoid resurfacing using three-dimensional computed tomography of the arthritic glenohumeral joint: the amount of glenoid retroversion that can be corrected. *J Should Elbow Surg.* 2009;18:680-688.
34. Walch G, Moraga C, Young A, Castellanos-Rosas J. Results of anatomic nonconstrained prosthesis in primary osteoarthritis with biconcave glenoid. *J Shoulder Elbow Surg.* 2012;21(11):1526-1533.
35. Orvets ND, Chamberlain AM, Patterson BM, et al. Total shoulder arthroplasty in patients with a B2 glenoid addressed with corrective reaming. *J Shoulder Elbow Surg.* 2018;27(6S):S58-S64.
36. Chin PC, Hachadorian ME, Pulido PA, Munro ML, Meric G, Hoenecke HR Jr. Outcomes of anatomic shoulder arthroplasty in primary osteoarthritis in type B glenoids. *J Shoulder Elbow Surg.* 2015;24(12):1888-1893.
37. Gillespie R, Lyons R, Lazarus M. Eccentric reaming in total shoulder arthroplasty: a cadaveric study. *Orthopedics.* 2009;32(1):21.
38. Walch G, Young AA, Boileau P, Loew M, Gazielly D, Mole D. Patterns of loosening of polyethylene keeled glenoid components after shoulder arthroplasty for primary osteoarthritis: results of a multicenter study with more than 5 years of follow-up. *J Bone Joint Surg Am.* 2012;94:145-150.
39. Strauss EJ, Roche C, Flurin PH, Wright T, Zuckerman JD. The glenoid in shoulder arthroplasty. *J Shoulder Elbow Surg.* 2009;18:819-833.
40. Sabesan V, Callanan M, Sharma V, Iannotti JP. Correction of acquired glenoid bone loss in osteoarthritis with a standard vs. an augmented glenoid component. *J Shoulder Elbow Surg.* 2014;23(7):964-973.

41. Cil A, Sperling J, Cofield R. Nonstandard glenoid components for bone deficiencies in shoulder arthroplasty. *J Shoulder Elbow Surg.* 2014;23:e149-e157.

42. Ghoraishian M, Abboud JA, Romeo AA, Williams GR, Namdari S. Augmented glenoid implants in anatomic total shoulder arthroplasty: review of available implants and current literature. *J Shoulder Elbow Surg.* 2019;28(2):387-395.

43. Johnson & Johnson Medical Device Companies. DePuy Global Steptech APG Shoulder System. Accessed April 10, 2020. https://www.jnjmedicaldevices.com/en-US/product/globalr-steptechr-apg-shoulder-system

44. Exachtech. Equinoxe Posterior Augment Glenoid Operative Technique. Accessed April 10, 2020. https://www.exac.com/wp-content/uploads/2020/10/718-01-32_RevD_Equinoxe_Posterior_Augment_Glenoid_Operative_Technique.pdf

45. Wright Medical. Aequalis Perform+. Surgical Technique. Accessed April 10, 2020. http://www.wrightemedia.com/ProductFiles/Files/PDFs/CAW-3876_EN_LR_LE.pdf

46. Kevin Ko JW, Syed UA, Barlow JD, et al. Comparison of asymmetric reaming versus a posteriorly augmented component for posterior glenoid wear and retroversion: a radiographic study. *Arch Bone Jt Surg.* 2019;7(4):307-313.

47. Stephens SP, Spencer EE, Wirth MA. Radiographic results of augmented all-polyethylene glenoids in the presence of posterior glenoid bone loss during total shoulder arthroplasty. *J Shoulder Elbow Surg.* 2017;26(5):798-803.

48. Grey SG, Wright TW, Flurin PH, Zuckerman JD, Roche CP, Friedman RJ. Clinical and radiographic outcomes with a posteriorly augmented glenoid for Walch B glenoids in anatomic total shoulder arthroplasty. *J Shoulder Elbow Surg.* 2020;29(5):e185-e195.

49. Das AK, Wright AC, Singh J, Monga P. Does posterior half-wedge augmented glenoid restore version and alignment in total shoulder arthroplasty for the B2 glenoid? *J Clin Orthop Trauma.* 2020;11(suppl 2):S275-S279.

50. Sabesan VJ, Lima DJL, Whaley JD, Pathak V, Zhang L. Biomechanical comparison of 2 augmented glenoid designs: an integrated kinematic finite element analysis. *J Shoulder Elbow Surg.* 2019;28(6):1166-1174.

51. Allred JJ, Flores-Hernandez C, Hoenecke HR, D'Lima DD. Posterior augmented glenoid implants require less bone removal and generate lower stresses: a finite element analysis. *J Shoulder Elbow Surg.* 2016;25(5):823-830.

52. Hermida JC, Flores-Hernandez C, Hoenecke HR, D'Lima DD. Augmented wedge-shaped glenoid component for the correction of glenoid retroversion: a finite element analysis. *J Shoulder Elbow Surg.* 2014;23(3):347-354.

53. Iannotti JP, Lappin KE, Klotz CL, Reber EW, Swope SW. Liftoff resistance of augmented glenoid components during cyclic fatigue loading in the posterior-superior direction. *J Shoulder Elbow Surg.* 2013;22(11):1530-1536.

54. Knowles NK, Ferreira LM, Athwal GS. Augmented glenoid component designs for type B2 erosions: a computational comparison by volume of bone removal and quality of remaining bone. *J Shoulder Elbow Surg.* 2015;24(8):1218-1226.

55. Knowles NK, Ferreira LM, Athwal GS. The arthritic glenoid: anatomy and arthroplasty designs. *Curr Rev Musculoskelet Med.* 2016;9(1):23-29.

56. Knowles NK, Langohr GDG, Athwal GS, Ferreira LM. A finite element analysis of augmented glenoid components. *J Shoulder Elbow Surg.* 2016;25(6): e166-e168.

57. Neer CS II, Morrison DS. Glenoid bone-grafting in total shoulder arthroplasty. *J Bone Joint Surg Am.* 1988;70A:1154-1162.

58. Steinmann SP, Cofield RH. Bone grafting for glenoid deficiency in total shoulder replacement. *J Shoulder Elbow Surg.* 2000;9:361-367.

59. Sabesan V, Callanan M, Ho J, Iannotti JP. Clinical and radiographic outcomes of total shoulder arthroplasty with bone graft for osteoarthritis with severe glenoid bone loss. *J Bone Joint Surg Am.* 2013;95:1290-1296.

60. Klika BJ, Wooten CW, Sperling JW, et al. Structural bone grafting for glenoid deficiency in primary total shoulder arthroplasty. *J Shoulder Elbow Surg.* 2014;23:1066-1072.

61. Nicholson GP, Cvetanovich GL, Rao AJ, O'Donnell P. Posterior glenoid bone grafting in total shoulder arthroplasty for osteoarthritis with severe posterior glenoid wear. *J Shoulder Elbow Surg.* 2017;26(10):1844-1853.

62. Papadonikolakis A, Neradilek MB, Matsen FA. Failure of the glenoid component in anatomic total shoulder arthroplasty: a systematic review of the English-language literature between 2006 and 2012. *J Bone Joint Surg Am.* 2013;95:2205-2212.

63. Gagliano JR, Helms SM, Colbath GP, Przestrzelski BT, Hawkins RJ, DesJardins JD. A comparison of onlay versus inlay glenoid component loosening in total shoulder arthroplasty. *J Shoulder Elbow Surg.* 2017;26(7):1113-1120.

64. Davis DE, Acevedo D, Williams A, Williams G. Total shoulder arthroplasty using an inlay mini-glenoid component for glenoid deficiency: a 2-year follow-up of 9 shoulders in 7 patients. *J Shoulder Elbow Surg.* 2016;25(8):1354-1361.

65. Cvetanovich GL, Naylor AJ, O'Brien MC, Waterman BR, Garcia GH, Nicholson GP. Anatomic total shoulder arthroplasty with an inlay glenoid component: clinical outcomes and return to activity. *J Shoulder Elbow Surg.* 2020;29(6):1188-1196.

66. Favorito PJ, Freed RJ, Passanise AM, Brown MJ. Total shoulder arthroplasty for glenohumeral arthritis associated with posterior glenoid bone loss: results of an all-polyethylene, posteriorly augmented glenoid component. *J Shoulder Elbow Surg.* 2016;25(10):1681-1689.

67. Priddy M, Zarezadeh A, Farmer KW. et al. Early results of augmented anatomic glenoid components. *J Shoulder Elbow Surg.* 2019;28(6S):S138-S145.

68. Iannotti JP, Jun BJ, Derwin KA, Ricchetti ET. Stepped augmented glenoid component in anatomic total shoulder arthroplasty for the B2 and B3 glenoid pathology: radiographic and clinical outcome (in prep).

69. Ricchetti ET, Jun BJ, Jin Y, Ho JC, Patterson TE, Dalton JE, Derwin KA, Iannotti JP. Three-dimensional computed tomography analysis of the relationship between glenoid component shift and osteolysis following anatomic total shoulder arthroplasty (Submitted to JBJS).

70. Ricchetti ET, Jun BJ, Jin Y, Entezari V, Patterson TE, Derwin KA, Iannotti JP. Three-dimensional computed tomography analysis of pathologic correction in total shoulder arthroplasty based on severity of preoperative pathology. *J Shoulder Elbow Surg.* 2020;S1058-2746(20)30628-5. doi:10.1016/j.jse.2020.07.033

71. Iannotti J, Baker J, Rodriguez E, Brems J, Ricchetti E, Mesiha M, Bryan J. Three-dimensional preoperative planning software and a novel information transfer technology improve glenoid component positioning. *J Bone Joint Surg Am.* 2014;96(9):e71.

72. Iannotti JP, Weiner S, Rodriguez E, et al. Three-dimensional imaging and templating improve glenoid implant positioning. *J Bone Joint Surg Am.* 2015;97(8):651-658.

73. Walch G, Vezeridis PS, Boileau P, Deransart P, Chaoui J. Three-dimensional planning and use of patient-specific guides improve glenoid component position: an in vitro study. *J Shoulder Elbow Surg.* 2015;24(2):302-309.

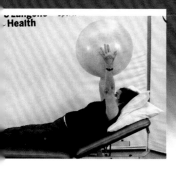

15 Postoperative Care and Rehabilitation

James Koo, PT, DPT and Laura Vasquez-Welsh, MS, OT/L, CHT

INTRODUCTION

Anatomic total shoulder arthroplasty (ATSA) has been well recognized as an excellent method of providing pain relief and improved function for glenohumeral (GH) osteoarthritis, inflammatory arthritis (eg, rheumatoid arthritis), and other arthropathies (eg, osteonecrosis).

The utilization of postoperative rehabilitation is often thought to be an important factor in the successful outcome of shoulder arthroplasty.[1-4] The physical or occupational therapists, in conjunction with input from the surgeon and patient, develop an individualized rehabilitation program consisting of a sequence of interventions to improve soft-tissue and joint mobility, dynamic GH joint stability, and strength around the shoulder complex.

The purpose of this chapter is to describe a phased progression of postoperative rehabilitation following ATSA to maximize the patient's ability to perform functional activities, and return to work (RTW), and recreational activities.

GENERAL REHABILITATION PRINCIPLES

While a consensus on general rehabilitation principles based on shoulder biomechanics, tissue healing times, and exercise loading strategies exists, there are several variations in the published protocols.[4-11] Ultimately, the goal of the rehabilitation process is to facilitate the patient's ability to return to full activities of daily living (ADLs), work and recreational activities, in a timely and safe manner. However, literature to support superior clinical outcomes of one rehabilitation protocol over another is limited. Therefore, the physical or occupational therapist must use the existing protocols as a general guide and work to individualize the rehabilitation progression to the patient.

The rehabilitation program involves a multiphased approach that progresses sequentially according to the principles of biological tissue healing, the surgical technique, and potential strain on the involved tissues. The protocol can be divided into five distinct phases, each with its own goals and objective criterion to progress to the next phase. Phase I focuses on the protection of the arthroplasty and initiation of passive range of motion (PROM). During this initial stage, the rehabilitation professional prioritizes the reduction of pain and inflammation along with the progressive restoration of PROM. Phase II advances the range of motion (ROM) from passive (PROM), to active-assisted (AAROM), to active (AROM) movements to allow for the gradual introduction of stress to the healing tissues. Treatment interventions focus on muscle activation, endurance, and neuromuscular control. When the patient can perform functional movement without compensation, the patient is ready to progress to the next phase. Improvements in AROM and function are contingent on improving the strength and control of the scapular muscles as well as the GH joint muscles. Phase III progresses periscapular and GH muscle strength by integrating resistance equipment such as dumbbells, elastic bands and cords, and manual resistance. Electromyography (EMG) studies have been used to identify exercises most appropriate for this phase of the rehabilitation. Once the patient achieves the necessary ROM and strength, advanced strengthening and activity-specific movements are performed to prepare the patients who plan to return to an occupation, activity, or sport with higher demands. Phase IV prepares the patient for return to their athletic activity or occupational demands by addressing deficits in power, agility, and speed. Phase V focuses on returning the athlete to preinjury sporting levels in a systematic method.

As the patient progresses through each phase, the exercises become more challenging and the stresses applied to the GH joint and shoulder complex are greater. The patient is reassessed at each therapy session to determine their response to the exercise progression, and when needed, the program is modified based on the patient's progress.

The time frames of each phase may vary depending on the patient's rate of progression. It is essential to manage expectations appropriately and continually involve the patient and their support team in decision-making to ensure high levels of motivation and engagement throughout the process.[12-14] Early in the rehabilitation process, physical or occupational therapists must educate patients on realistic time frames for improved function and return to work and sport. Steinhaus et al[15] reported that in 447 nonretired patients, approximately two-thirds (63.6%) of patients undergoing shoulder arthroplasty were able to RTW postoperatively. Patients returned at an average of 2.3 months postoperatively, with a wide range of 0.3 to 24 months. RTW was lower for patients with heavy-intensity occupations versus all intensity types (61.7% vs 67.6%). There was no significant difference in RTW among patients with ATSA (63.4%) and hemiarthroplasty (66.1%) or reverse total shoulder arthroplasty (61.5%).

If the patient is progressing slower than expected, the rehabilitation specialist should consider potential postoperative complications and be prepared to manage these problems swiftly should they arise. Westermann et al[16] reported that in a study of 2779 patients undergoing shoulder arthroplasty, 74 (2.66%) patients required unplanned readmissions within 30 days of surgery. The most common surgical causes for unplanned readmission were surgical site infections (18.6%), dislocations (16.3%), and venous thromboembolism (14.0%). Medical causes for readmission were responsible for 51% of unplanned readmissions. Therapists must continue to monitor for any signs and symptoms that may necessitate a referral back to the surgeon or primary care physician.[16,17]

POSTSURGICAL CONSIDERATIONS

An appropriate rehabilitation program accounts for the type of prothesis, surgical technique, and the information the surgeon provides regarding the intraoperative findings (eg, tissue status and ROM). This process is facilitated by an open line of communication between the surgeon and the rehabilitation professional. In addition, the surgeon and rehabilitation clinician should discuss any concomitant surgeries that may alter the standard protocol (eg, rotator cuff repair, biceps tenodesis) as well as any precautions before initiating treatment.

The therapist should be familiar with the referring surgeon's operative technique for shoulder arthroplasty, particularly as it pertains to gaining access to the GH joint. As described in previous chapters, surgeons generally use a deltopectoral approach and enter the GH joint through the subscapularis musculotendinous complex.[18-20] There are four common subscapularis management options: tenotomy, tendon peel, lesser tuberosity osteotomy, and subscapularis-sparing approaches.[18-20] When the subscapularis tendon or lesser tuberosity is involved, the therapist must take precautions to protect these structures during the postoperative rehabilitation process. To reduce stress on the healing tissues, the patient wears a sling to support the arm throughout the day. The clinician limits the external rotation (ER) ROM to a range based on what the surgeon determines to be safe based upon intraoperative assessment (typically less than 30°-40°). Internal rotation (IR) resistance exercises are avoided to minimize undue stress on the healing subscapularis.[2,4,5] Unfortunately, a potential negative outcome of approaches that detach and reattach the subscapularis is the potential for it not to heal.[21] Because the subscapularis has the largest force generating capacity of all the rotator cuff muscles, contributing to 53% of the cuff moment,[22] a compromised subscapularis will often result in decreased function. Common signs and symptoms of a compromised subscapularis include pain, IR weakness, and/or anterior GH instability.[23-26]

Lafosse et al[27] described a novel shoulder arthroplasty technique that preserves the subscapularis tendon by performing the procedure entirely through the rotator interval. Although more technically challenging, this subscapularis-sparing technique allows for the patient to initiate early AROM in all planes without restrictions.

Therefore, communication with the surgeon regarding the specific arthroplasty technique is essential to prescribe an individualized rehabilitation program.

EXAMINATION

The rehabilitation process typically begins on the day of surgery or the first postoperative day. The clinical examination begins with a thorough chart review of the patient's medical and surgical history. The clinician gathers any pertinent information that may affect the rehabilitation process and overall clinical outcome such as duration of impairments before surgery, preoperative quality of the rotator cuff, and the pre- and postoperative ROM of the shoulder. If unclear, it is important for the therapist to communicate with the surgeon to clarify their preferred time frames for progression and to understand if there are any precautions or ROM restrictions unique to the patient.

Upon meeting the patient, the therapist performs a thorough subjective history, including the events leading up to the surgery, their preoperative function, and their current pain and functional status. A standard upper quarter postoperative examination including observation, palpation, neurological status, ROM, joint mobility, flexibility, and strength of the proximal and distal joints should be performed. Patient-reported outcome measures provide insights into their perceived functional capacity. These baseline measures are captured at this visit and measured throughout the rehabilitation process. These outcome measures are described further in Chapter 21.

Throughout this interaction, the therapist also seeks to develop a therapeutic alliance to foster open communication and cooperation during the rehabilitation process.[28-31] The patient and their support team must be engaged as active participants in the rehabilitation process to ensure the best possible outcome.[14] The utilization of a biopsychosocial model allows the clinician to assess the patient holistically and further patient-centered care and outcomes.[31,32]

Page et al[33] described several themes that patients with shoulder pain experience: pain, physical function/activity limitations (eg, difficulties performing ADLs), participation restriction (eg, work disruption, limited recreation), sleep disruption (eg, difficulty falling and staying asleep, sleep positions), cognitive dysfunction (eg, poor concentration and memory), emotional distress (eg, frustration, anxiety, and depression), and impairment in musculoskeletal and movement-related functions (eg, loss of muscle strength). There can be many interactions between these themes, with certain experiences impacting on others (eg, pain leading to reduced activities and sleep disruption). Clinicians must seek to identify these themes in the context of the patient's specific experience and formulate strategies to address them.

Part of the initial discussion should also capture the patient's understanding of the rehabilitation process, expectations, and goals so that the therapist can clarify important points and align their rehabilitation program toward the achievement of the patient's goals.[12] Henn et al,[34] reported that preoperative patient expectations often included relief of daytime pain, relief of nighttime pain, and improvement in shoulder ROM. These themes were very important to 86%, 82%, and 84% of the patients, respectively. Younger patients had greater expectations for relief of nighttime pain, for an improved ability to interact with others, and for an improved ability to exercise or participate in sports. Reduced improvements in pain, function, and ROM increased the risk of dissatisfaction in patients 2 to 5 years after ATSA.[35]

The therapist then synthesizes all the findings and educates the patient on the rehabilitation plan of care, precautions, and expectations.

PHASES OF REHABILITATION

Phase I: Joint Protection and Early Passive Range of Motion (Table 15.1)

Phase I is initiated on postoperative day 0 or day 1. The goals of Phase I are to protect the integrity of the surgical reconstruction by minimizing inappropriate stress, decrease pain and inflammation, restore PROM to the shoulder to minimize stiffness, and initiate neuromuscular control exercises for the periscapular muscles.

To protect the healing tissues from excessive stress, the patient is instructed on supporting the surgical arm with a sling for the first 4 to 6 weeks. The patient is to immobilize the shoulder throughout the day and night, except during the therapy session, bathing, and home exercises.

Following ATSA and shoulder surgery in general, finding a position to sleep may be challenging for the patient. The patient may not sleep on the side of the affected shoulder, so the therapist must educate the patient on alternative positions of comfort and safety. If the patient prefers to sleep supine, the humerus should

TABLE 15.1 Phase I: Joint Protection and Range of Motion
Postoperative Day 0-Week 4

Goals

- Protect the integrity of tissues by minimizing inappropriate stress
- Diminish pain and inflammation
- Diminish swelling
- Independent with home program
- Initiate passive range of motion (PROM) exercises
- Initiate neuromuscular control exercises for the periscapular muscles

Patient education

- Rehabilitation plan of care
- Precautions
  - No weight bearing through the upper extremity
  - No lifting/carrying heavy objects with the arm
  - No sleeping onto the operated side
  - Avoid hand behind the back
  - Subscapularis (if applicable)
    - No forceful internal rotation contraction
    - No excessive external rotation (ER) range of motion (ROM) (typically less than 30°-40°)
- Signs and symptoms of infection and dislocation
- Sleeping positions
- General posture
- Sling immobilization except when bathing or performing exercises for recommended period (typically 4-6 wk)
- Home exercise program
  - Shoulder PROM within limits
  - ROM of the elbow, wrist, and hand
  - Pendulums or rock the baby
- Pain management
  - Timing of medication
  - Cryotherapy
- Edema control
  - Arm elevation
  - Sling readjustment
  - Ball squeezes
  - Cryotherapy

Range of motion

- Pendulums or rock the baby
- ROM of the elbow, wrist, and hand
- PROM: flexion to 90° and ER to 30°

Flexibility

- Cervical spine muscle stretch
- Levator scapula stretch
- Pectoralis minor stretch

Scapular neuromuscular reeducation

- Scapular clock
- Scapular retraction and depression
- Manually resisted scapular retraction and depression

Manual therapy

- Retrograde massage
- Passive range of motion
- Gentle scar mobilization once healed

Aerobic activities

- Recumbent bicycle while wearing the upper extremity sling

be supported using pillows, so that the arm is not in the extended position relative to the midline of the body. It is the author's clinical experience that patients are often most comfortable sleeping in a recliner or a semireclined position created by a wedge behind the thorax. The importance of protecting the healing tissues from excessive stress is emphasized to the patient throughout Phase I to ensure adherence.

To help manage pain that may limit the progression of therapy, it is recommended that patients utilize their prescribed analgesics half an hour to 1 hour before the start of therapy. Cryotherapy should be used following exercise and throughout the day to control pain and muscle spasm, suppress the inflammatory response, reduce swelling, and improve sleep patterns in the immediate postoperative period.[36-39] If excessive pain is limiting the progression of rehabilitation, the therapist should communicate these findings to the physician for further assessment and potential changes in the pain management program.

If excessive edema is noted, the patient is encouraged to elevate the arm throughout the day. The sling may need to be readjusted to minimize the dependent position of the hand relative to the elbow. The patient is encouraged to squeeze a ball to encourage forearm muscle contraction and improved circulation. Manual therapy techniques, such as retrograde lymphatic drainage, can be added with light compression bandages, sleeves, or gloves. If swelling persists or worsens or appears in conjunction with signs that may suggest infection, the therapist should communicate these findings with the physician as soon as possible.

Initiating PROM for the GH joint in the immediate postoperative period has remained a central principle in total shoulder arthroplasty rehabilitation protocols for many years.[3,7,40,41] Immediate motion helps minimize joint stiffness, assists in collagen synthesis and organization, and may promote a more rapid return of function compared to a protocol with a delayed initiation of ROM.[41-44] PROM exercises for the GH joint are performed in the scapular plane with limits of motion according to the referring physician's protocol (eg, 90° of shoulder flexion, 30° of ER in the scapular plane, and IR to the body). When performing the ROM exercises in the supine position, a rolled-up towel is placed under the humerus to raise it to the scapular plane, minimizing stress to the anterior tissues.

Active scapular movement (protraction, retraction, elevation, and depression) helps to facilitate early neuromuscular control. The side-lying scapular clock exercise is performed and then progressed to sitting or standing. Submaximal isometric contractions of the periscapular muscles, particularly into retraction and depression, are initiated to bridge the transition to Phase II.

To maintain the gains achieved in therapy, therapists should educate the patient on performing a daily home exercise program comprising AROM for the elbow, wrist, and hand; scapular clocks and isometric contractions; pendulum exercises; supine passive forward elevation; and passive ER within the range recommended by the surgeon.

Aerobic activity has been shown to improve overall health and fitness, psychological well-being, and quality of life in adults.[45-49] The American College of Sports Medicine recommends 150 minute of moderate-intensity aerobic activity per week or the amount of physical activity that one's abilities and conditions allow.[46] Therefore, in the latter part of Phase I, safe aerobic activities such as the stationary recumbent bicycle while wearing the sling are recommended.[50] Other forms of aerobic activity should be delayed until later phases to allow for sufficient tissue healing..

Phase II: ROM Progression and Neuromuscular Control (Table 15.2)

The goal of Phase II is to successfully advance the patient's PROM to AAROM and then to AROM. This is achieved by focusing on neuromuscular retraining to enhance muscle activation and endurance. By the end of this phase, the patient needs to demonstrate not only functional PROM but also functional AROM in the involved extremity without compensatory movements (eg, shoulder shrug).

TABLE 15.2 Phase II: Range of motion (ROM) and Neuromuscular Control

Postoperative Week 4-Week 8

Guideline for progression to Phase II

- Minimal pain and symptoms at rest
- Functional passive range of motion (PROM)
- Good scapular control

Goals

- Maintain reduced inflammation and pain
- Discontinue sling (typically at 4-6 wk postoperatively)
- Progressively introduce controlled tissue stress to promote healing
- Demonstrate good muscle activation
- Gradually progress full PROM
- Progress ROM from passive to active assisted
- Progress ROM from active assisted to active
- Active range of motion (AROM) to >120° of forward flexion and 30° of external rotation (ER) at the side
- Normalize arthrokinematics of shoulder complex
- Initiate muscular strength

Patient education

- Review Phase I education points
- Educate on new goals of Phase II
- Updated home exercise program to include neuromuscular retraining exercises

Modalities

- Cryotherapy to decrease pain and swelling
- Moist heat pack

TABLE 15.2 Phase II: Range of motion (ROM) and Neuromuscular Control (continued)

Postoperative Week 4-Week 8

ROM

- PROM initiated with no limitation in flexion or internal rotation (IR)
- IR initiated gently via PROM of other hand
- No excessive ER to protect the subscapularis repair
- Elbow, wrist, and forearm ROM and stretching
- Codman's pendulums, rock the baby
- Progress to active-assisted ROM
  - Using other hand
  - Using pulley in the scapular plane

Thoracic spine

- Manual therapy techniques to improve thoracic extension and rotation
- Patient extension mobilization techniques over a chair
- Patient rotation mobilization in side lying

Neuromuscular control

- Submaximal rotator cuff and deltoid isometrics
- Place and holds
- Gentle rhythmic stabilization
  - Open kinetic chain
  - Closed kinetic chain
- Isometric inferior glide
- Isometric low row
- Lawnmower

Active-assisted movement

- Therapist-assisted movements
- Equipment-assisted movements (<20% electromyographic maximum voluntary isometric contraction)
  - Foam roller
  - Dowel
  - Ball
  - Pulley
- Hydrotherapy

AROM in supine

- Exercises initially performed with elbow flexed and then extended position
- Exercises progressed from supine position to increasing degrees of incline

AROM in side lying

- Flexion
- Abduction
- Horizontal abduction (HABD)

AROM combined with neuromuscular retraining

- Inclined forward elevation with isometric ball compression
- Inclined forward elevation with isometric HABD
- Inclined forward elevation with isometric ER

The therapist continues to work on maximizing PROM in multiple planes **(FIGURES 15.1-15.6)**. Any continued mobility impairments can be addressed by modifying the frequency, duration, or intensity of the stretches, as well as performing manual therapy interventions to address

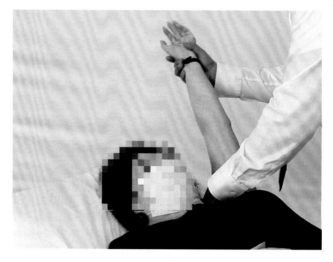

FIGURE 15.1 Passive range of motion flexion.

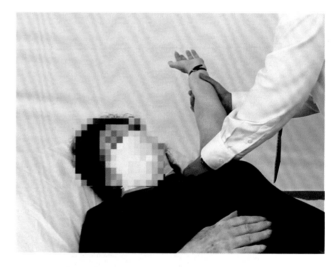

FIGURE 15.2 Passive range of motion abduction.

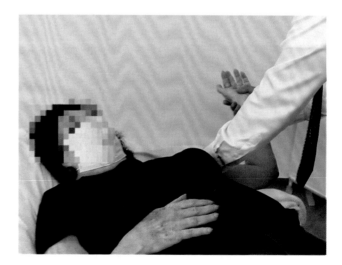

FIGURE 15.3 Passive range of motion external rotation in the scapular plane.

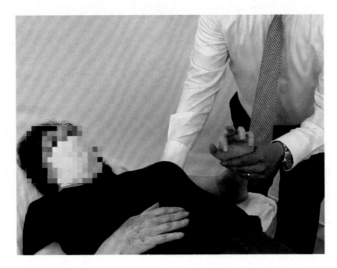

FIGURE 15.4 Passive range of motion internal rotation in the scapular plane.

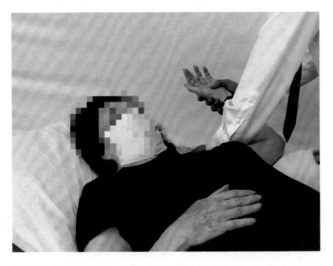

FIGURE 15.5 Passive range of motion external rotation at 90° abduction.

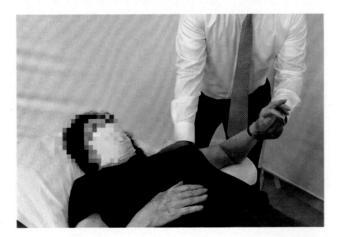

FIGURE 15.6 Passive range of motion internal rotation at 90° abduction.

any joint or muscle impairments. Factors such as the time from surgery, tissue irritability, and patient tolerance influence the decision-making process. Modalities such as a moist heat pack may be applied to muscles to promote relaxation as the patient performs their ROM exercises. As ROM targets are met, the focus of rehabilitation can shift to neuromuscular reeducation.

Early neuromuscular reeducation via submaximal isometrics and rhythmic stabilization is beneficial to enhance dynamic stabilization and improve proprioception, while providing an incremental increase in muscular demand to protect the healing structures. Patients are instructed on submaximal deltoid isometrics and periscapular muscle isometric contractions to stimulate muscle activation and minimize atrophy. The initial goal is to perform higher repetitions (15 or 20) of lower intensity contractions and then progress to a higher intensity of isometric contractions with fewer repetitions. To improve flexion neuromuscular control, the patient lies supine and places the arm to 90° and holds this position for a set period. As the patient develops strength, endurance, and control, the position is moved into further flexion or more challenging positions **(FIGURES 15.7-15.10)**. The therapist must regularly assess the response to strengthening by monitoring the patient-reported symptoms and for objective signs such as changes in motion or strength.

Rhythmic stabilization performed at varying shoulder angles helps prevent abnormal movement patterns from developing by enhancing stability and control into functional positions of the shoulder **(VIDEO 15.1)**. The patient is asked to hold shoulder positions in open or closed kinetic chain, and gentle oscillating manual perturbations facilitate low-level contractions of the periscapular and rotator cuff musculature[51] **(FIGURES 15.11-15.14)**.

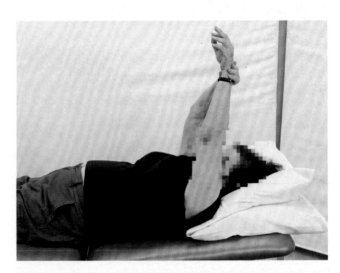

FIGURE 15.7 The patient begins the place and hold exercise by moving their arm with assistance to 90° of flexion.

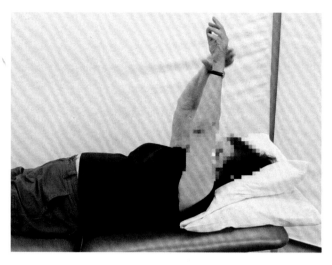

FIGURE 15.8 The patient then releases the assistance to promote an isometric contraction of the rotator cuff musculature.

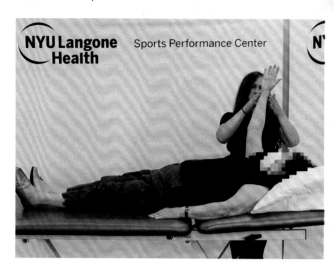

FIGURE 15.11 Rhythmic stabilization of flexion in supine.

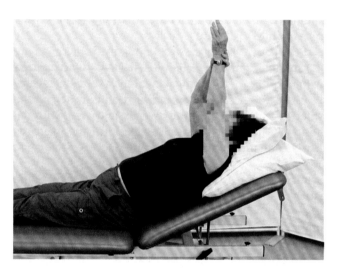

FIGURE 15.9 The therapist progresses the place and hold exercise to a more challenging position by raising the inclination of the trunk.

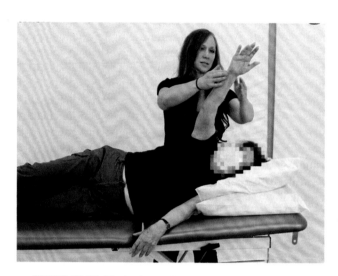

FIGURE 15.12 Rhythmic stabilization of flexion in side lying.

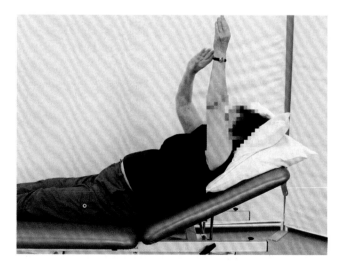

FIGURE 15.10 The patient moves their arm with assistance to the end of the range of motion and releases the assistance to promote an isometric contraction of the rotator cuff musculature.

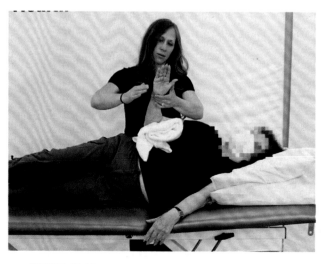

FIGURE 15.13 Rhythmic stabilization of external rotation.

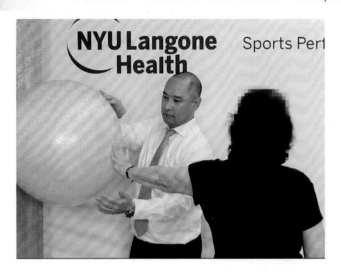

FIGURE 15.14 Rhythmic stabilization in closed kinetic chain with ball.

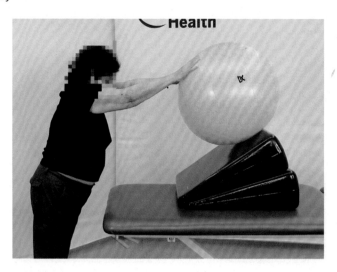

FIGURE 15.16 Active-assisted range of motion left shoulder flexion with a ball.

Once the patient demonstrates improved neuromuscular control, AAROM is initiated. As the clinician performs PROM, the patient may be asked to increase their participation in the movement. This active-assisted movement allows the clinician to gradually apply load without overstressing the healing structures during this phase. As the patient actively assists the action, the clinician provides accommodating support and gauges the patient's ability to support their arm. External support using a foam roller, stability ball, pulley, or dowel can be utilized to reduce the extremity weight while maintaining low muscle activation of the rotator cuff musculature (**FIGURES 15.15-15.17**).

EMG studies provide clinicians with evidence to guide early postoperative activities. A maximum voluntary isometric contraction (MVIC) of 20% or less during exercises is considered a safe loading range in the early stages following shoulder surgery.[52] **TABLE 15.2** contains common rehabilitation exercises that have been shown to have an MVIC of 20% or less.

If the patient has access to a pool, hydrotherapy may be a suitable option to facilitate AAROM.[53] Once cleared by the healthcare team, the patient may submerge themselves up to chest level to utilize the buoyancy of the water to reduce the extremity weight and assist with the motion. Care must be taken to perform the exercises slowly to minimize water resistance and excessive muscle strain.

Initiation of AROM should commence when the patient exhibits an effective isometric muscle contraction, acceptable PROM of the GH joint, and scapulothoracic articulation and good neuromuscular control with AAROM. If isotonic strengthening is initiated before proper mechanics are established, the patient is at risk for developing and reinforcing poor mechanics (eg, shoulder shrug) and thus increasing their risk for

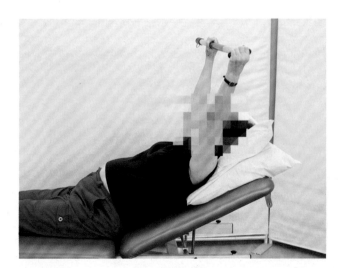

FIGURE 15.15 Active-assisted range of motion left shoulder flexion with a dowel.

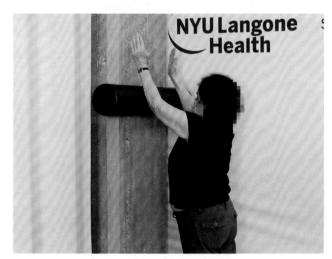

FIGURE 15.17 Active-assisted range of motion left shoulder flexion with a foam roller.

excessive soft tissue stress (eg, tendinitis). When starting isotonic strengthening, a low-weight, high-repetition program is recommended to mitigate these risks.

During this phase, the clinician determines how to best protect tissue from overloading by taking advantage of biomechanical principles such as short lever arms and positioning to minimize the effects of gravity. Initially, the exercises are performed with the elbow flexed in the supine position or side-lying position to minimize the torque and effects of gravity. The therapist then progresses to more functional and challenging positions by incrementally inclining the angle of the trunk from 0° to 30°, 45°, 60°, and then fully sitting upright or standing and performing the exercise with a straight elbow **(FIGURES 15.18-15.21)**.

Neuromuscular retraining of the rotator cuff muscles can be combined with AROM to facilitate force couples and improve the functional stability of the shoulder

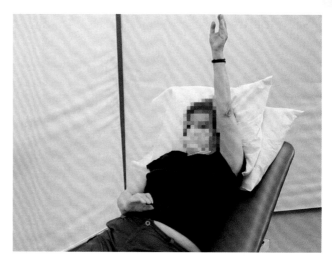

FIGURE 15.20 Active range of motion forward flexion with the head of the bed elevated to 60°.

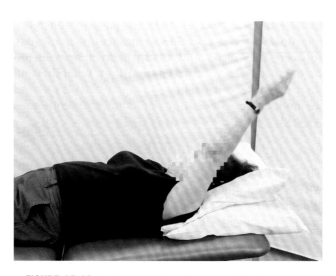

FIGURE 15.18 Active range of motion forward flexion supine.

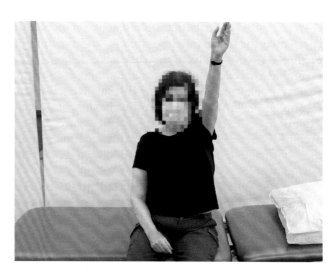

FIGURE 15.21 Active range of motion forward flexion in an upright position.

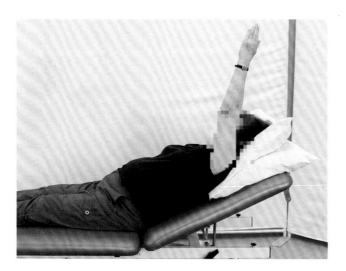

FIGURE 15.19 Active range of motion forward flexion with the head of the bed elevated to 45°.

complex. AROM, combined with isometric isolation of muscle groups, helps the patient elevate through challenging points of the ROM. For example, a ball can be squeezed to facilitate increased internal rotator muscle activation as elevation occurs. Because the subscapularis works in conjunction with the external rotators, it helps establish the internal/external rotator force couple that functions in concert with the deltoid. To minimize a shoulder flexion pattern with an overdominant humeral IR component, the therapist facilitates increased posterior cuff activation by asking the patient to maintain the hand position outside of the elbows. This can be progressed further by holding an elastic band isometrically into ER or horizontal abduction (HABD) during elevation[54] **(FIGURES 15.22-15.25)**.

The force couple from the upper, middle, and lower trapezius muscles combined with the serratus anterior muscle contributes to scapular stability and mobility.[55]

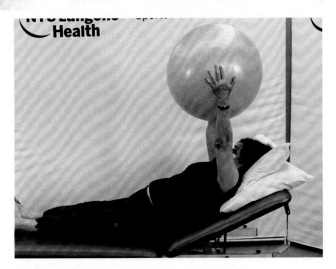

FIGURE 15.22 Forward elevation utilizing subscapularis facilitation via a ball squeeze.

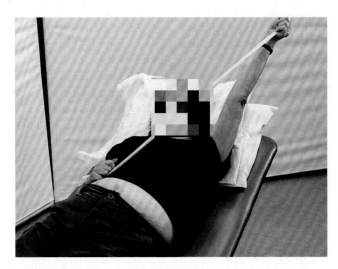

FIGURE 15.24 Forward elevation utilizing external rotator muscle facilitation finish position. While maintaining external rotation, the patient elevates in the scapular plane.

A synchronized contribution from scapular musculature is essential for the optimal positioning and functioning of the GH joint.[56,57] Exercises that have demonstrated favorable EMG activation ratios and timing for the trapezius complex include side-lying ER, side-lying forward flexion, prone HABD with ER, prone flexion, and prone extension.[56,57] Exercises that have demonstrated favorable EMG activation for the serratus anterior include the isometric inferior glide, isometric low row, and the lawnmower.[58-60]

This phase of rehabilitation can potentially require a significant amount of time to retrain the rotator cuff and periscapular musculature properly. Consequently, the healthcare team and patient must recognize that rehabilitation is an iterative process and not lose motivation or patience. It is incumbent upon the therapist

to determine if factors such as patient adherence, improper exercise selection or dosage, or inadequate recovery are contributing to any delay in progression. Before progressing into Phase III of rehabilitation, the patient needs to achieve adequate PROM as well as noncompensated shoulder and scapulothoracic AROM.

Phase III: Strengthening (Table 15.3)

The primary goal of Phase III is to regain full shoulder AROM in multiple directions and improve functional shoulder strength. The prerequisites to begin this phase include functional AROM, sound muscle activation, and endurance.

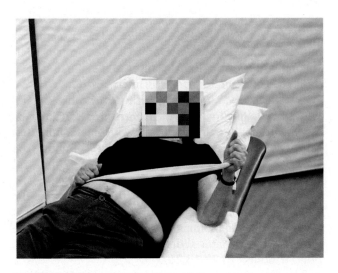

FIGURE 15.23 Forward elevation utilizing external rotator muscle facilitation start position. The patient begins by performing external rotation against resistance.

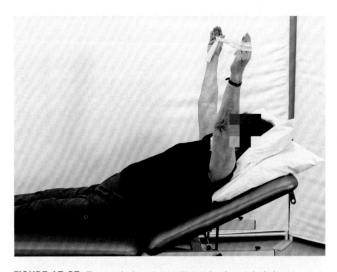

FIGURE 15.25 Forward elevation utilizing horizontal abductor muscle facilitation. The patient begins by performing horizontal abduction against resistance. While maintaining horizontal abduction, the patient elevates in the scapular plane.

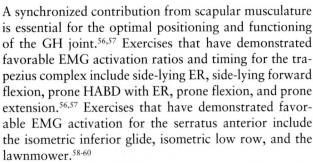

TABLE 15.3 Phase III: Late range of motion (ROM) and Early Strengthening

Postoperative Week 8-Week 12

Criteria to enter Phase III

- Full nonpainful active range of motion (AROM)
- Satisfactory stability
- Muscular strength (good grade or better)

Goals

- Establish and maintain full passive range of motion (PROM) and AROM
- Improve muscular strength
- Gradually increase functional activities

Patient education

- Precautions
  - No prolonged overhead activities
  - No lifting activities overhead
- Updated home exercise program to include strengthening

ROM

- Initiation of PROM and stretching beyond initial limits
- Passive hand behind back internal rotation (IR) stretching

Rhythmic stabilization

- Open and closed kinetic chain environments

Strengthening
Traditional rotator cuff and periscapular muscle isotonic exercise program
Exercises with maximum voluntary isometric contraction (MVIC) 21%-50%

- Supraspinatus
  - Wall walk
  - Standing-resisted shoulder extension
  - Standing external rotation (ER) in scapular plane
  - Seated row
- Infraspinatus
  - Active forward elevation
  - Low rows
  - High row
  - Standing ER with 0 of abduction (ABD) with towel
- Teres minor
  - Upright bar-assisted elevation
  - Standing ER 0° ABD
  - Prone horizontal abduction (HABD) 100°
  - Prone ER at 90°
- Subscapularis
  - Forward punch
  - IR at 0° ABD
  - IR at 45° ABD

Rotator cuff exercises with MVIC >50%

- Supraspinatus
  - Full can
  - Prone full can at 100°
  - Prone HABD at 90°
- Infraspinatus
  - ER with towel roll
  - Prone 90/90 ER
  - Full can ABD
  - Push-up plus

TABLE 15.3 Phase III: Late range of motion (ROM) and Early Strengthening   (continued)

Postoperative Week 8-Week 12

- Teres minor
  - Side-lying ER
  - Standing ER
  - Forward punches
  - Resisted shoulder flexion
- Subscapularis
  - IR diagonal pattern
  - Shoulder extension
  - High row
  - IR at 90° ABD

Scapular exercises with MVIC >50%

- Lower trapezius
  - Prone full can
  - Prone 90/90 ER
- Middle trapezius
  - Prone row
  - Prone HABD with ER
- Upper trapezius
  - Shrug
  - Prone row
  - Prone horizontal ABD with ER
- Rhomboids and levator scapulae
  - Prone row
  - Prone HABD with ER
  - Prone extension with ER
- Serratus anterior
  - Bear hug
  - Scapular protraction

Modalities

- PRN

Discharge planning if functional goals are met

ROM exercises are progressed to meet all functional demands, particularly for the hand behind back and hand behind head motions **(FIGURES 15.26** and **15.27)**. Functional use of the operative shoulder is demonstrated by a return to all ADLs and instrumental ADLs. Studies have reported that patients with an ATSA can achieve an average AROM of 146.4 (±27.6) degrees of forward elevation, 124.3 (±30.4) degrees of abduction, and 48.7 (±20.2) degrees of ER.[61]

The strengthening program targets the entire shoulder girdle with emphasis on increasing the intensity of the resistance exercises for the rotator cuff and periscapular musculature. The exercises previously prescribed in Phase II are made more challenging with the addition of dumbbells, elastic resistance bands or cords, strengthening machines, and manual resistance/perturbation. EMG studies may be used to identify exercises most appropriate for this phase of the rehabilitation. Exercises that have been shown to have EMG activation of 21% to 50% MVIC may be used initially. Later in the phase,

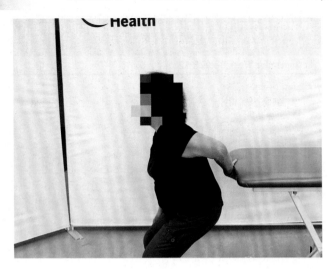

FIGURE 15.26 The patient grips a table or countertop and passively increases the hand behind the back motion by bending the knees.

strengthening exercises, with the highest EMG activations, should be chosen **(TABLE 15.3)**. Strengthening is progressed until the patient has reached a target strength ratio where the external rotator muscle strength is approximately 65% to 75% of the internal rotator muscles.[62-64]

If the patient has met the functional goals and does not have additional occupational or athletic needs requiring power and advanced movements, the patient may be discharged with an independent home exercise program. If the individual has functional demands beyond the performance of their ADLs, they will advance to the final phases of the rehabilitation program.

Phase IV: Advanced Strengthening and Return to Sport Preparation

In Phase IV, the primary objective is to prepare the patient for the return to high occupational and sports demands by addressing any deficits in shoulder strength,

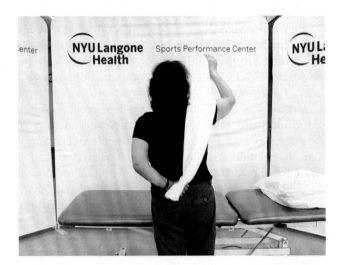

FIGURE 15.27 The patient utilizes a towel to passively increase the hand behind the back motion by pulling with the other arm.

TABLE 15.4 Phase IV: Advanced Strengthening and Return to Sport Preparation

Postoperative Week 12-16

Criteria to enter Phase IV

- Satisfactory static stability
- Full nonpainful active range of motion (AROM) at least 90% of contralateral side
- Muscular strength 80% of contralateral side
- External rotation (ER)/internal rotation (IR) ratio of at least 70%
- Communication with surgeon regarding plan to progress

Goals

- Enhance muscular strength, power, and endurance
- Improve neuromuscular control for sports-specific movements
- Maintain shoulder flexibility and range of motion (ROM)

ROM

- Continue all previous stretching and ROM exercises
- Normalize ER/IR at 90° of abduction
- Maintain posterior/inferior capsular mobility
- Maintain thoracic spine mobility

Strengthening

- Continue isotonic strengthening program with a progression in speed
- Plyometric strengthening
  - Bilateral overhead throw
  - Bilateral chest ball
  - Bilateral throws side to side
  - Bilateral ball slam
  - Unilateral ER ball flips in side lying and prone
  - Unilateral horizontal abduction ball flips in side lying and prone
  - Unilateral ER throw against trampoline at 0° and 90° of abduction
  - Unilateral IR throw against trampoline at 0° and 90° of abduction

Neuromuscular retraining

- Integrate sports specific movements during rehabilitation
- Identify sports-specific dysfunctional movement issues

endurance, power, and agility **(TABLE 15.4)**. In addition, impairments in other body regions that may hinder athletic ability, such as thoracic spine mobility, core strength, balance, and lower extremity mobility and strength are addressed **(FIGURES 15.28-15.31)**. The physical or occupational therapist continues to individualize the patient's program by incorporating sports-specific body positions and patterns of movement. The baseline criteria to progress to Phase IV include a satisfactory static stability of the shoulder, AROM of >90% of contralateral side, a limb symmetry index of 80% or greater, an ER/IR ratio of at least 70%, and communication with the surgeon regarding the plan to progress.

Strength testing periodically throughout this phase is vital to identify specific muscular deficits and to focus exercise prescriptions accordingly. Handheld dynamometry or the isometric function on an isokinetic

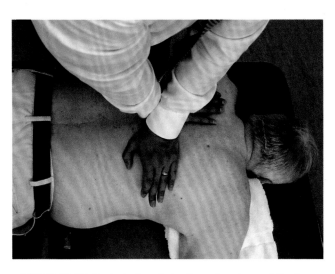

FIGURE 15.28 Posterior to anterior thoracic spine mobilization.

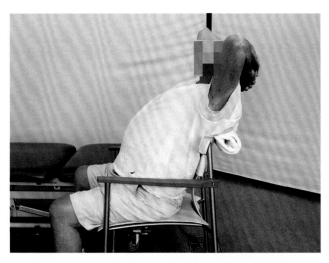

FIGURE 15.29 Seated thoracic spine extension mobilization.

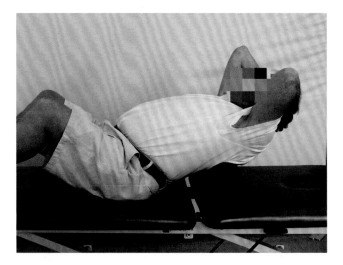

FIGURE 15.30 Supine thoracic spine extension mobilization with a foam roller.

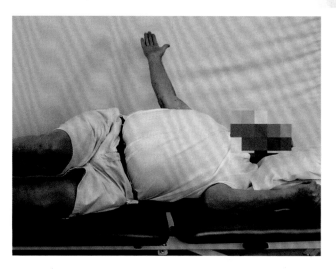

FIGURE 15.31 Side-lying thoracic spine rotation.

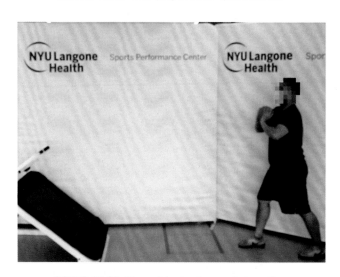

FIGURE 15.32 Plyometric chest pass start position.

dynamometer system offers an objective and reliable means of assessing muscle strength in a variety of positions.[65] Positions to assess include ER and IR at 0° abduction, ER and IR at 90° abduction, and scaption at 90°.

Plyometric exercises are utilized to increase power, endurance, and stability of the rotator cuff and periscapular musculature.[66,67] Bilateral upper extremity plyometric exercises, such as chest pass, overhead throws, side-to-side throws against a rebounder, and ball slams to the ground, are initially recommended **(FIGURES 15.32-15.39)**. These exercises are then progressed to single upper extremity plyometric exercises. The patient may continue with the previous isotonic strengthening program and add the variable of speed to each repetition. Other examples of unilateral plyometric exercises include ball flips into ER and HABD, and ER and IR throws against a trampoline. To mimic the demands of an overhead sport, the ER and IR exercises (prone 90/90 ER, supine 90/90 IR, IR wall dribbles) are advanced to 90° of GH joint abduction using a light handheld medicine ball **(FIGURES 15.40-15.44)**.

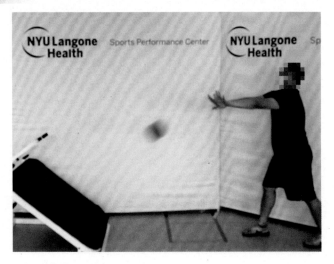

FIGURE 15.33 Plyometric chest pass finish position.

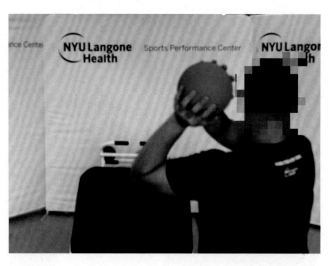

FIGURE 15.36 Plyometric side-to-side throw start position.

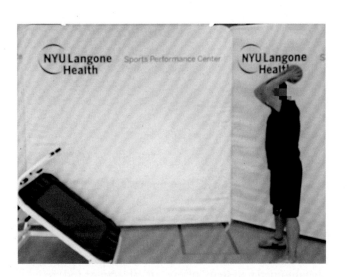

FIGURE 15.34 Plyometric overhead pass start position.

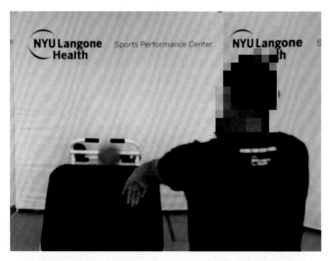

FIGURE 15.37 Plyometric side-to-side throw finish position.

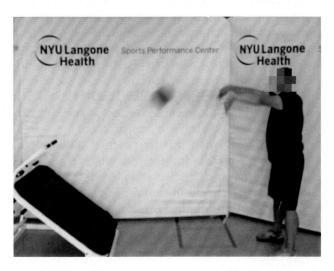

FIGURE 15.35 Plyometric overhead pass finish position.

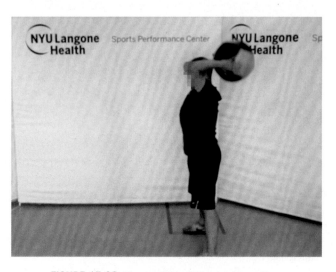

FIGURE 15.38 Plyometric ball slam start position.

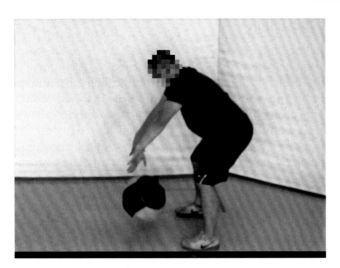

FIGURE 15.39 Plyometric ball slam finish position.

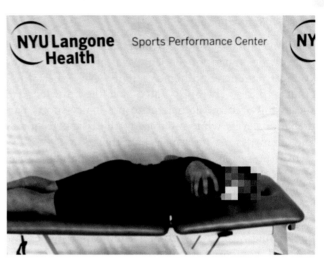

FIGURE 15.42 Plyometric horizontal abduction ball catches with a 2-lb ball start position.

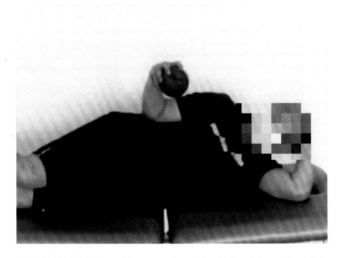

FIGURE 15.40 Plyometric external rotation ball catches with a 2-lb ball start position.

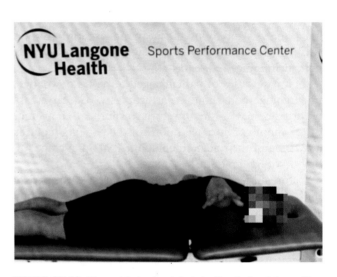

FIGURE 15.43 Plyometric horizontal abduction ball catches with a 2-lb ball. The patient releases and catches the ball repeatedly as quickly as possible.

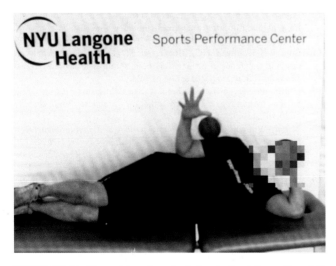

FIGURE 15.41 Plyometric external rotation ball catches with a 2-lb ball. The patient releases and catches the ball repeatedly as quickly as possible.

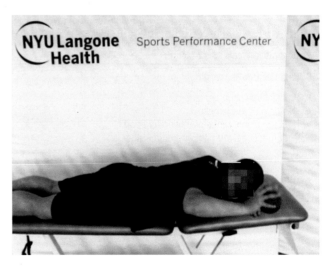

FIGURE 15.44 Plyometric 90/90 external rotation ball catches with a 2-lb ball.

Phase V: Return to Sport

Anatomic total shoulder arthroplasties are performed in a wide range of patient age groups, including younger patients with higher activity level expectations **(TABLE 15.5)**.[34] Therapists must have the knowledge to successfully return the patient to pre-injury sports participation levels while minimizing the risk of re-injury and compensatory movement patterns.

In their systematic review and meta-analysis, Liu et al[68] reported an overall rate of return to sports following shoulder arthroplasty of 85.1%, with 72.3% of patients returning to sports at an equivalent or improved level of play between 1 and 36 months postoperatively. Patients undergoing ATSA returned at a significantly higher rate (92.6%) compared to hemiarthroplasty (71.1%) or reverse total shoulder arthroplasty (74.9%). The most common sports were swimming, golf, fitness sports, and tennis.

Aim et al[69] also performed a systematic review and meta-analysis and found the mean rate of return to sport was 80.7%. The most common reported sports were golf, swimming, and tennis.

In a case series of patients aged 55 years or younger undergoing total shoulder arthroplasty, Garcia et al[70] reported a 96.4% rate of return to sports at an average of 6.7 months. Moreover, none of the patients required a revision of their glenoid component at an average follow-up of 61.0 months.

Before initiating this return to sport phase, the patient must meet the mobility and strength-based prerequisites. Exercise loading is further progressed toward the demands of the sport by manipulating the variables of speed, endurance, volume, and intensity. Sports-specific movements are simulated at a lower intensity to gauge the patient's physical readiness and overall confidence. The patient is then reintroduced slowly back into competitive sport, using the concepts of periodization and irritability to guide the progression.

TABLE 15.5 Phase V: Return to Sport

Postoperative Week 16-12 Months

Criteria to enter Phase V

- Satisfactory shoulder stability
- No pain or tenderness
- Full functional range of motion for sport
- Full functional strength and endurance

Goals

- Gradual return to sport activities
- Maintain strength, mobility, and stability via maintenance home exercise program

General guidelines

- Initiate interval sport program
- Monitor for symptoms of irritability and overuse

CONCLUSION

Rehabilitation after ATSA comprises a multiphased approach that progresses sequentially according to the principles of biological tissue healing, the surgical technique, and potential strain on the involved tissues. The protocol can be broken into five distinct phases, each with its own distinct goals and objective criterion to progress to the next phase. The clinical team must regularly assess and adjust the program based on the patient's individualized response and goals. As such, effective communication between the surgeon, therapist, and patient is essential during the rehabilitation process. Ultimately, the goal of the rehabilitation process is to maximize the patient's ability to return to full ADL, work, and recreational activities in a timely and safe manner.

REFERENCES

1. Wagner ER, Solberg MJ, Higgins LD. The utilization of formal physical therapy after shoulder arthroplasty. *J Orthop Sports Phys Ther.* 2018;48(11):856-863.
2. Brems JJ. Rehabilitation following total shoulder arthroplasty. *Clin Orthop Relat Res.* 1994;(307):70-85.
3. Hughes M, Neer CS II. Glenohumeral joint replacement and postoperative rehabilitation. *Phys Ther.* 1975;55(8):850-858.
4. Boardman ND III, Cofield RH, Bengtson KA, Little R, Jones MC, Rowland CM. Rehabilitation after total shoulder arthroplasty. *J Arthroplasty.* 2001;16(4):483-486.
5. Brown DD, Friedman RJ. Postoperative rehabilitation following total shoulder arthroplasty. *Orthop Clin North Am.* 1998;29(3):535-547.
6. Cahill JB, Cavanaugh JT, Craig EV. Total shoulder arthroplasty rehabilitation. *Tech Shoulder Elbow Surg.* 2014;15(1):13-17.
7. Bullock GS, Garrigues GE, Ledbetter L, Kennedy J. A systematic review of proposed rehabilitation guidelines following anatomic and reverse shoulder arthroplasty. *J Orthop Sports Phys Ther.* 2019;49(5):337-346.
8. Mulieri PJ, Holcomb JO, Dunning P, et al. Is a formal physical therapy program necessary after total shoulder arthroplasty for osteoarthritis? *J Shoulder Elbow Surg.* 2010;19(4):570-579.
9. Brameier DT, Hirscht A, Kowalsky MS, Sethi PM. Rehabilitation strategies after shoulder arthroplasty in young and active patients. *Clin Sports Med.* 2018;37(4):569-583.
10. Fusaro I, Orsini S, Stignani S, et al. Proposal for SICSeG guidelines for rehabilitation after anatomical shoulder prosthesis in concentric shoulder osteoarthritis. *Musculoskelet Surg.* 2013;97(suppl 1):31-37.
11. Etier BEJ, Pehlivan HC, Brockmeier SF. Postoperative rehabilitation and outcomes of primary anatomic shoulder arthroplasty. *Tech Shoulder Elbow Surg.* 2016;17(1):19-24.
12. Hoffmann TC, Lewis J, Maher CG. Shared decision making should be an integral part of physiotherapy practice. *Physiotherapy.* 2020;107:43-49.
13. Moody-Williams J. *Understanding patient and family engagement in health care.* In: *A Journey towards Patient-Centered Healthcare Quality: Patients, Families and Caregivers, Voices of Transformation.* Springer International Publishing; 2020:1-15.
14. Haverfield MC, Tierney A, Schwartz R, et al. Can patient–provider interpersonal interventions achieve the quadruple aim of healthcare? A systematic review. *J Gen Intern Med.* 2020;35(7):2107-2117.
15. Steinhaus ME, Gowd AK, Hurwit DJ, Lieber AC, Liu JN. Return to work after shoulder arthroplasty: a systematic review and meta-analysis. *J Shoulder Elbow Surg.* 2019;28(5):998-1008.
16. Westermann RW, Anthony CA, Duchman KR, Pugely AJ, Gao Y, Hettrich CM. Incidence, causes and predictors of 30-day readmission after shoulder arthroplasty. *Iowa Orthop J.* 2016;36:70-74.

17. Lung BE, Kanjiya S, Bisogno M, Komatsu DE, Wang ED. Preoperative indications for total shoulder arthroplasty predict adverse postoperative complications. *JSES Open Access.* 2019;3(2):99-107.

18. Shields E, Ho A, Wiater JM. Management of the subscapularis tendon during total shoulder arthroplasty. *J Shoulder Elbow Surg.* 2017;26(4):723-731.

19. Choate WS, Kwapisz A, Momaya AM, Hawkins RJ, Tokish JM. Outcomes for subscapularis management techniques in shoulder arthroplasty: a systematic review. *J Shoulder Elbow Surg.* 2018;27(2):363-370.

20. Louie PK, Levy DM, Bach BR Jr, Nicholson GP, Romeo AA. Subscapularis tenotomy versus lesser tuberosity osteotomy for total shoulder arthroplasty: a systematic review. *Am J Orthop (Belle Mead NJ).* 2017;46(2):E131-E138.

21. Ives EP, Nazarian LN, Parker L, Garrigues GE, Williams GR. Subscapularis tendon tears: a common sonographic finding in symptomatic postarthroplasty shoulders. *J Clin Ultrasound.* 2013;41(3):129-133.

22. Keating JF, Waterworth P, Shaw-Dunn J, Crossan J. The relative strengths of the rotator cuff muscles. A cadaver study. *J Bone Joint Surg Br.* 1993;75(1):137-140.

23. Armstrong A, Lashgari C, Teefey S, Menendez J, Yamaguchi K, Galatz LM. Ultrasound evaluation and clinical correlation of subscapularis repair after total shoulder arthroplasty. *J Shoulder Elbow Surg.* 2006;15(5):541-548.

24. Jackson JD, Cil A, Smith J, Steinmann SP. Integrity and function of the subscapularis after total shoulder arthroplasty. *J Shoulder Elbow Surg.* 2010;19(7):1085-1090.

25. Liem D, Kleeschulte K, Dedy N, Schulte TL, Steinbeck J, Marquardt B. Subscapularis function after transosseous repair in shoulder arthroplasty: transosseous subscapularis repair in shoulder arthroplasty. *J Shoulder Elbow Surg.* 2012;21(10):1322-1327.

26. Miller SL, Hazrati Y, Klepps S, Chiang A, Flatow EL. Loss of subscapularis function after total shoulder replacement: a seldom recognized problem. *J Shoulder Elbow Surg.* 2003;12(1):29-34.

27. Lafosse L, Schnaser E, Haag M, Gobezie R. Primary total shoulder arthroplasty performed entirely thru the rotator interval: technique and minimum two-year outcomes. *J Shoulder Elbow Surg.* 2009;18(6):864-873.

28. Taccolini Manzoni AC, Bastos de Oliveira NT, Nunes Cabral CM, Aquaroni Ricci N. The role of the therapeutic alliance on pain relief in musculoskeletal rehabilitation: a systematic review. *Physiother Theory Pract.* 2018;34(12):901-915.

29. Kidd MO, Bond CH, Bell ML. Patients' perspectives of patient-centredness as important in musculoskeletal physiotherapy interactions: a qualitative study. *Physiotherapy.* 2011;97(2):154-162.

30. Testa M, Rossettini G. Enhance placebo, avoid nocebo: how contextual factors affect physiotherapy outcomes. *Man Ther.* 2016;24:65-74.

31. Søndenå P, Dalusio-King G, Hebron C. Conceptualisation of the therapeutic alliance in physiotherapy: is it adequate? *Musculoskelet Sci Pract.* 2020;46:102131.

32. Babatunde F, MacDermid J, MacIntyre N. Characteristics of therapeutic alliance in musculoskeletal physiotherapy and occupational therapy practice: a scoping review of the literature. *BMC Health Serv Res.* 2017;17(1):375.

33. Page MJ, O'Connor DA, Malek M, et al. Patients' experience of shoulder disorders: a systematic review of qualitative studies for the OMERACT Shoulder Core Domain Set. *Rheumatology.* 2019;58(8):1410-1421.

34. Henn RF III, Ghomrawi H, Rutledge JR, Mazumdar M, Mancuso CA, Marx RG. Preoperative patient expectations of total shoulder arthroplasty. *J Bone Joint Surg Am.* 2011;93(22):2110-2115.

35. Jacobs CA, Morris BJ, Sciascia AD, Edwards TB. Comparison of satisfied and dissatisfied patients 2 to 5 years after anatomic total shoulder arthroplasty. *J Shoulder Elbow Surg.* 2016;25(7):1128-1132.

36. Osbahr DC, Cawley PW, Speer KP. The effect of continuous cryotherapy on glenohumeral joint and subacromial space temperatures in the postoperative shoulder. *Arthroscopy.* 2002;18(7):748-754.

37. Singh H, Osbahr DC, Holovacs TF, Cawley PW, Speer KP. The efficacy of continuous cryotherapy on the postoperative shoulder: a prospective, randomized investigation. *J Shoulder Elbow Surg.* 2001;10(6):522-525.

38. Speer KP, Warren RF, Horowitz L. The efficacy of cryotherapy in the postoperative shoulder. *J Shoulder Elbow Surg.* 1996;5(1):62-68.

39. Noyes MP, Denard PJ. Continuous cryotherapy vs ice following total shoulder arthroplasty: a randomized control trial. *Am J Orthop (Belle Mead NJ).* 2018;47(6):1-8.

40. Neer CS II, Watson KC, Stanton FJ. Recent experience in total shoulder replacement. *J Bone Joint Surg Am.* 1982;64(3):319-337.

41. Wilcox RB, Arslanian LE, Millett P. Rehabilitation following total shoulder arthroplasty. *J Orthop Sports Phys Ther.* 2005;35(12):821-836.

42. Boudreau S, Boudreau ED, Higgins LD, Wilcox RB III. Rehabilitation following reverse total shoulder arthroplasty. *J Orthop Sports Phys Ther.* 2007;37(12):734-743.

43. Wolff AL, Rosenzweig L. Anatomical and biomechanical framework for shoulder arthroplasty rehabilitation. *J Hand Ther.* 2017;30(2):167-174.

44. Denard PJ, Ladermann A. Immediate versus delayed passive range of motion following total shoulder arthroplasty. *J Shoulder Elbow Surg.* 2016;25(12):1918-1924.

45. Daimiel L, Martinez-Gonzalez MA, Corella D, et al. Physical fitness and physical activity association with cognitive function and quality of life: baseline cross-sectional analysis of the PREDIMED-Plus trial. *Sci Rep.* 2020;10(1):3472.

46. Chodzko-Zajko WJ, Proctor DN, Fiatarone Singh MA, et al. American College of Sports Medicine position stand. Exercise and physical activity for older adults. *Med Sci Sports Exerc.* 2009;41(7):1510-1530.

47. Piercy KL, Troiano RP, Ballard RM, et al. The physical activity guidelines for Americans. *J Am Med Assoc.* 2018;320(19):2020-2028.

48. Bauman A, Merom D, Bull FC, Buchner DM, Fiatarone Singh MA. Updating the evidence for physical activity: summative reviews of the epidemiological evidence, prevalence, and interventions to promote "active aging". *Gerontologist.* 2016;56(suppl 2):S268-S280.

49. O'Donovan G, Blazevich AJ, Boreham C, et al. The ABC of physical activity for health: a consensus statement from the British Association of Sport and Exercise Sciences. *J Sports Sci.* 2010;28(6):573-591.

50. Salamh PA, Speer KP. Post-rehabilitation exercise considerations following total shoulder arthroplasty. *Strength Condit J.* 2013;35(4):56-63.

51. Ellenbecker TS, Davies GJ, Bleacher J. 24 – proprioception and neuromuscular control. In: Andrews JR, Harrelson GL, Wilk KE, eds. *Physical Rehabilitation of the Injured Athlete.* 4th ed. W.B. Saunders; 2012:524-547.

52. Edwards PK, Ebert JR, Littlewood C, Ackland T, Wang A. A systematic review of electromyography studies in normal shoulders to inform postoperative rehabilitation following rotator cuff repair. *J Orthop Sports Phys Ther.* 2017;47(12):931-944.

53. Edwards T, Morris B. Rehabilitation after shoulder arthroplasty. In: *Shoulder Arthroplasty.* 2nd ed. Elsevier; 2019:461-464.

54. Lewis J, McCreesh K, Roy JS, Ginn K. Rotator cuff tendinopathy: navigating the diagnosis-management conundrum. *J Orthop Sports Phys Ther.* 2015;45(11):923-937.

55. Struyf F, Nijs J, Mottram S, Roussel NA, Cools AM, Meeusen R. Clinical assessment of the scapula: a review of the literature. *Br J Sports Med.* 2014;48(11):883-890.

56. Cools AM, Struyf F, De Mey K, Maenhout A, Castelein B, Cagnie B. Rehabilitation of scapular dyskinesis: from the office worker to the elite overhead athlete. *Br J Sports Med.* 2014;48(8):692-697.

57. Cools AM, Dewitte V, Lanszweert F, et al. Rehabilitation of scapular muscle balance: which exercises to prescribe? *Am J Sports Med.* 2007;35(10):1744-1751.

58. Kibler WB, Sciascia AD, Uhl TL, Tambay N, Cunningham T. Electromyographic analysis of specific exercises for scapular control in early phases of shoulder rehabilitation. *Am J Sports Med.* 2008;36(9):1789-1798.

59. Schory A, Bidinger E, Wolf J, Murray L. A systematic review of the exercises that produce optimal muscle ratios of the scapular stabilizers in normal shoulders. *Int J Sports Phys Ther.* 2016;11(3):321-336.

60. Cricchio M, Frazer C. Scapulothoracic and scapulohumeral exercises: a narrative review of electromyographic studies. *J Hand Ther.* 2011;24(4):322-334.

61. Simovitch RW, Friedman RJ, Cheung EV, et al. Rate of improvement in clinical outcomes with anatomic and reverse total shoulder arthroplasty. *J Bone Joint Surg Am.* 2017;99(21):1801-1811.

62. Wilk KE, Arrigo CA, Andrews JR. Current concepts: the stabilizing structures of the glenohumeral joint. *J Orthop Sports Phys Ther.* 1997;25(6):364-379.

63. Hughes RE, Johnson ME, O'Driscoll SW, An KN. Normative values of agonist-antagonist shoulder strength ratios of adults aged 20 to 78 years. *Arch Phys Med Rehabil.* 1999;80(10):1324-1326.

64. Ivey FM Jr, Calhoun JH, Rusche K, Bierschenk J. Isokinetic testing of shoulder strength: normal values. *Arch Phys Med Rehabil.* 1985;66(6):384-386.

65. Ellenbecker TS, Bailie DS. Chapter 26 – shoulder arthroplasty in the athletic shoulder. In: Wilk KE, Reinold MM, Andrews JR, eds. *The Athlete's Shoulder.* 2nd ed. Churchill Livingstone; 2009:315-324.

66. Wilk KE, Voight ML, Keirns MA, Gambetta V, Andrews JR, Dillman CJ. Stretch-shortening drills for the upper extremities: theory and clinical application. *J Orthop Sports Phys Ther.* 1993;17(5):225-239.

67. Maenhout A, Benzoor M, Werin M, Cools A. Scapular muscle activity in a variety of plyometric exercises. *J Electromyogr Kinesiol.* 2016;27:39-45.

68. Liu JN, Steinhaus ME, Garcia GH, et al. Return to sport after shoulder arthroplasty: a systematic review and meta-analysis. *Knee Surg Sports Traumatol Arthrosc.* 2018;26(1):100-112.

69. Aim F, Werthel JD, Deranlot J, Vigan M, Nourissat G. Return to sport after shoulder arthroplasty in recreational athletes: a systematic review and meta-analysis. *Am J Sports Med.* 2018;46(5):1251-1257.

70. Garcia GH, Liu JN, Sinatro A, et al. High satisfaction and return to sports after total shoulder arthroplasty in patients aged 55 years and younger. *Am J Sports Med.* 2017;45(7):1664-1669.

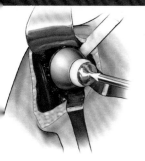

16 Resurfacing Shoulder Arthroplasty

Curtis R. Noel, MD

INTRODUCTION

Preserving humeral bone with short stems and stemless implants is a recent trend in total shoulder arthroplasty (TSA), but the first and most bone-conserving implant, the humeral head resurfacing (HHR), evolved from the hip resurfacing experience over 40 years ago.[1] Copeland's development of his humeral resurfacing design began in 1979, and it was first implanted in 1986.[2] Since then, a variety of systems and implants have been developed.

The benefits of HHR are well documented. It is the most bone conserving shoulder arthroplasty option, even with the development of newer stemless and short-stem implant designs. By eliminating humeral canal reaming, HHR is a more streamlined surgery with decreased blood loss and decreased operative time.[3] In addition, because the HHR avoids violating the canal, the threat of a periprosthetic humeral diaphyseal fracture is greatly diminished,[2] as is the threat of infection violating the humeral shaft. As HHR is not bound by the humeral canal, it has the freedom of expanded inclination and version options and potentially is a more anatomic shoulder replacement.[4] Finally, with minimal bone removal and with a less aggressive implant, revision of an HHR to a stemmed implant is much less complicated (VIDEO 16.1).

INDICATIONS

In general, HHR is indicated in many of the same cases considered for a hemiarthroplasty or TSA. These broad categories include primary and secondary osteoarthritis, rheumatoid and other inflammatory arthritis, posttraumatic and instability-related arthritis, osteonecrosis, and cuff tear arthropathy.[1-3] For those who cannot have a stemmed implant because of humeral deformity (genetic or posttraumatic) or previous surgery (elbow arthroplasty or previous open reduction internal fixation), HHR may also be the best option.

More specifically, HHR is often considered for the young, active patient with arthritis or osteonecrosis.[1,5] In these younger patients, conserving humeral bone for future surgeries and avoiding a glenoid implant that may eventually fail is often the most prudent option. Younger patients with significant Hill-Sachs impression fractures from shoulder dislocations may also benefit from HHR when other options are contraindicated. However, the HHR can also be considered in older patients with concentric osteoarthritis or with cuff tear arthropathy when a reverse total shoulder is contraindicated.[2]

Multiple comparative studies have reported superior outcomes with TSA over hemiarthroplasties.[6,7] Therefore, addressing the glenoid while performing an HHR is often desired. In HHR, the humeral head is reshaped and not resected, which makes exposure of the glenoid much more challenging. Success in performing a resurfacing TSA is increased by careful patient selection. Thinner patients with concentric glenoid wear (Walch A)[8] and whose shoulder range of motion is somewhat maintained are better candidates for a combined glenoid and humerus resurfacing. Having decreased soft tissue mass to retract, having absent or decreased glenoid retroversion, and having less joint stiffness allows for improved retraction of the humerus and better exposure of the glenoid.

CONTRAINDICATIONS

HHR is contraindicated in all circumstances in which a standard TSA is contraindicated; ie, active infections, nerve injury, and neuropathic arthropathy. In addition, HHR is contraindicated in cases where the proximal humerus bone will not support a nonstemmed implant owing to extreme proximal humeral bone loss (greater than 60% of the humeral head), excessively soft bone, or bone containing large cysts.[2] Those patients with acute proximal humerus fractures or chronic humeral neck fracture nonunions are also not candidates for HHR.[2,3,9]

Relative contraindications to preforming a resurfacing TSA include conditions that make glenoid exposure difficult or impossible. These conditions include patients with significant retroversion (Walch B or C glenoids),[8] obese or well-muscled patients, and patients with advanced arthritis with significant loss of motion and joint contracture.

Relative contraindications for an HHR include conditions that make hemiarthroplasties more likely to fail. These include excessive glenoid bone loss leading to instability or predisposing the glenoid to rapid medial wear. These are situations in which biconcave glenoids (Walch B2)[8] and posterior humeral head subluxation lead to decreased implant survival.[10]

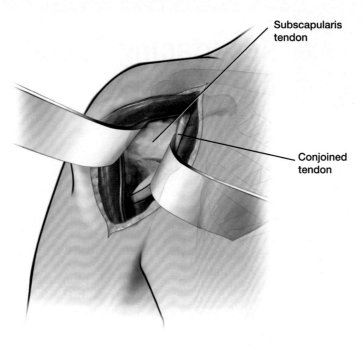

FIGURE 16.1 Exposure of the proximal humerus with a deltopectoral approach.

TECHNIQUE

The operating room setup and positioning for HHR is the same as that of any TSA. Unless contraindicated, all patients receive a regional block along with general anesthesia. In addition to the block, complete muscle paralysis may improve retraction and aid in difficult glenoid exposures. Once asleep, the patient is placed in the beach chair position with the head secured in the head rest and the operative arm freely mobile either on a Mayo stand or in an arm positioner.

A standard deltopectoral approach is routinely used **(FIGURE 16.1)**, but an anterosuperior approach, preferred by Copeland and Levy, could also be utilized.[11]

The subscapularis can be approached in a variety of ways. I prefer to do a subscapularis peel, but a tenotomy or lesser tuberosity osteotomy can also be performed with equal efficacy. Savoie has described a partial subscapularis sparing approach, which only releases the lower portion of the subscapularis.[5,12] In this approach, the tendinous portion of the upper subscapularis remains intact while the more muscular inferior portion of the subscapularis is removed along with the inferior capsule. The humerus is then abducted and externally rotated to slide under the intact upper subscapularis **(FIGURE 16.2)**. This approach can make visualizing the superior aspect of the humerus more challenging as the subscapularis lays across the top of the humerus, but it can allow for a more aggressive rehabilitation and quicker recovery because the important tendinous portion of the upper subscapularis remains intact.[5,12]

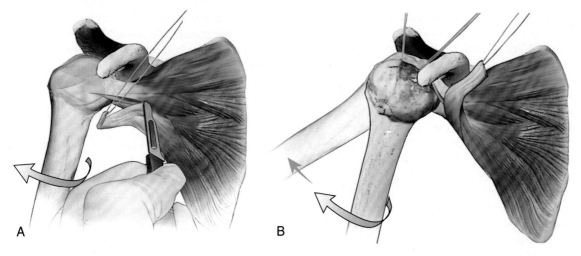

A   B

FIGURE 16.2 A and B, Savoie's subscapularis sparing approach: removing the bottom portion of the tendon and tucking the humeral head under the intact upper border of the subscapularis.

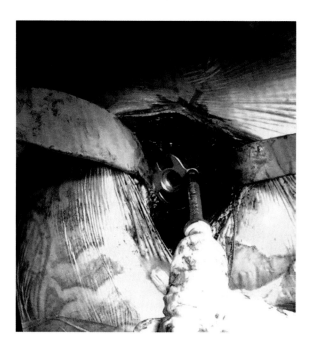

FIGURE 16.3 Adequate visualization allowing for glenoid preparation.

Regardless of how the subscapularis is addressed, it is critical to perform ample soft tissue releases, especially if the glenoid is going to be resurfaced. The subscapularis and capsular release must proceed down the inferior and medial aspect of the humeral neck continuing all the way to the posterior aspect of the humerus, making sure to protect the axillary nerve. Some authors prefer to excise the capsule, but I prefer to do an aggressive capsular release off the humerus and glenoid, leaving the remaining capsule attached to the undersurface of the subscapularis. I feel this decreases trauma to the subscapularis and adds mass to the tendon improving its repair.

Once the subscapularis and capsule are released, the humerus is externally rotated and extended to bring the humeral head into the wound. All osteophytes are removed from the humerus exposing the anatomic neck. At this point, if the glenoid is going to be resurfaced, it is prudent to attempt to retract the humerus posteriorly to assess the amount of glenoid exposure obtained with just the capsular release and osteophyte removal. A variety of retractors can be trialed to determine which provides the best exposure. If a full enface view of the glenoid is obtained, the glenoid can be prepared (**FIGURE 16.3**) and the glenoid component inserted. If the glenoid is visualized but removing some more humeral bone will improve the instrumentation of the glenoid, the humerus is then brought forward once again to prepare the humeral head for resurfacing. If it is determined that the glenoid cannot be safely prepared even with further bone preparation, then it is prudent to abandon the resurfacing and proceed with a humeral resection and an alternate arthroplasty option.

If continuation of the humeral resurfacing is still desirable, the humerus is extended and externally rotated into the wound and sizers are sequentially applied to the humeral head until the best fit is identified in the most anatomically correct position based on version and inclination. A pin is then inserted through the sizer, into the center of the humeral head, and just into the lateral humeral cortex (**FIGURE 16.4**). With the sizer removed, the pin is verified to be in the center of the humeral head. Reamers are then used to shape the humeral head (**FIGURE 16.5**). A significant pitfall in some humeral head replacement designs and techniques is the failure to remove enough bone for the thickness of metal being implanted. Alolabi et al reported that the humerus was improperly reamed in 89.3% of the cases in their series.[13] It may seem counterintuitive, since we are trying to maximize bone conservation, but if an inadequate amount of bone is removed, then depending on your implant design, the joint could be "overstuffed" (**FIGURE 16.6**). Similar to a standard TSA, the anatomic neck is key in determining the correct position of the humeral resurfacing. Inclination, version, and implant depth should be based upon the anatomic neck.[2] It is important not to damage the rotator cuff insertion, but at the same time, it is critical to ream to within a couple of millimeters of the anatomic neck to ensure the implant best recreates the center of rotation and to avoid overstuffing.[14] Another pitfall in HHR is the tendency to place the HHR into the varus.[15] Once again, identifying the anatomic neck can help to decrease these errors.

If the glenoid still needs to be addressed, then assessing the glenoid exposure at this point can be beneficial. The extra millimeters of exposure obtained from reaming the humerus, but before the final implant is applied, may maximize glenoid exposure. There is a concern that retracting on the reamed humeral head can damage the humerus. Personal experience has shown that, although the retractors can cause a small groove in the reamed humeral surface, it has not compromised the fixation or stability of the final implant. If good exposure is obtained, then glenoid preparation and implantation is performed (see **FIGURE 16.3**).

The humeral head is resized at this time to verify that the best fit is obtained (**FIGURE 16.7**). The central peg/cage is then drilled and tapped, and the final implant is inserted (**FIGURES 16.8** and **16.9**). If the glenoid still needs to be addressed, then the humerus is retracted posteriorly, once again, with the implant protecting the humeral bone from the retractors. The glenoid is then prepared and inserted. The risk of waiting until the final implant is inserted before assessing the glenoid exposure is twofold. First, retracting on the implant could scratch or damage the implant, and second, if the glenoid is inaccessible, then the humeral implant has just been wasted as conversion to a TSA becomes necessary.

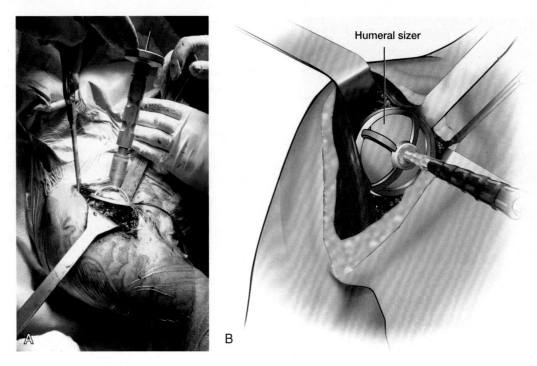

FIGURE 16.4 A and B, Placement of the humeral sizer paralleling the anatomic neck and K wire insertion making sure it is in the center of the humeral head.

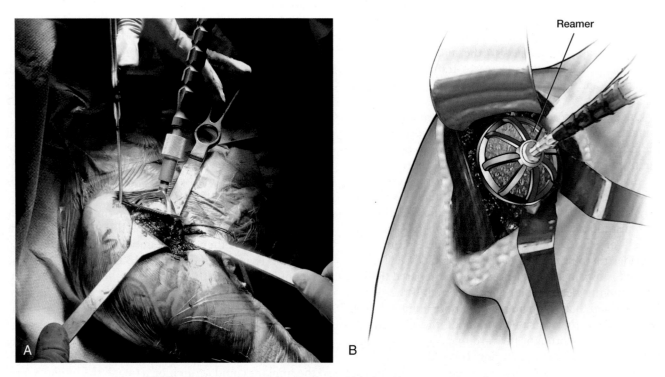

FIGURE 16.5 A and B, Reaming the humeral head making sure not to underream.

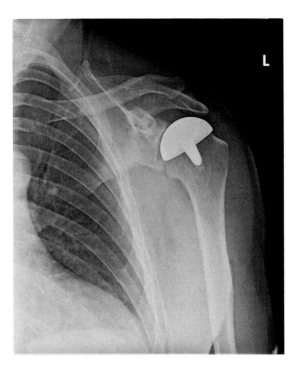

FIGURE 16.6 Overstuffing of the joint after humeral head resurfacing.

Range of motion and stability are assessed in the same manner as a standard hemiarthroplasty or TSA. After irrigating, the subscapularis is repaired. My current technique utilizes two triple-loaded suture anchors inserted in the lesser tuberosity near the bicipital groove.

Sutures are passed through the subscapularis in either a simple or modified Mason-Allen fashion and then tied incorporating the biceps tendon when possible. The final suture from the inferior anchor is then used to run up the subscapularis, into the rotator interval, and then back down, reinforcing the repair and the biceps tenodesis. Three to five nonabsorbable sutures are used to close the deltopectoral interval, and the skin is closed with running absorbable suture. I like to use a waterproof, silver ion–containing dressing that allows patients to shower within 24 to 48 hours after surgery and is kept on for a week. A sling is applied and used for 4 weeks, allowing the patient to remove to dress, shower, and do physical therapy, which starts on postoperative day #1.

RESULTS

HHR, either alone or as part of a TSA, has reported clinical outcomes equivalent to stemmed total shoulder and hemiarthroplasties.[2-5,9,16,17] Several studies by Levy and Copeland show improved shoulder function after HHR, with over 90% of their patients reporting improvement of their shoulders.[2-4,9] Age is not necessarily a predictor of poor outcomes. Iagulli et al showed that, in patients under the age of 60 years, 94% reported satisfaction with an HHR and the same percentage were able to return to sports or manual labor activities.[5] Levy and Copeland achieved a satisfaction score of 84% after HHR in patients over 80 years.[16] Like stemmed procedures, resurfacing total shoulders appear to have more

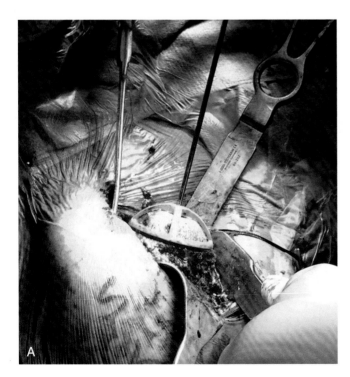

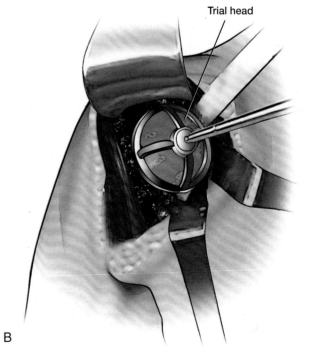

Trial head

FIGURE 16.7 A and B, Trial humeral head.

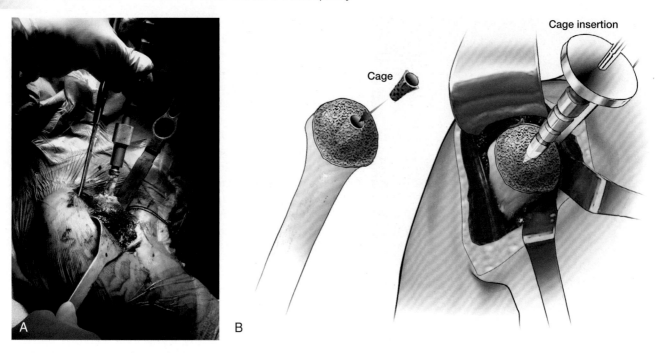

FIGURE 16.8 A and B, Humeral drilling and insertion of central cage implant.

favorable outcomes when compared with HHR alone. In their 2001 study, Levy and Copeland resurfaced both the glenoid and the humerus in 66% of their reported cases. Constant scores were better with a total shoulder (93.7%) versus HHR alone (73.5%) when performed for osteoarthritis.[2] As an alternative to a polyethylene glenoid component, other authors have reported on a variety of alternative, biologic resurfacing options for the glenoid but with mixed outcomes and inconsistent long-term results.[18-22] HHR can have good to excellent outcomes, but inferior outcomes are reported in patients with damaged or biconcave glenoids and in patients with posterior humeral head subluxation evident on preoperative axillary radiographs.[10,23,24]

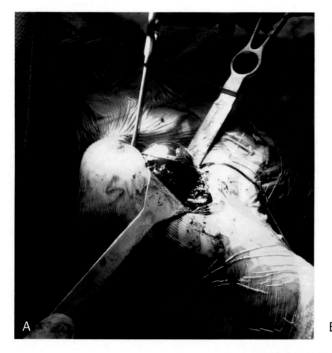

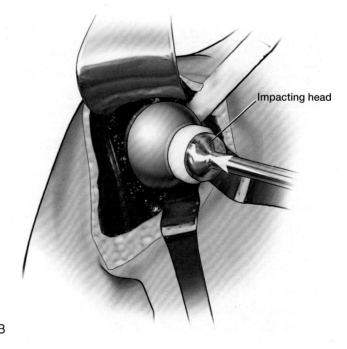

FIGURE 16.9 A and B, Final implant.

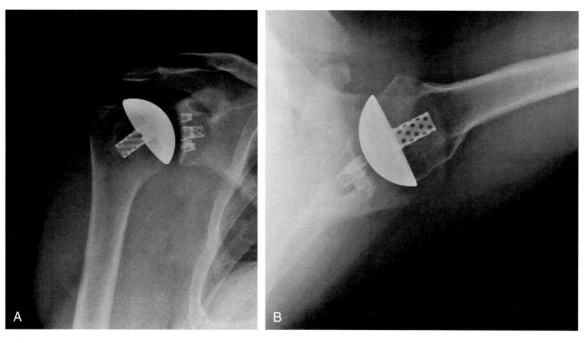

FIGURE 16.10 A and B, Appropriately sized total shoulder resurfacing.

Revision rates and complications, both intraoperative and postoperative, are low in HHRT, but revision rates increase with improper implant positioning and worsening glenoid deformity. Rai et al showed 95% survivorship at 18 years with the Copeland Mark III implant and had an 88% satisfaction in 46 shoulders.[25] Maier et al, however, reporting on their results using three different HHR systems, had a higher revision rate (24%) at 2.7 years. They reported that failure was related to a change in the Length of Glenohumeral Offset (LGHO).[26] Similarly, Mechlenburg and associates found that the Copeland resurfacing increased the postoperative LGHO and that this overstuffing of the joint led to a higher revision rate (14%).[27] These studies highlight the need to understand the system being used and the importance of properly implanting the HHR. Newer implant designs may allow for more anatomic reconstructions **(FIGURES 16.10** and **16.11).**[28]

CONCLUSION

HHR is an acceptable option for patients requiring shoulder replacement surgery. Excellent outcomes can be achieved with good survivorship if proper indications and techniques are followed. Glenoid resurfacing can be challenging but is possible, and results equivalent to stemmed implants can be obtained with the added benefit of increased bone preservation. Future improvements, including computer guidance, may lead to more accurate implantation and better soft tissue preserving approaches.

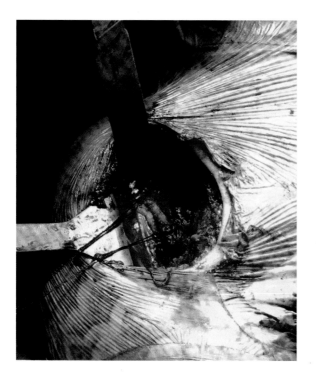

FIGURE 16.11 Subscapularis approximation for repair with little tension.

REFERENCES

1. Jensen KL. Humeral resurfacing arthroplasty: rationale, indications, technique, and results. *Am J Orthop.* 2007;36(12 suppl):4-8.
2. Levy O, Copeland SA. Cementless surface replacement arthroplasty of the shoulder. 5- to 10-year results with the Copeland Mark-2 prosthesis. *J Bone Joint Surg Br.* 2001;83:213-222.
3. Levy O, Funk L, Sforza G, Copeland SA. Copeland surface replacement arthroplasty of the shoulder in rheumatoid arthritis. *J Bone Joint Surg Am.* 2004;86:512-518.

4. Thomas SR, Sforza G, Levy O, Copeland SA. Geometrical analysis of Copeland surface replacement shoulder arthroplasty in relation to normal anatomy. *J Shoulder Elbow Surg.* 2005;14:186-192.

5. Iagulli ND, Field LD, Hobgodd ER, et al. Surface replacement arthroplasty of the humeral head in young, active patients. *Orthop J Sports Med.* 2014;2(1):2325967113519407. doi:10.1177/2325967113519407

6. Martin SD, Zurakowski D, Thornhill TS. Uncemented glenoid component in total shoulder arthroplasty. survivorship and outcomes. *J Bone Joint Surg Am.* 2005;87:1284-1292.

7. Norris BL, Lachiewicz PF. Modern cement technique and the survivorship of total shoulder arthroplasty. *Clin Orthop Relat Res.* 1996;(328):76-85.

8. Walch G, Badet R, Boulahia A, Khoury A. Morphologic study of the glenoid in primary glenohumeral osteoarthritis. *J Arthroplasty.* 1999;14:756-760.

9. Levy O, Copeland SA. Cementless surface replacement arthroplasty for osteoarthritis of the shoulder. *J Shoulder Elbow Surg.* 2004;13:266-271.

10. Smith T, Gettman A, Wellmann M, Pastor F, Struck M. Humeral surface replacement for osteoarthritis. *Acta Orthop.* 2013;84(5):468-472.

11. Mackenzie D. The antero-superior exposure for total shoulder replacement. *Orthop Traumatol.* 1993;2:71-77.

12. Routman HD, Savoie FH III. Subscapularis-sparing approaches to total shoulder arthroplasty: ready for prime time? *Clin Sports Med.* 2018;37(4):559-568.

13. Alolabi B, Youderian AR, Napolitano L, et al. Radiographic assessment of prosthetic humeral head size after anatomic shoulder arthroplasty. *J Shoulder Elbow Surg.* 2014;23:1740-1746.

14. Chen EJ, Simovitch R, Savoie FH, Noel CR. Assessment of the anatomic neck as an accurate landmark for humeral head resurfacing implant height placement. *Bull Hosp Jt Dis.* 2015;73(suppl 1):S28-S32.

15. Mansat P, Coutie AS, Bonnevialle N, Rongieres M, Mansat M, Bonnevialle P. Resurfacing humeral prosthesis: do we really reconstruct the anatomy? *J Shoulder Elbow Surg.* 2013;22(5):612-619.

16. Mullett H, Levy O, Raj D, Even T, Abraham R, Copeland SA. Copeland surface replacement of the shoulder. Results of an hydroxyapatite- coated cementless implant in patients over 80 years of age. *J Bone Joint Surg Br.* 2007;89:1466-1469.

17. Thomas SR, Wilson AJ, Chambler A, Harding I, Thomas M. Outcome of Copeland surface replacement shoulder arthroplasty. *J Shoulder Elbow Surg.* 2005;14:485-491.

18. Burkhead WZ Jr, Hutton KS. Biologic resurfacing of the glenoid with hemiarthroplasty of the shoulder. *J Shoulder Elbow Surg.* 1995;4(4):263-270.

19. Muh SJ, Streit JJ, Shishani Y, Dubrow S, Nowinski RJ, Gobezie R. Biologic resurfacing of the glenoid with humeral head resurfacing for glenohumeral arthritis in the young patient. *J Shoulder Elbow Surg.* 2014;23(8):e185-e190.

20. Bois AJ, Whitney IJ, Somerson JS, Wirth MA. Humeral head arthroplasty and meniscal allograft resurfacing of the glenoid: a concise follow-up of a previous report and survivorship analysis. *J Bone Joint Surg Am.* 2015;97(19):1571-1577.

21. Strauss EJ, Verma NN, Salata MJ, et al. The high failure rate of biologic resurfacing of the glenoid in young patients with glenohumeral arthritis. *J Shoulder Elbow Surg.* 2014;23(3):409-419.

22. Puskas GH, Meyer DC, Lebschi JA, Gerber C. Unacceptable failure of hemiarthroplasty combined with biological glenoid resurfacing the treatment of glenohumeral arthritis in the young. *J Shoulder Elbow Surg.* 2015;24(12):1900-1907.

23. Levine WN, Djurasovic M, Glasson JM, Pollock RG, Flatow EL, Bigliani LU. Hemiarthroplasty for glenohumeral osteoarthritis: results correlated to degree of glenoid wear. *J Shoulder Elbow Surg.* 1997;6:449-454.

24. Hettrich CM, Weldon E III, Boorman RS, Parsons IM IV, Matsen RD. Matsen FA III. Preoperative factors associated with improvements in shoulder function after humeral hemiarthroplasty. *J Bone Joint Surg Am.* 2004;86:1446-1451.

25. Rai P, Davies O, Wand J, Bigsby E. Long-term follow-up of the Copeland mark III shoulder resurfacing hemi-arthroplasty. *J Orthop.* 2016;13:52-56.

26. Maier MW, Hetto P, Raiss P, et al. Cementless humeral head resurfacing for degenerative glenohumeral osteoarthritis fails at a high rate. *J Orthop.* 2018;15:349-353.

27. Mechlenburg I, Amstrup A, Klebe T, Jacobsen SS, Teichert G, Stilling M. The Copeland resurfacing humeral head implant does not restore humeral head anatomy. A retrospective study. *Arch Orthop Trauma Surg.* 2013;133(5):615-619.

28. Hammond G, Tibbone JE, McGarry MH, Jun B, Lee TO. Biomechanical comparison of anatomic humeral head resurfacing and hemiarthroplasty in functional glenohumeral positions. *J Bone Joint Surg Am.* 2012;94:68-76.

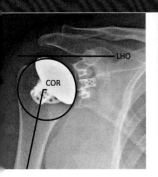

17

Stemless Total Shoulder Arthroplasty:
Indications and Technique

Jordan D. Walters, MD and Stephen F. Brockmeier, MD

INTRODUCTION

Shoulder arthroplasty has progressed from Péan's 1892 platinum and gum shoulder prosthesis to Neer's vitallium monoblock design in 1951 to the Neer II design with humeral and glenoid components in 1974 to second- and third-generation modular implants that typically rely on press-fit fixation rather than cementation.[1,2] Third-generation prostheses allow improved recreation of proximal humeral geometry including inclination, version, and diameter with variable stem lengths. However, the proximal portion of the implant was still bound by the stem. Now, a fourth generation of humeral implants for total shoulder arthroplasty (TSA) has been available since 2004, in which the humeral diaphyseal stem is no longer needed for fixation but, rather, the humeral implant is press-fit into the proximal humeral metaphysis. These stemless implants allow a more precise reconstruction of the proximal humeral geometry **(VIDEO 17.1)**.[2]

ADVANTAGES AND DISADVANTAGES

Several themes recur in the literature regarding the advantages of stemless humeral implants. These include bone stock preservation, humeral head anatomy recreation, ability to perform TSA in the setting of humeral deformity, facilitation of future implant revision, and avoidance of complications inherent with stemmed implants.[3,4] Stress shielding and humeral loosening are concerns for standard stemmed TSA implants, with reported loosening rates of 7% to 15%.[5] Compared to a standard stem system, in one report, the stemless implant had improved range of motion (ROM) and less radiolucent humeral lines.[2]

Stemless TSA has been reported to decrease operative time by 15 to 25 minutes compared to standard stemmed TSA, although one study compared stemless implants to cemented stemmed implants with limiting comparability.[6,7] In a study of a stemless reverse total shoulder arthroplasty (RTSA) implants versus a standard stemmed RTSA implant, the operative time in the stemless group averaged 30 minutes less. However, the stemless and stemmed implants were performed at different centers, making such a comparison difficult.[8]

Importantly, stemless TSA differs significantly from humeral head resurfacing. In stemless TSA, a humeral head resection is performed, which facilitates glenoid exposure and performance of the glenoid reconstruction. Humeral head resurfacing, in an effort to preserve as much bone as possible, only reshapes the humeral head, making glenoid exposure a challenge.[3,9] However, three-dimensional (3D) finite element modeling has shown that less bone stock loss occurs directly under the stemless TSA implant than under a resurfacing implant, suggesting better long-term fixation.[10]

Stemless TSA was developed with consideration of the need for future revision surgery. Revision surgery after stemless TSA compared with a standard stemmed TSA has been found to require cementation less often (27.8% vs 69.2%), require less OR time (84 vs 98 minutes), and have a higher postoperative Constant score (68 vs 51).[11]

With respect to blood loss, stemless implants avoid humeral endosteal canal reaming and the resultant bleeding. A study of 278 patients comparing stemless TSA, standard TSA, and standard RTSA showed a mean 100 mL less total blood loss for stemless patients compared to the other two groups.[12] No stemless TSA patients required a blood transfusion. These findings were corroborated by another study that also reported reduced blood loss of 100 mL in stemless versus stemmed arthroplasties.[5]

Ideally, humeral anatomy should be precisely restored to avoid alterations in capsular and myotendinous tissue balance and force dynamics. Because standard stemmed implants are bound by the relationship of the diaphyseal canal to the humeral head, they cannot always restore native humeral anatomy despite high degrees of modularity, although these differences may be small.[13] Lateral humeral offset (LHO), the distance from the medial side of the coracoid (a fixed structure) to the medial aspect of the greater tuberosity, is one parameter that quantifies overstuffing. Another parameter is the humeral head center of rotation (COR), measured as the distance from a line along the center of the humeral diaphysis perpendicularly to the center of a circle outlining the humeral head **(FIGURE 17.1)**. One study showed that with stemless TSA, LHO was restored to within 5 mm of the patient's

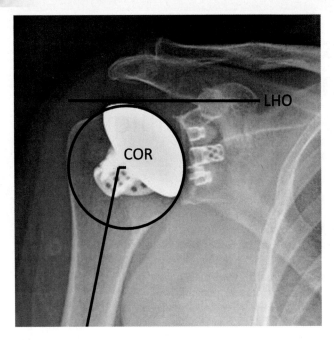

FIGURE 17.1 Lateral humeral offset (LHO) and center of rotation (COR) measurement for stemless total shoulder arthroplasty.

anatomy in 82% of cases, and COR was restored to within 3 mm of the patient's anatomy in 89% of cases.[14] Another study confirmed COR restoration to within 3 mm of original anatomy after stemless TSA in the majority of cases.[15] Other important restoration parameters include humeral head height and neck-shaft angle. Changes in these parameters of even several millimeters can be clinically significant, affecting shoulder ROM, glenoid component survival, and rotator cuff moment arms.[16] Generally, surgeons should avoid choosing the larger of two potential head sizes and avoid a varus head cut to minimize the risk of overstuffing.

Standard stemmed implants require greater bone removal from the proximal humerus, risk periprosthetic fractures during implantation, and limit the ability to achieve anatomic placement of the humeral head. One systematic review reported that 18% of all complications after standard stemmed TSA were related to the humeral side.[17] Treatment of periprosthetic fractures, humeral component revision, and management of infection can all be more difficult when a standard humeral implant is in place.[18] Shoulder arthroplasty performed for proximal humeral malunions can be more easily performed with a stemless humeral implant and can avoid the need for osteotomy.[19]

There are potential disadvantages with the use of a stemless humeral implant. First, there is no scientific method by which to definitively determine a patient's proximal humeral bone quality other than intraoperative assessment. The thumb assessment—attempting to press a thumb into the metaphyseal trabecular bone after the humeral head resection—and surgeon gestalt about the "feel" of the bone quality after osteotomy and implant

preparation are perhaps the best tools available. Second, it is also important for the surgeon to have a stemmed implant available in cases where metaphyseal bone will not support use of a stemless implant. Third, the surgeon should be completely knowledgeable about the stemless system being used and its capabilities. Most are not designed as platform systems to allow convertibility from anatomic total shoulder arthroplasty and RTSA can impact future revision procedures. Fourth, use of stemless implants can be more technically demanding because they rely on the surgeon's ability to reproducibly make an anatomic neck cut in appropriate version, inclination, and depth without the assistance of an intramedullary guide.[20] And lastly, every surgeon has to carefully asses the outcomes of any stemless system being considered to have confidence that patient satisfaction can be achieved. New implants are often industry driven, which requires each surgeon to be particularly focused on a careful and complete assessment of the technology before utilization.[21]

BIOMECHANICS

Wolff law guides stemless implant design. The bone remodels according to the load/stress placed upon it. Thus, areas of bone shielded by metal implants that share stress will resorb over time because of the lack of stimulation. This bone weakening can place implants that rely upon trabecular bone fixation at risk for loosening.[22] Since up to 82% of standard stemmed implants exhibit some degree of stress shielding, humeral stems have become progressively shorter in an effort to minimize this effect.[23] A finite element analysis showed that proximal humeral cortical stresses in stemless implants more closely matched those in the intact shoulder than did standard length or short-stem implants.[24] ACT study showed that below the plane of humeral head resection, the trabecular bone has greater density peripherally than centrally, suggesting a potential advantage of peripheral fixation stemless designs.[25] A 3D finite element model comparison of five implant types showed that the central screw design removed the least bone on insertion but upon loading led to the loss of bone mass.[26] The lateral quadrant of the implant/bone interface may be the most affected.[27] Additional research will undoubtedly lead to newer stemless implant designs that can address these areas of concern.

Another important factor is micromotion that can prevent bony ingrowth of the stemless implant. A finite element model of one stemless implant showed that 99% of the surface area had micromotion below the 150-μm threshold that defines whether bony ingrowth will occur during early rehabilitation ROM exercises.[28] Since SPECT/CT scan data have shown that osseointegrative metabolic activity is essentially complete 3 months after implantation,[29] limiting micromotion during early postoperative rehabilitation is essential to achieve bone ingrowth. This emphasizes the need for implant designs that minimize micromotion.

INDICATIONS

The ideal candidate for a stemless TSA is a young male or female (often less than 65 years old) with glenohumeral osteoarthritis and good-quality proximal humeral bone. Although younger age may increase the possibility of a revision procedure in the future, this is facilitated by the use of a stemless implant compared to stem designs. However, it is also important to note that in young patients with major chondral changes, the diagnosis is often osteonecrosis, inflammatory arthropathy, or other etiologies that may not be ideal for stemless implants.[30]

Stemless implants should not be used when the proximal humeral bone is compromised. This includes significant osteoporosis, metaphyseal cysts, acute fractures or chronic fracture sequelae that compromise the metaphyseal area, metabolic bone diseases, and revisions when a stemmed implant is in place.[3,8] Osteoporotic/osteopenic bone results in poor fixation and increased micromotion at the implant/bone interface, especially as the load increases.[31] Patients with rheumatoid arthritis should be carefully considered since one study showed proximal humeral bony changes in 33% of patients who underwent stemless TSA at only 2-year follow-up.[32]

CURRENT IMPLANT OPTIONS

Numerous implants have been developed with subtle variations for stemless metaphyseal fixation. Most implants involve either solid or open window fins that are impacted into the metaphysis to obtain press-fit fixation, although one design, the Eclipse, utilizes an open screw for initial fixation. The Eclipse, Simpliciti, and Sidus implants have collars. Most implants use metal heads, but the Affinis uses a ceramic head.[33] Each implant has some forms of coating material designed to promote either ingrowth or ongrowth.[34]

The first stemless implant to the European market in 2004 was the Biomet Total Evolutive Shoulder System (TESS). To enhance bony ingrowth, this three-component system has a six-arm porous corolla that is impacted into position.[3] The Biomet Nano system is the second generation of the TESS, which is a convertible system for revision to RTSA. It features a female Morse taper in the six-armed corolla that is impacted for press-fit fixation.[14] The Zimmer Biomet Sidus implant, a four-fin prosthesis with an ongrowth surface and large open windows, is also currently FDA approved.[23] In 2005, the Arthrex Eclipse stemless prosthesis was introduced in Europe. It has a cylindrical, open, fully threaded screw attached through a baseplate/trunnion. It is the only screw-in design that does not rely on impaction for fixation but instead relies on compression.[3]

Other options exist besides these two well-studied implants. The Mathys Affinis short stemless prosthesis was introduced in Europe in 2009. This two-component calcium phosphate–coated porous titanium component

with a ceramic head has four wings and is impacted into place.[3] The Simpliciti stemless prosthesis by Tornier/Wright first was first used in France in 2010. It is a tri-flanged porous-coated baseplate impacted into position. The Wright/Tornier Simpliciti is FDA approved in the United States.[3] The four-component Lima SMR has a trabecular ingrowth design that is impacted into place. It is a platform system that can be converted to RTSA. The FX solutions Easytech has three components and is also implanted via impaction.[34] The Exactech Equinoxe stemless implant consists of two components and is also impacted to gain initial fixation (**FIGURE 17.2**).

STEMLESS HUMERAL IMPLANTATION TECHNIQUE

Stemless TSA is performed in the standard beach chair position. A deltopectoral approach is typically utilized, taking care to limit bleeding and optimize visualization. Surgeon preference determines subscapularis management. Tenotomy, subscapularis peel, and lesser tuberosity osteotomy (LTO) are all effective with stemmed and stemless implants.[35] We prefer to create a thin wafer LTO of roughly 2 to 3 mm with a microsagittal saw and osteotome to avoid significant cortical disruption. After the humeral head is exposed, the surgeon should carefully identify the anatomic neck circumferentially by removing all osteophytes and ensuring visualization of the rotator cuff attachments. Intramedullary guides for the humeral head resection are not utilized in order to avoid disruption of metaphyseal bone. A majority of the available implants have some types of extramedullary guide instrumentation that can be used at the surgeon's discretion. A sagittal saw is used to carefully perform an anatomic neck cut maintaining the patient's natural humeral version and avoiding damage to the rotator cuff tendon insertions (**FIGURE 17.3**). Exacting technique should be used to ensure that a smooth plane is created. The thumb test is then used to press firmly into the metaphyseal trabecular bone to ensure that it is not easily depressed or indented and that a stemless implant is appropriate (**FIGURE 17.4**). If the bone is easily compressed with the thumb, then a stemless implant should not be attempted. The glenoid is then prepared and the glenoid component is inserted based upon the system being utilized.

The proximal humerus is again exposed with a combination of blunt retractors and arm positioning in external rotation/adduction/extension. Most stemless humeral implants are impacted into the proximal humeral metaphyseal bone. Guides are used initially to impact the center of the metaphyseal bone to prepare the flutes for the implant (**FIGURE 17.5**). Great care should be taken at this step to ensure that each impact with the cutting guide and then with the final implant is directly perpendicular to the plane of resection. Any twisting, angulation, or translation will disrupt the thin canals of the impacted trabecular bone and compromise the ultimate implant fixation. The surgeon should not

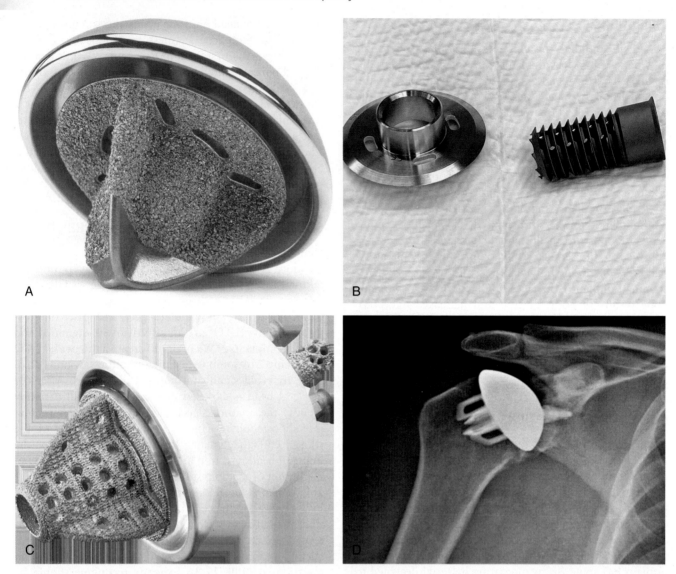

FIGURE 17.2 Various stemless humeral implants: **A**, Simpliciti (Published with permission from Tornier, Inc an indirect subsidiary of Wright Medial Group N.V.); **B**, Eclipse (Arthrex); **C**, Equinoxe stemless (Exactech); and **D**, Sidus (Zimmer Biomet). (A, Image reprinted with permission from Stryker Corporation. © 2021 Stryker Corporation. All rights reserved. B, This image provided courtesy of Arthrex®, Naples, Florida 2021. C, Used with permission from © Exactech, Inc. D, Used with permission from © Zimmer Biomet.)

simply rely on a guide pin to maintain relative alignment because it is often not stable or secure and allows excessive movement. If there is concern whether secure fixation is achieved, then conversion to a standard stemmed implant is necessary. Prior to final implantation, our technique for LTO fixation requires three 2-mm drill holes placed in the bicipital groove from proximal to distal, for placement of three #5 nonabsorbable sutures **(FIGURE 17.6)**. The sutures are brought from the anterior cortex through the impressions created by previous humeral preparation and looped through the final implant **(FIGURE 17.7)**. The humeral stemless implant is then impacted into final position. The humeral head that best matches the height and diameter of the resected head is chosen **(FIGURE 17.8)**. The concentric head with the smallest diameter that matches the anterior, posterior, and lateral surfaces is used. Residual medial

and inferior osteophytes can be removed to match the dimensions of the modular head rather than overstuffing with a larger size. After confirming the proper size based upon trial reductions, the head is impacted into position, and fixation is achieved by the Morse taper **(FIGURE 17.9)**. The shoulder is reduced and tension/stability is confirmed. The #5 sutures previously positioned are then used for the subscapularis/LTO repair with modified Mason-Allen sutures and secured so that the LTO wafer is compressed into its anatomic position **(FIGURE 17.10)**. Copious irrigation is followed by standard closure.

OUTCOMES

The TESS implant has been studied extensively. Early on, five cases of lateral cortical fracture occurred, but all healed within 2 months with no loss of fixation or need

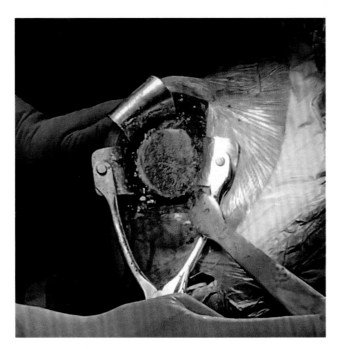

FIGURE 17.3 Humeral head osteotomy.

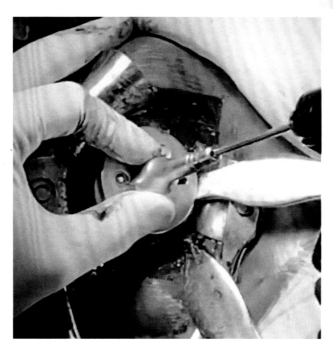

FIGURE 17.5 Preparation for stemless implant.

for intervention.[9,36] The TESS implant has good long-term follow-up, with one study having excellent clinical results with no humeral fixation problems with almost 8 years of follow-up.[37] Favorable results with low complication and revision rates have generally been reported with various implants as evidenced by improvement in patient-reported outcomes, ROM, and pain.[6,9,15,37-39] While many studies have been reported by implant developers, other unbiased study groups have corroborated these favorable results.[40]

Most studies have not reported humeral component loosening of a stemless TSA implant.[15,38,39] Radiolucent lines <2 mm around an Eclipse implant were observed in three out of 29 patients in one study, although this finding had no effect on patient outcomes.[41,42] This implant also showed decreased greater tuberosity cancellous bone density on radiographs in 35% of patients without loosening or an impact on clinical outcomes at a mean 6-year follow-up.[43] For the Eclipse, 9-year

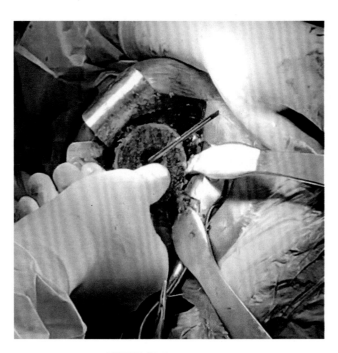

FIGURE 17.4 Thumb test.

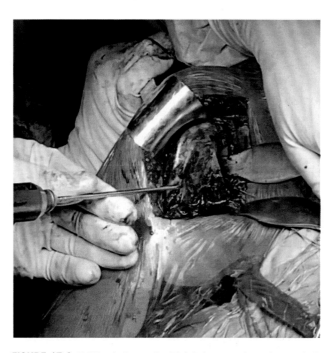

FIGURE 17.6 Drilling holes at the bicipital groove for subscapularis repair.

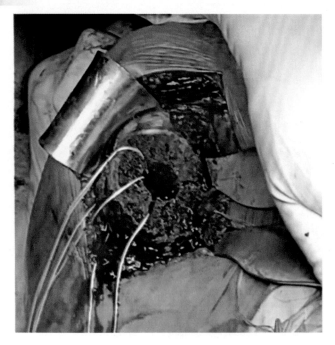

FIGURE 17.7 Sutures in place for subscapularis repair.

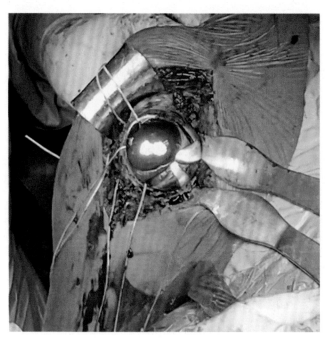

FIGURE 17.9 Humeral head after impaction.

follow-up data reported no humeral implant complications despite decreased radiographic bone mineral density being evident in 29.4% of patients.[44] Another study of 47 patients showed that 17 patients developed nonprogressive radiolucencies around the implant at short-term follow-up.[45] It is possible that radiolucencies may be artifacts due to radiation scatter causing a "halo effect" instead of being true stress shielding changes.[46] Long-term studies are needed to determine the significance of these radiographic findings.

With respect to complications, one concerning study reported an 11.2% infection rate for a series of stemless implants compared to a 4.3% infection rate for a standard stemmed implant.[47] Young males, the key demographic for stemless implants, are at higher risk for *Cutibacterium acnes* colonization, possibly placing these implants at slightly higher infection risk. However, most studies have not reported higher infection rates to date.

Regarding primary TSA outcomes, studies including a meta-analysis and a Nordic registry study have not

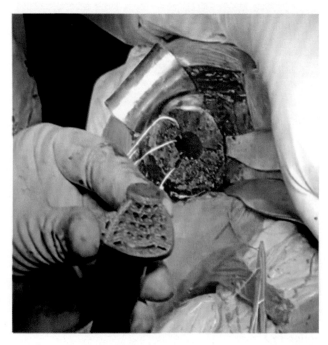

FIGURE 17.8 Humeral stemless implant.

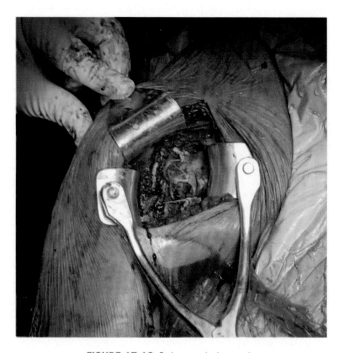

FIGURE 17.10 Subscapularis repair.

shown significant differences in Constant score, ROM, proprioception, or survival between stemless and standard TSA.[18,48-53] Another study reported no differences in neurologic complications, operative time, infection eradication, or ROM outcomes in revision surgeries performed for infection in either stemless or standard TSA implants.[54] Unfortunately, the literature lacks randomized controlled trials with sufficient patient numbers and long-term follow-up. Despite comparable clinical results, standard stemmed implants may have greater levels of tribocorrosion than stemless implants.[55] Long-term studies will determine whether such fretting will prove to be as significant as it has been for total hip arthroplasty.

STEMLESS IMPLANTS IN RTSA

The TESS is one of the few systems designed for both TSA and RTSA. One study reported good functional results at a follow-up of 39 months. However, two of the 16 displaced humeral implants occurred in the stemless RTSA group within 1 week of surgery.[56] Multiple studies show favorable short- to midterm clinical results with only one revision RTSA case required.[7,57,58] Another study reported no humeral implant–related issues at mean 8.4-year follow-up of the TESS stemless RTSA with an all-cause revision rate of 17.2%.[59] Stemless RTSA has not seen the same growth in surgeon acceptance as stemless TSA, but early results are encouraging.

CONCLUSION

Stemless humeral components in TSA have become a part of the armamentarium available to shoulder surgeons for the treatment of degenerative disorders of the glenohumeral joint. When the implant is appropriately matched to the patient, stemless components have shown excellent and enduring results. Research and implant design/development continues to improve our understanding of how best to recreate shoulder anatomy in the setting of shoulder arthroplasty.

REFERENCES

1. Lugli T. Artificial shoulder joint by Péan (1893): the facts of an exceptional intervention and the prosthetic method. *Clin Orthop Relat Res.* 1978;133:215-218.
2. Razmjou H, Holtby R, Christakis M, Axelrod T, Richards R. Impact of prosthetic design on clinical and radiologic outcomes of total shoulder arthroplasty: a prospective study. *J Shoulder Elbow Surg.* 2013;22:206-214.
3. Hawi N, Tauber M, Messina JM, Habermeyer P, Martetschlager F. Anatomic stemless shoulder arthroplasty and related outcomes: a systematic review. *BMC Musculoskelet Disord.* 2016;17:376.
4. Harmer L, Throckmorton T, Sperling JW. Total shoulder arthroplasty: are the humeral components getting shorter? *Curr Rev Musculoskelet Med.* 2016;9:17-22.
5. Lazarus MD, Cox RM, Murthi AM, Levy O, Abboud JA. Stemless prosthesis for total shoulder arthroplasty. *J Am Acad Orthop Surg.* 2017;25:e291-e300.
6. Berth A, Pap G. Stemless shoulder prosthesis versus conventional anatomic shoulder prosthesis in patients with osteoarthritis: a comparison of the functional outcome after a minimum of two years follow-up. *J Orthop Traumatol.* 2013;14:31-37.
7. Heuberer PR, Brandi G, Pauzenberger L, et al. Radiological changes do not influence clinical mid-term outcome in stemless humeral head replacements with hollow screw fixation: a prospective radiological and clinical evaluation. *BMC Musculoskelet Disord.* 2018;19:28.
8. Moroder P, Erustbrunner L, Zwelger C, et al. Short to mid-term results of stemless reverse shoulder arthroplasty in a selected patient population compared to a matched control group with stem. *Int Orthop.* 2016;40:2115-2120.
9. Huguet D, DeClercq G, Rio B, Teissier J, Zipoli B; the TESS Group. Results of a new stemless shoulder prosthesis: radiologic proof of maintained fixation and stability after a minimum of three years' follow-up. *J Shoulder Elbow Surg.* 2010;19:847-852.
10. Santos B, Quental C, Folgado J, Sarmento M, Monteiro J. Bone remodeling of the humerus after a resurfacing and a stemless shoulder arthroplasty. *Clin Biomech (Bristol, Avon).* 2018;59:78-84.
11. Holschen M, Franetzki B, Witt KA, Liem D, Steinbeck J. Is reverse total shoulder arthroplasty a feasible treatment option for failed shoulder arthroplasty? A retrospective study of 44 cases with special regards to stemless and stemmed primary implants. *Musculoskelet Surg.* 2017;101:173-180.
12. Malcherczyk D, Abelmoula A, Heyse TJ, et al. Bleeding in primary shoulder arthroplasty. *Arch Orthop Trauma Surg.* 2018;239:317-323.
13. Pinto MC, Archie AT, Mosher ZA, et al. Radiographic restoration of native anatomy: a comparison between stemmed and stemless shoulder arthroplasty. *J Shoulder Elbow Surg.* 2019;28:1595-1600.
14. Kadum B, Wahlstrom P, Khoschnau S, Sjoden G, Sayed-Noor A. Association of lateral humeral offset with functional outcome and geometric restoration in stemless total shoulder arthroplasty. *J Shoulder Elbow Surg.* 2016;25:e285-e294.
15. Gallacher S, Williams HLM, King A, et al. Clinical and radiologic outcomes following total shoulder arthroplasty using Arthrex Eclipse stemless humeral component with minimum 2 years' follow-up. *J Shoulder Elbow Surg.* 2018;27:2191-2197.
16. Kadum B, Hassany H, Wadsten M, Sayed-Noor A, Sjoden G. Geometrical analysis of stemless shoulder arthroplasty: a radiological study of seventy TESS total shoulder prostheses. *Int Orthop.* 2016;40:751-758.
17. Bohsali KI, Wirth MA, Rockwood CA Jr. Complications of total shoulder arthroplasty. *J Bone Joint Surg Am.* 2006;88(10):2279-2292.
18. Maier MW, Lauer S, Klotz MC, et al. Are there differences between stemless and conventional stemmed shoulder prostheses in the treatment of glenohumeral osteoarthritis? *BMC Musculoskelet Disord.* 2015;16:275.
19. Ballas R, Teissier P, Teissier J. Stemless shoulder prosthesis for treatment of proximal humeral malunion does not require tuberosity osteotomy. *Int Orthop.* 2016;40:1473-1479.
20. Brolin TJ, Cox RM, Abboud JA, Namdari S. Stemless shoulder arthroplasty: review of early clinical and radiographic results. *JBJS Rev.* 2017;5(8):e3-e9.
21. Routman HD, Becks L, Roche C. Stemless and short stem humeral components in shoulder arthroplasty. *Bull Hosp Jt Dis (2013).* 2015;73(suppl 1):S145-S147.
22. Denard PJ, Raiss P, Gobezie R, Edwards TB, Lederman E. Stress shielding of the humerus in press-fit anatomic shoulder arthroplasty: review and recommendations for evaluation. *J Shoulder Elbow Surg.* 2018;27:1139-1147.
23. Brabston EW, Fehringer EV, Owen MT, Ponce BA. Stemless humeral implants in total shoulder arthroplasty. *J Am Acad Orthop Surg.* 2020;28(7):e277-e287.
24. Razfar N, Reeves JM, Langohr DG, Willing R, Athwal GS, Johnson JA. Comparison of proximal humeral bone stresses between stemless, short stem, and standard stem length: a finite element analysis. *J Shoulder Elbow Surg.* 2016;25:1076-1083.
25. Reeves JM, Athwal GS, Johnson JA. An assessment of proximal humerus density with reference to stemless implants. *J Shoulder Elbow Surg.* 2018;27:641-649.

26. Comenda M, Quental C, Folgado J, Sarmento M, Monteiro J. Bone adaptation impact of stemless shoulder implants: a computational analysis. *J Shoulder Elbow Surg.* 2019;28:1886-1896.

27. Reeves JM, Langohr GDG, Athwal GS, Johnson JA. The effect of stemless humeral component fixation feature design on bone stress and strain response: a finite element analysis. *J Shoulder Elbow Surg.* 2018;27:2232-2241.

28. Favre P, Henderson AD. Prediction of stemless humeral implant micromotion during upper limb activities. *Clin Biomech (Bristol, Avon).* 2016;36:46-51.

29. Berth A, Marz V, Wissel H, et al. SPECT/CT demonstrates the osseointegrative response of a stemless shoulder prosthesis. *J Shoulder Elbow Surg.* 2016;25:e96-e103.

30. Tashjian RZ, Chalmers PN. Future frontiers in shoulder arthroplasty and the management of shoulder osteoarthritis. *Clin Sports Med.* 2018;37:609-639.

31. Favre P, Seebeck J, Thistlewaite PAE, et al. In vitro initial stability of a stemless humeral implant. *Clin Biomech (Bristol, Avon).* 2016;32:113-117.

32. Jordan RW, Manoharan G, Liefland MV, et al. Reliability of stemless shoulder arthroplasty in rheumatoid arthritis: observation of early lysis around the humeral component. *Musculoskelet Surg.* 2019. doi:10.1007/s12306-019-00629-8

33. Churchill RS. Stemless shoulder arthroplasty: current status. *J Shoulder Elbow Surg.* 2014;23:1409-1414.

34. Churchill RS, Athwal GS. Stemless shoulder arthroplasty-current results and designs. *Curr Rev Musculoskelet Med.* 2016;9:10-16.

35. Aibinder WR, Bicknell RT, Bartsch S, Scheibel M, Athwal GS. Subscapularis management in stemless total shoulder arthroplasty: tenotomy versus peel versus lesser tuberosity osteotomy. *J Shoulder Elbow Surg.* 2019;28:1942-1947.

36. Geurts GF, van Riet RP, Jansen N, Declercq G. Placement of the stemless humeral component in the total evolutive shoulder system (TESS). *Tech Hand Up Extrem Surg.* 2010;14:214-217.

37. Beck S, Beck V, Wegner A, et al. Long-term survivorship of stemless anatomical shoulder replacement. *Int Orthop.* 2018;42:1327-1330.

38. Churchill RS, Chuinard C, Wiater JM, et al. Clinical and radiographic outcomes of the Simpliciti canal-sparing shoulder arthroplasty system: a prospective two-year multicenter study. *J Bone Joint Surg Am.* 2016;98:552-560.

39. Sayed-Noor AS, Pollock R, Elhassan BT, Kadum B. Fatty infiltration and muscle atrophy of the rotator cuff in stemless total shoulder arthroplasty: a prospective cohort study. *J Shoulder Elbow Surg.* 2018;27:976-982.

40. Bulhoff M Spranz D, Maier M, et al. Mid-term results with an anatomic stemless shoulder prosthesis in patients with primary osteoarthritis. *Acta Orthop Traumatol Turc.* 2019;53:170-174.

41. Moursy M, Niks M, Kadavkolan AS, Lehmann LJ. Do the radiological changes seen at midterm follow up of stemless shoulder prosthesis affect outcome? *BMC Musculoskelet Disord.* 2019;20:490.

42. von Engelhardt LV, Manzke M, Breil-Wirth A, Filler TJ, Jerosch J. Restoration of the joint geometry and outcome after stemless TESS shoulder arthroplasty. *World J Orthop.* 2017;8(10):790-797.

43. Habermeyer P, Lichtenberg S, Tauber M, Magosch P. Midterm results of stemless shoulder arthroplasty: a prospective study. *J Shoulder Elbow Surg.* 2015;24:1463-1472.

44. Hawi N, Magosch P, Tauber M, Lichtenber S, Habermeyer P. Nine-year outcome after anatomic stemless shoulder prosthesis: clinical and radiologic results. *J Shoulder Elbow Surg.* 2017;26:1609-1615.

45. Collin P, Matsukawa T, Boileau P, Brunner U, Walch G. Is the humeral stem useful in anatomic total shoulder arthroplasty? *Int Orthop.* 2017;41:1035-1039.

46. Hudek R, Werner B, Abdelkawi AF, Schmitt R, Gohlke F. Radiolucency in stemless shoulder arthroplasty is associated with an imaging phenomenon. *J Orthop Res.* 2017;35:2040-2050.

47. Johansson L, Hailer NP, Rahme H. High incidence of periprosthetic joint infection with Propionibacterium acnes after the use of a stemless shoulder prosthesis with metaphyseal screw fixation – a retrospective cohort study of 241 patients propionibacter infections after eclipse TSA. *BMC Musculoskelet Disord.* 2017;18:203.

48. Rasmussen JV, Harjula J, Arverud ED, et al. The short-term survival of total stemless shoulder arthroplasty for osteoarthritis is comparable to that of total stemmed shoulder arthroplasty: a Nordic arthroplasty register association study. *J Shoulder Elbow Surg.* 2019;28:1578-1586.

49. Spranz DM, Bruttel H, Wolf SI, Zeifang F, Maier MW. Functional midterm follow-up comparison of stemless total shoulder prostheses versus conventional stemmed anatomic shoulder prostheses using a 3D-motion-analysis. *BMC Musculoskelet Disord.* 2017;18:478.

50. Uschok S, Magosch P, Moe M, Lichtenberg S, Habermeyer P. Is the stemless humeral head replacement clinically and radiographically a secure equivalent to standard stem humeral head replacement in the long-term follow-up? A prospective randomized trial. *J Shoulder Elbow Surg.* 2017;26:225-232.

51. Upfill-Brown A, Satariano N, Feeley B. Stemless shoulder arthroplasty: review of short and medium-term results. *JSES Open Access.* 2019;3:154-161.

52. Mariotti U, Motta P, Stucchi A, Ponti di Sant'Angelo F. Stemmed versus stemless total shoulder arthroplasty: a preliminary report and short-term results. *Musculoskelet Surg.* 2014;98:195-200.

53. Peng W, Ou Y, Wang C, et al. The short- to midterm effectiveness of stemless prostheses compared to stemmed prostheses for patients who underwent total shoulder arthroplasty: a meta-analysis. *J Orthop Surg Res.* 2019;14:469.

54. Padegimas EM, Narzikul A, Lawrence C, et al. Antibiotic spacers in shoulder arthroplasty: comparison of stemmed and stemless implants. *Clin Orthop Surg.* 2017;9(4):489-496.

55. Eckert JA, Mueller U, Jaeger S, Panzram B, Kretzer JP. Fretting and corrosion in modular shoulder arthroplasty: a retrieval analysis. *Biomed Res Int.* 2016;2016:1695906. doi:10.1155/2016/1695906

56. Kadum B, Mukka S, Englund E, Sayed-Noor A, Sjoden G. Clinical and radiological outcome of the Total Evolutive Shoulder System (TESS) reverse shoulder arthroplasty: a prospective comparative non-randomized study. *Int Orthop.* 2014;38:1001-1006.

57. Ballas R, Beguin L. Results of a stemless reverse shoulder prothesis at more than 58 months mean without loosening. *J Shoulder Elbow Surg.* 2013;22:e1-e6.

58. von Engelhardt LV, Manzke M, Filler TJ, Jerosch J. Short-term results of the reverse total evolutive shoulder system (TESS) in cuff tear arthropathy and revision arthroplasty cases. *Arch Orthop Trauma Surg.* 2015;135:897-904.

59. Beck S, Patsalis T, Busch A, et al. Long-term results of the reverse total evolutive shoulder system (TESS). *Arch Orthop Trauma Surg.* 2019;139:1039-1044.

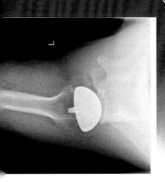

18 Shoulder Arthroplasty Using Inset and Inlay Glenoids

Kevin W. Farmer, MD

INTRODUCTION

Total shoulder arthroplasty (TSA) has become the gold standard treatment option for patients with glenohumeral osteoarthritis, an intact rotator cuff, and failed nonoperative management. In 1974, Charles Neer modified his Neer I prosthesis to add a cemented, keeled, onlay, polyethylene glenoid component, known as the Neer II prosthesis.[1] Early outcome studies demonstrated promising results but with a high level of radiographic glenoid loosening.[2] Since then, the use of TSA has continually increased over time, with good long-term survival outcomes. The glenoid component remains the "weak link" in the construct, with glenoid component loosening being one of the most common complications.[3] In a systematic review of 27 articles and 3853 TSA, authors found asymptomatic radiolucent lines occurred at 7.3% and symptomatic loosening at 1.2% per year following TSA, indicating the high prevalence of these findings.[4]

Glenoid loosening is an even more significant issue with worsening glenoid deformity. Increased incidence of radiolucent lines is observed in cases of posterior glenoid wear,[5] increased retroversion,[6] rotator cuff deficiency,[7] superior tilt, preoperative posterior subluxation, and excessive reaming[8] **(FIGURE 18.1)**. The preservation of subchondral bone is important for minimizing the risk of loosening and migration, thus limiting the amount of correction a surgeon can make during surgery. It is for these reasons that many surgeons choose to utilize a reverse total shoulder arthroplasty (RTSA) in cases of excessive glenoid wear.

The primary mechanism of failure of onlay glenoids in TSA is due to micromotion of the implant over time. This has been termed the "rocking-horse" phenomenon due to edge loading of the implant **(FIGURE 18.2)**.[7] Due to edge loading, there is microscopic compression of one end of the component, with subsequent elevation of the opposite side. Through repetitive cycles, the micromotion can lead to compromise of the polyethylene-cement-bone interface and subsequent loosening. Glenoid wear can compound this loosening through polyethylene debris, initiating a foreign body reaction with osteolysis.[1]

Early attempts to address glenoid loosening included metal-backed glenoids. Early versions eventually fell out of favor as a result of a high incidence of backside wear with 83% of glenoids demonstrating radiolucencies by 2 years.[9] More recently, newer designs of metal-backed implants are again being utilized in an effort to reduce the issues of loosening **(FIGURE 18.3)**. Other design features have also been employed to reduce the incidence of loosening, including pegged glenoids(with varying peg configurations), different glenoid shapes, and enhanced cementation technique.

INSET AND INLAY GLENOID RATIONALE

The notion of decreasing edge loading has led to the design of an "inset," in which part of the implant is inset within the glenoid, or an "inlay" glenoid, in which all of the implant is placed within the glenoid so that it is flush with the bone, with the hope of dispersing the contact forces between the implant and the native glenoid. In a biomechanical study of eight matched pairs of glenoids, authors looked at glenohumeral contact forces and fatigue testing at 4000 cycles using a cemented onlay glenoid and a cemented inlay glenoid. They found that the edge loading of the onlay glenoid increased compared to the native glenoid, presumably from lateralization of the contact area. In contrast, the inlay glenoid had a decrease in the edge-loading contact forces, as a result of the force being distributed between the implant and the native glenoid. With fatigue testing, all onlay glenoid components demonstrated loosening at a mean 1126 cycles (range 749-1838). None of the inlay glenoids demonstrated loosening at 4000 cycles[10] **(FIGURE 18.4)**.

In another biomechanical comparison of an inset glenoid compared to both a keel and pegged onlay glenoid, authors looked at displacement and loosening at 100,000 cycles. They found that an inset glenoid showed 87% less displacement compared to the pegged and keel onlay glenoids. They did not demonstrate a significant difference in loosening at 100,000 cycles.[11] These two studies provide strong biomechanical evidence that an inlay or inset glenoid has less micromotion and edge loading compared to an onlay glenoid.

Of course, the unanswered question is whether the biomechanical evidence translates to improved clinical outcomes and decreased loosening, especially in more active patients.

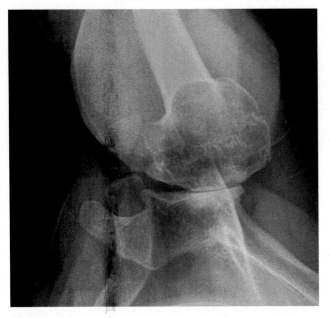

FIGURE 18.1 Axillary image of a B2 glenoid with posterior subluxation of the humeral head, both risk factors for glenoid implant loosening following anatomic total shoulder arthroplasty (TSA).

CLINICAL OUTCOMES

Based on the promising biomechanical evidence, there has been increased use of the inset or inlay glenoid, with midterm follow-up outcomes reported. Egger and Miniaci used the OVO total shoulder with an inlay glenoid (Arthrosurface, Franklin, MA) in 31 shoulders (29 patients; mean age 58.6 years). At an average 42.6-month follow-up, they reported no evidence of loosening or revision surgery, mean forward flexion of 167.3°, mean satisfaction of 8.4/10, and a visual analog scale (VAS) pain score of 0.9. Interestingly, 77.4% of the glenoids were considered "nonconcentric" or deficient. There were no differences in outcomes or lucency between concentric and nonconcentric glenoids.[12]

Using the same implant, Nicholson and colleagues looked at the outcomes in younger patients, with an average age of 52 years. They had 27 shoulders with a minimum of 2-year follow-up. The majority of the patients were type A or B1 glenoids, although there were a few B2 glenoids. There were no signs of loosening, with 93% returning to work, including 76% returning to the same level of work demand they had preoperatively. Interestingly, 75% returned to sport, with 50% at the same level or higher compared preoperatively.[13]

Gunther et al published short-term outcomes of an inset glenoid (Shoulder Innovations, Holland, MI) in seven patients with severe glenoid bone loss at an average 4.3-year

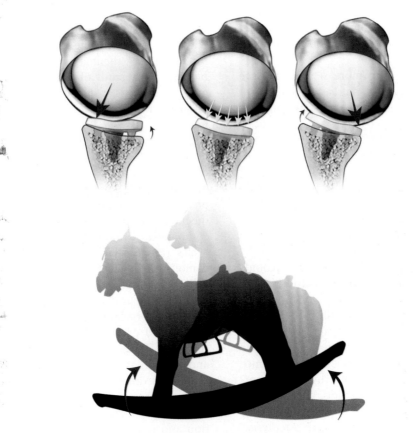

FIGURE 18.2 "Rocking-horse" micromotion of the glenoid component due to edge loading.

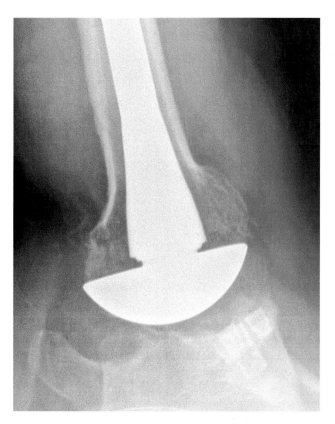

FIGURE 18.3 Metal-backed posterior augment glenoid used for the B2 glenoid shown in **FIGURE 18.1**. Metal cage and pegs designed to minimize glenoid loosening.

follow-up. They found no evidence of loosening of glenoids "at risk" and a statistically significant improvement in functional outcomes.[14] The same group also published a longer term follow-up of 21 patients with an average age of 68 years and with glenoid deficiency, defined by a glenoid vault less than 15 mm. At a mean follow-up of 8.7 years, there were statistically significant improvements in range of motion, VAS scores, and American Shoulder and Elbow Surgeons (ASES) scores. There was no evidence of glenoid loosening, and no revisions were performed. The authors concluded that an inset glenoid is a viable option in patients with a deficient glenoid vault that are not considered good candidates for a typical onlay glenoid.[15]

One particularly interesting finding of the above studies is the notion that the outcomes of an inlay or an inset glenoid are not dependent on glenoid shape or version. Both Gunther[14,15] and Miniaci[12] found good outcomes in nonconcentric or deficient glenoids. This has led to the idea of "playing it where it lies." This is a golf term, where you play your ball where it ends up rather than move it to a more desirable location. In the context of the glenoid, this phrase would mean to use an inlay glenoid in severe glenoid deformity without changing the version or anatomy. Authors have noted that some patients correct preoperative posterior subluxation by simply placing the inlay glenoid implant where the glenoid lies.[14] Williams and colleagues utilized an inlay glenoid (Arthrosurface, Franklin, MA) in

CONTACT FORCE - Inlay

Zone A2:	91.8N
Zone C:	73.3N
Zone D:	20.9N

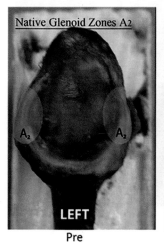
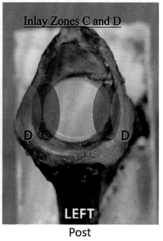

CONTACT FORCE - Onlay

| Zone A1: | 85.7N |
| Zone B: | 124.8N |

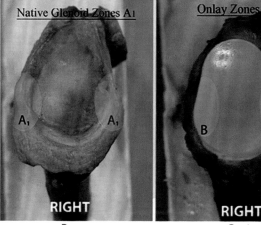
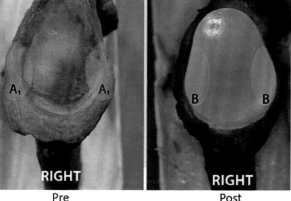

FIGURE 18.4 Edge-loading contact forces between the native glenoid, an inlay glenoid implant, and an onlay glenoid implant. (From Gagliano JR, Helms SM, Colbath GP, Przestrzelski BT, Hawkins RJ, DesJardins JD. A comparison of onlay versus inlay glenoid component loosening in total shoulder arthroplasty. *J Shoulder Elbow Surg.* 2017;26(7):1113-1120.)

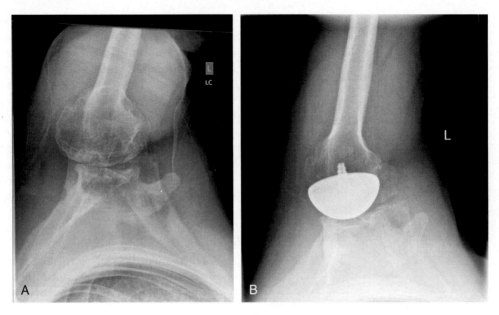

FIGURE 18.5 A, Preoperative axillary radiograph demonstrating a B2 glenoid with posterior subluxation of the humeral head. **B**, Postoperative axillary radiograph after a resurfacing humeral head and an inlay glenoid. Note the recentering of the humeral head without augments, bone graft, or capsulorrhaphy.

nine shoulders in patients with a mean age of 66 years and a mean follow-up of 34 months. Four glenoids were type B2, and two were type C; the others were not able to be classified. Pain scores decreased from 8 to 1, Sane scores increased from 32 to 90, and mean satisfaction was 8.6 on a 10 point scale.[16] These clinical studies demonstrate good functional outcomes, good pain improvement, low rates of loosening, and similar outcomes regardless of glenoid version and shape.

AUTHOR'S PREFERRED APPROACH

An inlay glenoid is my preferred option in younger, active patients. The typical age in my practice is around 50 years, and the more active they are, the more likely I am to use an inlay glenoid. I have used it in construction workers, weightlifters, and in the throwing shoulder of softball players. The glenoids in these patients have most commonly been of the B2 type **(FIGURE 18.5A and B)**. Thus far, I have not had any revisions or signs of loosening in these younger, more active patients.

I prefer a deltopectoral approach, using a slightly shorter incision than I would use for a standard TSA **(FIGURE 18.6; VIDEO 18.1)**. In these cases, I generally combine a humeral head resurfacing component with an inlay glenoid **(FIGURE 18.5B)**. I prefer a subscapularis tenotomy and leave approximately a 1-cm cuff of tissue on the lesser tuberosity. A biceps tenodesis is performed to the pectoralis tendon in most cases **(FIGURE 18.7)**.

A 30° offset guide is used to place a guide pin in the glenoid for reaming **(FIGURE 18.8A and B)**. It is important

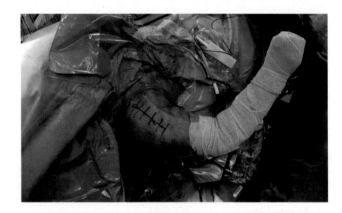

FIGURE 18.6 A deltopectoral incision is utilized for cases.

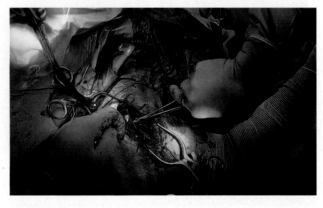

FIGURE 18.7 A biceps tenodesis to the pectoralis tendon is performed.

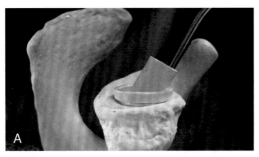
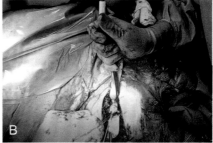

FIGURE 18.8 A and **B**, A 30° offset guide is utilized to place the guide pin for reaming. This offset allows you to work around the reamed humeral head.

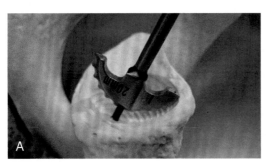
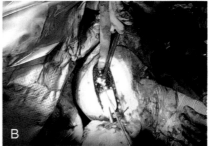

FIGURE 18.9 A and **B**, A 20-mm reamer is used over the guide wire to ream the socket for the inlay glenoid.

that the guide is placed as flat against the glenoid as possible. When a ridge is present on the glenoid as in a B2, I will smooth it to a flat surface with a Cobb elevator or curette. A 20-mm reamer (**FIGURE 18.9A** and **B**) is utilized, and the depth is checked with a trial until flush or slightly recessed (**FIGURE 18.10**). The implant is cemented in place (**FIGURE 18.11**).

Postoperative management includes a sling for 6 weeks. The rehabilitation program is somewhat more aggressive than a standard shoulder arthroplasty, in part, because of the patient population and a "return to sport" mentality. The subscapularis repair is protected for the first 3 months with external rotation limited to 30° for the first 6 weeks. Return to sport and manual labor is typically around 3 to 4 months.

CONCLUSION AND FUTURE DIRECTIONS

The desire to reduce glenoid radiolucent lines and glenoid loosening has led to the development of an inlay or inset glenoid, with the goal of reducing edge loading and the rocking-horse phenomenon. Biomechanical studies have validated these designs as viable options. Initial clinical studies with short- and midterm results demonstrate good outcomes, regardless of glenoid shape. Although, to date, there have been no revisions reported, the inevitable need for revisions in this setting is a concern because of the potential for further bone loss. Future studies looking at long-term follow-up, revisions, and noncemented options will determine whether this option will become more commonly utilized in the future.

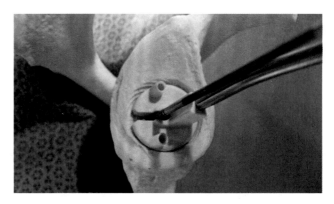

FIGURE 18.10 A trial implant is used to ensure the inlay glenoid is flush or slightly recessed.

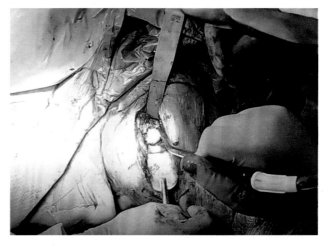

FIGURE 18.11 The final 20-mm inlay glenoid after cementing.

REFERENCES

1. Pinkas D, Wiater B, Wiater JM. The glenoid component in anatomic shoulder arthroplasty. *J Am Acad Orthop Surg.* 2015;23(5):317-326.
2. Cofield RH. Total shoulder arthroplasty with the Neer prosthesis. *J Bone Joint Surg Am.* 1984;66(6):899-906.
3. Gonzalez JF, Alami GB, Baque F, Walch G, Boileau P. Complications of unconstrained shoulder prostheses. *J Shoulder Elbow Surg.* 2011;20(4):666-682.
4. Papadonikolakis A, Neradilek MB, Matsen III FA. Failure of the glenoid component in anatomic total shoulder arthroplasty: a systematic review of the English-language literature between 2006 and 2012. *J Bone Joint Surg Am.* 2013;95(24):2205-2212.
5. Gallusser N, Farron A. Complications of shoulder arthroplasty for osteoarthritis with posterior glenoid wear. *Orthop Traumatol Surg Res.* 2014;100(5):503-508.
6. Ho JC, Sabesan VJ, Iannotti JP. Glenoid component retroversion is associated with osteolysis. *J Bone Joint Surg Am.* 2013;95(12):e82.
7. Franklin JL, Barrett WP, Jackins SE, Matsen III FA. Glenoid loosening in total shoulder arthroplasty. Association with rotator cuff deficiency. *J Arthroplasty.* 1988;3(1):39-46.
8. Walch G, Young AA, Boileau P, Loew M, Gazielly D, Molé D. Patterns of loosening of polyethylene keeled glenoid components after shoulder arthroplasty for primary osteoarthritis: results of a multicenter study with more than five years of follow-up. *J Bone Joint Surg Am.* 2012;94(2):145-150.
9. Tammachote N, Sperling JW, Vathana T, Cofield RH, Harmsen WS, Schleck CD. Long-term results of cemented metal-backed glenoid components for osteoarthritis of the shoulder. *J Bone Joint Surg Am.* 2009;91(1):160-166.
10. Gagliano JR, Helms SM, Colbath GP, Przestrzelski BT, Hawkins RJ, DesJardins JD. A comparison of onlay versus inlay glenoid component loosening in total shoulder arthroplasty. *J Shoulder Elbow Surg.* 2017;26(7):1113-1120.
11. Gunther SB, Lynch TL, O'Farrell D, Calyore C, Rodenhouse A. Finite element analysis and physiologic testing of a novel, inset glenoid fixation technique. *J Shoulder Elbow Surg.* 2012;21(6):795-803.
12. Egger AC, Peterson J, Jones MH, Miniaci A. Total shoulder arthroplasty with nonspherical humeral head and inlay glenoid replacement: clinical results comparing concentric and nonconcentric glenoid stages in primary shoulder arthritis. *JSES Open Access.* 2019;3(3):145-153.
13. Cvetanovich GL, Naylor AJ, O'Brien MC, Waterman BR, Garcia GH, Nicholson GP. Anatomic total shoulder arthroplasty with an inlay glenoid component: clinical outcomes and return to activity. *J Shoulder Elbow Surg.* 2020;29(6):1188-1196.
14. Gunther SB, Lynch TL. Total shoulder replacement surgery with custom glenoid implants for severe bone deficiency. *J Shoulder Elbow Surg.* 2012;21(5):675-684.
15. Gunther SB, Tran SK. Long-term follow-up of total shoulder replacement surgery with inset glenoid implants for arthritis with deficient bone. *J Shoulder Elbow Surg.* 2019;28(9):1728-1736.
16. Davis DE, Acevedo D, Williams A, Williams G. Total shoulder arthroplasty using an inlay mini-glenoid component for glenoid deficiency: a 2-year follow-up of 9 shoulders in 7 patients. *J Shoulder Elbow Surg.* 2016;25(8):1354-1361.

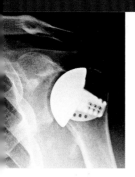

19 Hemiarthroplasty for Treatment of Glenohumeral Arthritis

Moby Parsons, MD

INTRODUCTION

Shoulder hemiarthroplasty (HA) began its modern development in 1951 when Neer designed his original monoblock prosthesis to address unsatisfactory results after operative fixation of complex proximal humerus fractures. His first published clinical series of 13 cases included one case for treatment of degenerative arthritis.[1] Several years after its introduction, the system was expanded to include multiple stem diameters, though there was only one humeral head diameter of 44 mm. Neer used this system for over 20 years and reported "When there was a good rotator cuff, a good deltoid muscle, and a good rehabilitation regimen, an excellent result could be obtained."[2]

Over the next 3 decades, humeral prosthesis design evolved to add progressive modularity and adaptability in an effort to better approximate proximal humeral anatomy.[3,4] Now in their fourth generation, systems have included the ability to independently adjust the anterior/posterior and medial/lateral head offset as well as platform stems that offer easy convertibility between anatomic and reverse arthroplasty. Resurfacing implants, developed originally in Scandinavia in the early 1980s and popularized by Copeland, have been used as an alternative to traditional stemmed implants for HA. They offer the advantages of bone preservation and the ability to address altered anatomy between the humeral head and shaft such as occurs in fracture malunions. Stemless implants have also been more recently introduced, also avoiding potential problems associated with stemmed implants including stress shielding, periprosthetic fracture, and the difficulty associated with stem removal at revision surgery. All of these design options can be applied to shoulder HA, and the advantages and disadvantages will be discussed.

The incidence of all shoulder arthroplasty has increased substantially over the past 20 years. Data from the Australian and New Zealand Joint Replacement Registries indicate that the number of shoulder replacement procedures has increased over 150% in the past 2 decades.[5,6] This growth is driven by several factors which include overall population growth, demographic changes, expanding indications, and improvements in implant design. The increased demand for treatment of arthritis in younger patients has also been documented. Padegimas et al have reported an 8% annual increase in shoulder arthroplasty in patients younger than 55 years and predicted a 333% increase in demand between 2010 and 2030.[7] Even Neer's original series of arthroplasty for treatment of glenohumeral arthritis, published in 1974, had an average age of 55 years at the time of surgery.[8]

During this same period, shoulder HA has seen a progressive decline in utilization. The Australian Registry reported that HA as a percentage of all shoulder replacement declined from 32% to 4% between 2008 and 2018 and that the percentage of HA performed for osteoarthritis has decreased from 60% to 25% over the same period.[5] **FIGURE 19.1** shows a histogram of arthroplasty type between 1999 and 2018 from the New Zealand Joint Registry. This shows a dramatic decline in HA and resurfacing arthroplasty from 47% to 7% of cases.[6] The Kaiser Permanente Registry has demonstrated that HA accounted for only 34% of all shoulder arthroplasty with only 38% (13% of the total) of these performed for arthritis.[9]

HA was traditionally used for a variety of diagnoses, including fractures, fracture sequelae, osteoarthritis, rheumatoid arthritis, osteonecrosis, and cuff tear arthropathy. Some portion of the decline in HA utilization is a result of the increasing use of reverse shoulder arthroplasty for several of the diagnoses for which HA is becoming more of a historical option or a salvage procedure. The use of HA for primary glenohumeral osteoarthritis has also declined based on literature suggesting superior pain relief and functional outcomes of total shoulder arthroplasty (TSA) as will be discussed further. Nevertheless, there are a subset of patients for whom HA may still be an appropriate treatment option in the management of degenerative joint disease. This chapter will focus on the role of HA for the treatment of glenohumeral osteoarthritis in this subset of patients. Biological resurfacing with HA will not be discussed since this technique has largely fallen out of favor.[10-12]

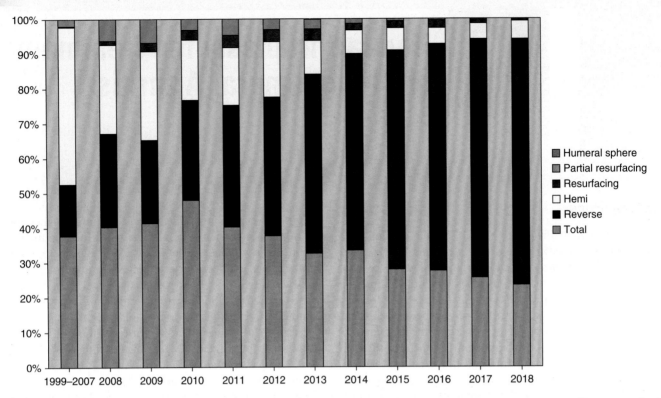

FIGURE 19.1 Histogram from the New Zealand Registry showing the progressive decline in prevalence of hemiarthroplasty with a concomitant substantial increase in reverse shoulder arthroplasty utilization. (Courtesy of the New Zealand Orthopaedic Association National Joint Registry.)

RATIONALE FOR HEMIARTHROPLASTY AS AN ALTERNATIVE TO TOTAL SHOULDER

In order to achieve a favorable outcome with HA, surgeons must adhere to principles and indications that recognize those clinical scenarios for which this option may be a comparable choice to TSA. The most common current indications for HA include select cases of primary osteoarthritis with an intact rotator cuff, atraumatic osteonecrosis, and select cases of secondary shoulder arthritis such as postcapsulorraphy arthropathy. In the cuff-intact shoulder, HA tends to be favored in younger patients or those with functional demands which may jeopardize the long-term survival of TSA.

Thus, a principle rationale for HA is the anticipation of glenoid implant failure and its consequences for salvage options in patients with a remaining life expectancy which is likely to exceed that of their implant. Several authors have noted a high frequency of radiolucent lines after TSA with a consequent negative impact on functional outcomes. Pfahler et al reported 68% glenoid radiolucent lines at an average 4-year follow-up,[13] while Galluser and colleagues noted 52% radiolucent lines with 11% recurrent posterior subluxation in patients with preoperative retroversion and decentering of the humeral head.[14] Roberson et al reported a 54% lucency rate in patients under age 65 with a 17.4% revision rate most commonly due to glenoid component loosening.[15] Similarly, Edwards reported 56% of glenoid implants with radiolucent lines

at midterm follow-up of TSA.[16] Schoch and coworkers found that increasing grade of radiolucency was significantly associated with worse postoperative function.[17] Walch et al have also noted worse outcomes when TSA is used to treat patients with B2 glenoids.[18,19]

These clinical findings are supported by biomechanical and finite element data. Farron et al showed that glenoid retroversion greater than 10° substantially increased stresses within the cement mantle and glenoid bone and resulted in increased micromotion at the bone-cement interface.[20] Nyffeler has also shown that retroversion is associated with posterior displacement of the humeral head and asymmetrical posterior loading of the glenoid implant which may result in loosening.[21] While the clinical implications of radiolucent lines around the glenoid implant remain debatable, the known association between radiolucencies and implant loosening in lower extremity arthroplasty would suggest that these glenoids are "at risk" of eventual failure. This information must be carefully considered when assessing patients' options for surgical management of glenohumeral osteoarthritis.

DELINEATING CAUSES OF POTENTIAL HEMIARTHROPLASTY FAILURE WITH A VIEW TOWARD PREVENTION

The most common reason for failure of HA is painful glenoid erosion. This has been documented in multiple clinical series, careful analysis of which may indicate an association with certain preoperative factors and other issues which can be addressed through surgical technique and perioperative management. Levine et al have noted a higher revision rate for HA in patients with eccentric versus concentric wear patters.[22,23] Norris and Iannotti also reported worse results with HA in patients with preoperative glenoid erosion and posterior humeral subluxation.[24] Hackett et al, reviewing a series of failed HA, also found that glenoid erosion was more common in decentered hemiarthroplasties and those positioned in valgus.[25] Herschel et al similarly found valgus implant position as a risk factor for postoperative glenoid erosion.[26]

Furthermore, while glenoid erosion after HA is linked to pain and poor outcomes, it is unclear from the literature if poor outcomes contribute to erosion or if erosion leads to poor outcomes. Neer observed, "Erosion of the glenoid does occur if the shoulder is stiff, causing the articular surfaces to bear constantly against each other in one area."[2] Sperling et al, in a long-term comparative analysis of HA and TSA, noted glenoid wear in 72% and further noted that stiffness was associated with unsatisfactory outcomes.[27] Getz and colleagues also reported worse functional results after HA in patients with residual stiffness, particularly loss of external rotation.[28] Because this is associated with obligate posterior humeral decentering in the native arthritic shoulder, postoperative external rotation stiffness may be associated with recurrent asymmetric posterior loading of the unresurfaced glenoid resulting in wear and pain.

Other authors have noted worse postoperative outcomes for HA in patients who have undergone prior surgical procedures.[25,29,30] Sperling noted a higher clinical failure and revision rate for patients with a preoperative diagnosis of posttraumatic arthritis or sequelae or trauma.[31] Hasan, characterizing risk factors for failed arthroplasty, noted fracture sequelae, prior surgery, implant malposition, and stiffness as causes of unsatisfactory outcomes.[32] The collective implication from analysis of these clinical series suggests that the characteristics of HA failure are often of the type that can be minimized by proper patient selection, optimal surgical technique, and perioperative management. Each of these factors will be considered.

PATIENT SELECTION

As Matsen has suggested, HA with or without nonprosthetic glenoid arthroplasty is "not for every surgeon, every patient, or every problem."[33] Achieving consistent outcomes requires a full understanding of the interplay between patient-specific variables and the underlying shoulder pathology. As most surgeons have come to understand, any well-done operation can be foiled by issues such as unmet expectations, poor compliance, psychosocial problems, and comorbid conditions. Shoulder HA is no exception to this rule.

- ***Surgeon factors***: HA for treatment of primary and secondary arthritis requires a thorough understanding of

the principles of HA as they apply to a given pathologic condition. Because many cases of HA failure can be attributed to avoidable causes, surgeons must understand the importance of the surgical technique and implant selection to the goals of recentering the head, providing distributed load transfer, balancing the soft tissues, and maximizing range of motion. Surgeons must also be willing to accept that recovery from HA can be much longer and more involved than TSA, and this requires a higher level of commitment to patient navigation through the episode of care in terms of education, expectation management, and postoperative follow-through.

- ***Patient factors***: Many patients may self-select for HA after carefully considering their surgical options in terms of their desired functional goals. Patients need to understand the importance of their commitment to an extended recovery that requires extensive motivation, persistence, and patience. As Neer has pointed out, "Patients should know that the arthroplasty simply sets the stage for them to do the exercises required to achieve the pain relief, motion and function desired."[2] If patients are unwilling to make this commitment, they are better served with glenoid resurfacing. While there are no specific age restrictions on the use of HA versus TSA, patients tend to present with moderate to severe osteoarthritis at a younger age when they are still participating in activities that risk premature glenoid implant loosening. Matsen has delineated selection criteria that lead to better results after ream and run arthroplasty. These include American Society of Anesthesiology Class 1, non–work-related etiology, lower baseline Simple Shoulder Test (SST) score, no prior surgery, and glenoid type other than A1.[34] Chronic pain, depression, active smoking, and psychosocial issues have also been found to negatively impact outcomes of HA.[35]

- ***Shoulder factors***: As mentioned, a history of prior surgery has been shown to negatively impact outcomes of HA.[25,29] This may be particularly true for any previous procedure on the rotator cuff indicating the possibility of suboptimal cuff function. Prior anatomy altering procedures, such as those which intentionally restricted external rotation for instability, may also risk poor outcomes due to the importance of restoring range of motion to HA biomechanics. Surgeons must carefully assess the status of the soft tissue envelope with a view toward the ability to balance the forces across the joint and recenter the humeral head. The quality of the glenoid bone must also be considered. Patients with inflammatory or erosive osteoarthritis often have substantial subchondral cyst formation. This can often be well seen on two-dimensional (2D) axial computed tomography (CT) cuts (**FIGURE 19.2**). In such cases, glenoid resurfacing should be considered.

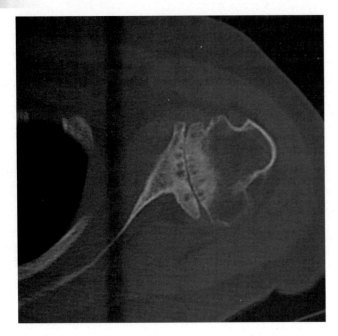

FIGURE 19.2 Axial two-dimensional computed tomography slice demonstrating subchondral cyst formation in the setting of advanced arthritis with glenoid wear.

PATIENT ASSESSMENT

As with any arthroplasty procedure, pertinent aspects of the history as they relate to the patient's development and experience of shoulder arthritis should be obtained. It is critical to understand the patient's desired activities after surgery and the degree to which the arthritis is currently disabling their participation. Furthermore, careful assessment of patient expectations for pain relief and function must be determined. Patients who are expecting complete pain relief may not be suitable candidates for this procedure. Alternatively, patients who are willing to accept some degree of residual discomfort in return for eliminating the risk of glenoid implant failure may be quite satisfied with their overall improvement despite some persistent symptoms. Thus, considering margin for improvement is essential as patients who have more preoperative functional disability are more likely to be satisfied than those who still maintain acceptable and manageable levels of discomfort and dysfunction prior to surgery. Matsen has shown that patients with lower baseline SST scores have better outcomes than those with higher baseline scores, which may indicate that patients with continued well-compensated comfort and function are less likely to be satisfied with the results of surgery.[34] Mahony and colleagues have also reported an association between higher preoperative ASES score and less satisfactory outcomes.[36]

Any history of prior surgery needs to be carefully evaluated in terms of its impact on anatomy, function, and surgical approach. The location of surgical incisions and their impact on the prospective arthroplasty should be noted. The presence of any existing hardware should be determined if special instruments are required to remove an implant. A history of prior injections should also be noted as both this and previous surgery may elevate a patient's risk for infection and *Cutibacterium acnes* colonization. Because conventional laboratory workup for infection is often normal in the case of *C. acnes*, an index of suspicion along with plans for intraoperative assessment is essential.

Physical examination should focus on preoperative range of motion and cuff integrity. Preoperative external rotation is perhaps the most important measure because of its effect on obligate posterior humeral decentering and the importance of being able to restore this range at the time of surgery. Examination of passive range of motion with the patient supine on the table eliminates some of the compensation for stiffness that can occur through the scapulothoracic articulation and may provide a more accurate delineation of isolated glenohumeral range. Visible and palpable cuff muscle atrophy without substitution patterns on manual resistance testing may indicate disuse weakness, which will require significant rehabilitation to overcome. Tenderness over the acromioclavicular (AC) joint should also be assessed as some patients presenting with glenohumeral arthrosis are also at risk for symptomatic AC arthrosis, particularly weightlifters.

IMAGING

Standard Radiographs

Standard radiographs should include, at a minimum, a Grashey and axillary lateral view (**FIGURE 19.3A** and **B**). Proper technique for these is critical to obtain images that are tangential to the joint line. With the arm in adduction, the Grashey view can provide information on the position of the humeral head on the glenoid in the superior/inferior plane and can show the presence of inferior humeral osteophytes which may be contacting the inferior glenoid. Other measurements can also help quantify the preoperative anatomy that will serve as the basis for anatomical reconstruction with the prosthesis. These include the humeral head diameter, the humeral head height, the humeral neck-shaft angle, the height of the humeral head above the tuberosity, and the lateral humeral offset (**FIGURE 19.4**).

The axillary lateral view is the most important for the assessment of glenohumeral arthritis and requires proper technique with the arm elevated to a position of function. A true axillary lateral demonstrates an "eye" sign posterior to the glenoid (**FIGURE 19.3B**), and the pathology seen on this view may not be readily visible on the true anteroposterior view. The key factors to assess on the axillary lateral include wear patterns on the glenoid face, pathologic retroversion, decentering of the humeral head, extent of medial erosion, and morphology of the

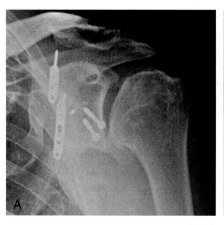
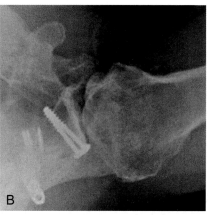
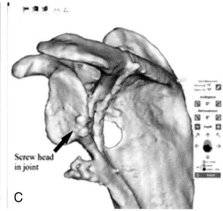

FIGURE 19.3 A and **B**, Preoperative Grashey and axillary lateral radiographs demonstrating the presence of glenoid fixation screws from prior scapular open reduction and internal fixation (ORIF) following a trauma. **C**, Computed tomography scan demonstrating exposure of the inferior screw head in the joint. This likely contributed to the progression of arthrosis and will require removal at the time of arthroplasty.

glenoid vault. This information provides the surgeon a better sense of the surgical goals that will be necessary to provide a stable and well-functioning HA.

CT Imaging

CT has become increasingly popular in the preoperative assessment of shoulder arthritis. A 2019 survey of the American Shoulder and Elbow Surgeons indicated that 67% of surgeons obtain a CT scan in a majority of patients and only 5% of surgeons rarely obtain one.[37] Their growing utility is based on the superior ability of three-dimensional CT scans to define pathologic

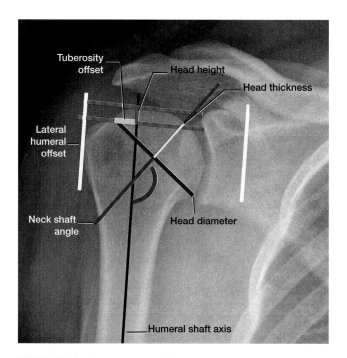

FIGURE 19.4 Measurements of proximal humeral anatomy pertinent to prosthetic shoulder reconstruction. These include head diameter, head thickness, neck-shaft angle, head height above the tuberosity, tuberosity offset, and lateral humeral offset.

retroversion and inclination and to correct for scapular plane alignment which can affect glenoid morphology assessment with 2D imaging studies (**FIGURE 19.3C**).[38-43] In recent years, CT imaging has fostered a better understanding of wear patterns in shoulder arthritis with respect to the Walch classification, and this information is critical in planning management of glenoid-sided pathology in the setting of HA.[44-46]

CT-based preoperative planning software is now available for many different implant systems and can allow for quantitative assessment glenoid retroversion, inclination, and posterior humeral decentering. In addition, detailed measurements can also be made of humeral head diameter and height with regard to implant planning (**FIGURE 19.5**). Determining the presence of biconcavity is particularly important. This Walch B2 morphology is common in patients who are suitable candidates for HA. In these cases, surgeons must carefully assess the balance between minimizing bone loss, restoring articular congruence, and addressing the combination of retroversion and decentering of the humeral head.

CT scans can also be used to assess rotator cuff muscle atrophy and fatty infiltration which may have implications for the postoperative rehabilitation necessary to regain strength and stability for the HA.[47] Chronic shoulder stiffness and disuse can lead to cuff weakness which may play a role in the postoperative discomfort encountered during HA rehabilitation and may explain why advocates such as Matsen have documented continued improvement in comfort and function up to 20 months following surgery.[29] **FIGURE 19.6** shows an oblique sagittal CT cut medial to the glenoid, which demonstrates supraspinatus atrophy. Donohue et al noted increasing cuff muscle fatty degeneration with increasing glenoid retroversion and increasing joint line medialization.[48] Sayed-Noor found that increasing fatty infiltration and atrophy on CT scans of arthritic shoulders led to increased weakness on postoperative follow-up.[49] To the

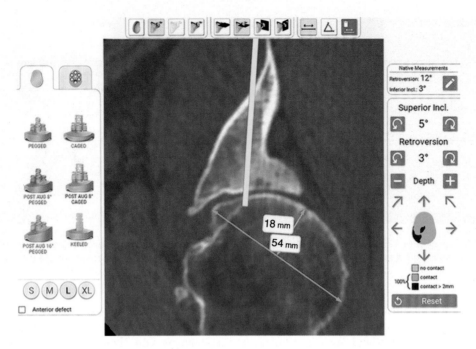

FIGURE 19.5 Computed tomography image from a preoperative planning software platform (Exactech GPS, Exactech Inc, Gainesville, FL). This demonstrates the pathologic glenoid version and inclination. Measurement has also been performed of the head diameter and height.

degree that a balanced cuff is necessary to centralize the humeral head in a concave glenoid, it may be important to inspect for cuff muscle atrophy or fatty degeneration on the oblique sagittal CT images so that patients may be appropriately counseled about the importance of persistent cuff strengthening to their functional recovery.

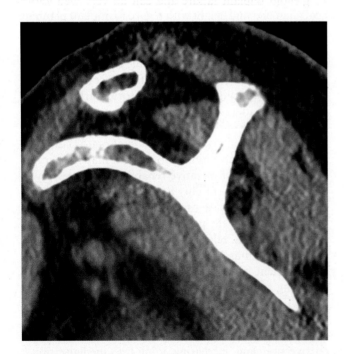

FIGURE 19.6 Oblique sagittal computed tomography slice medial to the glenoid demonstrating the rotator cuff muscles in cross section. These cuts can demonstrate disuse muscle atrophy due to long standing joint degeneration.

MAGNETIC RESONANCE IMAGING

While magnetic resonance imaging (MRI) can provide superior information about the rotator cuff, its ability to provide information about the bony anatomy is inferior to CT scanning. Given the relatively low frequency of cuff pathology in the setting of glenohumeral arthritis, MRI is generally not indicated on a routine basis. If the clinical examination suggests a potential rotator cuff tear, MRI could be obtained selectively. MRI may also be helpful in cases of osteonecrosis to determine staging, particularly in earlier cases prior to morphologic changes in the shape of the humeral head.

PRINCIPLES OF HEMIARTHROPLASTY FOR MANAGEMENT OF DEGENERATIVE JOINT DISEASE

Although HA is a humeral-sided operation, problems with HA most commonly result from failure to address glenoid-sided pathoanatomy. As discussed, this includes the shape of the surface, the preoperative retroversion and inclination, the dimensions of the glenoid vault, the degree of medial erosion, the presence of subchondral cysts, and any other indicator of the quality of the subchondral bone. These features can alert surgeons to strategies necessary to optimize glenohumeral load transfer and kinematics as well as risk factors for poor outcomes that may preclude the choice of HA over TSA. If there are pathologic changes on the glenoid which result in an eccentric erosion pattern, some type of nonprosthetic glenoid-sided arthroplasty must be performed in combination with humeral head resurfacing. This ream and run procedure has been pioneered and refined by

Dr Frederick A. Matsen, III. The principles outlined as follows are based the author's personal communication with Dr Matsen, as well as personal experience with this surgery.

Principle #1: A single glenoid concavity must be created to provide congruency with the resurfaced humeral head. This optimizes load transfer across the joint. Unlike TSA where several millimeters of mismatch have proven beneficial for long-term glenoid implant survival,[50-52] glenoid reshaping with the ream and run aims for 2 mm of mismatch to provide some degree of humeral translation without load concentration. This may require custom reamers with different diameters of curvature to correspond to the chosen head.

Principle #2: Recentering the humeral head in the concave glenoid is essential to optimize load transfer and prevent recurrent asymmetric posterior erosion. Recentering can be achieved through a combination of glenoid surface preparation, adjustment of implant configuration, and soft tissue balancing.

Principle #3: Bone stock must be preserved at all costs. To this end, version correction through high-side reaming is not undertaken as this may violate the subchondral bone and predispose to erosion. Persistent retroversion can be tolerated provided the head is recentered and a smooth concavity recreated.

Principle #4: The largest diameter humeral head should be chosen which does not overstuff the joint. Larger heads provide greater stability and surface area for load transfer. Adjustment of head height can offset a larger diameter to avoid overtensioning the soft tissue.

Principle #5: Recovery of joint range of motion is critical as stiffness has been associated with glenoid erosion and pain. As with recentering, this can include implant-related considerations as well as selective soft tissue release. Management of the postoperative recovery along with a commitment by the patient to a lengthy rehabilitation is imperative.

THE IMPACT OF PREOPERATIVE GLENOID EROSION

Several series have previously reported that preoperative eccentric glenoid wear patterns lead to worse functional outcomes and a higher risk of postoperative erosion.[22,23,25] These series, however, did not report on any surgical measures to correct the pathomechanics that result in such eccentric wear. Matsen pioneered the ream and run to address this problem by creating a single concavity that provides maximal glenohumeral contact to optimize load transfer and stability.

In considering HA according to the Walch Classification, A2 glenoids already have a centered head with a congruent wear pattern. Somerson et al have reported favorable results with the ream and run in patients with this glenoid morphology.[53] In contrast, patients with A1 glenoids, who often have minimal

glenoid-sided disease, are at a higher risk for glenoid-sided pain after HA.[34] This may indicate that these patients had less severe disease at presentation and, thus, their lower margin for improvement after surgery placed them at risk for worse self-reported outcomes.

B2 glenoids have traditionally presented the biggest challenge for both TSA and HA. These are marked by the triad of glenoid biconcavity, increased retroversion, and posterior head decentering. Hoenecke has suggested that head subluxation results more from the morphological biconcavity than the retroversion, suggesting that shape correction rather than version correction may be more important in the reconstruction.[54] Provided that a concavity can be restored with minimal bone removal and preservation of the subchondral bone, Matsen has shown that the ream and run can recenter the humeral head without significant version correction and yield durable functional results.[35] Similarly, because B3 glenoids already have a congruent articulation despite their substantial retroversion, they can be addressed with HA using measures to balance the soft tissues and restore external rotation range of motion.

Managing these challenging glenoids with HA and nonprosthetic glenoid arthroplasty is counterintuitive to current trends to use either augmented glenoids or reverse total shoulder in such cases; and these procedures may be appropriate in many cases. Nevertheless, as mentioned, there are select patients with very high functional ambitions who are motivated to avoid the long-term risk of glenoid implant failure and can do very well with a ream and run–type procedure provided that the surgical technique carefully addressed the aforementioned principles and the technical considerations that follow.

IMPLANT SELECTION

Shoulder HA can be performed with any type of humeral implant, including a standard-stem, short-stem, stemless, or resurfacing implant. The decision should be based on surgeon familiarity with the system in terms of the ability to restore proximal humeral anatomy in addition to features specific to the case that may favor one design over another. While the overarching goal of the reconstruction is to replicate native anatomy, there are instances where the impact of implant configuration on soft tissue balance and joint mechanics may take precedence over simple restoration of anatomical relationships.

There are some general principles that should be respected regardless of implant type. A head diameter that closely matches that of the native head can help prevent over- or understuffing of the joint. Where possible, the thickness of the humeral head should optimize soft tissue balance in a manner that provides stability without stiffness. Placement of the head flush with the insertion of the superior cuff is critical to recreate the normal head-tuberosity relationship. If the head is placed too high, it can tent and overtension the supraspinatus tendon predisposing to tendon failure. If the head sits too far below the cut surface, impingement of the tuberosity can occur with shoulder abduction.

There has been long-standing interest in the use of resurfacing implants in the setting of HA, particularly for younger patients who may have a higher risk of revision. These advantages include bone preservation, adaptability to altered anatomy, avoidance of medullary canalization which may cause less blood loss and less pain, less risk of fracture, and ease of revision.[55] While some series have reported excellent long-term outcomes of surface replacement arthroplasty, these results have not been consistent across the literature. Rai et al reported 95% survivorship of the Copeland Mark III implant at 18 years with an 88% patient satisfaction rate.[56] Bailie et al also reported high levels of patients satisfaction with cementless surface replacement in younger patients.[57]

Conversely, Verstaelen et al reported 54% risk of overstuffing and 45% rate of glenoid erosion at 7 years with the Copeland implant.[58] Lebon et al demonstrated that surface replacement HA had a higher revision rate than stemmed HA, which was felt to be due to a higher propensity toward overstuffing and erosion.[59] Geervliet and colleagues reported that deviation of the center of rotation of resurfacing implants by >5 mm from the native shoulder can lead to a higher incidence of glenoid erosion due to overstuffing the joint.[60] The New Zealand Joint Replacement Registry has also shown that resurfacing HA had twice the revision rate of stemmed HA.[6]

These results collectively imply that overstuffing and nonanatomic placement are risk factors for glenoid erosion with humeral resurfacing and that this tendency may be a matter of surgical technique and implant geometry **(FIGURE 19.7)**. This implies that some cases of failure are preventable by avoiding implant-related issues. If a resurfacing implant is chosen, sufficient humeral reaming must be performed to accommodate the thickness of the implant, and restoring the head tuberosity relationship relative to the cuff insertion is critical **(FIGURE 19.8)**.

In the absence of altered proximal humeral anatomy, such as in fracture malunion, stemmed HA has the advantage of humeral head modularity and adaptability. Systems that allow selection of different head heights for a given diameter, as well as independent adjustment of the medial and posterior head offset, can provide more on-table customization of soft tissue balance. Recentering the humeral head by allowing for alterations in the head position to accommodate glenoid retroversion is more critical in HA than TSA. Equally, it may provide for better balancing of surface contact versus range of motion. Harryman et al showed that increasing head height by 5 mm could decrease range of motion by 20° to 30° and result in earlier obligate translations of the humeral head. They equally demonstrated that smaller heads lead to decreased contact surface area and more concentrated loads that could result in glenoid erosion.[61] Because resurfacing implants only allow one head height per diameter, the ability to adapt the implant to correct arthritic pathomechanics may be more limited.

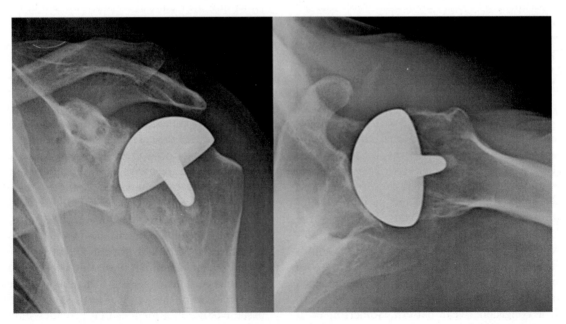

FIGURE 19.7 These x-rays demonstrate a humeral resurfacing implant which has been placed too high on the humeral neck. This results in a nonanatomic center of rotation, head-tuberosity relationships, and lateral glenohumeral offset. All of these pose a risk for stiffness and glenoid erosion. (Courtesy of Dr. Ryan Simovitch, HSS Florida.)

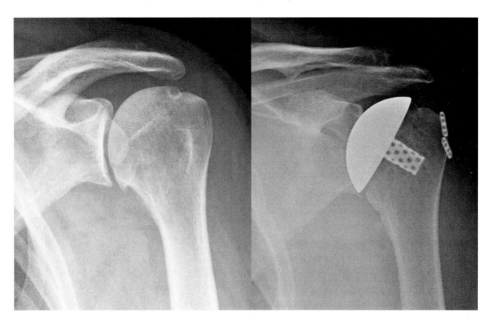

FIGURE 19.8 With sufficient humeral preparation and careful assessment of the neck-shaft angle, anatomic restoration is possible with resurfacing implants as shown in these pre- and postoperative Grashey radiographs. Their use may play a role in certain cases provided proper surgical technique to achieve appropriate implant-bone relationships.

Altering the head position to accommodate glenoid retroversion and preoperative posterior head decentering is an important consideration to prevent recurrent posterior subluxation after arthroplasty. Neer suggested that the combined retroversion of the glenoid and humeral implant should be around 40° and that increased anteversion of the humeral prosthesis should be added to account for residual glenoid retroversion after HA.[2] Matsen advocates shifting the head eccentrically anterior in such cases.[62] The net effect of both of these humeral prosthesis adjustments is to posteriorly shift the greater tuberosity to help tension the posterior soft tissues and resist recurrent subluxation of the humeral head as can occur in Walch B1, B2, and B3 glenoids.

Stemless implants are relatively newer and offer the advantages of bone preservation, avoidance of problems associated with medullary stem fixation, and improved exposure by resecting the humeral head **(FIGURE 19.9)**. While these systems do not offer the same degree of modularity as stemmed systems, some degree of anterior

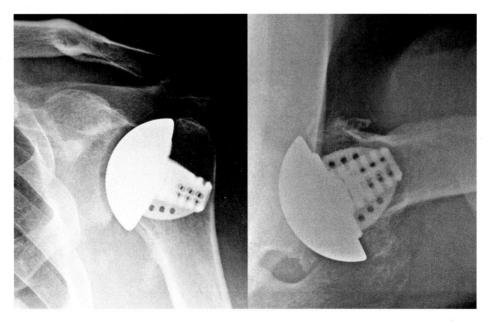

FIGURE 19.9 Postoperative x-rays of a stemless ream and run. These demonstrate key principles of the technique which include restoring a single congruent concavity and recentering the humeral head.

eccentricity can be accomplished by anterior placement of the humeral fixation device. Version and neck-shaft angle of the implant are entirely dependent on the humeral head cut, so surgeons must carefully plan this cut to avoid excessive humeral retroversion or valgus implant positioning. The author currently prefers the use of stemless implants for A2 and certain B2 glenoids if there is not excessive preoperative glenoid retroversion (maximum 12°-13°). B2 glenoids with significant retroversion and subluxation and B3 glenoids are likely better served with a stemmed implant to allow for increased on-table adjustment of the humeral prosthesis to optimize soft tissue balance.

TECHNICAL CONSIDERATIONS FOR THE REAM AND RUN PROCEDURE

The surgical approach is the same as a standard total or reverse shoulder arthroplasty (**VIDEO 19.1**). Management of the subscapularis is per the surgeon's discretion but must allow for a complete 360° release to restore external rotation range of motion. Failure to adequately release the subscapularis can result in persistent obligate posterior humeral translation and subsequent loss of a concentric glenohumeral relationship.

Preparation for the humeral component should also follow according to the chosen implant. If reaming of the glenoid is planned, an implant which resects the humeral head will provide better exposure. In general, the humeral component is placed in 30° to 35° of retroversion. As Neer pointed out, some additional anteversion can be added to offset severe glenoid retroversion, provided it does not compromise the head-tuberosity relationships.[2] Valgus positioning of the implant should be avoided and the largest head that covers the cut surface without significant overhang should be chosen.

Glenoid exposure should consider the preoperative anatomy. B2 and B3 glenoids generally have a patulous posterior capsule. In these cases, release of the inferior and posterior capsule should be avoided to prevent postoperative posterior humeral subluxation (**FIGURE 19.10A**). In cases with a centered wear pattern, such as A2 glenoids, an inferior and posterior release can be performed if necessary (**FIGURE 19.10B**). This is generally only the case in very tight shoulders such as those with a history chondrolysis. Releases should be performed in an extralabral fashion to preserve the contribution of the labrum to glenoid concavity and load sharing.

Preparation of the glenoid should focus on minimizing bone loss and preserving the subchondral plate. Any central ridge between the paleo- and neoglenoid can be smoothed with a burr prior to reaming and any remaining cartilage on the paleoglenoid can be removed with a curette (**FIGURE 19.11**). Depending on the system used, custom reamers may be necessary to achieve a mismatch of 2 mm between the chosen head diameter and glenoid curvature. This should be determined well in advance of the case as many systems have a single reamer radius of curvature regardless of the circumference. Reaming should be conservative with the aim of creating a smooth concavity. Correction of glenoid retroversion should only be performed to a degree that does not penetrate subchondral bone to minimize the risk of erosion (**FIGURE 19.12**).

Selection of the humeral implant should also consider the preoperative anatomy and goals necessary to rebalance the joint. In cases with significant posterior subluxation, the head can be dialed anteriorly eccentric to help tension the posterior capsule and resist recurrent decentering after arthroplasty (**FIGURE 19.13**). The height of the head should satisfy the 40/50/60 criteria as

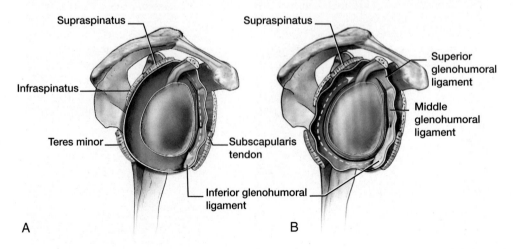

A   B

FIGURE 19.10 A, Capsular releases should be limited to the anterior-inferior glenohumeral ligament, avoiding an inferior and posterior release in shoulders with a patulous posterior capsule; (**B**) a complete circumferential release can be considered for tight shoulders with a concentric wear pattern, such as the A2 glenoid.

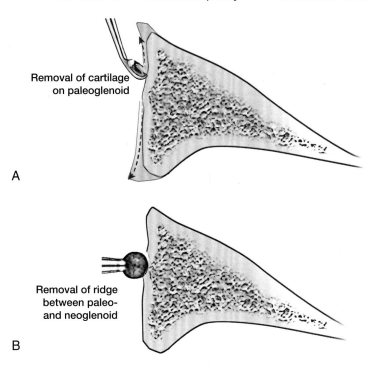

Removal of cartilage
on paleoglenoid

A

Removal of ridge
between paleo-
and neoglenoid

B

FIGURE 19.11 A, Any remaining cartilage on the paleoglenoid can be removed with a curette. **B**, The central ridge at the junction of the paleo-
and neoglenoid can be smoothed with a burr prior to reaming. This allows the reamer to reshape the surface into a smooth concavity with
minimal bone loss.

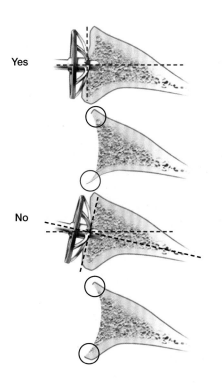

Yes

No

FIGURE 19.12 The principal goal of reaming is to reshape the glenoid and not to correct version. Corrective reaming to reduce retroversion will risk violation of the subchondral bone and resultant
glenoid erosion. Residual retroversion is acceptable provided the
humeral component is appropriately adjusted and soft tissue balance can address the tendency for posterior subluxation.

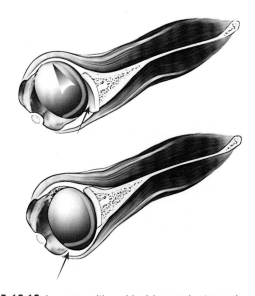

FIGURE 19.13 In cases with residual humeral retroversion and a
tendency toward posterior subluxation, the humeral implant can be
placed in an anteriorly eccentric position to shift the tuberosity posteriorly and help tension the patulous posterior capsule.

proposed by Matsen. This includes 40° of passive external rotation in adduction with the subscapularis reapproximated, 50% posterior translation of the head on the glenoid with a "bounce-back," and 60° of passive internal rotation in the abducted position.

If there is still a tendency toward posterior subluxation of the humeral implant, the rotator interval can be plicated after subscapularis repair. This plication should take into consideration that overtightening can restrict postoperative external rotation. Plication of the posterior capsule is an option but rarely necessary with appropriate soft tissue balancing, implant orientation and sizing, and interval plication. The subscapularis repair should be robust to allow for early passive range of motion exercises.

FIGURE 19.14 demonstrates the preoperative and postoperative axillary lateral radiographs of a patients with a B1 glenoid with recentering of the humeral head in a smooth and congruent concavity.

POSTOPERATIVE CARE

Because stiffness has been linked to poor outcomes and glenoid erosion, immediate range of motion must be instituted with the goal of achieving at least 40° of passive external rotation and 140° of passive forward elevation. Patients are instructed to perform self-directed exercises daily, and early referral to outpatient therapy should be arranged with an experienced shoulder arthroplasty therapist. It is imperative that the patient and the therapist both understand the importance of regaining and maintaining range of motion while protecting the subscapularis repair. Early external rotator

isometrics can also tension the posterior cuff and capsule and reduce the tendency toward posterior decentering.

If patients are showing early signs of stiffness, a manipulation under anesthesia should be considered around 6 weeks after surgery. By using Codman's paradox, external rotation range of motion can be achieved without applying torque on the humerus. This method can recover external rotation without applying stress to the subscapularis repair. If patients are already progressing on schedule, progressive range of motion can be added around 8 weeks along with progressive strengthening according to a standard TSA protocol.

Because of long standing stiffness and loss of function prior to surgery, improvement in shoulder comfort and function after the ream and run can continue for beyond a year after surgery. Patients who choose this procedure must understand the protracted nature of the recovery and that a substantial portion of the success comes from the active recovery assuming a well-done surgery. As previously mentioned, the arthroplasty simply sets the stage for what the patient can achieve through persistent and dedicated rehabilitation. Extensive preoperative patient education and postoperative stewardship are necessary to ensure a favorable result.

OTHER CONSIDERATIONS

Avoidance of infection is paramount in these cases. While a full review on the assessment, prevention, and management of infection is addressed in Chapter 32, surgeons should recognize that those patients who may be suitable candidates for HA may also present higher risk factors for *C. acnes* colonization or infection. This

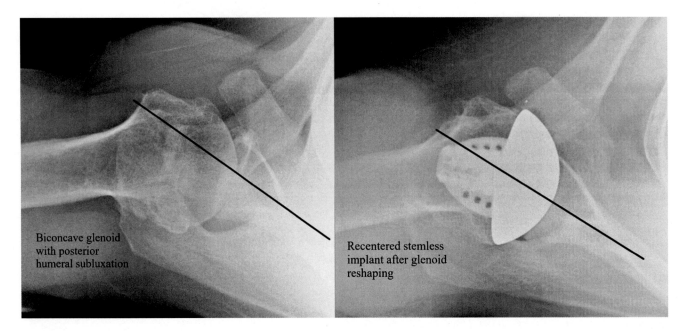

Biconcave glenoid
with posterior
humeral subluxation

Recentered stemless
implant after glenoid
reshaping

FIGURE 19.14 Pre- and postoperative axillary lateral radiographs demonstrating recentering of the posteriorly subluxated humeral head and reshaping of the glenoid into a stabilizing concavity.

includes male gender, younger age, and any history of injection therapy or prior surgery. In such cases, intraoperative assessments for infection along with aggressive measures to reduce contamination of the wound are essential.

RESULTS

Clinical results of the ream and run have shown improvement in self-reported outcome measures comparable to TSA in select patients.[53,63,64] Patients younger than 55 years and those with a previous surgery had a higher revision rate.[30] In the author's personal experience, failure of the ream and run typically occurs within the first 1 to 2 years postoperatively due to persistent glenoid-sided pain. Patients who achieve an excellent functional outcome within this time period generally have sustained results and do not require subsequent revision.

While the literature in general has demonstrated worse functional outcomes and a higher revision rate for HA versus TSA, a careful analysis paints a more nuanced picture of the comparative results. For instance, Sandow et al showed that while the early results of TSA are superior, the late results are not significantly different.[65] Gartsman demonstrated that TSA patients had better pain relief, but the overall patient satisfaction rate was not significantly different.[66] Lo and colleagues, in a prospective randomized trial, found no difference in disease-specific quality of life measures between HA and TSA for treatment of osteoarthritis.[67]

With regard to revision surgery, the literature consistently demonstrates a higher risk for HA, almost uniformly for glenoid-sided pain from erosion.[68-70] These findings must be balanced against the risk of the glenoid component loosening in patients undergoing TSA. For patients 60 years old or less, the life expectancy is now greater than 20 years, and many people continue to engage in physically demanding activities despite their age. Long-term results from the New Zealand Registry demonstrate that the survival curves of HA and TSA are relatively parallel and merge around 14 years after surgery **(FIGURE 19.15)**, suggesting that with time, failure due to glenoid implant loosening equals or exceeds failure due to native glenoid erosion.[6] Given that this data reflects the population average across all diagnoses, the risk for glenoid implant failure may be higher in those patients who choose HA to avoid this risk given their higher functional demands. In fact, Sperling noted a higher frequency of glenoid implant radiolucencies after TSA (76%) than glenoid erosion after HA (72%) in patients younger than 50 years who underwent

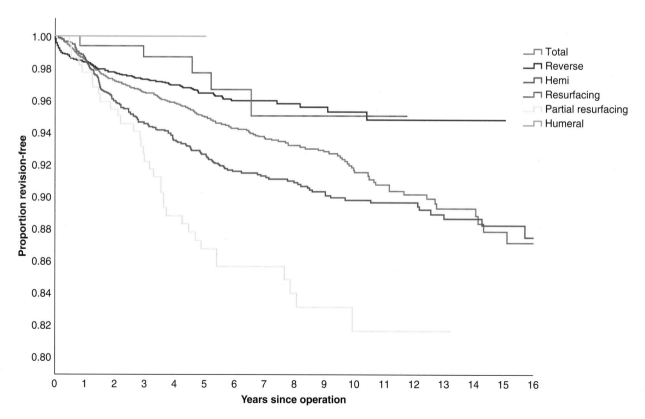

FIGURE 19.15 Survival curve graph from the New Zealand Joint Replacement Registry. This demonstrates that standard hemiarthroplasty and total shoulder have relatively parallel curves with a higher revision incidence for hemiarthroplasty until around 14 years when the curves merge. Note that resurfacing hemiarthroplasty has a markedly higher revision rate. (Courtesy of the New Zealand Orthopaedic Association National Joint Registry.)

shoulder arthroplasty.[31] Neyton et al also showed that for patients <55 years, HA and TSA had similar revision rates of 16% at long-term follow-up and that 88% of revised TSAs were for glenoid implant failure.[71]

Given that patients in this age category are at risk for revision for either failed HA or TSA, the question then becomes which mode of failure has greater morbidity. Failed HA due to glenoid side pain can often be revised by conversion to TSA, whereas failed TSA due to glenoid loosening is generally salvaged either by conversion to HA with or without bone grafting or full revision to reverse TSA. The author would contend that the former option offers less morbidity to the patient and burns fewer bridges for the prospects of the managing the patient's arthritic shoulder over the long term.

CONCLUSION

HA with or without nonprosthetic glenoid arthroplasty remains an acceptable treatment option for select patients with primary and secondary glenohumeral osteoarthritis for whom there is a substantial long-term risk of glenoid implant failure. As it has been shown that many cases of HA failure are attributable to preventable complications, durable results comparable to TSA can be achieved provided strict conditions are met. These include (1) adherence to the principles outlined above; (2) a standardized surgical technique that minimizes implant-related failures; (3) proper patient selection to avoid risk factors associated with poor outcomes; and (4) compliance with a longer rehabilitation regimen that emphasizes avoidance of stiffness. As part of a shared decision-making process, patients who elect to undergo HA as opposed to TSA must have a very clear understanding of the importance of their commitment to achieving the desire result as well as the acceptance that some degree of residual discomfort may be an acceptable alternative to the risk of glenoid implant failure.

REFERENCES

1. Neer CS. Articular replacement for the humeral head. *J Bone Joint Surg Am.* 1955;37-A:215-228.
2. Neer CS II. *Shoulder Reconstruction.* W.B. Saunders Company; 1990:551.
3. Boileau P, Walch G. The three-dimensional geometry of the proximal humerus. Implications for surgical technique and prosthetic design. *J Bone Joint Surg Br.* 1997;79:857-865. doi:10.1302/0301-620x.79b5.7579
4. Walch G, Boileau P. Prosthetic adaptability: a new concept for shoulder arthroplasty. *J Shoulder Elbow Surg.* 1999;8:443-451. doi:10.1016/s1058-2746(99)90074-5
5. Australian Orthopaedic Association National Joint Replacement Registry. *Hip, Knee and Shoulder Arthroplasty: 2019 Annual Report.* Australian Orthopaedic Association; 2019:270-292.
6. The New Zealand Joint Registry. *20 Year Report: January 1999 to December 2018.* New Zealand Orthopaedic Association; 2019:130-146.
7. Padegimas EM, Maltenfort M, Lazarus MD, et al. Future patient demand for shoulder arthroplasty by younger patients: national projections. *Clin Orthop Relat Res.* 2015;473:1860-1867. doi:10.1007/s11999-015-4231-z
8. Neer CS. Replacement arthroplasty for glenohumeral osteoarthritis. *J Bone Joint Surg Am.* 1974;56-A:1-13.
9. Dillon MT, Ake CF, Burke MF, et al. The Kaiser Permanente shoulder arthroplasty registry. *Acta Orthop.* 2015;86:286-292. doi:10.3109/17453674.2015.1024565
10. Strauss EJ, Verma NN, Salata MJ, et al. The high failure rate of biologic resurfacing of the glenoid in young patients with glenohumeral arthritis. *J Shoulder Elbow Surg.* 2014;23:409-419. doi:10.1016/j.jse.2013.06.001
11. Puskas GJ, Meyer DC, Lebschi JA, et al. Unacceptable failure of hemiarthroplasty combined with biological glenoid resurfacing in the treatment of glenohumeral arthritis in the young. *J Shoulder Elbow Surg.* 2015;24:1900-1907. doi:10.1016/j.jse.2015.05.037
12. Elhassan B, Ozbaydar M, Diller D, et al. Soft-tissue resurfacing of the glenoid in the treatment of glenohumeral arthritis in active patients less than fifty years old. *J Bone Joint Surg Am.* 2009;91:419-424. doi:10.2106/JBJS.H.00318
13. Pfahler M, Jena F, Neyton L, et al. Hemiarthroplasty versus total shoulder prosthesis: results of cemented glenoid components. *J Shoulder Elbow Surg.* 2006;15:154-163. doi:10.1016/j.jse.2005.07.007
14. Gallusser N, Farron A. Complications of shoulder arthroplasty for osteoarthritis with posterior glenoid wear. *Orthop Traumatol Surg Res.* 2014;100:503-508. doi:10.1016/j.otsr.2014.06.002
15. Roberson TA, Bentley JC, Griscom JT, et al. Outcomes of total shoulder arthroplasty in patients younger than 65 years: a systematic review. *J Shoulder Elbow Surg.* 2017;26:1298-1306. doi:10.1016/j.jse.2016.12.069
16. Edwards TB, Kadakia NR, Boulahia A, et al. A comparison of hemiarthroplasty and total shoulder arthroplasty in the treatment of primary glenohumeral osteoarthritis: results of a multicenter study. *J Shoulder Elbow Surg.* 2003;12:207-213. doi:10.1016/s1058-2746(02)86804-5
17. Schoch BS, Wright TW, Zuckerman JD, et al. Glenoid component lucencies are associated with poorer patient-reported outcomes following anatomic shoulder arthroplasty. *J Shoulder Elbow Surg.* 2019;28:1956-1963. doi:10.1016/j.jse.2019.03.011
18. Walch G, Moraga C, Young A, et al. Results of anatomic nonconstrained prosthesis in primary osteoarthritis with biconcave glenoid. *J Shoulder Elbow Surg.* 2012;21:1526-1533. doi:10.1016/j.jse.2011.11.030
19. Denard PJ, Raiss P, Sowa B, et al. Mid- to long-term follow-up of total shoulder arthroplasty using a keeled glenoid in young adults with primary glenohumeral arthritis. *J Shoulder Elbow Surg.* 2013;22:894-900. doi:10.1016/j.jse.2012.09.016
20. Farron A, Terrier A, Büchler P. Risks of loosening of a prosthetic glenoid implanted in retroversion. *J Shoulder Elbow Surg.* 2006;15:521-526. doi:10.1016/j.jse.2005.10.003
21. Nyffeler RW, Werner CML, Gerber C. Biomechanical relevance of glenoid component positioning in the reverse Delta III total shoulder prosthesis. *J Shoulder Elbow Surg.* 2005;14:524-528. doi:10.1016/j.jse.2004.09.010
22. Levine WN, Djurasovic M, Glasson J-M, et al. Hemiarthroplasty for glenohumeral osteoarthritis: results correlated to degree of glenoid wear. *J Shoulder Elbow Surg.* 1997;6:449-454. doi:10.1016/S1058-2746(97)70052-1
23. Levine WN, Fischer CR, Nguyen D, et al. Long-term follow-up of shoulder hemiarthroplasty for glenohumeral osteoarthritis. *J Bone Joint Surg Am.* 2012;94:e164. doi:10.2106/JBJS.K.00603
24. Norris TR, Iannotti JP. Functional outcome after shoulder arthroplasty for primary osteoarthritis: a multicenter study. *J Shoulder Elbow Surg.* 2002;11:130-135. doi:10.1067/mse.2002.121146
25. Hackett DJ, Hsu JE, Matsen FA. Primary shoulder hemiarthroplasty: what can be learned from 359 cases that were surgically revised? *Clin Orthop Relat Res.* 2018;476:1031-1040. doi:10.1007/s11999.0000000000000167
26. Herschel R, Wieser K, Morrey ME, et al. Risk factors for glenoid erosion in patients with shoulder hemiarthroplasty: an analysis of 118 cases. *J Shoulder Elbow Surg.* 2017;26:246-252. doi:10.1016/j.jse.2016.06.004
27. Sperling JW, Cofield RH, Rowland CM. Minimum fifteen-year follow-up of Neer hemiarthroplasty and total shoulder arthroplasty in patients aged fifty years or younger. *J Shoulder Elbow Surg.* 2004;13:604-613. doi:10.1016/S1058274604001296

28. Getz CL, Kearns KA, Padegimas EM, et al. Survivorship of hemiarthroplasty with concentric glenoid reaming for glenohumeral arthritis in young, active patients with a biconcave glenoid. *J Am Acad Orthop Surg.* 2017;25:715-723. doi:10.5435/JAAOS-D-16-00019

29. Gilmer BB, Comstock BA, Jette JL, et al. The prognosis for improvement in comfort and function after the ream-and-run arthroplasty for glenohumeral arthritis: an analysis of 176 consecutive cases. *J Bone Joint Surg Am.* 2012;94:e102. doi:10.2106/JBJS.K.00486

30. Saltzman MD, Chamberlain AM, Mercer DM, et al. Shoulder hemiarthroplasty with concentric glenoid reaming in patients 55 years old or less. *J Shoulder Elbow Surg.* 2011;20:609-615. doi:10.1016/j.jse.2010.08.027

31. Sperling JW, Cofield RH, Rowland CM. Neer hemiarthroplasty and Neer total shoulder arthroplasty in patients fifty years old or less. Long-term results. *J Bone Joint Surg Am.* 1998;80:464-473. doi:10.2106/00004623-199804000-00002

32. Hasan SS, Leith JM, Campbell B, et al. Characteristics of unsatisfactory shoulder arthroplasties. *J Shoulder Elbow Surg.* 2002;11:431-441. doi:10.1067/mse.2002.125806

33. Matsen FA. The ream and run: not for every patient, every surgeon or every problem. *Int Orthop.* 2015;39:255-261. doi:10.1007/s00264-014-2641-2

34. Matsen FA, Russ SM, Vu PT, et al. What factors are predictive of patient-reported outcomes? A prospective study of 337 shoulder arthroplasties. *Clin Orthop Relat Res.* 2016;474:2496-2510. doi:10.1007/s11999-016-4990-1

35. Matsen FA, Warme WJ, Jackins SE. Can the ream and run procedure improve glenohumeral relationships and function for shoulders with the arthritic triad? *Clin Orthop Relat Res.* 2015;473:2088-2096. doi:10.1007/s11999-014-4095-7

36. Mahony GT, Werner BC, Chang B, et al. Risk factors for failing to achieve improvement after anatomic total shoulder arthroplasty for glenohumeral osteoarthritis. *J Shoulder Elbow Surg.* 2018;27:968-975. doi:10.1016/j.jse.2017.12.018

37. Parsons M, Greene A, Rohrs E, et al. *Results of a Survey of the American Shoulder and Elbow Surgeons on Preoperative Planning of Anatomic and Reverse Shoulder Arthroplasty.* 2020.

38. Bryce CD, Davison AC, Lewis GS, et al. Two-dimensional glenoid version measurements vary with coronal and sagittal scapular rotation. *J Bone Joint Surg Am.* 2010;92:692-699. doi:10.2106/JBJS.I.00177

39. Budge MD, Lewis GS, Schaefer E, et al. Comparison of standard two-dimensional and three-dimensional corrected glenoid version measurements. *J Shoulder Elbow Surg.* 2011;20:577-583. doi:10.1016/j.jse.2010.11.003

40. Sabesan VJ, Callanan M, Youderian A, et al. 3D CT assessment of the relationship between humeral head alignment and glenoid retroversion in glenohumeral osteoarthritis. *J Bone Joint Surg Am.* 2014;96:e64. doi:10.2106/JBJS.L.00856

41. Hoenecke HR, Hermida JC, Flores-Hernandez C, et al. Accuracy of CT-based measurements of glenoid version for total shoulder arthroplasty. *J Shoulder Elbow Surg.* 2010;19:166-171. doi:10.1016/j.jse.2009.08.009

42. Fulin P, Kysilko M, Pokorny D, et al. Study of the variability of scapular inclination and the glenoid version – considerations for preoperative planning: clinical-radiological study. *BMC Muscoskel Disord.* 2017;18:16. doi:10.1186/s12891-016-1381-4

43. Gross DJ, Golijanin P, Dumont GD, et al. The effect of sagittal rotation of the glenoid on axial glenoid width and glenoid version in computed tomography scan imaging. *J Shoulder Elbow Surg.* 2016;25:61-68. doi:10.1016/j.jse.2015.06.017

44. Shukla DR, McLaughlin RJ, Lee J, et al. Intraobserver and interobserver reliability of the modified Walch classification using radiographs and computed tomography. *J Shoulder Elbow Surg.* 2019;28:625-630. doi:10.1016/j.jse.2018.09.021

45. Bercik MJ, Kruse K, Yalizis M, et al. A modification to the Walch classification of the glenoid in primary glenohumeral osteoarthritis using three-dimensional imaging. *J Shoulder Elbow Surg.* 2016;25:1601-1606. doi:10.1016/j.jse.2016.03.010

46. Walch G, Vezeridis PS, Boileau P, et al. Three-dimensional planning and use of patient-specific guides improve glenoid component position: an in vitro study. *J Shoulder Elbow Surg.* 2015;24:302-309. doi:10.1016/j.jse.2014.05.029

47. Goutallier D, Postel JM, Bernageau J, et al. Fatty muscle degeneration in cuff ruptures. Pre- and postoperative evaluation by CT scan. *Clin Orthop Relat Res.* 1994;(304):78-83.

48. Donohue KW, Ricchetti ET, Ho JC, et al. The association between rotator cuff muscle fatty infiltration and glenoid morphology in glenohumeral osteoarthritis. *J Bone Joint Surg Am.* 2018;100:381-387. doi:10.2106/JBJS.17.00232

49. Sayed-Noor AS, Pollock R, Elhassan BT, et al. Fatty infiltration and muscle atrophy of the rotator cuff in stemless total shoulder arthroplasty: a prospective cohort study. *J Shoulder Elbow Surg.* 2018;27:976-982. doi:10.1016/j.jse.2017.12.021

50. Schoch BS, Wright TW, Zuckerman JD, et al. The effect of radial mismatch on radiographic glenoid loosening. *JSES Open Access.* 2019;3:287-291. doi:10.1016/j.jses.2019.09.007

51. Schoch B, Abboud J, Namdari S, et al. Glenohumeral mismatch in anatomic total shoulder arthroplasty. *JBJS Rev.* 2017;5:e1. doi:10.2106/JBJS.RVW.17.00014

52. Walch G, Edwards TB, Boulahia A, et al. The influence of glenohumeral prosthetic mismatch on glenoid radiolucent lines: results of a multicenter study. *J Bone Joint Surg Am.* 2002;84-A:2186-2191.

53. Somerson JS, Matsen FA. Functional outcomes of the ream-and-run shoulder arthroplasty: a concise follow-up of a previous report. *J Bone Joint Surg Am.* 2017;99:1999-2003. doi:10.2106/JBJS.17.00201

54. Hoenecke HR, Tibor LM, D'Lima DD. Glenoid morphology rather than version predicts humeral subluxation: a different perspective on the glenoid in total shoulder arthroplasty. *J Shoulder Elbow Surg.* 2012;21:1136-1141. doi:10.1016/j.jse.2011.08.044

55. Widnall JC, Dheerendra SK, MacFarlane RJ, et al. The use of shoulder hemiarthroplasty and humeral head resurfacing: a review of current concepts. *Open Orthop J.* 2013;7:334-337. doi:10.2174/1874325001307010334

56. Rai P, Davies O, Wand J, et al. Long-term follow-up of the Copeland mark III shoulder resurfacing hemi-arthroplasty. *J Orthop.* 2016;13:52-56. doi:10.1016/j.jor.2015.09.003

57. Bailie DS, Llinas PJ, Ellenbecker TS. Cementless humeral resurfacing arthroplasty in active patients less than fifty-five years of age. *J Bone Joint Surg Am.* 2008;90:110-117. doi:10.2106/JBJS.F.01552

58. Verstraelen FU, Horta LA, Schotanus MGM, et al. Clinical and radiological results 7 years after Copeland shoulder resurfacing arthroplasty in patients with primary glenohumeral osteoarthritis: an independent multicentre retrospective study. *Eur J Orthop Surg Traumatol.* 2018;28:15-22. doi:10.1007/s00590-017-2023-8

59. Lebon J, Delclaux S, Bonnevialle N, et al. Stemmed hemiarthroplasty versus resurfacing in primary shoulder osteoarthritis: a single-center retrospective series of 78 patients. *Orthop Traumatol Surg Res.* 2014;100:S327-S332. doi:10.1016/j.otsr.2014.05.012

60. Geervliet PC, Willems JH, Sierevelt IN, et al. Overstuffing in resurfacing hemiarthroplasty is a potential risk for failure. *J Orthop Surg.* 2019;14:474. doi:10.1186/s13018-019-1522-1

61. Harryman DT, Sidles JA, Harris SL, et al. The effect of articular conformity and the size of the humeral head component on laxity and motion after glenohumeral arthroplasty. A study in cadavera. *J Bone Joint Surg Am.* 1995;77:555-563. doi:10.2106/00004623-199504000-00008

62. Matsen FA, Lippitt SB. Current technique for the ream-and-run arthroplasty for glenohumeral osteoarthritis. *JBJS Essent Surg Tech.* 2012;2:e20. doi:10.2106/JBJS.ST.L.00009

63. Clinton J, Franta AK, Lenters TR, et al. Nonprosthetic glenoid arthroplasty with humeral hemiarthroplasty and total shoulder arthroplasty yield similar self-assessed outcomes in the management of comparable patients with glenohumeral arthritis. *J Shoulder Elbow Surg.* 2007;16:534-538. doi:10.1016/j.jse.2006.11.003

64. Lynch JR, Franta AK, Montgomery WH, et al. Self-assessed outcome at two to four years after shoulder hemiarthroplasty with concentric glenoid reaming: *J Bone Joint Surg.* 2007;89:1284-1292. doi:10.2106/JBJS.E.00942

65. Sandow MJ, David H, Bentall SJ. Hemiarthroplasty vs total shoulder replacement for rotator cuff intact osteoarthritis: how do they fare after a decade? *J Shoulder Elbow Surg.* 2013;22:877-885. doi:10.1016/j.jse.2012.10.023

66. Gartsman GM, Roddey TS, Hammerman SM. Shoulder arthroplasty with or without resurfacing of the glenoid in patients who have osteoarthritis. *J Bone Joint Surg Am.* 2000;82:26-34. doi:10.2106/00004623-200001000-00004

67. Lo IKY, Litchfield RB, Griffin S, et al. Quality-of-life outcome following hemiarthroplasty or total shoulder arthroplasty in patients with osteoarthritis. A prospective, randomized trial. *J Bone Joint Surg Am.* 2005;87:2178-2185. doi:10.2106/JBJS.D.02198

68. Dillon MT, Inacio MCS, Burke MF, et al. Shoulder arthroplasty in patients 59 years of age and younger. *J Shoulder Elbow Surg.* 2013;22:1338-1344. doi:10.1016/j.jse.2013.01.029

69. Lapner PLC, Rollins MD, Netting C, et al. A population-based comparison of joint survival of hemiarthroplasty versus total shoulder arthroplasty in osteoarthritis and rheumatoid arthritis. *Bone Joint J.* 2019;101-B:454-460. doi:10.1302/0301-620X.101B4.BJR-2018-0620.R1

70. Rasmussen JV, Polk A, Brorson S, et al. Patient-reported outcome and risk of revision after shoulder replacement for osteoarthritis. 1,209 cases from the Danish Shoulder Arthroplasty Registry, 2006-2010. *Acta Orthop.* 2014;85:117-122. doi:10.3109/17453674.2014.893497

71. Neyton L, Kirsch JM, Collotte P, et al. Mid- to long-term follow-up of shoulder arthroplasty for primary glenohumeral osteoarthritis in patients aged 60 or under. *J Shoulder Elbow Surg.* 2019;28:1666-1673. doi:10.1016/j.jse.2019.03.006

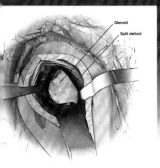

20 Subscapularis-Sparing Anatomic Total Shoulder Arthroplasty

Robert K. Fullick, MD and Christoph H. G. Fuchs, MD

INTRODUCTION

Surgery of the glenohumeral joint may be accomplished through multiple approaches. The deltopectoral, anterolateral, transacromial, and posterior approaches have all been described in the literature. The deltopectoral approach is the most commonly used approach in anatomic total shoulder arthroplasty (ATSA). This approach traditionally has required violating the subscapularis tendon by means of either tenotomy, tendon peel, or lesser tuberosity osteotomy. Anatomic repair and healing of subscapularis is critical to restore stability and adequate function following ATSA.[1] Postoperative subscapularis dysfunction, fatty atrophy, and incomplete or failed healing are commonly reported in the literature and can result in pain, poor function, instability, and early failure requiring revision surgery. A multitude of different techniques for repairing the subscapularis after tenotomy, peel, and lesser tuberosity osteotomy (LTO) have been developed[2-12] in order to improve postoperative subscapularis function. However, subscapularis dysfunction whether from partial or complete failure, weakness, or fatty atrophy continues to be an issue. Armstrong[13] used ultrasound to evaluate 30 patients following tenotomy for total shoulder arthroplasty (TSA) and found a 13% failure rate of their repair. Jackson found a 47% rate of subscapularis tenotomy repair failure on ultrasound examination in 15 patients and that these patients had significantly worse disabilities of the arm, shoulder, and hand (DASH) scores.[14] Miller found an abnormal lift-off and belly-press tests in 67% of patients.[15] Gerber found that 37 patients treated with LTO and repair during TSA had 100% healing of the osteotomy but only 89% had a normal belly-press test and 75% had a normal lift-off test.[16] Fatty infiltration was also noted to progress by one-stage in 24%, two stages in 15%, and three stages in 6% and was associated with poorer outcomes.[16] These findings were supported by Qureshi who found in a retrospective review of 30 patients following LTO that 40% of patients had an abnormal belly-press examination and 17% were unable to tuck their shirt in behind their back.[17] In a randomized, controlled trial of LTO versus subscapularis peel in shoulder arthroplasty, Laapner found no significant difference in functional outcomes.[8] Miller reported a 5.8% revision rate after total shoulder replacement (TSR) due to subscapularis repair failure in a study of 119 patients.[18] Due to these shortcomings, which persist despite numerous modifications of subscapularis management during ATSA, attention has recently been directed toward developing and modifying new approaches, which either minimize or completely avoid traumatizing the subscapularis tendon **(VIDEO 20.1)**.[1,19-22]

ANATOMY

Pertinent anatomy to understand and implement the approaches described in this chapter includes a detailed knowledge of the rotator interval, the subscapularis muscle, and the axillary nerve. Neer first named the triangular space between the subscapularis, the supraspinatus, and the coracoid as the "rotator interval."[23] The interval is bordered medially by the base of the coracoid process, superiorly by the anterior border of the supraspinatus, and inferiorly by the upper border of the subscapularis. Contents of the rotator interval include the superior and middle glenohumeral ligaments (SGHL and MGHL), the long head of the biceps tendon (LHBT), glenohumeral joint capsule, and the extra-articular coracohumeral ligament.[24] The rotator interval is an average of 414 mm[2]. in area. The capsule at the superior border of the subscapularis tendon at the glenoid is extremely thin, measuring only about 0.06 mm in thickness.[25]

The subscapularis muscle arises from the subscapularis fossa of the anterior scapula and is the most powerful rotator cuff muscle.[5] It constitutes 53% of all rotator cuff musculature, more than the other three parts of the rotator cuff combined[26] and constitutes the anterior portion of the transverse force couple that balances the glenohumeral joint. The upper two-thirds are tendinous and insert on the lesser tuberosity of the humerus. The lower one-third is muscular and inserts on the humeral metaphysis.[27] It is innervated by the upper (C5-C6) and lower (C5-7) subscapular nerves, which Checchia et al reported enter the muscle as close as 1 cm medial to the glenoid rim.[28] The axillary nerve is located 32.8 mm below the lower border of the subscapularis before it enters the quadrilateral space[29] but

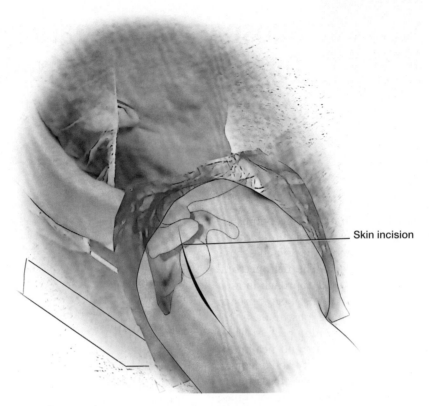

Skin incision

FIGURE 20.1 The Lafosse original superolateral skin incision is 8 cm long, located 1 cm anterior to the posterior margin of the acromioclavicular (AC) joint, and extends vertically down the lateral shoulder.

can move more proximally into the operative field with shoulder manipulation such as arm abduction, which tensions the nerve.

SUPEROLATERAL SUBSCAPULARIS-SPARING ROTATOR INTERVAL APPROACH

While some surgeons have been using a superior approach for reverse total shoulder arthroplasty (RTSA) for some time,[30] Lafosse was the first to describe a rotator interval technique for ATSA.[19] Designed to preserve the subscapularis, the approach consists of an anterolateral incision that angles down the lateral arm and utilizes a deltoid split and rotator interval approach to access the proximal humerus and glenoid **(FIGURES 20.1** and **20.2)**. He reported acceptable results in his published case series of 17 patients. However, several technical difficulties led him to abandon the technique. Commonly encountered problems included suboptimal inferior osteophyte resection (8/17 patients), difficulties judging head size (5/17 heads were deemed too small), and anatomic neck cuts that were either too proximal or distal (6/17). The technique also risked deltoid complications including dehiscence and potential anterior deltoid denervation. While these difficulties led Lafosse to develop a new technique, his superolateral rotator interval approach has been further utilized and refined by other surgeons including Adkison.[20]

Adkison modified the Lafosse subscapularis-sparing (SSS) superior approach via the rotator interval by changing the incision to a saber incision, which, in his opinion, not only allowed easier access to the proximal humerus but also made the approach extensile. He also had specialized instruments created, including special cutting blocks and angled drills and reamers, which allowed him to adopt the approach for almost all ATSAs. The subscapularis sparing approach was not utilized in cases with significant glenoid deformity or glenoid medialization. In these situations, a standard deltopectoral approach should be utilized.

TECHNIQUE

The patient is positioned in the beach chair position with a 45° incline and a folded sheet behind the ipsilateral scapula. Carefully position the patient at the edge of the bed to allow unrestricted shoulder extension. A 7 cm straight saber incision is made halfway between the anterolateral acromial margin and acromioclavicular joint **(FIGURE 20.3)**. Gelpi retractors are placed, and skin flaps are developed medially to the acromioclavicular joint and anterolaterally to expose the demarcation between the anterior and middle deltoid raphe. Stimulating the muscle with an electrocautery device can help identify this division in the deltoid. The deltoid is subperiosteally elevated off the anterior acromion

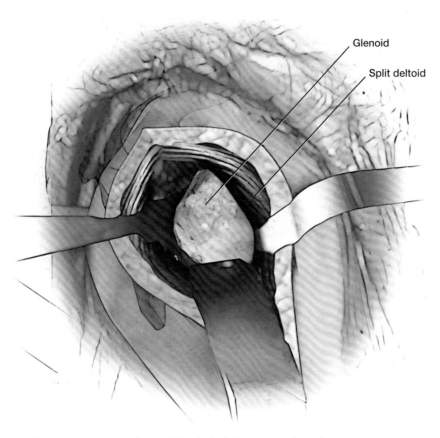

FIGURE 20.2 After osteotomizing and removing the humeral head, the Lafosse superolateral approach provides excellent glenoid visualization through the deltoid split and rotator interval.

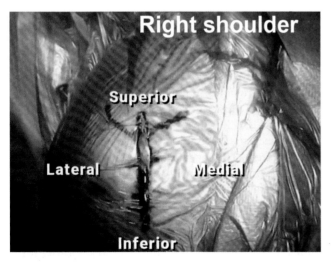

FIGURE 20.3 Superolateral incision for the Adkison modified superolateral technique. The incision begins 1 cm medial to the anterolateral acromial margin and extends anteroinferiorly approximately 7 cm.

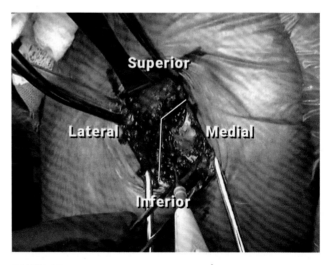

FIGURE 20.4 Deltoid split. The deltoid is released subperiosteally off the anterior aspect of the acromion and then split between its anterior and middle raphe. Care is taken not to release more than 3 to 4 cm below the acromial margin to avoid potential injury to the axillary nerve.

from the deltoid split approximately 1 cm medially. The deltoid is split distally, taking care not to extend past 3 to 4 cm distal to the acromion to minimize the risk of axillary nerve injury **(FIGURE 20.4)**. A stay suture can

be placed at the inferior margin of the split to minimize risk of propagation. The axillary nerve can be palpated through the deltoid split on the underside of the deltoid

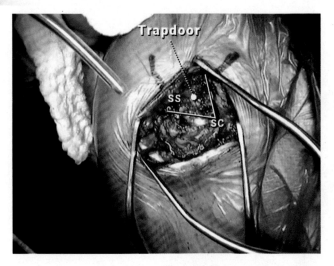

FIGURE 20.5 Trapdoor. After using the long head of the biceps tendon to identify the rotator interval, incise the interval tissue straight back to the glenoid margin along the rolled border of the subscapularis and to the supraspinatus articular insertion to create a trapdoor, which is then tucked in under the supraspinatus to allow for closure at the end of the case.

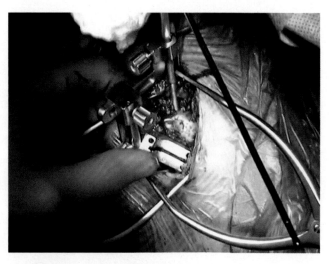

FIGURE 20.6 Intramedullary cut guide. A custom intramedullary guide is placed into the humerus, and then a safety saw is used to perform the osteotomy through the rotator interval.

muscle to confirm its location. Two blunt modified Kolbel self-retaining retractors are then inserted into the deltoid split, and subdeltoid adhesions are released digitally or with a Langenbeck elevator. The shoulder is then externally rotated to help identify the LHBT and define the borders of the rotator interval. The rotator interval tissue is incised starting from 5 mm posterior the biceps tendon, dividing the coracohumeral ligament, and exiting the shoulder joint anteriorly down to the upper border of the subscapularis tendon. Next, the arcuate artery is cauterized in the bicipital groove. The biceps tendon is tenotomized from its labral anchor and tenodesed at the transverse ligament. A biceps tenolysis may be done distal to the tenodesis to help ensure proper tension of the tendon. The rotator interval tissue is then incised posteriorly from the subscapularis upper edge back to the glenoid, creating a triangular flap of tissue that remains attached to the supraspinatus (**FIGURE 20.5**). The rotator interval tissue flap is tucked under the supraspinatus to protect it and allow for later closure at the conclusion of the procedure. The blunt modified Kolbel retractor is then placed into the rotator interval between the supraspinatus and subscapularis. A Darrach retractor may be inserted superiorly under the supraspinatus tendon to identify the insertion of the tendon. A second Darrach retractor may be inserted under the subscapularis to complete exposure. The humeral head cut is marked from the articular margin of the subscapularis to the supraspinatus articular margin with an electrocautery.

The medullary canal is opened with a rongeur posterior to the biceps tendon, approximately 5 mm from the supraspinatus insertion and at the highest point of the humeral head. An intramedullary guide is inserted into the humerus and is oriented such that the slotted

portion is placed into the gap between the supraspinatus and subscapularis (**FIGURE 20.6**). The cutting guide is pinned into position after appropriate placement is confirmed. The osteotomy is performed through the 132.5° neck-shaft angle cutting guide with an oscillating safety saw. Care should be taken not to damage the rotator cuff anteriorly or posteriorly and to protect critical medial and inferior neurovascular structures. After the resection is completed, it may sometimes be necessary to remove the head in two separate pieces. A curved osteotome and curette are used to free and remove the medial osteophytes. Adequate osteophyte removal may be confirmed by comparing the removed bone to the preoperative plan and by sliding an instrument back and forth along the medial calcar. During the learning curve for this approach, it may be helpful to use intraoperative fluoroscopy to confirm adequate osteophyte removal.

The Kolbel retractor blades are readjusted to access the glenoid (**FIGURE 20.7**). After confirming that the rotator cuff is intact, the labrum is circumferentially excised with electrocautery. The capsule is released around the inferior glenoid from approximately 10 o'clock to 2 o'clock in subperiosteal fashion to a depth of approximately 1 cm from the glenoid rim using electrocautery. The capsule on the undersurface of the subscapularis does not typically require release. Since the arm is adducted and the glenohumeral joint is not dislocated during this portion of the procedure, one can release the inferior capsule extending to the upper portion of the triceps insertion on the glenoid without significant risk of damaging the axillary nerve. The glenoid is prepared, and the glenoid component is inserted based upon the specific implant being utilized. Of note, angled glenoid reamers and an angled drill can be helpful during glenoid preparation.

After finishing the glenoid, the case transitions to humeral preparation. The head size is determined by

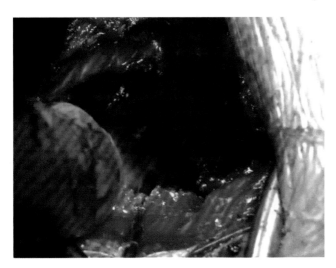

FIGURE 20.7 Glenoid preparation. After removing the osteotomized humeral head, retractors are readjusted deeper to allow for visualization of the glenoid.

measuring the medial to lateral distance across the resected surface. Alternatively, the removed humeral head may be measured or flat ring guides, which represent different head sizes, may also be overlaid on the cut surface. When in between sizes, Adkison chooses the larger head size to achieve on more medial metaphyseal coverage. The humeral canal is prepared by sequentially reaming and broaching based upon the technique for the implant system utilized. Trial implants are placed followed by a careful assessment of range of motion and stability. Trials are removed, the joint is irrigated, and one final check for osteophytes and loose bodies is performed. The humeral component is then assembled and implanted. A helpful trick to maintain correct humeral head rotation when inserting the implant is to place a steri-strip superiorly on the head and use this as a reference point to ensure that the implant does not rotate during insertion. The joint is irrigated one final time, and range of motion and stability are rechecked before proceeding to closure.

The rotator interval trapdoor is closed starting from posterior at the supraspinatus margin, proceeding anteriorly to the subscapularis, and then medially to the glenoid with interrupted #1 vicryl sutures. The deltoid is repaired back to the acromion with interrupted nonresorbable #2 transosseous sutures with knots placed deep to minimize the potential for prominence and patient discomfort. The deltoid split is repaired side to side with #1 vicryl. The subcutaneous tissue is closed in interrupted fashion, and the skin is sealed with a sealant.

POSTOPERATIVE PROTOCOL

The sling is removed the same evening of surgery for pendulums and passive range of motion, and then active elevation against gravity is initiated on postoperative day one. The sling may be discontinued all together as tolerated, which is typically between 1 and 7 days after surgery. Postoperative restrictions are designed to protect the deltoid repair. Early active elevation is permitted but resisted forward elevation, extension, and weight-bearing of greater than twenty pounds are delayed for 4 weeks.

RESULTS

There is a limited amount of reported results using this technique. Ransom et al compared radiographic results in 70 patients following ATSA using this SSS approach to 20 patients following ATSA using a deltopectoral (DP) approach.[31] The cases were all done by a single surgeon and were reviewed by an independent surgeon who was blinded to the technique. Humeral head height, humeral head medial offset, humeral head diameter, head-neck angle, humeral head centering, coracohumeral offset, and the anatomic reconstruction index (ARI) were used to evaluate overall reconstruction quality. The humeral head height, offset, coracohumeral offset, and ARI were the same between the two groups. The SSS group tended to be slightly undersized at 2.8 mm compared to slightly oversized by 1.4 mm in the DP group. Head-neck angle was 2° greater in the SSS group, and the humeral head centering was slightly improved in the DP group versus the SSS group. These three differences were all found to be below the measurement-error threshold. One significant difference that continued to be observed was that the superolateral approach consistently had a significantly smaller average decrease in osteophyte size from preoperative to postoperative radiographs and a significantly larger number of patients with osteophytes remaining postoperatively compared to the deltopectoral approach. There did not appear to be a notable clinically significant effect from residual osteophytes. The surgeon did note that his ability to resect these osteophytes had improved since these initial cases.

The principal advantage of the Adkison superolateral approach technique is the ability to immediately allow patients to perform active range of motion in all planes without concern of subscapularis repair failure. This early motion also theoretically decreases the risk of postoperative stiffness. There are no postoperative restrictions needed to protect a subscapularis repair; however, the amount of early-resisted shoulder elevation is at the discretion of the surgeon to protect the deltoid repair.

SSS DUAL-WINDOW APPROACH

The dual-window technique was initially developed by Lafosse due to difficulties encountered in the deltoid splitting rotator interval approach.[1] It uses a slightly lateralized deltopectoral incision with a superior rotator interval window and an inferior window below the subscapularis to facilitate capsular release and resection of osteophytes.

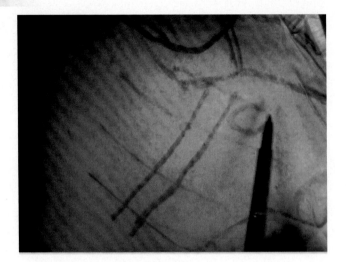

FIGURE 20.8 The dual-window skin incision is lateralized 1 cm from the standard deltopectoral incision to decrease soft tissue retraction and thus improve visualization.

CONTRAINDICATIONS

This approach is contraindicated in several situations including revision arthroplasty, morbid obesity, significant medial glenoid erosion, or deformity and situations that require glenoid bone grafting. Care must also be taken in patients with significant rotator cuff tendinopathy due to risk of iatrogenic rotator cuff injury from retraction.

TECHNIQUE

We prefer general anesthesia combined with a single-shot or indwelling interscalene block to maintain zero twitches of muscle relaxation when performing this procedure. We have found that this amount of relaxation to be both necessary and beneficial. The patient is positioned in the beach chair position at about 60° to 70° elevation. The incision is made approximately 1 cm lateral to the traditional deltopectoral incision to minimize the need for lateral soft tissue retraction (**FIGURE 20.8**). Full-thickness skin flaps are developed medially and laterally, and the coracoid and cephalic vein are used as landmarks to open the deltopectoral interval in standard fashion. The cephalic vein may be mobilized either laterally or medially, and care is taken to coagulate all bridging vessels. Subdeltoid and subacromial adhesions are released bluntly, and careful attention is paid to coagulate any bleeding vessels. A Brown shoulder retractor is placed. The clavipectoral fascia lateral to the conjoint tendon is incised, and the axillary nerve is palpated and protected with a blunt Hohmann retractor. If there is difficulty identifying the axillary nerve, the tug test can be helpful to confirm position of the nerve.[32] A sharp Hohmann retractor is positioned above the coracoid process, and the coracoacromial ligament is partially recessed to improve visualization of the rotator interval.

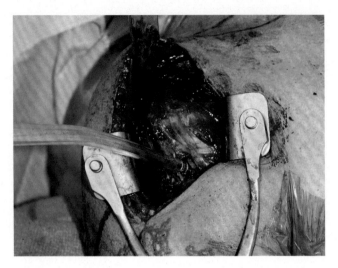

FIGURE 20.9 The inferior window is created by releasing approximately 5 mm of the muscular portion of the subscapularis from the humeral neck.

The anterior humeral circumflex artery and two veins are identified at the inferior portion of the subscapularis at the myotendinous junction and are either cauterized or ligated. The axillary nerve is palpated again to confirm protection with the blunt Hohmann retractor. The inferior capsule and approximately 5 mm of the inferior muscular portion of the subscapularis is released with electrocautery (**FIGURE 20.9**). The humerus is sequentially externally rotated, and subperiosteal dissection with electrocautery is performed to visualize the inferior and posteroinferior humeral neck and its osteophytes. A blunt Hohmann retractor is inserted into the joint at this time to aid in visualization of the inferior osteophytes. The osteophytes are removed with rongeurs and small curved osteotomes (**FIGURE 20.10**).

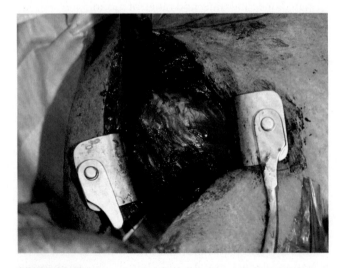

FIGURE 20.10 After releasing the inferior capsule, osteophytes are resected with small curved osteotomes and rongeurs while progressively externally rotating the arm.

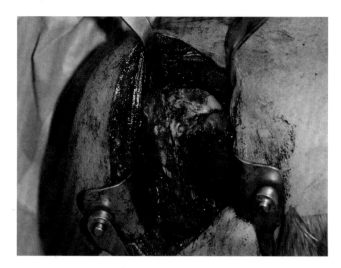

FIGURE 20.11 The superior window is created by excising the rotator interval tissue between the upper rolled border of the subscapularis and supraspinatus. Retractors are placed under the subscapularis and supraspinatus to facilitate exposure.

The focus is then shifted to the superior window. The bicipital sheath is identified and incised, and the biceps tendon is tenodesed to the pectoralis major tendon insertion with two nonabsorbable stitches. The biceps tendon is divided 1 cm above the level of the tenodesis and is unroofed proximally with electrocautery into the rotator interval. The upper rolled border of the subscapularis and the anterior border of the supraspinatus are identified, and the rotator interval tissue is excised from its lateral to medial to the superior glenoid **(FIGURE 20.11)**. The proximal biceps tendon is released at the glenoid margin. Specially designed spiked and angled Hohmann retractors are inserted anteriorly and posteriorly, one deep to the subscapularis tendon and one anterior to the posterior rotator cuff insertion along the anatomic neck of the humerus. Having secured visualization of the anatomic neck of the humerus, an extramedullary cutting guide that references off the bicipital groove is used to plan the humeral head resection. The guide is secured in place with several 2 mm Kirschner wires, and the head-cut angle is confirmed by palpating the humeral head/neck junction through the inferior window. The cut is then made with a microsagittal saw and is completed with a straight osteotome **(FIGURE 20.12)**. Care is taken to protect the axillary nerve with a blunt Hohmann retractor via the inferior window during resection. After completing the cut, the resected humeral head is removed and measured to assist in determining head size. The osteotomy is checked by visualizing it through the inferior window and/or using fluoroscopy, which the senior author recommends during the learning curve portion of your experience. Once satisfied with the humeral cut, the arm is adducted and extended to maximize exposure of the metaphyseal surface. A modified Gelpi or Hohman retractor is inserted to retract the anterior and posterior

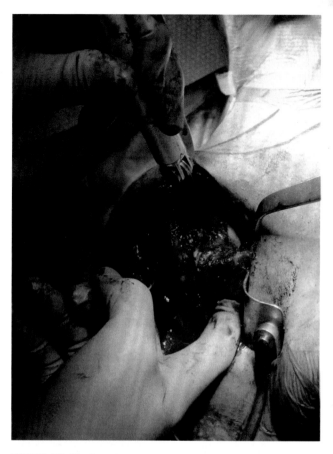

FIGURE 20.12 If performing the humeral head osteotomy free hand, a finger in the inferior window at the head-neck junction can help guide the cut angle.

cuff and widen the window of visualization through the interval. Next, the humeral canal is prepared in standard fashion before a head-cut protector is placed.

The arm is returned to neutral, and glenoid exposure is maximized by adjusting the amount of humeral external rotation. Typically, minimal external rotation provides the best view. Glenoid exposure is then completed by placing standard retractors anteriorly along the scapular neck and posteriorly on the glenoid. A rabbit ear retractor is frequently helpful on the inferior glenoid margin to depress the humeral head **(FIGURE 20.13)**. To improve exposure, a 360° capsular release and labral resection is performed while taking care to protect the axillary nerve when working inferiorly. The glenoid is prepared in the standard fashion dictated by the implant of choice. If a pegged glenoid is desired, a special angled drill can be helpful to improve access to the inferior peg if needed. The appropriately sized glenoid implant is cemented into place, and then attention is returned to the humerus **(FIGURE 20.14)**.

The arm is adducted and extended the arm to deliver the humeral cut surface, and the Gelpi is adjusted to retract the anterior and posterior rotator cuff. Humeral offset is judged by comparing the center of the trial

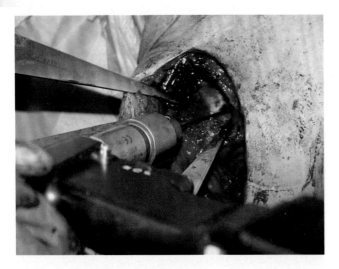

FIGURE 20.13 After removing the humeral head, readjustment of retractors allows for glenoid preparation.

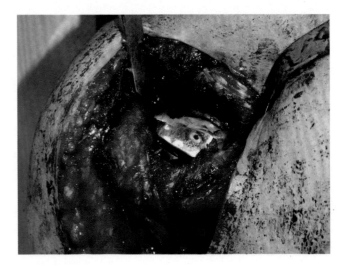

FIGURE 20.15 Final implant viewed through the rotator interval prior to closure.

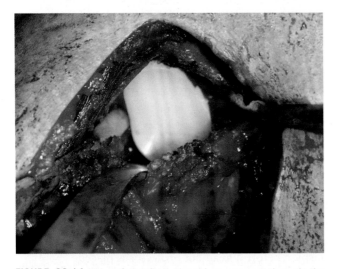

FIGURE 20.14 View of the final glenoid component through the rotator interval superior window.

prosthesis to the margins of the cut humeral surface. Trial components are placed as determined by the implant system being utilized, and stability and range of motion are assessed. When the proper implant sizes are selected, the trial is removed, the shoulder is irrigated, and the final assembled humeral component is inserted through the rotator interval (**FIGURE 20.15**). Prior to impacting the stem into the final position, the prosthesis rotation is checked to confirm that it is in correct orientation.

The shoulder is irrigated once more, and the wound is carefully inspected to confirm hemostasis. If the surgeon chooses to close the rotator interval, it is recommended to start laterally with the arm in slight external rotation to minimize overtightening and the potential for post-operative stiffness. The inferior muscular subscapularis portion, which was detached for inferior window exposure, does not require repair. A drain may be used at

the surgeon's discretion but is not required. The subcutaneous tissues are closed in standard fashion. The skin is closed with running #3 monocryl, and dermabond is applied.

POSTOPERATIVE PROTOCOL

Patients are placed in a sling for comfort for 10 to 14 days. Immediate passive, active-assisted, and active range of motion is allowed as tolerated. Strengthening is allowed when acceptable active range of motion and discomfort allow, usually between 2 and 6 weeks, and is advanced as tolerated.

RESULTS

Following the initial technique description by Simovitch et al[1] there have been only a few additional reports documenting the outcomes of this technique. Ding et al randomized 50 patients to standard deltopectoral approach with subscapularis tenotomy and 46 to the SSS dual-window technique.[33] Due to difficulties with visualization, seven patients (15.2%) were converted to subscapularis tenotomy intraoperatively. They found no significant difference in humeral head height, humeral head centering, humeral head medial offset, head-neck angle, humeral head diameter, and ARI between the two groups. However, there were significantly more post-operative osteophytes in the SSS TSA group, and subgroup analysis of humeral head diameter demonstrated that the SSS group also had more outliers with a >4 mm mismatch.

Kwon published a prospective, randomized clinical trial of 32 SSS versus 38 standard tenotomy TSAs with a minimum 2-year follow-up.[34] Nine patients (20%) in the SSS group had to be converted to tenotomy. There were no significant differences between the two groups with regards to American Shoulder and Elbow Surgeons (ASES) and visual analog scale (VAS) scores. Moreover, no significant difference was found in improvements of flexion and external rotation between the two techniques, and there was no significant difference in complications. It was noted that males with larger deltoid bulk frequently required crossover to the tenotomy group.

ADVANTAGES OF THE SSS DUAL-WINDOW TECHNIQUE

The main advantage of this technique is preservation of the subscapularis tendon. The inferior window also improves the surgeon's ability to resect osteophytes, plan and assess the humeral resection, and better appreciate humeral head sizing. This approach avoids the position of external rotation/abduction/extension during humeral preparation, which Nagda reported causes changes in intraoperative neuromonitoring.[35] Because the subscapularis tendon is not violated in this technique, the postoperative rehabilitation is accelerated, and the rate of subscapularis failure is theoretically lower. While postoperative rehabilitation has been accelerated for this technique, functional outcomes, thus far, have proven to be similar to standard shoulder arthroplasty techniques.

SUBSCAPULARIS-SPLITTING APPROACH

Savoie developed the subscapularis-splitting approach due to concerns regarding subscapularis tendon integrity following traditional techniques.[21,22] After multiple cadaver dissections, the following technique was developed to spare the more critical upper 50% to 70% of the subscapularis tendon attachment, given that approximately 60% of the tendon attaches to the upper third of the subscapularis footprint,[36] and this region experiences the greatest load transmission.[37]

TECHNIQUE

The patient is positioned in the beach chair position with general anesthesia and an interscalene nerve block. A folded sheet is placed just medial to the scapula to optimize glenoid access. A standard deltopectoral approach is utilized with a 5- to 7-cm vertical skin incision. After the deltopectoral interval is developed, the LHBT is identified and used as a landmark to help define the rotator interval. The LHBT is tenotomized and is tenodesed at the surgeon's discretion. The superior and inferior borders of the subscapularis tendon are identified. Gentle internal and external rotation can be helpful to define the tendon borders. The subscapularis is split with electrocautery approximately one-half to two-thirds inferior to the superior border of the tendon at the lower muscle-tendon raphe (**FIGURE 20.16**). Using electrocautery, the inferior 30% to 50% of the subscapularis tendon is released below the split. Care is taken to preserve some tissue laterally for repair during closure.

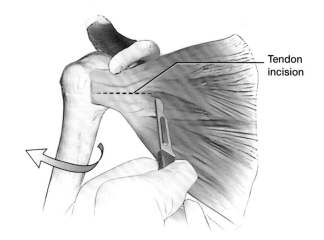

FIGURE 20.16 Subscapularis split. The subscapularis muscle is split at approximately the upper one-half or upper two-thirds with a knife while holding the arm externally rotated to keep the subscapularis on tension.

The subscapularis and capsule are elevated subperiosteally while slowly externally rotating the humerus. The release continues medially under any inferior humeral osteophytes. Care is taken to palpate and protect the axillary nerve. Once the posterior humeral neck is reached, the capsular release is continued under the teres minor and lower infraspinatus attachments with special attention not to damage the rotator cuff tendons. After this release is performed, a cobb retractor is used as a lever against the supraglenoid tubercle to flip the intact upper subscapularis tendon over the humeral head as the arm is abducted and externally rotated, allowing the shoulder to anteriorly dislocate under the intact upper subscapularis tendon (**FIGURE 20.17**).

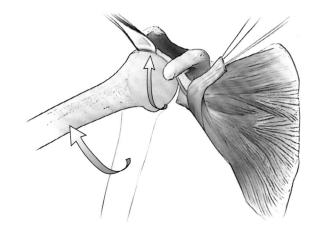

FIGURE 20.17 A retraction stitch is placed in the inferior portion of the subscapularis and retracted medially out of the field. A cobb retractor is placed under the upper intact subscapularis tendon and levered against the supraglenoid tubercle to flip the remaining subscapularis tendon over the humeral head while the arm is externally rotated and abducted.

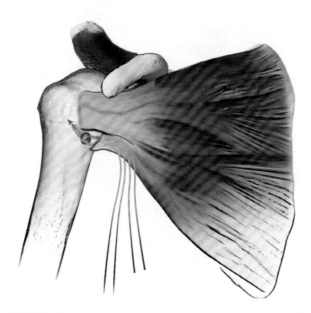

FIGURE 20.18 The inferior subscapularis tendon is reattached with one double-loaded suture anchor, and additional interrupted PDS reinforcement stitches are placed between the split raphe and at the distal tendon insertion.

After the shoulder is dislocated, a chandler retractor is placed medially and a Hohman retractor superiorly under the intact upper subscapularis tendon to fully expose the humeral head and protect surrounding soft tissues. Next, peripheral osteophytes are removed with an osteotome and rongeur to allow proper assessment of humeral head size. At this point, humeral preparation proceeds based on the implant being utilized. If performing a hemiarthroplasty, the final implant is placed, and the humerus is relocated under the upper border of subscapularis with the assistance of a Cobb retractor. The lower subscapularis is then repaired with either bugler #2 Orthocord or a double-loaded suture anchor with a double-row repair technique plus #2 polydioxanone (PDS) interrupted sutures **(FIGURE 20.18)**.

If performing an ATSA, two options are available for accessing the glenoid after preparing the humerus. The glenoid can be approached through either the rotator interval in which the humerus is dislocated anteroinferiorly through the lower subscapularis defect. Alternatively, a Fukuda or narrow bent Hohmann retractor is used to dislocate the humeral head either posteriorly or inferiorly to access the glenoid through the window below the intact upper subscapularis tendon. With the glenoid exposed, it can be prepared for component implantation. When this is completed, the humerus is redelivered anteriorly under the upper subscapularis tendon, and the final humeral implant is placed after trial reductions and assessment of range of motion and stability. Finally, the humerus is relocated under the subscapularis tendon, and the inferior portion of the subscapularis tendon is repaired as described.

POSTOPERATIVE PROTOCOL

Postoperatively, patients are maintained in a sling for 7 to 14 days. Passive range of motion and active external rotation are initiated during the first week. Active internal rotation is started at 3 weeks. The patient is allowed to progress as tolerated at 4 weeks, and most patients return to exercise activity by 8 weeks.

OUTCOMES

Two-year follow-up has been reported on 43 patients.[22] The subscapularis tendon was examined in 19 by magnetic resonance imaging (MRI) and in 24 by ultrasound. All 43 patients had imaging evidence of an intact subscapularis tendon, and none were noted to have fatty atrophy. On physical examination, all patients had subscapularis strength equal to the opposite side based upon lift-off, belly-press, and bear hug tests.

CONCLUSION

The orthopedic literature contains many examples of surgeons seeking to improve and innovate. While the standard deltopectoral trans-subscapularis approach for TSA is currently the standard of care, it does present some limitations related to subscapularis healing. This has led surgeon innovators to develop techniques that preserve the subscapularis during ATSA. The superolateral deltoid split approach allows a perpendicular view of the glenoid but has a more difficult learning curve and has the risk of deltoid dehiscence, anterior deltoid denervation, and some difficulties in recreating normal humeral anatomy and removing inferior humeral osteophytes. The SSS dual-window approach improves upon the visualization of the original Lafosse technique but requires a learning curve to assess anatomy and confirm removal of inferior osteophytes.[1] The subscapularis-splitting approach improves visualization but still requires violation of approximately 30% to 50% of the subscapularis and also shoulder dislocation. There have also been recent description of posterior approach for TSA with promising early outcomes.[38,39] Computer-guided navigation, which has been utilized widely in hip and knee arthroplasty, is becoming more common for shoulder arthroplasty. Navigation of the humerus and glenoid may allow surgeons to consistently recreate normal anatomy and further enhance the development and utilization of SSS surgical approaches to TSA.

REFERENCES

1. Simovitch R, FullickR, Kwon Y, Zuckerman JD. Use of the subscapularis preserving technique in anatomic total shoulder arthroplasty. *Bull Hosp Jt Dis (2013)*. 2015;73(suppl 1):S154-S160.
2. Ahmad CS, Wing D, Gardner TR, Levine WN, Biglani LU. Biomechanical evaluation of subscapularis repair used during shoulder arthroplasty. *J Shoulder Elbow Surg*. 2007;16(3 suppl):S59-S64.

3. Caplan JL, Whitfield B, Neviaser RJ. Subscapularis function after primary tendon to tendon repair in patients after replacement arthroplasty of the shoulder. *J Shoulder Elbow Surg.* 2009;18(2):193-196.

4. Ponce BA, Ahluwalia RS, Mazzocca AD, Gobezie RG, Warner JJP, Millett PJ. Biomechanical and clinical evaluation of a novel lesser tuberosity repair technique in total shoulder arthroplasty. *J Bone Joint Surg Am.* 2005;87(suppl 2):1-8.

5. DeFranco MJ, Higgins LD, Warner JJ. Subscapularis management in open shoulder surgery. *J Am Acad Orthop Surg.* 2010;18:707-717.

6. Giuseffi SA, Wongtriatanachai P, Omae H, et al. Biomechanical comparison of lesser tuberosity osteotomy vs subscapularis tenotomy in total shoulder arthroplasty. *J Shoulder Elbow Surg.* 2012;21(8):1087-1095.

7. Krishnan SG, Stewart DG, Reineck JR, Lin KC, Buzzell JE, Burkhead WZ. Subscapularis repair after shoulder arthroplasty: biomechanical and clinical validation of a novel technique. *J Shoulder Elbow Surg.* 2009;18(2):184-192.

8. Lapner PL, Sabri E, Rakhra K, Bell K, Athwal GS. Comparison of lesser tuberosity osteotomy to subscapularis peel in shoulder arthroplasty: a randomized controlled trial. *J Bone Joint Surg Am.* 2012;94(24):2239-2246.

9. Scalise JJ, Ciccone J, Iannotti JP. Clinical, radiographic, and ultrasonographic comparison of subscapularis tenotomy and lesser tuberosity osteotomy for total shoulder arthroplasty. *J Bone Joint Surg Am.* 2010;92(7):1627-1634.

10. Van den Berghe GR, Nguyen B, Patil S, et al. A biomechanical evaluation of three surgical techniques for subscapularis repair. *J Shoulder Elbow Surg.* 2008;17(1):156-161.

11. Choate WS, Kwapisz A, Momaya AM, Hawkins RJ, Tokish JM. Outcomes for subscapularis management techniques in shoulder arthroplasty: a systematic review. *J Shoulder Elbow Surg.* 2018;27(2):363-370.

12. Schrock JB, Kraeutler MJ, Crellin CT, McCarty EC, Bravman JT. How should I fixate the subscapularis in total shoulder arthroplasty? A systematic review of pertinent subscapularis repair biomechanics. *Shoulder Elbow.* 2017;9(3):153-159.

13. Armstrong A, Lashgari C, Teefey S, Menendez J, Yamaguchi K, Galatz LM. Ultrasound evaluation and clinical correlation of subscapularis repair after total shoulder arthroplasty. *J Shoulder Elbow Surg.* 2006;15:541-548.

14. Jackson JD, Cil A, Smith J, Steinmann SP. Integrity and function of the subscapularis after total shoulder arthroplasty. *J Shoulder Elbow Surg.* 2010;19:1085-1090.

15. Miller SL, Hafrzrati Y, Klepps S, Chiang A, Flatow EL. Loss of subscapularis function after total shoulder replacement: a seldom recognized problem. *J Shoulder Elbow Surg.* 2003;12:29-34.

16. Gerber C, Yan EH, Pfirrmann CA, Zumstein MAA, Werner CM. Subscapularis muscle function and structure after total shoulder replacement with lesser tuberosity osteotomy and repair. *J Bone Joint Surg Am.* 2005;87:1739-1745.

17. Qureshi S, Hsiao A, Klug RA, Lee E, Braman J, Flatow EL. Subscapularis function after total shoulder replacement: results with lesser tuberosity osteotomy. *J Shoulder Elbow Surg.* 2008;17:68-72.

18. Miller BS, Joseph TA, Noonan TJ, Horan MP, Hawkins RJ. Rupture of the subscapularis tendon after shoulder arthroplasty: diagnosis, treatment, and outcome. *J Shoulder Elbow Surg.* 2005;14:492-496.

19. Lafosse L, Schnaser E, Haag M, Gobezie R. Primary total shoulder arthroplasty performed entirely thru the rotator interval: technique and minimum two-year outcomes. *J Shoulder Elbow Surg.* 2009;18(6):864-873.

20. Adkison DP, Hudson PW, Worthen JV, et al. Subscapularis-sparing rotator interval approach for anatomic total shoulder arthroplasty. *JBJS Essent Surg Tech.* 2019;9(4):e42.1-e42.12.

21. Routman HD, Savoie FHB. Subscapularis-sparing approaches to total shoulder arthroplasty: ready for prime time? *Clin Sports Med.* 2018;37(4):559-568.

22. Savoie FHB, Charles R, Casselton J, O'Brien MJ, Hurt JA. The Subscapularis-sparing approach in humeral head replacement. *J Shoulder Elbow Surg.* 2015;24(4):606-612.

23. Neer CS. Displaced proximal humeral fractures. I. Classification and evaluation. *J Bone Joint Surg Am.* 1970;52:1077-1089.

24. Frank RM, Taylor D, Verma NN, Romeo AA, Mologne TS, Provencher MT. The rotator interval of the shoulder. Implications in the treatment of shoulder instability. *Orthop J Sports Med.* 2015;3(12):2325967115621494.

25. Plancher KD, Johnston JC, Peterson RK, Hawkins RJ. The dimensions of the rotator interval. *J Shoulder Elbow Surg.* 2005;14(6):620-625.

26. Keating JF, Waterworth P, Shaw-Dunn J, Crossan J. The relative strengths of the rotator cuff muscles. A cadaver study. *J Bone Joint Surg Br.* 1993;75(1):137-140.

27. Hinton M, Parker A, Drez D, Altcheck D. An anatomic study of the subscapularis tendon and myotendinous junction. *J Shoulder Elbow Surg.* 1994;3:224-229.

28. Checchia SL, Doncaux P, Martins MG, Meireles FS. Subscapularis muscle enervation: the effect of arm position. *J Shoulder Elbow Surg.* 1996;5(3):214-218.

29. Wright JM, Heavrin B, Hawkins RJ, Noonan T. Arthroscopic visualization of the subscapularis tendon. *Arthroscopy.* 2001;17(7):677-684.

30. Mole D, Wein F, Dezaly C, Valenti Philippe V, Sirveaux F. The anterosuperior approach for reverse shoulder arthroplasty. *Clin Orthop Relat Res.* 2011;469:2461-2468.

31. Ransom EF, Adkison DP, Woods DP, et al. Subscapularis sparing total shoulder arthroplasty through a superolateral approach: a radiographic study. *J Shoulder Elbow Surg.* 2020;29(4):814-820.

32. Flatow EL, Bigliani LU. Tips of the trade: locating and protecting the axillary nerve in shoulder surgery. The tug test. *Orthop Rev.* 1992;21(4):503-505.

33. Ding DY, Mahure SA, Aduoko JA, Zuckerman JD, Won YW. Total shoulder arthroplasty using a subscapularis-sparing approach: a radiographic analysis. *J Shoulder Elbow Surg.* 2015;24(6):831-837.

34. Kwon YW, Zuckerman JD. Subscapularis-sparing total shoulder arthroplasty: a prospective, double-blinded, randomized clinical trial. *Orthopedics.* 2019;42(1):e61-e67.

35. Nagda S, Rogers K, Sestokas A, Getz C. Neer Award 2005: peripheral nerve function during shoulder arthroplasty using intraoperative nerve monitoring. *J Shoulder Elbow Surg.* 2007;16(3 suppl):S2-S8.

36. Richards DP, Burkhart SS, Tehrany AM, Wirth MA. The subscapularis footprint: an anatomic description of its insertion site. *Arthroscopy.* 2007;23(3):251-254.

37. Halder A, Zobitz ME, Schultz E, An KN. Structural properties of the subscapularis tendon. *J Orthop Res.* 2000;18(5):829-834.

38. Amirthanayagam TD, Amis AA, Reilly P, Emery RJ. Rotator cuff-sparing approaches for glenohumeral joint access: an anatomic feasibility study. *J Shoulder Elbow Surg.* 2017;26(3):512-520.

39. Greiwe RM, Hill MA, Boyle MS, Nolan J. Posterior approach total shoulder arthroplasty: a retrospective analysis of short-term results. *Orthopedics.* 2020;43(1):e15-e20.

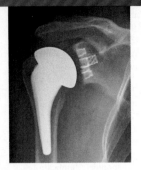

21 Clinical Outcomes of Anatomic Total Shoulder Arthroplasty

Ryan W. Simovitch, MD and Brent Mollon, MD, MSc

INTRODUCTION

Anatomic total shoulder arthroplasty (ATSA) involves the surgical replacement of the entire glenohumeral articulation with components designed to recreate native joint structure and kinematics. ATSA replaces the proximal humerus with a cobalt-chromium or titanium alloy component as in hemiarthroplasty (HA), but resurfaces the glenoid with a polyethylene component. This implant demands the presence of an intact and functional rotator cuff to appropriately balance and power shoulder movements. As a result, rotator cuff compromise (due to irreparable rotator cuff tears [RCTs], proximal humerus fractures, or functional attrition of the rotator cuff musculature) or situations where appropriate shoulder balance cannot be achieved (as in significant glenoid or humeral erosions) are being preferentially managed with reverse total shoulder arthroplasty (RTSA).

The first anatomic total shoulder prosthesis was designed by a dentist and implanted by French surgeon Jules Pean in 1893 for tuberculosis of the shoulder.[1] This implant, composed of a paraffin-coated ebonite glenoid and a leather/platinum humeral component, was ultimately removed 2 years later due to chronic infection.[2] Modern shoulder arthroplasty design is credited to Neer, who introduced a vitallium HA design to treat displaced proximal humerus fractures in the 1950s.[3] In 1976, ATSA became available after Stellbrink designed a polyethylene glenoid component to couple with the humeral heads designed by Neer.[2,4] ATSA has since evolved to become the standard of care for advanced glenohumeral arthritis with an intact rotator cuff and has been consistently found to offer superior clinical results to HA.[5,6]

ATSA is indicated in patients with glenohumeral arthritis who have failed nonoperative treatments or as a revision procedure for ongoing pain following shoulder HA. Contraindications include rotator cuff incompetency, severe bony abnormality, active infection, deltoid palsy, and inability to comply with postoperative instructions.

Fourth-Generation ATSA Design

While initial designs of ATSA prostheses consisted of monobloc humeral components and cemented all-polyethylene glenoid components, as was the case in Neer's initial design, modern fourth-generation implants have evolved significantly to provide additional options. Variability on the humeral and glenoid side allows multiple combinations to aid surgeons in providing their patients with an "anatomic" reconstruction. The prevalent thought of shoulder surgeons is that a more "anatomic reconstruction" will result in more durable and profound clinical improvements after surgery.

The factors that can be adjusted during the humeral reconstruction aspect of ATSA are head height, head thickness, head diameter, center of rotation (COR), neck-shaft angle, and humeral head offset.[7] In the initial monobloc humeral prostheses, the position of the humeral head was dictated by the stem position in the humeral intramedullary canal. Current ATSA prostheses now utilize modular components. The head and stem can be mated on the back table or in situ. Most systems utilize heads of varying diameters and thicknesses with eccentricity built into the head or head and stem, allowing the best anatomic coverage of the resected head independent of the position of the stem in the intramedullary canal. Double eccentricity has been shown to provide an anatomic reconstruction more often than single eccentricity, allowing medial and posterior offset to be corrected simultaneously and independently. The goal of modularity is to allow a humeral implant to restore the native humeral head size and COR in order to avoid overstuffing of the joint, which can result in loss of range of motion (ROM), attrition of the rotator cuff, edge loading of the glenoid, and subacromial impingement. A previous study by Flurin et al[8] demonstrated that improved anatomic reconstruction (optimizing humeral head height, humeral head centering, humeral head medial offset, humeral head diameter, and humeral neck angle) had a statistically significant positive effect on clinical outcomes.

Other aspects of the fourth-generation humeral component include methods of fixation as well as the shape and length of the stem. Fixation of humeral stems has largely evolved away from cementation, as methods of porous coating for fixation of the metaphyseal portion of the stem have been shown to provide reliable on-growth and in-growth. Fixation has predominantly been designed to be metaphyseal and not diaphyseal so as to reduce the rate of stress shielding. Furthermore, the trend has been away from large stems that result in three-point fixation in the diaphyseal bone, also in order to avoid stress shielding and difficult revision scenarios. Most recently, the concept of short stems and stemless humeral components has been introduced in an effort to further reduce stress shielding, minimize instrumentation of the intramedullary canal, and provide for an easier revision.

Similar to the evolution of humeral components in ATSA, glenoid implants have also dramatically evolved. Older generations of ATSA relied on pegged or keeled all-polyethylene components requiring cement fixation. These components fared well but demonstrated high rates of radiolucency over time. Fourth-generation prostheses now include hybrid polyethylene glenoid components capable of achieving initial fixation with cement but durable fixation with biologic on-growth, in-growth, and through growth **(FIGURE 21.1)**. Current glenoids are manufactured from ultrahigh molecular weight polyethylene that is highly cross-linked. Vitamin E[9] may be increasingly introduced to reduce oxidation as it has been shown to be effective in the lower extremity literature and early studies pertaining to the shoulder. Current ATSA systems rely on a radial mismatch (difference between radius of curvature of the humeral head and glenoid concave surface), with low or no mismatch having been shown to result in a higher incidence of radiolucent lines and loosening, whereas a higher mismatch can result in edge loading and instability.[10] A recent study by Schoch et al[11] has challenged the initial thinking that radial mismatch is optimized if kept between 6 and 10 mm as Walch et al[12] reported, noting that glenoid loosening as well as glenoid revision rates did not differ with radial mismatches between 3.4 and 7 mm.[11] Thus, radial mismatches below 5.5 mm may be acceptable and even desirable.

Trends in ATSA

The advent of fourth-generation prostheses has expanded the indications for ATSA. Modularity and innovation allow the implant to be adapted to a patient's anatomy, as opposed to adapting the individual patient anatomy to a fixed prosthesis, permitting surgeons to push the envelope in younger patients and patients with severe deformities. However, the frequency of utilization of ATSA has changed with the advent of the increasing popularity and durable outcomes of RTSA. In 2014, the use of RTSA surpassed the use of ATSA and this trend has continued.[13] The global shoulder replacement market has been estimated to increase at a compound annual growth rate of 7%, but RTSA growth is dwarfing that of ATSA. Despite the rapid growth of RTSA, ATSA will still account for a significant portion of the market share as HA has largely fallen out of favor for most conditions.

SURVIVORSHIP

Improvements in surgical technique, patient selection, and implant design have culminated in overall ATSA implant survivorship rates of 95% to 98% at 5 years, 93% to 97% at 10 years, 85% to 88% at 15 years, and 80% to 85% at 20 years.[14-17] Survivorship tends to be impacted by glenoid loosening, humeral stem loosening, infection, and rotator cuff dysfunction.

Overall survivorship has been most clearly linked to glenoid implant design. Historically, glenoid components could be broadly grouped into uncemented metal-backed polyethylene or cemented all-polyethylene components. All-polyethylene components could be further grouped according to how they are secured into the glenoid, either via a large central keel or through multiple pegs (both centrally and peripherally). Although overall glenoid survivorship across all implants is believed to be 96%, 96%, and 95% at 5 years, 10 years, and 15 years,[18] respectively, variability does exist across

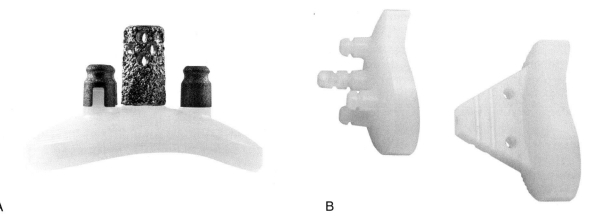

A   B

FIGURE 21.1 (A) Hybrid caged polyethylene glenoid implant compared to a **(B)** standard all-polyethylene pegged (left) implant and keeled (right) all-polyethylene implant.

component types. Independent of component type, it is recognized that an overall higher risk of failure has been identified in male patients and in those for whom the indication for surgery was posttraumatic osteoarthritis or osteonecrosis.[18]

The lowest rates of glenoid implant survivorship have been reported with uncemented metal-backed glenoid components, and this type of implant is now primarily of historical significance for that reason. Early randomized controlled trials compared these metal-backed implants to a cemented keeled all-polyethylene component and reported a 20% (4/20) loosening rate as well as a 15% revision rate in the metal-backed group compared with none of these complications in the all-polyethylene group. Despite this, the rate of radiolucent lines was much higher in the cemented component group at the time of final follow-up (85% compared with 25%).[19] Subsequent studies have reported failure rates of 5%, 11% and 54% at 5 years, 7.5 years, and 12 years, respectively, for metal-backed polyethylene glenoids.[15,20] Gauci et al[21] studied a cohort of patients younger than 60 years and noted a threefold greater rate of failure at 10.3 years with metal-backed components compared with cemented all-polyethylene components (70% vs 22%). Reported modes of failure in the above studies included loosening, polyethylene dissociation from the metal baseplate, and severe polyethylene wear. Although some studies have reported favorable outcomes[15] of newer generation metal-backed glenoids and current use of hybrid implants (distinct from historical metal-backed design) show promise,[22] cemented polyethylene components are still considered the current gold standard in ATSA.

In contrast to glenoid prostheses, humeral stem loosening is uncommon. According to a summary of 22 arthroplasty series published since 1980, humeral loosening occurred in only 4 of 1183 shoulders (0.3%) studied.[23] While the factors associated with humeral component failure include patient factors (young age, posttraumatic osteoarthritis, male gender) and the use of metal-backed glenoids,[22] no differences in failure rates between cemented and uncemented modern humeral components[24] have been noted.

Although a prerequisite for ATSA is an intact and functional rotator cuff, the integrity of the rotator cuff can change over time. The onset of rotator cuff dysfunction over time following ATSA has been termed secondary rotator cuff dysfunction. Young et al,[25] in a multicenter study examining 518 ATSAs performed for osteoarthritis with over 5-year follow-up, determined that the rate of survivorship free of secondary rotator cuff dysfunction was 100% at 5 years, 84% at 10 years, and 45% at 15 years. This is a common reason for revision of ATSA to RTSA.

It is possible that humeral component design may indirectly lead to glenoid failure due to nonanatomic prosthesis placement and improper soft tissue balance, resulting in edge loading as well as increased joint reaction forces. As a result, short and stemless humeral components are being evaluated for their ability to recreate humeral offset and restore COR while facilitating ease of revision surgery if required in the future.[24] Nonetheless, short stem and stemless humeral components represent the newest trends in ATSA design, and it remains to be seen if they have similar survivorship rates to standard length stems at longer-term follow-up.[26]

OUTCOME MEASURES

The remaining portion of this chapter will explore the clinical and radiographic results of ATSA prostheses and the factors that influence outcome. Some of the most common clinical metrics will be listed and briefly described, but a more in-depth analysis of these can be found in Chapter 27.

Patient-reported outcome measures (PROMs) that are often cited in the literature include the Simple Shoulder Test (SST), the American Shoulder and Elbow Surgeons (ASES) questionnaire, the Shoulder and Pain Disability Index (SPADI), the Oxford Shoulder Score (OSS), a pain Visual Analog Score (VAS), Single Assessment Numeric Evaluation (SANE), and Subjective Shoulder Value (SSV). These metrics utilize questions that are administered to the patient but do not have an examiner objective component. They are designed to allow a patient's clinical course to be longitudinally evaluated over time.

Other clinical metrics combine patient-reported measures and function with an examiner's objective findings such as ROM and strength. These include but are not limited to the University of California at Los Angeles (UCLA) score and the Constant score.

ROM assessment is an important metric that allows an objective comparison of outcomes. However, there is no standardized method for collecting ROM, so the variability of technique can influence direct comparison of outcome studies within the literature. In the future, digitized ROM assessment utilizing smart devices will likely impact the accuracy of these measurements in the clinical setting.

Other data collection tools that help to compare a cohort's improvement over time and also compare different cohorts within a single study as well as between studies are Health-Related Quality of Life (HRQOL) surveys. These include but are not limited to PROMIS-10, SF-36, SF-12, and VR-12. A more detailed explanation can also be found in Chapter 27.

MINIMAL CLINICALLY IMPORTANT DIFFERENCE AND SUBSTANTIAL CLINICAL BENEFIT

Historically, the clinical results of outcome studies have been reported by showing differences in means and recording statistical significance, generally shown as a *P*-value. Statistical significance denotes that a difference is not due to random chance. However, statistical significance does not equate to what a patient sees as a meaningful clinical change. One method to report whether or not a difference or improvement is clinically relevant to a patient is comparing it to the calculated minimal clinically important difference (MCID) or substantial clinical benefit (SCB) values. The concepts of MCID and SCB are explained in more detail in Chapter 27.

Values for MCID and SCB of common clinical metrics have previously been reported for ATSA **(TABLE 21.1)**.[27-29] Of note, studies by Simovitch et al[27,28] and Werner et al[29] both evaluated the MCID and SCB values for ASES after ATSA in distinct cohorts of patients and determined values that were nearly identical. MCID and SCB values after ATSA have been demonstrated to be higher than the values after RTSA. Furthermore, these values appear to be impacted by gender, length of follow-up, age at the time of surgery, and preoperative function.[27-29] MCID and SCB values can be used as additional means by which to evaluate clinical improvement following ATSA as opposed to solely statistical significance that can be influenced by a myriad of factors including sample size.

CLINICAL AND RADIOGRAPHIC RESULTS—STANDARD STEM ATSA

The majority of available clinical and radiographic data on ATSA pertains to a "standard" length modular humeral stem. As a result, it remains the most robustly studied in terms of clinical and radiographic results. For the purposes of the following discussion, we will consider the glenoid component in ATSA to be an all-polyethylene design unless otherwise stated.

Clinical Results of ATSA With Standard Stem

ATSA has been demonstrated to result in good to excellent clinical results in the context of implant survival with rates of 80% to 85% at 20 years as noted above.[17] Multiple series have documented statistically significant improvement in ROM, PROMs, and improved VAS pain scores in approximately 90% of patients or greater.[30-34] The authors reviewed a prospectively collected multicenter international database that utilizes a single-platform ATSA system with dual eccentricity (Equinoxe, Exactech, Gainesville, FL). After examining the results of 752 ATSAs with a minimum of 5-year follow-up (mean 87 ± 29 [SD] months), we determined a 94% satisfaction rate at the most recent follow-up. There was a statistically significant increase in ROM and PROMs (ASES, SST, Constant, UCLA, SPADI) scores as well as reduction in pain VAS scores from preoperative to postoperative time points. All-cause revision rate in this analysis was 5.6%.

Utilizing the same database percentage but applying the MCID and SCB value for metric analysis, Simovitch et al[28,29] noted that 92.7% of patients achieved MCID for ASES versus 79.5% achieving for SCB; 94.7% achieved MCID for the Constant score versus 84.9% achieving SCB; 90.8% achieved MCID for UCLA score versus 81.3% achieving SCB; 92% achieved MCID for SST score versus 81.7% achieving SCB; 91.5% achieved MCID for SPADI versus 73.4% achieving SCB; and 88.9% achieved MCID for pain VAS versus 71.6% achieving SCB. ROM was similar with 82.4% achieving MCID for active abduction versus 65.3% achieving SCB; 79.5% achieving MCID for active forward flexion

TABLE 21.1 Anatomic Total Shoulder Replacement Minimal Clinically Important Difference (MCID) and Substantial Clinical Benefit (SCB) Values for Common Metrics

Study	Metric	MCID	SCB
Simovitch et al,[27,28] 2018	ASES	17.0 ± 3.2	37.6 ± 2.6
	Constant	12.8 ± 2.5	25.4 ± 2.0
	UCLA	10.5 ± 0.8	15.0 ± 0.6
	SST	1.8 ± 0.4	3.7 ± 0.4
	SPADI	21.3 ± 3.5	48.3 ± 2.9
	Pain VAS	2.7 ± 1.4	3.8 ± 0.4
	Global function	1.7 ± 1.4	3.9 ± 0.3
	Abduction	13.9 ± 5.3	36.1 ± 4.3
	Flexion	23.1 ± 5.8	45.5 ± 4.6
	External rotation	14.5 ± 3.2	20.1 ± 2.5
Werner et al,[29] 2016	ASES	16.1 (5.4-26.7)[a]	37.4 (28.6-46.3)[a]

ASES, American Shoulder and Elbow Surgeons; SPADI, Shoulder and Pain Disability Index; SST, Simple Shoulder Test; UCLA, University of California at Los Angeles; VAS, Visual Analog Scale.
[a]95% confidence interval.

versus 62% achieving SCB; and 81.5% achieving MCID for active external rotation compared with 69.2% achieving SCB.

Radiographic Results of ATSA With Standard Stem

Radiographic evaluation of standard-stem humeral components has identified long-term humeral loosening rates to be as low as 0% for cemented prosthesis and as low as 1.5% for press-fit stems.[18,35-37] Despite this, the development of radiolucent lines and medial calcar osteolysis over time has been well documented. In uncemented press-fit standard-length stems, stress shielding of the medial calcar occurs as force is transferred distally to the metaphyseal/diaphyseal region of the humerus, leading to resorption of the bone in the unloaded proximal metaphyseal region. In contrast, osteolysis is also felt to occur through the generation of polyethylene wear particles from the glenoid, leading to bone resorption through a phagocytic response to these particles over time. A study by Verborgt et al[38] of 37 uncemented press-fit standard-length humeral components followed up over a mean of 9.2 years demonstrated radiolucency in 59%, with 14% demonstrating tilting not visualized on initial postoperative radiographs. Another study by Cole et al[39] evaluated 47 press-fit standard-length humeral stems utilized for ATSA with a minimum of 5-year follow-up and found a 43% rate of medial calcar osteolysis. The largest such study includes ATSA and HA, but similarly identified a 63% rate of stress shielding in uncemented stems and a 43% rate of proximal humeral osteolysis over a mean follow-up of 8.2 years.[40] Despite radiographic changes, an association between clinical metrics or ROM and the above radiographic findings has not been consistent and may be more related to glenoid component failure.[38-40] However, these radiographic changes reflect bone loss occurring and this deficiency can impact ease of revision surgery, need for bone grafting or bulk prostheses, and function after revision.

The rate of stress shielding likely differs with varying implant characteristics and technique of insertion. Stress shielding may be impacted by stem length, proximal coating, implant shape, absence of a collar, and the canal fill ratio. Nagels et al[41] examined a cohort of patients with and without stress shielding and noted that a higher canal filling ratio (ratio of stem width to the humeral intramedullary canal width) was associated with a higher rate of stress shielding. While the impact of humeral stress shielding on clinical results is not entirely understood, it is an undesirable result, potentially resulting in implant instability and complicated revisions because of bone loss.

Modularity in Current ATSA Designs

The humeral stem and head modular components work in tandem to reconstruct the humeral side of an ATSA. It is intuitive that a more anatomic reconstruction will result in improved clinical outcomes. Concerns that a humeral head component which fails to accurately reconstruct the COR and native offset will translate to poorer clinical outcomes have been evaluated in two case-control studies to date. Utilizing five radiographic parameters to obtain an Anatomic Reconstruction Index (ARI), Flurin et al[8] evaluated 49 ATSA patients with an average follow-up of 9.1 years. While the authors identified that more anatomic reconstructions trended toward better clinical results, the relatively low number of patients that were deemed to have a poor ARI ultimately limited the strength of their findings. In contrast, Chalmers et al[42] evaluated radiographic parameters in 95 patients with ATSA and a mean follow-up of 4.3 ± 1.7 years and found no statistical relationship with clinical outcomes in their series. While the bulk of literature pertains to the ability to achieve anatomic reconstruction in ATSA, there remains a paucity of literature regarding its effect on clinical outcomes.

SHORT STEM AND STEMLESS ATSA RESULTS

Due to concerns about stress shielding[43,44] as well as an effort to reduce blood loss,[45] decrease operative time,[45] limit instrumentation of the humeral intramedullary canal, and preserve bone if revision is needed, short stem and stemless humeral implants have been developed and are gaining in popularity. Early results are promising. Nonetheless, standard-length stems have performed well clinically with excellent long-term survivorship, so adoption of short stem and stemless components should proceed cautiously while long-term data are collected.

The clinical results of short stem and stemless ATSA have been favorable and similar to studies with standard-length stems. ATSA with these components has resulted in dramatic improvements of PROMs, pain, and ROM when utilized in patients with osteoarthritis.[46,47]

Finite Element Analysis of Short Stem and Stemless ATSA

Improvements in radiographic results are anticipated based on an expected reduction in stress shielding. Razfar et al[43] conducted a finite element analysis study examining proximal humeral bone stresses between stemless, short stem, and standard-length stem models. They noted that a reduction in stem length resulted in a progressive increase in proximal cortical stresses with the stemless model approximating the intact state of the proximal humerus. In addition, they found that stresses in the proximal trabecular bone increased with the use of a short stem or stemless device and that the stemless model demonstrated trabecular stresses that well exceeded the intact state. These findings, based on our understanding of bone remodeling, suggest that the frequency of stress shielding should decrease with short stem and stemless implants compared with their standard-length counterparts.

Radiographic Outcomes of Short Stem ATSA

The incidence of stress shielding has been examined in short stem humeral implants utilized for ATSA. Casagrande et al[48] reported a high rate of humeral bone adaptations with a first-generation short stem implant (Ascend Monolithic; Wright Medical, Memphis, TN, USA) in a cohort of 73 patients including calcar osteolysis (17%), radiolucency (71%), and condensation lines (19%). They determined that 10% of the stems were loose and 9% were "at risk"; ultimately, 12% were revised due to aseptic loosening. Another study utilizing the same prosthesis reported a high rate of humeral bone adaptations (52%). However, a subsequent study by Schnetzke et al[46] examined a cohort of patients undergoing ATSA with a second-generation short stem (Ascend Flex, Wright Medical, Memphis, TN, USA) modified to have a proximal plasma spray and different geometry, and this yielded a lower rate of bone adaptations (29%) and no stem loosening. Another study by Morwood et al[49] compared the first-generation Ascend Monolithic (Wright Medical, Memphis, TN, USA) with the second-generation Ascend Flex (Wright Medical, Memphis, TN, USA) and noted a dramatic reduction in humeral stem radiolucencies and stems at risk for loosening. A separate study that examined a cohort of patients with the Ascend Monolithic (Wright Medical, Memphis, TN, USA) and Ascend Flex (Wright Medical, Memphis, TN, USA) compared to a cohort with an Apex short stem (Arthrex, Naples, FL, USA) demonstrated that despite a higher filling ratio, the Apex (Arthrex, Naples, FL, USA) had a significantly lower rate of bone adaptations. These studies indicate that no one design or patient factor controls the propensity for stress shielding and bone adaptations. Rather it is a complex interplay of design parameters, patient anatomy, and implantation techniques. Multiple short stems have entered the market, many of which have been designed to maximize the ability to avoid stress shielding.

Radiographic Results of Stemless ATSA

Experience with stemless ATSA devices has more closely followed the predictions of bone adaptation according to the finite element analysis by Razfar et al.[43] Multiple studies with midterm and long-term follow-up have demonstrated a humeral lucency rate between 0% and 2.3% with the absence of signs of stress shielding or osteolysis.[47,50,51] These components hold promise to dramatically reduce bone adaptations and have demonstrated robust clinical improvement similar to ATSA with standard humeral stems. One concern voiced about stemless humeral components in ATSA is potentially their inability to recreate the patient's normal anatomy because of a lack of eccentricity. However, a radiographic study by Gallacher et al[52] demonstrated that a stemless device was able to recreate the humeral head size within 2 mm of normal anatomy and the COR within 3 mm of normal anatomy in 76% of the studied patients. Furthermore, in this series, the incidence of radiolucent lines was only 2.6%.

CLINICAL AND RADIOGRAPHIC RESULTS—GLENOID PROSTHESES

While the design of cemented all-polyethylene peg and keel glenoid components has evolved to include convex-backed components and partially cemented designs to achieve central peg or cage bony ingrowth, the clinical superiority of these designs continue to be debated. Radiographically, though, they show favorable results.

Polyethylene Keel Versus Peg Design

Keeled and pegged implants have primarily been compared by rates of radiolucent line formation at the bone/cement interface. Early concerns resulted from studies demonstrating high rates of radiolucent lines on the immediate postoperative radiographs of keeled designs (compared with pegged designs)[53] and were further supported by randomized controlled trials with follow-up radiographs at 2 years.[54,55] It remains unclear if the presence of immediate or the later development of radiolucencies translates into negative outcomes or clinical failure. In fact, overall survival rates for cemented keeled glenoid components have been favorable, with implant survival of 95% at 10 years and 92% at 15 years averaged across all keeled designs.[18] The long-term data for pegged implants are less robust, with the longest series reported by McLendon et al[56] demonstrating comparable survivorship (time to revision) of pegged compared with keeled implants at a mean 5-year follow-up.[18] However, this cohort of pegged polyethylene components demonstrated survival free of radiographic failure of 92% at 5 years and only 43% at 10 years. It is important to note that this study evaluated the Cofield 2 pegged prosthesis (Smith and Nephew), whose three inline peg configurations differ from more modern designs utilizing peripheral pegs placed in a nonlinear configuration. Aside from concerns for radiolucency, keeled components require more contiguous bone removal for implantation and hence may complicate revision compared with the standard nonlinear peripheral pegs in modern all-polyethylene glenoid implants.

Polyethylene Hybrid Glenoid

Pegged glenoid components have seen a more recent evolution toward a "biologic hybrid" design. In this design, a central peg or cage has an interface for bony ingrowth, with three smaller peripheral cemented pegs used to achieve initial stability. The proposed method of bone ingrowth for some implants that utilize a polyethylene three-dimensional surface for ingrowth is unclear, though others utilize porous three-dimensional tantalum or titanium surfaces with grit blast or plasma spray that encourages bone fixation. Regardless of specific hybrid design, short- to medium-term radiographic studies have been favorable. For example, radiographic follow-up across multiple designs has demonstrated bone ingrowth around the central peg to be between 68% and 91%, with osteolysis around the central peg to range from 7% to 25% in short- to medium-term follow-up.[53,57,58] A recent study by Friedman et al[59] compared a hybrid polyethylene glenoid with a central titanium grit blast cage and an all-polyethylene pegged glenoid component in age, gender, and length of follow-up matched study **(FIGURE 21.1)**. They found that the caged hybrid glenoid had significantly less ($P < 0.05$) radiolucent glenoid lines (9% vs 38%), aseptic glenoid loosening (1.3% vs 3.8%), glenoid revision (2.5% vs 6.9%), and associated radiolucent humeral lines (3% vs 9.1%).[59] Biologic fixation with hybrid components may result in improved glenoid survivorship.

In contrast to the robustness of radiographic studies, there is a paucity of clinical studies comparing keeled, pegged, and hybrid cemented components. The published survivorship data that exist do not demonstrate clinical superiority of any one design across comparable timeframes.[23] With the outcomes of the majority of modern generation implants being limited to medium-term follow-up, longer-term follow-up of modern cemented polyethylene and hybrid biologic designs is required to truly compare the clinical outcomes of the two designs. There is evidence that the overall risk of glenoid component failure is higher in male patients as well as in ATSA performed for posttraumatic osteoarthritis or osteonecrosis.[18]

Posterior Augmented Polyethylene Glenoid Implants

ATSA is predominantly performed in patients with Walch type A and B glenoids.[60] Given that the humeral head remains centered and glenoid retroversion changes and deformity are minimal with type A1, A2, and B1 glenoids, glenoid reconstruction is relatively straightforward and easily managed with standard glenoid implants. However, management of B2 glenoids (biconcave glenoid with posterior rim erosion and retroverted glenoid) as well as B3 glenoids (monoconcave and posterior wear with retroversion >15° or posterior humeral head subluxation >70% or both) poses particular challenges. Historically, eccentric reaming of the high side (anterior) of the glenoid or posterior bone grafting has been utilized but with the risks of vault narrowing, perforation, removal of subchondral bone support, medialization of the joint line, and complications relating to bone graft resorption or hardware loosening. This has led to the recent emergence of augmented polyethylene glenoid components for ATSA with the goal of restoring the joint line, restoring rotator cuff tension, correcting version, and recentering the humeral head in B2 and B3 glenoids by using an asymmetric polyethylene.

Posteriorly augmented polyethylene glenoids can be divided into full wedge, half wedge, and stepped polyethylene components.

Each design of posteriorly augmented polyethylene implants for ATSA aims to restore the joint line and recenter the humeral head while minimizing reaming and bone removal. However, the surgical preparation for each implant design is very different. A study by Knowles et al[61] evaluated all three designs with computational modeling and determined that in cases of B2 glenoids, the full wedge design removed a statistically significant less amount of bone than the half wedge design and the half wedge design removed a statistically significant less amount of bone than a stepped design. Thus, if the goal of bone preservation is prioritized, full wedge components are preferred.

Concerns about the use of posteriorly augmented glenoid components focus on the ability to provide favorable clinical and radiographic results as well as restore the humeral head to a centered position from a posteriorly subluxed position. Short-term clinical results of posteriorly augmented glenoid components, regardless of design, appear to be successful with low revision rates, but long-term survival rates are unknown and will need to be studied.[4,62-66] One study by Grey et al[66] evaluated a full wedge posterior augmented design with a minimum follow-up of 2 years but average follow-up of 4 years and noted that although the humeral head was posteriorly subluxated an average of 73% for each Walch B glenoid type preoperatively, all humeral heads were recentered at latest follow-up. Ho et al[67] evaluated the results of a stepped design and noted that 85% of the humeral heads were posteriorly subluxated prior to surgery while 85% of the humeral heads were centered postoperatively with 2-year minimum follow-up and a mean follow-up of 2.4 years. Future studies will evaluate if humeral head centering is maintained and if there is any impact on glenoid component lucency or loosening perhaps due to muscle forces and potential rim loading. However, radiographic results have been favorable with short- to midterm follow-up.

IMPACT OF AGE, GENDER, AND LENGTH OF FOLLOW-UP ON ATSA OUTCOMES

The clinical results of ATSA can be influenced by many patient factors outside of the control of the surgeon. It is important to understand the effect of each of these factors in order to educate patients regarding their expectations. Satisfaction after ATSA is ultimately predicated on patients surpassing their expectations for improvement.

Impact of Age at the Time of ATSA

A surge in demand for shoulder arthroplasty in patients younger than 55 years is projected to be on the order of 330% from 2011 to 2030,[68] thus codifying the importance of understanding the impact of a reduction in age at the time of surgery on short-term, midterm, and long-term outcomes. One concern about ATSA in young patients is a potentially heightened activity level which could have an impact on survivorship. Another concern is that young patients may not achieve as high satisfaction rates after surgery compared to their older counterparts. In fact, a systematic review published by Roberson et al[69] reviewed six pertinent studies in the literature and determined 10-year and 20-year survivorship rates of between 60% and 80% for ATSA in patients younger than 65 years. These survivorship rates compare unfavorably with the overall ATSA implant survivorship which is 93% to 97% at 10 years and 80% to 85% at 20 years. Clinical results were generally satisfactory but not excellent, reinforcing the concern that younger patients may not be as satisfied as older ATSA patients. One explanation for these findings may be the more severe pathology encountered in the younger population. Saltzman et al[70] compared a cohort of patients undergoing ATSA under the age of 50 years to a cohort above the age of 50 years and noted that the younger cohort had a complex diagnosis 74% of the time while the older cohort had a complex diagnosis 34% of the time. Thus, younger patients should be counseled regarding concerns for survivorship and clinical outcomes. Aligning expectations may actually improve their satisfaction.

In general, we prefer to postpone ATSA as long as possible to decrease the potential risk of mechanical failure of the implant, taking into account ongoing glenoid erosion and its impact on later glenoid reconstruction results. However, a clinician should also recognize when nonoperative modalities have been maximized or, as in severe glenohumeral arthritis, are unlikely to provide much benefit. In such instances, it is prudent to carefully and clearly explain and document treatment options, but not withhold treatment based on age alone, should all other options be exhausted.

Impact of Gender at the Time of Surgery

Although previous studies have reported that males and females have different expectations following ATSA, they both have similarly robust clinical improvement and satisfaction levels. A study by Jawa et al[71] noted that males more often value a return to sport while females more often value the ability to maintain their daily routine. Both males and females prioritize the ability to sleep throughout the night. Two previous studies also evaluated MCID and SCB values[27,28] for seven common shoulder outcome metrics as well as ROM and noted that females generally had lower values than their male counterparts meaning that smaller preoperative to postoperative improvements resulted in clinically meaningful improvements.

Impact of Length of Follow-Up on Outcomes After ATSA

It is important to clearly explain to patients what their expectations should be after surgery. Identifying the rate of expected improvement and return of function can help them plan appropriately and also improve ultimate satisfaction. Simovitch et al[72] determined that over 95% of patients reported clinical improvement in five common clinical metrics (ASES, SPADI, SST, Constant, and UCLA) by 6 months after the surgical procedures and maximum improvement was attained by approximately 24 months. ROM follows a similar trend. However, at approximately 72 months, there was a progressive decrease in magnitude of improvement for active abduction and flexion which was not identified for the clinical metrics. This may represent a generalized aging and deconditioning process or the onset of secondary rotator cuff dysfunction and will need to be further evaluated.

RETURN TO WORK AFTER ATSA

Return to work after ATSA is an aspect of shoulder arthroplasty that must be tailored to the individual patient. Timing of return to work as well as in what capacity is dependent on the type of vocation, patient characteristics, and the ability to return at modified capacity for limited or extended periods of time. Patients should be realistically counseled prior to surgery regarding the postoperative recovery and the postoperative restrictions and limitations once maximal clinical gains have been achieved.

A systematic review of seven studies by Steinhaus et al[73] suggests that the average return to work rate following ATSA is 63.4%.[73] They found that return to work was significantly lower in heavy-intensity occupations when compared with all intensity types (61.7% vs 67.6%, $P = 0.04$), but was not associated with the underlying diagnosis. Most patients were able to return to work in some capacity at an average of 2.3 months postoperatively.[73] One retrospective review focusing specifically on patients 55 years of age or younger found that 92% were able to return to work within 3 years (although only 64% returned to heavy tasks) at an average of 2.1 months postoperatively.[74]

Patients who undergo ATSA as a result of a Workers' Compensation claim pose additional challenges compared with patients who are not part of a Workers' Compensation claim. In general, shoulder surgery in this population is associated with lower return to work rates and lower patient surgical satisfaction rates when compared with those without active Workers' Compensation claims.[75] The reasons behind this are numerous and are likely multifactorial, but may include dissatisfaction with the place of work, dissatisfaction with Workers' Compensation processes, depression following injury, lack of transferable skills, more likely to be involved in manual labor tasks, younger age, and male gender.[75]

Interestingly, a meta-analysis by Steinhaus et al,[73] which reviewed the available literature, did not demonstrate lower return to work rates in this population when compared with non–Workers' Compensation claims.[73] However, a study by Cvetanovich et al[76] did determine that shoulder arthroplasty performed for Workers' Compensation claims resulted in a significantly higher reoperation rate as well as pain level and lower outcome scores such as ASES and SST scores. In this population, establishing clear postoperative goals prior to surgery and including return to work as part of the postoperative rehabilitation program help facilitate recovery. Preoperative worker buy-in with this approach, as well as a clear return to work plan, is thought to offer the best chance of returning these patients to some semblance of their preoperative tasks.

RETURN TO SPORT AFTER ATSA

Certain aspects of return to sport mimic those of return to work. Restrictions following ATSA are few, although patients may be counseled against intense upper extremity bearing exercises in the hopes of decreasing prosthesis wear under extreme conditions. Discussing the timing of return to sport is particularly important to patients, as some may choose to work around seasonal sports and activities in order to avoid missing out.

Available literature suggests that patients who were able to participate in sports within 5 years of an ATSA will likely return to sports postoperatively.[77] A systematic review by Liu et al[78] identified that the overall rate of return to sport at an equivalent or improved level of play within 36 months of undergoing ATSA was 92.6%. The most common sports included swimming, golf, fitness, and tennis.[78]

Based on the above data as well as personal experience, we inform patients who are interested in resuming athletics postoperatively that they have a high probability of doing so, although the overall trajectory of recovery may influence the timing of return.

SPECIAL CONSIDERATIONS

Posttraumatic Arthritis

Fractures of the proximal humerus and glenoid can lead to the development of accelerated degeneration of the glenohumeral joint. The location and severity of these fractures ultimately determines if an ATSA would be indicated. Complex proximal humeral fractures or those with significant glenoid bony deformities are most commonly managed with RTSA. As a result of the increasing utilization of RTSA, indications for ATSA for posttraumatic arthritis are narrowing, but ATSA can be effectively utilized in the correct circumstances. For example, Boileau et al[79] devised a radiographic classification of posttraumatic arthritis following proximal humerus fractures. They classified type 1 injuries to be

impacted fractures with humeral head collapse or necrosis; type 2 injures to be irreducible dislocations with or without fractures; type 3 injuries as nonunions of the surgical neck; and type 4 injuries to be severe tuberosity malunions. Their analysis suggests that ATSA can result in good outcomes for type 1 and type 2 fracture sequelae. A subsequent study by Audige et al[80] of 111 consecutive patients with posttraumatic arthritis treated with arthroplasty found that maximal gains occurred by 24 months, with type 1 fracture patterns having the best ROM gains following ATSA. This study is in keeping with previously published literature that suggested ATSA following type 2 fracture sequela patterns failed to achieve results similar to patients undergoing ATSA for osteoarthritis.[80]

There is scant literature on utilizing ATSA for posttraumatic arthritis following glenoid fractures since for most of these cases RTSA is preferred because of associated glenohumeral instability. Although open reduction internal fixation of the glenoid fracture with ATSA can be considered, practice trends suggest increasing utilization of RTSA for this indication.

For posttraumatic arthritis, preoperative stiffness and compromised function negatively correlate with maximal achievable outcomes following ATSA.[81] Thus, it is important to counsel these patients that their outcomes are not expected to achieve those attainable for other indications. ATSA for this diagnosis should be explained as a pain mitigating procedure with limited ability to improve ROM and function.

ATSA for Postcapsulorrhaphy Arthropathy or Instability

The patient with arthritis due to prior instability or instability surgery is more typically younger and more commonly male than the baseline ATSA population.[17] Osteoarthritis resulting as a sequela of recurrent instability or attempts at stabilization via capsulorrhaphy or nonanatomic procedures creates unique reconstructive challenges. Adhesions from postsurgical scaring and often underappreciated glenoid erosions require extensive soft tissue releases, eccentric reaming/glenoid augments, and meticulous soft tissue balancing with the added challenge that the subscapularis (SSC) is often deficient or poorly functioning. With this in mind, it is not surprising that the results of ATSA in this population are inferior to the cohort of patients that undergo ATSA for primary arthritis.

A recent systematic review by Cerciello et al[82] analyzed the results of 13 studies, which included 365 patients with an average of 53.4 months follow-up who underwent total shoulder arthroplasty (TSA) for anterior instability arthropathy. Although the authors reported significant increases in Constant (35.6-72.7) and ASES (35.7-77) scores, the overall complication rate was surprisingly high at 25.7%. Radiolucent lines were identified on 12.4% of humerus and 22.7% of glenoids on most recent radiographs. The reoperation rate in this population was 18.5%, a rate that was lower following RTSA than ATSA. These findings suggest that TSA for postcapsulorrhaphy arthropathy is a complex that is associated with a higher rate of reoperation and unsatisfactory outcomes. There is emerging evidence that suggests RTSA may be superior to ATSA for this unique population. In fact, a study by Cuff et al[83] showed similar clinical results after either ATSA or RTSA for postcapsulorrhaphy arthropathy. However, compared with the RTSA cohort, the ATSA cohort had a lower percentage of patients satisfied (84% vs 95%), a higher complication rate (21% vs 10%), and a higher revision rate (16% vs 0%). Future research may be directed at determining demographic or radiographic features predictive of success of ATSA over RTSA.

Osteoarthritis With Rotator Cuff Tear and Concurrent Repair

Although an irreparable or functionally deficient rotator cuff is a contraindication for ATSA, management of osteoarthritis with a small high-grade partial- or full-thickness RCT identified intraoperatively remains controversial. Advancing age and comorbid conditions may result in a decision to convert to an RTSA intraoperatively after recognizing a concomitant RCT. In instances where ATSA proceeds with a concomitant rotator cuff repair, the available literature suggests an overall acceptable clinical result though poorer than the population without RTC.

Studies regarding this topic are limited to small retrospective studies with short-term follow-up. For example, Livesey et al[84] analyzed 45 ATSA patients (22 high-grade partial-thickness and 23 full-thickness tears) with a minimum of 2-year follow-up by retrospective chart review. About 31% of their patients had a poor clinical result, with 18% of patients requiring revision during this short-term follow-up. Although all tears were deemed to be repairable, the authors found that a preoperative acromiohumeral distance less than 8 mm was predictive of a rotator cuff–related reoperation after ATSA. Simone et al[85] found that only 4.8% of 932 patients undergoing ATSA underwent concurrent rotator cuff repair in their sample. Of the 33 patients with ATSA and concomitant RCT repair available for analysis (follow-up 3 months to 13 years; mean 4.7 years), 6 developed radiographic evidence of instability and complications were noted in 5 patients (all of which had medium- to large-sized tears). And 12% of the sample required additional surgery. The authors concluded that in older and less active patients and those with larger tears, RTSA is the preferred procedure.

Surgeons should use judgment when assessing patients with osteoarthritis and concomitant RCTs. Although practice trends suggest increasing utilization of RTSA for RCTs with arthritis, variability in tear chronicity, morphology, and proximal migration of the humeral head must be weighed alongside patient age and activity requirements.[13] The ability to convert from an ATSA to an RTSA intraoperatively can be valuable, and we recommend that surgeons maintain this flexibility when an RCT is identified so that clinical judgment and not implant availability dictates arthroplasty choice.

Parkinson Disease and Other Related Neurologic Diagnoses

Parkinson disease (PD), along with related disorders to the neurologic system, deserves specific mention when discussing any form of shoulder arthroplasty. PD has been demonstrated to significantly increase the risk of nearly all forms of negative outcomes following ATSA.[86] While clinical outcomes following ATSA in those with neurologic conditions like PD have been mixed,[87-89] most studies suggest an acceptable reduction in pain but with poor functional results when compared to ATSA performed in non–Parkinson populations. The overall increase in perioperative and long-term complications warrants careful consideration before electing to perform an ATSA in the setting of PD. A study by Burrus et al[90] examined a large matched cohort of 3390 ATSAs in patients with PD matched to 47,034 ATSA controls. The authors found that PD was associated with a 1.5 greater odds of infection, 2.5 greater odds of dislocation, 1.7 greater odds of revision, 1.4 greater odds of systemic complications, 1.5 greater odds of fracture, and 1.5 greater odds of component loosening following ATSA when compared with those without a diagnosis of PD.

Inflammatory Arthritis

The most common type of inflammatory arthritis encountered in practice is rheumatoid arthritis (RA). There is a wide range of severity of this disease process, and the development of biologics and disease-modifying treatments has drastically changed the severity of disease encountered and the frequency that TSA is necessary. The inflammatory process also affects the periarticular soft tissues which increases the prevalence of rotator cuff insufficiency, leading to less predictable results following ATSA than for primary glenohumeral osteoarthritis.[17]

Historically, the management of RA only included HA and ATSA. Barlow et al[91] demonstrated that both HA and ATSA resulted in improved pain relief in the context of rotator cuff compromise. However, ATSA had superior improvements in pain, active abduction, and lower revision rates when compared with HA in RA patients. Lapner et al[92] later demonstrated no significant difference in implant survivorship when comparing HA with TSA for the management of RA in a large sample of 5777 patients.

Given concerns over the bone quality and soft tissue integrity, surgeons are increasingly utilizing RTSA to manage inflammatory arthritis in the United States and abroad.[13] Although early results have been promising, concern exists for intraoperative and postoperative complication rates that are higher than RTSA performed for other conditions.[93-95]

PREDICTORS OF CLINICAL SUCCESS

Factors Associated With Success or Failure of ATSA

While it can be expected that at least 90% of patients undergoing ATSA will be satisfied with the results, an understanding of the factors related to the success or failure of this procedure can help inform patient selection and guide both patient and surgeon expectations.[17]

A summary of the factors associated with failure of ATSA is listed in **TABLE 21.2**.[96,97] Although attempts have been made to predict postoperative outcomes following ATSA,[98] no robust scoring tool exists to quantify satisfaction with key patient-important outcomes prior to undertaking surgery to help guide preoperative decision-making. However, machine learning (ML) will likely play a role in the future.[99] Surgeons should be aware of these factors to help guide preoperative decisions and postoperative expectations, but not employ them as contraindications to ATSA in isolation.

The potential association between increasing number of medical comorbidities and negative outcomes

following ATSA should be considered prior to indicating a patient for surgery. It remains debatable if the number of medical comorbidities, often represented by a comorbidity index in large databases, has an independent association with ATSA outcomes. For example, an analysis of the National Surgical Quality Improvement Program (NSQIP) found that the Charlson Comorbidity Index had no greater association with adverse events following TSA than age or American Society of Anesthesiologist (ASA) classification alone.[100] In contrast, Holzgrefe et al[101] found that frailty (as identified with a five-item modified frailty index) predicted reoperation, readmission, postoperative complications, and increased hospital length of stay following ATSA. Thus, it is intuitive that increasing patient medical complexity translates into negative outcomes following ATSA to some degree, although how these factors interact together or with other nonmedical predictors of failure remains to be evaluated.

It should also be recognized that increased surgeon and institutional volume of ATSA has routinely been demonstrated to result in decreased complications and improved outcomes.[100] In the United States, a sample of Medical Provider Utilization and Payment Databases suggested that only 44.3% of surgeons who performed at least 1 TSA during the 3-year sample period performed 10 or more TSAs per year. Additionally, only 31.3% of surgeons performing TSA procedures were recognized as having subspecialty fellowship training in shoulder and elbow surgery.[102] Although minimum institutional and/or surgeon volume remains unclear, current literature suggests at least 15 TSAs per year are needed to optimize patient outcomes and decrease costs through economies of scale.[103]

Mental Health Diagnoses

Concomitant psychological diagnoses can impact results following ATSA. Although psychological diagnoses such as depression have been clearly linked to reduced clinical improvement following TSA,[104] these patients still realize clinical and functional benefits following surgery.

A review of the United Sates Nationwide Inpatient Sample (NIS) by Mollon et al[105] suggested that 12.4% of the 224,060 elective TSAs performed between 2002 and 2012 had a concomitant diagnosis of depression. The presence of depression was more frequent in low-income and in Medicaid-insured patients and was twice as common in women than in men (16.0% vs 8.0%). Depression was an independent risk factor for postoperative delirium, infection, and hospital discharge to a location other than home. A subsequent single-site prospective study evaluated the impact of depression, anxiety, schizophrenia, or bipolar disorder on outcomes following TSA. They identified mental health diagnoses in 37.5% (105/208) of their sample and did not find a significant difference in complication rates or outcomes in patients with and without mental health diagnoses.[106]

TABLE 21.2 Literature-Supported Factors Associated With Negative Outcomes Following Anatomic Total Shoulder Arthroplasty

Patient Factors
Diabetes
Female gender
Younger age
Inflammatory arthropathy
Prior substance/narcotic abuse
Mental health diagnoses
Parkinson disease/neurologic diagnoses
Medical frailty
Shoulder Factors
Previous surgery
Torn rotator cuff
Nondominant arm
Posttrauma/postfracture
Institutional Factors
Low surgeon volume
Low institutional volume

Despite the mixed results in the literature, the identification of mental health diagnoses should prompt preoperative optimization the same way that medical diagnoses do, with the ultimate goal of achieving the best possible TSA results in those indicated for the procedure.

The concept of resilience as a psychological/psychometric property is a noteworthy area of emerging research. Defined as the ability to recover from stress, resiliency may represent a bridge in the understanding of how psychology impacts both self-reported and physical outcomes following surgery. Most commonly quantified by the Brief Resilience Scale (BRS), patients identified as having low resilience have been associated with negative outcomes following other forms of orthopedic surgery.[107-110] Tokish et al[110] documented the BRS score in 70 patients undergoing all types of TSA and found that those classified as having low resilience had outcome scores 30 to 40 points lower across ASES, Penn, and SANE scores when compared with those identified as having high resilience. The concept of resiliency, its association with factors predictive of outcomes, and how it may be used to prognosticate results and improve outcomes following ATSA require further study.

Preoperative Opioid Use

Pain relief remains the primary reason that patients choose to undergo any form of shoulder arthroplasty. Although many patients have managed pain for an intermediate length of time, others have struggled with the physical and psychological effects of chronic pain. In the context of the global opioid crisis, more than 50% of patients have been reported to have had their pain managed with chronic opioid medications.[111,112] Preoperative narcotic medication use has been consistently shown to predict higher perioperative opioid consumption and higher VAS scores following surgery.[111-115] The association with hospital stay, perioperative complications, and readmission rates has been mixed across different series.[111,113,116] Due to higher opioid consumption and VAS pain scores, some have recommended that chronic pain patients should be weaned from their chronic opioids prior to surgery. Furthermore, regional anesthesia can be very helpful.

POSTOPERATIVE COMPLICATIONS

Complications that develop following ATSA can be categorized as intraoperative and postoperative. Postoperative complications can be further divided into surgical and medical. A review of 33 studies including 3360 ATSAs from 2006 to 2015 identified the most common surgical complications as component loosening (4%), instability (1%), RCT (0.9%), periprosthetic fracture (0.69%), neural injury (0.63%), infection (0.51%), hematoma (0.09%), deltoid injury (0.03%), and deep vein thrombosis (0.03%).[117] Based on this review, the overall surgical complication rate was 10%.

Glenoid Loosening

Glenoid component implantation for ATSA has historically relied on cement for fixation. The cement/component and cement/bone interfaces ultimately fail over time largely due to aseptic loosening. Recent implants have been developed to incorporate biologic fixation in the hope that radiolucency and aseptic loosening will dramatically decrease. Historically, glenoid loosening, whether or not it is symptomatic, has been expected to occur over the lifetime of an ATSA. One systematic review of the literature estimated that symptomatic glenoid loosening occurred at a rate of 1.2% per year and surgical revision occurred at a rate of 0.8% per year.[118] Previous studies have shown favorable results of pegged polyethylene and keeled components.[119] Hybrid components will continue to be evaluated and time will determine whether they represent an improvement.

Humeral Loosening

Though bony adaptations, especially after press-fit humeral stem implantation for ATSA is common, humeral component loosening is a rare occurrence. A systematic review of 3360 ATSAs demonstrated an incidence of 0.2%.[117] Most cases of aseptic humeral loosening are due to glenoid component wear or failure with polyethylene debris resulting in osteolysis around the stem.[40]

Instability

Shoulder instability following ATSA represents the spectrum from subluxation to frank dislocation.[120] The etiology of instability may relate to failure to adequately balance the shoulder intraoperatively, component loosening with bony erosions, or rotator cuff failure. Bohsali et al[117] performed a systematic analysis of the literature and determined the rate of instability after ATSA to be 1%.

Infection

Infection after ATSA has been reported with an incidence between 0.4% and 2.9%.[121] A deep infection is particularly troublesome as it often challenges implant retention and requires a one- or two-staged revision. Even with adequate treatment, a deep infection results in dissatisfaction.[122] A review of the Mayo Clinic Medical Center Total Joint Registry[123] including 2588 primary ATSAs demonstrated an infection incidence of 1.8%. Of the potential infections identified, 76% were confirmed deep periprosthetic joint infections (PJIs). Most of the deep infections were caused by *Staphylococcus* and *Propionobacterium* (*Cutibacterium*) *acnes*. The authors estimated time of survival free of deep PJI and found 5-, 10-, and 15-year rates of 99.3%, 98.5%, and 97.2%, respectively.

Subscapularis Failure

Multiple techniques are utilized to repair the SSC tendon during ATSA including a tendon peel, tenotomy, and lesser tuberosity osteotomy (LTO). A systematic review by Schrock et al[124] noted a higher load to failure for LTO compared to soft tissue repairs but no difference in cyclic displacement. Clinically, these three repair techniques seem comparable.

SSC insufficiency has been reported to occur in between 0% and 6% of patients.[125] Despite this incidence, several studies report a low incidence of reoperation that ranges from 0.3% to 3%[25,126] for SSC deficiency. These reoperations were predominantly necessary to treat anterior instability. SSC deficiency has been associated with poor tissue quality, oversizing of implants (overstuffing), technique of repair, lack of compliance, overly aggressive or premature therapy, and trauma.[125]

Secondary Rotator Cuff Dysfunction

Most patients undergoing ATSA will have an intact rotator cuff at the time of surgery. However, over time, ATSA patients can develop signs of rotator cuff insufficiency after, presenting with weakness, instability, or radiographic changes including cephalad migration of the prosthetic humeral head. Historically, this was seen in patients with RA who have a compromised soft tissue envelope inherent to the disease process. However, with the increased popularity of RTSA in the treatment of inflammatory arthritis, secondary rotator cuff dysfunction has become a problem encountered predominantly in ATSA performed for osteoarthritis. Secondary rotator cuff dysfunction can be described as the onset of rotator cuff tearing or functional deficiency subsequent to ATSA overt time. Young et al,[25] in a multicenter study examining 518 ATSAs performed for osteoarthritis with over 5-year follow-up, determined that the rate of survivorship free of secondary rotator cuff dysfunction was 100% at 5 years, 84% at 10 years, and 45% at 15 years. They determined secondary rotator cuff dysfunction by evaluating x-rays for superior head migration. The authors noted significantly worse clinical and radiographic outcomes in patients with secondary rotator cuff dysfunction. They also noted that implantation of the glenoid polyethylene component with a superior tilt and fatty infiltration of the infraspinatus muscle were risk factors for the development of secondary rotator cuff dysfunction.

Periprosthetic Fractures

Periprosthetic fractures can occur intraoperatively or postoperatively. A review of the Mayo Clinic Medical Center database[127] revealed that 2.8% of ATSAs were complicated by periprosthetic fractures. Of these fractures, 65% occurred intraoperatively and 35% postoperatively. Women had a higher risk of fracture than men and patients with the diagnosis of posttraumatic arthritis had a significantly higher risk of a periprosthetic fracture than other diagnoses. In addition, a higher burden of comorbidities as assessed by the Deyo-Charlson index was significantly associated with the occurrence of a periprosthetic fracture.

Neurologic Lesions

Neurologic injury during ATSA has been reported to occur with an incidence between 1% and 4.3%. These injuries include axillary nerve neurapraxias as well as brachial plexopathies. Despite this relatively low incidence, a study by Nagda et al[128] utilizing intraoperative nerve monitoring reported a nerve disturbance in up to 57% of patients undergoing ATSA. In this light, it may be due to human physiologic resiliency that we do not encounter a higher frequency of more severe or permanent neurologic impairments in the clinical setting. Interestingly, a study by Ladermann et al[129] examined ATSA patients prior to and following ATSA. They noted that 57% of the 23 patients studied demonstrated a preoperative nerve deficit based on electromyography. This was most commonly carpal tunnel syndrome followed by cervical radiculopathy and cubital tunnel syndrome. A careful neurologic examination of a patient's upper extremity is important to evaluate for and document any clinically relevant preoperative neurologic deficits.

Stiffness

Stiffness following ATSA likely represents an underreported complication. An aggregate of case series published since 1980 analyzed 1183 shoulder arthroplasties and identified only 1 (0.1%) arthroplasty classified as having isolated stiffness as a complication.[120] Our experience suggests that dissatisfied patients following ATSA often have some degree of postoperative stiffness but this may not be reported as a complication. A review of 4063 complications reported to the FDA database[130] from 2012 to 2016 identified pain/stiffness in 12.9% of cases, but did not separate the two symptoms. Although there are multiple factors that can contribute to stiffness following ATSA, one must be vigilant to recognize an indolent infection with *Cutibacterium acnes*, as this type of infection can present solely as pain and stiffness.

Medical Complications

Due to the relatively low incidence of medical complications following ATSA in distinction to the high volume of ATSAs performed, it is difficult to assess the incidence of complications in small studies. Therefore, analyses of larger databases are helpful. Anakwenze et al[131] examined the weighted NIS from 2006 to 2013 and determined the frequency of medical complications after TSA in 125,776 patients was 6.7%. The most common complications were respiratory (2.9%), renal (0.8%), and cardiac (0.8%). Pulmonary disorders and fluid and electrolyte disorders were the most common postoperative complications. Waterman et al[132] analyzed 2004 primary TSA patients in the NSQIP database recorded between 2006 and 2011 and documented a medical complication rate of 3.64%. They found that peripheral vascular disease and operative time over 174 minutes were associated with a statistically significant increase in complications. Thus, we report the risk of a medical complication to our patients undergoing ATSA as between 3% and 7%.

The overall postoperative mortality of hospitalized patients following TSA in the Anakwenze et al[131] study using the NIS database was 0.07%. Waterman et al[132] examined the 30-day mortality rate after primary TSA in 2004 patients recorded in the NSQIP database and noted it to be 0.25%. The primary risk factors for 30-day mortality were cardiac disease and increasing chronologic age.

More recently, as payers have begun to look closely at value and pay for performance, there has been a focus on 30- and 90-day readmission rates. Chung et al[133] examined the National Readmission Database including all patients who underwent an elective primary TSA in 2014 and noted the 30-, 60-, and 90-day readmission rates were 0.6%, 1.2%, and 1.7%, respectively. Medicare payer status, utilization of a skilled nursing facility, and chronic obstructive pulmonary disease were noted to be predictors of 90-day readmission.

RESULTS OF OUTPATIENT ATSA

Health care systems around the world are exploring ways to deliver efficient, cost-effective, and safe health care. In orthopedics, the value-driven health care movement is evolving into bundled-care and pay-for-performance programs that are designed to shift financial risk to health care institutions and providers if medical or surgical complications occur. Institutions and surgeons, in turn, are using this as an opportunity to innovate the care delivery models to drive cost savings. The perioperative delivery of ATSA is a natural choice for such an evolution, with standardized treatment protocols that can be efficiently operationalized through a systems approach to care delivery. The past decade has seen outpatient ATSA move from proof of concept to reality in the right circumstances.[134,135]

Early published results with ATSA have demonstrated what was previously reported in the hip and knee arthroplasty literature that care can be safely provided at home, after surgery, in select patient groups.[135-137] For example, Leroux et al[138] evaluated 41 TSAs (32 ATSAs and 9 RTSAs) performed in an outpatient ambulatory surgery center over a course of 60 weeks. The average reported age was 60.6 ± 4.8 years, with average ASA class to be 2.3 ± 0.6. They found a 97% patient satisfaction in those that completed the survey, with only

3 (7.3%) minor complications occurring in the cohort. They identified preoperative narcotic use to be a risk factor for dissatisfaction with outpatient TSA. The safety of outpatient TSA was further evaluated in a database review of Medicare subscribers between 2005 and 2012. Of the 123,347 patients identified, 2.8% had TSA performed as an outpatient. Those that did were more likely to be younger, male, and nonsmoker and less likely to have diabetes, congestive heart failure, coronary artery disease, and chronic kidney disease. After controlling for age, the authors found outpatient TSA patients to have lower rates of 30- and 90-day readmission and complication rates than inpatient TSA.[139]

In addition to excellent clinical outcomes, outpatient TSA has also been demonstrated to result in cost savings. Available economic models predict an approximately 750 to 15,500 USD savings per patient depending on local system factors and institutional volume.[140-142] Determining cost savings is a complicated matter due to variable implant costs and subtle market differences.

FUTURE OF ATSA

ATSA has largely evolved into a procedure used to treat osteoarthritis in younger healthy patients with an intact rotator cuff. Although modularity and innovation in ATSA implants have drastically changed our ability to reconstruct the shoulder joint, recent efforts to utilize computer navigation and patient-specific instrumentation has transcended implants and is allowing ATSA to be potentially performed with greater accuracy and precision relative to a preoperative plan. However, despite our basic understanding of the negative implications of aggressive glenoid reaming or implanting a glenoid component in superior tilt,[25] for example, we do not yet appreciate all of the intricacies of patient factors, radiographic factors, and technique that coalesce together to impact the outcome of ATSA. There are a multitude of variables that can contribute to clinical success and survivorship and undoubtedly no single study or human mind can contemplate all of these at the same time.

Recently, ML has been explored to harness its ability to understand the complex interplay of patient factors (ie, comorbidities, body mass index, gender, preoperative ROM, preoperative PROMs, VAS pain score) and radiographic factors (ie, glenoid version) that determine a patient's postoperative clinical outcomes with a high degree of accuracy. A recent study by Kumar et al[99] evaluated the accuracy of three different ML techniques to predict clinical outcomes after shoulder arthroplasty. The authors noted that these techniques were able to accurately predict outcome measures at each postoperative point utilizing preoperative values and patient attributes. In addition, the models were able to predict which patients would reach MCID for PROMs with 93% to 99% accuracy and also which patients would reach

SCB with 82% to 90% accuracy. A study by Gowd et al[143] compared the ability of supervised machine learning (SML) to predict postoperative complications after ATSA. The authors noted that SML accurately predicted postoperative complications utilizing routinely collected preoperative variables. The value of ML is in its ability to potentially identify how to optimize patients so they reach the best outcome possible, avoid complications, and identify variations in prosthesis choice and technique that might maximize outcomes and improve survivorship.

CONCLUSION

One can conceive of a time when ML is used to create a patient-specific operative plan utilizing even standard implants that can be executed using computer navigation and intraoperative real-time feedback. The strength of ML is its ability to learn and optimize algorithms with continued experience and processing of data.

REFERENCES

1. Lugli T. Artificial shoulder joint by Pean (1893): the facts of an exceptional intervention and the prosthetic method. *Clin Orthop Relat Res*. 1978;(133):215-218.
2. Iqbal S, Jacobs U, Akhtar A, Macfarlane RJ, Waseem M. A history of shoulder surgery. *Open Orthop J*. 2013;7:305-309.
3. Neer CS, Brown TH Jr, McLaughlin HL. Fracture of the neck of the humerus with dislocation of the head fragment. *Am J Surg*. 1953;85(3):252-258.
4. Engelbrecht E, Stellbrink G. Total shoulder endoprosthesis design St. Georg. *Chirurg*. 1976;47(10):525-530.
5. Singh JA, Sperling J, Buchbinder R, McMaken K. Surgery for shoulder osteoarthritis: a Cochrane Systematic Review. *J Rheumatol*. 2011;38(4):598-605.
6. Bryant D, Litchfield R, Sandow M, Gartsman GM, Guyatt G, Kirkley A. A comparison of pain, strength, range of motion, and functional outcomes after hemiarthroplasty and total shoulder arthroplasty in patients with osteoarthritis of the shoulder. A systematic review and meta-analysis. *J Bone Joint Surg Am*. 2005;87(9):1947-1956.
7. Keener JD, Chalmers PN, Yamaguchi K. The humeral implant in shoulder arthroplasty. *J Am Acad Orthop Surg*. 2017;25(6):427-438.
8. Flurin PH, Roche CP, Wright TW, Zuckerman JD. Correlation between clinical outcomes and anatomic reconstruction with anatomic total shoulder arthroplasty. *Bull Hosp Jt Dis (2013)*. 2015;73(suppl 1):S92-S98.
9. Alexander JJ, Bell SN, Coghlan J, Lerf R, Dallmann F. The effect of vitamin E-enhanced cross-linked polyethylene on wear in shoulder arthroplasty-a wear simulator study. *J Shoulder Elbow Surg*. 2019;28(9):1771-1778.
10. Schoch B, Abboud J, Namdari S, Lazarus M. Glenohumeral mismatch in anatomic total shoulder arthroplasty. *JBJS Rev*. 2017;5(9):e1.
11. Schoch BS, Wright TW, Zuckerman JD, et al. The effect of radial mismatch on radiographic glenoid loosening. *JSES Open Access*. 2019;3(4):287-291.
12. Walch G, Edwards TB, Boulahia A, Boileau P, Mole D, Adeleine P. The influence of glenohumeral prosthetic mismatch on glenoid radiolucent lines: results of a multicenter study. *J Bone Joint Surg Am*. 2002;84(12):2186-2191.
13. Palsis JA, Simpson KN, Matthews JH, Traven S, Eichinger JK, Friedman RJ. Current trends in the use of shoulder arthroplasty in the United States. *Orthopedics*. 2018;41(3):e416-e423.
14. Deshmukh AV, Koris M, Zurakowski D, Thornhill TS. Total shoulder arthroplasty: long-term survivorship, functional outcome, and quality of life. *J Shoulder Elbow Surg*. 2005;14(5):471-479.
15. Martin SD, Zurakowski D, Thornhill TS. Uncemented glenoid component in total shoulder arthroplasty. Survivorship and outcomes. *J Bone Joint Surg Am*. 2005;87(6):1284-1292.
16. Sperling JW, Cofield RH, Rowland CM. Neer hemiarthroplasty and Neer total shoulder arthroplasty in patients fifty years old or less. Long-term results. *J Bone Joint Surg Am*. 1998;80(4):464-473.
17. Austin LS, Williams GR, Iannotti JP. Unconstrained prosthetic arthroplasty for glenohumeral arthritis with an intact or repairable rotator cuff: indications, techniques and results. In: Iannotti JP, Williams GR, eds. *Disorders of the Shoulder Diagnosis and Management*. Lippincott Williams & Wilkins; 2014.
18. Fox TJ, Cil A, Sperling JW, Sanchez-Sotelo J, Schleck CD, Cofield RH. Survival of the glenoid component in shoulder arthroplasty. *J Shoulder Elbow Surg*. 2009;18(6):859-863.
19. Boileau P, Avidor C, Krishnan SG, Walch G, Kempf JF, Molé D. Cemented polyethylene versus uncemented metal-backed glenoid components in total shoulder arthroplasty: a prospective, double-blind, randomized study. *J Shoulder Elbow Surg*. 2002;11(4):351-359.
20. Boileau P, Moineau G, Morin-Salvo N, et al. Metal-backed glenoid implant with polyethylene insert is not a viable long-term therapeutic option. *J Shoulder Elbow Surg*. 2015;24(10):1534-1543.
21. Gauci MO, Bonnevialle N, Moineau G, Baba M, Walch G, Boileau P. Anatomical total shoulder arthroplasty in young patients with osteoarthritis: all-polyethylene versus metal-backed glenoid. *Bone Joint J*. 2018;100-B(4):485-492.
22. Panti JP, Tan S, Kuo W, Fung S, Walker K, Duff J. Clinical and radiologic outcomes of the second-generation Trabecular Metal glenoid for total shoulder replacements after 2-6 years follow-up. *Arch Orthop Trauma Surg*. 2016;136(12):1637-1645.
23. Sperling JW, Cofield RH. Complications of shoulder arthroplasty. In: Iannotti JP, Williams GR, eds. *Disorders of the Shoulder Diagnosis and Management*. Lippincott Williams & Wilkins; 2014.
24. Cil A, Veillette CJ, Sanchez-Sotelo J, Sperling JW, Schleck CD, Cofield RH. Survivorship of the humeral component in shoulder arthroplasty. *J Shoulder Elbow Surg*. 2010;19(1):143-150.
25. Young AA, Walch G, Pape G, Gohlke F, Favard L. Secondary rotator cuff dysfunction following total shoulder arthroplasty for primary glenohumeral osteoarthritis: results of a multicenter study with more than five years of follow-up. *J Bone Joint Surg Am*. 2012;94(8):685-693.
26. Beck S, Patsalis T, Busch A, et al. Long-term radiographic changes in stemless press-fit total shoulder arthroplasty. *Z Orthop Unfall*. 2020. doi:10.1055/a-1079-6549
27. Simovitch R, Flurin PH, Wright T, Zuckerman JD, Roche CP. Quantifying success after total shoulder arthroplasty: the minimal clinically important difference. *J Shoulder Elbow Surg*. 2018;27(2):298-305.
28. Simovitch R, Flurin PH, Wright T, Zuckerman JD, Roche CP. Quantifying success after total shoulder arthroplasty: the substantial clinical benefit. *J Shoulder Elbow Surg*. 2018;27(5):903-911.
29. Werner BC, Chang B, Nguyen JT, Dines DM, Gulotta LV. What change in American shoulder and elbow surgeons score represents a clinically important change after shoulder arthroplasty? *Clin Orthop Relat Res*. 2016;474(12):2672-2681.
30. Cofield RH. Total shoulder arthroplasty with the Neer prosthesis. *J Bone Joint Surg Am*. 1984;66(6):899-906.
31. Godeneche A, Boulahia A, Noel E, Boileau P, Walch G. Total shoulder arthroplasty in chronic inflammatory and degenerative disease. *Rev Rhum Engl Ed*. 1999;66(11):560-570.
32. Matsen FA III, Antoniou J, Rozencwaig R, Campbell B, Smith KL. Correlates with comfort and function after total shoulder arthroplasty for degenerative joint disease. *J Shoulder Elbow Surg*. 2000;9(5):465-469.
33. Norris TR, Iannotti JP. Functional outcome after shoulder arthroplasty for primary osteoarthritis: a multicenter study. *J Shoulder Elbow Surg*. 2002;11(2):130-135.
34. Torchia ME, Cofield RH, Settergren CR. Total shoulder arthroplasty with the Neer prosthesis: long-term results. *J Shoulder Elbow Surg*. 1997;6(6):495-505.

35. Gonzalez JF, Alami GB, Baque F, Walch G, Boileau P. Complications of unconstrained shoulder prostheses. *J Shoulder Elbow Surg.* 2011;20(4):666-682.

36. Sperling JW, Cofield RH, O'Driscoll SW, Torchia ME, Rowland CM. Radiographic assessment of ingrowth total shoulder arthroplasty. *J Shoulder Elbow Surg.* 2000;9(6):507-513.

37. Throckmorton TW, Zarkadas PC, Sperling JW, Cofield RH. Radiographic stability of ingrowth humeral stems in total shoulder arthroplasty. *Clin Orthop Relat Res.* 2010;468(8):2122-2128.

38. Verborgt O, El-Abiad R, Gazielly DF. Long-term results of uncemented humeral components in shoulder arthroplasty. *J Shoulder Elbow Surg.* 2007;16(3 suppl):S13-S18.

39. Cole EW, Moulton SG, Gobezie R, et al. Five-year radiographic evaluation of stress shielding with a press-fit standard length humeral stem. *JSES Int.* 2020;4(1):109-113.

40. Raiss P, Edwards TB, Deutsch A, et al. Radiographic changes around humeral components in shoulder arthroplasty. *J Bone Joint Surg Am.* 2014;96(7):e54.

41. Nagels J, Stokdijk M, Rozing PM. Stress shielding and bone resorption in shoulder arthroplasty. *J Shoulder Elbow Surg.* 2003;12(1):35-39.

42. Chalmers PN, Granger EK, Orvets ND, et al. Does prosthetic humeral articular surface positioning associate with outcome after total shoulder arthroplasty? *J Shoulder Elbow Surg.* 2018;27(5):863-870.

43. Razfar N, Reeves JM, Langohr DG, Willing R, Athwal GS, Johnson JA. Comparison of proximal humeral bone stresses between stemless, short stem, and standard stem length: a finite element analysis. *J Shoulder Elbow Surg.* 2016;25(7):1076-1083.

44. Santori FS, Manili M, Fredella N, Tonci Ottieri M, Santori N. Ultrashort stems with proximal load transfer: clinical and radiographic results at five-year follow-up. *Hip Int.* 2006;16(suppl 3):31-39.

45. Ballas R, Beguin L. Results of a stemless reverse shoulder prosthesis at more than 58 months mean without loosening. *J Shoulder Elbow Surg.* 2013;22(9):e1-e6.

46. Schnetzke M, Wittmann T, Raiss P, Walch G. Short-term results of a second generation anatomic short-stem shoulder prosthesis in primary osteoarthritis. *Arch Orthop Trauma Surg.* 2019;139(2):149-154.

47. Churchill RS, Athwal GS. Stemless shoulder arthroplasty-current results and designs. *Curr Rev Musculoskelet Med.* 2016;9(1):10-16.

48. Casagrande DJ, Parks DL, Torngren T, et al. Radiographic evaluation of short-stem press-fit total shoulder arthroplasty: short-term follow-up. *J Shoulder Elbow Surg.* 2016;25(7):1163-1169.

49. Morwood MP, Johnston PS, Garrigues GE. Proximal ingrowth coating decreases risk of loosening following uncemented shoulder arthroplasty using mini-stem humeral components and lesser tuberosity osteotomy. *J Shoulder Elbow Surg.* 2017;26(7):1246-1252.

50. Huguet D, DeClercq G, Rio B, Teissier J, Zipoli B; TESS Group. Results of a new stemless shoulder prosthesis: radiologic proof of maintained fixation and stability after a minimum of three years' follow-up. *J Shoulder Elbow Surg.* 2010;19(6):847-852.

51. Hawi N, Magosch P, Tauber M, Lichtenberg S, Habermeyer P. Nine-year outcome after anatomic stemless shoulder prosthesis: clinical and radiologic results. *J Shoulder Elbow Surg.* 2017;26(9):1609-1615.

52. Gallacher S, Williams HLM, King A, Kitson J, Smith CD, Thomas WJ. Clinical and radiologic outcomes following total shoulder arthroplasty using Arthrex Eclipse stemless humeral component with minimum 2 years' follow-up. *J Shoulder Elbow Surg.* 2018;27(12):2191-2197.

53. Lazarus MD, Jensen KL, Southworth C, Matsen FA III. The radiographic evaluation of keeled and pegged glenoid component insertion. *J Bone Joint Surg Am.* 2002;84(7):1174-1182.

54. Gartsman GM, Elkousy HA, Warnock KM, Edwards TB, O'Connor DP. Radiographic comparison of pegged and keeled glenoid components. *J Shoulder Elbow Surg.* 2005;14(3):252-257.

55. Edwards TB, Labriola JE, Stanley RJ, O'Connor DP, Elkousy HA, Gartsman GM. Radiographic comparison of pegged and keeled glenoid components using modern cementing techniques: a prospective randomized study. *J Shoulder Elbow Surg.* 2010;19(2):251-257.

56. McLendon PB, Schoch BS, Sperling JW, Sánchez-Sotelo J, Schleck CD, Cofield RH. Survival of the pegged glenoid component in shoulder arthroplasty: part II. *J Shoulder Elbow Surg.* 2017;26(8):1469-1476.

57. Arnold RM, High RR, Grosshans KT, Walker CW, Fehringer EV. Bone presence between the central peg's radial fins of a partially cemented pegged all poly glenoid component suggest few radiolucencies. *J Shoulder Elbow Surg.* 2011;20(2):315-321.

58. Wirth MA, Loredo R, Garcia G, Rockwood CA Jr, Southworth C, Iannotti JP. Total shoulder arthroplasty with an all-polyethylene pegged bone-ingrowth glenoid component: a clinical and radiographic outcome study. *J Bone Joint Surg Am.* 2012;94(3):260-267.

59. Friedman RJ, Cheung E, Grey SG, et al. Clinical and radiographic comparison of a hybrid cage glenoid to a cemented polyethylene glenoid in anatomic total shoulder arthroplasty. *J Shoulder Elbow Surg.* 2019;28(12):2308-2316.

60. Bercik MJ, Kruse K III, Yalizis M, Gauci MO, Chaoui J, Walch G. A modification to the Walch classification of the glenoid in primary glenohumeral osteoarthritis using three-dimensional imaging. *J Shoulder Elbow Surg.* 2016;25(10):1601-1606.

61. Knowles NK, Ferreira LM, Athwal GS. Augmented glenoid component designs for type B2 erosions: a computational comparison by volume of bone removal and quality of remaining bone. *J Shoulder Elbow Surg.* 2015;24(8):1218-1226.

62. Ghoraishian M, Stone MA, Elhassan B, Abboud J, Namdari S. Augmented glenoid implants in anatomic total shoulder arthroplasty: review of available implants and current literature. *J Shoulder Elbow Surg.* 2019;28(2):387-395.

63. Wright TW, Grey SG, Roche CP, Wright L, Flurin PH, Zuckerman JD. Preliminary results of a posterior augmented glenoid compared to an all polyethylene standard glenoid in anatomic total shoulder arthroplasty. *Bull Hosp Jt Dis (2013).* 2015;73(suppl 1):S79-S85.

64. Stephens SP, Spencer EE, Wirth MA. Radiographic results of augmented all-polyethylene glenoids in the presence of posterior glenoid bone loss during total shoulder arthroplasty. *J Shoulder Elbow Surg.* 2017;26(5):798-803.

65. Favorito PJ, Freed RJ, Passanise AM, Brown MJ. Total shoulder arthroplasty for glenohumeral arthritis associated with posterior glenoid bone loss: results of an all-polyethylene, posteriorly augmented glenoid component. *J Shoulder Elbow Surg.* 2016;25(10):1681-1689.

66. Grey SG, Wright TW, Flurin PH, Zuckerman JD, Roche CP, Friedman RJ. Clinical and radiographic outcomes with a posteriorly augmented glenoid for Walch B glenoids in anatomic total shoulder arthroplasty. *J Shoulder Elbow Surg.* 2020;29(5):e185-e195.

67. Ho JC, mini MH, Entezari V, et al. Clinical and radiographic outcomes of a posteriorly augmented glenoid component in anatomic total shoulder arthroplasty for primary osteoarthritis with posterior glenoid bone loss. *J Bone Joint Surg Am.* 2018;100(22):1934-1948.

68. Padegimas EM, Maltenfort M, Lazarus MD, Ramsey ML, Williams GR, Namdari S. Future patient demand for shoulder arthroplasty by younger patients: national projections. *Clin Orthop Relat Res.* 2015;473(6):1860-1867.

69. Roberson TA, Bentley JC, Griscom JT, et al. Outcomes of total shoulder arthroplasty in patients younger than 65 years: a systematic review. *J Shoulder Elbow Surg.* 2017;26(7):1298-1306.

70. Saltzman MD, Mercer DM, Warme WJ, Bertelsen AL, Matsen FA III. Comparison of patients undergoing primary shoulder arthroplasty before and after the age of fifty. *J Bone Joint Surg Am.* 2010;92(1):42-47.

71. Jawa A, Dasti U, Brown A, Grannatt K, Miller S. Gender differences in expectations and outcomes for total shoulder arthroplasty: a prospective cohort study. *J Shoulder Elbow Surg.* 2016;25(8):1323-1327.

72. Simovitch RW, Friedman RJ, Cheung EV, et al. Rate of improvement in clinical outcomes with anatomic and reverse total shoulder arthroplasty. *J Bone Joint Surg Am.* 2017;99(21):1801-1811.

73. Steinhaus ME, Gowd AK, Hurwit DJ, Lieber AC, Liu JN. Return to work after shoulder arthroplasty: a systematic review and meta-analysis. *J Shoulder Elbow Surg.* 2019;28(5):998-1008.

74. Liu JN, Garcia GH, Wong AC, et al. Return to work after anatomic total shoulder arthroplasty for patients 55 years and younger at average 5-year follow-up. *Orthopedics.* 2018;41(3):e310-e315.

75. Halpern M, Hurd JL, Zuckerman JB. Occupational shoulder disorders. In: Rockwood CA, Matsen F, eds. *The Shoulder.* 5th ed. Elsevier; 2016.

76. Cvetanovich GL, Savin DD, Frank RM, et al. Inferior outcomes and higher complication rates after shoulder arthroplasty in workers' compensation patients. *J Shoulder Elbow Surg.* 2019;28(5):875-881.

77. Bulhoff M, Sattler P, Bruckner T, Loew M, Zeifang F, Raiss P. Do patients return to sports and work after total shoulder replacement surgery? *Am J Sports Med.* 2015;43(2):423-427.

78. Liu JN, Steinhaus ME, Garcia GH, et al. Return to sport after shoulder arthroplasty: a systematic review and meta-analysis. *Knee Surg Sports Traumatol Arthrosc.* 2018;26(1):100-112.

79. Boileau P, Chuinard C, Le Huec JC, Walch G, Trojani C. Proximal humerus fracture sequelae: impact of a new radiographic classification on arthroplasty. *Clin Orthop Relat Res.* 2006;442:121-130.

80. Audige L, Graf L, Flury M, Schneider MM, Müller AM. Functional improvement is sustained following anatomical and reverse shoulder arthroplasty for fracture sequelae: a registry-based analysis. *Arch Orthop Trauma Surg.* 2019;139(11):1561-1569.

81. Wooten C, Klika B, Schleck CD, Harmsen WS, Sperling JW, Cofield RH. Anatomic shoulder arthroplasty as treatment for locked posterior dislocation of the shoulder. *J Bone Joint Surg Am.* 2014;96(3):e19.

82. Cerciello S, Corona K, Morris BJ, Paladini P, Porcellini G, Merolla G. Shoulder arthroplasty to address the sequelae of anterior instability arthropathy and stabilization procedures: systematic review and meta-analysis. *Arch Orthop Trauma Surg.* 2020. doi:10.1007/s00402-020-03400-y

83. Cuff DJ, Santoni BG. Anatomic total shoulder arthroplasty versus reverse total shoulder arthroplasty for post-capsulorrhaphy arthropathy. *Orthopedics.* 2018;41(5):275-280.

84. Livesey M, Horneff JG III, Sholder D, Lazarus M, Williams G, Namdari S. Functional outcomes and predictors of failure after rotator cuff repair during total shoulder arthroplasty. *Orthopedics.* 2018;41(3):e334-e339.

85. Simone JP, Streubel PH, Sperling JW, Schleck CD, Cofield RH, Athwal GS. Anatomical total shoulder replacement with rotator cuff repair for osteoarthritis of the shoulder. *Bone Joint J.* 2014;96-B(2):224-228.

86. Gerlach OH, Winogrodzka A, Weber WE. Clinical problems in the hospitalized Parkinson's disease patient: systematic review. *Mov Disord.* 2011;26(2):197-208.

87. Kryzak TJ, Sperling JW, Schleck CD, Cofield RH. Total shoulder arthroplasty in patients with Parkinson's disease. *J Shoulder Elbow Surg.* 2009;18(1):96-99.

88. Koch LD, Cofield RH, Ahlskog JE. Total shoulder arthroplasty in patients with Parkinson's disease. *J Shoulder Elbow Surg.* 1997;6(1):24-28.

89. Cusick MC, Otto RJ, Clark RE, Frankle MA. Outcome of reverse shoulder arthroplasty for patients with Parkinson's disease: a matched cohort study. *Orthopedics.* 2017;40(4):e675-e680.

90. Burrus MT, Werner BC, Cancienne JM, Gwathmey FW, Brockmeier SF. Shoulder arthroplasty in patients with Parkinson's disease is associated with increased complications. *J Shoulder Elbow Surg.* 2015;24(12):1881-1887.

91. Barlow JD, Yuan BJ, Schleck CD, Harmsen WS, Cofield RH, Sperling JW. Shoulder arthroplasty for rheumatoid arthritis: 303 consecutive cases with minimum 5-year follow-up. *J Shoulder Elbow Surg.* 2014;23(6):791-799.

92. Lapner PLC, Rollins MD, Netting C, Tuna M, Bader Eddeen A, van Walraven C. A population-based comparison of joint survival of hemiarthroplasty versus total shoulder arthroplasty in osteoarthritis and rheumatoid arthritis. *Bone Joint J.* 2019;101-B(4):454-460.

93. Young AA, Smith MM, Bacle G, Moraga C, Walch G. Early results of reverse shoulder arthroplasty in patients with rheumatoid arthritis. *J Bone Joint Surg Am.* 2011;93(20):1915-1923.

94. Rittmeister M, Kerschbaumer F. Grammont reverse total shoulder arthroplasty in patients with rheumatoid arthritis and non-reconstructible rotator cuff lesions. *J Shoulder Elbow Surg.* 2001;10(1):17-22.

95. Mangold DR, Wagner ER, Cofield RH, Sanchez-Sotelo J, Sperling JW. Reverse shoulder arthroplasty for rheumatoid arthritis since the introduction of disease-modifying drugs. *Int Orthop.* 2019;43(11):2593-2600.

96. Jacobs CA, Morris BJ, Sciascia AD, Edwards TB. Comparison of satisfied and dissatisfied patients 2 to 5 years after anatomic total shoulder arthroplasty. *J Shoulder Elbow Surg.* 2016;25(7):1128-1132.

97. Mahony GT, Werner BC, Chang B, et al. Risk factors for failing to achieve improvement after anatomic total shoulder arthroplasty for glenohumeral osteoarthritis. *J Shoulder Elbow Surg.* 2018;27(6):968-975.

98. Friedman RJ, Eichinger J, Schoch B, et al. Preoperative parameters that predict postoperative patient-reported outcome measures and range of motion with anatomic and reverse total shoulder arthroplasty. *JSES Open Access.* 2019;3(4):266-272.

99. Kumar V, Roche C, Overman S, et al. What is the accuracy of three different machine learning techniques to predict clinical outcomes after shoulder arthroplasty? *Clin Orthop Relat Res.* 2020;478:2351-2363

100. Fu MC, Ondeck NT, Nwachukwu BU, et al. What associations exist between comorbidity indices and postoperative adverse events after total shoulder arthroplasty? *Clin Orthop Relat Res.* 2019;477(4):881-890.

101. Holzgrefe RE, Wilson JM, Staley CA, Anderson TL, Wagner ER, Gottschalk MB. Modified frailty index is an effective risk-stratification tool for patients undergoing total shoulder arthroplasty. *J Shoulder Elbow Surg.* 2019;28(7):1232-1240.

102. Zmistowski B, Warrender W, Livesey M, Girden A, Williams GR Jr, Namdari S. The characteristics of surgeons performing total shoulder arthroplasty: volume consistency, training, and specialization. *Am J Orthop (Belle Mead NJ).* 2018;47(12).

103. Ramkumar PN, Navarro SM, Haeberle HS, Ricchetti ET, Iannotti JP. Evidence-based thresholds for the volume-value relationship in shoulder arthroplasty: outcomes and economies of scale. *J Shoulder Elbow Surg.* 2017;26(8):1399-1406.

104. Werner BC, Wong AC, Chang B, et al. Depression and patient-reported outcomes following total shoulder arthroplasty. *J Bone Joint Surg Am.* 2017;99(8):688-695.

105. Mollon B, Mahure SA, Ding DY, Zuckerman JD, Kwon YW. The influence of a history of clinical depression on peri-operative outcomes in elective total shoulder arthroplasty: a ten-year national analysis. *Bone Joint J.* 2016;98-B(6):818-824.

106. Wong SE, Colley AK, Pitcher AA, Zhang AL, Ma CB, Feeley BT. Mental health, preoperative disability, and postoperative outcomes in patients undergoing shoulder arthroplasty. *J Shoulder Elbow Surg.* 2018;27(9):1580-1587.

107. Magaldi RJ, Staff I, Stovall AE, Stohler SA, Lewis CG. Impact of resilience on outcomes of total knee arthroplasty. *J Arthroplasty.* 2019;34(11):2620-2623 e1.

108. Crijns TJ, Liu TC, Ring D, Bozic KJ, Koenig K. Influence of patient Activation, pain self-efficacy, and resilience on pain intensity and magnitude of limitations in patients with hip and knee arthritis. *J Surg Orthop Adv.* 2019;28(1):48-52.

109. Andrawis J, Akhavan S, Chan V, Lehil M, Pong D, Bozic KJ. Higher preoperative patient Activation associated with better patient-reported outcomes after total joint arthroplasty. *Clin Orthop Relat Res.* 2015;473(8):2688-2697.

110. Tokish JM, Kissenberth MJ, Tolan SJ, et al. Resilience correlates with outcomes after total shoulder arthroplasty. *J Shoulder Elbow Surg,* 2017;26(5):752-756.

111. Cheah JW, Sing DC, McLaughlin D, Feeley BT, Ma CB, Zhang AL. The perioperative effects of chronic preoperative opioid use on shoulder arthroplasty outcomes. *J Shoulder Elbow Surg.* 2017;26(11):1908-1914.

112. Berglund DD, Rosas S, Kurowicki J, Horn B, Mijic D, Levy JC. Preoperative opioid use among patients undergoing shoulder arthroplasty predicts prolonged postoperative opioid use. *J Am Acad Orthop Surg.* 2018;27(15):e691-e695.

113. Menendez ME, Lawler SM, Ring D, Jawa A. High pain intensity after total shoulder arthroplasty. *J Shoulder Elbow Surg.* 2018;27(12):2113-2119.

114. Curtis W, Rounds AD, Stone M, et al. Effect of preoperative opioid usage on pain after total shoulder arthroplasty. *J Am Acad Orthop Surg.* 2019;27(16):e734-e742.

115. Martusiewicz A, Khan AZ, Chamberlain AM, Keener JD, Aleem AW. Outpatient narcotic consumption following total shoulder arthroplasty. *JSES Int.* 2020;4(1):100-104.

116. Morris BJ, Sciascia AD, Jacobs CA, Edwards TB. Preoperative opioid use associated with worse outcomes after anatomic shoulder arthroplasty. *J Shoulder Elbow Surg.* 2016;25(4):619-623.

117. Bohsali KI, Bois AJ, Wirth MA. Complications of shoulder arthroplasty. *J Bone Joint Surg Am.* 2017;99(3):256-269.

118. Papadonikolakis A, Neradilek MB, Matsen FA III. Failure of the glenoid component in anatomic total shoulder arthroplasty: a systematic review of the English-language literature between 2006 and 2012. *J Bone Joint Surg Am.* 2013;95(24):2205-2212.

119. Vavken P, Sadoghi P, von Keudell A, et al. Rates of radiolucency and loosening after total shoulder arthroplasty with pegged or keeled glenoid components. *J Bone Joint Surg Am.* 2013;95(3):215-221.

120. Sperling JW, Hawkins RJ, Walch G, Mahoney AP, Zuckerman JD. Complications in total shoulder arthroplasty. *Instr Course Lect.* 2013;62:135-141.

121. Swanson AB, de Groot Swanson G, Sattel AB, Cendo RD, Hynes D, Jar-Ning W. Bipolar implant shoulder arthroplasty. Long-term results. *Clin Orthop Relat Res.* 1989;(249):227-247.

122. Mileti J, Sperling JW, Cofield RH. Reimplantation of a shoulder arthroplasty after a previous infected arthroplasty. *J Shoulder Elbow Surg.* 2004;13(5):528-531.

123. Singh JA, Sperling JW, Schleck C, Harmsen WS, Cofield RH. Periprosthetic infections after total shoulder arthroplasty: a 33-year perspective. *J Shoulder Elbow Surg.* 2012;21(11):1534-1541.

124. Schrock JB, Kraeutler MJ, Houck DA, Provenzano GG, McCarty EC, Bravman JT. Lesser tuberosity osteotomy and subscapularis tenotomy repair techniques during total shoulder arthroplasty: a meta-analysis of cadaveric studies. *Clin Biomech.* 2016;40:33-36.

125. Miller BS, Joseph TA, Noonan TJ, Horan MP, Hawkins RJ. Rupture of the subscapularis tendon after shoulder arthroplasty: diagnosis, treatment, and outcome. *J Shoulder Elbow Surg.* 2005;14(5):492-496.

126. Moeckel BH, Altchek DW, Warren RF, Wickiewicz TL, Dines DM. Instability of the shoulder after arthroplasty. *J Bone Joint Surg Am.* 1993;75(4):492-497.

127. Singh JA, Sperling J, Schleck C, Harmsen W, Cofield R. Periprosthetic fractures associated with primary total shoulder arthroplasty and primary humeral head replacement: a thirty-three-year study. *J Bone Joint Surg Am.* 2012;94(19):1777-1785.

128. Nagda SH, Rogers KJ, Sestokas AK, et al. Neer Award 2005: peripheral nerve function during shoulder arthroplasty using intraoperative nerve monitoring. *J Shoulder Elbow Surg.* 2007;16(3 suppl):S2-S8.

129. Ladermann A, Lübbeke A, Mélis B, Stern R, Christofilopoulos P, Bacle G, Walch G. Prevalence of neurologic lesions after total shoulder arthroplasty. *J Bone Joint Surg Am.* 2011;93(14):1288-1293.

130. Somerson JS, Hsu JE, Neradilek MB, Matsen FA III. Analysis of 4063 complications of shoulder arthroplasty reported to the US Food and Drug Administration from 2012 to 2016. *J Shoulder Elbow Surg.* 2018;27(11):1978-1986.

131. Anakwenze OA, O'Donnell EA, Jobin CM, Levine WN, Ahmad CS. Medical complications and outcomes after total shoulder arthroplasty: a Nationwide analysis. *Am J Orthop (Belle Mead NJ).* 2018;47(10).

132. Waterman BR, Dunn JC, Bader J, Urrea L, Schoenfeld AJ, Belmont PJ Jr. Thirty-day morbidity and mortality after elective total shoulder arthroplasty: patient-based and surgical risk factors. *J Shoulder Elbow Surg.* 2015;24(1):24-30.

133. Chung AS, Makovicka JL, Hydrick T, Scott KL, Arvind V, Hattrup SJ. Analysis of 90-day readmissions after total shoulder arthroplasty. *Orthop J Sports Med.* 2019;7(9):2325967119868964.

134. Fournier MN, Brolin TJ, Azar FM, Stephens R, Throckmorton TW. Identifying appropriate candidates for ambulatory outpatient shoulder arthroplasty: validation of a patient selection algorithm. *J Shoulder Elbow Surg.* 2019;28(1):65-70.

135. Brolin TJ, Throckmorton TW. Outpatient shoulder arthroplasty. *Orthop Clin North Am.* 2018;49(1):73-79.

136. Arshi A, Leong NL, Wang C, et al. Relative complications and trends of outpatient total shoulder arthroplasty. *Orthopedics.* 2018;41(3):e400-e409.

137. Nwankwo CD, Dutton P, Merriman JA, Gajudo G, Gill K, Hatch J. Outpatient total shoulder arthroplasty does not increase the 90-day risk of complications compared with inpatient surgery in prescreened patients. *Orthopedics.* 2018;41(4):e563-e568.

138. Leroux TS, Zuke WA, Saltzman BM, et al. Safety and patient satisfaction of outpatient shoulder arthroplasty. *JSES Open Access.* 2018;2(1):13-17.

139. Basques BA, Erickson BJ, Leroux T, et al. Comparative outcomes of outpatient and inpatient total shoulder arthroplasty: an analysis of the Medicare dataset. *Bone Joint J.* 2017;99-B(7):934-938.

140. Steinhaus ME, Shim SS, Lamba N, Makhni EC, Kadiyala RK. Outpatient shoulder arthroplasty: a cost-identification analysis. *J Orthop.* 2018;15(2):581-585.

141. Borakati A, Ali A, Nagaraj C, Gadikoppula S, Kurer M. Day case vs inpatient total shoulder arthroplasty: a retrospective cohort study and cost-effectiveness analysis. *World J Orthop.* 2020;11(4):213-221.

142. Gregory JM, Wetzig AM, Wayne CD, Bailey L, Warth RJ. Quantification of patient-level costs in outpatient total shoulder arthroplasty. *J Shoulder Elbow Surg.* 2019;28(6):1066-1073.

143. Gowd AK, Agarwalla A, Amin NH, et al. Construct validation of machine learning in the prediction of short-term postoperative complications following total shoulder arthroplasty. *J Shoulder Elbow Surg.* 2019;28(12):e410-e421.

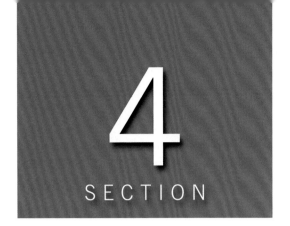

Reverse Total Shoulder Arthroplasty

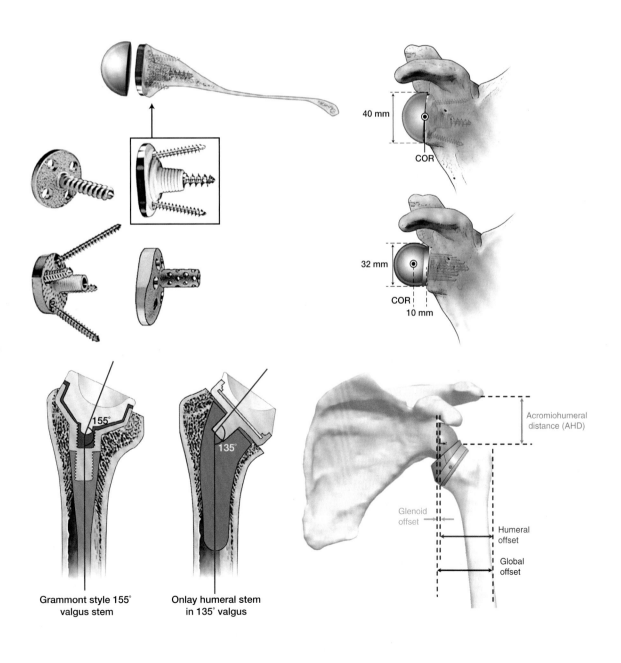

Grammont style 155° valgus stem

Onlay humeral stem in 135° valgus

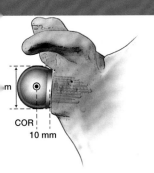

22

Implant Options:
Glenoid and Humerus

Georges Haidamous, MD and Mark A. Frankle, MD

INTRODUCTION

Reverse total shoulder arthroplasty (RTSA) is the most commonly performed shoulder replacement procedure in the United States.[1] New generation RTSA designs have revolutionized the treatment of various shoulder conditions beyond cuff tear arthropathy.[2-4] A variety of implant designs are available[5]; however, the clinical superiority of one over the other has not been established.[6-8] In the absence of well-defined criteria guiding implant choice, this process is still primarily surgeon dependent. Therefore, it is important to understand how different implant options affect the spatial positioning of the humerus with respect to the scapula and, in turn, shoulder biomechanics and postoperative outcomes.

ORIGINAL RTSA DESIGN CONCEPTS

In the early 1970s, Neer proposed the concept of reversing the ball and socket in cuff-deficient patients using a fixed-fulcrum design.[9] Three versions of this highly constrained system were developed, but the concept was abandoned because of early glenoid component failure.[10] Consequently, other design attempts were equally unsuccessful.[11-16] In 1985, Paul Grammont reintroduced Neer's concept, using (1) a two-thirds of a sphere ceramic glenoid component called the "glenosphere," and (2) a cemented 155° polyethylene (PE) stem.[17] The glenosphere shape was then modified by Baulot into a press-fit hemisphere, fixed by divergent superior and inferior screws,[18] also known as the Delta III glenosphere. The hemispheric design further medialized the center of rotation (COR) to the glenosphere/glenoid interface. Medialization of the COR, in addition to the 155° stem, placed the humerus in a more medial and distal position. This implant combination was thought to result in a more efficient deltoid lever arm compensating for the dysfunctional rotator cuff, as well as increased deltoid muscle tension that augmented joint compression forces and stabilized the construct.[19] Nevertheless, early outcome reports on the Delta III design have propagated an unsubstantiated causality between COR lateralization and increased glenoid loosening caused by increased torque on the fixation interface observed with previous (ie, more lateralized) designs.[20,21]

LIMITATIONS OF ORIGINAL RTSA DESIGN AND PROPOSED MODIFICATIONS

The original design, however, had its shortcomings, which included limited rotational range of motion (ROM) due to the reduced tension of the rotator cuff muscles as well as notching due to increased contact between the humeral component PE liner and the inferior scapular neck.[2,22-24] As such, changes were proposed with the goal of repositioning the COR closer to that of a normal shoulder and increasing the clearance distance between the humerus and the scapular neck.[25-29] This was achieved by (1) lateralizing the glenosphere's COR with metal[30] and bone graft augmented (BIO-RSA) constructs[31] and (2) lateralizing the humerus using an onlay stem design.[32] In addition, the latter was also achieved by decreasing the neck-shaft angle (NSA) from 155° to 135°.[28,32] This allowed for different implant combinations and has resulted in more than 29 implant designs that are available in the marketplace.[5] This multitude of designs have led researchers to attempt to understand which construct most closely replicates the normal shoulder and leads to optimal outcomes using classification systems based on glenosphere and stem lateralization.[24,33] However, the majority of the research comparing these configurations has been based on biomechanical and computer simulation studies,[24-29] whereas patient outcomes remain less well understood across designs[6-8] as they are influenced by several factors not assessed in biomechanical models, such as surgical technique, amount of bone resection and loss, and soft-tissue tension.

IS THERE AN IDEAL RTSA DESIGN?

Major advancements have been made in RTSA over the past 35 years after Grammont introduced his concept, allowing patients undergoing this procedure to experience improved outcomes.[2,34,35] Nevertheless, several challenges still exist, such as managing severe bone loss, improving implant stability and bone fixation, and surpassing the RTSA's expected "70% of a normal shoulder" functionality.[36] The ideal RTSA design would theoretically optimize muscular balance around the shoulder, reestablish anatomic force vectors across the COR, and maximize impingement-free ROM by restoring the native scapulohumeral positions, while simultaneously preserving the stability of the construct. In addition, components would have excellent bony fixation.

It is still uncertain whether the RTSA concept we know today will be capable of reproducing the normal shoulder function, especially with evidence of important kinematic differences.[37] Nevertheless, literature suggests that a particular component combination might be optimal for specific pathologies and outcomes.[6-8,38] For example, a computer modeling study investigated factors leading to the greatest impingement-free ROM in 126 RTSA implant combinations and showed that the hierarchy of implant and technique-related factors leading to an improvement in abduction ROM are different from those leading to an improvement in rotational ROM.[39] **TABLE 22.1** demonstrates how different component parameters can have different effects on outcomes.

GLENOID FIXATION

Achieving secure glenoid fixation is essential to minimize glenosphere failure, which has been attributed to the inability of the baseplate to overcome the forces exerted on the implant/bone interface before adequate bony ingrowth occurs.[49] To achieve bony ingrowth, it is important to minimize micromotion to less than 150 μm[50] between the baseplate and screws.[51] Increasing the length, diameter, and inclination of the peripheral screws can decrease micromotion,[51] which does not appear to be affected by hybrid screw use (ie, locking and nonlocking screws) as long as at least one locking screw is utilized.[52] The use of longer screws may compensate for the use of fewer screws[53,54] when bone quality or bone loss interferes with screw placement. In addition, fixation of the baseplate also depends greatly on the quality of the bone,[49,55] which becomes more challenging in the setting of severe glenoid bone loss.[56] Bone loss often results in reduced backside contact between the baseplate and glenoid bone, which further decreases the component's threshold for withstanding joint forces.[57]

Another essential requirement for achieving baseplate fixation is obtaining adequate baseplate compression via both the baseplate's central axis and peripheral screws.[58] Central axis fixation is usually in the form of a screw or a post **(FIGURE 22.1)**. Biomechanical evidence suggests that baseplates with central screws achieve a 10-fold increase in compression forces compared to posts (2000 vs 200 N), as well as a 2.3-fold increase in load to failure.[58] Adequate baseplate compression coupled with decreased micromotion at the peripheral screws is crucial to decreasing glenosphere failure. Earlier reports showed that the use of 3.5-mm nonlocking screws with a central screw baseplate resulted in a glenosphere failure rate of 10%.[31] Electron microscopy assessment of the retrieved components revealed that implant failure was due to decreased bone ingrowth.[59] A subsequent biomechanical evaluation comparing the use of peripheral 3.5-mm non-locking screws to 5.0-mm locking ones showed that the latter resulted in 29% less micromotion.[51] These benefits were also validated in a clinical study demonstrating a glenoid failure rate of 0.4% at 5-year follow-up.[60]

GLENOSPHERE LATERALIZATION

Regardless of implant design, the glenohumeral COR shifts medially and inferiorly compared to that of a normal shoulder following RTSA; however, the degree of this differs between designs.[61] Currently, there are two methods to achieve lateralization on the glenoid side. The first is through prosthetic lateralization of either the baseplate or the glenosphere. For the glenosphere, lateralization is dependent on the degree of sphericity rather than the size of the component **(FIGURE 22.2)**. The second method is by using bone graft augmentation (BIO-RSA). The two methods appear to have different biomechanical properties. A finite element analysis study comparing prosthetic to bony lateralization revealed that with BIO-RSA, only 5 mm of lateralization is mechanically acceptable as opposed to 10 mm with prosthetic lateralization and that baseplate stresses and displacement are increased with the former.[62] To decrease bony impingement, a glenosphere lateral offset of 5 mm or more has been shown to be ideal.[63,64] Gutierrez et al used computer simulation to examine the effects of different implant factors on abduction ROM.[27] They observed that impingement occurred at the acromion superiorly, at the glenoid and scapular neck inferiorly, and that the most important factor for maximizing ROM is the lateral COR offset of the glenosphere **(FIGURE 22.3C and D)**. A linear correlation was also detected between COR lateralization and abduction (ie, as COR lateralization increases, abduction increases).

Glenosphere lateralization also significantly increases anterior stability of the prosthetic construct[65] and restores the length of the internal and external rotators of the shoulder[7] **(FIGURE 22.3B)**. A biomechanical analysis evaluating changes in muscle lengths and moment arms from pre- to post-RTSA implantation using 8 mm of glenosphere lateral offset showed that the subscapularis and teres minor maintained their lengths and rotational moment arms and exhibited an increase in their flexion forces.[66] Likewise, findings from a computer modeling study demonstrated that an 8 mm increase in lateral glenosphere offset increased the length of the infraspinatus by 5%, the teres minor by 11%, and the teres major by 7%.[25] Clinical studies support these findings, particularly with respect to the improvement in external rotation (ER).[7,39] In a prospective randomized study, Grenier et al compared patients with 10-mm bone graft augmentation versus those who

TABLE 22.1 Studies Comparing the Effects of Different Reverse Shoulder Components on Range of Motion Outcomes

Variable	Author	Type of Study	Number of Shoulders	Follow-up	Implant	Abduction	Forward Flexion	External Rotation	Internal Rotation
Glenosphere lateralization	Gutiérrez et al,[27] 2007	Biomechanical	N/A	N/A	MG (0-mm offset) LG (10-mm offset)	67° 97°	N/A	N/A	N/A
	Gutiérrez et al,[29] 2008	Computer modeling	234 combinations	N/A	MG (0-mm offset) LG (10-mm offset)	54° 83°	N/A	N/A	N/A
	Virani et al,[39] 2012	Computer modeling	N/A	N/A	MG (0-mm offset) LG (5-mm offset) LG (10-mm offset)	70° arc 83° arc 85° arc	67° arc 89° arc 114° arc	67° arc 84° arc 88° arc	N/A
	Streit et al,[40] 2015	Clinical (prospective)	18	N/A	MG (155° inlay) LG (135° inlay)	N/A	144° 115°	28° 35°	N/A
	Collin et al,[41] 2018	Clinical (retrospective)	69	24 mo	MG BIO-RSA	N/A	138° 145°	No difference	No difference
Glenosphere size	Berhouet et al,[42] 2013	Biomechanical	40	N/A	36 mm 42 mm	N/A	N/A	31° 68°	34° 74°
	Virani et al,[39] 2012	Computer modeling	N/A	N/A	30 mm 36 mm 42 mm	79° arc 80° arc 82° arc	74° arc 98° arc 109° arc	52° arc 90° arc 102° arc	N/A
	Müller et al,[43] 2018	Clinical (retrospective)	68	60 mo	44 vs 36 mm	No difference	No difference	12° gain	No difference
	Mollon et al,[44] 2016	Clinical (prospective)	297	24 mo	38 mm (n = 160) 42 mm (n = 137)	N/A	44° 59°	18° 24°	No difference
	Schoch et al,[45] 2020	Clinical (retrospective)	589	24 mo	38 mm (n = 370) 42 mm (n = 219)	78° 76°	95°a 90°a	19°a 16°a	Sacrum L5

Continued

TABLE 22.1 Studies Comparing the Effects of Different Reverse Shoulder Components on Range of Motion Outcomes (continued)

Variable	Author	Type of Study	Number of Shoulders	Follow-up	Implant	Abduction	Forward Flexion	External Rotation	Internal Rotation
Glenosphere inferior position	Werner et al,[46] 2018	Computer modeling	21	N/A	2 mm eccentric > centered	N/A	N/A	N/A	9°
	Virani et al,[39] 2012	Computer modeling	N/A	N/A	Concentric / Eccentric	69° arc / 82° arc	131° arc / 87° arc	58° arc / 85° arc	N/A
	Gutiérrez et al,[29] 2008	Computer modeling	234 combinations	N/A	Concentric vs eccentric (0-mm offset) / Concentric vs eccentric (10-mm offset)	57° vs 100° / 85° vs 118°	N/A	N/A	N/A
	Choi et al,[47] 2017	Clinical (retrospective)	20	14 mo	Concentric (n = 9) / 5.8 mm eccentric (n = 11)	N/A	139° (gain 74°)[a] / 135° (gain 90°)[a]	24° (gain 13°) / 26° (gain 13°)	L4[a] / L3[a]
	De Biase et al,[48] 2013	Clinical	60	24 mo	Concentric (n = 31) / 4.3 mm eccentric (n = 29)	116° (gain 51°) / 115° (gain 55°)	129° (gain 67°) / 148° (gain 82°)	15° (gain 7°) / 16° (gain 11°)	L5 / L5
Humerus inlay versus onlay	Virani et al,[39] 2012	Computer modeling	N/A	N/A	Inlay / Onlay	80° arc / 81° arc	95° arc / 92° arc	81° arc / 81° arc	N/A
	Lädermann et al,[32] 2015	Computer modeling	N/A	N/A	Inlay (155°) / Onlay (145°)	78° / 65°	106° / 112°	16° / 28°	No difference
	Merolla et al,[6] 2018	Clinical (retrospective)	74	24 mo	Inlay (155°) / Onlay (145°)	131° / 131°	142° / 142°	30° / 32°	No difference

LG, lateralized glenosphere; MG, medialized glenosphere.
[a]Variables that have been statistically compared and showed nonsignificant differences ($P < 0.05$).

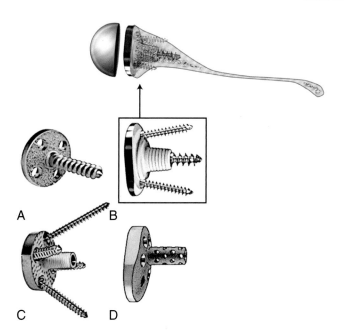

FIGURE 22.1 Commonly used baseplate central axis fixation: (**A**) RSP Monoblock baseplate (DJO Global), (**B**) Arthrex Universal Baseplate (Arthrex Inc), (**C**) Tornier Aequalis Reversed II baseplate (Wright Medical), (**D**) Equinoxe Baseplate (Exactech Inc). (A, DJO® is a registered trademark of DJO, LLC in the U.S. and/or other countries. © 2020 DJO, LLC. Used with permission from DJO, LLC. All rights reserved. B, This image provided courtesy of Arthrex®, Naples, Florida 2021. C, Image reprinted with permission from Stryker Corporation. © 2021 Stryker Corporation. All rights reserved. D, Used with permission from © Exactech, Inc.)

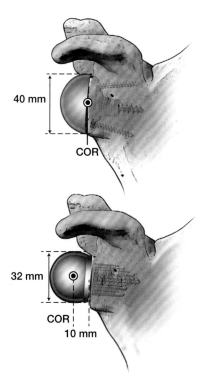

FIGURE 22.2 Illustrations demonstrating that a smaller glenosphere (32-mm diameter) has a 10-mm higher offset than the larger one (40-mm diameter), which has a 0-mm offset. A distinction should be made between the diameter and offset of glenosphere. COR, center of rotation.

did not.[7] They found a statistically significant improvement in ER in bone graft patients with an intact teres minor. In addition, there is evidence that patients with a severe ER deficit (<0°), who received glenospheres with 6 and 10 mm lateralization, experienced significant improvement in ER (>49°) without additional latissimus dorsi transfer.[67]

GLENOSPHERE INFERIOR OFFSET

Notching is a complication more commonly observed with earlier Grammont implants, with an incidence rate exceeding 50% in certain reports.[2,35,68-70] Increased awareness about this complication has led many surgeons to gravitate toward placing the glenosphere in an inferior position and at a 15° to 30° of inferior tilt/inclination, with the aim of increasing the impingement-free distance between the humeral component and scapular neck.[71] Although the effect of inferior glenosphere tilting on radiographic outcomes has not been supported clinically,[72] data suggest that an inferior COR position is associated with decreased scapular notching and improved adduction/abduction angles[48,73] (**FIGURE 22.4B** and **D**), as well as axial and sagittal ROM.[71] Gutierrez et al suggested that there is not one but several optimal glenosphere inclinations depending on the COR position of the component. For example, the most uniform distribution of forces (ie, the least baseplate rocking) for concentric (0 mm lateral, 0 mm inferior) and lateralized glenospheres was in inferior inclination, whereas it was in neutral for an inferiorly eccentric glenosphere.[74] Two studies evaluating the hierarchy of factors affecting impingement-free ROM demonstrated that inferior eccentricity was second only to glenosphere lateralization in maximizing abduction/adduction arc of motion.[27,30] In addition, radiographic evaluation comparing a 4-mm eccentric glenosphere to a concentric one showed that a 1-mm increase in inferior offset resulted in an improvement of 4° and 15° of ER and forward flexion (FF), respectively.[48] Nevertheless, the beneficial effects of inferior offset might level off after a certain degree of eccentricity.[47]

GLENOSPHERE SIZE

A larger glenosphere diameter may also improve functional outcomes. Berhouet et al examined ROM differences in 40 shoulder specimens following RTSA implantation with 36- and 42-mm glenospheres.[42] Their results indicated that the latter resulted in a 40° improvement in both ER and internal rotation (IR). Additionally, a computer modeling study assessing the effects of different implant configurations on impingement-free ROM showed that a larger glenosphere diameter was one of the factors that had the most significant effect on motion in all planes.[39] Clinical studies have demonstrated similar improvements in ROM. Müller et al reported that a 44-mm glenosphere size generated a 12° improvement in ER and an increase in abduction strength compared to the 36-mm size, at 1- and

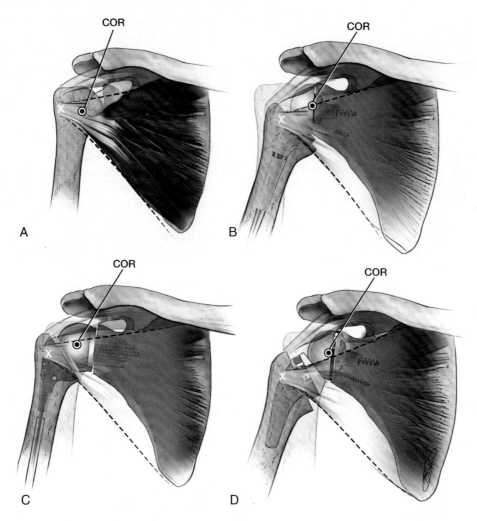

FIGURE 22.3 Illustration comparing the humerus position in different reverse shoulder arthroplasty designs to that in the normal shoulder. **A**, Normal shoulder; (**B**) Grammont-style design (medialized glenosphere and 155° stem); (**C**) lateralized glenosphere, 135° inlay stem; and (**D**) medialized glenosphere, 145° onlay stem. Note the change in position of the subscapularis muscle and deltoid wrapping with different designs. Design 2: The humerus is most medial and distal compared to the other designs. Design 3: The humerus is lateral (<than normal shoulder) but the least distalized among designs. Design 4: The humerus is lateral (<than normal shoulder) with a distalization between that of designs 2 and 3.

5-year follow-up intervals.[43] Furthermore, a study comparing functional scores and ROM differences between two groups of patients, one receiving a 42-mm glenosphere and the other a 38-mm glenosphere, found that the former experienced a 15° increase in FF and 6° increase in ER compared to the latter, with an overall improvement in pain scores.[44] In clinical practice, however, larger glenosphere diameters (ie, > 40 mm) are less commonly used, and the process of choosing the appropriate size is still surgeon dependent and is greatly influenced by patient sex and stature.[45] In addition, certain drawbacks have been described with larger glenospheres such as decreased IR[75] and higher PE volumetric wear rates.[76] On the other hand, ROM limitations associated with smaller glenosphere sizes may be offset by increased COR lateralization. A study evaluating the effect of smaller sized glenospheres in patients with severely limited ER < 0° showed that a size 32 mm (+10 mm lateralization) and size 36 mm (+6 mm lateralization) significantly improved ER.[68]

INLAY VERSUS ONLAY: LATERALIZATION

Stem design can be classified as either inlay or onlay depending on whether the humeral tray is inset in the proximal humeral metaphysis (inlay) or not (onlay). Nevertheless, this classification is not absolute and can be influenced by surgical technique (ie, an inlay stem may function as an inlay/onlay hybrid or onlay depending on how deep it is inset in the humeral metaphysis). The onlay stem was designed with the aim of preserving proximal humeral bone stock and increasing humeral lateralization,[33] which, in addition to that of the glenosphere, contributes to the global lateralization of the construct. This design, however, may also lead to humeral distalization[26] **(FIGURE 22.5)**. Another implication of lateralization is that it results in increased deltoid wrapping over the greater tuberosity, thereby increasing the joint compression forces on the construct, contributing to its stability.[27,61,77] In addition,

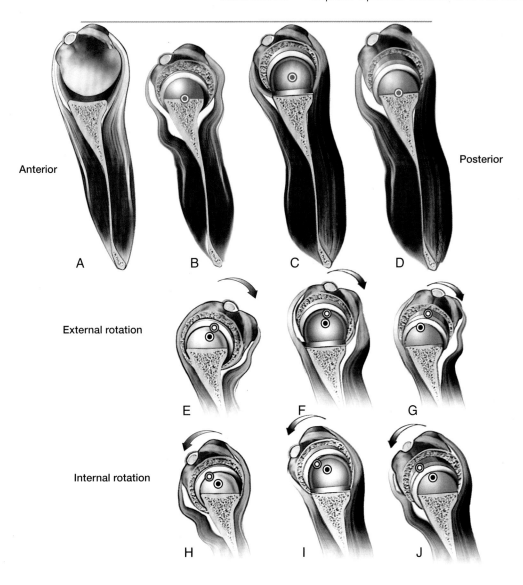

Anterior

Posterior

A   B   C   D

External rotation

E   F   G

Internal rotation

H   I   J

⊚ = Glenosphere center of rotation
◎ = Humeral center of rotation
⊙ = Stem center of rotation

FIGURE 22.4 Illustration showing how component lateralization improves rotator cuff tension. Compared to the normal shoulder (**A**), the least tension is observed with the medialized glenosphere and stem designs (**B**), whereas improved tension occurs with glenosphere (**C**) or glenosphere and stem lateralization (**D**). **E-J**, Demonstrate the effect of postoperative COR offset on rotator cuff balances during internal and external rotation. With an onlay stem, the humeral and stem COR are farther away from each other, resulting in a rotator cuff that is slack on one side and tight on the opposite side during rotational ROM (**G** and **J**). An inlay stem has a more anatomical COR offset (both the stem COR and humeral head COR overlap), resulting in balanced anterior and posterior cuff muscles during rotation when coupled with glenosphere lateralization (**F** and **I**). These benefits are lost with the use of a medialized glenosphere due to global slackening of the rotator cuff musculature (**E** and **H**).

humeral lateralization can increase rotator cuff muscle length and double the moment arm of the posterior rotator muscles[25] (**FIGURE 22.3D**).

Stem design also affects the positioning of the postoperative humeral COR (ie, its pivot point) relative to that of the native head, the distance between which is referred to as the COR offset.[78] With an inlay stem, the tray is inset within the proximal humeral metaphysis resulting in a more anatomical pivot point, closer to that of the native shoulder (**FIGURE 22.5**) As the distance

between the two pivot points increases (ie, with an onlay stem), the rotational arc of motion becomes nonanatomical, resulting in rotator cuff imbalances. **FIGURE 22.6** compares the effect of postoperative pivot point distance and location, from an axial view, of three different RSA constructs on rotator cuff balances during internal and external rotation. With an onlay stem, the two pivot points are farther away from each other resulting in a rotator cuff that is slack on one side and tight on the opposite side during rotational ROM. An inlay stem,

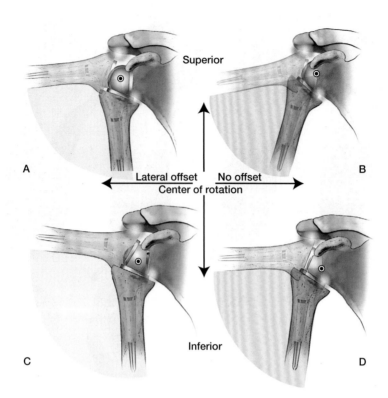

FIGURE 22.5 Illustration of the effects of glenosphere offset and positioning on impingement-free range of adduction/abduction motion for a 36-mm glenosphere diameter, a 150° humeral neck-shaft angle, and a neutral tilt. **A**, Superiorly positioned glenosphere with 10 mm of lateral offset. **B**, Superiorly positioned glenosphere with no offset. **C**, Inferiorly positioned glenosphere with 10 mm of lateral offset. **D**, Inferiorly positioned glenosphere with no offset. The shaded region represents impingement-free range of motion (ROM). The range of motion shown by the arrow represents the limits of the impingement-free ROM inferiorly and superiorly. Comparing the quadrants horizontally shows the effect of offset on arc of motion, whereas comparing quadrants horizontally shows the effect of superior inferior positioning of the center of rotation. Red zones are impingement locations between the humerus and scapula.

on the other hand, is expected to have a more anatomical pivot point and balanced anterior and posterior cuff muscles during rotation when it is coupled with glenosphere lateralization.

Clinical outcomes, on the other hand, have not shown a superiority of one stem design over the other. Merolla et al evaluated 2-year clinical and radiographic outcomes in 68 patients receiving either an inlay or an onlay stem design and observed that both implants provided similar postoperative clinical and functional outcomes.[6] The rates of radiographic risk factors such as scapular notching were higher with the inlay stem. However, this can be attributed to the fact that a 155° Grammont inlay stem was used in their study.

INLAY VERSUS ONLAY: DISTALIZATION

In addition to its lateralizing effect, stem design can also affect arm length[61,79,80] **(FIGURE 22.5D)**. Compared to the native shoulder, RTSA increases arm length by an average of 2.5 cm.[61,79] This increase, also reflected in an increase in acromiohumeral distance (AHD), may impact shoulder biomechanics. A computer simulation study evaluating the effects of different component configurations on muscle length showed that a 4.6-mm increase in AHD may double the length of the deltoid

muscle in abduction.[25] These results also showed that an additional 1 cm of lengthening was observed with the onlay stem compared to the inlay with the same NSA. When in excess, however, lengthening can increase the risk of iatrogenic nerve injuries and scapular spine fractures (SSFs).[78-80] A recent study evaluating the effect of stem design (inlay vs onlay) on the risk of SSF in 426 patients showed that lengthening, which was 10.4 mm higher in the onlay group, is a significant risk factor.[80] Radiographic measurements **(FIGURE 22.6)** from this study also demonstrate how implant design affects the spatial positioning of the humerus with respect to the scapula **(TABLE 22.2)**.

OTHER IMPLANT CONSIDERATIONS

Humeral Tray Offset

In addition to stem design, humeral tray offset may also influence ROM. A posterior offset position, which simulates the normal anatomical offset of the humeral head relative to the diaphysis in the anteroposterior plane, has been shown to maximize impingement-free ROM.[81] Berhouet et al evaluated the effects of five humeral tray positions (no offset and 5-mm offset in the anterior, posterior, medial, and lateral positions) on impingement-free ROM, as well as muscle lengths and moment arms.[82]

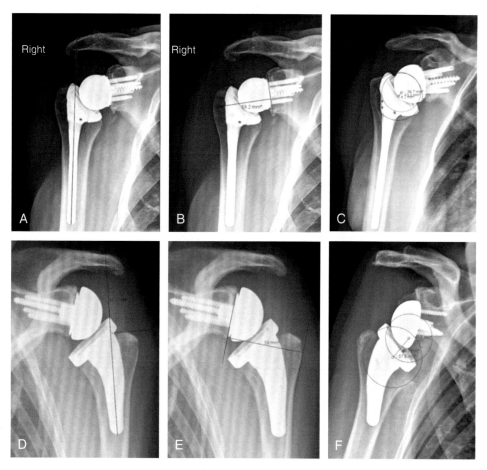

FIGURE 22.6 Radiographic measurements comparing distalization, lateralization, and center of rotation offset between inlay (**A-C**) and onlay designs (**D-F**). **A** and **D**, Acromiohumeral distance measured perpendicular to long axis of humerus. **B** and **E**, Lateralization of the humerus relative to the glenoid. **C** and **F**, Center of rotation offset.

They found that posterior tray offset decreases superior/inferior impingement and increases the subscapularis moment arm. Moreover, biomechanical evaluation also validated this improvement in ROM with posterior and posterolateral tray offset.[83] However, Dedy et al observed a 20° decrease in FF in three out of eight shoulders with a

posterior offset humeral cup and did not identify a difference between a concentric and posterior offset humeral tray.[84] This could possibly be explained, in part, by the fact that the authors used a medial glenosphere design with a 155° inlay stem compared to an onlay 135° stem used by Berhouet, indicating that the effects of tray offset may be influenced by stem design.

Cemented Versus Cementless Stems

Traditionally, RTSA implants were fixed using a cemented technique. Although the 10-year survival rate of cemented stems is 93%, a longer term complication with this type of fixation is stem loosening, which accounts for approximately 40% of revisions after 2 years.[85] In addition to the mechanical effects of loosening, it can also lead to decreased mid- to long-term functional outcomes. Our improved understanding of implant porous coating (ie, pore size: 100-400 μm, limits of micromotion: 150 μm), resulting in improved bony ingrowth, has limited the role of cemented stems in the primary setting.[86] Both cementless and cemented fixation appear to have comparable shorter term outcomes.[87] The advantages of cementless technique including less operative time, absence of cement-related complications,

TABLE 22.2 Radiographic Measurements for Inlay Versus the Onlay Stems

	AHD (mm)	Lateralization (mm)	Center of Rotation Offset (mm)
Inlay stem 1	31.4 ± 7.8	53.2 ± 6.2	12.5 ± 3.3
Inlay stem 2	31.5 ± 7.6	53.2 ± 7.4	8.6 ± 3.8
P-value	0.749	0.869	**<0.001**
Overall inlay	31.5 ± 7.7	53.1 ± 6.9	10.2 ± 4.0
Onlay stem	41.9 ± 9.9	57.0 ± 6.1	23.2 ± 3.8
P-value	**<0.001**	**<0.001**	**<0.001**

AHD, acromiohumeral distance; inlay stem 1 (Univers Revers; Arthrex, Inc); inlay stem 2 (AltiVate Reverse; DJO Inc; Dallas,TX).
P-values of <0.05 were considered significant (bold).

and the relative ease of revision support the use of this approach. Additionally, evidence suggests that there is no difference in terms of pain relief, tuberosity healing, component loosening, or notching between the two fixation methods when RTSA is used for the treatment of proximal humeral fractures.[88]

Long Stem Versus Short Stem

Earlier RTSA stem fixation relied on increased intramedullary diaphyseal purchase for stability. Advances in implant porous coating and improved bone ingrowth and fixation gave rise to newer short stems that rely more on metaphyseal fixation. The advantage of these stems is that they can be more bone preserving and have less risk of proximal humeral stress shielding.[89] Moreover, studies have demonstrated excellent survivorship of short-stemmed implants,[90] as well as lower incidences of revision and adverse radiographic outcomes with short porous-coated stems compared with long uncoated ones.[91] However, a main concern with short-stem RTSA is the potential for axial malalignment due to the mismatch in diameter between the humeral metaphysis and diaphysis, which makes it more challenging to achieve correct alignment along the humeral axis. A study evaluating the effect of short-stem RTSA implantation on the resultant NSA showed that 25% of stems were implanted with a NSA deviation of $> \pm 5°$ from the 145° NSA of the stem.[92] Eighty-five percent of malaligned stems were placed in valgus, corresponding to an NSA of $>150°$. This in turn can increase humeral medialization, thereby altering the biomechanics and outcomes that would be expected from a 145° stem.

Liner Constraint

RTSA is inherently more stable than a nonconstrained anatomic shoulder arthroplasty. Joint resistance measurements indicate that RTSA is more stable than both the intact shoulder and anatomic total shoulder arthroplasty, with a stability force ratio (maximum allowable subluxation force/joint compression force) that is more than twice that of the other two constructs.[26] RTSA stability appears to be multifactorial and is greatly affected by joint compression forces generated by passive and active stabilizers around the glenohumeral joint such as the rotator cuff and deltoid muscles.[26,58,93,94] Another important contributor to RTSA stability is liner constraint, defined as the ratio of liner depth to width. Constraint (ie, a deeper socket) can be achieved by either increasing the liner's peripheral rim thickness or by decreasing its central portion thickness, depending on design.[26] However, increasing liner constraint has been shown to have a variable impact on ROM. De Wilde et al showed that a 3-mm increase in PE depth resulted in 12° loss in ROM.[95] Conversely, another biomechanical

study indicated that maximal abduction ROM was not significantly different with varying degrees of constraint, signifying that terminal impingement might be tuberosity related rather than PE related.[96] While there has been conflicting data about the effects of constraint on impingement-free ROM, it has been suggested that combining constraint with glenosphere lateralization might improve the ROM that would be expected from constraint alone.[97] In addition, compared to nonconstrained liners, constraint does not appear to alter joint loads and deltoid forces.[96] As such, choosing constrained liners in the setting of RTSA instability is a viable option. Nevertheless, it should be noted that higher wear rates have been observed with these liners.[98]

CONCLUSION

RTSA is a versatile procedure that has become a very valuable part of our armamentarium for the treatment of glenohumeral pathologies. Many implant designs are available. However, the literature is still unclear about whether there is superiority of one design over another. It is probable that specific outcomes such as pain relief and ROM are impacted at the component level rather than across designs and that the best implant combination might be pathology specific. Consequently, understanding how these components affect outcomes is necessary for surgeons to develop the optimal surgical plan based upon the underlying pathology. The current literature related to the biomechanics and outcomes in patients undergoing RTSA emphasizes (1) the use of glenospheres with CORs closer to that of the normal shoulder (lateral offset) because they reduce the risk of notching as well as improve ROM and ER strength by retensioning the musculature around the shoulder leading to a more stable construct; (2) the use of a central lag screw to increase the baseplate compression in addition to the use of larger locking screws to improve glenosphere fixation; and (3) that the use of an onlay stem design may result in increased lengthening of the arm compared to an inlay stem design, which in turn may increase complications such as SSFs, and its use should be carefully evaluated in high-risk patients such as patients with osteoporosis.[99]

REFERENCES

1. Craig RS, Goodier H, Singh JA, Hopewell S, Rees JL. Shoulder replacement surgery for osteoarthritis and rotator cuff tear arthropathy. *Cochrane Database Syst Rev*. 2020;4(4):CD012879. doi:10.1002/14651858.CD012879.pub2
2. Boileau P, Watkinson D, Hatzidakis AM, Hovorka I. Neer Award 2005. The Grammont reverse shoulder prosthesis: results in cuff tear arthritis, fracture sequelae, and revision arthroplasty. *J Shoulder Elbow Surg*. 2006;15(5):527-540.
3. Donohue KW, Ricchetti ET, Iannotti JP. Surgical management of the biconcave (B2) glenoid. *Curr Rev Musculoskelet Med*. 2016;9(1):30-39.
4. Boileau P, Morin-Salvo N, Gauci MO, et al. Angled BIO-RSA (bony-increased offset–reverse shoulder arthroplasty): a solution for the management of glenoid bone loss and erosion. *J Shoulder Elbow Surg*. 2017;26(12):2133-2142.

5. Middernacht B, Van Tongel A, De Wilde L. A critical review on prosthetic features available for reversed total shoulder arthroplasty. *Biomed Res Int.* 2016;2016(2):1-9.

6. Merolla G, Walch G, Ascione F, et al. Grammont humeral design versus onlay curved-stem reverse shoulder arthroplasty: comparison of clinical and radiographic outcomes with minimum 2-year follow-up. *J Shoulder Elbow Surg.* 2018;27(4):701-710.

7. Greiner S, Schmidt C, Herrmann S, Pauly S, Perka C. Clinical performance of lateralized versus non-lateralized reverse shoulder arthroplasty: a prospective randomized study. *J Shoulder Elbow Surg.* 2015;24(9):1397-1404. doi:10.1016/j.jse.2015.05.041

8. Parry S, Stachler S, Mahylis J. Lateralization in reverse shoulder arthroplasty: a review. *J Orthop.* 2020;22:64-67.

9. Neer CI. *Shoulder reconstruction.* 1990:427-433.

10. Neer CS II, Watson KC, Stanton FJ. Recent experience in total shoulder replacement. *J Bone Joint Surg Am.* 1982;64(3):319-337.

11. Reeves BF, Jobbins B, Dowson D, Wright V. A total shoulder endo-prosthesis. *Eng Med.* 1972;1(3):64-67.

12. Reeves B, Jobbins B, Flowers F, Dowson D, Wright V. Some problems in the development of a total shoulder endo-prosthesis. *Ann Rheum Dis.* 1972;31(5):425.

13. Gérard Y, Leblanc JP, Rousseau B, Lannelongue J, Burdin P, Castaing J. Une prothèse totale d'épaule. *Chirurgie.* 1973;99(9):655-663.

14. Kölbel R, Friedebold G. Shoulder joint replacement. *Archiv fur Orthopadische und Unfall-chirurgie.* 1973;76(1):31-39.

15. Kolbel R, Rohlmann A, Bergmann G, Bayley I, Kessel L. *Biomechanical considerations in the design of a semi-constrained total shoulder replacement.* In: *Shoulder Surgery.* Springer; 1982:144-152.

16. Beddow FH, Elloy MA, Bayley I, Kessel L. *Clinical experience with the Liverpool shoulder replacement.* In: *Shoulder Surgery.* Springer; 1982:164-167.

17. Grammont P, Trouilloud P, Laffay JP, Deries X. Etude et réalisation d'une nouvelle prothèse d'épaule. *Rhumatologie.* 1987;39(10):407-418.

18. Baulot E, Sirveaux F, Boileau P. Grammont's idea: the story of Paul Grammont's functional surgery concept and the development of the reverse principle. *Clin Orthop Relat Res.* 2011;469(9):2425-2431.

19. Grammont PM, Baulot E. Delta shoulder prosthesis for rotator cuff rupture. *Orthopedics.* 1993;16(1):65-68.

20. Boulahia A, Edwards TB, Walch G, Baratta RV. Early results of a reverse design prosthesis in the treatment of arthritis of the shoulder in elderly patients with a large rotator cuff tear. *Orthopedics.* 2002;25(2):129-133.

21. Pupello D. *Origins of reverse shoulder arthroplasty and common misconceptions.* In: *Reverse Shoulder Arthroplasty.* Springer; 2016:3-18.

22. Guery J, Favard L, Sirveaux F, Oudet D, Mole D, Walch G. Reverse total shoulder arthroplasty: Survivorship analysis of eighty replacements followed for five to ten years. *J Bone Joint Surg Am.* 2006;88(8):1742-1747.

23. Zumstein MA, Pinedo M, Old J, Boileau P. Problems, complications, reoperations, and revisions in reverse total shoulder arthroplasty: a systematic review. *J Shoulder Elbow Surg.* 2011;20(1):146-157. doi:10.1016/j.jse.2010.08.001

24. Hamilton MA, Roche CP, Diep P, Flurin PH, Routman HD. Effect of prosthesis design on muscle length and moment arms in reverse total shoulder arthroplasty. *Bull Hosp Jt Dis (2013).* 2013;71(suppl 2):S31-S35.

25. Roche C, Flurin PH, Wright T, Crosby LA, Mauldin M, Zuckerman JD. An evaluation of the relationships between reverse shoulder design parameters and range of motion, impingement, and stability. *J Shoulder Elbow Surg.* 2009;18(5):734-741.

26. Gutiérrez S, Keller TS, Levy JC, Lee WE, Luo ZP. Hierarchy of stability factors in reverse shoulder arthroplasty. *Clin Orthop Relat Res.* 2008;466(3):670-676.

27. Gutiérrez S, Levy JC, Lee WE III, Keller TS, Maitland ME. Center of rotation affects abduction range of motion of reverse shoulder arthroplasty. *Clin Orthop Relat Res.* 2007;458:78-82.

28. Gutiérrez S, Levy JC, Frankle MA, et al. Evaluation of abduction range of motion and avoidance of inferior scapular impingement in a reverse shoulder model. *J Shoulder Elbow Surg.* 2008;17(4):608-615.

29. Gutiérrez S, Comiskey CA IV, Luo ZP, Pupello DR, Frankle MA. Range of impingement-free abduction and adduction deficit after reverse shoulder arthroplasty. Hierarchy of surgical and implant-design-related factors. *J Bone Joint Surg Am.* 2008;90(12):2606-2615.

30. Frankle M, Siegal S, Pupello D, Saleem A, Mighell M, Vasey M. The Reverse Shoulder Prosthesis for glenohumeral arthritis associated with severe rotator cuff deficiency: a minimum two-year follow-up study of sixty patients. *J Bone Joint Surg Am.* 2005;87(8):1697-1705.

31. Boileau P, O'Shea K, Moineau G, Roussane Y. Bony increased-offset reverse shoulder arthroplasty (BIO-RSA) for cuff tear arthropathy. *Operat Tech Orthop.* 2011;21(1):69-78.

32. Lädermann A, Denard PJ, Boileau P, et al. Effect of humeral stem design on humeral position and range of motion in reverse shoulder arthroplasty. *Int Orthop.* 2015;39(11):2205-2213. doi:10.1007/s00264-015-2984-3

33. Werthel JD, Walch G, Vegehan E, Deransart P, Sanchez-Sotelo J, Valenti P. Lateralization in reverse shoulder arthroplasty: a descriptive analysis of different implants in current practice. *Int Orthop.* 2019;43(10):2349-2360.

34. Sirveaux F, Favard L, Oudet D, Huquet D, Walch G, Mole D. Grammont inverted total shoulder arthroplasty in the treatment of glenohumeral osteoarthritis with massive rupture of the cuff: results of a multicentre study of 80 shoulders. *J Bone Joint Surg Br.* 2004;86(3):388-395. doi:10.1302/0301-620X.86B3.14024

35. Werner CM, Steinmann PA, Gilbart M, Gerber C. Treatment of painful pseudoparesis due to irreparable rotator cuff dysfunction with the Delta III reverse-ball-and-socket total shoulder prosthesis. *J Bone Joint Surg Am.* 2005;87(7):1476-1486. doi: 10.2106/JBJS.D.02342

36. Ernstbrunner L, Andronic O, Grubhofer F, Camenzind RS, Wieser K, Gerber C. Long-term results of reverse total shoulder arthroplasty for rotator cuff dysfunction: a systematic review of longitudinal outcomes. *J Shoulder Elbow Surg.* 2019;28(4):774-781.

37. Kwon YW, Pinto VJ, Yoon J, Frankle MA, Dunning PE, Sheikhzadeh A. Kinematic analysis of dynamic shoulder motion in patients with reverse total shoulder arthroplasty. *J Shoulder Elbow Surg.* 2012;21(9):1184-1190.

38. Helmkamp JK, Bullock GS, Amilo NR, et al. The clinical and radiographic impact of center of rotation lateralization in reverse shoulder arthroplasty: a systematic review. *J Shoulder Elbow Surg.* 2018;27(11):2099-2107. doi:10.1016/j.jse.2018.07.007

39. Virani NA, Cabezas A, Gutiérrez S, Santoni BG, Otto R, Frankle M. Reverse shoulder arthroplasty components and surgical techniques that restore glenohumeral motion. *J Shoulder Elbow Surg.* 2013;22(2):179-187.

40. Streit JJ, Shishani Y, Gobezie R. Medialized versus lateralized center of rotation in reverse shoulder arthroplasty. *Orthopedics.* 2015;38(12):e1098-e1103.

41. Collin P, Liu X, Denard PJ, Gain S, Nowak A, Lädermann A. Standard versus bony increased-offset reverse shoulder arthroplasty: a retrospective comparative cohort study. *J Shoulder Elbow Surg.* 2018;27(1):59-64.

42. Berhouet J, Garaud P, Favard L. Influence of glenoid component design and humeral component retroversion on internal and external rotation in reverse shoulder arthroplasty: a cadaver study. *Orthop Traumatol Surg Res.* 2013;99(8):887-894. doi:10.1016/j.otsr.2013.08.008

43. Müller AM, Born M, Jung C, et al. Glenosphere size in reverse shoulder arthroplasty: is larger better for external rotation and abduction strength? *J Shoulder Elbow Surg.* 2018;27(1):44-52. doi:10.1016/j.jse.2017.06.002

44. Mollon B, Mahure SA, Roche CP, Zuckerman JD. Impact of glenosphere size on clinical outcomes after reverse total shoulder arthroplasty: an analysis of 297 shoulders. *J Shoulder Elbow Surg.* 2016;25(5):763-771. doi:10.1016/j.jse.2015.10.027

45. Schoch BS, Vasilopoulos T, LaChaud G, et al. Optimal glenosphere size cannot be determined by patient height. *J Shoulder Elbow Surg.* 2020;29(2):258-265. doi:10.1016/j.jse.2019.07.003

46. Werner BS, Chaoui J, Walch G. Glenosphere design affects range of movement and risk of friction-type scapular impingement in reverse shoulder arthroplasty. *Bone Joint J.* 2018;100(9):1182-1186.

47. Choi CH, Kim SG, Lee JJ, Kwack BH. Comparison of clinical and radiological results according to glenosphere position in reverse total shoulder arthroplasty: a short-term follow-up study. *Clin Orthop Surg.* 2017;9(1):83-90. doi:10.4055/cios.2017.9.1.83

48. De Biase CF, Ziveri G, Delcogliano M, et al. The use of an eccentric glenosphere compared with a concentric glenosphere in reverse total shoulder arthroplasty: two-year minimum follow-up results. *Int Orthop.* 2013;37(10):1949-1955. doi:10.1007/s00264-013-1947-9

49. Chebli C, Huber P, Watling J, Bertelsen A, Bicknell RT, Matsen F III. Factors affecting fixation of the glenoid component of a reverse total shoulder prothesis. *J Shoulder Elbow Surg.* 2008;17(2):323-327.

50. Jasty M, Bragdon C, Burke D, O'Connor DA, Lowenstein J, Harris WH. In vivo skeletal responses to porous-surfaced implants subjected to small induced motions. *J Bone Joint Surg Am.* 1997;79(5):707-714.

51. Harman M, Frankle M, Vasey M, Banks S. Initial glenoid component fixation in "reverse" total shoulder arthroplasty: a biomechanical evaluation. *J Shoulder Elbow Surg.* 2005;14(1):S162-S167.

52. Formaini NT, Everding NG, Levy JC, Santoni BG, Nayak AN, Wilson C. Glenoid baseplate fixation using hybrid configurations of locked and unlocked peripheral screws. *J Orthop Traumatol.* 2017;18(3):221-228.

53. Lung TS, Cruickshank D, Grant HJ, Rainbow MJ, Bryant TJ, Bicknell RT. Factors contributing to glenoid baseplate micromotion in reverse shoulder arthroplasty: a biomechanical study. *J Shoulder Elbow Surg.* 2019;28(4):648-653.

54. Roche C, DiGeorgio C, Yegres J, et al. Impact of screw length and screw quantity on reverse total shoulder arthroplasty glenoid fixation for 2 different sizes of glenoid baseplates. *JSES Open Access.* 2019;3(4):296-303.

55. Humphrey CS, Kelly JD II, Norris TR. Optimizing glenosphere position and fixation in reverse shoulder arthroplasty, part two: the three-column concept. *J Shoulder Elbow Surg.* 2008;17(4):595-601.

56. Frankle MA, Teramoto A, Luo ZP, Levy JC, Pupello D. Glenoid morphology in reverse shoulder arthroplasty: classification and surgical implications. *J Shoulder Elbow Surg.* 2009;18(6):874-885.

57. Nigro PT, Gutiérrez S, Frankle MA. Improving glenoid-side load sharing in a virtual reverse shoulder arthroplasty model. *J Shoulder Elbow Surg.* 2013;22(7):954-962.

58. Frankle M. Rationale and biomechanics of the reverse shoulder prosthesis: the American experience. In: Frankle M, ed. *Rotator Cuff Deficiency of the Shoulder.* Thieme; 2008:76-104.

59. Gutiérrez S. *Reverse shoulder biomechanics: the research performed at the foundation for orthopaedic research and education (FORE).* In: *Reverse Shoulder Arthroplasty.* Springer; 2016:39-59.

60. Cuff D, Pupello D, Virani N, Levy J, Frankle M. Reverse shoulder arthroplasty for the treatment of rotator cuff deficiency. *J Bone Joint Surg Am.* 2008;90(6):1244-1251.

61. Roche CP, Diep P, Hamilton M, et al. Impact of inferior glenoid tilt, humeral retroversion, bone grafting, and design parameters on muscle length and deltoid wrapping in reverse shoulder arthroplasty. *Bull Hosp Jt Dis (2013).* 2013;71(4):284-293.

62. Denard PJ, Lederman E, Parsons BO, Romeo AA. Finite element analysis of glenoid-sided lateralization in reverse shoulder arthroplasty. *J Orthop Res.* 2017;35(7):1548-1555.

63. Keener JD, Patterson BM, Orvets N, Aleem AW, Chamberlain AM. Optimizing reverse shoulder arthroplasty component position in the setting of advanced arthritis with posterior glenoid erosion: a computer-enhanced range of motion analysis. *J Shoulder Elbow Surg.* 2018;27(2):339-349. doi:10.1016/j.jse.2017.09.011

64. Werner BS, Chaoui J, Walch G. The influence of humeral neck shaft angle and glenoid lateralization on range of motion in reverse shoulder arthroplasty. *J Shoulder Elbow Surg.* 2017;26(10):1726-1731. doi:10.1016/j.jse.2017.03.032

65. Ferle M, Pastor MF, Hagenah J, Hurschler C, Smith T. Effect of the humeral neck-shaft angle and glenosphere lateralization on stability of reverse shoulder arthroplasty: a cadaveric study. *J Shoulder Elbow Surg.* 2019;28(5):966-973.

66. Greiner S, Schmidt C, König C, Perka C, Herrmann S. Lateralized reverse shoulder arthroplasty maintains rotational function of the remaining rotator cuff. *Clin Orthop Relat Res.* 2013;471(3):940-946.

67. Berglund DD, Rosas S, Triplet JJ, Kurowicki J, Horn B, Levy JC. Restoration of external rotation following reverse shoulder arthroplasty without latissimus dorsi transfer. *JBJS Open Access.* 2018;3(2):e0054. doi:10.2106/JBJS.OA.17.00054

68. Farshad M, Gerber C. Reverse total shoulder arthroplasty – from the most to the least common complication. *Int Orthop.* 2010;34(8):1075-1082.

69. Lévigne C, Boileau P, Favard L, et al. Scapular notching in reverse shoulder arthroplasty. *J Shoulder Elbow Surg.* 2008;17(6):925-935.

70. Simovitch RW, Zumstein MA, Lohri E, Helmy N, Gerber C. Predictors of scapular notching in patients managed with the Delta III reverse total shoulder replacement. *J Bone Joint Surg Am.* 2007;89(3):588-600.

71. Li X, Dines JS, Warren RF, Craig EV, Dines DM. Inferior glenosphere placement reduces scapular notching in reverse total shoulder arthroplasty. *Orthopedics.* 2015;38(2):e88-e93.

72. Edwards TB, Trappey GJ, Riley C, O'Connor DP, Elkousy HA, Gartsman GM. Inferior tilt of the glenoid component does not decrease scapular notching in reverse shoulder arthroplasty: results of a prospective randomized study. *J Shoulder Elbow Surg.* 2012;21(5):641-646.

73. Nyffeler RW, Werner CM, Gerber C. Biomechanical relevance of glenoid component positioning in the reverse Delta III total shoulder prosthesis. *J Shoulder Elbow Surg.* 2005;14(5):524-528. doi:10.1016/j.jse.2004.09.010

74. Gutiérrez S, Walker M, Willis M, Pupello DR, Frankle MA. Effects of tilt and glenosphere eccentricity on baseplate/bone interface forces in a computational model, validated by a mechanical model, of reverse shoulder arthroplasty. *J Shoulder Elbow Surg.* 2011;20(5):732-739.

75. Langohr GD, Giles JW, Athwal GS, Johnson JA. The effect of glenosphere diameter in reverse shoulder arthroplasty on muscle force, joint load, and range of motion. *J Shoulder Elbow Surg.* 2015;24(6):972-979. doi:10.1016/j.jse.2014.10.018

76. Haggart J, Newton MD, Hartner S, et al. Neer Award 2017: wear rates of 32-mm and 40-mm glenospheres in a reverse total shoulder arthroplasty wear simulation model. *J Shoulder Elbow Surg.* 2017;26(11):2029-2037. doi:10.1016/j.jse.2017.06.036

77. Werthel JD, Schoch BS, van Veen SC, et al. Acromial fractures in reverse shoulder arthroplasty: a clinical and radiographic analysis. *J Shoulder Elbow Arthroplast.* 2018;2:2471549218777628.

78. Lädermann A, Lübbeke A, Mélis B, et al. Prevalence of neurologic lesions after total shoulder arthroplasty. *J Bone Joint Surg Am.* 2011;93(14):1288-1293. doi:10.2106/JBJS.J.00369

79. Lädermann A, Edwards TB, Walch G. Arm lengthening after reverse shoulder arthroplasty: a review. *Int Orthop.* 2014;38(5):991-1000. doi:10.1007/s00264-013-2175-z

80. Haidamous G, Lädermann A, Frankle MA, Gorman RA II, Denard PJ. The risk of postoperative scapular spine fracture following reverse shoulder arthroplasty is increased with an onlay humeral stem. *J Shoulder Elbow Surg.* 2020. doi:10.1016/j.jse.2020.03.036

81. Boileau P, Walch G. The three-dimensional geometry of the proximal humerus: implications for surgical technique and prosthetic design. *J Bone Joint Surg Br.* 1997;79(5):857-865. doi:10.1302/0301-620X.79B5.0790857

82. Berhouet J, Kontaxis A, Gulotta LV, et al. Effects of the humeral tray component positioning for onlay reverse shoulder arthroplasty design: a biomechanical analysis. *J Shoulder Elbow Surg.* 2015;24(4):569-577. doi:10.1016/j.jse.2014.09.022

83. Glenday J, Kontaxis A, Roche S, Sivarasu S. Effect of humeral tray placement on impingement-free range of motion and muscle moment arms in reverse shoulder arthroplasty. *Clin Biomech (Bristol, Avon).* 2019;62:136-143. doi:10.1016/j.clinbiomech.2019.02.002

84. Dedy NJ, Stangenberg M, Liem D, et al. Effect of posterior offset humeral components on range of motion in reverse shoulder arthroplasty. *Int Orthop.* 2011;35(4):549-554. doi:10.1007/s00264-010-1079-4

85. Bacle G, Nove-Josserand L, Garaud P, Walch G. Long-term outcomes of reverse total shoulder arthroplasty: a follow-up of a previous study. *J Bone Joint Surg Am.* 2017;99:454-461. doi:10.2106/JBJS.16.00223

86. Carpenter SR, Urits I, Murthi AM. Porous metals and alternate bearing surfaces in shoulder arthroplasty. *Curr Rev Musculoskelet Med.* 2016;9(1):59-66.

87. Wiater JM, Moravek JE Jr, Budge MD, Koueiter DM, Marcantonio D, Wiater BP. Clinical and radiographic results of cementless reverse total shoulder arthroplasty: a comparative study with 2 to 5 years of follow-up. *J Shoulder Elbow Surg.* 2014;23:1208-1214. doi:10.1016/j.jse.2013.11.032

88. Schoch B, Aibinder W, Walters J, et al. Outcomes of uncemented versus cemented reverse shoulder arthroplasty for proximal humerus fractures. *Orthopedics.* 2019;42(2):e236-e241.

89. Peduzzi L, Goetzmann T, Wein F, et al. Proximal humeral bony adaptations with a short uncemented stem for shoulder arthroplasty: a quantitative analysis. *JSES Open Access.* 2019;3(4):278-286.

90. Raiss P, Schnetzke M, Wittmann T, et al. Postoperative radiographic findings of an uncemented convertible short stem for anatomic and reverse shoulder arthroplasty. *J Shoulder Elbow Surg.* 2019;28(4):715-723.

91. Godenèche A, Garret J, Barth J, Michelet A, Geais L; Shoulder Friends Institute. Comparison of revision rates and radiographic observations of long and short, uncoated and coated humeral stem designs in total shoulder arthroplasty. *EFORT Open Rev.* 2019;4(2):70-76.

92. Abdic S, Athwal GS, Wittmann T, Walch G, Raiss P. Short stem humeral components in reverse shoulder arthroplasty: stem alignment influences the neck-shaft angle. *Arch Orthop Trauma Surg.* 2020:1-6. doi:10.1007/s00402-020-03424-4

93. Hansen ML, Routman H. The biomechanics of current reverse shoulder replacement options. *Ann Joint.* 2019;4:17.

94. Henninger HB, King FK, Tashjian RZ, Burks RT. Biomechanical comparison of reverse total shoulder arthroplasty systems in soft tissue–constrained shoulders. *J Shoulder Elbow Surg.* 2014;23(5):e108-e117.

95. De Wilde LF, Poncet D, Middernacht B, Ekelund A. Prosthetic overhang is the most effective way to prevent scapular conflict in a reverse total shoulder prosthesis. *Acta Orthopaedica.* 2010;81(6):719-726.

96. Abdulla I, Langohr DG, Giles JW, Johnson JA, Athwal GS. The effect of humeral polyethylene insert constraint on reverse shoulder arthroplasty biomechanics. *Shoulder Elbow.* 2018;10(1):25-31.

97. Gutiérrez S, Luo ZP, Levy J, Frankle MA. Arc of motion and socket depth in reverse shoulder implants. *Clin Biomech (Bristol, Avon).* 2009;24(6):473-479.

98. Carpenter S, Pinkas D, Newton MD, Kurdziel MD, Baker KC, Wiater JM. Wear rates of retentive versus nonretentive reverse total shoulder arthroplasty liners in an in vitro wear simulation. *J Shoulder Elbow Surg.* 2015;24(9):1372-1379.

99. Otto RJ, Virani NA, Levy JC, Nigro PT, Cuff DJ, Frankle MA. Scapular fractures after reverse shoulder arthroplasty: evaluation of risk factors and the reliability of a proposed classification. *J Shoulder Elbow Surg.* 2013;22(11):1514-1521.

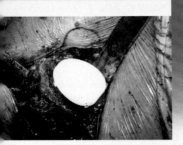

23 Operative Technique Using an Onlay Humeral Component

Kaveh R. Sajadi, MD

The reverse total shoulder arthroplasty (RTSA) designed in the 1980s by Dr. Paul Grammont medialized the center of rotation of the shoulder by moving it to the face of the glenoid. His design had three primary criteria—a medialized center of rotation, lengthening of the deltoid by lowering the humerus, and a convex glenoid (bearing side) with a concave supported humerus side. This design revolutionized the management of rotator cuff tear arthropathy. Problems with the design, however, began to appear with follow-up. The most common concerns with the original Grammont design have been scapular notching and instability. Scapular notching rates have been reported as high as 96%.[1] Though initially felt to be of unclear significance, numerous studies have associated notching with inferior clinical outcomes.[2-5] Instability, another common concern in RTSA, has been reported to occur at a rate between 1.5% and 31%.[6] Several modifications of Grammont's original design have been developed since, with most systems falling into three design categories, as described by Routman et al.[7] A prosthesis with the center of rotation 5 mm or less from the glenoid face was defined as a medialized glenoid, and those with the center of rotation more than 5 mm from the glenoid face were classified as lateralized glenoid (even with lateralized glenoids, the center of rotation is medial to a native shoulder). The three design categories are medialized glenoid and medialized humerus (original Grammont design); lateralized glenoid and medialized humerus; and medialized glenoid and lateralized humerus.

The medialized glenoid/lateralized humerus design offers several advantages. By medializing the glenoid, the center of rotation is placed on the face of the glenoid—allowing medialization of the center of rotation while minimizing glenoid shear forces, reducing the risk of loosening of the glenoid implant. By lateralizing the humerus, deltoid tension is optimized via the deltoid wrap angle. Deltoid wrapping refers to the wrapping of the middle deltoid around the greater tuberosity (**FIGURE 23.1**), resulting in increased humeral compression into the glenoid. This theoretically decreases the deltoid force needed to abduct the arm.[8] Humeral lateralization has also been shown in a cadaveric study to improve joint and muscle loading, by decreasing the

amount of deltoid force required for active abduction[9] while also improving tension on the remaining rotator cuff muscles, particularly with regard to external rotation. Humeral lateralization improves stability[10] as well as decreases scapular notching[11] and is achieved by decreasing the humeral neck angle from the Grammont design of 155° to a more anatomic humeral neck angle (145°). This allows an anatomic, bone-preserving osteotomy to be performed at the anatomic neck. Furthermore, an onlay design has a greater effect on humeral lateralization than modifying the humeral neck angle.[12] With use of an onlay prosthesis design, proximal humeral bone is preserved and lengthening of the humerus is achieved. In addition, with an onlay prosthesis, the glenosphere size is not limited to fitting within the proximal humerus as it is in an inlay system. Use of an onlay design makes a platform system ideal as well, making convertibility in a revision setting easier. In summary, an onlay, lateralized humerus design reverse system decreases scapular notching, improves stability, preserves proximal humeral bone, and allows for a platform stem while optimizing deltoid wrap, decreasing the deltoid force required to lift the arm, and maximizing tension on the remaining rotator cuff muscles (**VIDEO 23.1**).

EXPOSURE

Optimizing exposure does not start in the operating room. Preoperative factors to consider begin with the history and physical examination. Factors that make

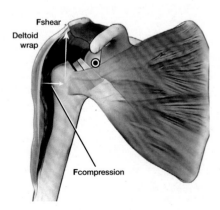

FIGURE 23.1 Illustration of deltoid wrap angle.

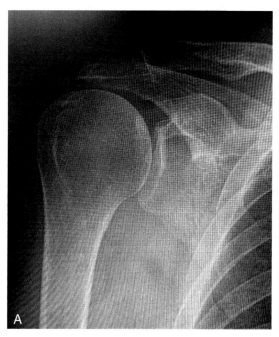
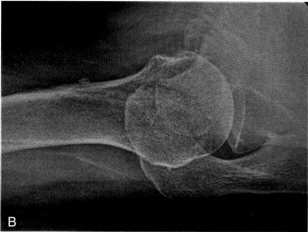

FIGURE 23.2 Preoperative radiographs of a 70-year-old man with long-standing shoulder pain and massive chronic rotator cuff tear. Patient is on chronic oral steroids and has failed nonoperative treatment including injections, medications, and physical therapy.

exposure more difficult or challenging include previous surgeries and scarring, altered postsurgical anatomy, and patient size. Previous operative reports should be reviewed for factors that could influence exposure. Truncal obesity can make adducting the arm difficult. Muscular patients can be challenging as well due to difficulty retracting the large, often noncompliant muscles.

Preoperative imaging should begin with standard radiographs, including an anteroposterior (AP) Grashey, a scapula lateral (Y or outlet view), and an axillary lateral/truth view **(FIGURE 23.2)**. At the discretion of the surgeon, a computed tomography (CT) scan in the plane of the scapula with 1 mm or less cuts with three-dimensional (3D) reconstruction can be beneficial, as it not only provides details of glenoid version and inclination but also allows assessment of bone stock and presence of bony defects or cysts which may require grafting. CT scan is also beneficial for templating and preoperative planning and/or navigation. Magnetic resonance imaging (MRI) can be beneficial to evaluate the rotator cuff preoperatively **(FIGURE 23.3)** but is not routinely ordered by the author. Routine laboratory studies are ordered, including hemoglobin A1c in diabetic patients. In addition, patients are given a preoperative prescription for topical benzoyl peroxide.

Operating room setup is critical for success. The operating table should be positioned such that the operative shoulder is rotated to the center of the room, allowing all surgical lights to be centered on the field. Adequate space for back table setup and position of assistants

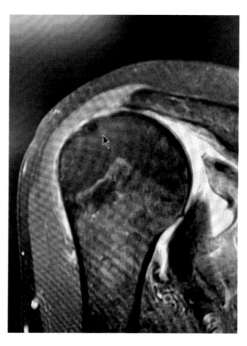

FIGURE 23.3 Preoperative magnetic resonance image (MRI) of the same patient confirming massive rotator cuff tear.

is essential **(FIGURE 23.4)**. Multiple commercial beach chair attachments are available, though not necessary. The head and neck must be positioned in neutral alignment, avoiding hyperextension or tilting of the neck, which may cause cervical nerve root compression. The patient is positioned in the beach chair position with their head/torso elevated approximately 30° and the

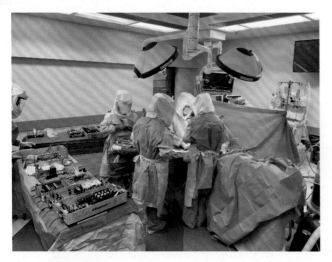

FIGURE 23.4 Operating room organization for reverse total shoulder arthroplasty (RTSA).

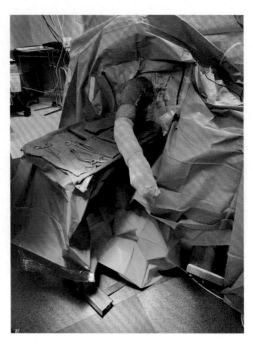

FIGURE 23.6 Arm prepped, draped, and positioned on padded Mayo stand.

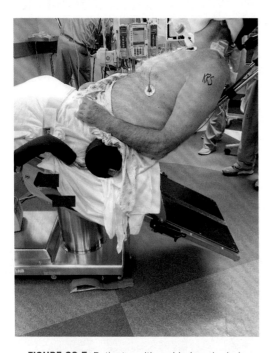

FIGURE 23.5 Patient positioned in beach chair.

lower extremities flexed at the hips and with a pillow under their knees to alleviate strain on the lumbar spine **(FIGURE 23.5)**. Using a Trendelenburg position, elevation of the head/torso, and flexion of the legs create a deep "V" which cradles the body and prevents sliding. If the patient is morbidly obese or has a large body habitus, the torso is elevated to a higher angle to ease positioning of the arm. A bolster may be placed under the medial scapula for support, and the arm should be completely free. It is essential to be able to extend, adduct, and externally rotate the humerus to allow vertical orientation of the humerus during humeral preparation and stem insertion. A body support or bolster placed on the operative side should be against the hip if possible so as

not to impede adduction/extension of the arm. Before prepping, the arm should be examined under anesthesia for range of motion and to ensure it can be positioned as necessary during the procedure. The entire arm should be prepped and draped. A pneumatic arm holder is helpful for positioning during the procedure, particularly if the surgeon has a limited number of surgical assistants. These arm holders, though expensive, have the advantage of not fatiguing and will also minimize crowding. When adequate assistants are present, the author prefers to use a padded Mayo stand, which should be draped to rest the arm upon during initial approach as well as glenoid exposure **(FIGURE 23.6)**.

Numerous skin preparation solutions are available. Patients are given a preoperative prescription for benzoyl peroxide to use for 3 to 5 days prior to the surgery.[13] On the day of surgery, the surgical area is shaved with electric clippers in the preoperative area. A chlorhexidine wipe is also administered to clean the surgical area. Anesthesia then performs the regional anesthetic. An indwelling interscalene catheter is utilized unless otherwise contraindicated. Once positioned in the operating room, the operative shoulder, axilla, and arm are wiped down with ethyl alcohol and then dried prior to prepping with chlorhexidine prep sticks. Recent studies suggest that the addition of hydrogen peroxide prior to chlorhexidine may reduce the *Cutibacterium acnes* load, though studies of the safety and efficacy of combinations of different preparation solutions are limited. Preoperative antibiotics are administered. The author's preference is appropriate weight-based first-generation cephalosporin followed by vancomycin to provide improved coverage of *C. acnes.* Prior to placement of surgical drapes, the indwelling interscalene nerve catheter is covered with a sterile blue towel to prevent drapes from adhering to it and causing it to be dislodged at the conclusion of the procedure. Draping should provide exposure from the area superior to the clavicle to several centimeters medial to the coracoid process anteriorly and allow posterior exposure to the medial edge of the scapula and full access to the arm. An iodine-impregnated drape is used to seal off the surgical field and to seal off the axilla.

The surgery can be performed with either general or regional anesthesia with sedation. The author's preferred technique is either general or sedation along with an indwelling interscalene catheter. Although paralytic agents may allow easier exposure, the author does not routinely use them but has anesthesia prepared to administer them, if necessary, in complicated or difficult exposures where complete muscle relaxation may be helpful.

The two most commonly performed surgical approaches are the superior approach and the deltopectoral approach. The superior approach, similar to an open rotator cuff approach, does allow for more direct glenoid exposure and potentially better stability through preservation of the subscapularis tendon if it is intact. However, it is not extensile and requires takedown and repair of the deltoid, which may compromise the deltoid if healing is impaired. The deltopectoral approach is the author's preferred approach for multiple reasons. First, it is more familiar to most orthopedic surgeons, especially with open rotator cuff repairs no longer routinely performed. Second, the approach is versatile, extensile, and revision friendly. Third, it does not compromise the deltoid origin or insertion, which is vital to the outcome of a reverse arthroplasty. Finally, if adjunctive muscle transfers are planned, they can be performed through the same incision.

The skin incision is made beginning at the lateral margin of the coracoid process and extends distally toward the deltoid insertion and 1 to 2 cm lateral to the axillary crease **(FIGURE 23.7)**. If extended, the incision should be on a path along the lateral edge of the biceps muscle, in line with the anterolateral approach to the humerus. Subcutaneous flaps are developed to create approximately 1.5 cm flaps on either side of the fat stripe **(FIGURE 23.8)**. The fat stripe may or may not contain or cover the cephalic vein due to variable anatomy. If the incision is made too lateral, one may be fooled by the fat stripe/raphe between the anterior and middle thirds of the deltoid. The correct fat stripe when followed proximally will lead to a trapezoidal area of fatty connective tissue that overlies the coracoid process. This location should be confirmed by palpation of the coracoid process, which has been referred to as the "lighthouse of the shoulder."[14] If the surgeon is having difficulty identifying the interval, it is best to begin at the coracoid process and progress

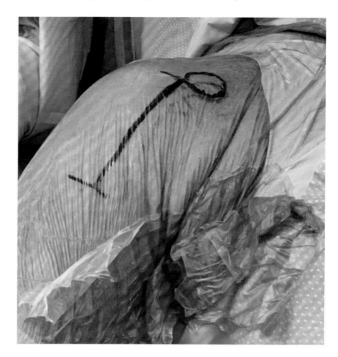

FIGURE 23.7 Surgical incision marked on iodine-impregnated drape.

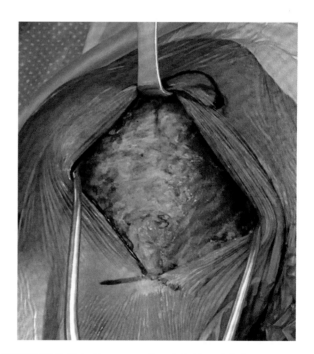

FIGURE 23.8 Fat stripe separating deltoid on left from pectoralis on right.

distally. Additionally, the deltoid and pectoralis muscles can be differentiated based on the direction of their muscle fibers, which can be accentuated by external rotation of the arm. The cephalic vein is exposed both to confirm its location and to protect it. It is then retracted either medially or laterally. Medial retraction has a decreased risk of injury as it crosses the interval proximally but

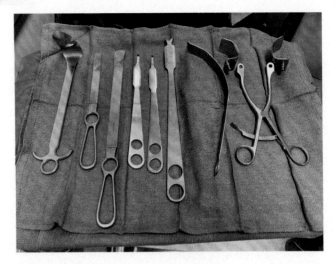

FIGURE 23.9 Common shoulder retractors, from left to right: Browne deltoid retractor; standard Darrach; extralarge Darrach; Hohmann retractors; forked-tip retractor; Bankart retractor; Kolbel self-retaining retractor with typical blades.

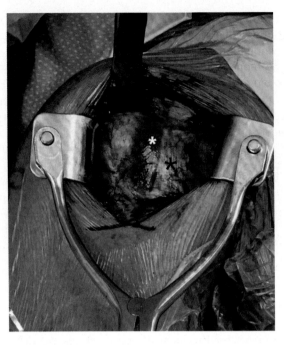

FIGURE 23.10 Retractors are deep to deltoid and pectoralis muscles. Black asterisk denotes the conjoined tendon. White asterisk denotes thin strip of muscle lateral to conjoined tendon and superficial to subscapularis.

requires more ligation of branches as there are more branches entering from the deltoid side. The vein actually often overlies the deltoid muscle and is not directly over the interval. This lends itself to mobilizing the vein laterally with the deltoid, which is the author's preferred approach. The deltopectoral interval is then developed by gentle dissection using Metzenbaum scissors with a gentle snipping technique to advance through the adventitial tissue separating the deltoid and pectoralis. Using this more precise method allows clearer differentiation of the interval with less muscular damage. A blunt elevator, such as a Cobb or Darrach **(FIGURE 23.9)**, is placed under the deltoid and over the proximal humerus. The subdeltoid and subpectoral spaces are bluntly developed to free adhesions. This mobilization is critical for improving mobility and for deep exposure to allow adequate mobilization of the humerus for later glenoid exposure. If a previous rotator cuff repair has been performed, particularly an open repair, extensive adhesions of the deltoid to the bursal tissue or proximal humerus may be present. Careful release of these adhesions is necessary for exposure and mobilization of the humerus. A blunt (Kolbel type) self-retaining retractor is placed under the deltoid and pectoralis muscles. Alternatively, a Browne deltoid retractor can be placed laterally under the deltoid, and a Richardson-type retractor is placed medially under the pectoralis muscle. Next, the clavipectoral fascia is opened on the lateral margin of the conjoined tendon. Often, a thin strip of muscle lies lateral to the tendon, and the fascia should be opened just lateral to this to preserve the muscle **(FIGURE 23.10)**. The fascia is opened proximally until reaching the coracoacromial (CA) ligament. It is the author's preference to preserve the CA ligament if possible. The Darrach or Cobb elevator is passed first over the supraspinatus fossa and

then over the infraspinatus fossa to release adhesions. It is then repositioned under the CA ligament, and the Kolbel retractor is then repositioned with the medial blade/retractor positioned deep to the conjoined tendon. Avoid excessive tension as this risks injury to the musculocutaneous nerve.

Next, the proximal ½ to 1 cm of pectoralis major tendon is released just medial to the long head of the biceps tendon. Pectoralis release allows exposure of the long head of the biceps and also facilitates posterior subluxation of the humerus during glenoid exposure. The biceps is then tenotomized or tenodesed based on surgeon preference. The author's preferred technique is soft-tissue tenodesis to the lateral edge of the pectoralis tendon using one to two figure-of-eight sutures with #2 braided nonabsorbable suture. If there is significant proximal migration of the humeral head, it may be necessary to release a little more pectoralis tendon to sufficiently mobilize the proximal humerus. Next, identify and cauterize the anterior humeral circumflex artery and its vena commitante (three sisters), which lie on the inferior margin of the subscapularis and serve as the dividing point between the upper two-third (tendinous portion) and the lower one-third (direct muscular insertion). The subscapularis may be chronically torn, but in many cases, the vessels and its inferior muscular portion remain intact.

The subscapularis, if present, may be released in three ways. A direct peel of the tendon allows for lengthening of the tendon if it is contracted and later repair is desired. Drill holes will need to be placed in the humerus prior

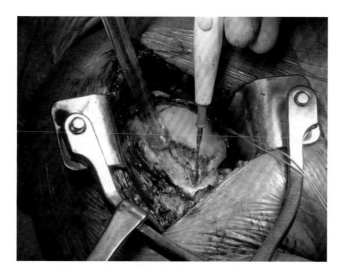

FIGURE 23.11 Release of inferior capsule on humerus.

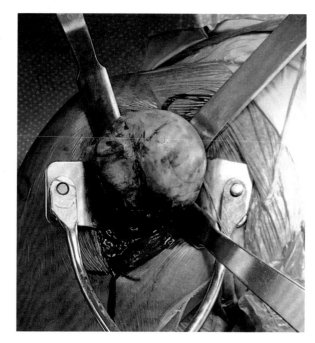

FIGURE 23.12 Dislocated humeral head ready for resection.

to stem placement if this is the desired technique. An osteotomy provides the theoretical advantage of bone to bone healing. If the osteotomy is too large, it may compromise metaphyseal stem fixation and stability. If it is too small, then it is similar to the peel technique. This technique also requires drill holes be placed prior to stem placement. Finally, tenotomy offers a reproducible technique with the ease of tendon to tendon repair. Outcomes of all three techniques are not significantly different in the literature[15]; therefore, the surgeon should use the same technique they utilize in anatomic total shoulder arthroplasty (ATSA). The author's preferred technique is a tenotomy performed approximately 1 to 1.5 cm medial to the lateral margin of the lesser tuberosity, leaving a robust cuff of tissue laterally for the repair while avoiding the musculotendinous junction medially. Tagging sutures are placed through the subscapularis tendon to control mobilization and later release of the anterior capsule. At least one suture is placed at the superior margin of the tendon to guide repair and restoration of anatomy. The rotator interval is then released in a lateral to medial direction to the anterosuperior glenoid and base of the coracoid process.

After release of the subscapularis tendon, the inferior capsule is released directly off the humerus. It is helpful to place a blunt retractor into the axillary recess to place the capsule under tension. Electrocautery is utilized to release the capsule directly off the inferior humeral neck while carefully externally rotating the arm to gain progressive posterior access **(FIGURE 23.11)**. The release is carried inferiorly to the superior edge of the latissimus tendon. The release is carried in a superior to inferior direction while an assistant progressively externally rotates the arm allowing the release to be carried from anterior/lateral to posterior/medial until at least 90° of external rotation is achieved. This is essential to allow posterior subluxation of the humerus for glenoid

exposure, to remove osteophytes, and to restore/improve postoperative range of motion. The axillary nerve is protected by use of the blunt retractor, use of electrocautery on coagulation setting, and keeping the electrocautery device directly on the humerus. Osteophytes should be removed from the anterior and inferior humerus to clearly identify the anatomic neck. Inferior and posterior osteophytes may also be removed after the humeral head osteotomy if they do not come off with the resected head.

The humeral head osteotomy may be performed with the humeral head reduced if there is adequate visualization of the entire humeral head, including the posterior insertion of the rotator cuff. For this technique, the arm is placed in a horizontal position, parallel to the floor, and the forearm is rotated to the desired degree of version (ie, 30° external rotation for a resection at 30° retroversion). The cut is then made perpendicular to the floor along the anatomic neck. The anatomic neck and angle can be identified with a guide specific to the implant system being used. The guide can be pinned to the humerus or used to mark the resection site with electrocautery.

The author's preferred technique is to dislocate the humeral head prior to osteotomy by bringing the humeral head anteriorly and extending, externally rotating, and adducting the arm **(FIGURE 23.12)**. The humerus should be oriented vertically at this point. The osteotomy may be carried out as above using a system-specific guide. Prior to performing the osteotomy, place a Hohmann-type retractor over the rotator cuff or more likely over the tuberosity if the rotator cuff is absent. A blunt extralarge Darrach-type retractor is placed on the posteromedial humeral neck and is used to lever the humeral head laterally. It is important to make certain any remaining bursa is removed and any adhesions in the subacromial space from previous surgeries, including rotator cuff repairs, are released to allow full mobility of the humerus. The supraspinatus is generally torn or absent when performing RTSA, and exploration and attempted repair is not indicated. However, it is important to preserve as much infraspinatus as possible to maximize postoperative external rotation function.

The humeral head should preferably be resected at the anatomic neck. If the osteotomy is too high, it will increase tension, overconstrain the joint, and limit glenoid exposure. Aggressive resection up to 5 mm distal to the anatomic neck will improve glenoid exposure, but care must be taken to avoid compromise of the posterior portion of the rotator cuff. The normal humeral version has been shown to vary from 10° to 50° of retroversion. Optimal version of the reverse implant has yet to be determined, but if the implant is placed in excessive retroversion, it may limit internal rotation; if placed in excessive anteversion, it may lead to instability. The author aims for approximately 20° to 30° retroversion to allow preservation of relatively normal anatomy while maximizing stability and postoperative internal rotation motion.

The normal humeral neck-shaft angle, the angle formed by the center line of the humeral head with the line of the humeral shaft, ranges from 115° to 148° with most falling between 130° and 140°.[16] RTSA humeral stems range from 135° to 155°. The original Grammont design utilized a 155° angle, but this design is associated with higher rates of scapular notching. Care should be taken to avoid an osteotomy that is too vertical to avoid loss of medial calcar support for the prosthesis. An excessive valgus cut may compromise the remaining rotator cuff. The author's preference for a lateralized onlay humerus system has been previously discussed. Therefore, a fixed-angle cutting guide (132.5°) is placed on the anatomic neck. Although the neck cut is 132.5°, the final construct once the implant is assembled is 145°. The guide has a version bar which is aligned with the forearm in the desired retroversion of approximately 20°. The guide is held or pinned, while the osteotomy is performed with a sagittal saw in an anterior to posterior direction. Once the head is resected, the author prefers to proceed with preparation and placement of the humeral implant or trial. However, the surgeon may elect to proceed to the humeral or glenoid side based on preference. If moving to the glenoid, a metaphyseal surface protector should be placed first.

The onlay humeral component technique is system specific. Choice of stem includes stemless (not currently available in the United States for reverse arthroplasty), short stem, and standard-length stem. Stems may be cemented or uncemented. Short humeral stems are bone

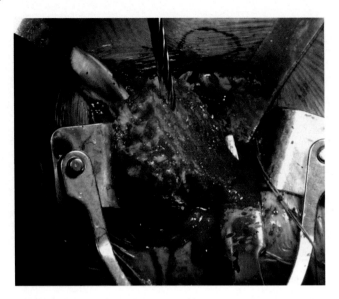

FIGURE 23.13 Humeral reamer entering in desired position, approximately 5 mm posterior and 5 mm medial to bicipital groove.

preserving and may prevent or minimize stress shielding leading to bone loss. The author utilizes short stems when bone quality permits, using an uncemented technique with occasional impaction bone grafting from the resected humeral head when necessary and very rarely will use cement.

The smallest available reamer is placed to enter the humeral canal. For ease of reaming and to minimize the risk of fracture, the humerus should be in as vertical a position as possible by a combination of adduction, extension, and external rotation. Proper patient positioning is essential to achieve this humeral position and to avoid excessive force on the humerus. The starting point is just posterior to the bicipital groove, approximately 5 mm medial to the supraspinatus tendon insertion **(FIGURE 23.13)**. The reamer should easily advance into the canal. Reaming is carried out by hand as power reamers increase the risk of fracture. When using a standard-length stem, reaming progresses until solid endosteal contact is made, with the reamer inserted to the appropriate depth as marked on the reamer. Reaming is followed by careful broaching up to the size of the largest reamer. With short humeral stems, generally only an initial reaming is performed followed by broaching to the appropriate size. The broach must be aligned with the desired implant version **(FIGURE 23.14)**. A version guide is available on the broach attachment. The final broach chosen should fit solidly in the metaphysis and achieve secure rotational stability. With the short stem, care should be taken to avoid varus or valgus seating of the implant. Once the appropriate size is chosen, a stem trial may be placed, but the author prefers to seat the final stem at this point **(FIGURE 23.15)**. If the humerus is between sizes, select the smaller size and consider impaction-grafting, utilizing cancellous autograft

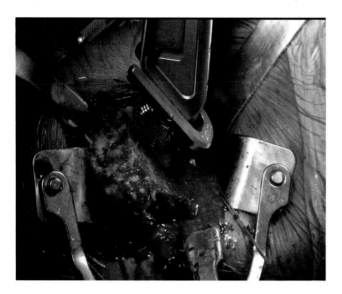

FIGURE 23.14 Humeral broaching.

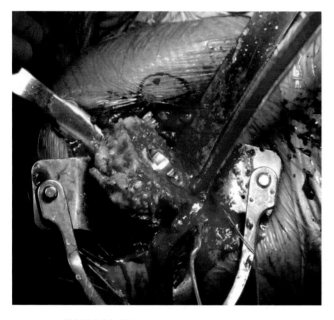

FIGURE 23.15 Final humeral stem in place.

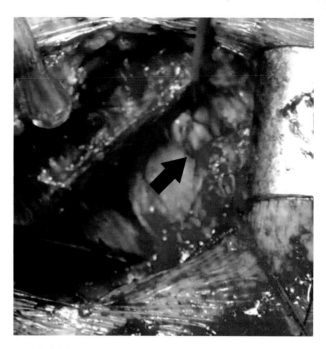

FIGURE 23.16 Anterior capsule reflection between the anterior labrum and subscapularis, marked with the arrow.

obtained from the resected humeral head. This can be obtained with a rongeur and placed along the medial calcar as the final stem is impacted. Rarely, if this is insufficient, cement can be used. In these situations, I prefer to place cement only around the proximal metaphyseal portion. Once the stem is seated, place a stem protector if moving to the glenoid component or begin trial reductions if the glenoid has already been placed.

Glenoid exposure begins with the steps previously mentioned during exposure, including positioning, skin incision, and the initial components of the deltopectoral approach. At this stage, a large, wide, blunt retractor (the author uses an extralarge Darrach because it is relatively straight, but alternatives include a Wolfe, Fukuda,

etc.) is placed over the cut humeral surface and placed around the posterior lip of the glenoid. It is helpful when performing this to bring the arm in a forward flexed position in relatively neutral rotation. This retractor is used to retract the proximal humerus posteriorly. The arm at this point is best rested on the padded Mayo stand. Next, a Hohmann-type retractor is placed over the superior labrum/biceps anchor, just posterior to the coracoid process. If not already done, the rotator interval should be released to the base of the coracoid process. The author prefers to use the bovie on coagulation setting due to the vascularity of the interval, particularly near the base of the coracoid. Pulling anteriorly and laterally on the subscapularis tendon tag sutures allows visualization of the anterior capsular reflection (**FIGURE 23.16**). The anterior capsule is then released along the entire anterior glenoid rim between the subscapularis and the anterior labrum to both mobilize the subscapularis tendon and to expose the anterior glenoid neck. By releasing just anterior to the labrum, capsule may be preserved on the undersurface of the subscapularis, which helps to thicken the tendon and improves suture pullout strength when repairing this tendon. After releasing the anterior capsule, gently slide a blunt flat retractor (Darrach) along the anterior neck of the scapula to release adhesions of the subscapularis muscle for additional mobilization. Place an anterior retractor, such as a Bankart-type pointed retractor, on the anterior glenoid (**FIGURE 23.17**). At this point, removing the Kolbel self-retaining retractor may be helpful, relieving tension from the deltoid and the conjoined tendon allowing greater posterior retraction of the proximal humerus

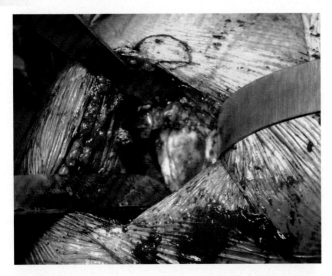

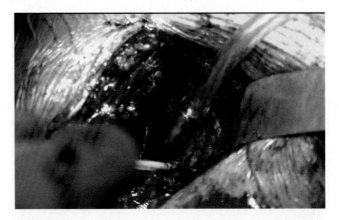

FIGURE 23.18 Inferior capsular release on glenoid with Darrach retractor depressing the inferior capsule and protecting the axillary nerve.

FIGURE 23.17 Placement of glenoid retractors, after removal of Kolbel retractor, prior to excision of labrum and capsular release.

and anterior retraction of the conjoined tendon, enhancing glenoid exposure. Elevate the operative table—this allows the arm/humerus to fall a little more posterior further facilitating glenoid exposure. However, if only the head of the bed is elevated, not the entire table, this may change the orientation of the glenoid, so maintain awareness of these changes to prevent malposition or malrotation of the glenoid implant.

Excise the labrum, including the biceps remnant. Generally, this is performed from superior to inferior, beginning anteriorly or posteriorly. I prefer to use the electrocautery for labrum excision, on "cut" above the equator of the glenoid and on "coag" below the equator to warn of proximity to the axillary nerve. The capsular release is generally more aggressive in RTSA than ATSA, particularly posteriorly. The inferior capsular release is also very important to allow visualization of the inferior glenoid margin for proper glenoid baseplate placement and to facilitate postoperative range of motion. A flat, blunt elevator (Darrach) is used to tension the inferior capsule, and the capsule is released with the electrocautery at the inferior glenoid margin from anterior to posterior (**FIGURE 23.18**). The capsular release should extend up to 1 cm along the inferior glenoid neck up to the insertion of the long head of the triceps tendon. The inferior glenoid must be fully visualized to ensure proper placement of the implant and minimize scapular notching. Excise any remaining bursal tissue as well as torn rotator cuff tendons to finalize the glenoid exposure.

At this time, the surgeon should be able to see the entire glenoid face and appreciate any wear pattern (**FIGURE 23.19**). Palpation of the anterior glenoid neck is useful for orientation and approximation of the version of the glenoid. If using navigation, once the glenoid exposure is complete, the necessary tracking components can be inserted. Navigation is described in Chapter 10.

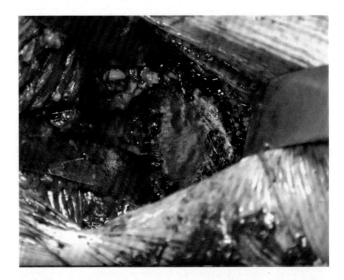

FIGURE 23.19 Desired glenoid exposure after capsular release.

If glenoid exposure is inadequate at this time, it should be addressed by rechecking each step above, beginning with adequate subdeltoid and subacromial mobilization and confirming adequate inferior humeral capsular release. These measures allow posterior retraction of the proximal humerus. Next, assess the humeral head resection to ensure it is adequate and all osteophytes have been removed. If necessary, an additional resection of the humerus of up to 5 to 10 mm below the anatomic neck may be performed if other steps are not successful in achieving the desired exposure. Additionally, ensure complete capsular release from the glenoid margin and reposition the glenoid retractors. Additional steps to improve glenoid exposure include release of additional pectoralis major tendon, particularly if there has been long-standing proximal humeral migration. Finally, if the patient is not already completely relaxed, anesthesia can use additional agents to relax muscle tension which will improve exposure.

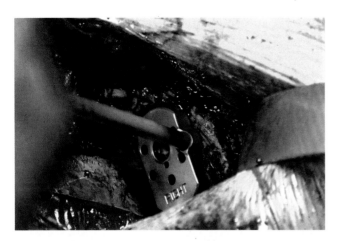

FIGURE 23.20 Proper placement of drill guide on glenoid face.

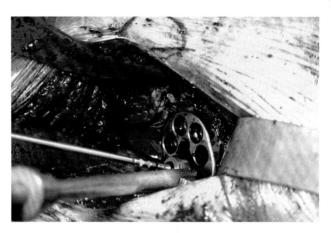

FIGURE 23.21 Drill trajectory for inferior screw placement on baseplate.

Glenoid preparation follows implant-specific instructions. The goal of baseplate positioning is to avoid superior tilt to minimize shear forces and achieve inferior overhang of the glenosphere to minimize scapular notching. Scapular notching has been a pervasive problem in RTSA, reported in up to 96% of cases.[1] Initially, it was not felt to be of clinical significance; however, recent studies[2-5] have shown it is associated with inferior outcomes. Although scapular notching can be related to implant design, it can be minimized by inferior tilt of the glenoid implant, inferior overhang of the glenosphere,[17] increased glenosphere size, or lateralization of the glenosphere either by implant design or placement. Of these measures, inferior overhang is the most effective.[18] To maximize inferior placement of the glenoid component and inferior overhang, it is essential to expose the inferior glenoid margin. This is facilitated by release of the inferior capsule. Careful assessment of preoperative imaging is critical to avoid inadvertent superior tilt of the glenoid implant due to unrecognized or unappreciated superior wear.

The drill guide for the glenoid is aligned so that the inferior margin of the prosthesis will sit at or 1 to 2 mm below the inferior margin of the glenoid to allow inferior overhang of the glenosphere **(FIGURE 23.20)**. The guide is utilized to drill a pilot hole to place glenoid reamers. Many systems allow both freehand and cannulated methods for glenoid preparation. The author prefers freehand in most situations. The glenoid is then gently reamed to a flat surface with care to preserve as much subchondral bone for support as possible. The goals of reaming are to remove any remaining articular cartilage, to create a flat surface to optimize contact with the backside of the baseplate, and to restore alignment. Palpation of the anterior neck of the glenoid can help with orientation for the appropriate angle of reaming. Due to the conical shape of the glenoid, aggressive reaming will quickly lead to insufficient bone for adequate implant support. It is safest to start the reamer slowly just prior to contacting the bone (ie, start just off the bone) to minimize fracture risk. Reaming begins with the smallest diameter reamer and proceeds to the anticipated diameter of the glenosphere. It is critical to ream to the diameter of the glenosphere to remove any osteophytes or other bony impingements that may prevent seating of the glenosphere. Further reaming is not possible once the glenoid base plate is seated.

Next, the baseplate is implanted on the glenoid. Numerous baseplate designs are available, with variations in baseplate shape (round vs oval), backside geometry (flat vs curved), central fixation (post vs screw), surface finish and coatings (grit-blasted, porous-coated), and position, diameter, and size of peripheral screws, as well as locking versus nonlocking compression screws. Regardless of the system used, it is essential to achieve proper position and to maximize glenoid bone support for the implant. The inferior margin of the baseplate should align with the inferior glenoid, allowing the glenosphere to overhang, minimizing scapular notching. An oval baseplate allows fixation of the central post or screw in the center of the glenoid vault, with the best bone, while still aligning the inferior baseplate with the inferior glenoid. Placement of screws further enhances the stability of the construct. The inferior screw is biomechanically the most important and is placed first.[19] It should be directed into the inferior neck/pillar of the scapula **(FIGURE 23.21)**. Placing the inferior screw first further minimizes the risk of superior tilt of the baseplate. The superior screw is directed toward the base of the coracoid. One anterior and one posterior screw are placed in a converging configuration to maximize bone purchase and length, with care to avoid the central post or screw. If the system has locking caps, these are placed next. If there are locking screws into the baseplate, these are secured. Next, the appropriate size glenosphere trial or definitive implant is placed and trialing proceeds. Full exposure of the glenoid is essential to ensure proper seating of the glenosphere. Repositioning of retractors

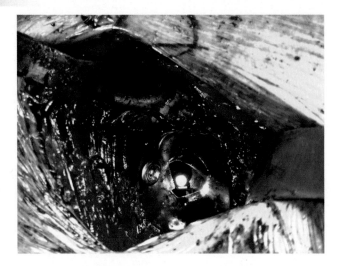

FIGURE 23.22 Final glenosphere in place.

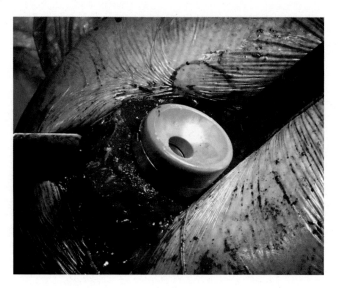

FIGURE 23.23 Trial humeral tray and polyethylene.

may be necessary to prevent the retractors from blocking seating. The final implant is secured with either a screw or via Morse taper, depending on the specific system utilized (**FIGURE 23.22**).

ASSESSING AND ACHIEVING STABILITY

Trialing is a critical step for ultimate success. If the construct is too loose, it may result in instability or inadequate tension to restore deltoid function. Instability has been one of the most common complications of RTSA.[6] If it is too tight, the risk of neurovascular complications increases, there is a possible increased risk of acromial or scapular spine stress fractures, and the increased tension could potentially cause pain in soft tissues, such as the conjoined tendon. I begin trialing with the shortest humeral trial (polyethylene and humeral liner tray) and begin with an unconstrained polyethylene (**FIGURE 23.23**).

After the trials are assembled, the shoulder is reduced (**FIGURE 23.24**). Ideally, this should require some distraction to reduce, often with an audible or palpable clunk. With the arm adducted at the side, there should be some tension on both the conjoined tendon and the deltoid. The arm is then taken through a range of motion to assess motion, stability, and impingement. The goal is to maximize passive impingement-free range of motion while maintaining stability. Begin with forward elevation and abduction, assessing maximal range and ensuring the joint is stable, and there is no impingement on the surrounding structures. Next, assess internal rotation and external rotation at both 0° and 90° for stability. Maximum external rotation may produce some posterior impingement but should not cause instability. Finally, adduct, extend, and externally rotate the arm. This is the position at highest risk of dislocation (ie, a patient pushing themselves out of bed or a chair), and the construct should remain stable.

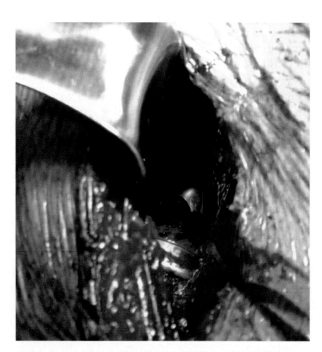

FIGURE 23.24 Trial humeral adaptor plate and polyethylene insert reduced onto the glenosphere.

If the trial construct is too loose or instability is a concern, additional length can be added to the polyethylene and liner tray sequentially until a stable construct is reached. Depending on the system utilized, lengthening of up to 17.5 mm can be obtained. This is another advantage of an onlay system, which is not limited by the proximal humeral anatomy. Length should be added prior to defaulting to a constrained liner. Constrained liners, although inherently more stable, may limit range of motion and increase stress on the glenoid implant-bone interface and may also increase the risk of scapular notching. If the construct is too loose, another option is to use a

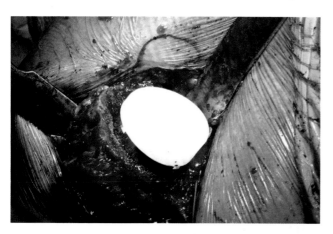

FIGURE 23.25 Final onlay humeral component.

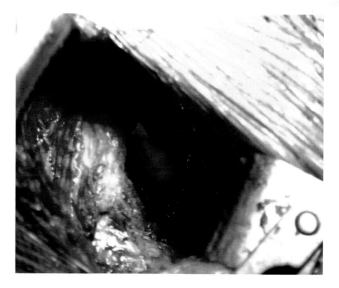

FIGURE 23.26 Final components reduced.

larger diameter glenosphere. Finally, if there is significant humeral bone loss or shortening, consider use of a tumor-type prosthesis or megaprosthesis to restore length and offset, though this is unlikely in the primary arthroplasty setting and more likely with revision surgery.

After reduction, if the trial construct is too tight, range of motion may be limited or excess tension may be placed on the deltoid, conjoined tendon, or neurologic structures. If the supraspinatus is intact, releasing the anterior margin may relieve some tension. A more extensive release of an intact supraspinatus tendon can be considered, but it is essential to avoid compromise of the infraspinatus insertion to preserve external rotation. If these soft-tissue releases do not adequately relieve tension, then it may be necessary to remove the stem or trial and resect additional proximal humerus. Another alternative is consideration of a smaller glenosphere if the final component has not yet been placed. It is essential that all necessary steps be taken to achieve a stable construct without excessive tension. Once trialing is complete, the final components are assembled. The humeral component may be assembled in situ or as a back-table assembly and then inserted en bloc. The author generally assembles the implant in situ **(FIGURES 23.25 and 23.26)**.

CLOSURE

The wound is copiously irrigated using either a bulb syringe or pulsatile lavage system. Sterile saline solution is utilized with the addition of Betadine.[20] Antibiotic-laden solutions have fallen out of favor with little evidence of efficacy. If repairable, the subscapularis is repaired at this time based on surgeon preference. Proponents of repair point to improvement in internal rotation as well as stability.[10,21] Those opposed to repair, or who debate its importance, note that it is often not repairable due to humeral lateralization or lengthening, and the vector of the subscapularis tendon has changed and may, in fact, inhibit deltoid function as it is now more of an adductor.[22] Lost in the discussion, however, is the role

of implant design. In the study by Edwards, the implant studied is a medialized glenoid and medialized humerus design with a 155° neck-shaft angle. In this study, subscapularis repair was significantly associated with less instability. In the meta-analysis by Matthewson et al, the overall pooled data found statistically significantly more dislocations in the group without subscapularis repair than with repair. When the data were stratified by implant design, however, the results varied. For medialized humerus/medialized glenoid designs, subscapularis repair decreased the dislocation rate. With lateralized implants, either humeral or glenoid lateralization, there was no difference in the dislocation rate with or without subscapularis repair. Furthermore, the lateralized implants showed fewer dislocations than the medialized design overall, whether the subscapularis was repaired or not. Finally, when the authors separated onlay design implants from inlay, the onlay design had a significantly lower risk of dislocation. In summary, subscapularis repair may only play a role in stability with medialized humerus/medialized glenoid designs. The author will repair the subscapularis only when it is robust and easily repairable in an effort to potentially improve internal rotation, though in his experience it is often not repairable or already torn.

The technique of subscapularis repair is based upon how it was released during exposure. Both subscapularis peel and lesser tuberosity osteotomy will require drill holes in the proximal humerus for repair, and these should be performed prior to final implant placement. It is also helpful to pass the sutures around the implant for added security. Mason-Allen suture technique provides increased pullout strength. When repaired, the author performs tendon-tendon repair using a combination of mattress and Mason-Allen sutures with braided nonabsorbable #2 sutures. Unlike in anatomic arthroplasty, the rotator interval is not closed.

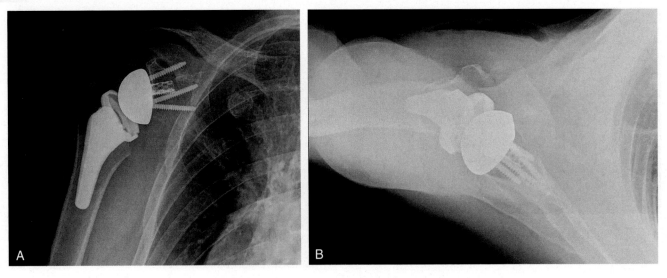

FIGURE 23.27 A and B, Postoperative radiographs.

Although blood transfusion after primary shoulder arthroplasty is uncommon, hematoma formation is a common complication after RTSA and may complicate wound healing and rehabilitation, as well as be a risk factor for infection. Tranexamic acid (TXA) has been shown to be a benefit in shoulder arthroplasty.[23-32] The most recent American Academy of Orthopaedic Surgeons (AAOS) Clinical guideline on glenohumeral joint arthritis found that clinical studies and meta-analyses "have concluded that administration of TXA was associated with a significant reduction in the postoperative change in hemoglobin concentration, drain output, total blood loss, and a trend toward reduction in rate of blood transfusions."[33] One of the referenced meta-analyses also found no difference in complication rates of thromboembolic events with use of TXA.[32] I prefer use of TXA as an intravenous dose before the procedure with a second dose as closure begins. Routine use of closed-suction drains is not utilized due to lack of evidence of benefit and evidence that shows an increased risk of transfusion and increased length of stay.[34] Vancomycin powder has not been well studied in the shoulder and is not routinely used but may be considered in high-risk patients.

Once the subscapularis repair (if performed) is complete, and the postoperative safe range of motion is assessed, the deltopectoral interval is loosely approximated with #0 absorbable suture, preferably under the cephalic vein to help with easier identification of the vein if revision surgery becomes necessary. The subcutaneous layer is closed with 2-0 absorbable suture, and the skin closed with a running subcuticular absorbable suture with fibrin glue to seal the wound. A waterproof, silver-impregnated bandage is applied. Patients may begin showering over the bandage once the indwelling nerve catheter is removed, which is usually 3 to 4 days after surgery. The bandage is removed at the first postoperative visit. Postoperative radiographs are obtained (**FIGURE 23.27**).

The procedure is performed as either an outpatient or overnight stay. Most patients spend one night in the hospital, and a very small percentage of patients, usually elderly patients that live alone, may go to a skilled nursing facility or rehabilitation facility. For the author's patients, rehabilitation begins on the day of surgery with instructions in sling management, activities of daily living, and exercises. A sling is worn for 6 weeks. Patients are allowed and encouraged to perform active range of motion exercises of the elbow, wrist, and hand, as well as active scapula retractions. Passive range of motion of the shoulder is performed by the patient and/or family support, with forward elevation in the plane of the scapula as tolerated, with no limit. Passive external rotation is allowed to 30° or the limits as determined by the subscapularis repair, if performed. Passive internal rotation is performed to the chest. At 6 weeks, the sling is discontinued and active range of motion of the shoulder is initiated along with formal outpatient physical/occupational therapy for range of motion, without limitations to the motion. At 12 weeks, a strengthening program is initiated. Patients are evaluated at 6 months follow-up with radiographs, then at 1 year, and then at 2-to 5-year intervals thereafter.

CONCLUSION

RTSA has revolutionized the management of rotator cuff tear arthropathy, as well as improved outcomes for many shoulder conditions with limited alternatives. Survival rates for RTSA now approach anatomic arthroplasty. Surgical exposure is key to optimal implant placement and reduction of complications and can be achieved with careful attention to the exposure steps above. Use of an onlay design prosthesis for the humerus offers several advantages. First, an onlay design allows a bone-preserving, anatomic neck cut with preservation of the metaphysis. Second, the onlay design has a greater effect on humeral lateralization than altering the neck-shaft angle, and humeral lateralization improves the deltoid wrap angle, decreasing the deltoid force required for abduction, and improves rotator cuff tension. Third, the glenosphere size is not limited to fitting within the proximal humerus anatomy, allowing potentially larger glenospheres, which may improve range of motion and stability. Fourth, it allows a platform stem, which can easily be converted in a revision setting. Fifth, again due to the humeral lateralization it provides, it reduces scapular notching, the most common complication of RTSA. Finally, also due to its humeral lateralization, the onlay design reduces instability independent of reparability of the subscapularis tendon. The onlay humeral design, along with a medialized glenosphere, allows optimal clinical outcomes while minimizing the two most common complications of RTSA, scapular notching and instability.

REFERENCES

1. Friedman RJ, Barcel DA, Eichinger JK. Scapular notching in reverse total shoulder arthroplasty. *J Am Acad Orthop Surg.* 2019;27(6):200-209.
2. Sirveaux F, Favard L, Oudet D, Huquet D, Walch G, Molé D. Grammont inverted total shoulder arthroplasty in the treatment of glenohumeral osteoarthritis with massive rupture of the cuff. Results of a multicentre study of 80 shoulders. *J Bone Joint Surg Br.* 2004;86(3):388-395.
3. Simovitch RW, Zumstein MA, Lohri E, Helmy N, Gerber C. Predictors of scapular notching in patients managed with the Delta III reverse total shoulder replacement. *J Bone Joint Surg Am.* 2007;89(3):588-600.
4. Wellmann M, Struck M, Pastor MF, Gettmann A, Windhagen H, Smith T. Short and midterm results of reverse shoulder arthroplasty according to the preoperative etiology. *Arch Orthop Trauma Surg.* 2013;133(4):463-471.
5. Mollon B, Mahure SA, Roche CP, Zuckerman JD. Impact of scapular notching on clinical outcomes after reverse total shoulder arthroplasty: an analysis of 476 shoulders. *J Shoulder Elbow Surg.* 2017;26(7):1253-1261.
6. Chae J, Siljander M, Wiater JM. Instability in reverse total shoulder arthroplasty. *J Am Acad Orthop Surg.* 2018;17:587-596.
7. Routman HD, Flurin PH, Wright TW, Zuckerman JD, Hamilton MA, Roche CP. Reverse shoulder arthroplasty design classification system. *Bull Hosp Jt Dis (2013).* 2015;73(suppl 1):S5-S14.
8. Hansen ML, Routman H. The biomechanics of current reverse shoulder replacement options. *Ann Joint.* 2019;4:17.
9. Giles JW, Langohr GDG, Johnson JA, Athwal GS. Implant design variations in reverse total shoulder arthroplasty influence the required deltoid force and resultant joint load. *Clin Orthop Relat Res.* 2015;473:3615-3626.
10. Matthewson G, Kooner S, Kwapisz A, Leiter J, Old J, MacDonald P. The effect of subscapularis repair on dislocation rates in reverse shoulder arthroplasty: a meta-analysis and systematic review. *J Shoulder Elbow Surg.* 2019;28(5):989-997.
11. Erickson BJ, Frank RM, Harris JD, Mall N, Romeo AA. The influence of humeral head inclination in reverse total shoulder arthroplasty: a systematic review. *J Shoulder Elbow Surg.* 2015;24(6):988-993.
12. Werthel JD. Humeral lateralization: what is it, is it really useful? In: Boileau P. ed. *Shoulder Concepts 2018: Arthroplasty for the Young Arthritic Shoulder.* Sauramps Médical; 2018:251-261.
13. Kolakowski L, Lai JK, Duvall GT, et al. Neer Award 2018: benzoyl peroxide effectively decreases preoperative Cutibacterium acnes shoulder burden. A prospective randomized controlled trial. *J Shoulder Elbow Surg.* 2018;27(9):1539-1544.
14. Neer CS II, Rockwood CA. Fractures and dislocations of the shoulder. In Rockwood CA, Green DP, eds. *Fractures in Adults.* JB Lippincott; 1984:675-985.
15. Choate WS, Kwapisz A, Momaya AM, Hawkins RJ, Tokish JM. Outcomes for subscapularis management techniques in shoulder arthroplasty: a systematic review. *J Shoulder Elbow Surg.* 2018;27(2):363-370.
16. Jeong J, Bryan J, Iannotti JP. Effect of a variable prosthetic neck-shaft angle and the surgical technique on replication of normal humeral anatomy. *J Bone Joint Surg Am.* 2009;91(8):1932-1941.
17. Roche CP, Marczuk Y, Wright TW, et al. Scapular notching in reverse shoulder arthroplasty: validation of a computer impingement model. *Bull Hosp Jt Dis (2013).* 2013;71(4):278-283.
18. Nyffeler RW, Werner CM, Gerber C. Biomechanical relevance of glenoid component positioning in the reverse Delta III total shoulder prosthesis. *J Shoulder Elbow Surg.* 2005;14:524-528.
19. Chebli C, Huber P, Watling J, Bertelsen A, Bicknell RT, Matsen F III. Factors affecting fixation of the glenoid component of a reverse total shoulder prothesis. *J Shoulder Elbow Surg.* 2008;17(2):323-327.
20. Cichos KH, Andrews RM, Wolschendorf F, Narmore W, Mabry SE, Ghanem ES. Efficacy of intraoperative antiseptic techniques in the prevention of periprosthetic joint infection: superiority of betadine. *J Arthroplasty.* 2019;34(7S):S312-S318.
21. Edwards TB, Williams MD, Labriola JE, Elkousy HA, Gartsman GM, O'Connor DP. Subscapularis insufficiency and the risk of shoulder dislocation after reverse shoulder arthroplasty. *J Shoulder Elbow Surg.* 2009;18(6):892-896.
22. Routman HD. The role of subscapularis repair in reverse total shoulder arthroplasty. *Bull Hosp Jt Dis (2013).* 2013;71(suppl 2):S108-S112.
23. Abildgaard JT, McLemore R, Hattrup SJ. Tranexamic acid decreases blood loss in total shoulder arthroplasty and reverse total shoulder arthroplasty. *J Shoulder Elbow Surg.* 2016;25(10):1643-1648.
24. Friedman RJ, Gordon E, Butler RB, Mock L, Dumas. Tranexamic acid decreases blood loss after total shoulder arthroplasty. *J Shoulder Elbow Surg.* 2016;25(4):614-618.
25. Gillespie R, Shishani Y, Joseph S, Streit JJ, Gobezie R. Neer Award 2015: a randomized, prospective evaluation on the effectiveness of tranexamic acid in reducing blood loss after total shoulder arthroplasty. *J Shoulder Elbow Surg.* 2015;24(11):1679-1684.
26. Kim SH, Jung WI, Kim YJ, Hwang DH, Choi YE. Effect of tranexamic acid on hematologic values and blood loss in reverse total shoulder arthroplasty. *Biomed Res Int.* 2017;2017:9590803-9590805.
27. Pauzenberger L, Domej MA, Heuberer PR, et al. The effect of intravenous tranexamic acid on blood loss and early post-operative pain in total shoulder arthroplasty. *Bone Joint J.* 2017;99-B(8):1073-1079.
28. Vara AD, Koueiter DM, Pinkas DE, Gowda A, Wiater BP, Wiater JM. Intravenous tranexamic acid reduces total blood loss in reverse total shoulder arthroplasty: a prospective, double-blinded, randomized, controlled trial. *J Shoulder Elbow Surg.* 2017;26(8):1383-1389.
29. Cvetanovich GL, Fillingham YA, O'Brien M, et al. Tranexamic acid reduces blood loss after primary shoulder arthroplasty: a double-blind, placebo-controlled, prospective, randomized controlled trial. *JSES Open Access.* 2018;2(1):23-27.
30. Box HN, Tisano BS, Khazzam M. Tranexamic acid administration for anatomic and reverse total shoulder arthroplasty: a systematic review and meta-analysis. *JSES Open Access.* 2018;2(1):28-33.
31. Kirsch JM, Bedi AB, Horner N, et al. Tranexamic acid in shoulder arthroplasty: a systematic review and meta-analysis. *JBJS Rev.* 2017;5(9):e3.
32. Kuo LT, Hsu WH, Chi CC, Yoo JC. Tranexamic acid in total shoulder arthroplasty and reverse shoulder arthroplasty: a systematic review and meta-analysis. *BMC Muscoskelet Disord.* 2018;19(1):60-13.
33. American Academy of Orthopaedic Surgeons. *Management of Glenohumeral Joint Osteoarthritis Evidence-Based Clinical Practice Guideline.* 2020. https://www.aaos.org/gjocpg
34. Chan JJ, Cirino CM, Huang HH, et al. Drain use is associated with increased odds of blood transfusion in total shoulder arthroplasty: a population-based study. *Clin Orthop Relat Res.* 2019;477(7):1700-1711.

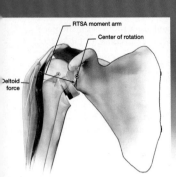

24 Operative Technique Using an Inlay Humeral Component

Charles M. Jobin, MD and William N. Levine, MD

INTRODUCTION

Reverse total shoulder arthroplasty (RTSA) was first approved by the Food and Drug Administration (FDA) in 2004 primarily for the treatment of rotator cuff tear arthropathy. RTSA indications have expanded and recently emerged as an alternative to anatomic total shoulder arthroplasty (ATSA) in patients with significant glenoid erosion with an intact rotator cuff. RTSA design principles have also evolved to accommodate these changing indications to allow improved preservation of the rotator cuff during reverse shoulder arthroplasty (RSA). This more "anatomic" reverse replacement with preserved rotator cuff is an emerging concept that utilizes RTSA component designs that lateralize the glenosphere center of rotation (COR) and inlay an anatomically inclined humeral stem to reduce humeral lengthening and achieve total lateralization that allows more normal cuff function. Preservation of the rotator cuff and a more normal excursion during RTSA is commonly achieved with humeral component inlay designs with a more lateralized glenosphere COR than the traditional Grammont style RTSA.[1] This combination of an inlay humeral stem and lateralized glenosphere avoids overlengthening the humerus and achieves RTSA stability while preserving more anatomic rotator cuff excursion and function (**FIGURE 24.1**).[2] In this chapter, we present our preferred techniques to perform an RTSA with an inlay humeral system (**VIDEO 24.1**). We present a case example of a patient with severe glenoid erosion and an intact rotator cuff (**FIGURE 24.2**) where an RTSA with an inlay humeral system was utilized, and we present our tips and tricks to optimize exposure, manage the subscapularis, prepare the humerus and glenoid, assess joint stability, and avoid complications to obtain a predictably successful outcome.

OPTIMIZING EXPOSURE

Our preferred exposure is the deltopectoral approach as this approach is more extensile, has less risk of injury to the axillary nerve on the undersurface of the deltoid, and represents an internervous plane. The anterosuperior approach that splits between the anterior and middle thirds of the deltoid is possible, and

we utilize this anterosuperior approach in patients on hemodialysis with an anteriovenous (AV) fistula and increased pressure, size, and flow in the cephalic vein so that it can be avoided during the surgical approach. In our experience, an anterosuperior approach may be more difficult to obtain interior or neutral tilt of the baseplate but is well suited for fracture RTSA as the tuberosities are retracted out of the way and glenoid exposure is not an issue.

SUBSCAPULARIS MANAGEMENT

The subscapularis is commonly peeled off the lesser tuberosity during RTSA. Tenotomy or lesser tuberosity osteotomy (LTO) are options, but we prefer a peel technique so that a subscapularis repair at the conclusion of the case is under less tension and can easily be medialized due to the peel technique preserving the entire length of the subscapularis tendon. We prefer to repair the subscapularis at the conclusion of the RTSA to increase internal rotation strength and potentially improve stability. In cases with significant external rotation (ER) lag and inability to externally rotate beyond neutral, the subscapularis may be left unrepaired to prevent it from providing an internal rotation tenodesis effect and relatively weakening the already weakened external rotators. An LTO is infrequently performed during RTSA as it may jeopardize the proximal humeral bone stock. This is especially relevant in an inlay humeral stem system in which metaphyseal reaming removes bone leaving an LTO without a medullary healing surface remaining.

PREPARATION OF THE HUMERUS

With an inlay humeral stem, the metaphyseal portion of the component is usually placed below or at the level of the humeral head resection, and the polyethylene is placed onto the humeral stem. In contrast, with an onlay humeral system, an anatomic neck cut is made, and then a humeral tray is placed on the stem that is flush with the resection. The polyethylene is then placed onto the humeral tray, which creates a "double stacking" of the components, which may add excessive length to the construct (**FIGURE 24.3**).[3] Depending

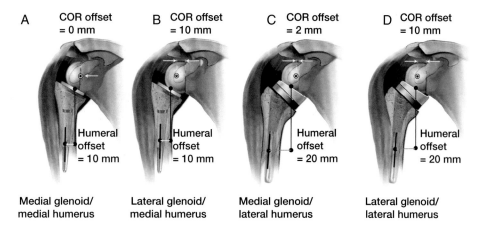

A | COR offset = 0 mm
B | COR offset = 10 mm
C | COR offset = 2 mm
D | COR offset = 10 mm

Humeral offset = 10 mm (A)

Humeral offset = 10 mm (B)

Humeral offset = 20 mm (C)

Humeral offset = 20 mm (D)

Medial glenoid/ medial humerus

Lateral glenoid/ medial humerus

Medial glenoid/ lateral humerus

Lateral glenoid/ lateral humerus

FIGURE 24.1 Comparison of reverse total shoulder arthroplasty (RTSA) total lateralization from humeral and glenoid contributions. The total lateralization of the RTSA construct is a combination of lateralization from the humeral design and the glenoid component design. A valgus 155° inlay stem tends to minimize the humeral offset (**A** and **B**), while an onlay humeral stem with an anatomic 135° neck-shaft angle creates more humeral offset (**C** and **D**). Glenosphere size, position, and design also affect the glenoid contribution to. COR, center of rotation and total RSA lateralization (Humeral offset + COR offset).

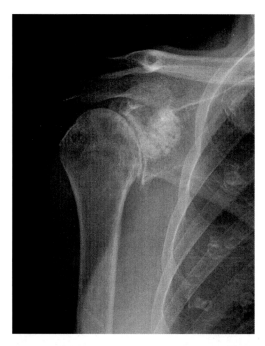

FIGURE 24.2 Preoperative inlay reverse total shoulder arthroplasty (RTSA) x-ray. Preoperative anteroposterior x-ray of the right shoulder with severe B3 glenoid erosion with medialization of the glenohumeral joint line and medialization of the proximal humerus beneath that lateral the acromion edge.

on the position of the humeral stem implant, the use of an inlay versus onlay design, the neck-shaft angle, the thickness of the polyethylene, differing amounts of deltoid tension, and joint compression can be applied to achieve stability and function. Onlay humeral designs tend to lengthen the humerus to tension the deltoid, while inlay humeral systems tend not to lengthen the humeral side but rather rely on glenosphere lateralization for appropriate joint tension and stability.

Humeral head resection depends on the RTSA system used and the inclination of the stem **(FIGURE 24.4)**. With inlay humeral components, a more anatomic head cut in 20° to 30° of retroversion helps preserve more anatomic rotator cuff excursion and function. The inclination of the head cut should match the stem and should exit superiorly at the junction of the greater tuberosity and articular surface margin **(FIGURE 24.5)**.[4] A head cut in an anatomic 135° inclination has been shown to have less notching in systems that do not solely utilize glenosphere lateralization to prevent notching.[5-7]

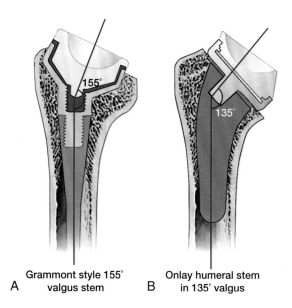

Grammont style 155° valgus stem (A)

Onlay humeral stem in 135° valgus (B)

FIGURE 24.3 Comparison of onlay verses inlay humeral designs. Humeral stem inclination effects humeral lateralization, with Grammont style 155° valgus inlay stems, cause less humeral lateralization and less lengthening (**A**), compared to an onlay humeral stem in 135° neck-shaft angle which causes more humeral lateralization and lengthening (**B**).

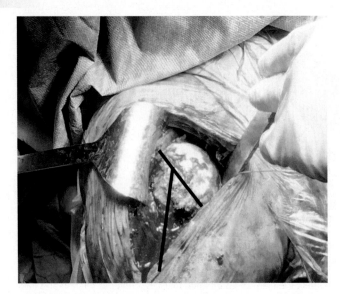

FIGURE 24.4 Humeral head resection inclination. The humeral head resection is planned to match the inclination of the inlay stem. The black lines drawn indicate the head osteotomy cut and the axis of the humeral shaft. A cutting guide or freehand technique may be utilized. Besides planning the inclination of the cut, retroversion must also be planned and typically is 20° to 30° retroverted to almost match the anatomic retroversion of the proximal humerus.

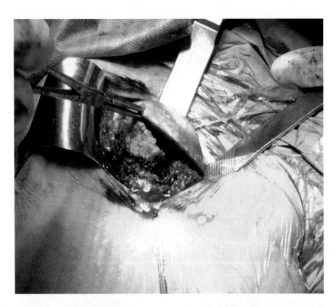

FIGURE 24.5 Humeral head resection. The amount of humeral head resection is important for glenoid exposure and preservation of remaining posterosuperior rotator cuff. Resecting too thin a head cut will make glenoid exposure difficult, while an aggressive head cut may remove remaining rotator cuff footprint.

After preparing the humerus for the inlay humeral stem with broaching and/or reaming, surgeons should focus on the integrity of the metaphyseal cortex **(FIGURES 24.6-24.8).** Aggressive metaphyseal bone removal may encroach on the cortex and weaken the proximal humerus. A weakened proximal humerus may get crushed and fragmented during glenoid preparation as a result of retraction of the proximal humerus for glenoid exposure. Insertion of the trial stem should

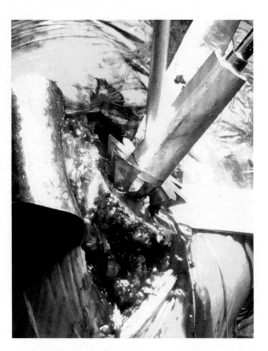

FIGURE 24.6 Humeral metaphyseal reamer. The proximal humerus metaphysis is prepared with a conical reamer that matches the geometry of the inlay stem. The metaphyseal reamer may be used by hand on forward for hard bone or on reverse by hand in the setting of osteoporotic bone to create an impaction-style bone preserving metaphyseal preparation. The reamer should be used at the desired retroversion.

ensure proper fit for the future final implantation of the humeral prosthesis **(FIGURE 24.9).** Leaving the stem trial in place **(FIGURE 24.10)** or using an osteotomy

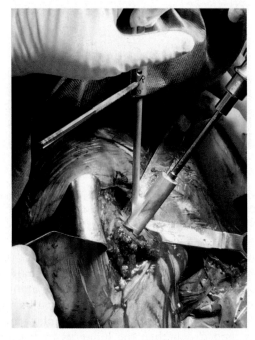

FIGURE 24.7 Completion of humeral metaphyseal preparation. Reaming the proximal humerus metaphysis is completed once the reamer matches the resection plane of the head. If a deeper seating of the inlay stem is desired in cases of stiffness or severe proximal migration, then the metaphyseal reamer may be brought a few millimeters below the head osteotomy plane.

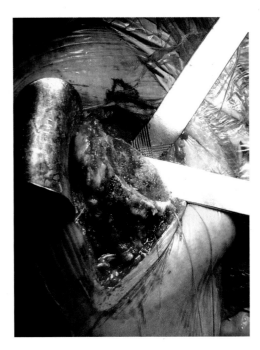

FIGURE 24.8 Completed proximal humerus preparation for inlay reverse total shoulder arthroplasty (RTSA). As depicted here, it is important to try to preserve the ring of cortical bone at the head osteotomy plane to help support the inlay stem. Likewise, it is critical to preserve the calcar bone, which will support the prosthesis. If a majority of the proximal cortical bone is lost from reaming or fracture, then the stem may require cementation for fixation.

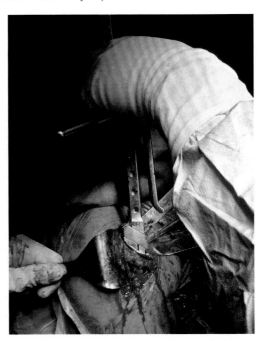

FIGURE 24.9 Trial of humeral inlay reverse total shoulder arthroplasty (RTSA) stem. The trial of humeral inlay RTSA stem is gently impacted into place ensuring the trial head surface seats at the level of the head osteotomy and is axially and rotationally stable to gentile manual forces. The trial inserter has a retroversion rod to ensure 20° to 30° of retroversion during trial insertion. It is critical not to impact the trail forcefully, but rather tap it into place, and if resistance is encountered, consider downsizing the stem size diameter to prevent iatrogenic humeral shaft fracture.

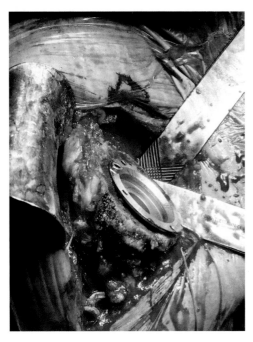

FIGURE 24.10 Inserted trial of humeral inlay reverse total shoulder arthroplasty (RTSA) stem. The appropriately inserted trial of humeral inlay RTSA stem is pictured here with preservation of the superior rotator cuff and trail seating against the humeral calcar. Also evident is the intact cortical ring of bone at the head osteotomy plane without apparent iatrogenic fracture. Overimpaction of the trial (or real prosthesis) risks "log splitting" the proximal humerus, so gentle insertion with tapping lightly is recommended, and if resistance is encountered, then downsizing the trial is recommended.

surface metal protector helps share the load during glenoid retractor use and prevents damage to the proximal humeral cortex.

HUMERAL LATERALIZATION VERSUS GLENOID LATERALIZATION

When using an inlay humeral system, the humeral lateral offset is often set by the design of the stem and humeral polyethylene socket as inlay humeral designs do not allow adjustment from intercalary modular components. Therefore, lateralization of the inlay RTSA is obtained primarily by baseplate and glenosphere configurations and less so from altering humeral stem positioning.[8] Humeral lateralization has many theoretic and biomechanical advantages to deltoid efficiency at arm elevation forces; glenosphere lateralization tends to reduce deltoid efficiency[9] and jeopardize glenoid fixation but may improve rotator cuff function.[10-12] Progressively thicker humeral polyethylene inserts produce both humeral lateralization and distalization which can overlengthen.[13] Humeral anteroposterior offset is another factor that can affect rotator cuff moment arms and excursion, but during inlay humeral stem usage, there are less options to adjust this factor as the stem position within the humeral metaphysis determines this anteroposterior offset.[14] Total combined humeral and glenoid offset can significantly affect deltoid lever arm mechanics.[15]

PREPARATION OF THE GLENOID

Visualizing and preparing the glenoid for baseplate implantation is critical to a successful and durable RTSA. The arm is typically in ER and mild abduction to allow the proximal humerus to slide posteriorly. An adequate humeral head resection optimizes exposure and provides the path to work on the glenoid. ER and abduction have been shown to place the brachial plexus on stretch, and prolonged positioning and forceful retraction may stretch the plexus. When glenoid exposure is inadequate, then repeating soft-tissue releases and removing any remaining osteophytes, rather than retracting with more force, is typically required. These releases commonly include the subacromial space, releasing the upper 1 cm of the pectoralis major tendon, and a complete inferior capsular release off the proximal humerus from anterior to posterior extending to the insertion of the teres minor. The anterior supraspinatus may often be released, if intact, which may assist in exposure during RTSA. An inferior capsulotomy directed toward the posteroinferior glenoid, while protecting the axillary nerve either digitally or with blunt retractor, is critical for improved glenoid exposure. Subperiosteal dissection around the inferior half of the glenoid from three to nine o'clock may also facilitate glenoid exposure by improving retractor placement and allowing the humerus to be retracted posteriorly. If glenoid exposure remains inadequate despite confirming all soft-tissue releases and ensuring removal of all osteophytes, then resecting additional proximal humerus by revising the head resection to a deeper level or considering isolated lesser tuberosity resection with rongeurs can be performed to provide the necessary glenoid exposure.

Glenoid retractors placement and selection are also important for glenoid exposure. Typically, a Fakuda, or two Bankart retractors, or one Bankart posteroinferiorly and one Homan posterosuperiorly are adequate for glenoid exposure. The length and rigidity of the retractor affect the assistant's ability to lever the humerus posteriorly and glenoid anteriorly for exposure. The anterior retractor commonly utilized is a wide Bankart retractor. Self-retaining retractors on the glenoid are less often utilized because they risk prolonged or excessive retraction force that may cause unappreciated brachial plexus stretch and injury. Manually held retractors have the tactile feedback of the assistant and can be adjusted constantly during preparation of the glenoid.

Positioning of the glenoid baseplate depends on the system utilized and the availability of eccentric and lateral offset glenosphere placement relative to the baseplate. Typically, the entire baseplate/glenosphere construct should have a 2 to 3 mm overhang on the inferior glenoid if a 155° humeral implant is utilized to prevent adduction impingement and notching. In systems with significant glenosphere lateralization and/or humeral inclination angles near 135°, inferior glenosphere overhang may not be as critical to prevent mechanical impingement and notching. Therefore, the baseplate location on the glenoid face is impacted by baseplate/glenosphere design and options for glenosphere size, eccentricity, and offset. Nevertheless, baseplate implantation position should avoid superior tilt to improve the mechanics of bone ingrowth on the baseplate. Using an inlay humeral stem allows more anatomic rotator cuff length-tendon relationships and vectors of pull. With the use of this design, RTSA stability is obtained with lateralization of the glenosphere rather than humeral lengthening. Lateralization of the glenoid component may be obtained with an intercalary structural bone graft between the native glenoid and baseplate often referred to as a "bony increased-offset reverse shoulder arthroplasty (BIO-RSA)" **(FIGURE 24.11).**[16] Glenoid component lateralization may also be obtained from component design either from the baseplate (thickness) or the glenosphere (lateral expansion).[17-19]

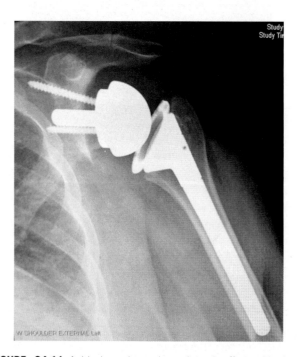

FIGURE 24.11 Achieving glenosphere lateral offset with bony increased-offset reverse shoulder arthroplasty (BIO-RSA). This anteroposterior x-ray demonstrates a structural bone autograft (BIO-RSA) that increases the glenosphere center of rotation (COR) lateral offset, and in combination with the inlay humeral stem, a combined offset improves posterior cuff function and reduces humeral distalization.

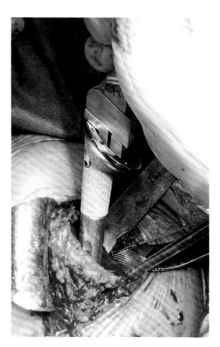

FIGURE 24.12 Implanting the final prosthesis of the humeral inlay reverse total shoulder arthroplasty (RTSA) stem. The real final stem is impacted in line with the humeral shaft at the appropriate retroversion. The prosthesis is placed while ensuring no contact with the skin or gloved hands to minimize any risk of seeding bacteria onto the prosthesis. The stem is inserted with gentle tapping to prevent iatrogenic periprosthetic fracture.

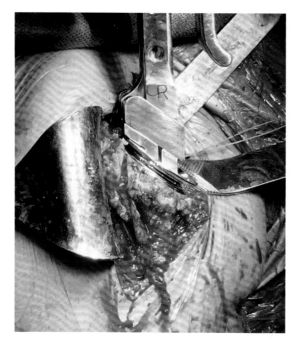

FIGURE 24.13 Final seating of the inlay reverse total shoulder arthroplasty (RTSA) humeral prosthesis. The final seating of the prosthesis is shown here, demonstrating the inlay seating within the proximal humerus. Axial and rotational fixation is ensured with gentle manual force on the inserter handle. Press fit fixation with the ingrowth stem design is nearly always achievable, and if fixation is poor at this stem, cementation of the stem should be performed rather than upsizing the stem diameter as this risks humeral shaft fracture.

ASSESSING RANGE OF MOTION AND ACHIEVING STABILITY

After glenoid baseplate and glenosphere final prosthetic implantation, the final humeral stem is implanted with press fit technique **(FIGURE 24.12)**. The final humeral inlay stem is inserted to the depth of the humeral trail stem **(FIGURE 24.13)**. Then the tension and stability of the RTSA is assessed with polyethylene implant trialing **(FIGURE 24.14)**. Once the appropriate polyethylene thickness is determined, the final component is implanted **(FIGURES 24.15 and 24.16)**; the shoulder should again be assessed for stability and impingement which can limit range of motion (ROM) and predispose to instability.[20] Detecting impingement can often be a subtle examination finding. In addition to limited passive motion, we find that one reliable finding of impingement is gapping of the component articulation that is observed when the mechanical impingement causes the joint surface to lever open. This "gapping" of the articulation can be identified by palpation during ROM or visualized directly. If gapping occurs and is believed to be from bony impingement with the humeral side (despite adequate osteophyte removal) and not from joint laxity, then the implants should be adjusted to reduce impingement. These steps

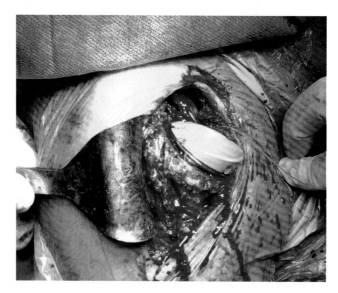

FIGURE 24.14 Polyethylene trialing for appropriate tension and stability. The various sizes of trail poly liners are inserted, and the joint is reduced and then checked for appropriate joint tension, impingement range of motion, and stability. With an inlay reverse total shoulder arthroplasty (RTSA) stem in the setting of an intact rotator cuff, the RTSA is not overtensioned for stability as the rotator cuff will provide dynamic stability to the RTSA. Retentive liners are rarely, if not ever, used for RTSA in the setting of an intact rotator cuff.

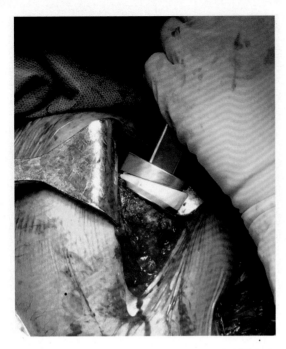

FIGURE 24.15 Final impaction of polyethylene humeral liner. The final polyethylene is impacted into the inlay humeral stem until engaged. The seating of the polyethylene is double checked to ensure proper engagement. If the bone is weak then the polyethylene may be engaged to the stem with a tool that compresses the poly to the stem without impaction.

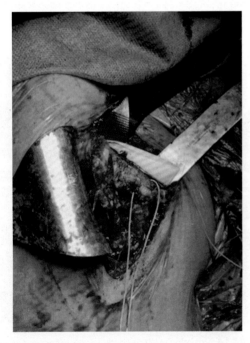

FIGURE 24.16 Final inlay humeral stem and polyethylene position relative to humeral head resection. After insertion of the final inlay humeral stem and appropriate polyethylene liner, the humeral stem sits flush with the level of the humeral head resection and only the polyethylene is proud to the bone resection plane. A #2 nonabsorbable transosseous suture has been placed through the lesser tuberosity in preparation for subscapularis repair. If the lesser tuberosity bone is weak or will not hold sutures reliably, then the sutures may be passed through suture holes in the prosthesis.

may include altering the direction of eccentric glenosphere, increasing glenosphere size and/or lateral offset,[21] or utilizing a nonretentive polyethylene liner. If the greater tuberosity is impinging on the acromion or the coracoid, then lengthening the arm with a prouder humeral stem, increasing the humeral offset, or resecting portions of the greater tuberosity may alleviate the impingement. We do not recommend resecting portions of the acromion or coracoid as this will likely predispose to acromial or coracoid fracture in the early postoperative months. The design of the humeral stem inclination and the position of the glenoid component construct are critical to understanding and addressing RTSA impingement.[22,23]

Assessment of RTSA stability can be performed by assessing the force needed to dislocate the articulation in various positions including maximal shoulder adduction, ER, and abduction. Commonly, the surgeon places a finger on the humeral calcar and applies lateral- and/or anterior-directed digital pressure to assess the force required to dislocate the prosthesis. Axial shuck testing is also helpful with downward pressure on the arm in neutral shoulder position while noting and palpating any gapping of the articulation The RTSA articulation should not gap more than a few millimeters when stable. Other tests of stability include palpating the tension in the strap tendons and axillary nerve with the arm in extension or other positions. Utilization of lateral offset of the combined humeral and glenoid components can help provide more dynamic stability with deltoid wrapping and rotator cuff tensioning. Overlengthening the arm should not be the intraoperative solution to instability of the RTSA as >2 cm of humeral lengthening places the brachial plexus at risk **(FIGURE 24.17)**.[24,25] Similarly,

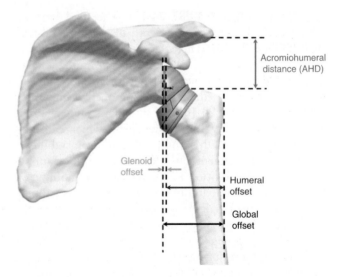

FIGURE 24.17 Components of humeral distalization measured by acromiohumeral distance. Distalization of the humerus, also known as lengthening, has contributions from humeral and glenoid component design. Specifically, humeral inclination, onlay humeral designs, and glenosphere size/eccentricity/offset.

overlengthening the humerus increases the risk of acromial fracture, while glenosphere lateralization does not appear to increase the risk of brachial plexus injury.[26]

Common complications of RTSA overlengthening are acromial and scapular spine fractures, stretch nerve injury, and intraoperative fracture due to a difficult and "too tight" reduction. These complications are more common with onlay humeral RTSA designs but occur with inlay systems also. A recent article by Ascione et al examined 485 primary onlay RTSAs and identified a 4.3% scapular spine fracture rate.[27] Acromial fracture after RTSA negatively affects the final outcome.[28]

Onlay implant systems tend to have a higher rate of postoperative acromial fractures when compared to inlay implant systems. Acromial fracture complications[29] occur more often in elderly females with low body mass index (BMI) (under 30) and some degree of osteopenia or osteoporosis.[27] In addition, the amount of lengthening and lateralization,[7,18] rotator cuff tension,[4] and deltoid tension[24,30,31] can contribute to the incidence of acromial fractures. We suggest that surgeons should carefully consider the RTSA implant system design when treating patients at increased risk of acromial fracture including those with significant acromial erosion from acetabularization in cuff tear arthropathy.[32] We feel that these considerations favor the use of an inlay humeral design based on the reduced lengthening achieved.

CLOSURE AND AFTERCARE

During closure, the subscapularis is often repaired to the lesser tuberosity **(FIGURE 24.18)** especially if the patient has expectations of higher level activities requiring internal rotation strength like wood cutting, if there is concern about RTSA instability, and in patients who have cuff-intact arthritis and significant glenoid erosion requiring RTSA.[33] In patients with retracted complete subscapularis tears, we do not routinely attempt repair. The deltopectoral interval is closed with a few nonabsorbable sutures to reduce space for a potential hematoma and to help identify the interval if revision surgery required in the future. Postoperatively, radiographs are performed in the recovery room to ensure no unexpected periprosthetic fractures or prosthetic dislocation **(FIGURE 24.19)** occured. Postoperative immobilization is typically performed with a pillow abduction sling for 2 to 4 weeks depending on intraoperative stability testing and subscapularis repair.

EXPECTED OUTCOMES

Patients who undergo RTSA with an inlay humeral stem can expect reliably excellent results.[34,35] ER and forward elevation are predictably improved, pain is reduced to very low levels, functional outcome scores improve, and a majority of patients return to sport-like activity especially if they were active in sports prior to

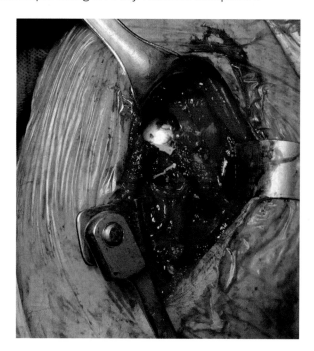

FIGURE 24.18 Final repair of the subscapularis to the lesser tuberosity. Final repair of the subscapularis to the lesser tuberosity is depicted here with a Mason-Allen-type repair and is performed with the arm in 30° of external rotation to ensure the subscapularis has enough excursion to allow external rotation. Overtightening the subscapularis may limit external rotation. We prefer the subscapularis peel during initial exposure to ensure the adequate length of the subscapularis. A medialized subscapularis repair is also possible if excursion is poor.

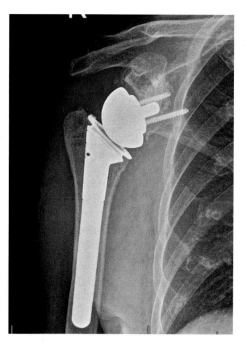

FIGURE 24.19 Postoperative radiographs after inlay reverse total shoulder arthroplasty (RTSA). The postoperative anteroposterior x-ray demonstrates an inlay humeral stem that is positioned at the level of the humeral head resection at the junction of the greater tuberosity and superior edge of the humeral head.

the deterioration of their shoulder condition. Functional outcomes are typically more improved in patients with better functional scores preoperatively. Satisfaction often depends on preoperative expectations of outcome. It is critical for surgeons to appropriately indicate patients for RTSA. Patients with irreparable cuff tears without arthritis may not experience the same high level of satisfaction after RTSA, especially if overhead motion was preserved preoperatively, if their preoperative pain levels were not as high, and the strength achieved after RSA does not live up to their expectations.

REFERENCES

1. Hansen ML, Routman H. The biomechanics of current reverse shoulder replacement options. *Ann Joint*. 2019;4(2):1-7.
2. Routman HD, Flurin PH, Wright TW, Zuckerman JD, Hamilton MA, Roche CP. Reverse shoulder arthroplasty prosthesis design classification system. *Bull Hosp Jt Dis (2013)*. 2015;73(suppl 1):S5-S14.
3. Middernacht B, Van Tongel A, De Wilde L. A critical review on prosthetic features available for reversed total shoulder arthroplasty. *BioMed Res Int*. 2016;2016:3256931.
4. Roche CP, Diep P, Hamilton MA, et al. Impact of posterior wear on muscle length with reverse shoulder arthroplasty. *Bull Hosp Jt Dis (2013)*. 2015;73(suppl 1):S63-S67.
5. Erickson BJ, Frank RM, Harris JD, Mall N, Romeo AA. The influence of humeral head inclination in reverse total shoulder arthroplasty: a systematic review. *J Shoulder Elbow Surg*. 2015;24(6):988-993.
6. Gutierrez S, Levy JC, Frankle MA, et al. Evaluation of abduction range of motion and avoidance of inferior scapular impingement in a reverse shoulder model. *J Shoulder Elbow Surg*. 2008;17(4):608-615.
7. Merolla G, Walch G, Ascione F, et al. Grammont humeral design versus onlay curved-stem reverse shoulder arthroplasty: comparison of clinical and radiographic outcomes with minimum 2-year follow-up. *J Shoulder Elbow Surg*. 2018;27(4):701-710.
8. Churchill JL, Garrigues GE. Current controversies in reverse total shoulder arthroplasty. *JBJS Rev*. 2016;4(6):e4.
9. Hettrich CM, Permeswaran VN, Goetz JE, Anderson DD. Mechanical tradeoffs associated with glenosphere lateralization in reverse shoulder arthroplasty. *J Shoulder Elbow Surg*. 2015;24(11):1774-1781.
10. Elwell J, Choi J, Willing R. Quantifying the competing relationship between adduction range of motion and baseplate micromotion with lateralization of reverse total shoulder arthroplasty. *J Biomech*. 2017;52:24-30.
11. Hamilton MA, Diep P, Roche C, et al. Effect of reverse shoulder design philosophy on muscle moment arms. *J Orthop Res*. 2015;33(4):605-613.
12. Streit JJ, Shishani Y, Gobezie R. Medialized versus lateralized center of rotation in reverse shoulder arthroplasty. *Orthopedics*. 2015;38(12):e1098-e1103.
13. Giles JW, Langohr GD, Johnson JA, Athwal GS. Implant design variations in reverse total shoulder arthroplasty influence the required deltoid force and resultant joint load. *Clin Orthop Relat Res*. 2015;473(11):3615-3626.
14. Dedy NJ, Stangenberg M, Liem D, et al. Effect of posterior offset humeral components on range of motion in reverse shoulder arthroplasty. *Int Orthop*. 2011;35(4):549-554.
15. Walker DR, Kinney AL, Wright TW, Banks SA. How sensitive is the deltoid moment arm to humeral offset changes with reverse total shoulder arthroplasty? *J Shoulder Elbow Surg*. 2016;25(6):998-1004.
16. Boileau P, Morin-Salvo N, Gauci MO, et al. Angled BIO-RSA (bony-increased offset-reverse shoulder arthroplasty): a solution for the management of glenoid bone loss and erosion. *J Shoulder Elbow Surg*. 2017;26(12):2133-2142.
17. Collin P, Liu X, Denard PJ, Gain S, Nowak A, Ladermann A. Standard versus bony increased-offset reverse shoulder arthroplasty:

18. Greiner S, Schmidt C, Herrmann S, Pauly S, Perka C. Clinical performance of lateralized versus non-lateralized reverse shoulder arthroplasty: a prospective randomized study. *J Shoulder Elbow Surg*. 2015;24(9):1397-1404.
19. Werthel JD, Walch G, Vegehan E, Deransart P, Sanchez-Sotelo J, Valenti P. Lateralization in reverse shoulder arthroplasty: a descriptive analysis of different implants in current practice. *Int Orthop*. 2019;43(10):2349-2360.
20. Tashjian RZ, Burks RT, Zhang Y, Henninger HB. Reverse total shoulder arthroplasty: a biomechanical evaluation of humeral and glenosphere hardware configuration. *J Shoulder Elbow Surg*. 2015;24(3):e68-77.
21. Werner BS, Chaoui J, Walch G. The influence of humeral neck shaft angle and glenoid lateralization on range of motion in reverse shoulder arthroplasty. *J Shoulder Elbow Surg*. 2017;26(10):1726-1731.
22. Chan K, Langohr GDG, Mahaffy M, Johnson JA, Athwal GS. Does humeral component lateralization in reverse shoulder arthroplasty affect rotator cuff torque? Evaluation in a cadaver model. *Clin Orthop Relat Res*. 2017;475(10):2564-2571.
23. Ladermann A, Denard PJ, Boileau P, et al. Effect of humeral stem design on humeral position and range of motion in reverse shoulder arthroplasty. *Int Orthop*. 2015;39(11):2205-2213.
24. Ladermann A, Edwards TB, Walch G. Arm lengthening after reverse shoulder arthroplasty: a review. *Int Orthop*. 2014;38(5):991-1000.
25. Ladermann A, Denard PJ, Collin P, et al. Effect of humeral stem and glenosphere designs on range of motion and muscle length in reverse shoulder arthroplasty. *Int Orthop*. 2020;44(3):519-530.
26. Lowe JT, Lawler SM, Testa EJ, Jawa A. Lateralization of the glenosphere in reverse shoulder arthroplasty decreases arm lengthening and demonstrates comparable risk of nerve injury compared with anatomic arthroplasty: a prospective cohort study. *J Shoulder Elbow Surg*. 2018;27(10):1845-1851.
27. Ascione F, Kilian CM, Laughlin MS, et al. Increased scapular spine fractures after reverse shoulder arthroplasty with a humeral onlay short stem: an analysis of 485 consecutive cases. *J Shoulder Elbow Surg*. 2018;27(12):2183-2190.
28. Teusink MJ, Otto RJ, Cottrell BJ, Frankle MA. What is the effect of postoperative scapular fracture on outcomes of reverse shoulder arthroplasty? *J Shoulder Elbow Surg*. 2014;23(6):782-790.
29. Levy JC, Anderson C, Samson A. Classification of postoperative acromial fractures following reverse shoulder arthroplasty. *J Bone Joint Surg Am*. 2013;95(15):e104.
30. Jobin CM, Brown GD, Bahu MJ, et al. Reverse total shoulder arthroplasty for cuff tear arthropathy: the clinical effect of deltoid lengthening and center of rotation medialization. *J Shoulder Elbow Surg*. 2012;21(10):1269-1277.
31. Marcoin A, Ferrier A, Blasco L, De Boissieu P, Nerot C, Ohl X. Reproducibility of a new method for measuring lowering and medialisation of the humerus after reverse shoulder arthroplasty. *Int Orthop*. 2018;42(1):141-147.
32. Wong MT, Langohr GDG, Athwal GS, Johnson JA. Implant positioning in reverse shoulder arthroplasty has an impact on acromial stresses. *J Shoulder Elbow Surg*. 2016;25(11):1889-1895.
33. Keener JD, Patterson BM, Orvets N, Aleem AW, Chamberlain AM. Optimizing reverse shoulder arthroplasty component position in the setting of advanced arthritis with posterior glenoid erosion: a computer-enhanced range of motion analysis. *J Shoulder Elbow Surg*. 2018;27(2):339-349.
34. Boutsiadis A, Lenoir H, Denard PJ, et al. The lateralization and distalization shoulder angles are important determinants of clinical outcomes in reverse shoulder arthroplasty. *J Shoulder Elbow Surg*. 2018;27(7):1226-1234.
35. Helmkamp JK, Bullock GS, Amilo NR, et al. The clinical and radiographic impact of center of rotation lateralization in reverse shoulder arthroplasty: a systematic review. *J Shoulder Elbow Surg*. 2018;27(11):2099-2107.

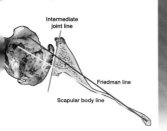

25 Addressing Glenoid Deformity in Reverse Total Shoulder Arthroplasty

Michael A. Boin, MD and Mandeep Singh Virk, MD

INTRODUCTION

Glenoid deformity in shoulder arthritis presents significant challenges for surgeons performing total shoulder arthroplasty (TSA). The etiology of glenoid deformity can be acquired or, less commonly, congenital in nature. Acquired glenoid deformity is commonly present in arthritic shoulders in the form of glenoid wear or glenoid erosion. Other less common causes of acquired glenoid deformity include shoulder trauma (glenoid fracture), infection, or prior shoulder surgery (Latarjet or Bristow procedure). In this chapter, we will focus on treatment of glenoid deformity in the setting of primary reverse total shoulder arthroplasty (RTSA). The treatment of glenoid bone loss in revision RTSA is covered in Chapter 43.

The location of glenoid wear in glenohumeral arthritis is dictated by the underlying pathology. Posterior glenoid wear is commonly encountered in primary glenohumeral arthritis; superior glenoid wear is encountered in the setting of rotator cuff tear arthropathy; anterior glenoid wear is encountered in association with anterior instability, and concentric glenoid wear is encountered in inflammatory arthritis. However, these specific patterns are not exclusive to the aforementioned individual pathologies, and combination patterns (posterior-superior) of glenoid wear are often present.

Pathologic glenoid wear, if not corrected during RTSA, can result in implant malposition, which has the potential to affect stability, function, and implant longevity. Excessive superior tilt of the glenosphere predisposes to dislocation, subacromial impingement, scapular notching, and excessive shear forces resulting in baseplate loosening and failure. Excessive medialization of the glenoid component can lead to decreased rotator cuff muscle tension, inferior-medial impingement with scapular notching, and polyethylene wear; abnormal version of the glenosphere can lead to decreased internal or external rotation.[1-6]

There is considerable variation in the physiologic version and inclination of the native, nonarthritic glenoid. Therefore, correction of the morphometric glenoid anatomy to neutral in TSA may not necessarily be patient specific in every case. The end point of correction of glenoid wear during shoulder arthroplasty is unclear at this time. Placing the glenoid component within 10° of Freidman axis for correction of posterior glenoid wear and within 10° of neutral tilt is considered acceptable in RTSA although further research with long-term data is required to confirm that these end points for correction of glenoid wear are truly acceptable. RTSA is a constrained arthroplasty design, and consequently, the acceptable limits for correction of glenoid wear and glenoid component placement are less stringent compared to anatomic total shoulder arthroplasty (ATSA).

There are several recognized techniques that can be used to correct glenoid wear during RTSA. These techniques include eccentric glenoid reaming, glenoid bone grafting, use of augmented baseplates, and combinations of these aforementioned techniques. However, the indications and end point of deformity correction varies among surgeons. In this chapter, we will present our strategy for the evaluation and treatment of glenoid wear when performing RTSA.

HOW DO I TREAT GLENOID DEFORMITY IN RTSA?

Imaging Studies

All patients undergoing RTSA obtain standard radiographs that include true anterior-posterior (AP; Grashey), axillary, and outlet (scapular Y) views. Superior glenoid wear and posterior or anterior glenoid wear patterns can be visualized on true AP and axillary views, respectively. We routinely obtain computed tomography (CT) with three-dimensional (3D) reconstruction on patients undergoing shoulder arthroplasty. This allows for accurate classification of glenoid wear patterns and is used for preoperative planning for guided shoulder arthroplasty (computer-assisted navigation [CAN] or with patient-specific instrumentation [PSI] guides). Three-dimensional computed tomography (3D CT) has been shown to be superior to two-dimensional computed tomography (2D CT) when critically evaluating the degree and location of glenoid deformity.[7] As 3D CT is not affected by the scapular position in the CT scanner, it can reliably and accurately determine glenoid anatomy.

TABLE 25.1 Computer Navigation System and Patient-Specific Instrumentation Guides With Three-Dimensional Computer Planning Software Commonly Used in the United States

Proprietary Name	Company	Guidance Technology	Features
Blueprint	Wright Medical/Tornier	PSI (single use)	3D planning software with templating for glenoid and humerus in ATSA and RTSA available 3D bone model of glenoid provided PSI guide arms (4) rests on the glenoid edge
ExactechGPS	Exactech	Computer-assisted navigation surgery	3D planning software + Glenoid navigation for ATSA and RTSA Intraoperative modification of plan permissible Templating for augments available
Match Point System	DJO Surgical	PSI (single use)	3D planning software with templating for glenoid for ATSA and RTSA available 3D bone model of glenoid provided PSI guide arm rests on the coracoid
Signature Personalized Patient Care Glenoid System	Zimmer-Biomet	PSI (single use)	3D planning software with templating for glenoid for ATSA and RTSA available 3D bone model of glenoid provided Pin placement guide for glenoid for ATSA and RTSA present in a single PSI guide PSI guide rests directly on the glenoid face and anterior glenoid rim
TrueSight	Stryker	PSI (singe use)	3D planning software with templating for glenoid for RTSA available 3D bone model of glenoid provided PSI guide arm rests on the coracoid and can be pinned with a K-wire
TruMatch	DePuy Synthes	PSI (singe use)	3D planning software with templating for glenoid for ATSA and RTSA available 3D bone model of glenoid provided PSI guide arm rests on the coracoid and can be pinned with a K-wire
Virtual Implant Positioning (VIP) system	Arthrex	PSI (reusable)	3D planning software with templating for glenoid for ATSA and RTSA available 3D bone model of glenoid provided Reusable glenoid targeter with arms (4) resting on the glenoid face and anterior glenoid rim
Zimmer PSI Shoulder System	Zimmer	PSI (single use)	3D planning software with templating for glenoid for RTSA available 3D bone model of glenoid provided PSI guide rests directly on the glenoid face and anterior glenoid rim; separate guides are available for glenoid pin placement, depth of reaming, screw placement, and implant positioning on the glenoid

3D, three dimensional; ATSA, anatomic total shoulder arthroplasty; K-wire, Kirschner wire; PSI, patient-specific instrumentation; RTSA, reverse total shoulder arthroplasty.

PREOPERATIVE PLANNING

We routinely use a preoperative computer-planning tool for RTSA. Different preoperative planning software programs that utilize manufacturer-specific implant simulation are commercially available in the United States **(TABLE 25.1)**. These preoperative planning tools are typically based on 3D CT imaging of the glenohumeral joint and require thin cuts, which are typically 0.6 mm or less with slice increments of 0.6 mm or less of the entire scapula. The raw CT images are transferred to a computer application, which generates a 3D image of the glenoid and is uploaded into the preoperative planning software for planning. The planning software provides automated measurements of glenoid version and inclination using the scapular plane method, and if the surgeon disagrees with the measurements, there is an option to obtain manual measurements.

We preoperatively plan all of our shoulder arthroplasties with planning software irrespective of our decision to use computer navigation, PSI guides, or standard instrumentation. The software allows us to determine

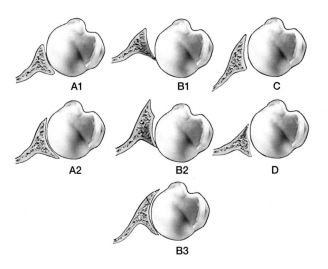

Modified Walch classification

FIGURE 25.1 Walch classification of glenoid deformity. (Redrawn with permission from Bercik, Michael J, et al. A modification to the Walch classification of the glenoid in primary glenohumeral osteoarthritis using three-dimensional imaging. *J Shoulder Elbow Surg.* 2016;25(10):1601-1606.)

the extent of glenoid wear in a 3D plane, size the implants, and choose the final position of the implant with respect to the glenoid axis. The preoperative planning software, by default, places the selected glenoid implant neutral to Freidman axis. The inclination and version of the selected glenoid implant is then changed to match the patient's anatomy using computer controls on a 3D and 2D CT image interface. The preoperative planning software provides real-time feedback during manipulation of the glenoid component with respect to changes in the version and inclination. During simulation of the surgical plan, we evaluate for critical findings like peg perforation of the glenoid (in ATSA) or wall/vault perforation by the central peg or post (ATSA and RTSA) and adjust the implant position and/or implant size accordingly. The extent of reaming and implant stability is determined virtually using the assessment of backside contact of the implant with the glenoid. The size of the augmented components and their position on the glenoid can be determined preoperatively, and the degree of correction achieved can be visualized in real time. The preoperative plan, once finalized by the surgeon, is transferred to the computer station to be used intraoperatively if computer navigation is being utilized.

CLASSIFICATION OF GLENOID WEAR

Classification of glenoid wear patterns in arthritis is presented in detail in Chapters 5 and 6. We use the modified Walch classification for documenting glenoid wear in the axial plane **(FIGURE 25.1)**, and we classify superior glenoid wear using the classification by Favard et al **(FIGURE 25.2)**.[8-11] More recently, we have found the use of classification systems to be less helpful as a

result of the development of preoperative planning software, which provides the opportunity to both assess the degree of deformity and determine the necessary correction. However, classifying glenoid wear is important for understanding the impact of glenoid wear on outcomes of reconstructive techniques and for education and research purposes.

TREATMENT OPTIONS

Eccentric Reaming

Eccentric or "high side" reaming refers to reaming of the nondeformed/less deformed part of the glenoid (paleoglenoid and intermediate glenoid) to meet the level of the worn glenoid (neoglenoid). It is usually performed for mild degrees of glenoid wear which require less than 10° to 15° of correction in coronal or axial plane with removal of a limited amount of bone.[5,12-14] Eccentric reaming is technically easy to perform and is preferred for correction of mild glenoid deformity. However, use of eccentric reaming to completely correct severe asymmetric glenoid wear can result in considerable iatrogenic bone loss, especially of the subchondral bone, which is critical to long-term stability of fixation of the glenoid component[5,12,15] **(FIGURE 25.3)**. Eccentric reaming for severe glenoid wear also results in excessive joint-line medialization, which results in loss of rotator cuff tension/function and predisposes to impingement and instability.[4] Furthermore, excessive reaming and medialization results in downsizing of the glenoid face and loss of glenoid neck predisposing to scapular notching and baseplate overhang at the anterior or posterior margin.

Glenoid Bone Grafting

Glenoid bone grafting is an option in severe glenoid erosion where accepting the deformity or eccentric reaming alone is not a reasonable approach. The major benefit of glenoid bone grafting is the ability to restore bone stock. Another benefit is the ability to customize each graft to fit the unique bone-loss pattern in each specific patient. Glenoid bone grafting is better tolerated in RTSA than in ATSA because the graft fixation is more secure in RTSA. The graft is secured using the baseplate post and/or screws, which can also provide compression across the bone graft as well as secure fixation.[11,16-19]

There have been several different graft sources described in the literature. In primary RTSA cases, humeral head autograft is a popular graft choice.[2,11,16,17,20] This graft has the benefit of autograft properties without any additional donor-site morbidity. It can also be used as both a structural and nonstructural graft. If the resected humeral head bone quality or size is not adequate to correct the glenoid defect, other autograft options (iliac crest) or allografts (femoral head allograft) can be used.[2,11,17,20,21] Although concern has been expressed regarding the ability of allograft to

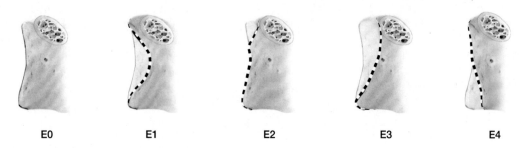

EO   E1   E2   E3   E4

FIGURE 25.2 Favard classification of glenoid deformity. (Redrawn with permission from Sirveaux, Favard, et al. Grammont inverted total shoulder arthroplasty in the treatment of glenohumeral osteoarthritis with massive rupture of the cuff. *J Bone Joint Surg Br.* 2004;86(3):388-395.)

incorporate compared to autograft, there is growing evidence of equivalent patient outcomes and graft incorporation when the two graft choices are compared.[2]

There are limitations to using bone graft for correcting glenoid wear regardless of the graft choice. Shaping of the graft to perfectly match the deformity and fixation of the graft to the glenoid is technically demanding and adds to the surgical time.[1] The outcome of RTSA with glenoid bone grafting is dependent on the graft incorporating into the native scapula. Graft resorption, nonunion, and fracture can compromise fixation over a period of time resulting in baseplate failure.[1]

Augmented Glenoid Baseplate

Advances in implant technology have led to the development of augmented glenoid baseplates. These augmented baseplates offer a simpler solution for dealing with moderate and severe glenoid deformity.[15] There are many different options for augment glenoid baseplates. These can vary in location of the augment (superior, posterior, superior-posterior), size, and shape of the augment. Augment shapes include lateralized, half-wedge, and full-wedge designs, each of which can be used for unique glenoid wear patterns[6] **(FIGURE 25.4)**.

The obvious benefit of using augmented baseplates is the relative technical simplicity compared to bone grafting.

Eccentric reaming

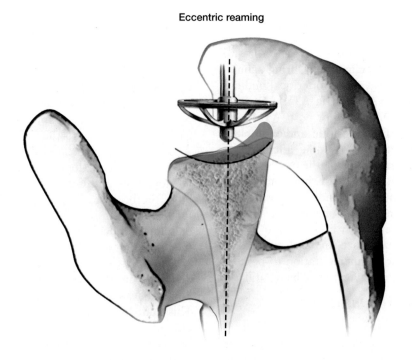

FIGURE 25.3 Technique of eccentric reaming.

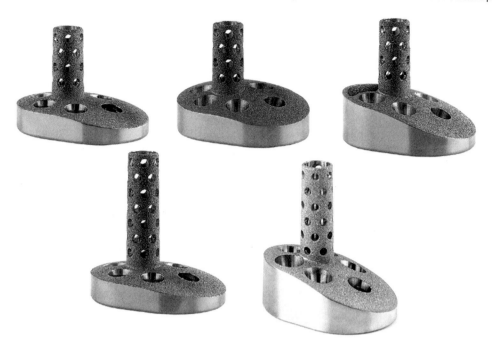

FIGURE 25.4 Augmented baseplates available to correct glenoid deformity including standard baseplate, 8° posterior augment, 10° superior augment, extended bone cage, and combined posterosuperior augmented baseplate. (Used with permission from © Exactech, Inc.)

Augmented baseplate utilization also preserves bone stock if an off-axis reaming technique is used to remove the intermediate glenoid[6,15] **(FIGURE 25.5)**. Unlike bone grafting for glenoid defects, RTSA outcomes with augmented baseplates are not dependent on graft incorporation, thereby avoiding the potential problems of graft resorption, nonunion, and fracture. Limited reports in the literature demonstrate that the use of augmented baseplates compared to glenoid bone grafting have lower surgical times, lower complication rates, and equivalent clinical outcomes.[1]

Off axis

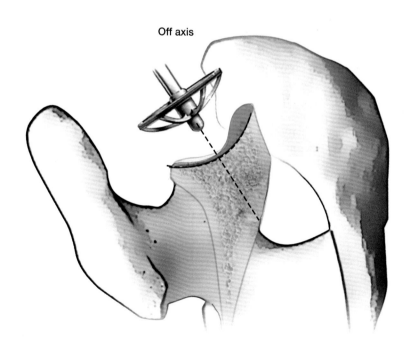

FIGURE 25.5 Technique of off-axis reaming.

Augmented baseplate limitations include their expense and the requirement for special instrumentation. Unlike bone grafting, they do not restore glenoid bone stock. The use of navigation technology can facilitate placement of augmented glenoid baseplates in cases of severe glenoid deformity.

In cases with extremely severe glenoid bone loss in which conventional or augmented baseplates cannot obtain secure glenoid fixation, custom implants can be considered. These implants are associated with a high cost and have limited track record in the literature. Of the few studies reporting outcomes of custom glenoid implants for severe bone loss, the results in the short and medium term have been mixed with a high incidence of loosening and reoperation.[22,23]

There is paucity of studies reporting midterm or long-term results of augments, bone grafting, and custom-made glenoid implants. Results of recent studies using bone grafts and augments are encouraging, although long-term studies are necessary to determine the cost-effectiveness of these techniques.

PRINCIPLES OF TREATMENT

The glenoid could very well be the most valuable "real estate" in total shoulder arthroplasty surgery. Our goal is to correct glenoid wear in shoulder arthroplasty with minimal removal of native bone (paleoglenoid). The goal during surgery is to correct the glenoid wear and achieve a final version within 10° of neutral and a final inclination within 10° of neutral. Additionally, our goal is to have at least 70% backside contact of the glenoid baseplate with the glenoid and no wall perforation to optimize stability of the baseplate construct. However, a minimum of 50% backside contact has been shown to provide sufficient stability, but studies with long-term data are lacking.[24,25]

To achieve this goal, we rely on preoperative planning software and use of computer navigation to reliably determine the true glenoid axis (Friedman axis) or the "alternate glenoid axis." Establishing the glenoid axis is critically important because it provides guidance for the proper reaming and implanting of the glenoid component based on the preoperative plan. We define "alternate glenoid axis" as an axis that is within 10° of Friedman axis, as determined on preoperative planning, that allows us to position the baseplate with maximal backside contact, no violation of the glenoid walls (vault containment), and minimal removal of glenoid bone. This is utilized for all the corrective techniques including eccentric reaming, glenoid bone grafting, and augmented glenoid components. In the absence of guidance technology, the glenoid axis in the axial plane can be determined intraoperatively by different techniques. The palpation technique consists of triangulation with the surgeon's finger placed along the anterior glenoid neck.

Alternatively, glenoid drill guides can be used which rest either directly on the face of the glenoid or have an extension (targeting guides) that can slide along the anterior neck. In absence of considerable glenoid wear, these techniques can be used to establish the glenoid axis within acceptable range. However, we do not think these manual techniques provide the precision, accuracy, and reproducibility necessary to guide reconstructive procedures in the context of severe glenoid deformity when use of an augmented baseplate, bone grafting, or accurate eccentric reaming is required.

The current implant system that we use (Exactech Inc.) has two glenoid sizes (~34 × 25.4 and 30 × 24) with different post lengths (13.1, 16.6, 23.1, and 26.6 mm) and three different types of augments (8-degree posterior, 10-degree superior, and 8/10-degree posterosuperior). This multitude of options provides us with the versatility to adapt to virtually all glenoids of different sizes and address glenoid deformity to achieve the aforementioned goals.

Depending on the degree of glenoid wear, typical scenarios that are encountered are as follows:

Scenario 1: Mild glenoid wear (<10° of version or <10° of inclination)

In mild glenoid wear patterns, we use high side reaming to correct the glenoid wear. Preoperatively, we use either the true glenoid axis or the alternate glenoid axis to determine the extent of high side reaming and the final implant position such that least amount of glenoid bone is reamed, but at the same time, there is containment of the baseplate post in the vault (no wall perforation), and there is maximum possible baseplate contact with the glenoid.

Scenario 2: Moderate glenoid wear (10°-20° of version or 10°-15° of inclination)

We typically use augmented glenoid baseplates (8-degree posterior, 10-degree superior or 8/10-degree posterosuperior) with or without eccentric reaming to achieve the desired implant position that meets our preoperative goals of correction of glenoid wear (minimal removal of bone, containment of the post in the wall, maximum back side contact). Although, bone grafts can be used for correcting moderate glenoid wear, we prefer to correct moderate glenoid wear with an augmented baseplate.

Scenario 3: Severe glenoid wear (>20° of version or >15° of inclination)

We use an augmented glenoid baseplate and bone graft alone or in combination to correct severe glenoid wear. Choosing an alternate glenoid axis instead of Friedman axis allows us to combine eccentric reaming with the use of a glenoid baseplate and bone grafts to improve backside contact with native glenoid. This precise planning requires use of preoperative planning software and intraoperative navigation. In glenoids with severe deformity, custom-made implants are an additional option but are less commonly used.

SURGICAL TECHNIQUE

Patient-Specific Instrumentation

Patient-specific instrumentation (PSI) in RTSA refers to patient-specific guides that are determined by a preoperative plan and patient-specific CT images. Preoperative imaging and planning are performed as previously described. Once the preoperative plan is finalized, the manufacturer creates a glenoid model and corresponding guides. The model and guides can then be sterilized and used intraoperatively.

PSI guides vary in design depending on the manufacturer, but in general, these guides use the patient's specific bony landmarks to help seat the guide in order to place the guidewire in an accurate position.[26] Because each PSI guide references CT images, it is imperative to remove all soft tissue from the glenoid including the labrum and remaining cartilage while preserving all bone including osteophytes as these are important reference landmarks. Once the glenoid is adequately exposed and all soft tissue has been removed, the guide is placed on the face of the glenoid with the arms of the guide placed on the predetermined bony landmarks (glenoid rim, coracoid, osteophyte) to achieve a stable fit. The guidewire is then inserted through the center of the guide into the glenoid. After the guidewire is placed, the glenoid is prepared for reaming and drilling of the central peg for baseplate implantation. Some systems have specific guides to set the depth of reaming and guide placement of baseplate screws in predetermined location. PSI can be used in cases utilizing either standard or augmented baseplates. Care must be taken to ensure that the guidewire remains stable throughout glenoid preparation, as any toggle or loosening of the wire prior to drilling for the central peg/screw can result in inaccurate baseplate placement.

Computer-Assisted Navigation

Computer-assisted navigation (CAN) provides the surgeon with real-time visual feedback during shoulder arthroplasty surgery. This technology uses the previously discussed CT imaging and preoperative planning to precisely execute the preoperative plan. This is achieved by use of intraoperative trackers, which provide intraoperative positional information relative to the anatomic glenoid axis when reamers and drills are being used.

Shoulder-specific CAN systems consist of a computer station with a monitor, a camera with infrared sensor, and a set of three trackers.[27] The computer station is mounted across the operative shoulder so that the camera has a clear and unobstructed view of the shoulder. There are typically three types of trackers used in

shoulder arthroplasty. The glenoid (G) tracker is place on a coracoid block, which is secured to the coracoid bone with the help of two screws. The probe (P) tracker is a handheld probe that is used to register bony acquisition points on the glenoid. The tool (T) tracker is attached in order to provide real-time feedback of the position of the tool relative to the glenoid.

During the glenoid exposure, the soft tissues and labrum are removed but glenoid osteophytes should be preserved prior to the acquisition of bony landmarks. After this, the soft tissue on the top of the coracoid is cleared and the coracoid block is secured onto the coracoid with two screws. The G tracker is then mounted on the coracoid block and its signal confirmed on the monitor screen. After this, the P tracker is used to probe the acquisition bony points, and once this registration process is completed, the computer generates a 3D image of the face of glenoid and 2D images in the coronal and axial planes. The starting point for the drill, as per the preoperative plan, is shown on the computer screen with a blue dot on the face of glenoid. The T tracker is then mounted on the modular driver and used to provide real-time feedback of version and inclination for determining the preplanned glenoid axis, and perform glenoid reaming, drilling of the central cage/peg, and screw placement for baseplate implantation and fixation. The position of the tip of the drill is shown as a yellow dot on the computer screen, and the goal is to overlay this yellow dot (signifying user's tool) onto the blue dot (starting point as per the preoperative plan) on the face of glenoid in order to achieve correct starting point. The orientation of the modular driver is guided version and inclination measurements as well as by the circular crosshair indicator on the computer screen in real time fashion. This allows the user to prepare the glenoid for both standard or augmented baseplate implantation and translate the preoperative plan inside the operating room with precision and accuracy. Furthermore, CAN also allows the user to make changes to the preoperative plan real time in the operative room.

The screws used to fix the coracoid block can create a stress riser predisposing to coracoid fracture. CAN is contraindicated in patients with previous Latarjet procedure, and presence of intraoperative coracoid fracture necessitates aborting the navigation procedure.[27]

Eccentric or Asymmetric Reaming

The amount of glenoid reaming and the axis of reaming are determined preoperatively on the planning software. If the true glenoid axis (Friedman axis) is used for eccentric reaming, more glenoid is reamed compared to when an alternate glenoid axis is used (**FIGURE 25.6**).

Prior to addressing the glenoid deformity, the surgical steps for an RTSA are completed as described in Chapters 23 and 24. After the glenoid is exposed, we use

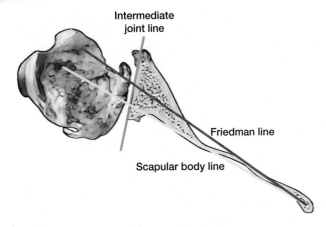

FIGURE 25.6 Comparison of alternate glenoid axis with Friedman line.

computer navigation to determine either the true glenoid axis or alternate glenoid axis based on our preoperative planning. In absence of intraoperative guidance technology (computer navigation or PSI), manual targeting guides can be used to determine the true glenoid axis. Asymmetric reaming of the paleoglenoid surface—ie, the premorbid glenoid surface or the nonworn portion of the native glenoid—is performed to reach a neutral joint line (perpendicular to Friedman line) or a joint line with some degree of residual version if an alternate axis is selected. It is important that minimal or no reaming be performed on the "low side" or the neoglenoid to preserve the already compromised bone stock and avoid excessive medialization of the glenoid component. Once the planned degree of correction is achieved drilling is performed for the post of the baseplate using computer guidance to assure proper placement for both correction of the deformity and vault containment. The baseplate is then placed and fixed based upon the system being utilized (**CASE 25.1**).

Glenoid Bone Grafting

Correcting glenoid deformity with bone grafting is a reasonable option in moderate to severe glenoid wear patterns. Glenoid bone grafting can be performed in either a single-stage or two-stage technique. For the purposes of this chapter, we will focus on single-stage bone grafting techniques. For a patient to be a candidate for a single-stage technique, they must have enough native glenoid bone stock to support a baseplate.

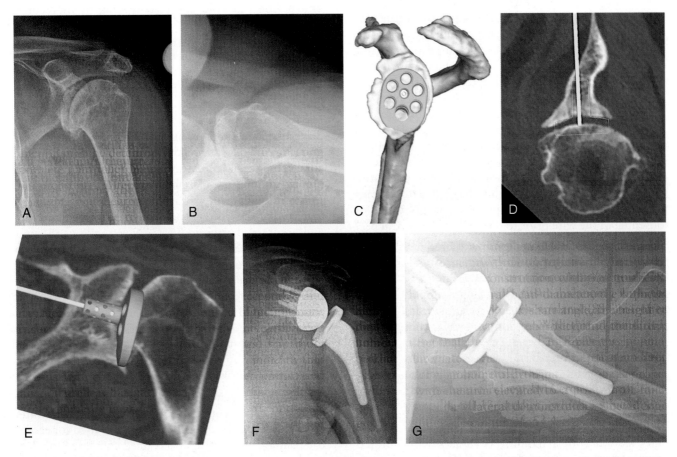

CASE 25.1 Reverse total shoulder arthroplasty (RTSA) with standard glenoid baseplate and eccentric reaming for treatment of mild posterior glenoid wear (<10°). **A,** preoperative anteroposterior view (AP view); (**B**) preoperative axillary view; (**C-E**) computed tomography (CT)–based preoperative planning tool templating for eccentric reaming of the anterior glenoid (**C**) and placement of standard glenoid component in neutral version (**D**) and inclination (**E**); (**F**) postoperative AP view; and (**G**) postoperative axillary view.

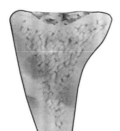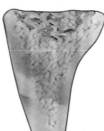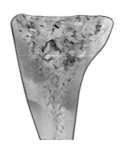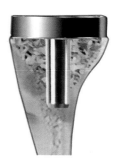

FIGURE 25.7 Impaction Grafting.

For central-contained glenoid defects, impaction grafting can be performed **(FIGURE 25.7)**. With this technique, cancellous autograft from the humeral head is preferred or cancellous allograft (off shelf freeze-dried or from frozen cancellous allograft bone) mixed with bone marrow aspirate (from humeral medullary canal or iliac crest) can also be utilized. The remaining glenoid bone surrounding the defect is then prepared for grafting using curettes, burr, and/or a drill in order to obtain bleeding bone surfaces with care taken to minimize any bone removal. The hole for the cage post is drilled and the drill bit is left in place. Impaction grafting is then performed until the defect is adequately filled with cancellous bone around the drill. The baseplate post is filled with the graft also if the design allows. After this, the drill bit is carefully removed and replaced with the baseplate making sure that the graft does not fall into prepared hole. The baseplate is fixed with screws as per the preoperative plan. Typically, three to four screws are used for fixation.

Structural bone grafting to correct glenoid deformity can be technically challenging and requires additional operating room time. In primary reverse arthroplasty, we prefer humeral head as the bone graft, and in revision cases, we use femoral head allograft. Determining the appropriate size of the bone graft can be challenging, but preoperative planning can be beneficial for this also.

Depending on the size and location of the defect and the degree of planned correction, we use either hemispherical or full-wedge grafts. Typically for moderate size posterior and/or superior glenoid wear patterns, we use hemispherical grafts obtained from patient's humeral head. The humeral head-neoglenoid contact relationship is used as a guide for determining the shape and size of the defect. After the humeral head is osteotomized, the osteotomized head piece is placed in the neoglenoid defect to determine the graft size. The graft is fixed with a Kirschner wire (K-wire) and cut in situ with a saw. A right-angled saw is used to mark out the proper resection location on the graft surface parallel to the paleoglenoid. Final shaping of the graft is performed on the back table. A hole is drilled for the post, and articular side of the graft is debrided of any remaining cartilage. Drill holes are then created with a K-wire. The neoglenoid

surface is debrided, and a bleeding surface is obtained by drilling the surface with a K-wire. After preparation of the graft, the final graft position and location of the drill hole for cage post is determined. The graft is fixed with a K-wire out of plane with the baseplate insertion. This K-wire along with a solid retractor (like Darrach) positioned posterosuperiorly prevents escape of the graft during baseplate impaction. The screws for baseplate fixation (posterior, posterosuperior and superior) are passed through the graft to achieve compressive fixation of the graft to the native articular surface.

In severe degrees of glenoid wear, we prefer full-wedge-shaped bone grafts. Typically, this requires allograft, and our graft of choice is femoral head and neck allograft. We prefer a standard, nonaugmented large baseplate with a long post, but an augmented baseplate with a longer post (posterior-superior augment) can also be used. When correcting severe glenoid wear patterns/defects, the stability of the graft-implant composite in the native glenoid is very critical for long-term success of the RTSA.

The femoral allograft is cut perpendicular to its axis. The baseplate is used to shape the graft surface that will be in contact with the glenoid component. The articular side of the graft and thickness of the graft are shaped based on the glenoid defect and preoperative plan. After the graft is shaped, a drill hole for the baseplate is marked and drilled. The baseplate and graft construct is then impacted into the glenoid and fixed with screws through the baseplate and graft and into the native glenoid. In severe glenoid wear patterns, an alternate glenoid axis (within 10° of neutral version) is selected to allow at least a 10 mm depth of circumferential baseplate-post contact with the native glenoid so as to allow sufficient stability of the cage in glenoid vault.

Augmented Glenoid Baseplate

We use an augmented baseplate with or without bone graft for correction of moderate to severe glenoid deformity. The size and type of augmented baseplate required for correcting the glenoid wear pattern is determined and planned preoperatively using the planning software. Although, manual guides are available for using augmented glenoid baseplates, the key step of surgery is establishing the glenoid axis. This step can be precisely done with computer navigation

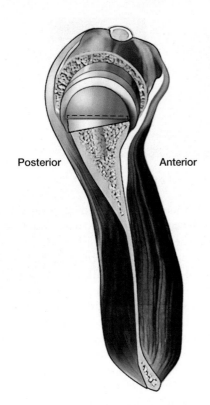

Posterior   Anterior

FIGURE 25.8 Off-axis reaming with insertion of an augmented baseplate to correct deformity.

or using patient-specific instrument guides. The subsequent steps of reaming and baseplate implantation are based upon the glenoid axis. Reaming when using an augmented baseplate is performed with an off-axis technique. The off-axis technique is performed by reaming in-line with the face of the glenoid rather than reaming in-line with the glenoid axis, as performed with an on-axis technique **(FIGURE 25.8)**. The off-axis technique preserves glenoid bone stock by only removing the minimum amount of bone

necessary to seat the augmented baseplate (intermediate glenoid). Both half-wedge and full-wedge augmented baseplates are available, but we prefer full-wedge augments. Once reaming is completed, the baseplate is placed with the augment flush with the defect. Screws are then used to fixate the baseplate in the usual fashion **(CASES 25.2 and 25.3)**.

CONCLUSION

Correction of glenoid wear in conjunction with reverse shoulder arthroplasty is important to achieve in order to improve the function and longevity of RTSA. The end point of correction of glenoid deformity in conjunction with RTSA is still a matter of ongoing debate. Implanting the glenoid component within 10° of Freidman' axis and 10° of neutral tilt in coronal plane with minimal glenoid bone removal and maximum possible backside contact is currently an acceptable standard for RTSA. Mild degrees of glenoid wear can be corrected by high side reaming of the glenoid to achieve a neutral axis or by minimal reaming of glenoid in line with the alternate glenoid axis. Moderate or severe degrees of glenoid wear can be addressed with high side reaming, bone grafting of glenoid, and augmented glenoid components. Use of CT-based preoperative planning software along with patient-specific instrumentation guides or computer-assisted navigation allows the surgeon to address moderate-severe glenoid deformities with higher degrees of precision and accuracy. However, cost-effectiveness and long-term survival advantage of RTSA with the use of guidance technology have not been established yet.

VIDEO 25.1: Treatment of severe glenoid deformity using bone graft and reverse total shoulder arthroplasty with intraoperative computer-assisted navigation (CAN).

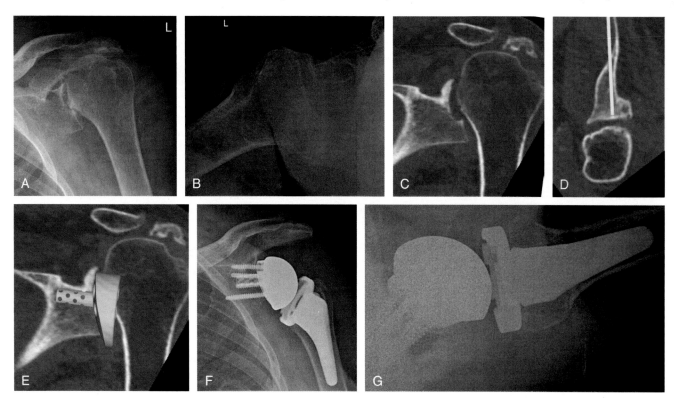

CASE 25.2 Reverse total shoulder arthroplasty (RTSA) with superior augmented baseplate for treatment of moderate superior glenoid wear (Favard E2 glenoid). **A**, Preoperative anteroposterior view (AP view); (**B**) preoperative axillary view; (**C-E**) computed tomography (CT)–based preoperative planning tool templating for superior glenoid wear (Favard E2; **C**) and Walsh B1 glenoid and placement of 10° superior augmented baseplate RTSA; (**F**) postoperative AP view; and (**G**) postoperative axillary view showing degree of correction achieved postoperatively.

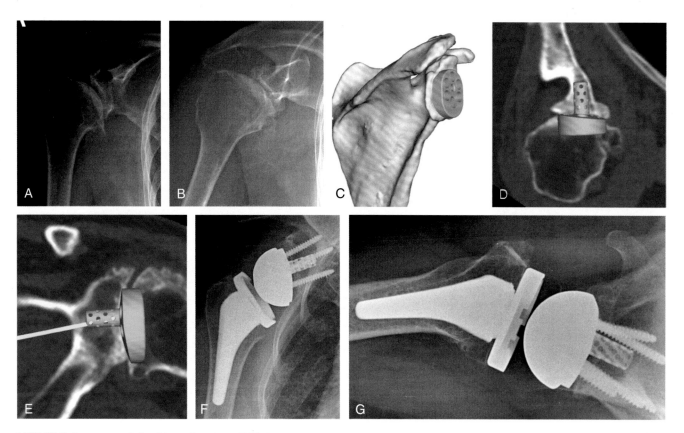

CASE 25.3 Reverse total shoulder arthroplasty (RTSA) with posterior augmented baseplate for correction of moderate posterior glenoid wear (B2 glenoid). **A**, Preoperative anteroposterior view (AP view); (**B**) preoperative axillary view; (**C-E**) computed tomography (CT)–based preoperative planning tool templating for posterior glenoid wear (Walsh B2) and placement of 8-degree posterior augmented baseplate RTSA; (**F**) postoperative AP view and (**G**) postoperative axillary view showing degree of correction achieved postoperatively.

REFERENCES

1. Jones RB, Wright TW, Roche CP. Bone grafting the glenoid versus use of augmented glenoid baseplates with reverse shoulder arthroplasty. *Bull Hosp Jt Dis (2013)*. 2015;73(suppl 1):S129-S135.

2. Jones RB, Wright TW, Zuckerman JD. Reverse total shoulder arthroplasty with structural bone grafting of large glenoid defects. *J Shoulder Elbow Surg*. 2016;25(9):1425-1432.

3. Lopiz Y, García-Fernández C, Arriaza A, Rizo B, Marcelo H, Marco F. Midterm outcomes of bone grafting in glenoid defects treated with reverse shoulder arthroplasty. *J Shoulder Elbow Surg*. 2017;26(9):1581-1588.

4. Roche CP, Diep P, Hamilton MA, et al. Impact of posterior wear on muscle length with reverse shoulder arthroplasty. *Bull Hosp Jt Dis (2013)*. 2015;73(suppl 1):S63-S67.

5. Friedman R, Stroud N, Glattke K, et al. The impact of posterior wear on reverse shoulder glenoid fixation. *Bull Hosp Jt Dis (2013)*. 2015;73(suppl 1):S15-S20.

6. Virk M, Yip M, Liuzza L, et al. Clinical and radiographic outcomes with a posteriorly augmented glenoid for Walch B2, B3, and C glenoids in reverse total shoulder arthroplasty. *J Shoulder Elbow Surg*. 2020;29(5):e196-e204.

7. Frankle MA, Teramoto A, Luo ZP, Levy JC, Pupello D. Glenoid morphology in reverse shoulder arthroplasty: classification and surgical implications. *J Shoulder Elbow Surg*. 2009;18(6):874-885.

8. Bercik MJ, Kruse K, Yalizis M, Gauci MO, Chaoui J, Walch G. A modification to the Walch classification of the glenoid in primary glenohumeral osteoarthritis using three-dimensional imaging. *J Shoulder Elbow Surg*. 2016;25(10):1601-1606.

9. Sirveaux F, Favard L, Oudet D, Huquet D, Walch G, Molé D. Grammont inverted total shoulder arthroplasty in the treatment of glenohumeral osteoarthritis with massive rupture of the cuff. *J Bone Joint Surg Br*. 2004;86(3):388-395.

10. Walch G, Badet R, Boulahia A, Khoury A. Morphologic study of the glenoid in primary glenohumeral osteoarthritis. *J Arthroplasty*. 1999;14(6):756-760.

11. Bateman E, Donald SM. Reconstruction of massive uncontained glenoid defects using a combined autograft-allograft construct with reverse shoulder arthroplasty: preliminary results. *J Shoulder Elbow Surg*. 2012;21(7):925-934.

12. Gilot GJ. Addressing glenoid erosion in reverse total shoulder arthroplasty. *Bull Hosp Jt Dis (2013)*. 2013;71(suppl 2):S51-S53.

13. Nowak DD, Bahu MJ, Gardner TR, et al. Simulation of surgical glenoid resurfacing using three-dimensional computed tomography of the arthritic glenohumeral joint: the amount of glenoid retroversion that can be corrected. *J Shoulder Elbow Surg*. 2009;18(5):680-688.

14. Youderian AR, Iannotti JP. Preoperative planning using advanced 3-dimensional virtual imaging software for glenoid component in anatomic total shoulder replacement. *Tech Shoulder Elbow Surg*. 2012;13(4):145-150.

15. Wright TW, Roche CP, Wright L, Flurin PH, Crosby LA, Zuckerman JD. Reverse shoulder arthroplasty augments for glenoid wear. Comparison of posterior augments to superior augments. *Bull Hosp Jt Dis (2013)*. 2015;73(suppl 1):S124-S128.

16. Boileau P, Morin-Salvo N, Gauci MO, et al. Angled BIO-rsa (Bony-Increased offset-reverse shoulder arthroplasty): a solution for the management of glenoid bone loss and erosion. *J Shoulder Elbow Surg*. 2017;26(12):2133-2142.

17. Ernstbrunner L, Werthel JD, Wagner E, Hatta T, Sperling JW, Cofield RH. Glenoid bone grafting in primary reverse total shoulder arthroplasty. *J Shoulder Elbow Surg*. 2017;26(8):1441-1447.

18. Klein SM, Dunning P, Mulieri P, Pupello D, Downes K, Frankle MA. Effects of acquired glenoid bone defects on surgical technique and clinical outcomes in reverse shoulder arthroplasty. *J Bone Joint Surg Am*. 2010;92(5):1144-1154.

19. Tashjian RZ, Granger E, Chalmers PN. Structural glenoid grafting during primary reverse total shoulder arthroplasty using humeral head autograft. *J Shoulder Elbow Surg*. 2018;27(1):e1-e8.

20. Neyton L, Boileau P, Nové-Josserand L, Edwards TB, Walch G. Glenoid bone grafting with a reverse design prosthesis. *J Shoulder Elbow Surg*. 2007;16(3 suppl):S71-S78.

21. Gupta A, Thussbas C, Koch M, Seebauer L. Management of glenoid bone defects with reverse shoulder arthroplasty-surgical technique and clinical outcomes. *J Shoulder Elbow Surg*. 2018;27(5):853-862.

22. Cil A, Sperling JW, Cofield RH. Nonstandard glenoid components for bone deficiencies in shoulder arthroplasty. *J Shoulder Elbow Surg*. 2014;23(7):e149-e157.

23. Chammaa R, Uri O, Lambert S. Primary shoulder arthroplasty using a custom-made hip-inspired implant for the treatment of advanced glenohumeral arthritis in the presence of severe glenoid bone loss. *J Shoulder Elbow Surg*. 2017;26(1):101-107.

24. Formaini NT, Everding NG, Levy JC, et al. The effect of glenoid bone loss on reverse shoulder arthroplasty baseplate fixation. *J Shoulder Elbow Surg*. 2015;24(11):e312-e319.

25. Werner BS, Böhm D, Abdelkawi A, Gohlke F. Glenoid bone grafting in reverse shoulder arthroplasty for long-standing anterior shoulder dislocation. *J Shoulder Elbow Surg*. 2014;23(11):1655-1661.

26. Walch G, Vezeridis PS, Boileau P, Deransart P, Chaoui J. Three-dimensional planning and use of patient-specific guides improve glenoid component position: an in vitro study. *J Shoulder Elbow Surg*. 2015;24(2):302-309.

27. Virk M, Steinmann SP, Romeo AA, Zuckerman JD. Managing glenoid deformity in shoulder arthroplasty: role of new technology (computer-assisted navigation and patient-specific instrumentation). *Instr Course Lect*. 2020;69:583-594.

28. Rouleau K, Kidder JF, Pons-Villanueva J, Dynamidis S, Defranco M, Walch G. Glenoid version: how to measure it? Validity of different methods in two-dimensional computed tomography scans. *J Shoulder Elbow Surg*. 2010;19:1230-1237.

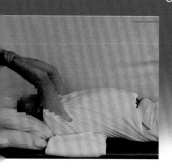

26 Postoperative Care and Rehabilitation

Laura Vasquez-Welsh, MS, OT/L, CHT and James Koo, PT, DPT

INTRODUCTION

Although initially designed as a salvage procedure to manage arthritis in the rotator cuff (RC)–deficient shoulder, the indications for use of reverse total shoulder arthroplasty (RTSA) have expanded over the years. As discussed in previous chapters, there are multiple clinical indications for RTSA including management of massive irreparable RC tears in the absence of osteoarthritis, primary osteoarthritis with excessive posterior glenoid erosion, and complex fractures of the humerus.[1] Due to the growing acceptance of this procedure to treat a variety of conditions, there has been a concomitant increase in the number of RTSAs performed in the United States.[2] With greater utilization of this technique, it is undeniable that an understanding of proper postoperative care and rehabilitation has become increasingly imperative for rehabilitation professionals.

REHABILITATION: RTSA VERSUS ATSA

The primary goal of RTSA is to decrease pain and increase functional elevation of the shoulder as the deltoid becomes the primary mover of the arm. While similarities do exist between RTSA and anatomic total shoulder arthroplasty (ATSA) rehabilitation, the postoperative course is different. One of the inherent reasons for this difference lies within the newly established mechanics of the glenohumeral joint. The RTSA design reverses the orientation of the glenohumeral joint by replacing the glenoid fossa with a glenoid base plate and glenosphere and the humeral head with a stem and concave cup.[3] This design moves the center of rotation of the shoulder joint medially and inferiorly. As a result, the deltoid moment arm and deltoid tension both increase to enhance the torque and line of pull produced by the deltoid.[4,5] Since the deltoid now acts as the prime elevator of the shoulder, it is able to substitute for a deficient RC. Due to this newly established anatomy, there are certain differences in postoperative precautions as well as therapist focus when selecting specific therapeutic interventions.

Another procedural difference that alters the therapeutic approach is that unlike ATSA, RTSA is much less reliant on an intact subscapularis tendon. Naturally,

the rehabilitation protocol reflects this. A 2017 study that compared RTSA outcomes with and without subscapularis repair found that all patients showed significant improvements in pain and function after treatment with RTSA regardless of whether a subscapularis repair was performed.[6] When rehabilitating a shoulder following RTSA, quite often protection of the subscapularis is unnecessary, unless indicated by the surgeon. This is contrary to the protocol followed for a patient who has undergone ATSA. As discussed in Chapter 15, if the surgeon does not utilize a subscapularis-sparing technique for ATSA, protection of the subscapularis becomes a priority during the early postoperative period. As a result, external rotation (ER) is progressed more slowly and cautiously as detailed in Chapter 15. Following RTSA, protocols can be much more liberal with the progression of ER, which can often be progressed as tolerated.

The concept that the RC is either absent or minimally functional after RTSA also alters the therapeutic approach.[3] Although some believe that this reduced need to protect healing structures justifies a faster, more aggressive rehabilitation protocol, the complication rates following this operation including risk for dislocation and stress fracture are higher.[7] Therefore, rehabilitation professionals must rely on their clinical judgment and close communication with the surgeon in order to advance this patient population appropriately.

ENGAGING THE PATIENT AS A PARTNER/ PSYCHOSOCIAL IMPLICATIONS

When possible, prehabilitation sessions with an occupational or physical therapist can be valuable to begin to establish expectations as well as to engage the patient as a partner in the rehabilitation process. When meeting the patient for the first time, the clinician is able to establish a preoperative baseline for range of motion (ROM) and function, review expectations, and promote an environment in which the patient is able to practice exercises prior to surgery. During this session, the therapist should place emphasis on a few key components. These include protecting the newly established joint from dislocation, emphasizing the role of the deltoid, and establishing realistic ROM and functional expectations.[4] There is a link between setting patient expectations early in the process and successful outcomes following shoulder arthroplasty.[8] If the therapist and surgeon clearly define realistic expectations for recovery prior to the operation, patient-reported outcomes may be more favorable.[1]

The role that the patient plays in the rehabilitation process is not to be underemphasized. Patients who are active participants in their recovery tend to achieve optimal results and are more satisfied with their outcome overall.[1] It can also be beneficial to highlight that, ultimately, the patient and multidisciplinary team's goals are the same—to relieve pain and return the patient to an independent lifestyle safely.

POSTOPERATIVE PRECAUTIONS AND FUNCTIONAL IMPLICATIONS

The primary precaution following RTSA is to avoid combined shoulder extension and adduction (ADD), ER, and also to avoid placing the hand behind the back for approximately 4 to 6 weeks postoperatively as these are positions of potential instability. In rehabilitation, it is a common misconception that the risk for dislocation after RTSA is greatest with internal rotation (IR) of the shoulder. However, these replacements are most unstable and likely to dislocate anteriorly with shoulder hyperextension or with end-range ER in either an adducted or abducted position (J. D. Zuckerman, personal communication, May 28, 2020). Nevertheless, clearance from and close communication with the surgeon is always required prior to initiating these motions and positions, especially if initiated prior to 6 weeks postoperatively. Though temporary, the functional impairments that often stem from this precaution may include difficulty with clothing management, especially upper body dressing behind the back (ie, garment fastening, tucking in shirts, donning a belt, and reaching for items in a back pocket), eating, bathing, grooming, and toileting. In order to provide comprehensive care, the therapist should be prepared to discuss strategies for activities of daily living (ADLs) following such an operation. Accounting for and discussing the functional impact that this operation has on the patient's quality of life in the early phases of rehabilitation can help to enhance the therapeutic alliance, guiding the patient through this phase of the process on both a personal and psychological level.

Strategies for Self-Care

In the immediate postoperative phase, it is helpful to educate the patient so that they are equipped with strategies for self-care. As mentioned, the therapist should be prepared to discuss considerations for dressing **(FIGURES 26.1-26.5; VIDEO 26.1)**, sling management **(FIGURES 26.6-26.10; VIDEO 26.1)**, eating, bathing, grooming,

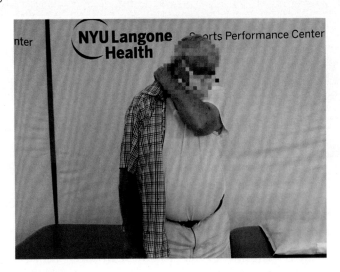

FIGURE 26.1 The patient dresses the operative arm first.

toileting, sleep positioning **(FIGURES 26.11 and 26.12)**, and home management in order to improve the patient's quality of life in the first few weeks following surgery **(TABLE 26.1)**. Toileting is one of the most commonly reported impairments in the immediate weeks following surgery. This fundamental ADL significantly affects a patient's sense of independence and quality of life. The therapist should reassure the patient that after primary RTSA, over 90% of patients are able to manage toileting following the procedure and that toileting inability after the procedure is rare at 1.3%.[9]

INITIATION OF REHABILITATION FOLLOWING SURGERY

Timeline for patient examination by the therapist following surgery can vary. Some hospitals have moved to a same-day discharge model in which the therapist's main contact with the patient is prior to surgery in the form of a prehabilitation session and then potentially not again until

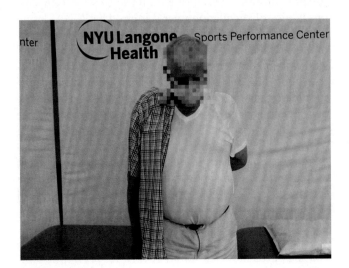

FIGURE 26.2 The nonoperative arm is used to dress the operative arm.

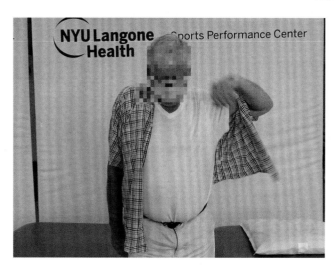

FIGURE 26.3 The nonoperative arm is used to pull the shirt around the back and onto the nonoperative arm.

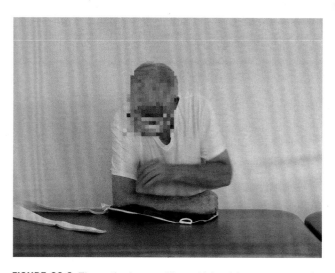

FIGURE 26.6 The patient may utilize a high table as a strategy for donning a sling without putting weight through the operative arm.

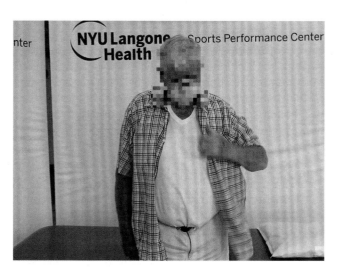

FIGURE 26.4 The nonoperative arm is used to make adjustments as necessary.

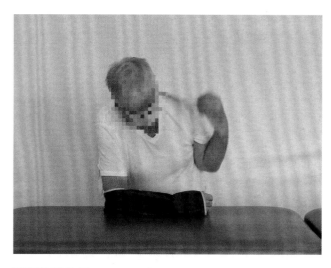

FIGURE 26.7 The nonoperative arm is used to position the strap around the neck and back.

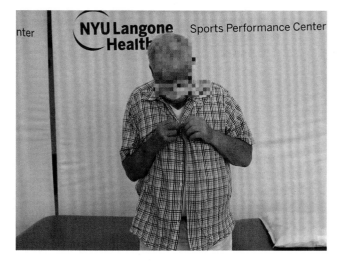

FIGURE 26.5 The patient keeps the operative arm close to the body while assisting the nonoperative arm with buttons.

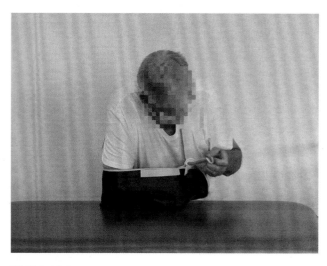

FIGURE 26.8 The nonoperative arm is used to thread the strap through the loops.

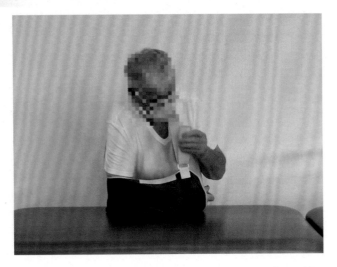

FIGURE 26.9 The nonoperative arm is used to adjust the position of the velcro strap so that the operative arm is positioned properly.

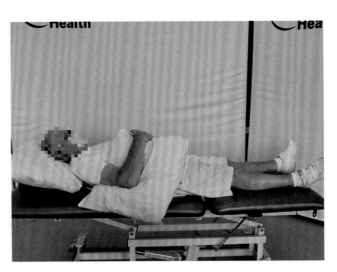

FIGURE 26.11 Supine sleeping position.

they are ready to begin formal outpatient therapy. Outside of a same-day discharge program, patient examination by the therapist will typically begin on postoperative day zero (POD #0). At this phase, rehabilitation goals include protection of healing structures, pain control, functional mobility, independence with basic ADLs, patient education, and independence with a home exercise program (HEP). Under the discretion of the surgeon, passive range of motion (PROM) of the operative upper extremity (UE) typically begins on POD #0 or #1 with a progression to self-assisted or caregiver-assisted ROM exercises **(FIGURES 26.13-26.16)**. Following discharge from the hospital, a period of immobilization may continue for 2 to 6 weeks. The patients continue with their home exercises during this period until they are ready to begin a formal outpatient therapy program **(TABLE 26.2; VIDEO 26.2)**.

When arriving to outpatient therapy, clinical examination will begin with a thorough chart review as described in Chapter 15. The patient relays subjective history including events leading up to surgery, prior and current level of function, and pain levels. A standard postoperative examination is then performed, which includes palpation, visual inspection, bilateral ROM assessment, strength testing of noninvolved joints as appropriate, postural alignment, neurological assessment, and assessment of pain and function.

PHASES OF REHABILITATION

For RTSA rehabilitation, the literature does not support one standardized protocol. Most protocols described in the literature include three to four phases of rehabilitation. There are significant differences in protocols specifically for initiation of exercises, the degree of shoulder motion permitted, the timing of resisted exercises, and the long- and short-term precautions.[1] Collaboration

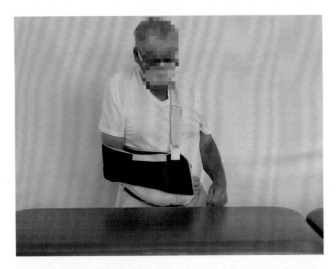

FIGURE 26.10 When the patient returns to a standing position, the elbow should sit at the back corner of the sling and remain at a 90° angle.

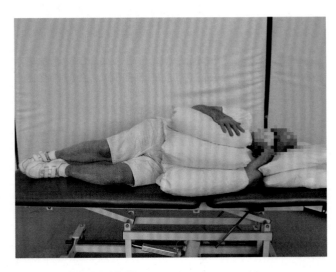

FIGURE 26.12 Side-lying sleeping position.

TABLE 26.1 Strategies for Independence With ADLs

ADL	Tip
Upper body dressing	• Select loose-fitting clothing • Always dress the operative arm *first* • Use the nonoperative arm to pull the shirt onto the operative arm, pulling the shirt as far up the arm as possible. Use the nonoperative arm to pull the shirt over your head or behind your back and down your body. The nonoperative arm goes into the shirt last • Always undress the operative arm *last* • Consider shirts with buttons or zippers in the first few weeks following surgery (remember to keep your operative arm close to your body while assisting with buttoning or zipping) • Females may consider wearing a camisole or tank top as an alternative to a bra following surgery. If a bra is preferred, consider sports bras that zip or close in the front or a strapless bra to avoid irritation at the incision site
Lower body dressing	• Utilize your nonoperative arm to thread both feet into pants while sitting. Stand up to pull pants up past your hips using your nonoperative arm. When securing pants, the operative arm may assist, but be sure to keep it close to your body • Consider pants with elastic
Sling management	• Wear your sling at all times as instructed by the physician (this includes sleeping). You may remove the sling when sitting and at rest. During this time, you may allow your elbow to straighten • Make sure your elbow remains at a 90° angle while in the sling. If your hand becomes swollen, it may be a sign that your elbow is too straight and that the elbow position is not 90°. Discuss additional options for edema control with your therapist as needed • While in the sling, remember to move your wrist and fingers • Continue to wear sling until further instruction from your physician
Eating	• It is permitted to bend at the elbow and bring food to your mouth • Be careful not to initiate movement from the shoulder • Begin with foods that do not require cutting
Bathing	• To wash and clean the underarm of your surgical arm, bend at the waist and let the arm passively move away from your body as you bend forward (as in a pendulum exercise) • Consider purchasing a bath mat for prevention of falls while showering
Grooming	• Bend forward from your trunk (as in pendulum exercise) to move your arm away from your body for activities such as bathing, deodorant application, shaving underarms
Toileting	• Use your nonoperative arm • Place toilet paper on your nonoperative side • Consider use of toileting aid
Sleeping	• Keep sling on for sleeping • Consider sleeping on nonoperative side, on your back or in a semireclined position • While lying on your back, place a small pillow behind your operative arm so that it stays aligned with your body **(FIGURE 26.11)** • While lying on your nonoperative arm, stack pillows in front of your body so that you can prop your operative arm on top keeping it in a slightly abducted position **(FIGURE 26.12)** • Consider sleeping in a recliner if available
Home management	• Consider preparing meals and freezing them prior to surgery • Temporarily move frequently use items from higher shelves to counter top level
Driving	• Consult your physician before resumption of driving

ADLs, activities of daily living.

between the surgeon and occupational or physical therapist is therefore essential to ensure optimal patient outcomes and appropriate rehabilitation following RTSA. In order to individualize the program to best suit the patient's needs, the therapist should be aware of the patient's preoperative status, bone quality, the integrity of the remaining or repaired RC, and the overall stability achieved intraoperatively.[4] When progressing treatment, it is important that the therapist meet the patient at the current level of need rather than relying solely on protocol alone. For example, if a patient begins therapy at 6 weeks following surgery and has 70° of passive forward elevation, the therapist must have the wherewithal to hold progression to the next phase of rehabilitation until PROM goals are achieved and communicate findings to the physician. It is imperative that the clinician

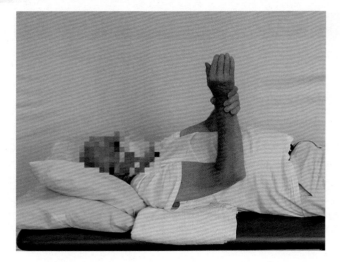

FIGURE 26.13 Passive forward elevation (start position).

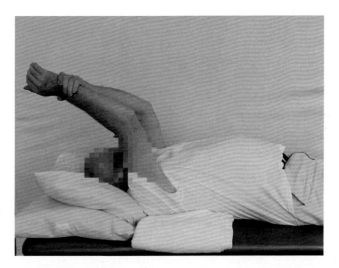

FIGURE 26.14 Passive forward elevation (end position).

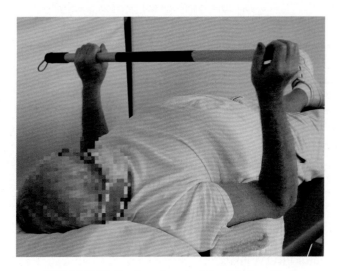

FIGURE 26.15 Passive external rotation (start position).

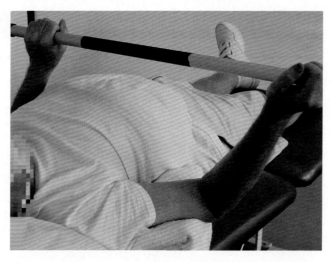

FIGURE 26.16 Passive external rotation (end position).

TABLE 26.2 Initial HEP
Initial HEP Following Discharge From Hospital

Precautions:

- All shoulder exercises are to be performed *passively*

Exercises:

- Passive forward elevation supine
- Passive external rotation supine
- Passive elbow flexion supine
- Active elbow extension supine
- AROM of forearm and wrist
- AROM of hand (including thumb opposition)

Frequency:

- Perform two sets of 10 repetitions of all of the above exercises three times per day

AROM, active range of motion; HEP, home exercise program.

calls upon their knowledge of the underlying biomechanics, physiological healing process, and the patient's preexisting pathology and tolerance for exercise and activity in order to progress the patient appropriately.[7]

Phase I: Immediate Postoperative Phase (Table 26.3)

The first phase of rehabilitation is the immediate postoperative phase, which occurs between 0 and 6 weeks. Therapeutic interventions should aim to reduce pain and inflammation, promote healing, and achieve the ROM goals for this stage. Early in the rehabilitation process, pendulum exercises are typically included as part of the HEP. When performed correctly, movement of the hips and trunk creates secondary movement of the postsurgical limb. If the patient has difficulty initiating the pendulum motion passively, the therapist may consider teaching a modification of this exercise sometimes referred to as "rock the baby." In this variation, the nonoperative arm is utilized to assist the operative arm

TABLE 26.3 Phase I

Phase I: Immediate Postoperative Phase (0-6 wk)

Goals:

- Protect healing structures
- Reduce pain and inflammation
- Scar management
- Establish PROM goals and initiate AAROM of the shoulder joint at the end of this phase

Precautions:

- Avoid combined shoulder extension and ADD, ER, and hand behind the back
- Avoid shoulder hyperextension
- No weight bearing through the postsurgical upper extremity (ie: pushing up from a chair or bed; pushing through arm to use an assistive device such as a cane)
- No lifting/carrying/pulling/pushing

General principles:

- Sling immobilization for 2-6 wk per MD orders
- Modality use (heat/cryotherapy) PRN

Therapeutic exercises:

- Pendulum exercises
- PROM of shoulder (to approximately 90° forward elevation and 20°-30° ER by week 3 and progress gradually to 120° forward elevation and 30°-40° ER by week 6)
- Submaximal pain-free deltoid and periscapular isometrics within first 3 wk
- Consider gentle scapular retraction/postural exercises
- Scapular neuromuscular reeducation (ie: scapular clocks)
- Gentle rhythmic stabilization by therapist
- AROM of elbow wrist and hand
- Consider gentle grip strengthening with putty or foam sponge

Patient education:

- Instruction to always be able to visualize the elbow no matter what the task
- Frequency of HEP: three times per day
- Signs of infection
- Self-care/ADLs

AAROM, active-assisted range of motion; ADD, adduction; ADLs, activities of daily living; AROM, active range of motion; ER, external rotation; HEP, home exercise program; PROM, passive range of motion.

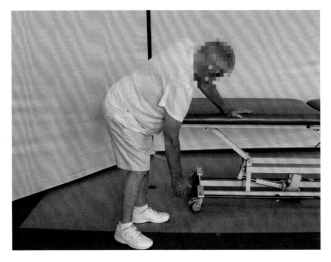

FIGURE 26.17 Pendulum exercises.

overload the acromion and put the patient at risk for a stress fracture.[11] Over these 6 weeks, ROM is gradually progressed from PROM to active-assisted range of motion (AAROM) to active range of motion (AROM) under the skilled guidance of a therapist and is never forceful or aggressive in nature. Progression of PROM within weeks 1 to 3 proceeds as tolerated to at least 90° of elevation and 20° to 30° of ER with both in the scapular plane. It is also beneficial to initiate submaximal and pain-free deltoid and periscapular isometrics within the first 3 weeks to assist in restoring deltoid function and provide stability to the glenohumeral joint.[3] Gentle rhythmic stabilization exercises can also be beneficial to promote dynamic stability. By week 6 of this phase, PROM goals include the progression of elevation to approximately 120° and ER between 30° and 40°.

Generally, all patients who undergo RTSA discontinue sling use completely by week 6. However, this element varies greatly, and therefore open dialogue between

through gentle PROM (**FIGURES 26.17** and **26.18; VIDEO 26.3**). The benefits of these exercises include gentle joint distraction, stretching of the capsule, pain relief, and the initiation of secondary ROM of the shoulder without active muscular contraction at the shoulder joint.[10]

As mentioned, it is important to avoid the combined movement of shoulder extension and ADD, excessive ER, and hand behind the back positioning for the first 4 to 6 weeks. The rehabilitation professional must emphasize this to avoid potential instability. In order to make this position clear to the patient, the therapist may instruct the patient to make sure that they can always visualize their elbow, no matter the task. During the course of this phase, the therapist must also keep in mind that the nature of the newly placed tension on the deltoid can

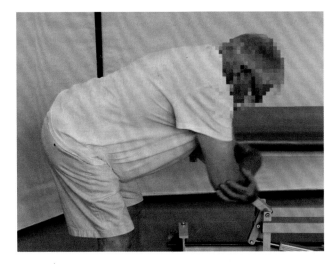

FIGURE 26.18 Variation of pendulum exercises—"rock the baby."

the therapist, patient, and physician is key. Some surgeons may promote the use of a sling for comfort only. Still others allow the patient to wean from its use as early as 2 to 4 weeks, wearing it only for protection while standing and moving about or when out in public.

Phase II: Early AROM and Strengthening (Table 26.4)

Weeks 6 through 12 mark the early AROM and strengthening phase of rehabilitation. In order to progress to this phase, the patient should be able to achieve passive forward elevation and ER in the previously mentioned ranges. At this point, the therapist may initiate passive IR in a protected position of at least 60° of abduction in the scapular plane. The therapist may also initiate AAROM and AROM for elevation in a supine position for scapular stabilization. During this phase, it is important to challenge the shoulder musculature at an appropriate level to avoid development of poor mechanics, unnecessary pain, and compromised joint integrity.[3] To do so, the therapist initiates both ROM and early strengthening in gravity-reduced positions with assistance or support and progresses to more functional and challenging positions.[12] By week 8, the therapist begins

to introduce submaximal ER and IR isometrics to respect the soft-tissue integrity of the teres minor and subscapularis if repaired or intact. In order to begin to reestablish scapulohumeral rhythm, incorporation of isotonic periscapular and deltoid exercises between week 6 and 8 is encouraged.[13] With clearance from the physician, the therapist may also initiate gentle resistive therapeutic exercise with bands by week 8. The therapist must also ensure that the patient avoids shoulder hyperextension during this phase to prevent undue stress on the anterior shoulder (ie, with posterior deltoid strengthening).

Phase III: Resistance Strengthening and Proprioception Phase (Table 26.5)

Phase III of the rehabilitation process is the resistance strengthening and proprioception phase. Progression to this phase is appropriate once the patient achieves ROM goals from the previous phases as well as "good" muscle strength. The goal of this phase is to advance strengthening and functional use of the operative UE. Therapy emphasizes low weight and high repetitions.

Phase IV: Advanced Goal-specific Strengthening and Proprioception Phase (Table 26.6)

The final phase of rehabilitation is the advanced goal-specific strengthening and proprioception phase. The goal is functional, pain-free shoulder AROM and independence with HEP. In 2018, Liu et al published a systematic review indicating that patients who undergo RTSA do return to sports at a rate of approximately 75%.[14] Therefore, this phase of rehabilitation can

---

TABLE 26.4 Phase II

Phase II: Early ROM and Strengthening Phase (6-12 wk)

Criteria for progression:

- Shoulder PROM to 120° of forward elevation and 30° ER
- Adequate mechanics and acceptable AROM prior to initiating isotonic strengthening

Goals:

- Progress pain-free shoulder PROM to tolerance (typically maximum of 140°)
- Initiate shoulder AAROM and progress to AROM
- AROM of shoulder to 90° of forward elevation and 30° of ER without substitution patterns

Precautions:

- Continue to avoid shoulder hyperextension

General principles:

- Initiate shoulder AAROM for elevation and progress to AROM (beginning in supine)
- Initiate passive IR (protected position of at least 60° of abduction in the scapular plane)

Therapeutic exercises:

- Incorporate isotonic periscapular and deltoid exercises at week 6-8 (include prone and side-lying therapeutic exercise)
- Initiate submaximal IR and ER isometrics by week 8
- Begin light resistive exercises with band by week 8 and progress to light dumbbells
- Begin short arc PNF patterns

AAROM, active-assisted range of motion; AROM, active range of motion; ER, external rotation; HEP, home exercise program; IR, internal rotation; PNF, proprioceptive neuromuscular facilitation; PROM, passive range of motion; ROM, range of motion.

TABLE 26.5 Phase III

Phase III: Resistance Strengthening and Proprioception Phase (12-16 wk)

Criteria for progression:

- Achievement of shoulder ROM goals from previous phase
- "Good" or better muscle strength

Goals:

- Increase AROM: 100°-120° elevation (emphasize stability over mobility)
- Increase strength of deltoid and scapular stabilizers
- Increase functional independence

Precautions:

- Guided by patient tolerance

General principles:

- Emphasize low resistance and high repetitions
- Continue modalities per therapist discretion

Therapeutic exercises:

- Initiate advanced resisted scapular exercises
- Incorporate gentle closed chain proprioception exercises

AROM, active range of motion; ROM, range of motion.

TABLE 26.6 Phase IV

Phase IV: Advanced Goal-Specific Strengthening and Proprioception Phase (16 wk+)

Criteria for progression:

- Functional and pain-free shoulder AROM

Goals:

- Functional, pain-free shoulder AROM
- Independence with HEP
- Dependent on patient's activity and demand level

Precautions:

- Discourage participating in heavy work or recreational activities that result in high loading of the shoulder
- A 10-15 lb bilateral UE lifting limit should be followed indefinitely

General principles:

- Modalities per therapist discretion

Therapeutic exercises:

- Advance strengthening as tolerated—remaining RC, deltoid, and scapular stabilizers
- Initiate plyometric and open chain exercises
- Incorporate increased range PNF patterns into strengthening program

Patient education:

- Regarding safe return to prior activity level (including work and sports) at the discretion of the physician

AROM, active range of motion; HEP, home exercise program; PNF, proprioceptive neuromuscular facilitation; RC, rotator cuff; UE, upper extremity.

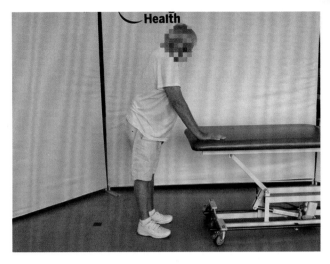

FIGURE 26.19 Variation of passive elevation—walk backs (start position).

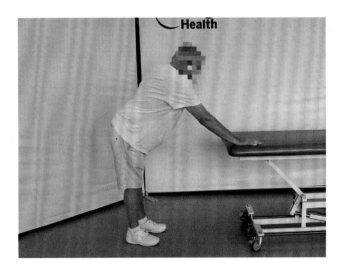

FIGURE 26.20 Variation of passive elevation—walk backs (end position).

incorporate gradual resumption of their previous sport, with modifications as necessary, at the discretion of both their physician and body's tolerance.

CLINICAL PEARLS BY PHASE

Phase I

Early on in the rehabilitation process, it can be quite difficult for patients to perform passive forward elevation of the shoulder in the supine position. There a few modifications to this exercise that have proven to be beneficial if the patient is unable to perform it in a supine position due to pain or contralateral shoulder pathology. The therapist can teach a variation of this exercise utilizing a chair or tabletop. For this exercise, the patient places the operative UE on the stable surface while standing and carefully walks back while bending over **(FIGURES 26.19 and 26.20; VIDEO 26.4).**[12] As an alternative, while seated, patients may also place their operative UE on a foam roller on the table. The therapist then instructs the patient to use trunk flexion to initiate movement of the foam roller on the table, thus bringing the operative extremity through gentle forward elevation. It is important to instruct the patient to keep the operative UE completely relaxed during this variation **(FIGURES 26.21 and 26.22; VIDEO 26.4).**

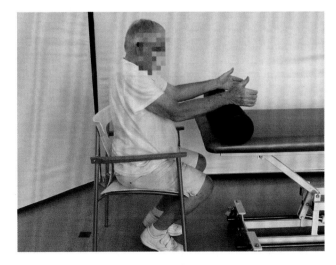

FIGURE 26.21 Variation of passive elevation—foam roller on table (start position).

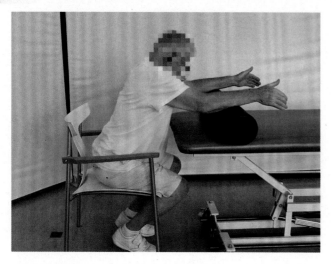

FIGURE 26.22 Variation of passive elevation—foam roller on table (end position).

During the initial phase of rehabilitation, the therapist must also recognize that pain and reflexive muscle guarding is a natural response following surgery.[12] In order to earn the patient's confidence, it is important that the therapist respect the patient's response to initiation of movement by avoiding any forceful PROM. It can be helpful to apply heat for 10 minutes prior to the initiation of ROM to promote muscle relaxation. Incorporation of scapular mobilization can also be beneficial to aid in patient relaxation and help to facilitate early neuromuscular control of the scapula. The patient can also continue to utilize cryotherapy for pain control following therapy sessions and throughout the day as needed.

Phase II

When transitioning from Phase I to Phase II of rehabilitation, it is important that the therapist continue to protect tissue healing while advancing exercise intensity. Progression of active-assisted and active elevation from supine and side lying to positions of sitting and standing against gravity can prove challenging if not progressed strategically. In order to do so effectively, the therapist must take advantage of short lever arms, positioning the arm relative to gravity, and using simple equipment such as a ball or incline board.[12] Research has demonstrated that "closed chain" or supported active-assisted exercise (SAAE) requires less RC activity than "open chain" exercises.[15] This fact can be beneficial in this patient population as the status of their RC muscles is often unknown or the muscles themselves are nonexistent. Therapists should begin with supported AROM exercises before advancing to more demanding unsupported or open kinetic chain AROM exercises. There is an art to strategically utilizing different surfaces or equipment to successfully progress elevation **(VIDEOS 26.5 and 26.6)**.

Phase II to IV

Shoulders that have undergone RTSA show kinematics that are significantly different from the kinematics of normal shoulders. Research has shown that patients with RTSA use more scapulothoracic motion and less glenohumeral motion to elevate the arm.[13] It is for this reason that protocols focus on reestablishing proper scapulohumeral rhythm throughout the course of rehabilitation in order to optimize functional outcomes for this patient population.

Abnormal scapular motion has been linked to excess activation of the upper trapezius, combined with decreased control of the lower trapezius (LT), and the serratus anterior (SA). When attempting to enhance scapulothoracic motion following RTSA, it is beneficial to select strengthening exercises that promote the optimal activation of the LT, middle trapezius, and SA muscles.[17] These exercises include side-lying ER, prone abduction with ER, side-lying forward elevation, and prone extension (with care to limit hyperextension of the shoulder with this patient population). When properly conditioned, these periscapular muscles assist in providing stability to the shoulder by promoting smooth upward rotation of the scapula and preventing scapular winging.[16] Strengthening of the SA muscle in isolation is also especially helpful. When functioning efficiently, it produces upward rotation of the scapula, posterior tipping and ER and helps to preserve the subacromial space **(FIGURES 26.23-26.32)**.[16]

OUTCOMES

There are multiple factors that affect patient outcomes following RTSA. These include preexisting pathology, implant design and placement, quality of the remaining soft tissue, quality of the rehabilitation program, and

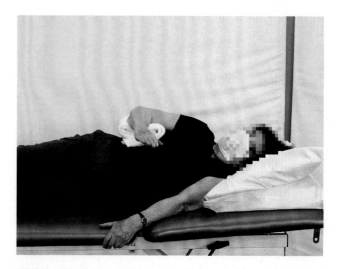

FIGURE 26.23 Shoulder external rotation in side lying (start position).

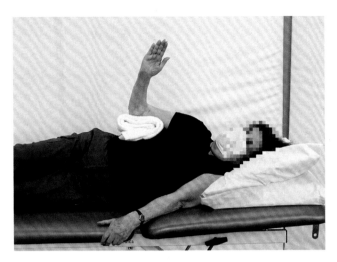

FIGURE 26.24 Shoulder external rotation in side lying (end position).

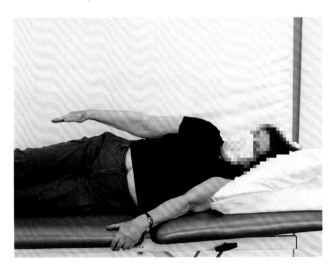

FIGURE 26.27 Side-lying forward elevation (start position).

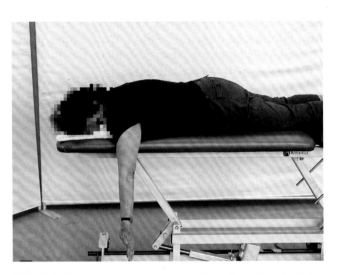

FIGURE 26.25 Prone horizontal abduction with external rotation (start position).

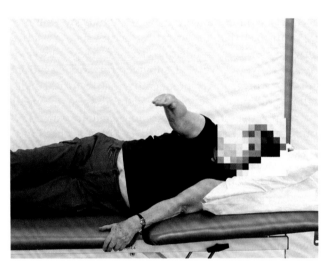

FIGURE 26.28 Side-lying forward elevation (end position).

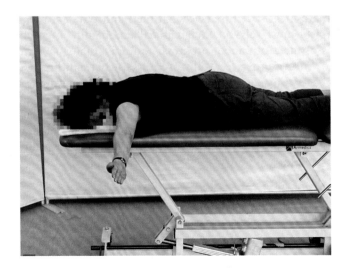

FIGURE 26.26 Prone horizontal abduction with external rotation (start position).

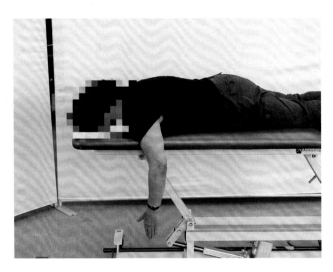

FIGURE 26.29 Prone extension (start position).

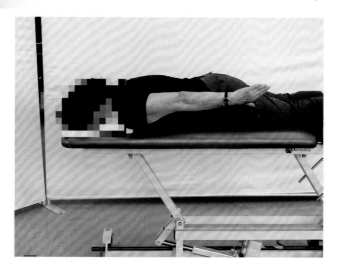

FIGURE 26.30 Prone extension (end position).

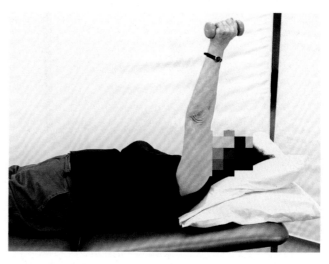

FIGURE 26.32 Serratus strengthening supine (end position).

overall patient compliance.[7] A 2017 study by Collin et al. confirmed that preoperative factors such as active forward elevation and deltoid strength are predictive of postoperative recovery of shoulder forward elevation. In other words, lower preoperative active forward elevation and poor preoperative deltoid strength yields poorer postoperative outcomes for active forward flexion.[18] In a 2014 study, Schwartz et al found that intraoperative forward flexion was the strongest predictor of final postoperative ROM, followed by gender and preoperative ROM. Final functional outcome is therefore directly dependent on motion achieved in the operating room.[19]

In general, patients undergoing primary RTSA have been shown to gain about 105° or greater of active shoulder elevation and about 15° of active ER if the teres minor is intact.[3] Return of active shoulder rotation is dependent upon the postoperative condition of the teres minor. Boudreau et al reported that patients with a negative ER lag sign during the initial strengthening phase progress more rapidly in terms of strength, function, and active elevation of the operative UE.

In terms of overall long-term outcome after RTSA, despite promising results in early and midterm follow-up, a 2018 study does describe long-term compromise of shoulder function. A lack of exercise in elderly patients may be one reason for this loss in function. Future studies would be beneficial to examine whether a return to therapy is able to prevent a decrease in long-term shoulder function.[20]

CONCLUSION

Although currently there is not one standardized protocol for RTSA, it is essential to apply the basic principles of shoulder rehabilitation. These principles may be similar for RTSA and ATSA, but rehabilitation following RTSA is unique due to the newly established anatomical structure. Occupational and physical therapists must rely on their clinical judgment, on-going assessment of patient progress, and open dialogue with the surgeon to successfully progress the patient through phases of rehabilitation at the appropriate rate. In order to increase patient satisfaction with their overall outcome, it is important to engage the patient as a partner in the rehabilitation process and to take a holistic approach considering both their physical and psychological needs.

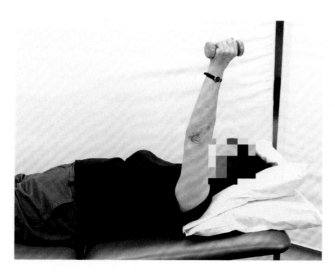

FIGURE 26.31 Serratus strengthening supine (start position).

REFERENCES

1. Bullock GS, Garrigues GE, Ledbetter L, Kennedy J. A systematic review of proposed rehabilitation guidelines following anatomic and reverse shoulder arthroplasty. *J Orthop Sports Phys Ther.* 2019;49(5):337-347.
2. Schairer WW, Nwachukwu BU, Lyman SL, Craig EV, Gulotta LV. National utilization of reverse total shoulder arthroplasty in the United States. *J Shoulder Elbow Surg.* 2015;24(1):91-97.

3. Boudreau S, Boudreau E, Higgins LD, Wilcox RB III. Rehabilitation following reverse total shoulder arthroplasty. *J Orthop Sports Phys Ther.* 2007;32(12):734-743.

4. Ellenbecker TS, Wilcox RB III. Rehabilitation following total shoulder and reverse total shoulder arthroplasty. In: Giangarra CE, Manske RC, Brotzman SB, eds. *Clinical Orthopaedic Rehabilitation: A Team Approach.* 4th ed. Elsevier; 2018:181-188.

5. Kontazis A, Johnson GR. The biomechanics of reverse anatomy shoulder replacement – a modelling study. *Clin Biomech (Bristol, Avon).* 2009;24(3):254-260.

6. Friedman RJ, Flurin PH, Wright TW, Zuckerman JD, Roche CP. Comparison of reverse total shoulder arthroplasty outcomes with and without subscapularis repair. *J Shoulder Elbow Surg.* 2017;26(4):662-668.

7. Wolff AL, Rosenzweig L. Anatomical and biomechanical framework for shoulder arthroplasty rehabilitation. *J Hand Ther.* 2017;30:167-174.

8. Swarup I, Henn CM, Nguyen JT, et al. Effect of pre-operative expectations on the outcomes following total shoulder arthroplasty. *Bone Joint J.* 2017;99(9):1190-1196.

9. Rojas J, Bitzer A, Joseph J, Srikumaran U, McFarland EG. Toileting ability of patients after primary revers total shoulder arthroplasty. *JSES Int.* 2020;4:174-181.

10. Sebelski CA, Guanche CA. Total shoulder arthroplasty. In: Maxey L, Magnusson J, eds. *Rehabilitation for the Post-surgical Orthopedic Patient.* 3rd ed. Elsevier; 2013:118-143.

11. Farshad M, Gerber C. Reverse total shoulder arthroplasty – from the most to the least common complication. *Int Orthop.* 2010;34:1075-1082.

12. Ellenbecker TS, Manske RC, Kelley M. *The shoulder: physical therapy patient management using current evidence.* In: *Current Concepts for Orthopaedic Physical Therapy.* 4th ed. Orthopaedic Section, APTA Inc; 2016:54-69.

13. Walker D, Matsuki K, Struk AM, Wright TW, Banks SA. Scapulohumeral rhythm in shoulders with reverse shoulder arthroplasty. *J Shoulder Elbow Surg.* 2015;24(7):1129-1134.

14. Liu JN, Steinhaus ME, Garcia GH, et al. Return to sport after shoulder arthroplasty: a systematic review and meta-analysis. *Knee Surg Sports Traumatol Arthrosc.* 2018;26:100-112.

15. Wise MB, Uhl TL, Mattacola CG, Nitz AJ, Kibler WB. The effect of limb support on muscle activation during shoulder exercises. *J Shoulder Elbow Surg.* 2004;13(6):614-620.

16. Cricchio M, Frazer C. Scapulothoracic and scapulohumeral exercises: a narrative review of electromyographic studies. *J Hand Ther.* 2011;24:322-334.

17. Cools AM, Dewitte V, Lanszweert F, et al. Rehabilitation of scapular muscle balance: which exercises to prescribe? *Am J Sports Med.* 2007;35(10):1744-1751.

18. Collin P, Matsukawa T, Denart PJ, Gain S, Ladermann A. Pre-operative factors influence the recovery of range of motion following reverse shoulder arthroplasty. *Int Orthop.* 2017;41:2135-2142.

19. Schwartz DG, Cottrell BJ, Teusink MJ, et al. Factors that predict postoperative motion in patients treated with reverse shoulder arthroplasty. *J Shoulder Elbow Surg.* 2014;23(9):1289-1295.

20. Uschok S, Herrmann S, Pauly S, Perka C, Greiner S. Reverse shoulder arthroplasty: the role of physical therapy on the clinical outcome in the mid-term to long-term follow-up. *Arch Orthop Trauma Surg.* 2018;138:1347-1352.

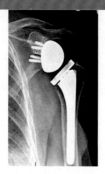

27 Clinical Outcomes of Reverse Total Shoulder Arthroplasty

Ryan W. Simovitch, MD and Richard J. Friedman, MD

INTRODUCTION

Reverse total shoulder arthroplasty (RTSA) designs came into clinical use in the early 1970s. However, the early designs were fraught with many complications, and most failed within 2 to 3 years, as the glenoid component often loosened due to the high forces present, especially in cases where the rotator cuff was absent. As a result of this, combined with the early success of Neer's anatomic total shoulder arthroplasty (ATSA), RTSA fell out of favor.[1]

While ATSA provided excellent pain relief and restoration of function in patients with an intact rotator cuff, those with a cuff-deficient shoulder did not do as well. Patients with glenohumeral arthritis and massive rotator tearing developed instability in a superior or anterior-superior direction because the absent rotator cuff could not provide a fixed fulcrum for the humeral head against the glenoid. Patients with glenohumeral arthritis and massive rotator cuff tears, referred to as cuff tear arthropathy (CTA), exhibited shoulder weakness, incongruous joints surfaces, instability, and bone loss. The promise of RTSA was that it could restore glenohumeral joint stability, provide smooth articulating surfaces, replace bone loss, and optimize the remaining rotator cuff muscles and deltoid to improve strength and function.

It was not until the middle 1980s when Paul Grammont in France developed and articulated his principles of RTSA that clinical interest in the prosthesis emerged.[2] Grammont proposed moving the center of rotation (COR) medially and distally, thereby protecting the glenoid component from early failure and providing stability for the prosthetic construct. The glenoid had a convex weight-bearing portion matching up with a concave humeral cup, and the center of the glenoid sphere (glenosphere) was at or within the glenoid neck. His original prosthesis, first implanted in 1985, underwent further development and design changes in 1991 and 1994, and each redesign showed clinical promise and avoided the failures of earlier designs.[3] This was the catalyst that led to the development of the modern RTSA.

Initial reports on the clinical outcomes of RTSA were from Europe, given the fact that the current design originated there and was not released for use in the United

States until 2003. Published studies showed significant clinical improvements in a very difficult patient population, but the complication rates were significantly higher than those reported for ATSA. These included hematoma formation,[4] infection,[4,5] scapular notching,[6,7] instability,[8,9] acromial insufficiency,[4,10] and glenoid component failures.[11,12] However, prosthetic designs have evolved, surgical techniques have improved, and surgical experience has increased, and as a result, the complication rate for RTSA is now similar to and, in fact, may be less than ATSA.[13]

The original indication for RTSA when it was first approved by the United States Food and Drug Administration in December 2003 was CTA. The indications have expanded significantly since that time, as the clinical outcomes and survivorship have been favorable and remained so over time. Current indications for RTSA include CTA, massive irreparable cuff tear with osteoarthritis, irreparable massive rotator cuff tear, primary osteoarthritis in older patients with an intact rotator cuff, rheumatoid arthritis and other inflammatory arthropathies, proximal humerus fractures, sequelae of proximal humerus fractures such as nonunions and malunions, revision total shoulder arthroplasty, chronic dislocations, periprosthetic fractures, tumors, infection sequelae, severe glenoid deformity with or without an intact rotator cuff, and severe posterior subluxation with posterior glenoid erosion.

Given the expanding indications for RTSA, one could argue that there is one indication for ATSA and all other patients would be candidates for an RTSA. The indication for an ATSA is a patient with osteoarthritis who is relatively young, has no severe systemic illnesses, has no significant glenoid deformity, has an intact functional rotator cuff, and has not had any previous open shoulder surgery that violated the subscapularis. This makes for a very homogeneous group with consistent and reliable outcomes. RTSA is done for many different indications, and therefore the clinical outcome and survivorship vary based upon the underlying pathology. One must be careful when comparing the results of ATSA and RTSA to make sure the comparison is between similar groups with similar indications.

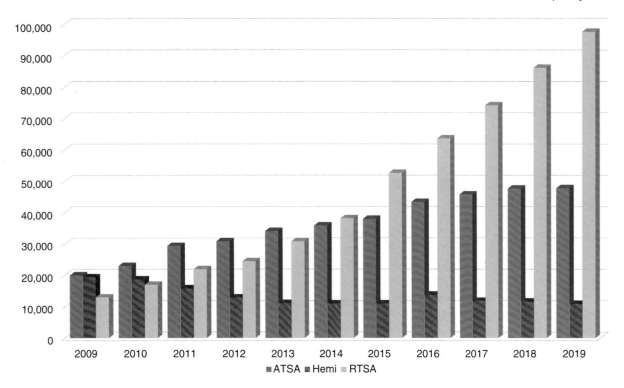

FIGURE 27.1 Shoulder arthroplasty usage from 2009 to 2019 in the United States, demonstrating the increase in reverse total shoulder arthroplasty (RTSA) and decrease in hemiarthroplasty over that time. Note that 2014 was the year that RTSA outnumbered anatomic total shoulder arthroplasty (ATSA).

With the expanding indications for RTSA, the clinical volume has grown exponentially over the past 15 years, far surpassing the growth of ATSA.[14] There has been a 17-fold increase in the use of RTSA over the past 15 years, compared to a 3-fold increase in ATSA **(FIGURE 27.1)**. In 2014, the use of RTSA surpassed that of ATSA in the United States for the first time and has continued to do so.[15] It is projected that RTSA utilization will increase 122% over the next 5 years.

In this chapter, we will explore the various indications for RTSA, the clinical outcomes achieved, and the factors that can influence outcomes and survivorship.

INFLUENCE OF BIOMECHANICS ON OUTCOMES

Initial early success with the use of a traditional Grammont-style RTSA spawned the development of multiple reverse shoulder implant designs and implantation techniques that are utilized today. Variations in implant design and implantation techniques have been shown to impact clinical and radiographic results.

Implant variability includes both glenoid- and humeral-sided considerations. Different RTSA designs utilize glenospheres of varying spherical radii and thickness, which together influence the COR.[16] Altering the COR can influence rotator cuff and soft-tissue tension, thus impacting range of motion (ROM), strength, and stability.

Furthermore, the COR influences the deltoid moment arm, whereby a medialized COR results in a greater moment arm in turn providing the deltoid with greater efficiency in elevating the arm during abduction. The converse is true in the case of a glenosphere with a lateralized COR.[16-20]

Humeral-sided design variability includes neck-shaft angle, inlay versus onlay design, stem shape, and humeral tray offset, all of which result in a specific amount of humeral-sided lateralization. The degree of humeral-sided lateralization influences soft-tissue tensioning and deltoid wrapping, which can influence both strength and stability. Other design characteristics that can influence clinical and radiographic outcomes after RTSA are polyethylene depth and constraint as well as stem length. A combination of glenoid- and humeral-sided design attributes has been shown to influence the rate of scapula notching, impingement-free arc of motion, active ROM, acromial fracture rate, and stability.[21-33]

Routman et al[16] first described a classification system that categorized various RTSA prosthesis designs based on their glenoid- and humeral-sided design attributes. Specifically, this classification stratified prostheses into those with a glenosphere with a COR of 5 mm or less lateral to the glenoid face labeled as a medialized glenoid (MG) or with a COR greater than 5 mm lateral to the glenoid labeled as a lateralized glenoid (LG). Similarly, they classified humeral prostheses according to the degree of offset, which was defined based on the horizontal distance between the humeral stem axis and the center of the humeral liner. It was stipulated that a humeral implant with an offset of 15 mm or less was a medialized humerus (MH) and a humeral implant with an offset greater than 15 mm was a lateralized humerus (LH). Different implant systems combine a specific glenoid design with a specific humerus design, thus yielding three general design combinations: MG/MH, MG/LH, and LG/MH. Each design has various advantages and disadvantages specific to its biomechanical design.

Werthel et al[34] attempted to stratify RTSA prosthesis designs by considering combined global implant lateralization. The measurement of humeral lateralized offset was similar to the technique employed by Routman et al[16]; however, the contribution from glenoid lateralization included the sum of the offset contributed by the COR offset in addition to the perceived radius of the glenosphere. The quantitative global implant lateralization was then fit into five categories relative to the Delta III prosthesis (Grammont design): medialized reverse shoulder arthropathy (RSA), minimally lateralized RSA, lateralized RSA, highly lateralized RTSA, and very highly lateralized RSA.

The classification systems of both Routman et al[16] and Werthel et al[34] help to lay the framework for understanding the biomechanical differences in various RTSA implant designs. Understanding the various biomechanical attributes of each implant system can help predict their strengths and weaknesses and can also help to avoid potential pitfalls. While specific implants have defined biomechanical properties, the technique of implantation and hence surgeon choices can alter the biomechanical principles and expected outcomes. For example, it has been demonstrated that the position of glenosphere implantation matters greatly. Based on previous studies, a position biased inferiorly[6,35] and posteriorly[36] is associated with reduced rates of scapula notching. Thus, the increased rates of scapular notching in Grammont-style prostheses (MG/MH) can be mitigated, but not eliminated, by lowering the position of the glenoid baseplate[6] or augmenting the glenoid bone with autograft such as in the BIO-RSA.[37] Other implants reduce the rate of scapula notching through the implant design attributes alone or in combination such as the MG/LH and LG/MH designs. Another example of a technique variation that impacts outcome is the decision to repair the subscapularis after RTSA. Repair of this tendon may result in certain limitations and certain benefits depending on the implant utilized.[38] This confirms the connected interplay between implant choice and surgical technique. This complex interplay should be appreciated when reviewing the literature and the results of RTSA. Implant designs are vividly different, and thus comparing results among different cohorts in the literature can be deceiving or, at best, confusing.

SURVIVORSHIP

When RTSA was introduced in the United States, many surgeons recommended avoiding the procedure in patients younger than 70 years because survivorship was unknown. Over time, however, it has become clear that the survivorship is similar to that reported following ATSA. Given the fact that the glenoid component in RTSA relies on bone ingrowth and not methyl methacrylate as with an ATSA for long-term fixation, the survivorship of RTSA could surpass that of an ATSA as we acquire longer term follow-up.

Earlier studies utilizing a first-generation Grammont-style prosthesis reported survivorship of 89% at 10 years, but the clinical outcomes deteriorated over that time period.[39] This was likely related to the high incidence of scapular notching in these patients, which is much less frequent now with more contemporary designs and compensatory surgical techniques. While previous studies suggested that scapular notching did not affect the clinical outcome, more recent articles have shown that the clinical results deteriorate over time if scapular notching is present when compared to those without scapular notching.[22] Another early study looking at the 10-year results of RTSA performed in patients younger than 65 years for massive irreparable rotator cuff tears showed that the significant clinical improvements were maintained out to 10 years, but there was a high complication rate.[40] A large multicenter study utilizing the same first-generation RTSA prosthesis with a minimum follow-up of 10 years showed that survivorship depended on the underlying diagnosis.[41] The overall survivorship was 92% at a minimum of 10 years. RTSAs performed for osteoarthritis with or without rotator cuff disease had a 97% survivorship, while those performed for revision of a previously placed prosthesis, such as conversion of a hemiarthroplasty (HA) to an RTSA or revision of an ATSA to an RTSA, had a survivorship of 88%.

Time and experience have demonstrated that this procedure has excellent outcomes and survivorship even in younger patients using contemporary prosthetic designs. Otto et al reported on 67 patients younger than 55 years undergoing RTSA for a variety of diagnoses and reported 91% survivorship at a mean follow-up of 5 years, with the range being from 2 to 12 years. Patients undergoing a primary RTSA had significantly better outcomes compared to those who had a failed previous arthroplasty revised to RTSA.[42]

Two early studies looking at the long-term survivorship of RTSA for osteoarthritis and/or rotator cuff disease both found survival rates of 95% at 8 and 12 years, respectively.[5,9] Bacle et al found an implant survival rate of 93% at a minimum of 10 years for multiple indications using what would be considered second-generation implant designs.[43] Another more recent study looking at the 10-year minimum survivorship of a contemporary design performed only for the treatment of rotator cuff deficiency showed 91% survivorship.[24]

These survivorship results, for both first-generation designs and more contemporary implants, are excellent and compare favorably with those for ATSA. This is true for both primary RTSA done for arthritis and/or rotator cuff disease and for multiple other indications, including revision arthroplasty. Torchia et al reviewed the results of 113 first-generation Neer ATSAs performed for a variety of indications, such as osteoarthritis, rheumatoid arthritis, and posttraumatic arthritis, and reported 93% survivorship at 10 years and 87% survivorship at 15 years.[44] Another study of survivorship of a Neer total shoulder arthroplasty in patients with both osteoarthritis and rheumatoid arthritis showed similar results, with survivorship of 93% at 10 years, 88% at 15 years, and 85% at 20 years.[45] This is the standard to which RTSA needs to be compared and, at this time, appears to be similar.

National registry databases from countries where all arthroplasties are entered into a national registry also provide valuable information on survivorship. The 2019 Annual Report from the Australian Orthopaedic Association National Joint Replacement Registry documents a survivorship of approximately 91% for ATSA and 94% for RTSA at 10 years of follow-up for all patients, and this difference is statistically significant ($P < 0.001$).[46] Survivorship data for ATSA from the 2019 Swedish Shoulder and Elbow Registry Annual Report showed that for the 1999-2003 cohort, the survivorship was 92%, and for the 2003-2008 cohort, it was 96% at 15 years.[47] For RTSA, the 15-year survivorship was 89% for the 1999-2003 cohort and 93% for the 2003-2008 cohort, showing, once again, a favorable comparison.

OUTCOME MEASURES

A variety of shoulder outcome metrics exist within the literature and are utilized to evaluate outcomes following RTSA. Some of these metrics rely only on patient reporting. These are called patient-reported outcome measures (PROMs). Other outcome metrics involve patient reporting and objective measures quantified by an examiner. These may have a PROM component but are not purely patient reported. For brevity, only the most common measures will be detailed.

Scoring metrics can generally be divided into those that are purely patient reported and hence PROMs and those that have an examiner component. The Simple Shoulder Test (SST) is a PROM composed of 12 questions that assess pain and function of the shoulder. The maximum score is 12 and pain is weighted 20% while function is weighted 80%.[48] The American Shoulder and Elbow Surgeons (ASES) score is a PROM that combines questions related to function and pain, each weighted 50%, to generate a maximum score of 100.[49] The Shoulder Pain and Disability Index (SPADI) is a PROM that evaluates pain (38%) and disability (62%). The maximum score for SPADI is 130.[48,50] Unlike most other metrics, a low score denotes a better clinical state. The Oxford Shoulder Score (OSS) is also a PROM that utilizes 12 multiple choice questions to evaluate pain (33%) and function (67%). The maximum score is 60. In 2009, a change was made to the scoring methodology of the OSS. Prior to that date, a higher score denoted a worse disease state; following that date, a higher score denoted a reduced disease state. The rank of the questions was inverted though the content remained the same.[51] A visual analog scale (VAS) for pain is a PROM that asks a patient to rate their pain numerically between 0 and 10.[52] Similarly, a Single Assessment Numeric Evaluation (SANE) metric is a PROM that requires a patient to evaluate the shoulder as a percent of normal between 0 and 100. A score of 100 is considered a "normal" shoulder.[53] Similar to the SANE, the subjective shoulder value (SSV) is a PROM that asks a patient to rate the shoulder as a percent of normal between 0% and 100%.

The following scoring metrics combine patient-reported measures and examiner contributions, typically with an assessment of ROM and/or strength. The University of California at Los Angeles (UCLA) Shoulder metric assimilates a score based on a combination of ROM, strength, function, satisfaction, and pain. The maximum score is 35.[54,55] The Constant metric assesses strength (25%), pain (15%), sleeping comfort, and activity level (20%) as well as ROM (40%).[56]

There is a group of data collection tools called health-related quality of life (HRQoL) surveys. These are increasingly utilized in the shoulder arthroplasty literature allowing the comparison of results of different cohorts as well as to follow the effect of the intervention (shoulder arthroplasty) on a patient's general quality of health. These surveys include but are not limited to Patient-Reported Outcomes Measurement Information System (PROMIS) 10, 36-Item Short Form (SF-36), 12-Item Short Form (SF-12), and Verterans Rand 12 (VR-12). The PROMIS-10 allows the measurement of symptoms, function, and HRQoL for chronic diseases and conditions such as arthritis using 10 questions. It can be separated into physical (global physical health) and mental (global mental health) components. The SF-36 relies on 36 questions to evaluate physical function, role limitations due to physical health, role limitations due to emotional problems, energy and fatigue, emotional well-being, social functioning, general health, and pain. The SF-12 and SF-8 are shorter but similar surveys. The VR-12 examines health domains similar to the SF-36 but is summarized into a Physical Component Score (PCS) and a Mental Component Score.

Radiographic evaluation of RTSA centers on the evaluation of inferior scapula notching. The degree of inferior notching is measured according to the method of Sirveaux and Nerot. grade 0 notching denotes the absence of a notch, grade 1 denotes involvement of the inferior pillar, grade 2 describes a defect that reaches the inferior screw, grade 3 describes a defect that rises above the inferior screw, and grade 4 denotes a notch extending underneath the baseplate.

MCID AND SCB

Historically, the clinical results of outcome studies were reported by showing differences in means and recording statistical significance, generally represented as a *P*-value. Statistical significance denotes that a difference is not due to random chance. However, statistical significance does not equate to meaningful clinical change. Otherwise stated, statistical significance does not mean a change from preoperative to postoperative would be considered meaningful by a patient. Toward that end, the concepts of the minimal clinically important difference (MCID) and substantial clinical benefit (SCB) are becoming more popular. There are a variety of methods that can be utilized to calculate MCID and SCB, although a comprehensive discussion of these techniques is outside the scope of this chapter.[57] MCID has been defined as "the smallest difference in score in the domain of interest which patients perceive as beneficial and which would mandate, in the absence of troublesome side-effects and excessive cost, a change in the patient's management."[58] SCB has been defined as the smallest difference in score in the domain of interest that exceeds the minimum threshold of improvement—a value that surgeons would choose to aim for.[59] The difference between statistical significance and reaching MCID is illustrated in a study by Torrens et al,[60] which studied 60 patients undergoing RTSA for rotator cuff insufficiency and found that improvement in the lateral rotation and strength components of the Constant score reached statistical significance but failed to reach the MCID, indicating that despite reaching a level of statistical significance, these values were not clinically relevant to patients.

Values for MCID and SCB of common clinical metrics have previously been reported for RTSA **(TABLE 27.1)**. MCID and SCB values after RTSA have been demonstrated to be lower than the values after ATSA. Furthermore, these values appear to be impacted by gender, length of follow-up, age at time of surgery, and preoperative function.[57,59,61] These reported MCID and SCB values can be used as an additional lens by which to evaluate clinical improvement after RTSA as opposed to relying solely on statistical significance that can be influenced by a myriad of factors including sample size.

TABLE 27.1 MCID and SCB Values for Common Metrics

Study	Metric	MCID	SCB
Simovitch et al,[57,59] 2018	ASES	10.3 ± 3.3	25.9 ± 2.9
	Constant	−0.3 ± 2.8	13.6 ± 2.6
	UCLA	7.0 ± 0.8	10.4 ± 0.7
	SST	1.4 ± 0.5	3.2 ± 0.5
	SPADI	20.0 ± 3.9	42.7 ± 3.4
	Pain VAS	1.4 ± 0.4	2.6 ± 0.4
	Global function	1.0 ± 0.4	2.4 ± 0.3
	Abduction	−1.9 ± 4.9	19.6 ± 4.3
	Flexion	−2.9 ± 5.5	22.3 ± 4.8
	ER	−5.3 ± 3.1	3.6 ± 2.7
Werner et al,[61] 2016	ASES	8.4 (2.8-14)[a]	32.1 (26.9-37.2)[a]

ASES, American Shoulder and Elbow Surgeons; ER, external rotation; MCID, minimal clinically important difference; SCB, substantial clinical benefit; SPADI, Shoulder Pain and Disability Index; SST, Simple Shoulder Test; UCLA, University of California at Los Angeles; VAS, visual analog scale.
[a]95% confidence intervals.

RESULTS OF RTSA BY DIAGNOSIS

Rotator Cuff Tear Arthropathy

Rotator CTA can be defined as severe arthritis of the glenohumeral joint with a high-riding humeral head resulting in acetabularization of the undersurface of the acromion and femoralization of the humeral head, glenoid bone loss, massive tearing of the rotator cuff tendons, and muscle changes including atrophy and fatty infiltration.[62] Prior to RTSA, standard surgical treatment included an attempt at repair of part of the rotator cuff along with a standard head size HA or a large head size HA. While patients experienced pain relief and improvement in function, these did not approximate the improvement reported after ATSA and for glenohumeral arthritis with an intact rotator cuff.[63,64]

With the introduction of RTSA in the United States in 2003, CTA was the sole indication for this procedure. Since then, as the indications have expanded, it has revolutionized the ability to manage complex problems about the shoulder, including CTA. Studies have shown that RTSA far outperforms HA for CTA.[65-68] ROM, pain relief, and functional outcomes documented by PROM were all significantly better in patients who underwent RTSA compared to those who underwent an HA. Other studies have documented the pain relief, superior functional outcomes, and improved ROM in patients with CTA treated with RTSA, which has become the procedure of choice in these patients.[66,68-73] Studies have shown that these outcomes can be expected in both younger and older patients.[74]

Inflammatory Arthropathies

Inflammatory arthropathies, the most common being rheumatoid arthritis, frequently affect the periarticular soft tissues. For the shoulder, this represents a high incidence of rotator cuff disease including attenuation, dysfunction, or full-thickness tearing. While the incidence of rotator cuff involvement has decreased with the use of biologics over the past 20 years, it is still an issue that has to be addressed in the face of disabling arthritic changes about the glenohumeral joint. ATSA used to be the procedure of choice, but patients would often develop cuff failure after arthroplasty, leading to poor function, increased pain, and early failure. With the availability of RTSA, the condition or subsequent viability of the rotator cuff is no longer an issue that will affect the patient's outcome.

Studies have shown similar results for RTSA performed in the setting of inflammatory arthropathy compared to RTSA performed for other diagnoses. Patients experience predictable, consistent, and significant pain relief and improvements in ROM and function.[72,75-77] Complication rates are similar to RTSA performed for other indications, and recent studies have shown complication rates of RTSA to be similar to those reported for ATSA.[38,78]

Osteoarthritis With Rotator Cuff Tear

RTSA has also been utilized in patients with osteoarthritis and rotator cuff tears of varying sizes without CTA. Significant improvements in overhead function and improvements in pain, ROM, and PROM have been documented with follow-up of 20 years without significant deterioration over time.[24,79]

The use of RTSA in patients with an intact rotator cuff and severe glenoid bone loss has been reported and is growing in frequency. The surgeon has more reconstruction options in patients with a B2-, B3-, or C-type glenoid when using a reverse prosthesis, with or without bone graft. Glenoid bone grafting is also a much easier procedure with an RTSA baseplate and screw fixation compared to an ATSA with screw fixation and the use of methyl methacrylate cement for implant fixation. Mizuno et al reported on deformities with a mean retroversion of 32° and mean posterior subluxation of 87% with excellent clinical outcomes and no recurrences of posterior subluxation with follow-up of 5 years.[80] Other subsequent studies have also shown excellent clinical results in these patients with or without bone grafting.[81,82]

More recently, RTSA has been used in older patients with severe osteoarthritis and an intact rotator cuff, as

our comfort level with the procedure has grown and the longer term results have shown favorable survivorship compared to ATSA. In fact, in some countries such as Australia and South Korea, 78% to 90% of all total shoulder arthroplasties are performed using a reverse prosthesis regardless of the indication or condition of the rotator cuff.[46] Studies have shown similar outcomes when comparing RTSA performed with an intact rotator cuff compared to ATSA performed for osteoarthritis with an intact cuff.[83,84] A retrospective cohort study looked at 135 patients who underwent either ATSA or RTSA, and all had an intact rotator cuff confirmed with advanced imaging.[83] There were no significant differences in pain relief, ROM including internal rotation, or patient-reported outcomes. Satisfaction was very high in both groups, and complications and revision rates were similar.

Most surgeons have the impression that their best ATSA outcome is better than their best RTSA outcome. However, most of the time, they are not looking at comparable groups. ATSA is performed for one indication—osteoarthritis with an intact rotator cuff. RTSA is performed for many different indications, and the outcomes will depend on the underlying pathology and indication. A patient with a locked posterior dislocation for 5 years who undergoes an RTSA is not going to have the same clinical outcome as someone with osteoarthritis and an intact cuff. When looking at comparable groups, that is, ATSA and RTSA performed in patients with an intact rotator cuff, the results are quite comparable. As mentioned, 78% of total shoulder arthroplasties performed in Australia in 2018 used a reverse prosthesis, and their registry results suggest outcomes similar to other countries with a lower usage of RTSA.[46]

Even in studies that do a direct comparison of ATSA and RTSA for all indications, similar clinical outcomes with regard to pain relief, ROM, and functional outcomes are reported at 2 to 4 years of follow-up.[78,85] Even though the reverse patients have worse clinical outcome scores and ROM preoperatively, at follow-up statistically significant improvements are observed with regard to outcome metrics, pain relief, and motion. Complication and revision rates were similar between the two groups.

Post-Capsulorrhaphy Arthropathy

Post-capsulorrhaphy arthropathy, also known as arthritis of dislocation, is a long-term complication that can develop years after a surgical stabilization procedure for recurrent instability. This typically occurs in young males in their 40s and 50s, and in addition to having severe arthritic changes, there is marked limitation in ROM, especially rotation, due to the distorted anatomy. Historically, they have been treated with ATSA, but this is fraught with increased complications and revision rates, often due to the fact that the subscapularis fails as a result of the previous procedures.[86] Recently, Cuff and Santoni showed that the use of RTSA for these patients resulted in higher patient satisfaction scores, a lower complication rate, and lower revision rate.[87] ROM and functional outcome score improvements were similar between ATSA and RTSA.

Irreparable Rotator Cuff Tears

As the use of RTSA for CTA has demonstrated durable positive results, surgeons have increasingly utilized RTSA to manage patients with irreparable rotator cuff tears or failed rotator cuff repair surgery in the absence of significant arthritis. RTSA has rivaled tendon transfers and partial rotator cuff repairs to manage these patients. For the purpose of this section, the discussion will be confined to the situation where rotator cuff deficiency exists as the primary pathology and the joint surfaces are either normal or minimally worn. This is in contradistinction to osteoarthritis in the setting of a full-thickness rotator cuff tear and CTA, which are different pathologies and detailed elsewhere.

The utilization of RTSA to treat patients with irreparable rotator cuff tears or failed previous rotator cuff repairs has been associated with positive and durable outcomes.[4,88-90] An early study by Werner et al[4] examined the results of RTSA with an MG/MH prosthesis for massive irreparable rotator cuff tears and found favorable clinical results. However, the authors reported a high complication rate of 50% and an exceedingly high notching rate of 96%. It should be noted that they included patients with a primary operation as well as those that were revisions following previous shoulder surgery or arthroplasty. Despite a high complication rate, only 21% of the shoulders with complications (10% of the patients) required explant of the prosthesis or conversion to an HA. Patients with a prior surgery had a significantly higher rate of reoperation than those patients in whom the RTSA was the primary surgery (50% vs 18%; $P = 0.005$). Aside from patients who required explant, complications postoperatively did not affect overall patient satisfaction. Interpretation of the high scapular notching rate is nuanced. This study, published in 2005, preceded the valuable knowledge acquired later on emphasizing inferior position of the glenosphere to avoid inferior notching, which may have compounded the predisposition to notching inherent to a MG/MH (Grammont) design.

Boileau et al[89] examined patients who underwent an RTSA after failed rotator cuff surgery. They found significant clinical improvement following surgery in the entire cohort of patients, but when they compared patients with and without pseudoparalysis (<90° of anterior active elevation with preserved passive ROM), they found a statistically significant difference

in pre- to postoperative improvement for the Constant score, adjusted Constant score, activity, mobility, and anterior active elevation, with the preoperative pseudoparalysis cohort more improved. There were two other important findings. First, patients without pseudoparalysis (>90° of anterior active elevation) preoperatively lost an average of 24° of anterior active elevation following surgery compared to an average gain of 67° in the patients with pseudoparalysis (<90° of anterior active elevation with preserved passive ROM) preoperatively; pain was similarly improved in both cohorts. This illustrates that patients who retain overhead function should be counseled that they may lose ROM after RTSA for recurrent irreparable rotator cuff tears. Second, the existence of a preoperative hornblower sign was correlated with postoperative active external rotation (ER). Active ER increased by 17° in the absence of a hornblower sign, while it decreased by an average of 12° when a preoperative hornblower sign was present ($P = 0.005$). These findings, once again, can help counsel patients.

Similar to the findings by Boileau et al,[89] Mulieri et al[90] identified a very high satisfaction rate (>85%) and profound clinical improvement following RTSA for irreparable rotator cuff repairs. They noted that patients who had <90° of active shoulder flexion preoperatively had a higher complication rate (50% vs 25%) than those with >90° of active shoulder flexion preoperatively. However, patients with >90° of preoperative active flexion still had overall clinical improvement and a high satisfaction rate. In addition, when comparing patients with an irreparable rotator cuff tear and no prior surgery on the operative shoulder to those with a history of failed rotator cuff repair, there was no statistically significant difference in clinical outcome.

Despite the overall efficacy of RTSA to treat irreparable rotator cuff tears, certain risk factors exist for poor functional improvement. Specifically, Hartzler et al[91] examined a subset of patients who did not meet or exceed the MCID for SST and compared these patients to a cohort who did achieve or exceed the MCID. They determined that young age, high preoperative function, and neurologic dysfunction were associated with poor functional improvement.

RTSA for Proximal Humerus Fractures

RTSA has also dramatically changed the manner in which we are able to handle acute fractures as well as malunions and nonunions of the proximal humerus. RTSA has been demonstrated to surpass the clinical outcomes of HA for three- and four-part proximal humerus fractures.[92] In addition, greater tuberosity healing has generally been demonstrated to be less important following RTSA than HA for proximal humerus fractures, although some studies have shown that tuberosity healing can be important for ER-type tasks.[93] Several studies have also demonstrated favorable clinical improvement after the use of RTSA for malunion or nonunion of the tuberosities, reporting satisfaction rates that exceed 98%.[94,95] The use of RTSA to manage proximal humerus fractures will be discussed in greater detail in Chapter 29.

Revision Shoulder Arthroplasty

RTSA has evolved into a powerful tool that has dramatically changed the approach to patients with a failed shoulder arthroplasty due to its ability to provide favorable outcomes. ATSA and HA can fail for a variety of reasons including, but not limited to, rotator cuff dysfunction, infection, and loosening. Failure can lead to glenoid and humeral bone loss as well as loss of supportive soft tissues, all of which complicate revision procedures. RTSA is able to both address and circumvent bone and soft-tissue deficiencies in a relatively straightforward manner that previously required extensive and unpredictable bone grafting, the use of methyl methacrylate, and limited gains salvage procedures with little expectation for functional recovery.

A multicenter retrospective analysis by Wagner et al[96] compared the utilization of RTSA for revision surgery between the 2005 to 2010 and 2011 to 2016. They noted that the incidence of revision arthroplasty with RTSA grew from 51% to 78% in those respective time periods. Furthermore, a recent systematic review of the literature[97] noted that 54% of all revision shoulder arthroplasties in North America and Europe utilized an RTSA. The mean age at revision was 66 years, and the most common indications for revision were rotator cuff insufficiency followed by glenoid loosening. The overall complication rate was 17%, and 74% of complications led to reoperation with instability or dislocation being the primary indications followed by glenoid loosening, infection, and humeral loosening in order of frequency. Of concern is the finding that revisions were performed at a mean of only 4 years from the index primary procedure.

Patients who undergo revision RTSA from a failed ATSA or HA have been shown to have worse preoperative shoulder function but can expect similar improvements to primary RTSA performed for other etiologies.[88] Studies by Kelly et al[98] and Patel et al[99] demonstrated statistically significant improvements in clinical outcomes and ROM but a widely disparate complication and revision rate. There was a fivefold and a threefold difference in the complication and revision rates, respectively, between the studies. The higher complication and revision rates in the study by Kelly et al[98] may be related to the use of a structural (tricortical iliac crest bone graft) composite graft in 40% of the shoulders (compared to 6% in Patel et al[99]) due to glenoid bone loss as well as some patients requiring that the implant be positioned in the subcoracoid region of the scapula (because the native vault was so severely worn). However, only 2 of the 15 complications pertained to the glenoid. There are likely other differences in the study cohorts or complexity of the revisions that may account for this disparity.

As the frequency of shoulder arthroplasty continues to grow so too will the frequency of revision arthroplasty in the elderly population. Undoubtedly, in an aging and active population, the need for revision RTSA in elderly patients will pose complexities of risk and surgical challenges that may not exist in a younger population. Alentorn-Geli et al[100] studied a cohort of patients younger than 80 years (mean age = 84 years) who underwent revision RTSA for rotator cuff insufficiency after ATSA or HA (32%), glenoid wear after HA (26%), glenoid loosening (18%), instability (11%), pain (5%), implant loosening/fracture (5%), and infection (3%). The majority of patients were American Society of Anesthesiologists II and III. These patients had significant clinical improvement with a medical complication rate of 8% and surgical complication rate of 13%. The 90-day mortality rate was 3%, with 1-year mortality being 5%. Only one death occurred within the 90-day period following surgery and was due to stroke. The authors reported a cumulative incidence of revision of 11% at 2 years and 16% at 5 years. Based on the low risk of serious complications, mortality, and revision rates as well as recognized clinical improvement, the authors concluded that revision RTSA should not be avoided, when indicated, in patients older than 80 years. Little additional data exist regarding clinical outcomes of revision RTSA in the aged population as well as where these surgeries may fall on the value-based medicine continuum.

Perhaps one of the greatest challenges stems from revision RTSA in the case of a failed RTSA. Common reasons for RTSA failure are instability, baseplate failure, infection, fracture, and humeral loosening.[76,101,102] Boileau et al[102] reported on a series of 37 patients who underwent revision RTSA for a failed RTSA predominantly due to instability, humeral loosening, and infection. Subsequent to revision RTSA, 30% of the cohort required an additional operation due to a complication. At an average of 3 years of follow-up, 86% of revised patients retained their prosthesis, 6% required conversion to HA, and 8% had a resection arthroplasty. Despite the 30% reoperation rate, the authors reported that 89% of patients were satisfied or very satisfied and demonstrated that patients had a statistically significant improvement in their Constant score, reported a mean SSV of 50%, and achieved an average of 111° of active anterior elevation.

Black et al[101] analyzed 16 patients who underwent revision RTSA for a failed RTSA mostly due to instability and glenoid baseplate failure and found a similar reoperation rate (38%) after revision RTSA in the setting of a 56% major complication rate. Clinical results were favorable, and 88% of the cohort indicated they felt "better" after revision. Holcomb et al[76] reported on 14 patients with baseplate failure after RTSA with an LG/MH design. Subsequent to revision, 86% of patients reported excellent or good satisfaction. The complication rate was 21%, and the reoperation rate was 14%. Nonetheless, there remains a paucity of literature regarding revision of failed RTSA to RTSA.

Revision RTSA has demonstrated favorable clinical outcomes regardless of conversion from HA, ATSA, or RTSA. Still, complication rates and reoperation rates remain a concern. Revision RTSA after ATSA and HA are associated with lower complication and revision rates than revision RTSA after RTSA, although the etiology of failure of HA and ATSA likely has an impact on these rates with greater bone loss and soft tissue compromise resulting in higher rates of failure.

IMPACT OF AGE, GENDER, AND LENGTH OF FOLLOW-UP ON RTSA OUTCOMES

Understanding the effect of gender and age on RTSA outcomes can help a surgeon counsel the patients regarding expectations and also lays the foundation for understanding subtle differences between outcomes studies that may differ in cohort selection. A surge in demand for shoulder arthroplasty in patients younger than 55 years is projected to be on the order of 330% from 2011 to 2030,[103] thus codifying the importance of understanding the impact of a reduction in age at the time of surgery on short-, mid-, and long-term outcomes.

Impact of Age at the Time of RTSA

Multiple studies have demonstrated statistically significant improvement in clinical metrics as well as ROM after RTSA in patients younger than 65 years for multiple different etiologies.[69,104-109] A study by Monir et al[106] examined RTSA in patients younger than 65 years with a minimum of 5-year follow-up. They determined that all five metrics were studied (Constant, ASES, SPADI, SST, and UCLA), and all ROM measurements and pain VAS not only improved with statistical significance but also exceeded SCB with the exception of ER, which only exceeded MCID. Despite very favorable clinical results, Matthews et al[105] noted lower postoperative functional scores and worse perceived outcome (SF-12 and ASES) in gender- and diagnosis-matched patients younger than 65 years compared to their counterparts older than 70 years.

Just as the impact of young age on RTSA is of interest, so is the impact of advancing age. Friedman et al[50] determined in a cohort of RTSA patients, when controlling for gender, that every 1-year increase in age was associated with a mean improved ASES score of 0.19 points ($P = 0.011$) and a mean decrease in abduction by 0.26° ($P = 0.007$) and flexion by 0.39° ($P = 0.001$).

Complication rates for RTSA in patients younger than 65 years have been reported between 5% and 39%.[69,104-109] However, gender- and diagnosis-matched cohorts of patients younger than 65 years compared to patients older than 70 years failed to demonstrate a statistically significant difference in complication rates.[105] Reoperation rates have been reported between 0% and 25%, while revision rates are between 0% and 15%.[69,104-109] Survivorship rates free of reoperation for any complication have been reported to be between 82% and 88% at 5 years and 74% to 76% at 10 years.[69,104] Survivorship rates free of revision (removal or conversion) have been reported to be between 96% and 98% at 5 years and 88% to 92% at 10 years.[69,104] Thus, RTSA in younger patients appears to be commensurate in outcome with RTSA in older individuals, perhaps dispelling the concerns about the impact of increased activity and young age on durability.

Despite favorable results overall, several studies have reported that previous surgery and smoking in young patients can be risk factors for complications and worse clinical outcomes. Ek et al[69] reported a higher complication rate (47% vs 30%) in patients with a history of at least one prior surgery compared to no prior surgery, although this was not statistically significant. Ernstbrunner et al[104] showed a correlation between the number of surgical procedures preceding RTSA and postoperative pain level ($r = 0.59$; $P = 0.005$) as well as SSV ($r = -0.51$; $P = 0.019$). Monir et al[106] illustrated that a history of prior surgery impacted postoperative satisfaction in 95% of patients without a history of prior surgery reported being much better or somewhat better compared to 75% in those with prior surgery. Samuelsen et al[107] observed the effect of smoking on outcomes and noted that smoking in patients undergoing RTSA under the age of 65 years was associated with an increased rate of complication ($P = 0.01$) and revision surgery ($P < 0.0001$).

Impact of Gender on RTSA

The effect of gender on RTSA outcome is less well studied and less understood compared to age. Nonetheless, gender does appear to influence outcomes following RTSA, and Friedman et al[50] demonstrated it has a greater impact on outcome than age. When controlling for age, male gender had a statistically significant improvement in SST, Constant, UCLA, ASES, SPADI, flexion, abduction, and passive ER compared to their female counterparts. Wong et al[110] also confirmed that males achieved higher ASES function ($P = 0.009$) and also noted that they fared better than females for the physical component summary of SF-12 (SF-12 PCS) ($P = 0.008$). Specifically, as it relates to SF-12 PCS, females improved 69% and 42% as much as their male counterparts at 1 year and 2 years, respectively. Similarly, in regard to ASES functional scores, women improved 94% and 75% as much as their male counterparts at 1 and 2 years, respectively. Despite better functional results in males, gender difference did not impact length of stay, in-hospital opiate use, pain VAS, or the mental component summary of SF-12.

Impact of Length of Follow-Up on Outcomes After RTSA

Few studies have evaluated the rate of improvement and the potential effect of length of follow-up on outcomes. Studies by Simovitch et al[48] and Friedman et al[50] determined that most improvement after ATSA occurs in the first 6 months after surgery according to five common clinical metrics (ASES, SPADI, SST, Constant, and UCLA), and full improvement is attained by approximately 24 months. ROM follows a similar trend. However, at approximately 72 months, there was a progressive decrease in magnitude of improvement for active abduction and flexion, which is not seen for the clinical metrics. This may represent a generalized aging and deconditioning process or a sign that deltoid fatigue is an entity that arises over time after RTSA.

ACTIVITY LEVEL AFTER RTSA

As surgeons continue to broaden the indications and extend the age limits for RTSA, it is becoming increasingly important to be able to counsel patients on expected and suggested activity level after surgery. In particular, it is important to provide guidance toward expectations of return to sport and work.

A meta-analysis by Steinhaus et al[111] tabulated that the rate of return to work is 62% following RTSA and did not differ significantly from the rate of return following ATSA or HA. Intensity of work did influence the rate of return. Underlying diagnosis or workers' compensation status did not influence the rate of return to work. Mean time to return to work has been reported to be between 2.3[112] and 3.1[113] months after RTSA.

The ability to return to sport and do so safely has been examined after RTSA. In 2012, a study by Golant et al[114] surveyed 310 members of the American Shoulder and Elbow Surgeons regarding return to sport after RTSA. They reported that 72% of respondents allowed a return to low-impact sports, 36.2% allowed a return to high-impact sports, and only 18% allowed a return to contact sports. It is unknown if these practices may have evolved over the ensuing years. In a study of 41 patients older than 65 years, Simovitch et al[115] identified that 95% of RTSA patients were able to return to sport at the same or higher level than before surgery and had favorable clinical outcomes without a novel mode of failure. The cohort also had low complication (7%) and notching (7%) rates. Kurowicki et al[116] compared the ability of patients to return to sports requiring shoulder function and found that ATSA outperformed RTSA.

Furthermore, Bulhoff et al[117] demonstrated that the majority of their RTSA patients required between 1 and 2 years to return to sports at their normal level.

SPECIAL CONSIDERATIONS

RTSA in Parkinson Disease

Patients with Parkinson disease have always presented a challenge when they require shoulder arthroplasty. Previous treatment with either an HA or ATSA has resulted in an increased incidence of infection, dislocation, component loosening, periprosthetic fracture, revision arthroplasty, and systemic complications when compared with matched controls. With the use of RTSA in this difficult patient group, the incidence of periprosthetic fracture and component loosening are less than following ATSA or HA, but the other complications remain increased compared to matched controls.[118] While patients achieve significant improvements in pain and functional outcome scores, the gains in PROM are not as great as those for matched controls.[119] Patients with Parkinson disease undergoing RTSA had less predictable improvements in ROM and significantly higher complication rates.

Bilateral RTSA

With first-generation reverse prostheses, the humeral head was medialized and distalized and often coupled with putting the humeral component in zero degrees of retroversion. As a result, the remaining rotator cuff muscles were not under optimum tension, and rotation, especially internal, was less than that reported for ATSA. As a result, many surgeons recommended not performing bilateral RTSA in patients due to the loss of internal rotation. However, this has not been borne out in the literature, particularly with more recent studies using more contemporary prosthetic designs that have more global lateralization, thus putting the remaining cuff muscles under better tension to obtain improved ROM. Mellano et al[120] reported on 50 patients who underwent staged bilateral RTSA and, at a mean follow-up of 5 years, found significant improvements in pain relief, clinical outcome scores, and ROM, including rotation. Welborn et al[121] compared 13 patients with bilateral ATSA to 13 patients with bilateral RTSA and found no differences in functional outcome scores or patient satisfaction between the two groups.

RTSA With Massive Glenoid Bone Loss

In patients with significant glenoid bone loss such as encountered in B2-, B3-, and C-type glenoids, autogenous bone graft has been used in primary ATSA with variable clinical results due to high complication and failure rates. A recent systematic review showed a 29% complication rate, 14% revision rate, 17% graft failure rate, and 35% recurrence of posterior humeral head subluxation.[122] Larger bone defects are even more difficult to address with ATSA due to the lack of secure fixation of the cemented polyethylene glenoid component into host bone.

RTSA has recently been used to address glenoid bone loss from both posterior glenoid wear and the massive bone loss encountered in primary and revision cases. The glenoid baseplate is able to secure both small and large bone grafts under compression with the screws used for baseplate fixation that also reach into good-quality host bone by at least 1 cm **(FIGURE 27.2)**. Also, there is no need for methyl methacrylate that can impede graft incorporation. One can treat posterior defects, superior defects, combined posterior-superior defects, and anterior defects by customizing the allograft or autogenous bone graft as needed to fill the defect, in combination with an augmented glenoid component. Often, augmented glenoid baseplates and large glenospheres (42 and 46 mm) can be used even without bone grafting to address large glenoid bone defects.

The results to date are encouraging and appear to be far superior to those following ATSA with a cemented polyethylene glenoid. Studies of glenoid bone grafting in RTSA with or without an intact rotator cuff with follow-up of 3 to 4 years show significant clinical improvements in ROM and outcome metrics, good graft incorporation, and low complication rates, with failure rates and revision rates comparable to ATSA. Lorenzetti et al followed up 57 patients who underwent RTSA with structural bone grafting for severe glenoid bone loss for a mean of 46 months and found significant clinical improvements with a 7% major complication rate but no baseplate failures.[123] Ernstbrunner et al reported on 41 patients followed up for a mean of 3 years after RTSA with glenoid bone grafting and found significant improvements in pain, motion, and outcome scores.[104] All patients with structural grafts showed incorporation with no signs of glenoid lucency and no revision surgery.

A systematic review looked at glenoid bone grafting in RTSA with 3- to 5-year follow-up. While all studies reported significant clinical improvements for both

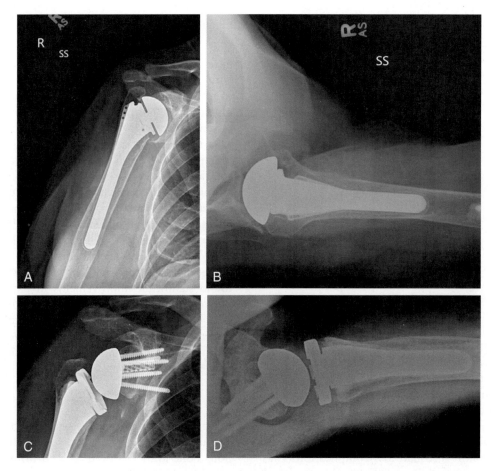

FIGURE 27.2 A and **B**, Sixteen years after a hemiarthroplasty in a 48-year-old man with rheumatoid arthritis, the implant is loose and has migrated medially with significant glenoid bone loss. **C** and **D**, Three years following revision to a reverse total shoulder arthroplasty with a large bulk humeral head allograft, showing good fixation of the screws and central cage into host bone and full incorporation of the graft.

primary and revision RTSA, the revision rate was 3% in primary RTSA but rose to 21% in revision cases.[124] While the procedure is clearly successful in primary RTSA, further studies are needed to determine the optimal allograft material for massive grafts and the best surgical techniques to lower the failure rate in revision RTSA.

Perhaps the greatest power of RTSA in addressing the challenge of massive glenoid bone loss and severe retroversion deformities is its ability to often be used without structural bone autografts or allografts. Jones et al[125] compared the use of structural bone graft behind a standard baseplate to the use of augmented baseplates for posterior and superior defects and found similar favorable clinical results but a higher complication (14% vs 0%; $P = 0.0126$) and notching rate in the structural bone graft cohort. Several studies have reported favorable outcomes with the use of augmented baseplates without bone graft in Walch B2, B3, C, and Favard E2 glenoids. Virk et al[126] reported on 67 patients who received an 8° posterior augmented full-wedge baseplate utilized to correct the glenoid to within 10° of neutral version as measured by Friedman axis[127] and found that 90% of patients exceeded the MCID for clinical metrics and a low 4.5% complication rate. No complications were related to the glenoid. A study by Abdic et al[128] quantified bone preservation in type E2 glenoids from patient-matched glenoid augments and concluded that a full-wedge design provided the best reconstruction with dramatically less bone removal than standard designs.

RTSA With Massive Humeral Bone Loss

RTSA has also been used to treat massive bone loss on the humeral side. There has been debate as to whether an allograft-prosthesis composite (APC) is necessary for a successful clinical outcome, and the literature would suggest that it is not. Cox et al reported on their experience with 2- to 15-year follow-up using an APC for humeral bone loss and RTSA.[129] At a mean of almost 6 years, they reported good to excellent clinical results in 70% of the patients. The reoperation-free survivorship was 88% at 5 years and 78% at 10 years. While the use of an APC provided reliable pain relief and improved motion, the authors concluded that the ultimate function is limited but patient satisfaction is high. The Mayo Clinic experience in 26 patients with an APC in both primary and revision RTSA showed similar outcomes, with significant improvements in pain and motion at a mean of 4 years follow-up.[100] The revision-free survival rate was 96% at 5 years.

Other studies have shown significant clinical improvements with high patient satisfaction without the use of allograft augmentation. Budge et al reported significant improvements in the clinical outcome scores with 87% patient satisfaction in patients with proximal humeral

bone loss secondary to a failed shoulder arthroplasty.[130] Stephens et al reported on 16 patients followed up for a mean of 4 years and found that revision RTSA can provide successful outcomes in the presence of proximal humeral bone loss without the use of an APC.[131]

Still in cases of severe bone loss in RTSA, the lack of a tuberosity and tenting of the deltoid can affect stability and muscle moment arms. Therefore, utilizing an APC may be desirable. The risks inherent to APC are lack of integration of host to grafted bone, bone resorption, and infection. An alternative has recently been introduced with prostheses that can act in place of an allograft proximal humerus, substituting a metal proximal humerus in place of a cadaveric allograft. Outcome studies regarding the use of these humeral reconstruction prostheses will be forthcoming.

PREDICTORS OF CLINICAL SUCCESS

Successful clinical outcomes following RTSA depend greatly on meeting patient expectations and matching these expectations with what is possible for each patient given their specific clinical situation. While the surgeon can control all of the factors related to the surgery, we have a much better understanding now about controlling other factors, both preoperatively and postoperatively, that can affect the clinical outcome and minimize complications and unsatisfactory results. Something that is very difficult for surgeons to learn, and comes only with a great deal of experience, is how to say no to a patient who may not be a good candidate for an RTSA due to either physical or psychological issues. Optimizing patient selection improves patient outcomes and leads to higher patient satisfaction rates. We have a better understanding today of modifiable versus nonmodifiable risk factors, and while delaying surgery for modifiable risk factors can be a difficult conversation to have with the patient, it is in everyone's interest to optimize the patient prior to surgery to ensure the best outcome possible.

Psychosocial Factors

Psychiatric comorbidities have been associated with poor clinical outcomes in a number of settings, including surgery. Bot et al showed that the influence of psychiatric conditions such as depression, anxiety, dementia, or schizophrenia on the outcomes of shoulder arthroplasty is significant.[132] Patients undergoing shoulder arthroplasty with preoperative psychiatric illness are at risk for increased perioperative morbidity and readmission rates. Werner et al looked at depression and patient-reported outcomes following total shoulder arthroplasty and found that while they experience significant clinical improvements from their baseline status, they are less than those without depression.[133] They identified depression to be an independent predictor of significantly less improvement in the ASES scores following total shoulder arthroplasty. Following RTSA specifically, they found that depression correlated with poor postoperative improvement.

Resiliency, defined as the ability to recover from a stress, is increasingly recognized as something that can affect surgical outcomes and patient satisfaction. A study looking at the correlation between resiliency and total shoulder arthroplasty showed that there was a direct relationship between resilience and outcomes.[134] Patients with lower resilience had lower outcome scores postoperatively. Resilience is now recognized as a major predictor of postoperative outcomes following total shoulder arthroplasty.

A systematic review looking at how psychosocial factors affect outcome following both ATSA and RTSA showed that these factors may play just as important a role in the patients' outcome as the technical factors of total shoulder arthroplasty.[135] Patients with anxiety and depression disorders had an increased risk of perioperative complications and lower functional outcome scores. Patients with worker's compensation had lower satisfaction and outcome scores compared to those without claims. However, patients with higher confidence and preoperative expectations were correlated with better outcomes.

Chronic Opioid Use

Chronic opioid use for the treatment of end-stage osteoarthritis of the shoulder by physicians other than orthopedic surgeons has increased significantly over the last 10 years as part of the opioid epidemic and should be considered a modifiable risk factor. As a result, just as in patients undergoing total hip and knee arthroplasty, the use of chronic opioids preoperatively has profound effects on the outcomes following RTSA. Morris et al followed up 60 patients with a preoperative history of opioid use for 2 to 5 years.[136] While these patients had significant improvements in PROMs and patient satisfaction, they had significantly lower baseline outcome scores and achieved significantly lower outcome scores postoperatively compared to a comparison group with no history of preoperative opioid use. Another study by Vajapey et al showed that the preoperative use of opioids was associated with lower outcome scores and satisfaction rate.[135] Cheah et al, however, found that unlike total hip and knee arthroplasty patients, preoperative opioid use was not associated with increased hospital stay, perioperative complications, or readmission rates following ATSA and RTSA.[137]

BMI and Smoking

Other modifiable risk factors that negatively affect the clinical outcome and patient satisfaction following RTSA are body mass index (BMI) and smoking. While there have been conflicting data regarding the exact effects of obesity on the outcomes of RTSA, a negative effect exists. Obese patients achieve significant improvements in ROM following RTSA but are at increased risk for complications, both surgical (including dislocation, blood loss) and medical.[138,139] Morbidly obese patients had less gains on the Medical Outcomes SF-12 scores and had less rotation likely due to body habitus.[140]

More recent studies have shown that the risk of infection[141] and dislocation[142] increases as the BMI increased in RTSA. An additional study has shown that the clinical outcomes are adversely affected by increasing BMI, but the incidence of scapular notching and the scapular notch grade are less in morbidly obese patients, likely due to their body habitus and the fact that they cannot adduct their arm as much as normal BMI patients.[143]

Smoking has been documented to be a significant risk factor for increased complication rates (particularly infection) and decreased clinical outcomes following total hip and knee arthroplasty. Data that show similar results for both ATSA and RTSA are now emerging. While earlier studies did not show an increased risk of infection following RTSA, they were likely not sufficiently powered.[144] A more recent study that was sufficiently powered showed smokers had significantly higher risks of periprosthetic joint infection and postoperative fractures and concluded that smoking is a significant risk factor for complications following both ATSA and RTSA.[104] Smoking cessation programs preoperatively should be considered very beneficial and will improve outcomes.

Surgeon and Hospital Volume

Just as in lower extremity total joint arthroplasty, high-volume surgeons or high-volume hospitals, or the combination of the two, lead to improved clinical outcomes and lower complication rates. Hospital volume was inversely correlated with blood loss and operative time, and surgeon volume was inversely related to operative time for RTSA.[145] Higher surgeon and hospital volumes led to improved perioperative metrics for both ATSA and ATSA, and surgeon volume had a greater effect than hospital volume. Another study looked at both the short-term and long-term outcomes as they relate to surgical volume. For RTSA, lower surgical volume was associated with higher all-cause revision rates throughout the follow-up period.[146] In both the United States and Australia, the majority of RTSA are performed by surgeons who do less than one per month, despite significant growth in the utilization of RTSA.

FUTURE OF RTSA

Although the future of RTSA may be refined by prosthesis and surgical technique development, the ability to utilize machine learning (ML), patient-specific guides, robotics, and computer navigation holds promise to be disruptive to the status quo.

A recent study by Kumar et al[147] evaluated the accuracy of three different ML techniques to predict clinical outcomes following shoulder arthroplasty. The authors noted that these techniques were able to accurately predict outcome measures at each postoperative point utilizing preoperative values and patient attributes. In addition, the models were able to predict which patients would reach MCID for PROMs with 93% to 99% accuracy and also which patients would reach SCB with 82% to 90% accuracy. The value of ML is in its ability to potentially identify how to optimize patients so that they reach the best outcome possible as well as identify variations in prosthesis choice and technique that might maximize outcomes.

As ML improves our ability to understand the impact of variation in implant choice and surgical techniques of implantation, it will become increasingly important to ensure accuracy of preparation and implantation of an RTSA in the operating room. Three recent methods to help improve accuracy include three-dimensional (3D) preoperative planning, patient-specific instrumentation (PSI), and computer navigation.

3D CT scan preoperative planning has been identified as a valuable resource in helping to achieve accurate glenoid reconstruction in RTSA. A study by Werner et al[148] demonstrated that the accuracy of measuring glenoid version and inclination on 3D preoperative planning software is significantly more accurate than measuring from 2D-reformatted CT scans. Berhouet et al[149] demonstrated that the use of 3D CT preoperative planning with the entire scapula visualized compared to a "blind technique" without the entire scapula visually resulted in statistically significant differences in version, tilt, and vault perforation. This understanding has led to the evolution of multiple 3D preoperative planning software options.

3D preoperative planning allows virtual implantation, which enables a surgeon to determine the best choice of implants and position for implantation. Several implant systems have the ability to utilize PSI with custom 3D printed or reusable intraoperative guides to execute the preoperative virtual plan in surgery. The ability for PSI to achieve templated version and inclination is variable. Cadaveric studies report variability in accuracy of achieving planned glenoid version (range of mean: 1.6°-5°) and inclination (range of mean: 0.9°-3.0°).[150-152] In vivo studies report variability in achieving planned glenoid version (range of mean: 1.1°-10°) and inclination (range of mean: 1.0°-1.6°) as well.[140,153-156]

Some of this inconsistency may be due to the different types of guides as well as different combinations of glenoid morphology. It may also be due to human error as the guides must be positioned in surgery and are fixed—they cannot be adapted intraoperatively. Another technology that has emerged more recently than PSI is intra-operative computer navigation. This allows execution of a 3D preoperative plan as well as real-time feedback to the surgeon and the ability to alter the plan during the surgery. A recent study noted that computer navigation of the glenoid resulted in a statistically significant improvement in alignment toward what was planned for both inclination and version compared to a matched cohort with standard glenoid preparation and implantation. Computer navigation allowed glenoid implantation within 5° of the surgical plan in 70% of the cases, and there were no detectable differences between plan and execution in 40% of cases.[157] These technologies, along with ML, will enable customized treatment of patients and a better understanding of the impact of subtle positional changes.

REFERENCES

1. Neer CS II. Replacement arthroplasty for glenohumeral osteoarthritis. *J Bone Joint Surg Am*. 1974;56(1):1-13.
2. Grammont P, Trouilloud P, Laffay J, Deries X. Concept study and realization of a new total shoulder prosthesis. *Rhumatologie*. 1987;39:407-418.
3. Flatow EL, Harrison AK. A history of reverse total shoulder arthroplasty. *Clin Orthop Relat Res*. 2011;469(9):2432-2439.
4. Werner CM, Steinmann PA, Gilbart M, Gerber C. Treatment of painful pseudoparesis due to irreparable rotator cuff dysfunction with the Delta III reverse-ball-and-socket total shoulder prosthesis. *J Bone Joint Surg Am*. 2005;87(7):1476-1486.
5. Sirveaux F, Favard L, Oudet D, Huquet D, Walch G, Molé D. Grammont inverted total shoulder arthroplasty in the treatment of glenohumeral osteoarthritis with massive rupture of the cuff. Results of a multicentre study of 80 shoulders. *J Bone Joint Surg Br*. 2004;86(3):388-395.
6. Simovitch RW, Zumstein MA, Lohri E, Helmy N, Gerber C. Predictors of scapular notching in patients managed with the Delta III reverse total shoulder replacement. *J Bone Joint Surg Am*. 2007;89(3):588-600.
7. Levigne C, Garret J, Boileau P, Alami G, Favard L, Walch G. Scapular notching in reverse shoulder arthroplasty. *J Shoulder Elbow Surg*. 2008;17(6):925-935.
8. Wierks C, Skolasky RL, Ji JH, McFarland EG. Reverse total shoulder replacement: intraoperative and early postoperative complications. *Clin Orthop Relat Res*. 2009;467(1):225-234.
9. Guery J, Favard L, Sirveaux F, Oudet D, Mole D, Walch G. Reverse total shoulder arthroplasty. Survivorship analysis of eighty replacements followed for five to ten years. *J Bone Joint Surg Am*. 2006;88(8):1742-1747.
10. Frankle M, Siegal S, Pupello D, Saleem A, Mighell M, Vasey M. The Reverse Shoulder Prosthesis for glenohumeral arthritis associated with severe rotator cuff deficiency. A minimum two-year follow-up study of sixty patients. *J Bone Joint Surg Am*. 2005;87(8):1697-1705.
11. Gristina A, Webb L. The Trispherical total shoulder replacement. In: Bayley I, Kessel L, eds. *Shoulder Surgery*. Springer-Verlag; 1982:153-157.
12. Reeves B, Jobbins B, Flowers F, Dowson D, Wright V. Biomechanical problems in the development of a total shoulder endo-prosthesis. *Ann Rheum Dis*. 1972;31(5):425-426.
13. Parada SA, Flurin PH, Wright TW, Zuckerman JD, Elwell J, Roche CP, Friedman RJ. Comparison of complication types and rates associated with anatomic and reverse total shoulder arthroplasty. *J Shoulder Elbow Surg*. 2020. doi:10.1016/j.jse.2020.07.028.
14. Botros M, Curry E, Yin J, Jawa A, Eichinger J, Li X. Reverse shoulder arthroplasty has higher perioperative implant complications and transfusion than total shoulder arthroplasty. *J Shoulder Elbow Surg Int*. 2019;3(2):108-112.
15. Palsis JA, Simpson KN, Matthews JH, Traven S, Eichinger JK, Friedman RJ. Current trends in the use of shoulder arthroplasty in the United States. *Orthopedics*. 2018;41(3):e416-e423.
16. Routman HD, Flurin PH, Wright TW, Zuckerman JD, Hamilton MA, Roche CP. Reverse shoulder arthroplasty prosthesis design classification system. *Bull Hosp Jt Dis (2013)*. 2015;73(suppl 1):S5-S14.

17. Roche CP, Hamilton MA, Diep P, et al. Optimizing deltoid efficiency with reverse shoulder arthroplasty using a novel inset center of rotation glenosphere design. *Bull Hosp Jt Dis (2013)*. 2015;73(suppl 1):S37-S41.

18. Hamilton MA, Roche CP, Diep P, Flurin PH, Routman HD. Effect of prosthesis design on muscle length and moment arms in reverse total shoulder arthroplasty. *Bull Hosp Jt Dis (2013)*. 2013;71(suppl 2):S31-S35.

19. Hansen ML, Routman H. The biomechanics of current reverse shoulder replacement options. *Annals of Joint*. 2019;4(17):8-14.

20. Sheth U, Saltzman M. Reverse total shoulder arthroplasty: implant design considerations. *Curr Rev Musculoskelet Med*. 2019;12(4):554-561.

21. Mollon B, Mahure SA, Roche CP, Zuckerman JD. Impact of scapular notching on clinical outcomes after reverse total shoulder arthroplasty: an analysis of 476 shoulders. *J Shoulder Elbow Surg*. 2017;26(7):1253-1261.

22. Simovitch R, Flurin PH, Wright TW, Zuckerman JD, Roche C. Impact of scapular notching on reverse total shoulder arthroplasty midterm outcomes: 5-year minimum follow-up. *J Shoulder Elbow Surg*. 2019;28(12):2301-2307.

23. Cuff D, Clark R, Pupello D, Frankle M. Reverse shoulder arthroplasty for the treatment of rotator cuff deficiency: a concise follow-up, at a minimum of five years, of a previous report. *J Bone Joint Surg Am*. 2012;94(21):1996-2000.

24. Cuff DJ, Pupello DR, Santoni BG, Clark RE, Frankle MA. Reverse shoulder arthroplasty for the treatment of rotator cuff deficiency: a concise follow-up, at a minimum of 10 years, of previous reports. *J Bone Joint Surg Am*. 2017;99(22):1895-1899.

25. Torrens C, Guirro P, Miquel J, Santana F. Influence of glenosphere size on the development of scapular notching: a prospective randomized study. *J Shoulder Elbow Surg*. 2016;25(11):1735-1741.

26. Mollon B, Mahure SA, Roche CP, Zuckerman JD. Impact of glenosphere size on clinical outcomes after reverse total shoulder arthroplasty: an analysis of 297 shoulders. *J Shoulder Elbow Surg*. 2016;25(5):763-771.

27. Lädermann A, Denard PJ, Boileau P, et al. Effect of humeral stem design on humeral position and range of motion in reverse shoulder arthroplasty. *Int Orthop*. 2015;39(11):2205-2213.

28. Lädermann A, Denard PJ, Collin P, et al. Effect of humeral stem and glenosphere designs on range of motion and muscle length in reverse shoulder arthroplasty. *Int Orthop*. 2020;44(3):519-530.

29. Gobezie R, Shishani Y, Lederman E, Denard PJ. Can a functional difference be detected in reverse arthroplasty with 135° versus 155° prosthesis for the treatment of rotator cuff arthropathy: a prospective randomized study. *J Shoulder Elbow Surg*. 2019;28(5):813-818.

30. Glenday J, Kontaxis A, Roche S, Sivarasu S. Effect of humeral tray placement on impingement-free range of motion and muscle moment arms in reverse shoulder arthroplasty. *Clin Biomech (Bristol, Avon)*. 2019;62:136-143.

31. Berhouet J, Kontaxis A, Gulotta LV, et al. Effects of the humeral tray component positioning for onlay reverse shoulder arthroplasty design: a biomechanical analysis. *J Shoulder Elbow Surg*. 2015;24(4):569-577.

32. de Wilde LF, Poncet D, Middernacht B, Ekelund A. Prosthetic overhang is the most effective way to prevent scapular conflict in a reverse total shoulder prosthesis. *Acta Orthop*. 2010;81(6):719-726.

33. King JJ, Dalton SS, Gulotta LV, Wright TW, Schoch BS. How common are acromial and scapular spine fractures after reverse shoulder arthroplasty?: a systematic review. *Bone Joint J*. 2019;101-B(6):627-634.

34. Werthel JD, Walch G, Vegehan E, Deransart P, Sanchez-Sotelo J, Valenti P. Lateralization in reverse shoulder arthroplasty: a descriptive analysis of different implants in current practice. *Int Orthop*. 2019;43(10):2349-2360.

35. Nyffeler RW, Werner CM, Gerber C. Biomechanical relevance of glenoid component positioning in the reverse Delta III total shoulder prosthesis. *J Shoulder Elbow Surg*. 2005;14(5):524-528.

36. Kolmodin J, Davidson IU, Jun BJ, et al. Scapular notching after reverse total shoulder arthroplasty: prediction using patient-specific osseous anatomy, implant location, and shoulder motion. *J Bone Joint Surg Am*. 2018;100(13):1095-1103.

37. Athwal GS, MacDermid JC, Reddy KM, Marsh JP, Faber KJ, Drosdowech D. Does bony increased-offset reverse shoulder arthroplasty decrease scapular notching? *J Shoulder Elbow Surg*. 2015;24(3):468-473.

38. Friedman RJ, Flurin PH, Wright TW, Zuckerman JD, Roche CP. Comparison of reverse total shoulder arthroplasty outcomes with and without subscapularis repair. *J Shoulder Elbow Surg*. 2017;26(4):662-668.

39. Favard L, Levigne C, Nerot C, Gerber C, De Wilde L, Mole D. Reverse prostheses in arthropathies with cuff tear: are survivorship and function maintained over time? *Clin Orthop Relat Res*. 2011;469(9):2469-2475.

40. Brunner U, Ruckl K, Fruth M. Cuff tear arthropathy - long-term results of reverse total shoulder arthroplasty. Article in German. *Orthopä*. 2013;42(7):522-530.

41. Favard L, Young A, Alami G, et al. Survivorship of the reverse shoulder arthroplasties (RSA) with a minimum follow up of 10 years. *Orthopaedic Proceedings*. 2012;94-B(suppl 37):24.

42. Otto RJ, Clark RE, Frankle MA. Reverse shoulder arthroplasty in patients younger than 55 years: 2- to 12-year follow-up. *J Shoulder Elbow Surg*. 2017;26(5):792-797.

43. Bacle G, Nové-Josserand L, Garaud P, Walch G. Long-term outcomes of reverse total shoulder arthroplasty: a follow-up of a previous study. *J Bone Joint Surg Am*. 2017;99(6):454-461.

44. Torchia ME, Cofield RH, Settergren CR. Total shoulder arthroplasty with the Neer prosthesis: long-term results. *J Shoulder Elbow Surg*. 1997;6(6):495-505.

45. Deshmukh AV, Koris M, Zurakowski D, Thornhill TS. Total shoulder arthroplasty: long-term survivorship, functional outcome, and quality of life. *J Shoulder Elbow Surg*. 2005;14(5):471-479.

46. Australian Orthopaedic Association National Joint Replacement Registry (AOANJRR). *Hip, Knee & Shoulder: 2019 Annual Report*. Australian Orthopaedic Association; 2019.

47. Swedish Shoulder and Elbow Registry. *Annual Report*. 2019. http://www.ssas.se/files/docs/rapp19.pdf

48. Simovitch RW, Friedman RJ, Cheung EV, et al. Rate of improvement in clinical outcomes with anatomic and reverse total shoulder arthroplasty. *J Bone Joint Surg Am*. 2017;99(21):1801-1811.

49. Michener LA, McClure PW, Sennett BJ. American shoulder and elbow surgeons standardized shoulder assessment form, patient self-report section: reliability, validity, and responsiveness. *J Shoulder Elbow Surg*. 2002;11(6):587-594.

50. Friedman RJ, Cheung EV, Flurin PH, et al. Are age and patient gender associated with different rates and magnitudes of clinical improvement after reverse shoulder arthroplasty? *Clin Orthop Relat Res*. 2018;476(6):1264-1273.

51. Dawson J, Rogers K, Fitzpatrick R, Carr A. The Oxford shoulder score revisited. *Arch Orthop Trauma Surg*. 2009;129(1):119-123.

52. Scott J, Huskisson EC. Graphic representation of pain. *Pain*. 1976;2(2):175-184.

53. Gowd AK, Charles MD, Liu JN, et al. Single Assessment Numeric Evaluation (SANE) is a reliable metric to measure clinically significant improvements following shoulder arthroplasty. *J Shoulder Elbow Surg*. 2019;28(11):2238-2246.

54. Amstutz HC, Sew Hoy AL, Clarke IC. UCLA anatomic total shoulder arthroplasty. *Clin Orthop Relat Res*. 1981;155:7-20.

55. Nutton RW, McBirnie JM, Phillips C. Treatment of chronic rotator-cuff impingement by arthroscopic subacromial decompression. *J Bone Joint Surg Br*. 1997;79(1):73-76.

56. Constant CR, Murley AH. A clinical method of functional assessment of the shoulder. *Clin Orthop Relat Res*. 1987;214:160-164.

57. Simovitch R, Flurin PH, Wright T, Zuckerman JD, Roche CP. Quantifying success after total shoulder arthroplasty: the minimal clinically important difference. *J Shoulder Elbow Surg*. 2018;27(2):298-305.

58. Jaeschke R, Singer J, Guyatt GH. Measurement of health status. Ascertaining the minimal clinically important difference. *Contr Clin Trials*. 1989;10(4):407-415.

59. Simovitch R, Flurin PH, Wright T, Zuckerman JD, Roche CP. Quantifying success after total shoulder arthroplasty: the substantial clinical benefit. *J Shoulder Elbow Surg.* 2018;27(5):903-911.

60. Torrens C, Guirro P, Santana F. The minimal clinically important difference for function and strength in patients undergoing reverse shoulder arthroplasty. *J Shoulder Elbow Surg.* 2016;25(2):262-268.

61. Werner BC, Chang B, Nguyen JT, Dines DM, Gulotta LV. What change in American shoulder and elbow surgeons score represents a clinically important change after shoulder arthroplasty? *Clin Orthop Relat Res.* 2016;474(12):2672-2681.

62. Rugg CM, Gallo RA, Craig EV, Feeley BT. The pathogenesis and management of cuff tear arthropathy. *J Shoulder Elbow Surg.* 2018;27(12):2271-2283.

63. Goldberg SS, Bell JE, Kim HJ, Bak SF, Levine WN, Bigliani LU. Hemiarthroplasty for the rotator cuff-deficient shoulder. *J Bone Joint Surg Am.* 2008;90(3):554-559.

64. Sanchez-Sotelo J, Cofield RH, Rowland CM. Shoulder hemiarthroplasty for glenohumeral arthritis associated with severe rotator cuff deficiency. *J Bone Joint Surg Am.* 2001;83(12):1814-1822.

65. Barlow JD, Jamgochian G; Wells Z, et al. Reverse shoulder arthroplasty is superior to hemiarthroplasty for cuff tear arthropathy with preserved motion. *Arch Bone Jt Surg.* 2020;8(1):75-82.

66. Ashford W, Eichinger JK, Friedman RJ. Outcomes of reverse total shoulder arthroplasty. *Med Res Arch.* 2016;4(7):1-15.

67. Leung B, Horodyski M, Struk AM, Wright TW. Functional outcome of hemiarthroplasty compared with reverse total shoulder arthroplasty in the treatment of rotator cuff tear arthropathy. *J Shoulder Elbow Surg.* 2012;21(3):319-323.

68. Baker MP, Crosby LA. Cuff tear arthropathy is best treated with a reverse total shoulder arthroplasty. *Semin Arthroplasty.* 2014;25(1):7-12.

69. Ek ETH, Neukom L, Catanzaro S, Gerber C. Reverse total shoulder arthroplasty for massive irreparable rotator cuff tears in patients younger than 65 years old: results after five to fifteen years. *J Shoulder Elbow Surg.* 2013;22(9):1199-1208.

70. Al-Hadithy N, Domos P, Sewell MD, Pandit R. Reverse shoulder arthroplasty in 41 patients with cuff tear arthropathy with a mean follow-up period of 5 years. *J Shoulder Elbow Surg.* 2014;23(11):1662-1668.

71. Familiari F, Rojas J, Nedim Doral M, Huri G, McFarland EG. Reverse total shoulder arthroplasty. *EFORT Open Rev.* 2018;3(2):58-69.

72. Lindbloom BJ, Christmas KN, Downes K, et al. Is there a relationship between preoperative diagnosis and clinical outcomes in reverse shoulder arthroplasty? An experience in 699 shoulders. *J Shoulder Elbow Surg.* 2019;28(6 suppl):S110-S117.

73. Petrillo S, Longo UG, Papalia R, Denaro V. Reverse shoulder arthroplasty for massive irreparable rotator cuff tears and cuff tear arthropathy: a systematic review. *Musculoskelet Surg.* 2017;101(2):105-112.

74. Chelli M, Lo Cunsolo L, Gauci MO, et al. Reverse shoulder arthroplasty in patients aged 65 years or younger: a systematic review of the literature. *JSES Open Access.* 2019;3(3):162-167.

75. Gee EC, Hanson EK, Saithna A. Reverse shoulder arthroplasty in rheumatoid arthritis: a systematic review. *Open Orthop J.* 2015;9:237-245.

76. Holcomb JO, Cuff D, Petersen SA, Pupello DR, Frankle MA. Revision reverse shoulder arthroplasty for glenoid baseplate failure after primary reverse shoulder arthroplasty. *J Shoulder Elbow Surg.* 2009;18(5):717-723.

77. Postacchini R, Carbone S, Canero G, Ripani M, Postacchini F. Reverse shoulder prosthesis in patients with rheumatoid arthritis: a systematic review. *Int Orthop.* 2016;40(5):965-973.

78. Flurin PH, Roche CP, Wright TW, Marczuk Y, Zuckerman JD. A comparison and correlation of clinical outcome metrics in anatomic and reverse total shoulder arthroplasty. *Bull Hosp Jt Dis (2013).* 2015;73(suppl 1):S118-S123.

79. Ernstbrunner L, Andronic O, Grubhofer F, Camenzind RS, Wieser K, Gerber C. Long-term results of reverse total shoulder arthroplasty for rotator cuff dysfunction: a systematic review of longitudinal outcomes. *J Shoulder Elbow Surg.* 2019;28(4):774-781.

80. Mizuno N, Denard PJ, Raiss P, Walch G. Reverse total shoulder arthroplasty for primary glenohumeral osteoarthritis in patients with a biconcave glenoid. *J Bone Joint Surg Am.* 2013;95(14):1297-1304.

81. Hyun YS, Huri G, Garbis NG, McFarland EG. Uncommon indications for reverse total shoulder arthroplasty. *Clin Orthop Surg.* 2013;5(4):243-255.

82. McFarland EG, Huri G, Hyun YS, Petersen SA, Srikumaran U. Reverse total shoulder arthroplasty without bone-grafting for severe glenoid bone loss in patients with osteoarthritis and intact rotator cuff. *J Bone Joint Surg Am.* 2016;98(21):1801-1807.

83. Wright MA, Keener JD, Chamberlain AM. Comparison of clinical outcomes after anatomic total shoulder arthroplasty and reverse shoulder arthroplasty in patients 70 years and older with glenohumeral osteoarthritis and an intact rotator cuff. *J Am Acad Orthop Surg.* 2020;28(5):e222-e229.

84. Streit JJ, Clark JC, Allert J, et al. Ten years of reverse total shoulder arthroplasty performed for osteoarthritis and intact rotator cuff: indications and outcomes. *J Shoulder Elbow Surg.* 2017;26(5):e159.

85. Kiet TK, Naimark M, Gajiu T, Hall SL, Chung TT, Ma CB. Outcomes after shoulder replacement: comparison between reverse and anatomic total shoulder arthroplasty. *J Shoulder Elbow Surg.* 2015;24(2):179-185.

86. Cerciello S, Corona K, Morris BJ, Paladini P, Porcellini G, Merolla G. Shoulder arthroplasty to address the sequelae of anterior instability arthropathy and stabilization procedures: systematic review and meta-analysis. *Arch Orthop Trauma Surg.* 2020;140(12):1891-1900.

87. Cuff DJ, Santoni BG. Anatomic total shoulder arthroplasty versus reverse total shoulder arthroplasty for post-capsulorrhaphy arthropathy. *Orthopedics.* 2018;41(5):275-280.

88. Wall B, O'Connor DP, Edwards TB, Nové-Josserand L, Walch G. Reverse total shoulder arthroplasty: a review of results according to etiology. *J Bone Joint Surg Am.* 2007;89(7):1476-1485.

89. Boileau P, Gonzalez JF, Chuinard C, Bicknell R, Walch G. Reverse total shoulder arthroplasty after failed rotator cuff surgery. *J Shoulder Elbow Surg.* 2009;18(4):600-606.

90. Mulieri P, Dunning P, Klein S, Pupello D, Frankle M. Reverse shoulder arthroplasty for the treatment of irreparable rotator cuff tear without glenohumeral arthritis. *J Bone Joint Surg Am.* 2010;92(15):2544-2556.

91. Hartzler RU, Steen BM, Hussey MM, et al. Reverse shoulder arthroplasty for massive rotator cuff tear: risk factors for poor functional improvement. *J Shoulder Elbow Surg.* 2015;24(11):1698-1706.

92. Cuff DJ, Pupello DR. Comparison of hemiarthroplasty and reverse shoulder arthroplasty for the treatment of proximal humeral fractures in elderly patients. *J Bone Joint Surg Am.* 2013;95(22):2050-2055.

93. Simovitch RW, Roche CP, Jones RB, et al. Effect of tuberosity healing on clinical outcomes in elderly patients treated with a reverse shoulder arthroplasty for 3- and 4-Part Proximal humerus fractures. *J Orthop Trauma.* 2019;33(2):e39-e45.

94. Raiss P, Edwards TB, Collin P, et al. Reverse shoulder arthroplasty for malunions of the proximal part of the humerus (Type-4 fracture sequelae). *J Bone Joint Surg Am.* 2016;98(11):893-899.

95. Dezfuli B, King JJ, Farmer KW, Struk AM, Wright TW. Outcomes of reverse total shoulder arthroplasty as primary versus revision procedure for proximal humerus fractures. *J Shoulder Elbow Surg.* 2016;25(7):1133-1137.

96. Wagner ER, Chang MJ, Welp KM, et al. The impact of the reverse prosthesis on revision shoulder arthroplasty: analysis of a high-volume shoulder practice. *J Shoulder Elbow Surg.* 2019;28(2):e49-e56.

97. Knowles NK, Columbus MP, Wegmann K, Ferreira LM, Athwal GS. Revision shoulder arthroplasty: a systematic review and comparison of North American vs. European outcomes and complications. *J Shoulder Elbow Surg.* 2020;29(5):1071-1082.

98. Kelly JD II, Zhao JX, Hobgood ER, Norris TR. Clinical results of revision shoulder arthroplasty using the reverse prosthesis. *J Shoulder Elbow Surg.* 2012;21(11):1516-1525.

99. Patel DN, Young B, Onyekwelu I, Zuckerman JD, Kwon YW. Reverse total shoulder arthroplasty for failed shoulder arthroplasty. *J Shoulder Elbow Surg.* 2012;21(11):1478-1483.

100. Alentorn-Geli E, Clark NJ, Assenmacher AT, et al. What are the complications, survival, and outcomes after revision to reverse shoulder arthroplasty in patients older than 80 years? *Clin Orthop Relat Res.* 2017;475(11):2744-2751.

101. Black EM, Roberts SM, Siegel E, Yannopoulos P, Higgins LD, Warner JJP. Failure after reverse total shoulder arthroplasty: what is the success of component revision? *J Shoulder Elbow Surg.* 2015;24(12):1908-1914.

102. Boileau P, Melis B, Duperron D, Moineau G, Rumian AP, Han Y. Revision surgery of reverse shoulder arthroplasty. *J Shoulder Elbow Surg.* 2013;22(10):1359-1370.

103. Padegimas EM, Maltenfort M, Lazarus MD, Ramsey ML, Williams GR, Namdari S. Future patient demand for shoulder arthroplasty by younger patients: national projections. *Clin Orthop Relat Res.* 2015;473(6):1860-1867.

104. Ernstbrunner L, Suter A, Catanzaro S, Rahm S, Gerber C. Reverse total shoulder arthroplasty for massive, irreparable rotator cuff tears before the age of 60 years: long-term results. *J Bone Joint Surg Am.* 2017;99(20):1721-1729.

105. Matthews CJ, Wright TW, Farmer KW, Struk AM, Vasilopoulos T, King JJ. Outcomes of primary reverse total shoulder arthroplasty in patients younger than 65 years old. *J Hand Surg Am.* 2019;44(2):104-111.

106. Monir JG, Abeyewardene D, King JJ, Wright TW, Schoch BS. Reverse shoulder arthroplasty in patients younger than 65 years, minimum 5-year follow-up. *J Shoulder Elbow Surg.* 2020;29(6):e215-e221.

107. Samuelsen BT, Wagner ER, Houdek MT, et al. Primary reverse shoulder arthroplasty in patients aged 65 years or younger. *J Shoulder Elbow Surg.* 2017;26(1):e13-e17.

108. Sershon RA, Van Thiel GS, Lin EC, et al. Clinical outcomes of reverse total shoulder arthroplasty in patients aged younger than 60 years. *J Shoulder Elbow Surg.* 2014;23(3):395-400.

109. Walters JD, Barkoh K, Smith RA, Azar FM, Throckmorton TW. Younger patients report similar activity levels to older patients after reverse total shoulder arthroplasty. *J Shoulder Elbow Surg.* 2016;25(9):1418-1424.

110. Wong SE, Pitcher AA, Ding DY, et al. The effect of patient gender on outcomes after reverse total shoulder arthroplasty. *J Shoulder Elbow Surg.* 2017;26(11):1889-1896.

111. Steinhaus ME, Gowd AK, Hurwit DJ, Lieber AC, Liu JN. Return to work after shoulder arthroplasty: a systematic review and meta-analysis. *J Shoulder Elbow Surg.* 2019;28(5):998-1008.

112. Garcia GH, Taylor SA, Mahony GT, et al. Reverse total shoulder arthroplasty and work-related outcomes. *Orthopedics.* 2016;39(2):e230-e235.

113. Hurwit DJ, Liu JN, Garcia GH, et al. A comparative analysis of work-related outcomes after humeral hemiarthroplasty and reverse total shoulder arthroplasty. *J Shoulder Elbow Surg.* 2017;26(6):954-959.

114. Golant A, Christoforou D, Zuckerman JD, Kwon YW. Return to sports after shoulder arthroplasty: a survey of surgeons' preferences. *J Shoulder Elbow Surg.* 2012;21(4):554-560.

115. Simovitch RW, Gerard BK, Brees JA, Fullick R, Kearse JC. Outcomes of reverse total shoulder arthroplasty in a senior athletic population. *J Shoulder Elbow Surg.* 2015;24(9):1481-1485.

116. Kurowicki J, Rosas S, Law TY, Levy JC. Participation in work and sport following reverse and total shoulder arthroplasty. *Am J Orthop (Belle Mead NJ).* 2018;47(5):1-15.

117. Bulhoff M, Sowa B, Bruckner T, Zeifang F, Raiss P. Activity levels after reverse shoulder arthroplasty. *Arch Orthop Trauma Surg.* 2016;136(9):1189-1193.

118. Burrus MT, Werner BC, Cancienne JM, Gwathmey FW, Brockmeier SF. Shoulder arthroplasty in patients with Parkinson's disease is associated with increased complications. *J Shoulder Elbow Surg.* 2015;24(12):1881-1887.

119. Cusick MC, Otto RJ, Clark RE, Frankle MA. Outcome of reverse shoulder arthroplasty for patients with Parkinson's disease: a matched cohort study. *Orthopedics.* 2017;40(4):e675-e680.

120. Mellano CR, Kupfer N, Thorsness R, et al. Functional results of bilateral reverse total shoulder arthroplasty. *J Shoulder Elbow Surg.* 2017;26(6):990-996.

121. Welborn BT, Butler RB, Dumas BP, Mock L, Messerschmidt CA, Friedman RJ. Patient reported outcome measures of bilateral reverse total shoulder arthroplasty compared to bilateral anatomic total shoulder arthroplasty. *J Orthop.* 2020;17:83-86.

122. Gates S, Cutler H, Khazzam M. Outcomes of posterior glenoid bone-grafting in anatomical total shoulder arthroplasty: a systematic review. *JBJS Rev.* 2019;7(9):e6.

123. Lorenzetti A, Streit JJ, Cabezas AF, et al. Bone graft augmentation for severe glenoid bone loss in primary reverse total shoulder arthroplasty: outcomes and evaluation of host bone contact by 2D-3D image registration. *JBJS Open Access.* 2017;2(3):e0015.

124. Malahias MA, Chytas D, Kostretzis L, et al. Bone grafting in primary and revision reverse total shoulder arthroplasty for the management of glenoid bone loss: a systematic review. *J Orthop.* 2020;20:78-86.

125. Jones RB, Wright TW, Roche CP. Bone grafting the glenoid versus use of augmented glenoid baseplates with reverse shoulder arthroplasty. *Bull Hosp Jt Dis (2013).* 2015;73(suppl 1):S129-S135.

126. Virk M, Yip M, Liuzza L, et al. Clinical and radiographic outcomes with a posteriorly augmented glenoid for Walch B2, B3, and C glenoids in reverse total shoulder arthroplasty. *J Shoulder Elbow Surg.* 2020;29(5):196-204.

127. Friedman RJ, Hawthorne KB, Genez BM. The use of computerized tomography in the measurement of glenoid version. *J Bone Joint Surg Am.* 1992;74(7):1032-1037.

128. Abdic S, Knowles NK, Walch G, Johnson JA, Athwal GS. Type E2 glenoid bone loss orientation and management with augmented implants. *J Shoulder Elbow Surg.* 2020;29(7):1460-1469.

129. Cox JL, McLendon PB, Christmas KN, Simon P, Mighell MA, Frankle MA. Clinical outcomes following reverse shoulder arthroplasty-allograft composite for revision of failed arthroplasty associated with proximal humeral bone deficiency: 2- to 15-year follow-up. *J Shoulder Elbow Surg.* 2019;28(5):900-907.

130. Budge MD, Moravek JE, Zimel MN, Nolan EM, Wiater JM. Reverse total shoulder arthroplasty for the management of failed shoulder arthroplasty with proximal humeral bone loss: is allograft augmentation necessary? *J Shoulder Elbow Surg.* 2013;22(6):739-744.

131. Stephens SP, Paisley KC, Giveans MR, Wirth MA. The effect of proximal humeral bone loss on revision reverse total shoulder arthroplasty. *J Shoulder Elbow Surg.* 2015;24(10):1519-1526.

132. Barlow JD, Yuan BJ, Schleck CD, Harmsen WS, Cofield RH, Sperling JW. Shoulder arthroplasty for rheumatoid arthritis: 303 consecutive cases with minimum 5-year follow-up. *J Shoulder Elbow Surg.* 2014;23(6):791-799.

133. Werner BC, Wong AC, Chang B, et al. Depression and patient-reported outcomes following total shoulder arthroplasty. *J Bone Joint Surg Am.* 2017;99(8):688-695.

134. Tokish JM, Kissenberth MJ, Tolan SJ, et al. Resilience correlates with outcomes after total shoulder arthroplasty. *J Shoulder Elbow Surg.* 2017;26(5):752-756.

135. Vajapey SP, Cvetanovich GL, Bishop JY, Neviaser AS. Psychosocial factors affecting outcomes after shoulder arthroplasty: a systematic review. *J Shoulder Elbow Surg.* 2020;29(5):e175-e184.

136. Morris BJ, Sciascia AD, Jacobs CA, Edwards TB. Preoperative opioid use associated with worse outcomes after anatomic shoulder arthroplasty. *J Shoulder Elbow Surg.* 2016;25(4):619-623.

137. Cheah JW, Sing DC, McLaughlin D, Feeley BT, Ma CB, Zhang AL. The perioperative effects of chronic preoperative opioid use on shoulder arthroplasty outcomes. *J Shoulder Elbow Surg.* 2017;26(11):1908-1914.

138. Beck JD, Irgit KS, Andreychik CM, Maloney PJ, Tang X, Harter GD. Reverse total shoulder arthroplasty in obese patients. *J Hand Surg Am.* 2013;38(5):965-970.

139. Gupta AK, Chalmers PN, Rahman Z, et al. Reverse total shoulder arthroplasty in patients of varying body mass index. *J Shoulder Elbow Surg.* 2014;23(1):35-42.

140. Dallalana RJ, McMahon RA, East B, Geraghty L. Accuracy of patient-specific instrumentation in anatomic and reverse total shoulder arthroplasty. *Int J Shoulder Surg.* 2016;10(2):59-66.

141. Anakwenze O, Fokin A, Chocas M, et al. Complications in total shoulder and reverse total shoulder arthroplasty by body mass index. *J Shoulder Elbow Surg.* 2017;26(7):1230-1237.

142. Kusin DJ, Ungar JA, Samson KK, Teusink MJ. Body mass index as a risk factor for dislocation of total shoulder arthroplasty in the first 30 days. *JSES Open Access.* 2019;3(3):179-182.

143. Theodoulou A, Krishnan J, Aromataris E. Risk of poor outcomes in patients who are obese following total shoulder arthroplasty and reverse total shoulder arthroplasty: a systematic review and meta-analysis. *J Shoulder Elbow Surg.* 2019;28(11):e359-e376.

144. Morris BJ, Haigler RE, Laughlin MS, Elkousy HA, Gartsman GM, Edwards TB. Workers' compensation claims and outcomes after reverse shoulder arthroplasty. *J Shoulder Elbow Surg.* 2015;24(3):453-459.

145. Singh A, Yian EH, Dillon MT, Takayanagi M, Burke MF, Navarro RA. The effect of surgeon and hospital volume on shoulder arthroplasty perioperative quality metrics. *J Shoulder Elbow Surg.* 2014;23(8):1187-1194.

146. Brown JS, Gordon RJ, Peng Y, Hatton A, Page RS, Macgroarty KA. Lower operating volume in shoulder arthroplasty is associated with increased revision rates in the early postoperative period: long-term analysis from the Australian Orthopaedic Association National Joint Replacement Registry. *J Shoulder Elbow Surg.* 2020;29(6):1104-1114.

147. Kumar V, Roche C, Overman S, et al. What is the accuracy of three different machine learning techniques to predict clinical outcomes after shoulder arthroplasty? *Clin Orthop Relat Res.* 2020;478(10):2351-2363.

148. Werner BS, Hudek R, Burkhart KJ, Gohlke F. The influence of three-dimensional planning on decision-making in total shoulder arthroplasty. *J Shoulder Elbow Surg.* 2017;26(8):1477-1483.

149. Berhouet J, Gulotta LV, Dines DM, et al. Preoperative planning for accurate glenoid component positioning in reverse shoulder arthroplasty. *Orthop Traumatol Surg Res.* 2017;103(3):407-413.

150. Levy JC, Everding NG, Frankle MA, Keppler LJ. Accuracy of patient-specific guided glenoid baseplate positioning for reverse shoulder arthroplasty. *J Shoulder Elbow Surg.* 2014;23(10):1563-1567.

151. Throckmorton TW, Gulotta LV, Bonnarens FO, et al. Patient-specific targeting guides compared with traditional instrumentation for glenoid component placement in shoulder arthroplasty: a multi-surgeon study in 70 arthritic cadaver specimens. *J Shoulder Elbow Surg.* 2015;24(6):965-971.

152. Walch G, Vezeridis PS, Boileau P, Deransart P, Deransart P. Three-dimensional planning and use of patient-specific guides improve glenoid component position: an in vitro study. *J Shoulder Elbow Surg.* 2015;24(2):302-309.

153. Hendel MD, Bryan JA, Barsoum WK, et al. Comparison of patient-specific instruments with standard surgical instruments in determining glenoid component position: a randomized prospective clinical trial. *J Bone Joint Surg Am.* 2012;94(23):2167-2175.

154. Suero EM, Citak M, Lo D, Krych AJ, Craig EV, Pearle AD. Use of a custom alignment guide to improve glenoid component position in total shoulder arthroplasty. *Knee Surg Sports Traumatol Arthrosc.* 2013;21(12):2860-2866.

155. Heylen S, Van Haver A, Vuylsteke K, Declercq G, Verborgt O. Patient-specific instrument guidance of glenoid component implantation reduces inclination variability in total and reverse shoulder arthroplasty. *J Shoulder Elbow Surg.* 2016;25(2):186-192.

156. Lau SC, Keith PPA. Patient-specific instrumentation for total shoulder arthroplasty: not as accurate as it would seem. *J Shoulder Elbow Surg.* 2018;27(1):90-95.

157. Nashikkar PS, Scholes CJ, Haber MD. Computer navigation re-creates planned glenoid placement and reduces correction variability in total shoulder arthroplasty: an in vivo case-control study. *J Shoulder Elbow Surg.* 2019;28(12):e398-e409.

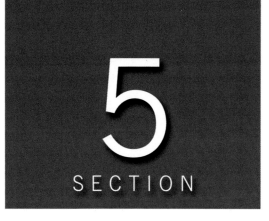

Shoulder Arthroplasty for Fracture

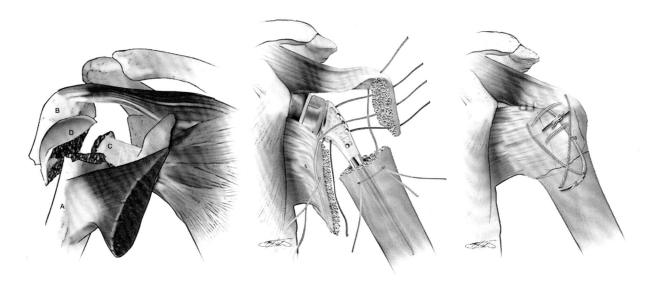

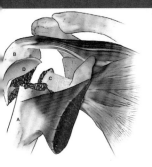

28 Hemiarthroplasty:
Indications and Technique

Blake J. Schultz, MD and Kenneth A. Egol, MD

INTRODUCTION

Fractures involving the proximal humerus account for approximately 4% to 5% of all fractures.[1-3] They occur in a bimodal distribution and are the second most common upper extremity fracture in patients older than 65 years.[4] While the majority of proximal humerus fractures, especially in the elderly, can be treated nonoperatively,[5,6] three- and four-part fractures and fracture-dislocations are often indicated for surgery. The popularization of locking plate technology has expanded the indications for open reduction and internal fixation (ORIF) of proximal humerus fractures,[7-14] but locked plating of the proximal humerus has its own set of complications.[15-20] Arthroplasty remains an option when there is concern about the viability of the humeral head or the ability to achieve an acceptable reduction and secure fixation. Hemiarthroplasty has proven to reliably reduce pain, but postoperative functional outcomes have been less predictable.[21-27] More recently, reverse total shoulder arthroplasty (TSA) has been proven to be a safe and effective option for restoration of motion and function in elderly patients who sustain a proximal humerus fracture,[28-33] but there is still a role for hemiarthroplasty in select patients. This chapter reviews the indications for shoulder hemiarthroplasty in the setting of proximal humerus fractures, including fracture pattern and pertinent patient factors, as well as surgical techniques to optimize outcomes.

FRACTURE CLASSIFICATION

The Neer classification classically used to describe proximal humerus fractures is based on the number of distinct fracture parts and their displacement.[34] The four potential parts include the humeral articular surface, greater tuberosity, lesser tuberosity, and humeral shaft **(FIGURE 28.1)**. Traditionally, displacement was defined as fragments with angulation of >45° or >1 cm of separation. In addition, literature suggests that only 5 mm of displacement of the greater tuberosity specifically should be accepted, but this is also based on the direction of fragment displacement.[15,35,36] Fractures are described as two-, three- and four-part fractures with or without dislocations. Proximal humerus fractures can also be described according to the AO Foundation/Orthopaedic

Trauma Association classification, which focuses on the extra- versus intra-articular location of the fracture[37] **(FIGURE 28.2)**. The Hertel classification is also used, noting specific fracture characteristics to predict the risk of fracture-induced humeral head ischemia.[38] Fractures through the anatomic neck, metaphyseal extension less than 8 mm, loss of the medial hinge, and displacement of the humeral head all increase the risk of humeral head ischemia.[38]

Indications for hemiarthroplasty are discussed in detail below. However, they generally include certain classic four-part fractures, select three-part fractures, three- and four-part fracture-dislocations, and head-splitting fracture patterns with substantial articular involvement that are not amenable to ORIF.

EVALUATION

Proximal humerus fractures typically occur in a bimodal distribution, with young patients often involved in high-energy trauma and elderly patients via low-energy mechanisms. Low-energy mechanism proximal humerus fractures should raise concern for poor bone quality. These fractures in the elderly are considered a "fragility fracture" and should lead to the implementation of appropriate medical care for the treatment of osteoporosis. As with any fracture, it is important to assess for any medical comorbidities or risk factors that could affect bone healing potential.

SOCIAL HISTORY

There is a wide range of treatment options for proximal humerus fractures, so a detailed social history is important, including occupation, handedness, activity level, and social habits including alcohol and drug use. Baseline functional status and activities of daily living goals (patient expectations) are particularly important to understand when considering hemiarthroplasty. Additionally, any conditions that predispose the patient to seizures (medications, trauma, strokes, etc) are important to document when considering any type of arthroplasty. The patient's cognitive and physical ability to follow a structured postoperative rehabilitation course should also be considered.[21,39,40]

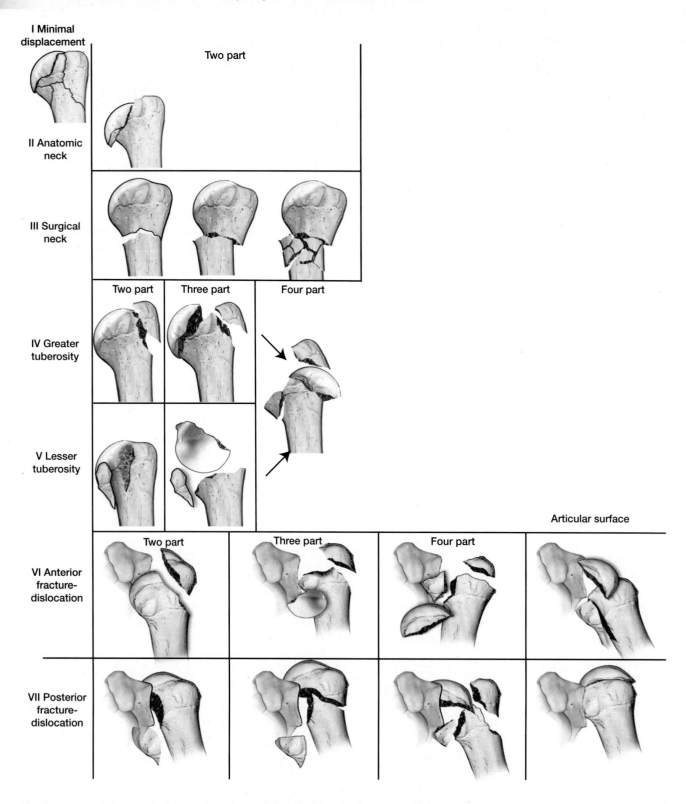

FIGURE 28.1 Neer took Codman's original classification of proximal humerus fractures that divided the proximal humerus into the greater tuberosity, lesser tuberosity, humeral head, and shaft and expanded it to include fracture displacement (>1 cm) and angulation (>45°). General indications for hemiarthroplasty according to the Neer classification include select three-part fractures, classic four-part fractures, and fracture-dislocations. (Reprinted with permission from Jones CB. Proximal humeral fractures. In: Boyer MI, ed. *AAOS Comprehensive Orthopaedic Review 2*. American Academy of Orthopedic Surgeons; 2014:293-302.)

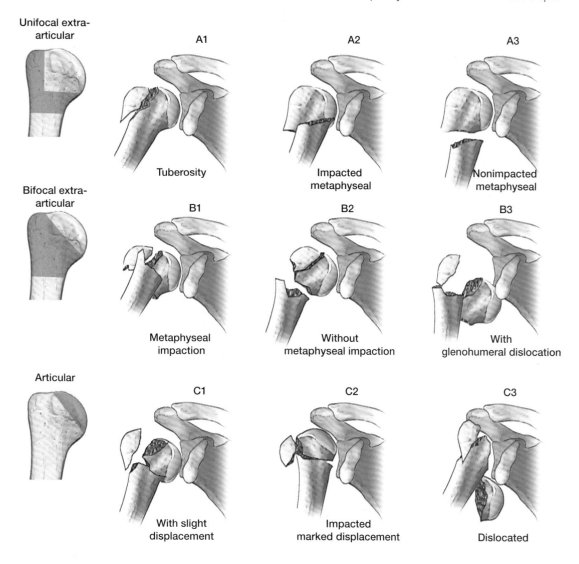

FIGURE 28.2 The AO Foundation/Orthopaedic Trauma Association classification focuses on the extra- versus intra-articular location of the fracture. Specific fracture patterns indicated for hemiarthroplasty including head-splitting and those with substantial articular involvement. (Redrawn with permission from Cadet ER, Ahmad CS. Hemiarthroplasty for three- and four-part proximal humerus fractures. *J Am Acad Orthop Surg.* 2012;20(1):17-27, Figure 3.)

PHYSICAL EXAMINATION

Patients with a proximal humerus fracture will have swelling, tenderness, and ecchymosis about the shoulder girdle and extending into the arm and forearm and often to the chest wall **(FIGURE 28.3)**. They will have limited active and passive range of motion (ROM) secondary to pain or loss of rotator cuff function. Assessment for signs of anterior or posterior dislocation, including the ability to palpate the humeral head, may guide the need to assist or utilize alternative radiographic views. Overall, up to 90% of proximal humerus fractures are isolated injuries.[41] However, in the elderly population, up to 16% of patients will have an associated fracture, with distal radius and proximal femur being the two most common fractures, so a thorough musculoskeletal examination is necessary.

It is essential to document a careful neurologic examination, especially axillary and musculocutaneous nerve function, as neurologic injury may be present in up to 45% of these injuries.[39] Assessing deltoid motor function to evaluate axillary nerve function is particularly important when considering different arthroplasty options. While this can be difficult in the acute setting, assessing all three heads of the deltoid is essential. A vascular examination, both at the fracture site and distally in the hand, is also important to obtain. Any palpable thrill or bruit necessitates a vascular surgery consult.

Though it will be difficult to assess in an acute fracture due to pain, rotator cuff function should be evaluated in all patients with proximal humerus fracture, especially the elderly, because of the risk for associated injury.[42] Previous studies have demonstrated that rotator

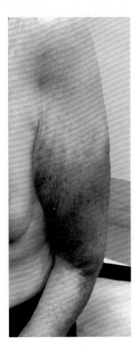

FIGURE 28.3 Patients may have ecchymosis and swelling through the shoulder girdle extending into the axilla and down the humeral shaft.

cuff tears may be present in up to 50% of patients who sustain proximal humerus fractures. This incidence increases to over 60% in patients older than 60 years.[43-46] However, rotator cuff compromise is often present prior to the injury as a result of age-related degeneration, making it difficult to discern if a rotator cuff deficit is acute, chronic, or an acute exacerbation of a chronic problem. Regardless, rotator cuff function is an important factor to consider when determining a treatment plan and implant options. Concomitant injuries to the shoulder

are also particularly important to diagnose and understand since they may dictate treatment. Patients with fracture-dislocations may have associated glenoid rim or neck fractures (especially in the elderly), so a thorough radiographic assessment is important.

RADIOGRAPHIC/IMAGING STUDIES

A standard shoulder trauma series should be obtained, including an anteroposterior (AP), lateral scapula, and axillary view (**FIGURE 28.4**). The axillary view is critical to evaluate the position of the humeral head on the glenoid and to assess for an associated glenohumeral dislocation. If the patient cannot tolerate positioning for the axillary view, a Velpeau axillary view can be obtained.[47] Computed tomography (CT) scans can be helpful to assess tuberosity displacement, as well as to assess involvement of the humeral head, including head-splitting components (**FIGURE 28.5**). The soft-tissue window in the axial and sagittal views provides information about rotator cuff degeneration, including muscle atrophy or fatty infiltration, which can affect surgical decision-making.[48] Three-dimensional reconstruction with glenoid subtraction can also be helpful to understand the tuberosity fracture lines.[23]

The four rotator cuff muscles attach to the proximal humerus and are responsible for the direction of fracture fragment displacement. The supraspinatus, infraspinatus, and teres minor attach to the greater tuberosity and displace the fragment superiorly or posteriorly, depending on the portion of the greater tuberosity involved. The subscapularis attaches to the lesser tuberosity and will displace this fragment anteromedially. The humeral shaft is also displaced medially and anteriorly by the pectoralis major[49] (**FIGURE 28.6**). The articular segment is

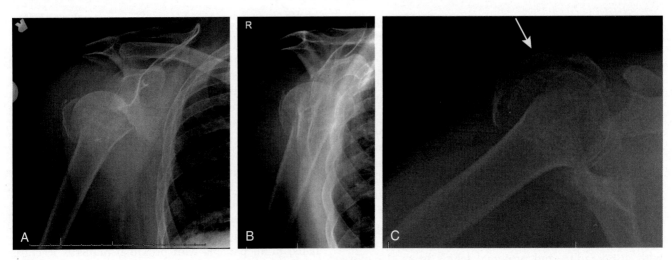

FIGURE 28.4 A 64-year-old woman following a ground-level fall. **A,** Anteroposterior view of the right shoulder showing a four-part proximal humerus fracture involving the anatomic neck and greater and lesser tuberosities. There is inferior subluxation of the humeral head in relation to the glenoid. **B,** Lateral scapula view. **C,** Axillary view showing the glenohumeral joint is reduced.

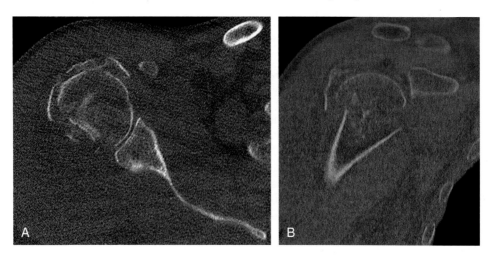

FIGURE 28.5 A 64-year-old male patient who fell down the stairs with isolated right shoulder pain. **A**, Axial CT images showing involvement of the greater and lesser tuberosity fragments adjacent to the bicipital groove. Also confirms the glenoid is intact. **B**, Coronal CT cut showing the anatomic neck fracture with significant comminution and the displaced greater tuberosity fragment. Intraoperatively, the articular surface was rotated 180° away from the glenohumeral joint with extensive comminution of the anatomic neck fracture. Because of concern regarding the viability of the humeral head and ability to maintain an accurate reduction, the plan was changed from open reduction and internal fixation to arthroplasty. The patient's main complaint preoperatively was pain control, so the decision was made to proceed with hemiarthroplasty.

typically displaced and rotated laterally, but this can be variable. The loss of soft-tissue attachments to the articular segment can significantly affect the blood supply to the humeral head, putting it at risk for osteonecrosis (ON). The length of medial humeral calcar involvement (<8 mm) is also a risk factor for head ischemia.[38]

SURGICAL INDICATIONS

Indications for prosthetic replacement include the significantly displaced four-part fractures (excluding the valgus impacted), four-part fracture-dislocations, select three-part fractures and fracture-dislocations, and

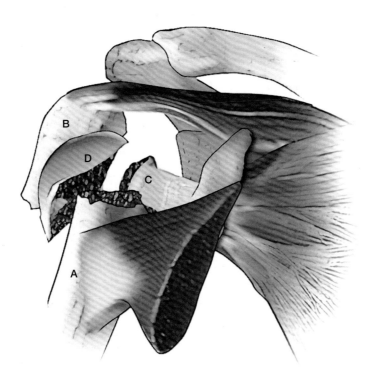

FIGURE 28.6 Classic four-part fracture characterized by anterior and medial displacement of the shaft caused by the pull of the pectoralis major (**A**), posterior/superior displacement of the greater tuberosity caused by the supraspinatus, infraspinatus, and teres minor (**B**), antero-medial displacement of the lesser tuberosity caused by the pull of the subscapularis (**C**), and lateral displacement of the articular segment (**D**).

specific fracture patterns including head-splitting fractures and head depression fractures involving more than 40% of the articular surface.[23,35]

Locked plating technology has expanded the indications for ORIF for most three-part and even some four-part fractures, especially in young patients with good bone stock and an intact rotator cuff.[7-10] However, patients with severe osteopenia or inadequate bone stock may be better candidates for arthroplasty than for internal fixation.[49,50] ON of the humeral head is a known sequelae of certain proximal humerus fracture patterns and may guide treatment toward arthroplasty rather than ORIF in high-risk patients or fracture patterns. ON after surgical fixation is generally a predictor of poor outcomes.[51] However, some authors have found that patients with ON after proximal humerus fixation had comparable functional outcomes to patients with hemiarthroplasty, which may indicate that the risk of ON should not necessarily be an absolute indication for hemiarthroplasty.[52]

Four-part fractures and fracture-dislocations occur more commonly in elderly patients.[53] The deforming muscle forces causing displacement of each part make adequate closed reduction difficult to maintain.[34,53] In addition, closed reduction of fracture-dislocations specifically has an increased risk of neurovascular injury secondary to traction and manipulation attempts.[49] Increasing displacement also impacts the blood supply to the humeral head, with four-part fractures having the highest risk of developing ON[23] with a reported incidence of 20% to 30%.[54] Patients with selected three-part fractures, including fracture-dislocations, head-splitting fractures, or compression fractures of 40% or more of the humeral head may also be candidates for hemiarthroplasty.[23,24]

When deciding between anatomic TSA, reverse TSA, and shoulder hemiarthroplasty, it is important to consider rotator cuff integrity since rotator cuff compromise is a contraindication to hemiarthroplasty and anatomic TSA. In addition, patient-specific social and functional factors need to be noted. Hemiarthroplasty has been shown to reliably reduce pain, but functional outcome has been less predictable.[1,21-23,52] With this in mind, the patient's age, baseline functional status, and activity goals will all play significant roles in treatment choice. If the initial decision is ORIF, the surgeon should still be prepared to change plans intraoperatively to a hemiarthroplasty if the humeral head is not reconstructable or to a reverse TSA if there is concern for rotator cuff dysfunction. While there has been a shift away from hemiarthroplasty toward reverse TSA,[11] the issues surrounding glenoid bone stock and the potential for future revision surgery allow hemiarthroplasty to remain a viable option in select patients such as younger patients with unreconstructable fractures, those with an axillary nerve injury that compromises deltoid function, or those with compromised glenoid bone stock not amenable to glenoid resurfacing.

CONTRAINDICATIONS

Contraindications for hemiarthroplasty include patients with global neurologic injury that limits use of the involved upper extremity and those with known rotator cuff dysfunction.[23] Reverse shoulder arthroplasty is a better option for patients with significant preexisting rotator cuff compromise as long as deltoid function is intact. As with all arthroplasty procedures, contraindications include patients not medically stable for surgery and those with active infections.

SURGICAL TECHNIQUE

Implant Options

Manufacturers have developed fracture-specific stems to help address the traditional pitfalls of hemiarthroplasty, including component malposition and tuberosity reduction, fixation, and healing.[55]

To address tuberosity reduction, stems have strategically placed slots for suture fixation and keel cutouts for tuberosity fragment placement (**FIGURE 28.7**). To facilitate tuberosity healing, there are various implant coating options as well as fenestrations in the stem to allow for bone grafting. For stem positioning, there are temporary intra- and extramedullary fixation jigs that allow for provisional assessment of stem placement, as well as various stem size and shape options to optimize canal fit. To enhance stability, there is a range of head sizes available, and some systems have radiopaque trial heads that allow for intraoperative fluoroscopy to assess stem position and greater tuberosity to head height.

Newer stems also have the ability to convert a well-fixed hemiarthroplasty to a reverse TSA, which is an important benefit should a revision be necessary.[56] Surgeons should be familiar with the specific design characteristics and stem options of whichever implant system they use to optimize outcomes.[23]

APPROACH

We prefer that the patient be seated in the beach chair position with the head firmly secured in the head rest, similar to that for anatomic or reverse TSA described in Chapters 13 and 23 (**FIGURE 28.8**). For hemiarthroplasty, it is important to be able to fully adduct and extend the arm for canal preparation. Hemiarthroplasty is most often performed through a deltopectoral approach, but the anterolateral deltoid-splitting approach is an acceptable alternative, and may have some advantage for addressing posterior fracture fragments and managing rotator cuff issues.[57,58] The anterior branch of the axillary nerve traverses the deltoid 4 to 6 cm distal to the edge of the acromion,[59,60] so particular attention is needed to identify and protect the nerve throughout the procedure.[58] The deltopectoral approach is our preferred approach and is described here.

A standard deltopectoral approach is made starting at the tip of the coracoid process (**FIGURE 28.9; VIDEO 28.1**).

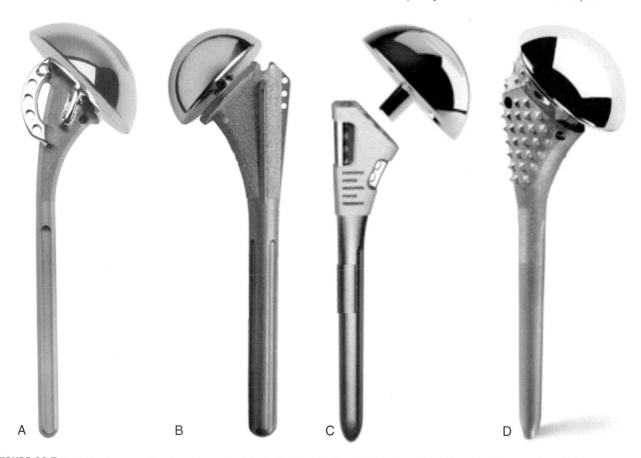

FIGURE 28.7 A-C, Fracture-specific stems have struts to facilitate reduction of the tuberosities with suture. Fenestrations in the stem to allow for bone grafting and various implant coating options facilitate bony growth. **A**, Equinoxe Fracture System, Exactech, Gainesville, FL. **B**, Global Foundation Shoulder System, DJO Lewisville, TX. **C**, ReUnion RFX Reversible Fracture System, Stryker, Kalamazoo, MI. **D**, Anatomical Shoulder Fracture System, Zimmer, Warsaw, IN. (A, Used with permission from © Exactech, Inc. B, DJO® is a registered trademark of DJO, LLC in the U.S. and/or other countries. © 2020 DJO, LLC. Used with permission from DJO, LLC. All rights reserved. C, Image reprinted with permission from Stryker Corporation. © 2021 Stryker Corporation. All rights reserved. D, Used with permission from © Zimmer Biomet.)

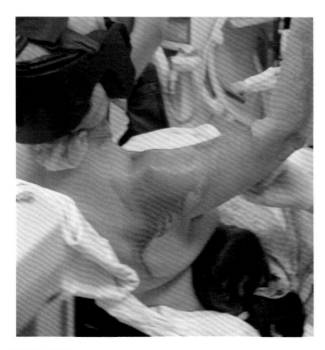

FIGURE 28.8 Beach chair position with the head secured. The lateral kidney positioner is important to secure the trunk in position and allow for proper position of the arm during humeral shaft preparation.

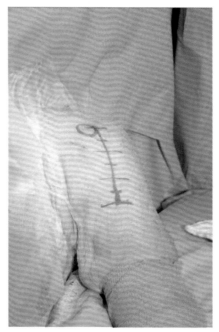

FIGURE 28.9 A standard deltopectoral approach is made from the tip of the coracoid process toward the deltoid insertion on the humerus. If the fracture extends into the humeral shaft, the incision can be extended distally into an extensile approach.

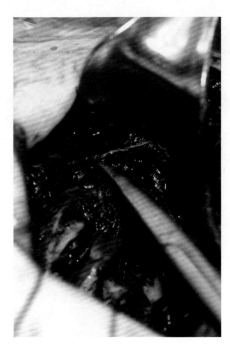

FIGURE 28.10 Intraoperative view of a left shoulder demonstrating preservation of the coracoacromial ligament.

Unlike for elective arthroplasty, patients undergoing arthroplasty for fracture often have diffuse swelling, so meticulous surgical dissection is necessary to avoid iatrogenic damage to the neurovascular structures. Fracture hematoma is usually identified after dividing the clavipectoral fascia. Evacuation of the hematoma will expose the deeper structures. Care should be taken

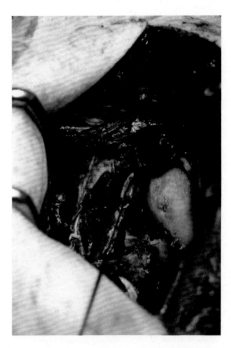

FIGURE 28.11 In the left shoulder, the long head of the biceps is identified and tagged with a suture. This is key to identifying the tuberosity fracture fragments that are located on each side.

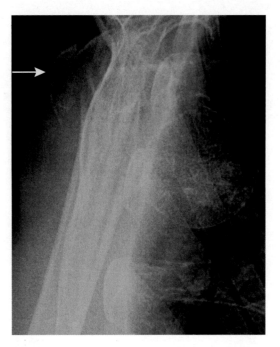

FIGURE 28.12 Scapular lateral radiograph of a right shoulder anterior fracture-dislocation. Note the large greater tuberosity fragment that is displaced posteriorly (yellow arrow). This piece can be difficult to reduce from the standard deltopectoral approach.

to preserve the coracoacromial ligament because it contributes to the anterosuperior stability of the prosthetic construct[61] **(FIGURE 28.10)**. If more exposure is needed, 1 cm of the ligament may be released. If additional exposure is needed distally, 1 to 2 cm of the pectoralis major tendon can also be released.[35] It is important to identify and tag the biceps tendon because it will provide orientation to the displaced greater and lesser tuberosities[49] **(FIGURE 28.11)**. Some surgeons choose to tenodese the biceps tendon to the pectoralis major. The benefit of tenodesis is a reported decrease in pain, likely secondary to pathology of the long head of the biceps.[62] The benefit of keeping a healthy biceps tendon intact is added soft-tissue restraint to prevent superior migration of the humeral head and as an additional anatomic landmark to judge implant height.[63] The greater tuberosity fracture bed is usually located approximately 1 cm posterior to the area of the bicipital groove although the fragment may be more widely displaced[23] **(FIGURE 28.12)**.

The tuberosities are tagged with a large braided traction suture to assist in mobilizing the fragments throughout the procedure **(FIGURE 28.13)**. The sutures are placed at the bone-tendon junction to maximize pullout strength and to avoid fragmentation of tuberosity fragments, which may have preexisting comminution. The main difference in technique for approaching three-part versus four-part fractures is the need to osteotomize the intact tuberosity from the articular segment if needed.[64] There may be nondisplaced fractures present, which can facilitate this step. The bone quality of the tuberosity is

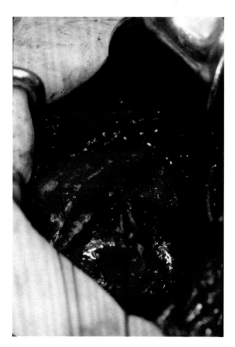

FIGURE 28.13 Intraoperative views of a left shoulder demonstrating sutures placed in the greater and lesser tuberosities. It is important to place the sutures at the bone-tendon junction to maximize pullout strength and avoid fragmentation of tuberosity fragments.

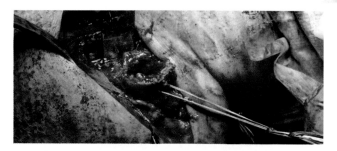

FIGURE 28.14 The humerus is extended and adducted to expose the humeral canal for broaching. This view is looking down onto a right shoulder. The head is out of the image on the upper left and the abdomen is on the top right.

important to note because of the implications for secure tuberosity reattachment and bone healing. Once the tuberosities are tagged, visualization of the articular surface can be increased by retracting the greater tuberosity fragment superiorly and laterally and the lesser tuberosity fragment medially. These fragments are of varying size and may have articular cartilage attached. One should avoid resizing the tuberosities until ready for fixation so that adequate bone stock is maintained.

In four-part fractures, the articular segment is usually devoid of soft-tissue attachments or may be impacted into the shaft segment. Once removed, it can be measured and used as a reference for the humeral head size. The cancellous bone from the head will also be utilized to bone graft the tuberosities at final fixation. With the humeral head removed, the glenoid can be easily visualized and should be inspected for degenerative changes, rim fractures, or other acute injuries.

HUMERAL SHAFT PREPARATION

Placing the humerus in extension will allow easy access to the humeral shaft for preparation **(FIGURE 28.14; VIDEO 28.2)**. Depending on the fracture pattern, you may need to freshen up the humeral neck cut with a sagittal saw or rongeur. It is important to preserve as much bone stock as possible to avoid seating the implant too inferior, which could cause instability. The canal is prepared with sequential intramedullary reamers and broaches until there is good cortical contact. If an additional

fracture line is present, which extends down the shaft, prophylactic cabling should be performed to prevent displacement during preparation and stem placement.

IMPLANT POSITIONING

Implant malposition is a common pitfall in shoulder hemiarthroplasty that can compromise postoperative functional outcomes. Specific attention needs to be given to restoring appropriate height and version. Because of the proximal bone loss associated with the fracture, the prosthesis often has to sit "proud," making it difficult to maintain the position of the prosthesis and control rotation during trial reductions. Murray et al recommend using a surgical sponge wrapped around the prothesis to fill the canal and maintain proper position[49] **(FIGURE 28.15)**. The goal is for the ultimate humeral head level to re-create the anatomic head height.[65] Cadaver studies have demonstrated that the average distance between the top of the humeral head to the upper border of the pectoralis muscle insertion is 5.6 cm.[66] This measurement can be used to approximate the appropriate humeral height if there is concern about malposition.

Since the normal version of the proximal humerus is approximately 30° of retroversion (see Chapter 2), placing the humeral head into 20° to 40° of retroversion is the recommended position.[64] Excessive retroversion or inadequate retroversion/anteversion of the component may lead to postoperative instability. There are many methods available to confirm retroversion. Using the transepicondylar axis as a guide is one option. This can be supplemented with system-specific alignment rods, including intramedullary position guides or extramedullary jigs[67,68] **(FIGURE 28.16)**. Additionally, on specific implants, the lateral fin of the stem can also be used as a guide by lining it up with the bicipital groove. The set retroversion may differ between implant systems, so it is important for the surgeon to be familiar with the selected implant. The position of the anterior or lateral flange should be marked on the humeral cortex so that it can be used as a reference for final positioning during

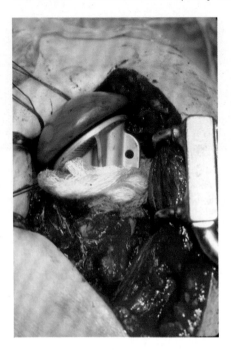

FIGURE 28.15 Proximal bone loss often seen with fractures makes it is difficult to maintain implant position during trialing. A sponge placed around the trial implant can maintain the component in proper position for trial reduction.

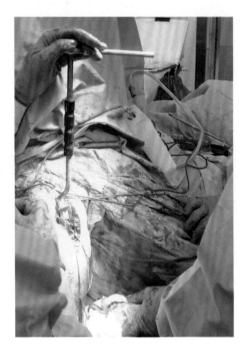

FIGURE 28.16 An intramedullary guide can be used to assess the version of the humeral stem implant. The proximal aiming arm should be parallel to the patient's forearm as a method of achieving the desired position of retroversion.

cementing. Intraoperative fluoroscopy can also be used to assess implant position.

MYOFASCIAL TENSIONING AND TRIAL REDUCTION

Inadequate tension in the myofascial sleeve is often due to bone loss, but can also be the result of the stem being seated too low, or choosing a humeral head that is too small. An improper length-tension relationship can result in an unstable construct. To avoid this, assessment of the humeral height and head size is critical. Adjusting the size of the humeral head is an option to address either excess laxity or excessive soft-tissue tensioning. Trial reduction is especially important in fracture cases because it assesses the stability of the construct. Reconstructing the bone and soft-tissue anatomy as much as possible, including reducing the tuberosities onto the implant, gives the best sense of final stability **(FIGURE 28.17)**. Intraoperative fluoroscopy can be used to evaluate stem height and tuberosity reduction. The tuberosities should be reduced anatomically to the shaft with minimal overlap, and the head-to-tuberosity distance should be less than 1 cm.[23] When testing stability clinically, up to 25% of anterior translation and up to 50% of posterior translation and inferior translation of the head relative to the glenoid can be accepted.[64]

Once the trial reduction is deemed to be acceptable, the trial implant can be removed. Two drill holes should be placed through the lateral humeral cortex approximately 1.5 to 2 cm distal to the surgical neck and on either side of the bicipital groove **(FIGURE 28.18)**. These

will be used to pass sutures for tuberosity fixation after cementing.

CEMENTING

While press-fit stems are effectively used in shoulder arthroplasty for osteoarthritis, the poor bone stock and bone quality often present in proximal humerus fractures make noncemented fixation more difficult to achieve and also increase the risk of fracture propagation during stem insertion and stem loosening over time. These factors have made cement fixation a more attractive option.[69-73] In addition to the technical considerations, cement fixation has been associated with better patient-reported satisfaction scores.[74] There are some recent literature demonstrating similar functional and radiographic outcomes in cemented versus uncemented reverse TSA for fracture,[75] but these results have not been reported following hemiarthroplasty. Therefore, cement fixation remains our preference.

Prior to cementing, the medullary canal should be prepared with brushing and irrigation, and any loose cancellous bone should be removed. A cement restrictor can be used to improve cement distribution. The canal should be packed with a sponge to ensure it is clean and dry. Cement can be mixed in a syringe and injected into the canal. Formal pressurization of the cement is avoided, especially in osteoporotic bone, to avoid humeral shaft fractures. When cementing, make sure to leave the implant "proud" and with the same retroversion that was marked during trialing. The stem should

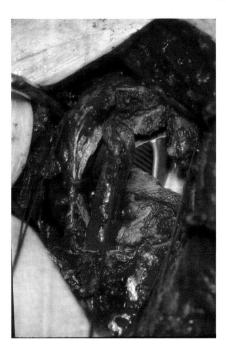

FIGURE 28.17 During trial reduction, reduce the humeral head onto the glenoid and pull the tuberosities into position. The biceps tendon should fall into place between the tuberosities.

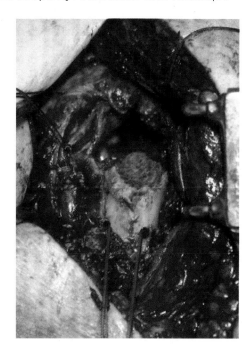

FIGURE 28.18 Two drill holes placed through the lateral humeral cortex approximately 1.5 to 2 cm distal to the surgical neck and on either side of the bicipital groove. Sutures placed here will provide longitudinal fixation of the tuberosities.

be held in position until the cement is hardened. It is essential to make certain that no cement has extruded from the canal through the fracture site into the soft tissue as this can be symptomatic and risk nerve injury[76] **(VIDEO 28.2)**.

TUBEROSITY REDUCTION AND FIXATION

Repair of the tuberosities to the humeral shaft, to the implant, and to each other is critical, and failure to do so will result in pain, instability, weakness, and decreased ROM.[25,77-81] Accurate reduction is critical, especially of the greater tuberosity, which should be placed approximately 1 cm below the humeral head.[82] To ensure adequate repair, follow the principles of tuberosity fixation, which include (1) longitudinal sutures to bring the tuberosities into a position below the prosthetic articular surface to help avoid subacromial impingement and into contact with the humeral shaft and (2) transverse suture fixation that brings the tuberosities into contact with each other **(FIGURE 28.19; VIDEO 28.3)**. Longitudinal fixation is achieved using the sutures passed through the humeral shaft and into each tuberosity. Transverse fixation is achieved by fixation of the reduced tuberosities to the implant and to each other. Closure of the rotator interval will further enhance fixation. The addition of two cerclage sutures around the entire construct adds further stability **(FIGURE 28.19)**. Heavy, nonabsorbable braided sutures should be used to ensure adequate suture strength. Sequential tightening of the sutures brings the tuberosities to the stem **(FIGURE 28.20)**. If intact, the biceps tendon can be secured in between the tuberosities

to provide a restraint to superior displacement.[49,63] This tuberosity reduction and fixation should occur with the arm in 20° abduction, neutral flexion, and 10° to 20° of external rotation. In addition, morselized cancellous bone from the humeral head may be placed between the tuberosity fragments and the shaft as needed to fill any bony voids and to enhance tuberosity healing.

Intraoperative fluoroscopy or standard films can be used to assess final implant height and positioning prior to closing. Placement of a drain is based on surgeon preference. If the surgeon chooses to place a drain, make sure it is placed at the inferior aspect of the incision and exits the skin in the lateral arm to avoid the anterior branch of the axillary nerve. Drains can generally be removed when output is less than 30 mL per shift. The deltopectoral incision can be closed in a standard manner and the patient's arm can be placed in a standard sling. Final radiographs include an AP view with external rotation and an axillary view. It is important to visualize the distal aspect of the stem to assess for any intraoperative periprosthetic fractures **(FIGURE 28.21)**.

POSTOPERATIVE REHABILITATION

Early ROM improves final outcomes and minimizes shoulder stiffness, but it must occur in a stepwise fashion. The general postoperative rehabilitation plan should be early passive ROM of the shoulder. Passive internal rotation should be limited to the chest wall. Limits for forward elevation and external rotation should be determined intraoperatively based on the security of the

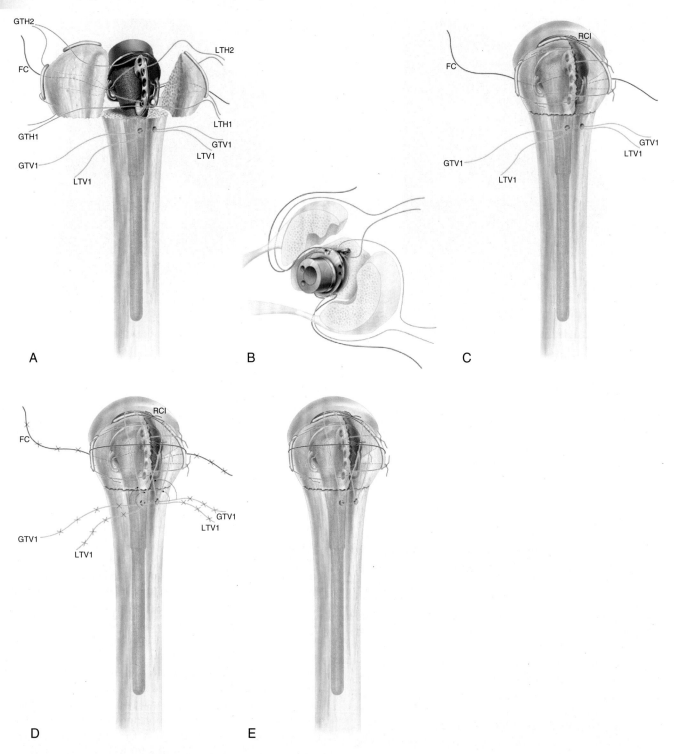

FIGURE 28.19 Technique for suture fixation reduction with a fracture-specific stem. **A-B**, Horizontal sutures GTV1 and LTV1 are passed through the drill holes in the humeral shaft on either side of the bicipital groove. GTH1 and GTH2 are passed through the inferior and superior aspects of the infraspinatus tendon attached to the greater tuberosity and through the posterior stem handle and sutures holes in the lateral fin. LTH1 and LTH2 are similarly passed through the subscapularis tendon attached to the lesser tuberosity and through the anterior stem handle and suture holes in the lateral fin. FC is passed through the middle of the subscapularis tendon and around the medial portion of the stem and out through the infraspinatus tendons. **C-E**, The horizontal sutures are tied first, starting with GTH1 and GTH2. Externally rotate the arm to relieve tension on the suture. LTH1 and LTH2 are tied with the arm in neutral rotation. The rotator interval is closed in external rotation with heavy, nonabsorbable suture. The vertical sutures are then tied by passing LTV1 through the subscapularis and GTV1 through the supraspinatus. The final cerclage sutures are then secured. FC, final cerclage; GTH, greater tuberosity horizontal; GTV, Greater greater tuberosity vertical; LTH, lesser tuberosity horizontal; LTV, lesser tuberosity vertical; RCI, rotator cuff interval.

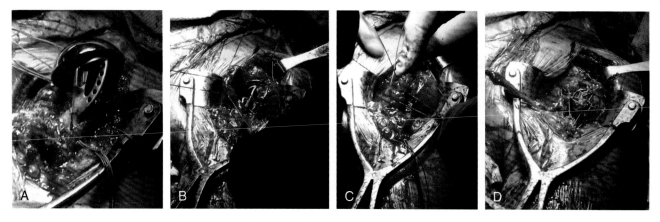

FIGURE 28.20 A, Intraoperative images of a left shoulder showing sutures tagging the tuberosities. **B**, Suture passage through the fenestrations in the fracture-specific stem. **C**, Sequential tightening of the sutures bring the tuberosities to the stem. **D**, Definitive suture fixation.

fixation. Active ROM of the elbow, wrist, and hand can be performed immediately postoperatively, but active ROM of the shoulder should be delayed 6 to 8 weeks to allow adequate tuberosity healing[24] **(FIGURE 28.22)**. At this time, the sling can be discontinued and an active-assisted ROM program can be started, limited to neutral rotation and 90° of forward flexion. At 8 to 10 weeks, patients can begin isometric deltoid and internal and external rotation strengthening exercises.[78,79] Resistive strengthening exercises should be avoided until at least 3 months postoperatively.[49] Patients typically take up to a full year to reach a plateau in their recovery and can expect to have mild to no pain with forward flexion around 100° to 110°.[1,21,23]

OUTCOMES

In a systematic review of over 800 hemiarthroplasties for proximal humerus fractures, Kontakis et al showed reliable pain relief, with 80% to 90% of patients reporting no pain or only mild pain at final follow-up.[21,24] Restoration of ROM and functional outcomes have been less predictable, and patients rarely regain preinjury

function.[21-25] Across studies, mean active forward elevation was approximately 105°, external rotation was 30°, and abduction was approximately 90°.[24] These ranges of motion are more limited than those in patients with similar fractures treated with ORIF.

Similar to ROM, functional outcomes are unpredictable. Across 560 patients, the mean constant score was 56 out of 100. Various functional outcome scores were used across studies, but three reports found excellent and satisfactory results in only 40% of patients.[25,78,79] Results were considered excellent if patients had only slight or no pain, active anterior elevation >140°, and external rotation >50% and were satisfied or very satisfied with the results. Satisfactory results required patients to have no, slight, or moderate pain only with vigorous activity, active anterior elevation >90°, and external rotation >50% of the contralateral side and to be satisfied with the results. The literature is mixed when comparing functional outcomes between ORIF and hemiarthroplasty, though the general consensus is that functional outcome scores are better in patients undergoing ORIF.[1,52]

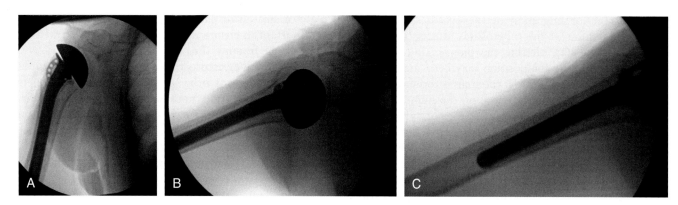

FIGURE 28.21 Intraoperative fluoroscopy is used to assess implant position. **A**, External rotation view showing restoration of the "gothic arch" formed by the lateral border of the scapular body and the medial aspect of the proximal humerus shaft. The head-to-tuberosity distance is also ~1 cm as desired. **B**, Axillary view showing symmetric reduction of the glenohumeral joint. **C**, Additional image showing the tip of the stem to assess for any intraoperative periprosthetic fractures.

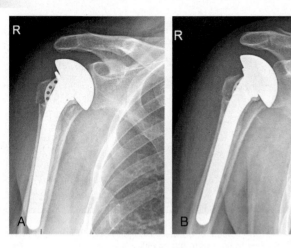
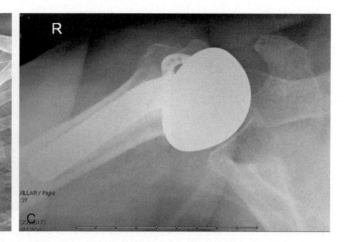

FIGURE 28.22 A, Scapular anteroposterior (AP) view in external rotation 2 months following right shoulder cemented hemiarthroplasty. Note the greater tuberosity is reduced, but still not fully healed. **B,** Scapular AP with internal rotation. **C,** Axillary radiograph.

Overall patient satisfaction following hemiarthroplasty has been reported to be between 54% and 75%.[24,26,80,83] Satisfaction is likely related to the severity of the injury. In a review of four-part fractures and fracture-dislocations in 207 patients, Murray et al found that 79% of patients treated with hemiarthroplasty achieved satisfactory or better results.[49] One study showed that satisfaction was more dependent on patient's reported pain relief than on restoration of function.[26]

COMPLICATIONS

Tuberosity Nonunion/Malunion

Successful tuberosity reconstruction is the key to a successful hemiarthroplasty. Tuberosity-related complications have been reported in 18% of patients,[24,52] making them the most common cause of failed shoulder hemiarthroplasty, persistent pain, and patient dissatisfaction.[25,78,79] Tuberosity complications are more common in patients older than 70 years,[25,26] which should be a consideration in patient selection.[80] Tuberosity nonunion or resorption can lead to weakness, instability, and superior migration of the prosthesis **(FIGURE 28.23).** Malunion of the tuberosities affects the head-to-tuberosity height, altering the biomechanics of the shoulder. Tuberosity malposition may be related to the height of the humeral stem. If the stem is too proud, the tuberosities will be relatively low on the humeral head and place increased stress across the rotator cuff, resulting in dysfunction and gradual degeneration. Placing the humeral component too low may result in tuberosities that are above the level of the humeral head, which can cause subacromial impingement. Inappropriate myofascial tensioning—that is, an overstuffed joint—can also affect the biomechanics of the glenohumeral joint, leading to progressive glenoid erosion.[35] The complications and pitfalls associated with tuberosity fixation have

been the driving force in the shift to reverse TSA for fractures.[84] Reverse TSA implants rely on deltoid function to drive ROM, so while tuberosity fixation can still be important for shoulder stability, it is not as important for functional outcomes.

PERIPROSTHETIC FRACTURE

Intraoperative periprosthetic fractures in all shoulder arthroplasty are reported between 0.6% and 3%.[85-88] Most fractures occur while attempting to gain access to the glenoid,[86] so intraoperative fractures during hemiarthroplasty are less common than in TSA. In hemiarthroplasty for fracture, they can occur with extension of the fracture into the shaft or from propagation of the drill holes used for tuberosity fixation.[89] Excessive cement pressurization or arm manipulation to gain exposure can also cause intraoperative fractures, especially in osteoporotic bone. If the fracture does not extend past the distal aspect of the humeral stem, it can often be treated with cerclage fixation. If there is extension past the tip of the stem, a long stemmed component with cerclage wiring can be utilized. If this is not available, a plate or strut graft past the fracture site can be used. It is important to ensure that cement does not extravasate through the fracture site.

Postoperative periprosthetic fractures often occur as a result of a fall or other traumatic event. Treatment is based on location and extension of the fracture and whether the implant is stable. Fractures into the humeral shaft can be addressed with the same principles as periprosthetic fractures following TSA (Chapter 40). Most postoperative periprosthetic fractures will extend beyond the tip of the stem. In general, if the implant is not loose and has overall acceptable alignment, nonoperative management with a fracture orthosis can be considered, especially in elderly, low-demand patients.[89]

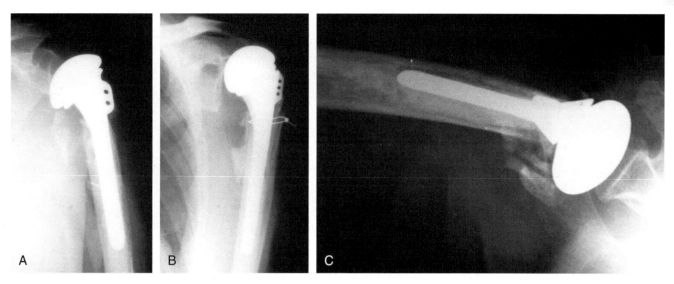

FIGURE 28.23 A, Displacement of the lesser tuberosity leads to anterior instability. **B,** Displacement of the greater tuberosity leads to superior migration of the humeral head. **C,** Posterior displacement of the greater tuberosity creates a mechanical block to external rotation.

LOOSENING

Loosening is uncommon following hemiarthroplasty for fracture, likely due to the lower demand nature of the patients undergoing this treatment and the use of cement fixation.[77,90] Diagnosis is based upon progressive radiolucency at the bone-cement interface of at least 1.5 mm in diameter in multiple zones of the humeral stem[89,91] **(FIGURE 28.24).** It is important to rule out other causes of postoperative shoulder pain and confirm that humeral loosening is the etiology of the symptoms. If revision is necessary, reverse TSA may be preferred especially if there is associated tuberosity dysfunction or glenoid erosion.

INFECTION

In their systematic review of multiple series, Kontakis et al documented a 1.6% superficial infection rate and a 0.6% deep infections rate in 771 hemiarthroplasties. The treatment algorithm is similar to that for anatomic and reverse TSA (Chapter 32). If explantation is required, it is

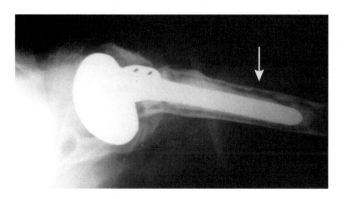

FIGURE 28.24 Radiolucency around the bone-cement interface indicates possible stem loosening (yellow arrow).

important to remove all cement. Antibiotic-impregnated cement spacers are an excellent option with staged revision arthroplasty as necessary.

Glenoid wear requiring revision surgery is uncommon. Risk factors include preoperative degenerative changes, unrecognized glenoid injury, and component malpositioning **(FIGURE 28.25).** An intra-articular lidocaine injection can be helpful to confirm that glenoid wear is the cause of the symptoms. If symptoms do not resolve with activity modification and anti-inflammatory medication, revision arthroplasty with insertion of a glenoid component can be considered.[92]

STIFFNESS

Limited ROM is a common outcome of hemiarthroplasty, and patients should be thoroughly counseled on this preoperatively. Stiffness can be the result of many of the complications above, specifically tuberosity malunion or nonunion. Heterotrophic ossification, which is reported in up to 8.8% of cases, can also contribute to postoperative stiffness.[24]

If there are passive and active ROM restrictions with an obvious etiology evident on imaging, arthroscopic or open soft-tissue releases can be considered. However, this is rarely necessary in this patient population.

Cumulative revision rates are relatively low, with up to 97% survivorship at 5 years and 94% at 10 years.[25,27] Reverse TSA is an important option for failed hemiarthroplasty secondary to tuberosity-related complications, rotator cuff failure, and glenoid erosion. The functional outcomes of reverse TSA for failed hemiarthroplasty are worse than those of reverse TSA performed as the index procedure.[93] Techniques for these often complex revisions are addressed in detail in Chapter 30.

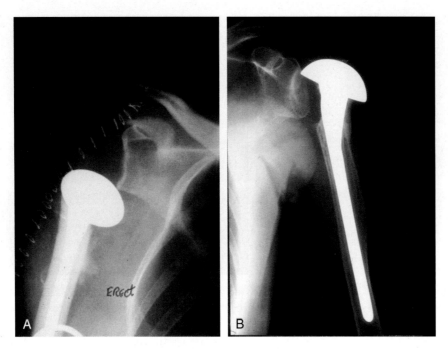

FIGURE 28.25 Examples of component malposition. **A,** Inadequate restoration of humeral length resulting in inferior subluxation. **B,** Improper version leads to unintended rotation of a noncemented humeral stem resulting in instability.

CONCLUSION

While the majority of proximal humerus fractures can be treated nonoperatively, there are more complex fracture patterns, including many four-part fractures, fracture-dislocations, and select three-part fracture and fracture-dislocations that should be considered for operative intervention. Although reverse shoulder arthroplasty is becoming an increasingly popular treatment option for these injuries in elderly patients,[11,28] hemiarthroplasty remains a reliable treatment option in select patients. When performed for fracture management, hemiarthroplasty has its own set of challenges, including tuberosity repair, proper component positioning, and tensioning of the myofascial sleeve,[16] but it remains a valuable tool, especially in low-demand patients whose primary goal is a relatively pain-free shoulder.[24,26,27]

REFERENCES

1. Khurana S, Davidovitch RI, Kwon YK, Zuckerman JD, Egol KA. Similar function and improved range of shoulder motion is achieved following repair of three- and four-part proximal humerus fractures compared with hemiarthroplasty. *Bull Hosp Jt Dis (2013)*. 2016;74(3):212-218.
2. Palvanen M, Kannus P, Niemi S, Parkkari J. Update in the epidemiology of proximal humeral fractures. *Clin Orthop Relat Res*. 2006;442:87-92. doi:10.1097/01.blo.0000194672.79634.78
3. Shukla DR, McAnany S, Kim J, Overley S, Parsons BO. Hemiarthroplasty versus reverse shoulder arthroplasty for treatment of proximal humeral fractures: a meta-analysis. *J Shoulder Elbow Surg*. 2016;25(2):330-340. doi:10.1016/j.jse.2015.08.030
4. Baron JA, Karagas M, Barrett J, et al. Basic epidemiology of fractures of the upper and lower limb among Americans over 65 years of age. *Epidemiology*. 1996;7(6):612-618. doi:10.1097/00001648-199611000-00008
5. Bell J-E, Leung BC, Spratt KF, et al. Trends and variation in incidence, surgical treatment, and repeat surgery of proximal humeral

6. fractures in the elderly. *J Bone Joint Surg Am*. 2011;93(2):121-131. doi:10.2106/JBJS.I.01505
6. Zyto K. Non-operative treatment of comminuted fractures of the proximal humerus in elderly patients. *Injury*. 1998;29(5):349-352. doi:10.1016/s0020-1383(97)00211-8
7. Solberg BD, Moon CN, Franco DP, Paiement GD. Locked plating of 3- and 4-part proximal humerus fractures in older patients: the effect of initial fracture pattern on outcome. *J Orthop Trauma*. 2009;23(2):113-119. doi:10.1097/BOT.0b013e31819344bf
8. Sproul RC, Iyengar JJ, Devcic Z, Feeley BT. A systematic review of locking plate fixation of proximal humerus fractures. *Injury*. 2011;42(4):408-413. doi:10.1016/j.injury.2010.11.058
9. Shulman BS, Egol KA. Open reduction internal fixation for proximal humerus fractures indications, techniques, and pitfalls. *Bull Hosp Jt Dis (2013)*. 2013;71(suppl 2):54-59.
10. Robinson CM, Stirling PHC, Goudie EB, MacDonald DJ, Strelzow JA. Complications and long-term outcomes of open reduction and plate fixation of proximal humeral fractures. *J Bone Joint Surg Am*. 2019;101(23):2129-2139. doi:10.2106/JBJS.19.00595
11. Khatib O, Onyekwelu I, Yu S, Zuckerman JD. Shoulder arthroplasty in New York State, 1991 to 2010: changing patterns of utilization. *J Shoulder Elbow Surg*. 2015;24(10):e286-e291. doi:10.1016/j.jse.2015.05.038
12. Goch AM, Christiano A, Konda SR, Leucht P, Egol KA. Operative repair of proximal humerus fractures in septuagenarians and octogenarians: does chronologic age matter? *J Clin Orthop Trauma*. 2017;8(1):50-53. doi:10.1016/j.jcot.2017.01.006
13. Shulman BS, Ong CC, Lee JH, Karia R, Zuckerman JD, Egol KA. Outcomes after fixation of proximal humerus (OTA type 11) fractures in the elderly patients using modern techniques. *Geriatr Orthop Surg Rehabil*. 2013;4(1):21-25. doi:10.1177/2151458513498597
14. Broder K, Christiano A, Zuckerman JD, Egol K. Management of proximal humerus fractures with the Equinoxe® locking plate system. *Bull Hosp Jt Dis (2013)*. 2015;73(suppl 1):S107-S110.
15. Egol KA, Patel D. Open reduction, internal fixation of proximal humerus fractures: indications, techniques, outcomes and complications. In: Iannotti JP, Williams GR Jr, Miniaci A, Zuckerman JD, eds. *Disorders of the Shoulder: Diagnosis & Management*. 3rd ed. Wolters Kluwer/Lippincott Williams & Wilkins; 2014.
16. Egol KA, Jazrawi L, Zuckerman JD, Koval KJ. Proximal humerus fractures: Pitfalls in diagnosis and management. *J Musculoskelet*

Med. 1999;16(4):245-257. Accessed January 12, 2020. https://link.galegroup.com/apps/doc/A55491975/AONE?sid=lms

17. Kavuri V, Bowden B, Kumar N, Cerynik D. Complications associated with locking plate of proximal humerus fractures. *Indian J Orthop.* 2018;52(2):108-116. doi:10.4103/ortho.IJOrtho_243_17

18. Ong CC, Kwon YW, Walsh M, Davidovitch R, Zuckerman JD, Egol KA. Outcomes of open reduction and internal fixation of proximal humerus fractures managed with locking plates. *Am J Orthop.* 2012;41(9):407-412.

19. Ong C, Bechtel C, Walsh M, Zuckerman JD, Egol KA. Three- and four-part fractures have poorer function than one-part proximal humerus fractures. *Clin Orthop Relat Res.* 2011;469(12):3292-3299. doi:10.1007/s11999-011-1864-4

20. Egol KA, Ong CC, Walsh M, Jazrawi LM, Tejwani NC, Zuckerman JD. Early complications in proximal humerus fractures (OTA Types 11) treated with locked plates. *J Orthop Trauma.* 2008;22(3):159-164. doi:10.1097/BOT.0b013e318169ef2a

21. Goldman RT, Koval KJ, Cuomo F, Gallagher MA, Zuckerman JD. Functional outcome after humeral head replacement for acute three- and four-part proximal humeral fractures. *J Shoulder Elbow Surg.* 1995;4(2):81-86. doi:10.1016/s1058-2746(05)80059-x

22. Skutek M, Fremerey RW, Bosch U. Level of physical activity in elderly patients after hemiarthroplasty for three- and four-part fractures of the proximal humerus. *Arch Orthop Trauma Surg.* 1998;117(4-5):252-255. doi:10.1007/s004020050239

23. Wiesel BB, Nagda S, Williams GR. Technical pitfalls of shoulder hemiarthroplasty for fracture management. *Orthop Clin North Am.* 2013;44(3):317-329. doi:10.1016/j.ocl.2013.03.006

24. Kontakis G, Koutras C, Tosounidis T, Giannoudis P. Early management of proximal humeral fractures with hemiarthroplasty: a systematic review. *J Bone Joint Surg Br.* 2008;90(11):1407-1413. doi:10.1302/0301-620X.90B11.21070

25. Antuña SA, Sperling JW, Cofield RH. Shoulder hemiarthroplasty for acute fractures of the proximal humerus: a minimum five-year follow-up. *J Shoulder Elbow Surg.* 2008;17(2):202-209. doi:10.1016/j.jse.2007.06.025

26. Valenti P, Aliani D, Maroun C, Werthel JD, Elkolti K. Shoulder hemiarthroplasty for proximal humeral fractures: analysis of clinical and radiographic outcomes at midterm follow-up. A series of 51 patients. *Eur J Orthop Surg Traumatol.* 2017;27(3):309-315. doi:10.1007/s00590-017-1927-7

27. Robinson CM, Page RS, Hill RMF, Sanders DL, Court-Brown CM, Wakefield AE. Primary hemiarthroplasty for treatment of proximal humeral fractures. *J Bone Joint Surg Am.* 2003;85(7):1215-1223. doi:10.2106/00004623-200307000-00006

28. McLean AS, Price N, Graves S, Hatton A, Taylor FJ. Nationwide trends in management of proximal humeral fractures: an analysis of 77,966 cases from 2008 to 2017. *J Shoulder Elbow Surg.* 2019;28(11):2072-2078. doi:10.1016/j.jse.2019.03.034

29. Peters P-M, Plachel F, Danzinger V, et al. Clinical and radiographic outcomes after surgical treatment of proximal humeral fractures with head-split component. *J Bone Joint Surg Am.* 2020;102(1):68-75. doi:10.2106/JBJS.19.00320

30. Valenti P, Katz D, Kilinc A, Elkholti K, Gasiunas V. Mid-term outcome of reverse shoulder prostheses in complex proximal humeral fractures. *Acta Orthop Belg.* 2012;78(4):442-449.

31. Bufquin T, Hersan A, Hubert L, Massin P. Reverse shoulder arthroplasty for the treatment of three- and four-part fractures of the proximal humerus in the elderly: a prospective review of 43 cases with a short-term follow-up. *J Bone Joint Surg Br.* 2007;89(4):516-520. doi:10.1302/0301-620X.89B4.18435

32. Cazeneuve JF, Cristofari D-J. The reverse shoulder prosthesis in the treatment of fractures of the proximal humerus in the elderly. *J Bone Joint Surg Br.* 2010;92(4):535-539. doi:10.1302/0301-620X.92B4.22450

33. Acevedo DC, Vanbeek C, Lazarus MD, Williams GR, Abboud JA. Reverse shoulder arthroplasty for proximal humeral fractures: update on indications, technique, and results. *J Shoulder Elbow Surg.* 2014;23(2):279-289. doi:10.1016/j.jse.2013.10.003

34. Neer CS II. Displaced proximal humeral fractures. Part I. Classification and evaluation. *Clin Orthop Relat Res.* 1987;223:3-10.

35. Streubel P, Sanchez-Sotelo J, Steinmann S. *Proximal humerus fractures.* In: *Rockwood and Green's Fractures in Adults.* 6th ed. Lippincott Williams & Wilkins; 2006:1341-1425.

36. Warner JJP, Costouros JG, Gerber C. *Fractures of the proximal humerus.* In: *Rockwood and Green's: Fractures in Adults.* 6th ed. Williams & Wilkins; 2006:1161-1209.

37. Sidor M, Koval K, Zuckerman JD. The radiographic evaluation and classification of proximal humerus fractures. In: Flatow E, Ulrich C, eds. *Musculoskeletal Trauma.* Butterworth-Heinemann; 1996.

38. Hertel R, Hempfing A, Stiehler M, Leunig M. Predictors of humeral head ischemia after intracapsular fracture of the proximal humerus. *J Shoulder Elbow Surg.* 2004;13(4):427-433. doi:10.1016/j.jse.2004.01.034

39. Stableforth PG. Four-part fractures of the neck of the humerus. *J Bone Joint Surg Br.* 1984;66(1):104-108.

40. Green A, Barnard WL, Limbird RS. Humeral head replacement for acute, four-part proximal humerus fractures. *J Shoulder Elbow Surg.* 1993;2(5):249-254. doi:10.1016/S1058-2746(09)80084-0

41. Court-Brown CM, Cattermole H, McQueen MM. Impacted valgus fractures (B1.1) of the proximal humerus. The results of non-operative treatment. *J Bone Joint Surg Br.* 2002;84(4):504-508. doi:10.1302/0301-620x.84b4.12488

42. Yamaguchi K, Ditsios K, Middleton WD, Hildebolt CF, Galatz LM, Teefey SA. The demographic and morphological features of rotator cuff disease. A comparison of asymptomatic and symptomatic shoulders. *J Bone Joint Surg Am.* 2006;88(8):1699-1704. doi:10.2106/JBJS.E.00835

43. Gallo RA, Sciulli R, Daffner RH, Altman DT, Altman GT. Defining the relationship between rotator cuff injury and proximal humerus fractures. *Clin Orthop Relat Res.* 2007;458:70-77. doi:10.1097/BLO.0b013e31803bb400

44. Nanda R, Goodchild L, Gamble A, Campbell RSD, Rangan A. Does the presence of a full-thickness rotator cuff tear influence outcome after proximal humeral fractures? *J Trauma.* 2007;62(6):1436-1439. doi:10.1097/TA.0b013e3180514ce2

45. Wilmanns C, Bonnaire F. Rotator cuff alterations resulting from humeral head fractures. *Injury.* 2002;33(9):781-789. doi:10.1016/s0020-1383(02)00088-8

46. Schai PA, Hintermann B, Koris MJ. Preoperative arthroscopic assessment of fractures about the shoulder. *Arthroscopy.* 1999;15(8):827-835. doi:10.1053/ar.1999.v15.015082

47. Bloom MH, Obata WG. Diagnosis of posterior dislocation of the shoulder with use of Velpeau axillary and angle-up roentgenographic views. *J Bone Joint Surg Am.* 1967;49(5):943-949.

48. Goutallier D, Postel JM, Gleyze P, Leguilloux P, Van Driessche S. Influence of cuff muscle fatty degeneration on anatomic and functional outcomes after simple suture of full-thickness tears. *J Shoulder Elbow Surg.* 2003;12(6):550-554. doi:10.1016/s1058-2746(03)00211-8

49. Murray D, Zuckerman JD. Four-part fractures and fracture-dislocations. In: Zuckerman JD, Koval KJ, eds. *Shoulder Fractures: The Practical Guide to Management.* Thieme; 2005:3.

50. Resch H, Beck E, Bayley I. Reconstruction of the valgus-impacted humeral head fracture. *J Shoulder Elbow Surg.* 1995;4(2):73-80. doi:10.1016/s1058-2746(05)80071-1

51. Belayneh R, Lott A, Haglin J, Konda S, Zuckerman JD, Egol KA. Osteonecrosis after surgically repaired proximal humerus fractures is a predictor of poor outcomes. *J Orthop Trauma.* 2018;32(10):e387-e393. doi:10.1097/BOT.0000000000001260

52. Solberg BD, Moon CN, Franco DP, Paiement GD. Surgical treatment of three and four-part proximal humeral fractures. *J Bone Joint Surg Am.* 2009;91(7):1689-1697. doi:10.2106/JBJS.H.00133

53. Horak J, Nilsson BE. Epidemiology of fracture of the upper end of the humerus. *Clin Orthop Relat Res.* 1975;(112):250-253.

54. Hagg O, Lundberg A. Aspects of prognostics factors in comminuted and dislocated proximal humerus fracture. In: Batenab J, Welsh R, eds. *Surgery of the Shoulder.* BC Decker; 1984.

55. Krishnan SG, Reineck JR, Bennion PD, Feher L, Burkhead WZ. Shoulder arthroplasty for fracture: does a fracture-specific stem make a difference? *Clin Orthop Relat Res.* 2011;469(12):3317-3323. doi:10.1007/s11999-011-1919-6

56. Crosby LA, Wright TW, Yu S, Zuckerman JD. Conversion to reverse total shoulder arthroplasty with and without humeral stem retention: the role of a convertible-platform stem. *J Bone Joint Surg Am.* 2017;99(9):736-742. doi:10.2106/JBJS.16.00683

57. Chou YC, Tseng IC, Chiang CW, Wu CC. Shoulder hemiarthroplasty for proximal humeral fractures: comparisons between the deltopectoral and anterolateral deltoid-splitting approaches. *J Shoulder Elbow Surg.* 2013;22(8):e1-e7. doi:10.1016/j.jse.2012.10.039

58. Robinson CM, Murray IR. The extended deltoid-splitting approach to the proximal humerus. *J Bone Joint Surg Br.* 2011;93(3):387-392. doi:10.1302/0301-620X.93B3.25818

59. Burkhead WZ, Scheinberg RR, Box G. Surgical anatomy of the axillary nerve. *J Shoulder Elbow Surg.* 1992;1(1):31-36. doi:10.1016/S1058-2746(09)80014-1

60. Cetik O, Uslu M, Acar HI, Comert A, Tekdemir I, Cift H. Is there a safe area for the axillary nerve in the deltoid muscle? A cadaveric study. *J Bone Joint Surg Am.* 2006;88(11):2395-2399. doi:10.2106/JBJS.E.01375

61. Lee TQ, Black AD, Tibone JE, McMahon PJ. Release of the coracoacromial ligament can lead to glenohumeral laxity: a biomechanical study. *J Shoulder Elbow Surg.* 2001;10(1):68-72. doi:10.1067/mse.2001.111138

62. Soliman OA, Koptan WMT. Proximal humeral fractures treated with hemiarthroplasty: does tenodesis of the long head of the biceps improve results? *Injury.* 2013;44(4):461-464. doi:10.1016/j.injury.2012.09.012

63. Kido T, Itoi E, Konno N, Sano A, Urayama M, Sato K. The depressor function of biceps on the head of the humerus in shoulders with tears of the rotator cuff. *J Bone Joint Surg Br.* 2000;82(3):416-419. doi:10.1302/0301-620x.82b3.10115

64. Egol KA, Koval KJ. Three-Part Fractures and fracture-dislocations. In: Zuckerman JD, Koval KJ, eds. *Shoulder Fractures: The Practical Guide to Management.* Thieme; 2005:86-98.

65. Kancherla VK, Singh A, Anakwenze OA. Management of acute proximal humeral fractures. *J Am Acad Orthop Surg.* 2017;25(1):42-52. doi:10.5435/JAAOS-D-15-00240

66. Murachovsky J, Ikemoto RY, Nascimento LGP, Fujiki EN, Milani C, Warner JJP. Pectoralis major tendon reference (PMT): a new method for accurate restoration of humeral length with hemiarthroplasty for fracture. *J Shoulder Elbow Surg.* 2006;15(6):675-678. doi:10.1016/j.jse.2005.12.011

67. Dines D, Warren R, Craig E, Lee D, Dines J. Intramedullary fracture positioning sleeve for proper placement of hemiarthroplasty in fractures of the proximal humerus. *Tech Shoulder Elbow Surg.* 2007;8(2):69-74. doi:10.1097/bte.0b013e318039bb1e

68. Boileau P, Pennington SD, Alami G. Proximal humeral fractures in younger patients: fixation techniques and arthroplasty. *J Shoulder Elbow Surg.* 2011;20(2 suppl):S47-S60. doi:10.1016/j.jse.2010.12.006

69. Sanchez-Sotelo J, Wright TW, O'Driscoll SW, Cofield RH, Rowland CM. Radiographic assessment of uncemented humeral components in total shoulder arthroplasty. *J Arthroplasty.* 2001;16(2):180-187. doi:10.1054/arth.2001.20905

70. Torchia ME, Cofield RH, Settergren CR. Total shoulder arthroplasty with the Neer prosthesis: long-term results. *J Shoulder Elbow Surg.* 1997;6(6):495-505. doi:10.1016/s1058-2746(97)90081-1

71. Litchfield RB, McKee MD, Balyk R, et al. Cemented versus uncemented fixation of humeral components in total shoulder arthroplasty for osteoarthritis of the shoulder: a prospective, randomized, double-blind clinical trial-A JOINTs Canada Project. *J Shoulder Elbow Surg.* 2011;20(4):529-536. doi:10.1016/j.jse.2011.01.041

72. Athwal GS, Sperling JW, Rispoli DM, Cofield RH. Periprosthetic humeral fractures during shoulder arthroplasty. *J Bone Joint Surg Am.* 2009;91(3):594-603. doi:10.2106/JBJS.H.00439

73. Werthel J-D, Lonjon G, Jo S, Cofield R, Sperling JW, Elhassan BT. Long-term outcomes of cemented versus cementless humeral components in arthroplasty of the shoulder: a propensity score-matched analysis. *Bone Joint J.* 2017;99-B(5):666-673. doi:10.1302/0301-620X.99B5.BJJ-2016-0910.R1

74. Schoch B, Aibinder W, Walters J, et al. Outcomes of uncemented versus cemented reverse shoulder arthroplasty for proximal humerus fractures. *Orthopedics.* 2019;42(2):e236-e241. doi:10.3928/01477447-20190125-03

75. Youn SM, Deo S, Poon PC. Functional and radiologic outcomes of uncemented reverse shoulder arthroplasty in proximal humeral fractures: cementing the humeral component is not necessary. *J Shoulder Elbow Surg.* 2016;25(4):e83-e89. doi:10.1016/j.jse.2015.09.007

76. Fram B, Elder A, Namdari S. Periprosthetic humeral fractures in shoulder arthroplasty. *JBJS Rev.* 2019;7(11):e6. doi:10.2106/JBJS.RVW.19.00017

77. Hawkins RJ, Switlyk P. Acute prosthetic replacement for severe fractures of the proximal humerus. *Clin Orthop Relat Res.* 1993;(289):156-160.

78. Boileau P, Krishnan SG, Tinsi L, Walch G, Coste JS, Molé D. Tuberosity malposition and migration: reasons for poor outcomes after hemiarthroplasty for displaced fractures of the proximal humerus. *J Shoulder Elbow Surg.* 2002;11(5):401-412. doi:10.1067/mse.2002.124527

79. Demirhan M, Kilicoglu O, Altinel L, Eralp L, Akalin Y. Prognostic factors in prosthetic replacement for acute proximal humerus fractures. *J Orthop Trauma.* 2003;17(3):181-188. doi:10.1097/00005131-200303000-00004

80. Kralinger F, Schwaiger R, Wambacher M, et al. Outcome after primary hemiarthroplasty for fracture of the head of the humerus. A retrospective multicentre study of 167 patients. *J Bone Joint Surg Br.* 2004;86(2):217-219. doi:10.1302/0301-620x.86b2.14553

81. Wiesel BB, Gartsman GM, Press CM, et al. What went wrong and what was done about it: pitfalls in the treatment of common shoulder surgery. *Instr Course Lect.* 2014;63:85-93.

82. Loebenberg MI, Jones DA, Zuckerman JD. The effect of greater tuberosity placement on active range of motion after hemiarthroplasty for acute fractures of the proximal humerus. *Bull Hosp Jt Dis (2013).* 2005;62(3-4):90-93.

83. Grönhagen CM, Abbaszadegan H, Révay SA, Adolphson PY. Medium-term results after primary hemiarthroplasty for comminute proximal humerus fractures: a study of 46 patients followed up for an average of 4.4 years. *J Shoulder Elbow Surg.* 2007;16(6):766-773. doi:10.1016/j.jse.2007.03.017

84. Sebastiá-Forcada E, Cebrián-Gómez R, Lizaur-Utrilla A, Gil-Guillén V. Reverse shoulder arthroplasty versus hemiarthroplasty for acute proximal humeral fractures. A blinded, randomized, controlled, prospective study. *J Shoulder Elbow Surg.* 2014;23(10):1419-1426. doi:10.1016/j.jse.2014.06.035

85. Chin PYK, Sperling JW, Cofield RH, Schleck C. Complications of total shoulder arthroplasty: are they fewer or different? *J Shoulder Elbow Surg.* 2006;15(1):19-22. doi:10.1016/j.jse.2005.05.005

86. Worland RL, Kim DY, Arredondo J. Periprosthetic humeral fractures: management and classification. *J Shoulder Elbow Surg.* 1999;8(6):590-594. doi:10.1016/s1058-2746(99)90095-2

87. Wright TW, Cofield RH. Humeral fractures after shoulder arthroplasty. *J Bone Joint Surg Am.* 1995;77(9):1340-1346. doi:10.2106/00004623-199509000-00008

88. Cameron B, Iannotti JP. Periprosthetic fractures of the humerus and scapula: management and prevention. *Orthop Clin North Am.* 1999;30(2):305-318. doi:10.1016/s0030-5898(05)70085-7

89. Zuckerman J, Murray D. Complications of proximal humerus fractures. In: Zuckerman J, Koval K, eds. *Shoulder Fractures: The Practical Guide to Management.* Thieme; 2005:146-180.

90. Compito CA, Self EB, Bigliani LU. Arthroplasty and acute shoulder trauma. Reasons for success and failure. *Clin Orthop Relat Res.* 1994;(307):27-36.

91. Muldoon MP, Cofield RH. Complications of humeral head replacement for proximal humeral fractures. *Instr Course Lect.* 1997;46:15-24.

92. Mighell MA, Kolm GP, Collinge CA, Frankle MA. Outcomes of hemiarthroplasty for fractures of the proximal humerus. *J Shoulder Elbow Surg.* 2003;12(6):569-577. doi:10.1016/s1058-2746(03)00213-1

93. Levy J, Frankle M, Mighell M, Pupello D. The use of the reverse shoulder prosthesis for the treatment of failed hemiarthroplasty for proximal humeral fracture. *J Bone Joint Surg Am.* 2007;89(2):292-300. doi:10.2106/JBJS.E.01310

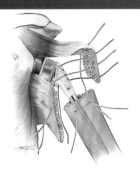

29 Reverse Total Shoulder Arthroplasty for Acute Fracture

Toufic R. Jildeh, MD and Stephanie J. Muh, MD

INTRODUCTION AND HISTORICAL PERSPECTIVE

Proximal humerus fractures account for 5% of all fractures and are increasing in frequency,[1] particularly among the elderly. It remains the second most common fracture of the upper extremity and third most common fracture in patients older than 65 years. Current research suggests an approximate threefold increase in the incidence of proximal humerus fractures, concomitant with the aging population.[2] While a majority of proximal humerus fractures are minimally displaced and have acceptable clinical results with nonoperative treatment,[3] for fractures with significant displacement, operative intervention is often indicated. Displaced three- and four-part fractures, treated nonoperatively, can result in chronic pain and loss of function. Unsurprisingly, due to the bone morphological changes associated with aging, elderly patients sustaining lower energy injuries often present with more complicated fracture patterns than the younger population[1] and, as a result, can present a formidable challenge. Locked plating for proximal humerus fractures has been associated with high rates of osteonecrosis, intra-articular screw penetration, and loss of fracture reduction, resulting in inconsistent results. Shoulder hemiarthroplasty (HA) has shown reliable outcomes with respect to pain, but has been associated with unpredictable results for range of motion and function, likely due to tuberosity displacement, nonunion or resorption, and rotator cuff dysfunction.[4]

Traditionally, reverse total shoulder arthroplasty (RTSA) has been used to manage cuff tear arthropathy and other glenohumeral disorders in the setting of irreparable rotator cuff tears or insufficiency. However, with increasing experience, the indications have been expanding. Due to the unpredictable results of operative management of proximal humerus fractures with open reduction and internal fixation (ORIF) and HA, RTSA has become a reliable and predictable alternative in appropriately selected patients **(VIDEO 29.1)**.

PROXIMAL HUMERUS ANATOMY

There have been numerous classification systems developed for proximal humeral fractures due, in part, to the difficulty of defining the fracture patterns. Codman first attempted to classify these fractures in the 1930s by dividing the proximal humerus into four parts: the greater tuberosity, the lesser tuberosity, the head, and the shaft based upon the epiphyseal segments. Neer built upon this scheme in an effort to better define fracture displacement, which he defined as angulation >45° or greater than 1 cm of separation. Despite being the most commonly used classification system, studies have found the Neer classification to have relatively poor interobserver reliability ($\kappa = 0.52$).[5] The AO classification of proximal humerus fractures places emphasis on the blood supply to the articular surface and divides these fractures into three groups, with increasing rates of osteonecrosis: A (extra-articular, unifocal), B (extra-articular, bifocal), and C (extra-articular with compromise to the vascular supply).[6] Hertel devised a system for reading proximal humerus fractures where classifications are classified using a binary description system used to classify the four fracture parts and five basic planes of fracture.[7] Despite these various classification systems **(FIGURE 29.1)**, no one system has shown accuracy in predicting the development of osteonecrosis in the setting of acute proximal humerus fractures.

A special consideration for proximal humerus fractures of the three- and four-part variety in the elderly are that these fractures are often associated with a high incidence of osteonecrosis and poor bone healing.[1,2] Multiple factors have been associated with increased osteonecrosis and complications including loss of the medial hinge, four-part fracture patterns, posteromedial metaphyseal head extension of less than 8 mm, angular displacement of the head greater than 45°, and fracture displacement greater than 1 cm.[7] Treated nonoperatively, these fractures can result in debilitating malunion and poor function.[3] A recent review article by Iyengar et al found that three- and four-part proximal humerus fractures reached a 98% rate of radiographic union; however, they were associated with highest overall complication rate at 48% (23% rate of varus malunion and 14% rate of osteonecrosis).[3] ORIF with locked plating was initially a promising treatment modality for proximal humerus fractures. However, multiple studies have demonstrated high complication rates due to loss of reduction, screw cutout of up to 67%, postoperative stiffness, and osteonecrosis

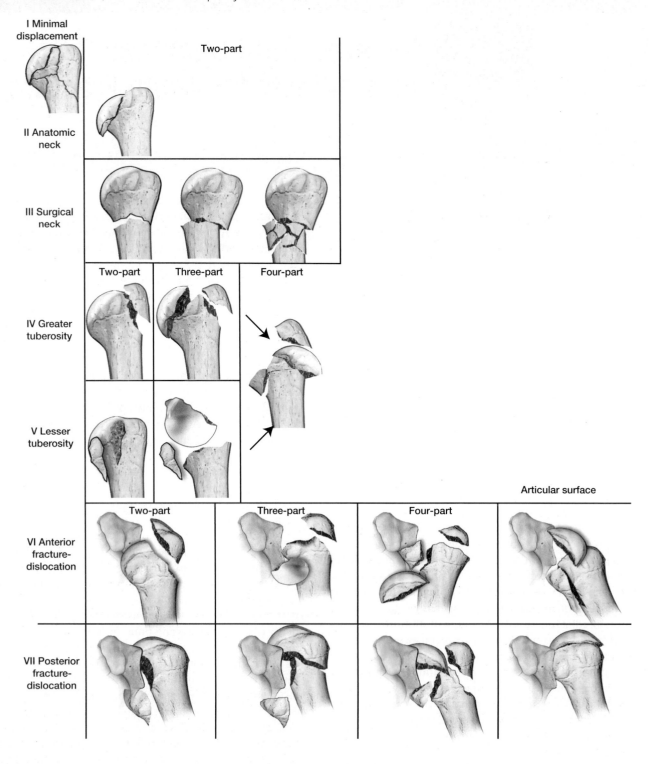

FIGURE 29.1 The Neer four-segment classification system and AO Foundation/Orthopaedic Trauma Association classification system for proximal humerus fractures. (Reproduced from Neer CS II. Displaced proximal humeral fractures. I. Classification and evaluation. *J Bone Joint Surg [Am]*. 1970;52(6):1077-1089.)

in up to 55% of cases.[4,7] Studies have shown that poor bone quality is associated with a significantly increased failure rate with ORIF.[6,8] HA alleviates the threat of osteonecrosis and screw cutout; however, the functional outcomes are completely dependent on tuberosity union, and multiple studies have demonstrated postoperative tuberosity osteolysis and displacement with subsequent loss of motion and function and poor patient satisfaction.[5,9-13] Additionally, fractures with non reconstructable tuberosities have been associated with poor outcomes following ORIF and HA. Concern for humeral head osteonecrosis, poor bone quality, compromised healing capacity, and poor functional outcomes following treatment of three- and four-part fractures has made RTSA a favorable treatment option.

PATIENT EVALUATION

When evaluating any patient with an acute proximal humerus fracture, it is important to appropriately assess the patient's general health status. This includes an assessment of the patients' medical comorbidities, cognitive status, functional demands, and expectations. A patient unable to comply with a postoperative rehabilitation program or restrictions will compromise the outcome of the surgery. A history of previous shoulder injury or surgery should be identified since it may factor into the selected treatment plan. Neurological status must be accurately documented, particularly axillary nerve function, which has been reported to be injured in up to 67% of patients with low energy proximal humerus fractures.[9] Although deltoid function is considered essential for a successful RTSA, Ladermann et al in a retrospective study of 49 patients undergoing RTSA with deltoid dysfunction reported a 98% patient satisfaction rate based upon increases in forward elevation and Constant scores.[10] Nonetheless, careful examination of deltoid function is imperative and is performed by assessing for contraction of all three portions in an isometric assessment of elevation, abduction, and extension. Assessment of deltoid function in a patient with an acute proximal humerus fracture can be a challenge but is essential. If contraction is confirmed, the function of the muscle is thought to be adequate. If a contraction is not confirmed, then an electromyography and further workup is required.

Radiographs should include a standard shoulder trauma series. This includes a scapular anterior-posterior or Grashey, axillary, and scapular-Y view. Images of the contralateral shoulder may be useful for templating purposes. A CT scan is useful for more precisely defining bone and fracture morphology including tuberosity comminution and displacement, articular segment involvement, degree of osteopenia, and possible glenoid fracture. If preoperative planning software is utilized, then thin slice CT scans of less than 1 mm are necessary.

OPERATIVE INDICATIONS

Due to the unpredictable results of ORIF and HA and the successful results of RTSA for an expanding spectrum glenohumeral pathologies, RTSA has become an attractive option for the treatment of complex proximal humerus fractures. Our indications include displaced four-part fractures and fracture-dislocations; displaced three-part fractures and fracture-dislocations in selected patients with poor bone quality that is not amenable to ORIF; fractures involving a head split in the elderly; proximal humerus fractures with associated glenoid fractures compromising glenohumeral joint stability; fractures with significant tuberosity comminution not amenable to ORIF; and elderly patients requiring early mobility and function of injured arm such as wheelchair dependence or contralateral paralysis.

Contraindications to RTSA for fracture include an associated brachial plexopathy and open fractures. Isolated axillary nerve compromise is a not an absolute contraindication since the vast majority resolve over time. However, it should be closely monitored both preoperatively and postoperatively. Associated injuries to the glenoid and acromion, although very uncommon, require careful assessment to determine if it will impact the outcome of RTSA. Since the proximal humerus is a common site for primary and metastatic oncologic lesions, if there is suspicion for a pathologic fracture, further preoperative evaluation is required including consultation with an orthopedic oncologist before proceeding with RTSA.[11,12]

OPERATIVE TECHNIQUE

The surgeon's preference is to use general anesthesia without a regional anesthetic. This allows for an immediate postoperative neurological examination. A periarticular infiltration of a pain cocktail is also used for postoperative pain control at the conclusion of the procedure, which will be described. Patients are positioned in the beach chair position with the operative arm secured to an arm positioner **(FIGURE 29.2)**. Ensure the endotracheal tube is secured on the opposite side of the operative arm. A standard deltopectoral approach is utilized, with care taken not to compromise the deltoid muscle because of its importance in postoperative stability, range of motion, and overall function.

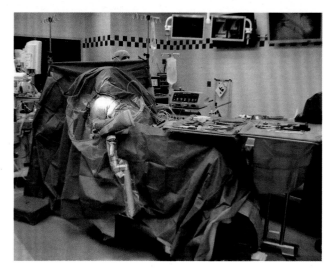

FIGURE 29.2 Preoperative photograph shows the patient positioning for the reverse shoulder arthroplasty. The patient is in a standard beach chair position with the operative arm secured to an arm positioner.

Once the deltopectoral interval is identified, the cephalic vein is most commonly mobilized lateral with the deltoid. There are several soft-tissue considerations to be mindful of which drastically improves surgical exposure. If necessary, the pectoralis major tendon insertion can be released approximately 1 cm from its insertion onto the humerus to aid in exposure. Subacromial and subdeltoid adhesions, hematoma, and any early callus must also be released to allow adequate visualization. At this time, the biceps tendon is usually identified at the bicipital groove and tenotomized with a 2-0 Vicryl suture.

This gives the surgeon exposure to the greater and lesser tuberosities. In three-part fractures, an osteotome is often necessary to separate the greater and lesser tuberosity at the bicipital groove. Once the tuberosities are isolated, they are secured using two braided, non-absorbable #5 heavy sutures at the tendon-bone interface evenly spaced to allow control of the tuberosity fragments. They are then mobilized to allow the fracture morphology to be assessed **(FIGURE 29.3)**. If there is comminution of the tuberosities present, it is suggested

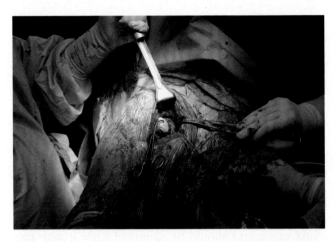

FIGURE 29.4 Intraoperative photograph of humeral head extraction.

that the comminution remain attached to the rotator cuff. At this point, the humeral head should be extracted and saved to be used for bone grafting **(FIGURE 29.4)**. The status of the humeral neck/calcar, the quality of cancellous and cortical bone, and additionally comminution should be assessed at this time.

Once the humeral head has been extracted, it is the surgeon's preference to first prepare the glenoid. In the context of proximal humerus fracture, glenoid exposure is generally more easily achieved due to capsular injury and loss of proximal humeral bone from the trauma. The proximal biceps stump as well as the labrum must be completely excised from the glenoid face. Care should be taken during the inferior capsulolabral resection to avoid injury to the axillary nerve **(FIGURE 29.5)**. It is recommended to detach the capsule directly off the glenoid bone to avoid neurologic injury. Once glenoid exposure is achieved, placement of a central pin perpendicular to the glenoid allows for reaming, which is particularly important in setting of acute fracture due to the abundant articular cartilage that may be present **(FIGURE 29.6)**. If preoperative templating identifies significant glenoid deformity or version, glenoid reaming can be adjusted to allow either bone or metal augments to be utilized. Once the glenoid is reamed, either a central screw or post is prepared, and the glenoid baseplate is inserted and should sit flush with the bone. Peripheral screws are used to further secure the baseplate to the scapula. A glenosphere is then applied onto the baseplate in the standard fashion **(FIGURE 29.7)**. Depending on the amount of proximal humeral comminution, consideration for a lateralized or larger glenosphere should be given to improve postoperative stability.

The humeral canal is then exposed **(FIGURE 29.8)** and prepared using hand reaming to prevent perioperative fracture in osteoporotic bone. Using trial components, the humeral prosthesis height and version of the implant is measured relative to the normally intact humeral calcar. If significant comminution of the humeral canal is

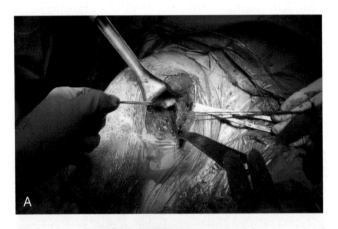

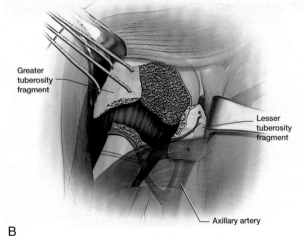

FIGURE 29.3 Intraoperative photograph (**A**) and illustration (**B**) of suture fixation of greater and lesser tuberosities with a heavy #5 braided suture.

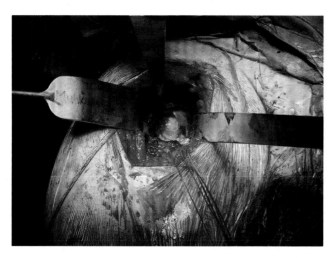

FIGURE 29.5 Intraoperative photograph of glenoid exposure with retractors.

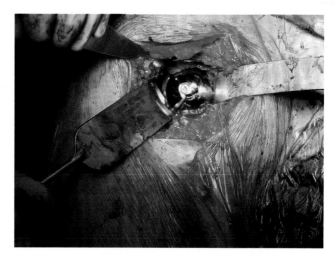

FIGURE 29.7 Intraoperative photograph of glenosphere attachment.

present, the superior border of the pectoralis tendon is utilized, and a distance of 5.0 cm is used to identify the most superior aspect of the humeral prosthesis.[14] Alternatively, radiographs of the contralateral unaffected shoulder can be obtained to better approximate humeral height.[15] The proper humeral height is critical to retain appropriate soft-tissue tensioning, with instability being the major consequence of inappropriate tensioning. A version rod is generally used to guide the amount of planned version for the humeral stem. It is our preference to place the humeral stem in 20° to 30° of retroversion, as these values have been found to provide optimal stability and minimal scapular notching.[16,17] Often, a surgical sponge (raytec) is used to help insert humeral trial implants to control rotation, and a trial reduction is performed and stability assessed **(FIGURE 29.9)**. The reduction of the tuberosity fragments must be assessed at this time as well as tuberosity healing is critical for optimal postoperative function.

Prior to implanting final humeral components, the surgical site is irrigated and a two 3.2 mm drill holes should be made through the humerus on either side of the bicipital groove and a heavy #5 nonabsorbable

suture should be used to facilitate tuberosity repair to the humeral shaft **(FIGURE 29.10)**. Additionally, a cement restrictor should be placed approximately 1 to 1.5 cm below the distal aspect of the prosthesis to allow for adequate cement mantle. Once the final implants are cemented with antibiotic-loaded cement, and the shoulder is reduced, the tuberosities are repaired to the prosthesis **(FIGURE 29.11 + drawing)**.

First, the #5 sutures used to secure the greater tuberosity are cerclaged around the humeral stem and passed through the implant fin, allowing for greater tuberosity reduction. At this time, if necessary, a rectangular portion of autograft from the humeral head is placed between the tuberosity and implant to provide support, improve deltoid wrap over the tuberosity, and promote healing. The tuberosity is secured to the implant at this time. Second, the #5 sutures securing the lesser tuberosity are reduced in a similar fashion around the humeral stem. Finally, the vertical suture through the humeral shaft is passed through the

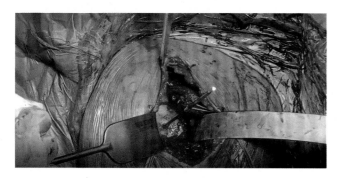

FIGURE 29.6 Intraoperative photograph of guide pin placement into the glenoid.

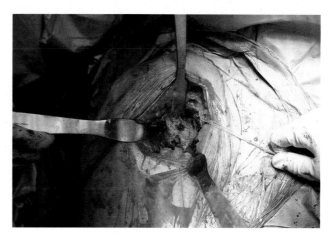

FIGURE 29.8 Intraoperative photograph of humeral canal exposure to prepare for reaming.

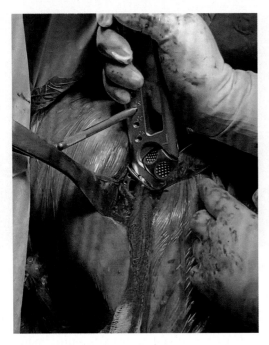

FIGURE 29.9 Intraoperative photograph of placement of trial humeral stem wrapped with a raytec sponge to aid in rotational control during trialing.

greater and lesser tuberosity. This suture is then tightened to reduce the tuberosities to the humeral shaft.

The operative arm is then taken through a range of motion and stability assessed. The wound is thoroughly irrigated. The pain cocktail consisting of 300 mg of 0.5% ropivacaine (60 mL), 1 mg epinephrine (1 mL), and 30 mg ketorolac (1 mL) is injected to provide adequate postoperative pain control in addition to a multimodal oral pain regimine.[13,18] A 60 mL syringe is used to administer the cocktail in the periarticular region prior to closure. Of the total, 15 mL is injected into the periosteum surrounding the glenoid and spinoglenoid notch targeting the suprascapular nerve, 15 mL into the deltoid muscle administered in 2 mL increments in a fan-shaped pattern staying close to the muscle origin, 10 mL into the remaining rotator cuff and capsule in 2 mL increments, 10 mL into the pectoralis major muscle in 2 mL increments, and the final 10 mL is injected evenly into the subcutaneous tissues along the incision. The biceps tendon is tenodesed to the pectoralis major muscle at its insertion and the deltopectoral interval is loosely reapproximately with two to three interrupted 2-0 Vicryl sutures to decrease the dead space. The subcutaneous

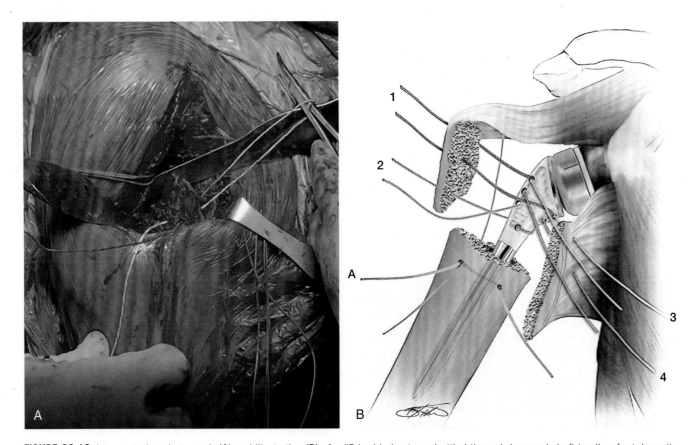

FIGURE 29.10 Intraoperative photograph (**A**) and illustration (**B**) of a #5 braided suture shuttled through humeral shaft to allow for tuberosity fixation to humeral shaft.

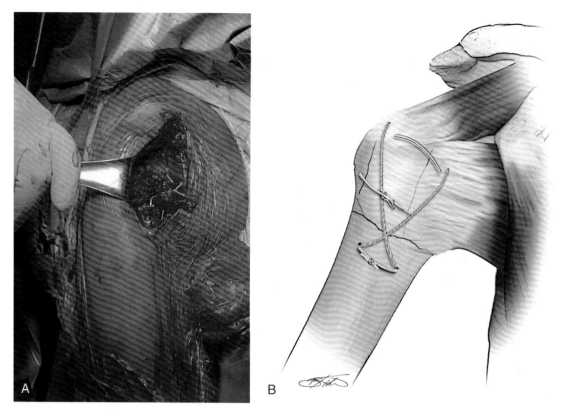

FIGURE 29.11 Intraoperative photograph (**A**) and illustration (**B**) of final tuberosity fixation to humeral stem and shaft.

tissue is closed in layers with 2-0 Vicryl and the skin is closed with a 4-0 running Monocryl barbed suture. The arm is placed in a shoulder immobilizer.

SPECIAL CONSIDERATIONS FOR RTSA IN ACUTE FRACTURES

The Tuberosities

The primary advantage of RTSA is that shoulder function does not solely rely on a functioning rotator cuff and healing of the tuberosities, both of which may become compromised in a patient with fracture.[19-21] However, healed tuberosities in RTSA, defined as the healing of the tuberosities in an anatomical position around a humeral stem, have been shown to have improved outcomes (**FIGURE 29.12A** and **B**). Tuberosity healing rates were reported to be lower with first-generation, Grammont-style designed humeral stems, due to the bulkier nature of the metaphyseal component and the associated difficulty with reconstruction of the tuberosities.[22] However, humeral fracture–specific stem modifications have been made to include lower profile metaphyseal regions, fins that resist rotational forces and act as a scaffold for tuberosity reconstruction, large surfaces for bone grafting, and prosthetic bone windows that promote improved tuberosity fixation and healing.[23,24] Contemporary designs report rates for tuberosity

healing after RTSA for proximal humerus fracture from 36.8%[25] to 84.6%[26] with an average tuberosity healing rate of 68.3% ± 15.9%.[27]

There have also been significant advances in surgical technique and the utilization of bone grafts that facilitate more anatomic tuberosity positioning and healing. This includes use of structural cancellous bone graft from the humeral head under the greater tuberosity and lesser tuberosity,[28] the "black and tan method" which is a hybrid cementation-impaction grafting technique that uses cancellous bone graft to create an interface between a cement mantle and area of tuberosity repair, thereby providing a buffer for thermal necrosis and the usage of a horseshoe graft.[20] The use of bone grafts is thought to enlarge the area for tuberosity repair and improve healing potential.

Healed tuberosities in the setting of RTSA for fractures have been correlated to improved outcomes. In a systematic review of nine studies reporting on tuberosity repair in RTSA performed for fracture, Anakwenze et al found significant improved forward elevation (126° vs 112°, $P < 0.0001$) and external rotation at neutral (24° vs 15°, $P = 0.003$) and external rotation at 90° (38° vs 4°, $P < 0.0001$) when the greater tuberosity is repaired as compared to when it is not repaired.[29] In a retrospective study of 38 displaced three- and four-part proximal humerus fractures and fracture-dislocations treated with

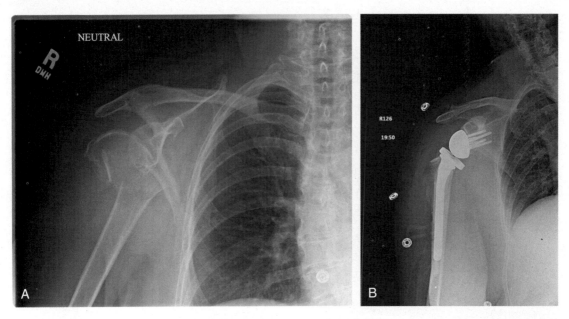

FIGURE 29.12 A, Preoperative radiograph demonstrating comminuted four-part proximal humerus fracture. **B**, Postoperative radiograph demonstrating cemented reverse total shoulder arthroplasty with reduction of greater tuberosity around the humeral prosthesis.

RTSA in which the tuberosities were reattached, healed greater tuberosities were associated with significantly higher subjective results (Subjective Shoulder Value of 83% vs 65%, $P = 0.029$), forward elevation ($141° ± 25°$ vs $115° ± 26°$, $P = 0.023$), and external rotation ($27° ± 12°$ vs $11° ± 12°$, $P = 0.010$).[30] In another systematic review, Jain et al[27] investigated the outcomes of seven studies investigating 382 RTSAs after proximal humerus fractures in the elderly and found that the weighted mean Constant-Murley Shoulder Outcome Score consistently improved in patients with a healed tuberosity as compared to patients with a nonhealed tuberosity (63.54 vs 56.60, $P < 0.05$). No significant differences were found among American Shoulder and Elbow Surgeons (ASES), Disabilities of the Arm, Shoulder, and Hand (DASH), Visual Analog Scale (VAS), and Simple Shoulder Test (SST) scores. It is thought that tuberosity reconstruction has three advantages: (1) restoration of the soft-tissue envelope and humeral length, which enhances stability to the articulation; (2) decreased periprosthetic dead space, thereby minimizing infection risk; and (3) decreased humeral implant loosening due to both proximal and distal points of fixation.

Prosthetic Considerations

RTSA was originally designed to provide function in rotator cuff–deficient shoulders that lost the essential transverse plane force coupling required for proper shoulder motion and function. Due to the biomechanical advantage of medializing the center of rotation and distalizing the humerus, the RTSA is able to better utilize the deltoid for forward elevation and abduction. Although this biomechanical design was also advantageous for the

treatment of proximal humerus fractures, it was also recognized that the humeral stem could be redesigned to be better suited for this indication. These design changes included a low profile metaphyseal body, rotational fin, suture attachment sites, and a fenestration for placement of bone graft **(FIGURE 29.13)**. The results of the use of these fracture-specific designs have been variable. In an observational study of 87 patients undergoing RTSA with a fracture-specific stem, Garofalo et al found favorable

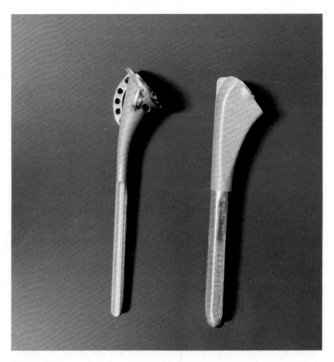

FIGURE 29.13 Photograph demonstrating difference between fracture stem and primary stem.

clinical results, with a radiographic tuberosity healing rate of 75%.[31] In a cohort of 48 patients comparing a fracture stem and a nonfracture stem, Jeong et al were unable to identify significant clinical or radiographic differences between the two groups.[32] It is evident that more experience will be needed to determine if fracture-specific stems can consistently result in improved outcomes in this challenging patient group.

CEMENTING

Cementing the humeral component is usually needed to achieve stable fixation because the extent of the metaphyseal bone loss compromises rotational and length stability. The remaining intact humerus is not sufficient to provide stability for a traditional press fit. In a retrospective study of 38 proximal humerus fractures treated with RTSA, Schoch et al compared 19 patients with a cemented stem to 19 patients with a noncemented stem.[33] They reported similar VAS scores, postoperative range of motion, and DASH scores between the two cohorts. However, ASES scores and satisfaction scores were higher with cemented humeral fixation (76.3 vs 48.0, $P = 0.005$; 1.2 vs 1.8, $P = 0.04$).[33] Radiographically, there was no difference in terms of tuberosity healing, component loosening, or notching ($P > 0.05$). A level IV study of RTSA for comminuted proximal humerus fractures demonstrated 97% stable uncemented humeral stem fixation with a 70% tuberosity healing rate, with acceptable motion and outcome scores.[34] Clinical experience provides support for both cemented and noncemented fixation. Press fit stems also provide other potential advantages. Modular systems allow for press fit stem fixation within the humeral canal with variable proximal body sizes to allow for optimal tuberosity repair. The addition of proximal porous coatings also facilitates press fit fixation and tuberosity healing. Press fit fixation also avoids the potential morbidity of using cement, which can include cardiopulmonary events, cytotoxicity, difficulty with revision surgery, and inhibition of a bony healing due to cement interposition between the tuberosities.[34] It should also be noted that the risk of iatrogenic fracture is greater with the use of noncemented stems. It is evident that there are advantages and disadvantages with the use of both cemented and noncemented stems. As clinical experience expands, a preference for one approach may become more conclusive. At present, cemented fixation continues to be our preference when performing RTSA for proximal humerus fractures.

POSTOPERATIVE MANAGEMENT

To date, there is little or no consensus regarding the postoperative management of patients undergoing RTSA after proximal humerus fractures due to the lack of high-level evidence. It is our practice to have the patient utilize a shoulder immobilizer postoperatively that allows

immediate elbow, wrist, and hand range of motion. On postoperative day #1, patients may begin passive forward flexion in a supine position to tolerance, passive internal rotation to the abdomen, and passive external rotation in the scapular plane to 15° as the patient tolerates. The next part of recovery is separated into four phases. Phase I, the passive phase, is implemented during weeks 1 to 3. The goal of this phase is to allow for the soft tissues to heal, maintain integrity of the joint, and decrease pain and inflammation. This phase consists of pendulums and passive range of motion as tolerated (forward flexion to 100°, abduction to 100°, and external rotation to 20°). Phase II is considered the active-assisted phase and should take place from weeks 3 to 6. The goals of this phase are to gradually restore full passive range of motion (forward flexion to 140°, external rotation to 45°, abduction to 100°, and internal rotation to buttock), gradually restore active motion, and reestablish dynamic shoulder stability. During phase II, active-assistive range of motion with passive stretch is emphasized.

The goal of phase III, the active phase, is to restore strength, power, and endurance during weeks 6 to 12. Patients work on optimizing their neuromuscular control, and a graduated return to functional activities. During this phase, scapular mobilization, deltoid strengthening, and periscapular strengthening are emphasized. Phase IV, the strengthening phase, begins at week 12. The goals of this phase are to maintain full, nonpainful active range of motion, maximize the use of the upper extremity, and maximize strength, power, and endurance. Patients will emphasize home exercises and a gradual progression in strengthening programs. The ultimate goal is for patient to resume recreational hobbies by postoperative months 4 to 6 following proximal humerus fractures with maximal improvements expected approximately 1 year after surgery.

In a cadaveric study by Hawthorn et al, placing shoulders in a sling with a small abduction pillow reduced the tension on the supraspinatus 27% anteriorly and 55% posteriorly compared to placing the shoulder in a sling without an abduction pillow. A large abduction pillow caused a further reduction in supraspinatus tension of 42% anteriorly and 56% posteriorly.[35] The use of an abduction pillow postoperatively can be considered if there is concern about tuberosity fixation and position.

OUTCOMES

While there is a relative paucity of long-term outcome data regarding RTSA for proximal humerus fractures, short-term outcomes have shown that RTSA is an encouraging option for these complex fractures. RTSA appears to provide reliable motion, pain relief, and function when used for the treatment of complex, acute proximal humerus fractures. A number of case series evaluating the outcomes of RTSA for proximal humerus fractures have shown favorable results.[19,36-39] In a case series of 43 patients with an average age of 78 years (range 65-97 years) and an average follow-up of 22 months, Bufquin et al found that patients were able to reach an average of 97° forward elevation (35°-160°) and 30° external rotation (0°-80°) with acceptable Constant, ASES, and DASH scores.[37] Lenarz was able to further substantiate these findings in a case series of 30 patients with an average age of 77 years (range 65-94 years) and an average follow-up of 23 months (12-36 months). They reported an average forward elevation of 138° (90°-180°) and external rotation of 27° (0°-45°) with a 10% complication rate.[19] These studies illustrated acceptable outcomes for treatment of proximal humerus fractures using RTSA and were followed by comparative studies of RTSA versus HA and RTSA versus ORIF for proximal humerus fractures.

In a systematic review of 17 studies (1346 patients, 322 undergoing RTSA and 1024 undergoing HA for acute proximal humerus fracture), Ferrel et al found that patients undergoing RTSA experienced a significant increase in mean forward flexion (118° vs 108°, $P < 0.01$) but less external rotation (20° vs 30°, $P < 0.01$) as compared to HA. There was no difference in ASES. Constant score was lower following HA (58.0 vs 54.6, $P < 0.01$).[40] The authors found significantly fewer complications following HA as compared to RTSA (4.1% vs 9.6%, $P < 0.01$). However, the revision rate was higher following HA (4.0% vs 0.93%). In a case-control study of 27 patients (9 RTSA, 9 HA, 9 ORIF), Chalmers et al found that significantly more patients achieved >90 degrees of forward flexion after RTSA as compared to the HA or ORIF groups and significantly more patients in the RTSA group reached 30° of external rotation than in the HA or ORIF groups. There were no differences in SST, ASES, or 12-Item Short Form Survey scores. These findings suggest that RTSA appears to provide superior range of motion more predictably with equivalent outcomes and a lower revision rate as compared to HA.

COMPLICATIONS

Complications are not uncommon for proximal humerus fractures treated with RTSA. The complications of instability and infection are particularly worrisome and range from 4% to 11% and 2% to 10%, respectively.[41] Radiographic signs of glenoid loosening and scapular notching are also of concern; however, their full clinical implications in this patient population have not been definitively assessed.[41] The surgeon must be mindful of these complications.

In an analysis of 146 patients with proximal humerus fractures treated with RTSA, Klug et al found a complication rate of 22.0% with a revision rate of 5.1%. Risk factors for higher complication rates were identified in

patients with higher Charlson comorbidity indices, and diabetes. The Neer classification was not predictive of complications.[42] A BMI >35 kg/m² was associated with a higher complication rate primarily as a result of the added medical and surgical complexity.[42] A review of the literature shows that other pertinent complications include complex sympathetic dystrophy (1.7%), instability (3.5%), infection (2.9%), and deltoid paresis, acromion fracture, lower extremity deep vein thrombosis, and lymphedema (0.6%, each). Minimizing complications is the goal when RTSA is performed for complex proximal humerus fractures. Careful patient selection, meticulous surgical technique, and close postoperative follow-up are important steps to minimize the risk of complications.

Case Presentation

A 71-year-old, right-hand-dominant woman presented 3 days after sustaining a right proximal humerus fracture after falling off a deck. She was initially evaluated and treated in the emergency department including radiographs and a computerized axial tomography (CAT) scan. She was placed in a sling and instructed to follow up as an outpatient. Relevant history included a previous left proximal humerus fracture treated nonoperatively with a moderate loss of active range of motion. Her current activities included playing golf and gardening. Radiographs demonstrated a three-part fracture of the proximal humerus **(FIGURE 29.14A-C)**. CAT scan confirmed a comminuted three-part proximal humerus fracture **(FIGURE 29.15A-C)**.

The patient's physical examination demonstrated bruising of the affected extremity with an intact neurovascular examination including deltoid activation and sensation. Given the limitations in function on her left upper extremity from the previous left proximal humerus fracture and the degree of comminution and displacement, a discussion was held with the patient regarding surgical options. After a lengthy discussion, the patient elected to proceed with an RTSA.

Intraoperatively, a three-part comminuted proximal humerus fracture was confirmed. The rotator cuff remained intact and attached to the greater and lesser tuberosities. A standard RTSA was performed as previously. The glenoid consisted of a standard baseplate and 36 mm glenosphere; an 8.5 mm cemented fracture stem placed in 20° of retroversion with a +2.5 mm polyethylene liner was used. The tuberosities were repaired utilizing the technique described. Cancellous bone graft was used between the tuberosities and the fracture stem and humeral shaft. Intraoperative examination demonstrated full arc of motion without signs of impingement. The patient was placed in an immobilizer for 1 week postoperatively **(FIGURE 29.16)**. At 8 months follow-up, the patient had no pain in the

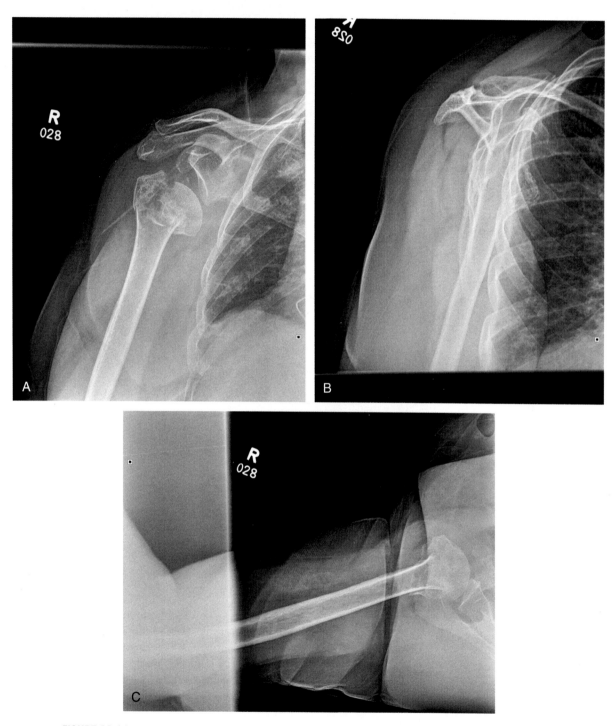

FIGURE 29.14 A, Preoperative Grashey view. **B**, Preoperative scapular-Y view. **C**, Preoperative axillary view.

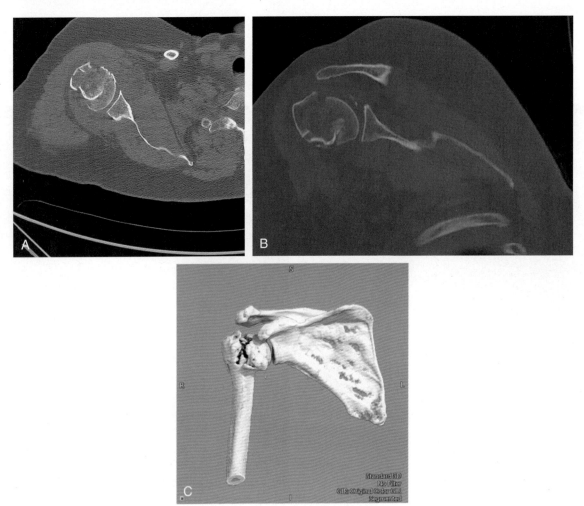

FIGURE 29.15 A, Preoperative axillary CT image. **B**, Preoperative coronal CT image. **C**, Preoperative three-dimensional reconstruction of the proximal humerus fracture.

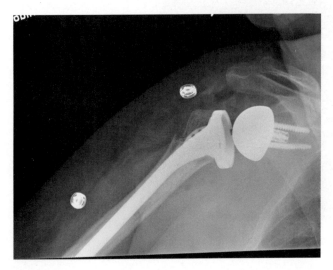

FIGURE 29.16 Postoperative Grashey view demonstrating reverse total shoulder with a fracture stem and well-reduced greater tuberosity fracture.

shoulder and demonstrated active forward elevation of 150°, internal rotation to T10, and external rotation of 30°. She has returned to all of her activities including golfing and gardening.

CONCLUSION

RTSA shows significant potential as a beneficial treatment option for patients who sustain complex proximal humerus fractures. The outcomes are superior to HA, and it provides an excellent option when ORIF is not considered to be desirable because of comminution and bone quality. Careful patient selection is important. Several modifiable and nonmodifiable factors contribute to improved results. Meticulous surgical technique with particular emphasis on tuberosity reduction and fixation is essential including bone grafting to enhance healing. Currently, cemented stem fixation is preferred, but this may change as new technology is developed for noncemented fixation.

REFERENCES

1. Gupta AK, Harris JD, Erickson BJ, et al. Surgical management of complex proximal humerus fractures-a systematic review of 92 studies including 4500 patients. *J Orthop Trauma.* 2015;29(1):54-59.

2. Kannus P, Palvanen M, Niemi S, Parkkari J, Jarvinen M, Vuori I. Osteoporotic fractures of the proximal humerus in elderly Finnish persons: sharp increase in 1970-1998 and alarming projections for the new millennium. *Acta Orthop Scand.* 2000;71(5):465-470.

3. Hanson B, Neidenbach P, de Boer P, Stengel D. Functional outcomes after nonoperative management of fractures of the proximal humerus. *J Shoulder Elbow Surg.* 2009;18(4):612-621.

4. Greiner SH, Diederichs G, Kroning I, Scheibel M, Perka C. Tuberosity position correlates with fatty infiltration of the rotator cuff after hemiarthroplasty for proximal humeral fractures. *J Shoulder Elbow Surg.* 2009;18(3):431-436.

5. Hettrich CM, Boraiah S, Dyke JP, Neviaser A, Helfet DL, Lorich DG. Quantitative assessment of the vascularity of the proximal part of the humerus. *J Bone Joint Surg Am.* 2010;92(4):943-948.

6. Marongiu G, Leinardi L, Congia S, Frigau L, Mola F, Capone A. Reliability and reproducibility of the new AO/OTA 2018 classification system for proximal humeral fractures: a comparison of three different classification systems. *J Orthop Traumatol.* 2020;21(1):4.

7. Hertel R, Hempfing A, Stiehler M, Leunig M. Predictors of humeral head ischemia after intracapsular fracture of the proximal humerus. *J Shoulder Elbow Surg.* 2004;13(4):427-433.

8. Solberg BD, Moon CN, Franco DP, Paiement GD. Surgical treatment of three and four-part proximal humeral fractures. *J Bone Joint Surg Am.* 2009;91(7):1689-1697.

9. Visser CP, Coene LN, Brand R, Tavy DL. Nerve lesions in proximal humeral fractures. *J Shoulder Elbow Surg.* 2001;10(5):421-427.

10. Ladermann A, Walch G, Denard PJ, et al. Reverse shoulder arthroplasty in patients with pre-operative impairment of the deltoid muscle. *Bone Joint J.* 2013;95-B(8):1106-1113.

11. Bonnevialle N, Mansat P, Lebon J, Laffosse JM, Bonnevialle P. Reverse shoulder arthroplasty for malignant tumors of proximal humerus. *J Shoulder Elbow Surg.* 2015;24(1):36-44.

12. De Wilde L, Boileau P, Van der Bracht H. Does reverse shoulder arthroplasty for tumors of the proximal humerus reduce impairment? *Clin Orthop Relat Res.* 2011;469(9):2489-2495.

13. Okoroha KR, Lynch JR, Keller RA, et al. Liposomal bupivacaine versus interscalene nerve block for pain control after shoulder arthroplasty: a prospective randomized trial. *J Shoulder Elbow Surg.* 2016;25(11):1742-1748.

14. Cagle PJ, Reizner W, Parsons BO. A technique for humeral prosthesis placement in reverse total shoulder arthroplasty for fracture. *Shoulder Elbow.* 2019;11(6):459-464.

15. Boileau P, Walch G, Krishnan SG. Tuberosity osteosynthesis and hemiarthroplasty for four-part fractures of the proximal humerus. *Tech Shoulder Elbow Surg.* 2000;1(2):96-109.

16. Favre P, Sussmann PS, Gerber C. The effect of component positioning on intrinsic stability of the reverse shoulder arthroplasty. *J Shoulder Elbow Surg.* 2010;19(4):550-556.

17. Berhouet J, Garaud P, Favard L. Evaluation of the role of glenosphere design and humeral component retroversion in avoiding scapular notching during reverse shoulder arthroplasty. *J Shoulder Elbow Surg.* 2014;23(2):151-158.

18. Sicard J, Klouche S, Conso C, et al. Local infiltration analgesia versus interscalene nerve block for postoperative pain control after shoulder arthroplasty: a prospective, randomized, noninferiority study involving 99 patients. *J Shoulder Elbow Surg.* 2019;28(2):212-219.

19. Lenarz C, Shishani Y, McCrum C, Nowinski RJ, Edwards TB, Gobezie R. Is reverse shoulder arthroplasty appropriate for the treatment of fractures in the older patient? Early observations. *Clin Orthop Relat Res.* 2011;469(12):3324-3331.

20. Levy JC, Badman B. Reverse shoulder prosthesis for acute four-part fracture: tuberosity fixation using a horseshoe graft. *J Orthop Trauma.* 2011;25(5):318-324.

21. Martin TG, Iannotti JP. Reverse total shoulder arthroplasty for acute fractures and failed management after proximal humeral fractures. *Orthop Clin North Am.* 2008;39(4):451-457.

22. Routman HD. Indications, technique, and pitfalls of reverse total shoulder arthroplasty for proximal humerus fractures. *Bull Hosp Jt Dis (2013).* 2013;71(suppl 2):64-67.

23. Krishnan SG, Reineck JR, Bennion PD, Feher L, Burkhead WZ Jr. Shoulder arthroplasty for fracture: does a fracture-specific stem make a difference? *Clin Orthop Relat Res.* 2011;469(12):3317-3323.

24. Li F, Zhu Y, Lu Y, Liu X, Wu G, Jiang C. Hemiarthroplasty for the treatment of complex proximal humeral fractures: does a trabecular metal prosthesis make a difference? A prospective, comparative study with a minimum 3-year follow-up. *J Shoulder Elbow Surg.* 2014;23(10):1437-1443.

25. Chun YM, Kim DS, Lee DH, Shin SJ. Reverse shoulder arthroplasty for four-part proximal humerus fracture in elderly patients: can a healed tuberosity improve the functional outcomes? *J Shoulder Elbow Surg.* 2017;26(7):1216-1221.

26. Grubhofer F, Wieser K, Meyer DC, et al. Reverse total shoulder arthroplasty for acute head-splitting, 3- and 4-part fractures of the proximal humerus in the elderly. *J Shoulder Elbow Surg.* 2016;25(10):1690-1698.

27. Jain NP, Mannan SS, Dharmarajan R, Rangan A. Tuberosity healing after reverse shoulder arthroplasty for complex proximal humeral fractures in elderly patients-does it improve outcomes? A systematic review and meta-analysis. *J Shoulder Elbow Surg.* 2019;28(3):e78-e91.

28. Krishnan SG, Bennion PW, Reineck JR, Burkhead WZ. Hemiarthroplasty for proximal humeral fracture: restoration of the Gothic arch. *Orthop Clin North Am.* 2008;39(4):441-450.

29. Anakwenze OA, Zoller S, Ahmad CS, Levine WN. Reverse shoulder arthroplasty for acute proximal humerus fractures: a systematic review. *J Shoulder Elbow Surg.* 2014;23(4):e73-e80.

30. Boileau P, Alta TD, Decroocq L, et al. Reverse shoulder arthroplasty for acute fractures in the elderly: is it worth reattaching the tuberosities? *J Shoulder Elbow Surg.* 2019;28(3):437-444.

31. Garofalo R, Flanagin B, Castagna A, Lo EY, Krishnan SG. Reverse shoulder arthroplasty for proximal humerus fracture using a dedicated stem: radiological outcomes at a minimum 2 years of follow-up-case series. *J Orthop Surg Res.* 2015;10:129.

32. Jeong JJ, Kong CG, Park SE, Ji JH, Whang WH, Choi BS. Non-fracture stem vs fracture stem of reverse total shoulder arthroplasty in complex proximal humeral fracture of asian elderly. *Arch Orthop Trauma Surg.* 2019;139(12):1649-1657.

33. Schoch B, Aibinder W, Walters J, et al. Outcomes of uncemented versus cemented reverse shoulder arthroplasty for proximal humerus fractures. *Orthopedics.* 2019;42(2):e236-e241.

34. Wright JO, Ho A, Kalma J, et al. Uncemented reverse total shoulder arthroplasty as initial treatment for comminuted proximal humerus fractures. *J Orthop Trauma.* 2019;33(7):e263-e269.

35. Hawthorne JR, Carpenter EM, Lam PH, Murrell GAC. Effects of abduction pillows on rotator cuff repair: a biomechanical analysis. *HSS J.* 2018;14(2):114-122.

36. Klein M, Juschka M, Hinkenjann B, Scherger B, Ostermann PA. Treatment of comminuted fractures of the proximal humerus in elderly patients with the Delta III reverse shoulder prosthesis. *J Orthop Trauma.* 2008;22(10):698-704.

37. Bufquin T, Hersan A, Hubert L, Massin P. Reverse shoulder arthroplasty for the treatment of three- and four-part fractures of the proximal humerus in the elderly: a prospective review of 43 cases with a short-term follow-up. *J Bone Joint Surg Br.* 2007;89(4):516-520.

38. Gallinet D, Clappaz P, Garbuio P, Tropet Y, Obert L. Three or four parts complex proximal humerus fractures: hemiarthroplasty versus reverse prosthesis. A comparative study of 40 cases. *Orthop Traumatol Surg Res.* 2009;95(1):48-55.

39. Cazeneuve JF, Cristofari DJ. The reverse shoulder prosthesis in the treatment of fractures of the proximal humerus in the elderly. *J Bone Joint Surg Br.* 2010;92(4):535-539.

40. Ferrel JR, Trinh TQ, Fischer RA. Reverse total shoulder arthroplasty versus hemiarthroplasty for proximal humeral fractures: a systematic review. *J Orthop Trauma.* 2015;29(1):60-68.

41. Chalmers PN, Slikker W III, Mall NA, et al. Reverse total shoulder arthroplasty for acute proximal humeral fracture: comparison to open reduction-internal fixation and hemiarthroplasty. *J Shoulder Elbow Surg.* 2014;23(2):197-204.

42. Klug A, Wincheringer D, Harth J, Schmidt-Horlohe K, Hoffmann R, Gramlich Y. Complications after surgical treatment of proximal humerus fractures in the elderly-an analysis of complication patterns and risk factors for reverse shoulder arthroplasty and angular-stable plating. *J Shoulder Elbow Surg.* 2019;28(9):1674-1684.

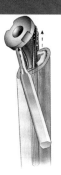

30 Reverse Total Shoulder Arthroplasty After Failed Fracture Hemiarthroplasty

Surena Namdari, MD and Gerald R. Williams Jr, MD

INTRODUCTION

Hemiarthroplasty for the diagnosis of proximal humerus fracture is less commonly performed. Rates of hemiarthroplasty utilization have declined and are projected to decline further due to the expanding indications for reverse shoulder arthroplasty. While satisfactory results can be achieved with hemiarthroplasty for fracture, the technical demands of the operation and the unpredictability with regards to tuberosity healing and rehabilitation potential can compromise results. When hemiarthroplasty for fracture fails, unique challenges are encountered, including proximal humeral deformity, glenoid and humeral bone loss, and prosthetic loosening. The purpose of this chapter is to discuss the evaluation and complex management of the failed hemiarthroplasty for fracture with focus on conversion to reverse total shoulder arthroplasty.

EVALUATION

Patients present with dissatisfaction following hemiarthroplasty for fracture because of a number of reasons. Most often, the last recollection they have of their shoulder, before they broke it, is that it was normal. Therefore, a certain amount of dissatisfaction occurs even in patients who have a good result because of the lack of prior disability. Patient complaints usually center around pain and restricted function. Although both complaints are usually present to some degree, determining which is most prominent is important from a prognostic perspective. Pain is more responsive than function to revision surgery. Once the most prominent chief complaint has been identified, the remainder of the evaluation includes history, physical examination, and imaging. In addition, based on the presentation, other studies may be indicated. Finally, an attempt should be made to attain the prior operative report, as it can yield information regarding the specific implant used, whether or not cement was used, and specific surgical technique details that might impact the revision.

A thorough history will help elucidate shoulder complaints that were present before the fracture, the severity of the trauma that caused the injury, the presence of concomitant injuries, the presence of patient comorbidities that may affect outcome, as well as the postoperative course following the hemiarthroplasty. The presence of numbness or paresthesia, either at the time of the original injury or at presentation for revision, may be indicative of a brachial plexus or other nerve injury that likely will affect the outcome. Finally, the patient should be questioned about whether or not there were any wound healing issues such as drainage or redness that prompted temporary antibiotic treatment.

Careful physical examination will provide information that is helpful in determining the cause(s) of the patient's complaints as well as potential strategies for surgical intervention. The location and physical characteristics of the scar should be noted. The presence of actively draining or apparently healed sinus tracts, widened scars, or hypertrophic scars should also be noted. In addition, all three heads of the deltoid should be inspected for atrophy. Observable atrophy of all three heads may indicate complete axillary nerve palsy; while individual atrophy of the anterior deltoid may indicate partially recovered axillary nerve injury, local trauma to the anterior deltoid muscle, or denervation of the anterior deltoid from the surgical approach. Specific atrophy of the supraspinatus or infraspinatus may suggest preexisting cuff tear, greater tuberosity nonunion, or suprascapular nerve injury.

Active and passive range of motion should be measured and compared to the opposite, normal side. Patients presenting for revision rarely have good motion, unless they are presenting with late pain following a good functional result. Most often, the shoulder is stiff with equal or nearly equal loss of active and passive range of motion in virtually all planes. Alternatively, patients with tuberosity nonunion may present with relatively preserved passive range of motion but poor active motion. This may be accompanied by the presence of a positive external rotation lag sign, a positive abdominal compression test, or anterosuperior humeral head escape with attempted elevation. It is also possible to have combined severe stiffness as well as cuff insufficiency, particularly with fibrous union or malunion of the greater tuberosity.

Identification of localized tenderness is also important. Tenderness over the tip of the coracoid process is common and may represent abnormal contact between the coracoid and the humeral head, especially if the humeral head has been placed too superiorly or the subscapularis has failed. Tuberosity failure may result in proximal humeral migration which, if severe and prolonged, may result in acromial erosion with subsequent stress fracture. This may present with direct acromial tenderness. Finally, symptomatic acromioclavicular arthropathy may rarely present concomitantly with painful hemiarthroplasty. Tenderness over the acromioclavicular joint should be noted.

Initial imaging should include anteroposterior views in internal rotation and external rotation, an axillary lateral view, and a trans-scapular Y view. All images should include the tip of the prosthesis. In addition, an attempt should be made to attain all preoperative images, including computed tomographic (CT) and magnetic resonance imaging (MRI) scans. The preoperative and serial postoperative radiographs may yield information with regard to the presence of dislocation, the type of fracture, the amount of comminution, as well as the size and quality of the tuberosity fragments, especially the greater tuberosity.

Plain radiographic examination most often reveals enough information to formulate a diagnosis and initial plan. Important findings include proximal humeral migration (**FIGURE 30.1**), tuberosity position, tuberosity union, presence or absence of cement, the size of the distal cement plug, humeral component loosening, endosteal humeral erosion or resorption, humeral head subluxation, and glenoid erosion. If proximal humeral migration is absent or mild, it suggests that rotator cuff function is reasonable. When proximal migration is severe, it is often associated with anterosuperior glenoid erosion. The greater tuberosity, especially if it is ununited, may be positioned severely posteriorly (**FIGURE 30.2**). This is often not seen well except on the axillary view. It is also commonly associated with anterior humeral subluxation and anterior glenoid erosion. The presence of severe endosteal erosion of the humerus is usually a sign that the component is loose. In addition, this should raise the suspicion for infection. However, cemented stems that are smooth and cylindrical and not supported by adequate proximal bone can loosen early in the absence of infection.[1,2] If substantial proximal humeral bone loss is present, full-length views of both humeri with magnification markers should be attained to accurately measure the amount of humeral bone loss and shortening.[3]

Advanced imaging is performed in most patients who are being considered for revision of hemiarthroplasty following fracture to reverse total shoulder arthroplasty. The presence of the metal humeral head can make the recognition of glenoid erosion difficult on plain radiographs. CT scan is indicated in most cases to assess glenoid morphology tuberosity position (**FIGURE 30.3**).

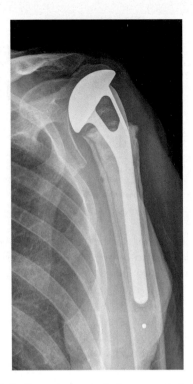

FIGURE 30.1 Radiograph demonstrating a cemented hemiarthroplasty with greater tuberosity resorption and proximal humeral migration.

Three-dimensional reconstruction and metal suppression techniques are typically used. Although intra-articular contrast is helpful for determining cuff integrity, if the decision has already been made to convert to reverse arthroplasty, this information may not be as relevant. Although some centers have found postarthroplasty MRI scanning to be helpful, we prefer to add contrast to the CT if we are concerned about rotator cuff integrity rather than use MRI scanning.[4]

Additional studies may be indicated, depending on the presentation. Infection workup is performed in every case and is described in another chapter. Electromyography and nerve conduction velocity (EMG/NCV) studies are performed if there is suspicion of persistent nerve injury on physical examination. We have a low threshold for attaining EMG/NCV studies because patients with completely or incompletely recovered nerve injuries may be more susceptible to recurrent nerve injury at the time of revision. Finally, arteriography is rarely used and is reserved for patients with diminished pulses or abnormal Allen tests, especially if they complain of cold intolerance or forearm cramping.

SURGICAL MANAGEMENT

The decision to revise a painful, dysfunctional hemiarthroplasty that was placed for humeral fracture to a reverse total shoulder arthroplasty should be made carefully and with considerable discussion with the patient. Preoperative planning is critical in all revisions. In almost

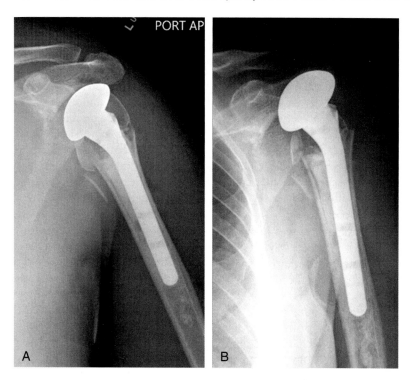

FIGURE 30.2 Radiographs demonstrating a hemiarthroplasty performed for acute fracture indication (**A**) followed by greater tuberosity displacement and resorption (**B**).

all cases, it is possible to know the implant manufacturer. The prior operative report is extremely helpful. In addition, the appearance of the stem may be recognized by the surgeon. There is also a library of common implants with radiographic examples that was created by the University of Washington Shoulder Service and can be accessed at this link: http://faculty.washington.

edu/alexbert/Shoulder/CommonUSShoulderProstheses. htm.

Knowledge of the specific implant will allow the surgeon to have the implants at surgery if the stem is convertible and instruments to facilitate extraction if they are needed. Assuming the stem is going to be replaced, the surgeon should have short, standard, and long-stem

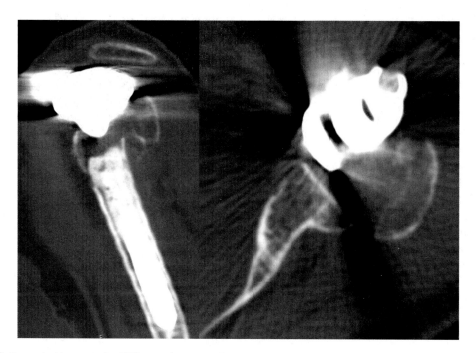

FIGURE 30.3 Computed tomography (CT) scan demonstrating posteriorly displaced and nonunited greater tuberosity fragment.

implants available. A dedicated shoulder revision instrument set or a hip revision set should be available in addition to a C-arm, microsagittal saw, complete set of osteotomes, pencil-tipped burr, and cables. In cases with a large distal cement plug, ultrasonic cement removal devices may be helpful, particularly if the plan is to convert to a long-stemmed device.[5] Structural proximal humeral allografts—with attached rotator cuff tendons, if possible—allograft struts, and nonstructural cancellous allograft chips should be available. Finally, metal-augmented humeral and glenoid components can be used as an alternative to allograft in cases with humeral or glenoid bone loss.[6,7]

SURGICAL TECHNIQUE

Revisions are always more complicated than primary procedures. These revisions are among the most challenging. The surgeon should take a systematic approach to all portions of the procedure and attempt to make each step as similar as possible to a primary reverse arthroplasty. Important principles include adequate development of all soft-tissue planes from the skin all the way to the glenoid, identification and protection of neurovascular structures, adequate capsular release or excision, avoidance of bone impingement, and reestablishment of adequate soft-tissue tension. Some cases will be more challenging than others, but the important steps in all include anesthesia and patient positioning, skin incision and superficial dissection, deep dissection, humeral exposure, greater tuberosity assessment, glenoid exposure, humeral stem extraction, humeral component placement, stability assessment, final implant placement, and subscapularis closure.

The ultimate choice of anesthesia is made by the patient in consultation with the anesthesiologist. Most often, a combination of general and regional anesthesia is chosen. After induction of anesthesia, the patient is placed in a beach chair position with the shoulder positioned over the edge of the table allowing unencumbered adduction and extension of the arm. The head and neck are stabilized in a neutral position and, all bony and neurological prominences are padded appropriately. The C-arm is positioned on the opposite side of the table, and verification of adequate x-ray visualization is performed. The shoulder is then prepared and draped in normal sterile fashion. A mechanical arm holding device is used to stabilize the arm throughout the procedure. Alternatively, a padded Mayo stand can be used.

The previous skin incision is often slightly vertical and lateral in comparison to the normal deltopectoral incision. This may be the result of the incision having been made on an extremely swollen shoulder and arm. However, in almost all cases, the previous incision can be utilized. If necessary, full-thickness subcutaneous flaps can be undermined superomedially and inferolaterally to expose the deltopectoral interval. The incision may need to be extended distally to facilitate an anterolateral approach to the humerus, especially if a humeral split or window is required for stem removal. The cephalic vein may not be easily identified. Rather than trying to dissect in a scarred deltopectoral interval, identify the tip of the coracoid and expose it by incising over it with an electrocautery. This allows taking a small (5 mm) strip of the pectoralis major laterally with the scarred deltopectoral interval and the remaining portion of the pectoralis major medially. This interval is dissected proximally to the clavicle and distally to the deltoid tubercle.

The superficial layers are typically scarred to one another because of the soft-tissue injury associated with the fracture as well as the prior surgery. There are usually dense adhesions between the pectoralis major and the conjoined tendon, the deltoid and underlying humerus, and within the subacromial space. Starting at the tip of the coracoid, dissect between the deep surface of the pectoralis muscle and the underlying conjoined tendon, from proximal to distal. The glistening fibers of the conjoined tendon are clearly discernible from the muscular pectoralis muscle. This interspace should be dissected completely to the pectoralis insertion. After identifying the pectoralis insertion on the humerus, dissect between it and the tendon of the deltoid until a space is created between the deltoid tendon and the humeral shaft. Place a blunt Hohmann retractor in this space and retract the anterior deltoid insertion laterally. Proceed to dissect the deltoid away from the humeral shaft from distal to proximal until a point just distal to the metaphyseal flare of the humerus to avoid injuring the axillary nerve. The subacromial space can be identified by palpating the coracoacromial ligament attachment on the exposed coracoid tip and dissecting bluntly under it with a curved Mayo scissors. A blunt Hohmann retractor is placed in this interval, and the adhesions in the lateral portion of the subacromial space are released. The arm is then slightly abducted and progressively internally rotated so that the adhesions between the proximal humerus and the deltoid can be released. Care is taken to keep the dissection on bone to protect the axillary nerve. With the superficial layers mobilized, the pectoralis major is retracted medially and the deltoid is retracted laterally with a self-retaining Koebel retractor. The anterosuperior deltoid is retracted superolaterally with a blunt Hohmann or Brown Deltoid retractor within the subacromial space.

Deep dissection is comprised of developing the layer between the posterior surface of the conjoined tendon and the anterior surface of the subscapularis in addition to biceps exposure and tenodesis. The easiest and safest place to start the dissection deep to the conjoined tendon is superiorly, just distal to the base of the coracoid. In almost all cases, the space deep to the coracoid elbow and tip, and distal to the coracoid base is relatively devoid of adhesions. Blunt dissection is performed with a curved Mayo scissors in this area from lateral to medial. Once this space has been enlarged, digital palpation can usually identify the axillary nerve, and occasionally, the axillary artery. Distal and lateral dissection can then proceed until the axillary nerve can be palpated at the inferior aspect of the joint progressing into the quadrilateral space. The surgeon should also palpate for the musculocutaneous nerve, which, if present in the surgical field, will be slightly lateral and anterior to the axillary nerve. All neurovascular structures should be protected throughout the procedure. In some cases, the subscapularis and anterior capsule may be deficient. The process of finding the neurovascular structures is the same, but the surgeon should proceed with even greater caution.

A special mention should be made regarding the course of the musculocutaneous nerve and axillary artery in these cases. As the dissection is carried distally, along the lateral aspect of the conjoined tendon, the musculocutaneous nerve can occasionally be found in an extremely lateral and anterior location. Utilization of an electrocautery to dissect slowly along the lateral aspect of the conjoined tendon while mobilizing it away from the subscapularis can provide the surgeon a warning when the nerve is getting close to the dissection plane. One can then proceed with blunt dissection to identify and protect the nerve. The axillary artery can be scarred into the subscapularis and be damaged, even with blunt dissection. When this happens, the rate of blood loss is substantial. The situation can be stabilized with application of direct pressure. Exposure of the axillary artery can be gained quickly by releasing the conjoined tendon origin and the pectoralis minor tendon insertion from the coracoid.[8] Occasionally, release of the pectoralis major tendon from the humerus is also required.[8] These maneuvers allow immediate and extensile visualization of the axillary artery. Vessel loops can be passed around the artery, proximal and distal to the injury, to gain control. Definitive management may require vascular consult. This is a rare event but one that requires quick recognition and management.

After complete mobilization of the conjoined tendon, it is retracted medially. The arm is placed in slight internal rotation using the mechanical arm holder. An attempt is made to aspirate the joint for fluid to send for culture. The biceps tendon is palpated slightly superior to the upper border of the pectoralis major tendon. It is then exposed by incising the sheath from the upper border of the pectoralis tendon proximally, through the bicipital groove, and across the rotator interval to the supraglenoid tubercle. This rotator interval incision is often made parallel to the upper border of the subscapularis, leaving the rotator interval tissue with the supraspinatus. Our preference is to angle slightly more posteriorly, along the anterior edge of the supraspinatus, so that the rotator interval stays with the subscapularis.

This helps with visualization of the greater tuberosity junction with the prosthetic head. The long head of the biceps, when present, is then tenodesed to the upper border of the pectoralis major tendon with two nonabsorbable sutures and excised proximally. Soft-tissue cultures are sent from the bicipital groove area and the rotator interval.

The humerus is exposed by releasing and reflecting the subscapularis and capsule from the anterior humerus. The method of releasing the subscapularis depends on the condition of the lesser tuberosity and the subscapularis tendon. The subscapularis tendon is released with the lesser tuberosity if the tuberosity is ununited or malunited. In addition, if the tuberosity is anatomic, the subscapularis is released with a lesser tuberosity osteotomy so long as its tendinous attachment is relatively anatomic and the muscle is in good condition.[9,10] Under any of these circumstances, the lesser tuberosity is reflected independent from the underlying capsule and 2 to 3 heavy nonabsorbable tapes are passed through the bone tendon junction. The arm is then externally rotated slightly, the interval between the subscapularis muscle and underlying capsule is identified inferiorly, this interval is developed proximally with a Cobb or other elevator, and the subscapularis is released sharply from the underlying capsule. The subscapularis and lesser tuberosity are then retracted medially. The capsule is then released from the humerus, starting superiorly and extending inferomedially. Capsular release is facilitated by progressively externally rotating and flexing the humerus. The release must be taken past the 6 o'clock position posteriorly in order to facilitate glenoid exposure. Care should be taken to protect the axillary nerve during this extensive posteromedial capsular release.

Subscapularis reflection with the lesser tuberosity is not performed if its tendinous attachment is not adequate or if the quality of the muscle and tendon is poor. Under these circumstances, the subscapularis and capsule are reflected in a single layer off the lesser tuberosity. Two or three heavy, nonabsorbable tapes are passed through the lateral subscapularis tendon in a Mason-Allen configuration.[11] Once the tendon and capsule have been reflected, an assessment of the subscapularis muscle belly is made. If it is good quality and reasonable thickness, the underlying capsule can be separated from the subscapularis muscle using blunt dissection medially. The capsule can then be sharply released from the overlying tendon, leaving the previously placed tapes intact. If the surgeon judges the subscapularis muscle and tendon to be of questionable quality and thickness, the layers are left intact and retracted medially as one unit.

Attempted delivery of the humerus out of the glenoid can now be performed. This is done by adducting, extending, and externally rotating the arm. Care should be taken not to place undue torque on the elbow in these typically elderly, osteoporotic individuals. Typically, a

Brown deltoid or blunt Hohmann retractor is within the subacromial space and can be used to help push the humerus anteriorly. However, excess levering should be avoided, as it can result in acromial fracture. A large Darrach or blunt Hohmann retractor is placed between the glenoid and humerus and can help guide the head out of the glenoid. Greater tuberosity malunion can interfere with humeral head delivery. In most cases, with placing a bone hook around the surgical neck to pull the humerus laterally, in combination with gentle leverage from the subacromial Brown deltoid or blunt Hohmann retractor and guidance from the intra-articular large Darrach, the head can be delivered.

Most humeral prostheses are modular. Therefore, with the humerus delivered, the modular humeral head is removed from the stem. This can be done with the removal instrument contained in the instrument set of the specific prosthesis. Alternatively, a small or large Cobb elevator can be placed between the head and the underlying humerus laterally and driven medially with taps from a mallet. This can be performed superior and inferior to the taper. Do not lever the Cobb into the proximal bone. When the head is removed, a piece of the soft-tissue membrane that invariably forms between the head and the native bone is excised and sent for culture. The modular stem is left in place to protect the humerus during glenoid exposure and instrumentation. In some situations, the humeral prosthesis is cemented proud, has a male taper, or otherwise obstructs adequate glenoid exposure. Under these circumstances, it is best to remove the stem before exposing the glenoid. Details regarding stem extraction are discussed below. After removing the stem, a slightly undersized broach from whichever system will be used is placed in the humeral canal to protect it during glenoid exposure and instrumentation.

Prior to exposing the glenoid, the greater tuberosity should be assessed. Unless absolutely necessary for delivery of the humerus, greater tuberosity osteotomy is avoided. Greater tuberosity nonunion with substantial displacement is usually characterized by the tuberosity being positioned at the posterior glenoid surrounded by a large amount of scar. Placing a humeral head retractor (eg, Fukuda) behind the glenoid only makes exposure and mobilization more difficult. The humeral head can be pulled laterally with a bone hook, or a laminar spreader can be placed with one arm of the retractor placed on the glenoid rim and the other on the humeral broach to push the humerus laterally. The superior and posterior capsules are then released deep to the displaced and ununited greater tuberosity, and a Cobb elevator is placed through the resultant capsulotomy to create a space between the posterior glenoid and the tuberosity. Two to three heavy, nonabsorbable tapes are passed through the bone tendon junction of the tuberosity for lateral traction and later repair.

Malunion of the greater tuberosity can be managed in one of two ways, depending on how much displacement there is. The major problem with malunion of the greater tuberosity with severe displacement is the potential for impingement and subsequent instability. In the majority of cases, a small stem can be cemented with a posterior offset so that the shell for the polyethylene cup can be placed into the displaced tuberosity. Occasionally, the displacement is so severe that this is not possible. This determination is most easily made during humeral preparation and will be explained below. In short, if after reaming the humeral shaft and epiphysis, including the displaced tuberosity, the trial cannot be positioned with the shell in the tuberosity, osteotomy is performed.

After assessment and management of the greater tuberosity has been completed, the glenoid is exposed for preparation and placement of the glenoid component. If the posterior capsule has not yet been incised, a bone hook is used to pull the humerus laterally and the posterior capsule is released from the glenoid. A humeral head retractor (eg, Fukuda retractor) is placed within this capsulotomy, and the humerus is retracted posteriorly. If the anterior capsule and subscapularis were reflected independently, the anterior and inferior capsule is completely excised, taking care to protect the axillary nerve. The inferior capsule is often thickened and scarred and can lead to instability if not excised. A reverse double-pronged Bankart retractor is then placed on the anterior neck of the scapula. The labrum is excised circumferentially and any remaining posterior or superior capsule is released. It is important that no capsular attachment remains on any portion of the glenoid. A blunt Hohmann retractor is placed posterosuperiorly. If the anterior capsule is not going to be excised, it is critical to release the residual anterior capsule completely from the glenoid.

There are many implant systems available for reverse shoulder arthroplasty. A discussion of all of them is beyond the scope of this chapter. The surgeon should know the characteristics and technique for whichever system he or she is using. Our preference is a system that has a screw-in, circular baseplate with four peripheral locking screws and a variably lateralized glenosphere.[12] The glenoid is prepared with a cannulated reamer over a tap. Prior to placing the central drill hole for glenoid preparation, an assessment is made of the glenoid surface, in combination with review of the preoperative radiographic studies, for substantial bone loss. If it is present and not amenable to asymmetric reaming, the defect can be managed with structural allograft or an augmented glenoid baseplate (**FIGURE 30.4**). A discussion of the specific details of these techniques is beyond the scope of this chapter and can be found in other portions of this text.

In general, we match the glenosphere to the size of the patient and select no more than 6 mm of lateralization. Therefore, a 32 to 4 sphere (6 mm of lateralization) is

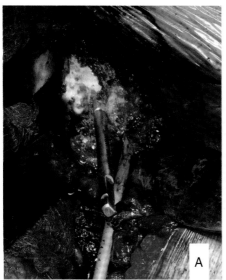 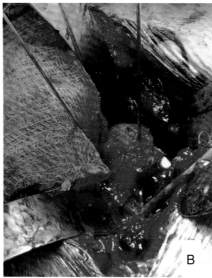 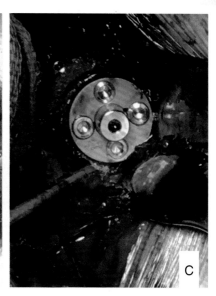

FIGURE 30.4 A, Intraoperative image demonstrating severe posterior superior glenoid erosion. **B,** Placement of structural allograft provisionally fixed with Kirschner wires around a central tap. **C,** Final baseplate utilized to compress and fixate graft to native glenoid.

used in small individuals, a 36 standard sphere (6 mm of lateralization) is used in medium-sized individuals, and a 40 standard sphere (4 mm of lateralization) is used in large individuals. Trialing is not always necessary when selecting the glenosphere. However, in revisions, especially those performed for fracture sequelae, the abnormal bony anatomy as well as the scarred soft-tissue envelope may result in having to use different sizes from the ones predicted by patient size. Therefore, the trial size that we think is appropriate is placed on the baseplate, and the humerus is redelivered into the wound.

Stems that can be converted to a reverse configuration without removing the entire stem have been available for 10 years, and a discussion of their design principles is beyond the scope of this chapter. Regardless of the method of convertibility, If the first stem is malpositioned, it must be removed, regardless of whether or not it is convertible to a reverse. It is important to know the shell and glenosphere options available for all convertible stems. There may be a reason to use a different (eg, smaller or with lateral offset) glenosphere than is available in the system that is being converted. It is possible to get the manufacturer to make a cup that fits on their stem and fits the favored sphere. This is an off-label use that must be discussed with the patient but can be preferable to removing a well-fixed stem in osteoporotic bone.

Assuming the original humeral stem was modular and the head has been removed, the method of stem removal depends on whether the implant was placed with or without cement, whether it has a collar, and whether or not it is porous coated. If the greater tuberosity has been osteotomized and reflected or was ununited and mobilized enough for repair, access to the prosthesis-bone or prosthesis-cement interface is much easier. If the greater

tuberosity is still intact, the first step is to use curettes and rongeurs to remove the bone superior to any fins on the prosthesis. In addition, the sutures that were used to repair the tuberosities to the prosthesis should be removed. If these two steps are not taken, when the prosthesis is removed, the fins or the sutures may cause a fracture of the proximal humerus.

When removing a cementless prosthesis, the general principle is to create a circumferential gap between the prosthesis and the remaining bone **(FIGURE 30.5)**. This can be done using a series of small osteotomes or a pencil-tipped burr.[13] If no collar is present, this is a relatively straightforward process. We prefer small osteotomes and pass them directly on the margin of the prosthesis, parallel to the long axis of the humerus, using a mallet. Medially, a curved osteotome is often required to follow the curvature of the prosthesis. The osteotomes should be passed slightly distal to the level of any porous coating. If the implant has a collar, a small v-shaped piece of bone is removed from the medial calcar so that an osteotome can be used to access the proximal portion of the stem immediately under the collar.[14] If one is methodical in accessing the entire circumference of the prosthesis to a depth that is beyond the level of the porous coating, the stem almost always comes out easily. This can be done using the extracting device supplied by the manufacturer and a mallet. If this is not available, a square-shaped tamp placed medially under the collar will work. If there is no collar, a high-speed specialized burr can be used to create a slot at the medial prosthetic neck, and the tamp can then be used. It is always best to know the manufacturer and have extraction instruments available.

Removal of cemented prostheses can be more difficult than their cementless counterparts. The same general approach is utilized, except that the gap is created

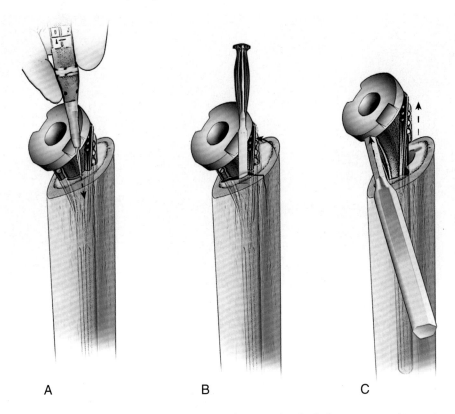

A   B   C

FIGURE 30.5 A, Pencil tip bur used to create a gap between stem and bone proximally. **B**, Osteotome used to create a gap between ingrowth surface and bone. **C**, Square-shaped tamp placed at medial collar and used to extract stem.

between the metal and the cement rather than the metal and the bone. The osteotomes should be passed to a depth that exceeds the metaphyseal flair of the proximal portion of the implant. The same approach to the most proximal portion of the stem under a collar that was used above for cementless implants is also used here. Most implants can be extracted at this point using either the extraction instrument supplied by the manufacturer or a medial tamp. The cement that is stable and left in the canal can be used to cement in a smaller stem[1] **(FIGURE 30.6)**. This may be preferable to trying to remove all the cement because of the potential of causing substantial humeral damage.

Very occasionally, the stem is still fixed after these maneuvers. Under these circumstances, a cut is made in the humerus slightly lateral to the bicipital groove using a microsagittal saw. The cut should start at the most superior extent of the humerus and end slightly distal to the tip of the prosthesis and should be made to a depth of at least the cement mantel or, preferably, to the actual prosthesis. A small drill hole is placed at the very distal extent of the cut to decrease risk of distal extension. A large, straight osteotome is then placed in the cut and is driven into the metal prosthesis for the full length of the saw track. Unless the stem was porous coated and cemented, it almost always is extractable after this maneuver **(FIGURE 30.7)**. A cortical window is also an option, and the details of this technique are beyond the

scope of this chapter but can be found elsewhere.[15] The very next step after component removal is placement of cables to protect the humerus.

HUMERAL COMPONENT PLACEMENT

After implant removal, there are several considerations that need to be made for revising the humeral side. In general, the goal is to preserve bone stock and to achieve stable fixation of a revision implant. Hemiarthroplasty for the indication of acute fracture is commonly performed using a cemented humeral component. Unfortunately, when revising a failed cemented humeral component, complete removal of cement within the humeral canal can lead to significant intraoperative bone loss. Because of this, unless there are gross signs of infection, our preference is to utilize an undersized humeral component cemented within a retained cement mantle.[16] If the original stem was cementless, a cementless revision stem can commonly be utilized using a combination of impaction grafting, a larger stem, and/or a longer stem. If cement is required, a small amount is placed distally in combination with a proximally coated stem and proximal impaction grafting with allograft cancellous chips.

Proximal humeral bone loss is commonly a problem when revising a failed hemiarthroplasty for fracture. Bone loss can result from resorption of the greater and/or lesser tuberosity, proximal stress shielding or osteolysis, and iatrogenically during stem extraction. Greater

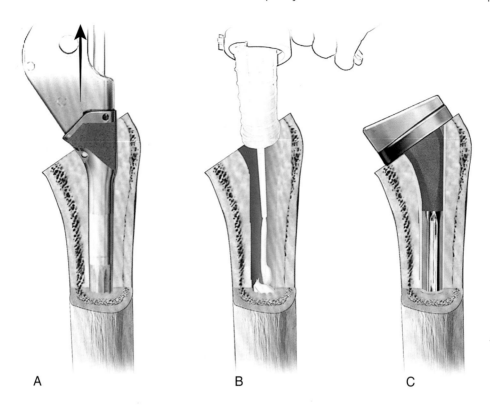

A   B   C

FIGURE 30.6 A, Cemented hemiarthroplasty explanted with retained cement mantle. **B**, Cement being pressurized into preexisting cement mantle (blue). **C**, Final placement of reverse arthroplasty stem using a cement-in-cement technique.

degrees of bone loss have implications for both function and implant stability and longevity. As bone loss extends distally, violation of the deltoid insertion is associated with poorer functional results. Additionally, the proximal humerus adds stability to the fixation of a humeral implant, and loss of bone leads to greater rotational stress.[17] While the amount of bone loss that requires use of a proximal humeral allograft or a metalloprosthesis is controversial, 5 cm is a reasonable threshold in the absence of clinical or biomechanical data.[2,18]

In cases with proximal bone loss that do not require a proximal humeral allograft **(FIGURE 30.8)** or metalloprosthesis, assessment of humeral height and version can be challenging. We aim for 30° of retroversion with reference to the forearm. A sponge can be used within the canal to gain some stability of the trial component so that tension can be assessed. In addition, several anatomic checks can be utilized. If the calcar is present, the inferior aspect of the cup of an inlay humeral prosthesis should rest on the calcar or within 2 to 3 mm of it; the distance between the superior pectoralis insertion and the top of the cup should be 5 to 6 cm[19]; and with the trial prosthesis reduced, the top of the greater tuberosity (assuming it was not excised) should be even with the top of the cup.

In cases of substantial proximal humeral bone loss, a proximal humeral allograft or metalloprosthesis may be required. Our preference currently is a proximal

humeral allograft **(FIGURE 30.9)**. The details of the technique can be found elsewhere and are beyond the scope of this chapter.

STABILITY ASSESSMENT

With the trial humerus reduced, an assessment of soft-tissue tension and bony impingement is made. The shoulder is ranged in forward elevation, abduction, external rotation, internal rotation, and extension while checking for bone contact against the scapula or limits to motion due to soft tissue contracture. If gapping between the trial liner and the glenosphere occurs in external rotation, it is typically a sign of posterior impingement. Soft tissue tension is first assessed by placing a downward force on the arm in order to assess separation between the trial liner and the glenosphere. If greater than 1 to 2 mm of translation is palpable, the liner should be upsized. Subsequently, the tension in the conjoined tendon and the axillary nerve is palpated and compared subjectively to the tension palpated at the start of the procedure. Finally, the humerus is laterally translated with two fingers on the medial calcar to determine the ease with which it can be dislocated. Stability can be modified through glenosphere lateralization, glenosphere diameter, or by adding humeral thickness (polyethylene or metal). Once the final components have been chosen, the trials are removed. The glenoid is reexposed, the taper is cleaned and dried,

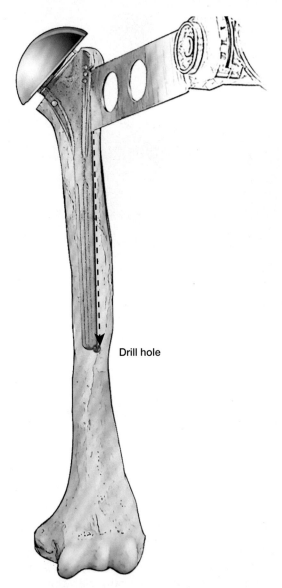

FIGURE 30.7 Illustration demonstrating osteotomy line created lateral to the bicipital groove and extending to the distal extent of the stem.

Drill hole

and the final sphere is inserted. The humerus is redelivered, and the final component is placed. The humerus is reduced, and stability and lack of impingement are confirmed. If the greater tuberosity fragment is present and able to be mobilized and repaired to the implant, it can improve stability and function, particularly external rotation. We consider adequate tuberosity excursion to exist when the medial border of the tuberosity can be pulled at least 3 to 4 cm lateral to the posterior glenoid rim without undue tension. If the tuberosity fragment is contracted and displaced posteriorly, it can cause posterior impingement and instability. In these cases, the tuberosity is excised.

SUBSCAPULARIS CLOSURE

If the subscapularis can be reapproximated to the proximal humerus with the arm in 30 or more degrees of external rotation, it may be repaired. There is data to support both subscapularis repair[20,21] and to support leaving the subscapularis unrepaired.[22-24] In the authors experience, subscapularis repair aids in the identification of the axillary nerve if reoperation is required. If the decision to repair has been made, the technique is determined by how it was released and is beyond the scope of this chapter.

REHABILITATION

In general, the primary goal for revision to reverse from hemiarthroplasty for fracture is pain relief. In addition, instability, poor bone quality, and need for grafting are more common in this scenario than it is for other diagnoses. Therefore, rehabilitation is slower in comparison to primary reverse. We assign rehabilitation based on what is found at surgery. Patients are generally divided into two categories based on general tissue quality, stability, and implant fixation: early versus delayed rehabilitation. In the early rehabilitation group, immediate prelabor rupture of membranes (PROM) (elevation to 130, ER to 30) is initiated during the hospital admission, and table glides begin at 2 weeks after surgery. Overhead pulleys are initiated at 4 to 6 weeks with progression of active-assisted and active range of motion. Strengthening is initiated at 8 to 10 weeks. In the delayed group, a sling is continued for 6 weeks. Range of motion exercises are initiated at 6 weeks with progression of passive, active-assisted, and active motion. Strengthening is initiated at 12 weeks.

OUTCOMES

Results of revision of hemiarthroplasty to reverse arthroplasty are unpredictable. While the primary surgical goal is pain relief, improvements in range of motion and strength are common patient expectations that must be managed. Franke et al evaluated results of revision hemiarthroplasty to reverse arthroplasty based on etiology.[25] Compared with failed hemiarthroplasty performed for cuff tear arthropathy or osteoarthritis, conversion of failed hemiarthroplasty performed for fracture to reverse arthroplasty resulted in less improvements in range of motion and functional scores. In general, outcomes were modest with a mean American Shoulder and Elbow Surgeons (ASES) score of 58 and a mean active forward elevation of 95°. Similarly, Dezfuli et al[26] reported a mean ASES score of 54 and a mean active forward elevation 103°, and Merolla et al[27] reported a median ASES score of 60 and a mean abduction of 100°. In general, we counsel patients that pain is highly likely to improve after surgery and that achieving active

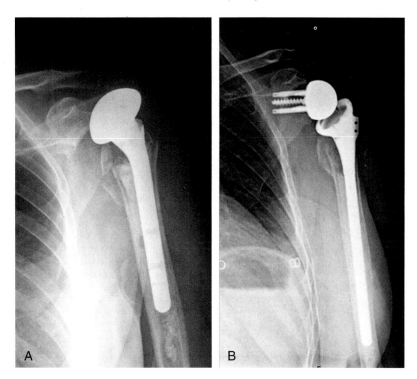

FIGURE 30.8 Revision of hemiarthroplasty (**A**) to long-stem reverse arthroplasty with less than 5 cm of proximal humeral bone loss (**B**).

motion between 90° to 100° is considered a satisfactory result for this complex operation.

COMPLICATIONS

Complication rates after conversion of a failed hemiarthroplasty for fracture to reverse arthroplasty are common. Intraoperative complications include periprosthetic

fracture and nerve injury. Due to soft tissue contracture, tuberosity malunion, and weakened bone from stress shielding or osteolysis, the risk of fracture is greatest during humeral exposure and during implant explantation. Early postoperative complications include instability and acute infection. Late postoperative complications implant loosening, chronic infection, and fracture.

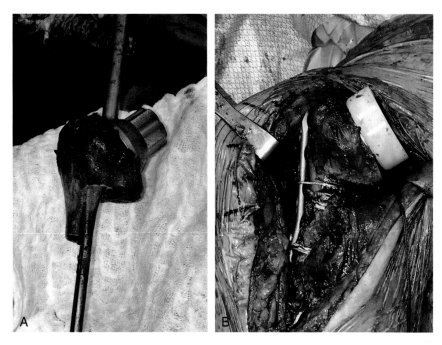

FIGURE 30.9 Intraoperative picture demonstrating proximal humeral alloprosthesis preparation (**A**) and placement (**B**).

Management of these complications are more comprehensively discussed in other chapters. Franke et al[25] reported a reoperation rate of 14%, and Merolla et al[27] reported a reoperation rate of 7% after revision of failed hemiarthroplasty for fracture to reverse arthroplasty with implant loosening and infection being the most common etiologies.

CONCLUSION

While hemiarthroplasty for proximal humerus fracture is less commonly performed, revision of a failed hemiarthroplasty for fracture remains a common indication for reverse arthroplasty. Revision of the failed hemiarthroplasty presents unique challenging due to alterations in proximal humeral anatomy, cemented humeral components, and bone loss. While following the surgical pearls discussed in this chapter can lead to a technically well-performed revision surgery, functional outcomes are modest, and complications are common.

REFERENCES

1. McLendon PB, Cox JL, Frankle MA. Humeral bone loss in revision shoulder arthroplasty. *Am J Orthop (Belle Mead NJ)*. 2018;47(2).
2. Chacon A, Virani N, Shannon R, Levy JC, Pupello D, Frankle M. Revision arthroplasty with use of a reverse shoulder prosthesis-allograft composite. *J Bone Joint Surg Am*. 2009;91(1):119-127.
3. Boileau P, Melis B, Duperron D, Moineau G, Rumian AP, Han Y. Revision surgery of reverse shoulder arthroplasty. *J Shoulder Elbow Surg*. 2013;22(10):1359-1370.
4. Koff MF, Burge AJ, Potter HG. Clinical magnetic resonance imaging of arthroplasty at 1.5 T. *J Orthop Res*. 2020;38:1455-1464.
5. Giannotti S, Bottai V, Dell'Osso G, Bugelli G, Guido G. Cement extractor device in revision prosthesis of the humerus. *Surg Technol Int*. 2014;25:246-250.
6. Grey SG, Wright TW, Flurin P-H, Zuckerman JD, Roche CP, Friedman RJ. Clinical and radiographic outcomes with a posteriorly augmented glenoid for Walch B glenoids in anatomic total shoulder arthroplasty. *J Shoulder Elbow Surg*. 2020;29(5):e185-e195.
7. Duquin TR, Matthews JR, Dubiel MJ, Sperling JW. Running out of room: managing humeral and glenoid bone loss in shoulder arthroplasty. *Instr Course Lect*. 2019;68:79-90.
8. Padegimas EM, Schoch BS, Kwon J, DiMuzio PJ, Williams GR, Namdari S. Evaluation and management of axillary artery injury: the orthopaedic and vascular surgeon's perspective. *JBJS Rev*. 2017;5(6):e3.
9. Gerber C, Pennington SD, Yian EH, Pfirrmann CAW, Werner CML, Zumstein MA. Lesser tuberosity osteotomy for total shoulder arthroplasty. Surgical technique. *J Bone Joint Surg Am*. 2006;88(suppl 1 pt 2):170-177.
10. Qureshi S, Hsiao A, Klug RA, Lee E, Braman J, Flatow EL. Subscapularis function after total shoulder replacement: results with lesser tuberosity osteotomy. *J Shoulder Elbow Surg*. 2008;17(1):68-72.
11. Gerber C, Schneeberger A, Beck M, Schlegel U. Mechanical strength of repairs of the rotator cuff. *J Bone Joint Surg Br*. 1994;76(3):371-380.
12. Cuff DJ, Pupello DR, Santoni BG, Clark RE, Frankle MA. Reverse shoulder arthroplasty for the treatment of rotator cuff deficiency: a concise follow-up, at a minimum of 10 years, of previous reports. *J Bone Joint Surg Am*. 2017;99(22):1895-1899.
13. Kang JR, Logli AL, Tagliero AJ, Sperling JW. The router bit extraction technique for removing a well-fixed humeral stem in revision shoulder arthroplasty. *Bone Joint Lett J*. 2019;101-B(10):1280-1284.
14. Sperling JW, Cofield RH. Humeral windows in revision shoulder arthroplasty. *J Shoulder Elbow Surg*. 2005;14(3):258-263.
15. Sahota S, Sperling JW, Cofield RH. Humeral windows and longitudinal splits for component removal in revision shoulder arthroplasty. *J Shoulder Elbow Surg*. 2014;23(10):1485-1491.
16. Wagner ER, Houdek MT, Hernandez NM, Cofield RH, Sánchez-Sotelo J, Sperling JW. Cement-within-cement technique in revision reverse shoulder arthroplasty. *J Shoulder Elbow Surg*. 2017;26(8):1448-1453.
17. Cuff D, Levy JC, Gutiérrez S, Frankle MA. Torsional stability of modular and non-modular reverse shoulder humeral components in a proximal humeral bone loss model. *J Shoulder Elbow Surg*. 2011;20(4):646-651.
18. Levy J, Frankle M, Mighell M, Pupello D. The use of the reverse shoulder prosthesis for the treatment of failed hemiarthroplasty for proximal humeral fracture. *J Bone Joint Surg Am*. 2007;89(2):292-300.
19. Murachovsky J, Ikemoto RY, Nascimento LGP, Fujiki EN, Milani C, Warner JJP. Pectoralis major tendon reference (PMT): a new method for accurate restoration of humeral length with hemiarthroplasty for fracture. *J Shoulder Elbow Surg*. 2006;15(6):675-678.
20. Edwards TB, Williams MD, Labriola JE, Elkousy HA, Gartsman GM, O'Connor DP. Subscapularis insufficiency and the risk of shoulder dislocation after reverse shoulder arthroplasty. *J Shoulder Elbow Surg*. 2009;18(6):892-896.
21. Matthewson G, Kooner S, Kwapisz A, Leiter J, Old J, MacDonald P. The effect of subscapularis repair on dislocation rates in reverse shoulder arthroplasty: a meta-analysis and systematic review. *J Shoulder Elbow Surg*. 2019;28(5):989-997.
22. Clark JC, Ritchie J, Song FS, et al. Complication rates, dislocation, pain, and postoperative range of motion after reverse shoulder arthroplasty in patients with and without repair of the subscapularis. *J Shoulder Elbow Surg*. 2012;21(1):36-41.
23. Roberson TA, Shanley E, Griscom JT, et al. Subscapularis repair is unnecessary after lateralized reverse shoulder arthroplasty. *JB JS Open Access*. 2018;3(3):e0056.
24. Werner BC, Wong AC, Mahony GT, et al. Clinical outcomes after reverse shoulder arthroplasty with and without subscapularis repair: the importance of considering glenosphere lateralization. *J Am Acad Orthop Surg*. 2018;26(5):e114-e119.
25. Franke KJ, Christmas KN, Downes KL, Mighell MA, Frankle MA. Does the etiology of a failed hemiarthroplasty affect outcomes when revised to a reverse shoulder arthroplasty? *J Shoulder Elbow Surg*. 2020;29:S149-S156.
26. Dezfuli B, King JJ, Farmer KW, Struk AM, Wright TW. Outcomes of reverse total shoulder arthroplasty as primary versus revision procedure for proximal humerus fractures. *J Shoulder Elbow Surg*. 2016;25(7):1133-1137.
27. Merolla G, Wagner E, Sperling JW, Paladini P, Fabbri E, Porcellini G. Revision of failed shoulder hemiarthroplasty to reverse total arthroplasty: analysis of 157 revision implants. *J Shoulder Elbow Surg*. 2018;27(1):75-81.

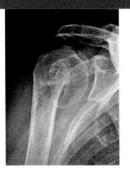

31 Arthroplasty for Postfracture Sequelae and Failed Open Reduction and Internal Fixation

Rick F. Papandrea, MD and Christopher M. Kilian, MD

INTRODUCTION

Proximal humerus fractures continue to be an enigma for the shoulder surgeon. Advanced arthroscopic and percutaneous fixation of fractures are technically demanding techniques and have yet to show superiority to other options. Despite advances in fixation, including locking and anatomically shaped plates, open reduction and internal fixation has, in some studies, demonstrated equivalence to nonoperative treatment.[1-4]

Primary operative treatment of proximal humerus fractures with arthroplasty is an important treatment option. Hemiarthroplasty (HA) had been the mainstay for prosthetic replacement, especially in three- and four-part fractures, and still has a role.[5,6] Reverse total shoulder arthroplasty (RTSA) has recently shown promise for acute treatment of complex fractures but is not without its complications.[5-10] Acute treatment of proximal humerus fractures with arthroplasty is covered in Chapters 28 and 29. Surgeons treating proximal humeral fractures understand the equivalence of fixation and nonoperative treatment is not because both give excellent outcomes. On the contrary, the current treatment options for proximal humerus fractures provide surgeons, and more importantly patients, with less than optimal outcomes, often not exceeding nonoperative management.[1,4,11,12]

Although some studies demonstrate worse outcomes with delayed arthroplasty in proximal humerus fractures, other studies have demonstrated equivalency in outcomes for delayed treatment of fractures with RTSA.[13,14] This equivalence in delay, combined with the equivalence in some studies of intervention with nonoperative treatment, gives credence to a thoughtful approach for intervention of acute proximal humerus fractures, especially in the elderly.

Following proximal humerus fracture, patients should maximize the use of rest, anti-inflammatories, physical therapy, and corticosteroid injections (if appropriate), in order to maximize recovery of their premorbid shoulder function. Patients should recognize that following fracture healing their range of motion most likely will be decreased compared to the uninvolved side. However, often the degree of loss is accommodated very well. Mild to moderate malunions of the proximal humerus can be tolerated. However, when range of motion is less than 120° of forward elevation and 30° of external rotation, it has been suggested that osteotomies should be considered to address the mechanical block.[15] After adequate time, many patients with a proximal humerus fracture have reasonable return of function, and additional treatment is no longer needed.[3,16,17]

While there may be a small amount of continued improvement from 6 to 12 months after fracture, it tends to be insignificant, with most of the perceived improvement in this period coming from accommodation and acceptance by the patient of their new level of function. If this new "normal" is accompanied with significant pain or dysfunction, reconstruction should be considered. This chapter will address shoulder arthroplasty for postfracture sequelae (PFS), including failed open reduction and internal fixation (ORIF). Revision of initial arthroplasty for fracture is covered in Chapter 30. Delayed arthroplasty treatment can consist of HA, anatomic total shoulder replacement (ATSA), or RTSA.

POSTFRACTURE SEQUELAE

Despite a growing body of evidence suggesting that ORIF of proximal humeral fractures may not result in improvement compared with nonoperative treatment, fixation is still often performed. As surgeons, we are accustomed to restoration of function following anatomic fracture fixation. Unfortunately, this is not always the case with proximal humerus fractures. Arthritis from hardware complications, nonunions, malunions, and osteonecrosis (ON) are all potential sequelae from fracture fixation in the proximal humerus, which may be treated with arthroplasty. Shannon et al has shown a higher *complication* rate following RTSA for failed ORIF compared to primary RTSA for fracture.[18] However, the revision rate and clinical outcomes were similar. Similarly, Nowak et al found the *reoperation* rate following arthroplasty for failed ORIF to be significantly higher compared to primary arthroplasty. The higher rate of revision for arthroplasty after failed ORIF has also been documented by the Danish shoulder arthroplasty registry.[19] Thus, the decision to undergo primary ORIF should be made with

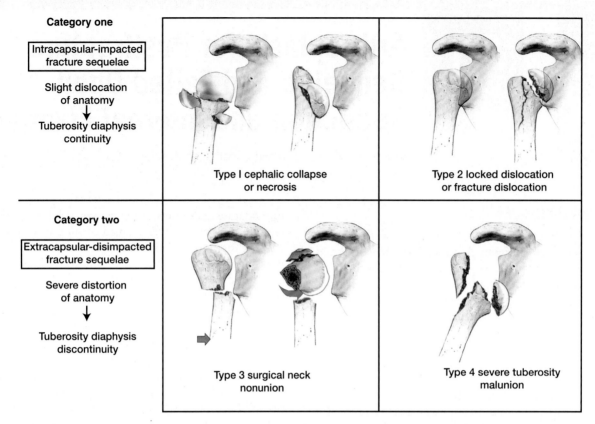

FIGURE 31.1 Boileau classification for proximal humeral fracture sequelae or postfracture sequelae (PFS). **Type 1** consists of impaction of the humeral head, while the tuberosities remain attached. There may be varus or valgus position of the humeral head, the head may be split. **Type 2** injuries include locked dislocations or fracture dislocations. These are both in **category one** and are considered intracapsular. **Category two** injuries are extracapsular with tuberosities that are dissociated or severely displaced from the proximal humerus: type 3 includes surgical neck nonunion; type 4 are those proximal humerus fractures with severe tuberosity malunion, which are **type 4**. While the original classification recommended anatomic hemiarthroplasty (HA) or total shoulder arthroplasty (ATSA) for category one and reverse total shoulder arthroplasty (RTSA) for type two injuries, current literature and experiences demonstrate the recommended treatment for PFS may be more nuanced.

caution a full understanding of the outcomes and the risk of complications and reoperations.

Multiple classifications for PFS exist, but none are comprehensive.[20-23] Despite this, the Boileau classification is both simple and practical, providing the surgeon with some guidance for treatment **(FIGURE 31.1)**.[21,22]

Boileau et al. originally classified nonunion and malunion depending on whether the injury was intracapsular (category 1, type 1 and 2) or extracapsular (category 2, type 3 and 4). Type 1 fractures are characterized by humeral head ON or impaction, and type 2 are chronic dislocations or fracture-dislocations. They recommended ATSA without greater tuberosity osteotomy for these injuries. Category 2 includes the sequelae of extracapsular/disimpacted fractures. These include type 3 fractures with nonunion of the surgical neck and type 4 fractures characterized by severe malunion of the tuberosities. They recommended RTSA for these fracture sequelae. (See text below for current recommendations, especially for type 3 and 4.)

The Boileau classification has been utilized in multiple studies but has not undergone a formal, peer-reviewed validation process for inter- and intra-observer reliability.[21,24-30] PFS of proximal humerus fractures includes pathology that is not specified in any of the four types

in Boileau classification. Additionally, advances in prosthetic design and surgeon experience have provided additional options for treatment.

EVALUATION OF THE POSTFRACTURE PATIENT

To consider an orthopedic intervention, one must obtain a relevant history, physical examination, imaging studies, and any special testing needed. Fractures affect more than the skeletal structures, and the reconstruction of the proximal humerus post fracture requires attention to more than just the bone. When evaluating the patient who is having difficulties after proximal humerus fracture treatment, one must evaluate the soft tissue envelope and consider its status and function before finalizing a treatment plan. Additionally, pain, nerve deficits, and rotator cuff functional status are all important factors, which must be considered when discussing the potential for reconstruction.

HISTORY

Understanding the patient's premorbid health, activities, avocations, and occupation are paramount to formulating a plan for treatment of any PFS of the proximal humerus. This is especially true in the low demand, elderly, and often frail, patient. Handedness should be understood by the surgeon because depending on the length of time since the injury, many patients may have made some changes in dexterity, such that hand dominance is a less important factor to consider.

The physician should inquire with the patient as to why they are presenting for evaluation. There are the occasional patients who present for evaluation solely because they were told to do so by another provider or family member. They may feel as though they have equilibrated to a tolerable level of comfort and function and feel no desire to proceed with additional treatment. The treatment focus should be on the patient, not the radiograph or the limited range of motion. When queried, some patients will give very specific functional needs. These should be acknowledged, addressed, and documented. If patients have expectations that are not likely to be met by reconstruction, it is important to emphasize this to the patient and anyone accompanying them. This should be recorded in the medical record, and the patient should be reminded of this again preoperatively. Surgeon understanding of the patient's needs and desires is the basis for the shared decision-making to be made with the patient.

The mechanism of injury which caused the proximal humerus fracture may impart an understanding of the amount of energy applied, as well as provide insights as to other potential injuries that may have been sustained. More critical factors are typically related to the soft tissue envelope and any confirmed or potential nerve injury. The patient should be asked about bleeding from the shoulder around the time of the injury or if any treating providers felt the fracture was open or "compound" or if they were placed on antibiotics around the time of treatment.

Further questioning should include any sensory or motor disturbances noticed by the patient, family, physician, or therapist. If any neurologic deficits were noted, the length of time until resolution or any persistent symptoms should be recorded. Even though the shoulder is the focus of the injury and reconstruction, a detailed examination of the function of the hand should be recorded such that any prereconstruction brachial plexus pathology is identified, recorded, and discussed.

PHYSICAL EXAMINATION

The detailed physical examination of the shoulder will not be reviewed here. The aspects of the physical examination that are critical to patient education and shared decision-making for PFS will be emphasized.

Both active and passive range of motion should be assessed in the PFS patient. Deficits should be pointed out to patients, with further discussion as to perceived potential for change with intervention. This will provide patients with realistic expectations following

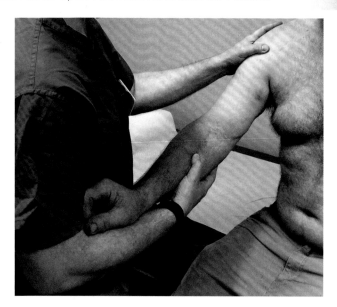

FIGURE 31.2 Examination of the function of the deltoid in a patient with limited motion and pain: The patient's forearm is cradled in the examiner's hand and forearm. The opposite hand rests on the uncovered deltoid. By having the patient withdraw, the posterior head is palpated to assess for contraction; the lateral head is felt when the patient attempts abduction; by pushing the hand forward (as to put keys in a cars ignition) the anterior head is palpated to assess for contraction.

any proposed surgical procedure. Previous surgical approaches should be noted in the context of additional surgery. These incisions can be utilized, partially incorporated into an approach, or ignored due to the excellent vascularity about the shoulder.

Regardless of the arthroplasty option being considered, a functional deltoid is necessary. Examination should first include visual inspection of the deltoid to evaluate for atrophy. The shoulder should be examined with direct comparison to the contralateral side.

Assessment for disuse atrophy should be made while the examiner inspects the anterior, lateral, and posterior heads of the deltoid. If previous surgery has been performed, any relationship of atrophy to previous incisions should be noted. If a surgical approach included a deltoid split, it is possible that the portion anterior to the split could be denervated with selective atrophy noted.

During the palpation portion of the physical examination, the deltoid should be examined for contraction with use. Even a poorly functioning shoulder can typically be examined for function of all three portions of the deltoid. The examiner can place one hand over the deltoid while using the other hand to support the forearm **(FIGURE 31.2)**. From this position, the patient may extend, abduct, and flex to assess the posterior, middle, and anterior deltoid, respectively. The examiner should also assess sensation over the lateral deltoid, although that is not always reliable to confirm axillary nerve function. When there is a question or concern for an axillary nerve injury, electrodiagnostic studies should be obtained.

If there is concern about the status of the deltoid after the physical examination, additional imaging such as ultrasound or magnetic resonance imaging (MRI) may be considered to visualize the muscle itself. Nerve conduction studies (NCS) and electromyograms (EMGs) can be performed to assess muscle and nerve function. Even though these tests may provide more information about the deltoid, the surgeon should consider treatment options other than arthroplasty if the deltoid demonstrates severe dysfunction upon inspection and physical examination.[31-33]

A patient with tuberosity malunion or nonunion will likely show deficits during the physical examination. The tuberosity position and examination findings help determine possible future interventions. Patients with greater tuberosity malunion or nonunion will likely show weakness on resisted external rotation with the arm at the side. Additionally, an external rotation lag sign may be present with severe malposition or nonunion of the greater tuberosity. These patients will usually lack active external rotation, and passive external rotation may be limited by the blocking effect of the greater tuberosity malposition. Those with lesser tuberosity malunion generally show weakness with internal rotation based upon assessment by the belly-press maneuver, bear hug test, and lift-off test. These findings may be difficult to distinguish clinically from rotator cuff compromise.

Depending on a patient's ability to compensate with their deltoid, the loss of the posterior or posterior-superior rotator cuff may also cause a loss of active external rotation. If this is severe, there can be significant difficulties getting the hand to the mouth with the arm at the side, as neutral rotation cannot be maintained and the hand "falls" to the abdomen. If possible, a patient may accommodate this by hyperabducting the shoulder, such that the rotation "bottoms out" with gravity and the hand can reach the mouth. This posturing forms the position of the "hornblower sign." Even with this accommodation, patients find it difficult to eat, especially with a spoon, as the utensil cannot be held horizontal.

IMAGING

The standard radiographic evaluation of the shoulder includes a Grashey view, scapular Y, and an axillary view. These images will provide reasonable visualization of most proximal humeral anatomy including malunions and nonunions. The glenoid can also be visualized although less well.

If surgical intervention is being considered, a three-dimensional (3D) computed tomography (CT) scan of the shoulder is very important. This study allows for a more thorough evaluation of the fracture fragments, as well as the position of the tuberosities and articular surface. It also provides some information of the rotator cuff musculature and often provides a good indication of rotator cuff tendon status. A standard CT scan may be performed without 3D reconstructions. However, the 3D reconstruction provides a more thorough understanding of the relevant anatomy. If metallic hardware is in place, Metal Artifact Reduction Software (MARS) is essential for proper visualization of the shoulder. This algorithm is sometimes both hardware and software dependent and cannot be done after the study is acquired. It is important that the ordering physician understand these constraints so that MARS is ordered and utilized when needed to avoid the need for a second study with the associated additional cost and radiation exposure.

While most facilities completing a CT scan will create selected 3D images for the study, it is more valuable for the surgeon to be able to choose the perspective and "drive" the 3D reconstructions themselves. This can be done on some workstations but often is difficult and/or requires the surgeon to be at the main facility where the study was done. A simpler and yet more powerful way to select the perspective of the 3D images is for the surgeon to perform the reconstruction on their own. All CT scanners can export the raw axial data in Digital Imaging and Communication in Medicine (DICOM) format. The highest quality (thinnest cut) data should be obtained by the surgeon and can be manipulated in a DICOM viewer. If there is data with MARS, it should be utilized. Open-source software for both PCs (Radiant: www.radiantviewer.com) and Mac (Horos: www.horosproject.org) are available. The DICOM data can be uploaded to these programs, and 3D reconstructions can be created and manipulated. Experienced users will be able to subtract bone, change perspective, and make measurements on their personal computers.

MRI is not always needed, even when surgery is planned, but may be considered to better evaluate for ON and rotator cuff tendon and muscle compromise.

Nuclear medicine studies may be considered but typically do not add to the treatment plan. Three-phase bone scans will show nonunion and degenerative changes postoperatively, but these are typically well understood from standard radiographs and CT scans. Indolent infections are not readily diagnosed with a three-phase bone scan, and the addition of indium labeling of the white blood cells does not add enough specificity or sensitivity to make it valuable.[34]

LABORATORY STUDIES

Routine laboratory studies prior to arthroplasty reconstruction are typically performed at the surgeon's discretion. Modern arthroplasty techniques, especially the use of tranexamic acid, have nearly eliminated the need for transfusions during or after even extensive arthroplasty reconstructions. Despite this, it is typically advisable to have a preoperative complete blood count (hemoglobin/hematocrit), in case blood loss exceeds expectations.

When previous fracture surgery is being evaluated for reconstruction with a shoulder arthroplasty, one does need to consider that there may be an indolent infection. Laboratory evaluation with an erythrocyte sedimentation rate (ESR), C-reactive protein (CRP), and white blood count (WBC) with differential will provide a baseline but typically are normal, especially when an indolent infection is present.[34]

The most common postoperative infections in the shoulder are from *Cutibacterium acnes* (approximately 39%) and are notoriously difficult to diagnose, especially preoperatively.[34-36] As noted, standard laboratory tests are typically normal. Aspiration of the joint may show high specificity and positive predictive value (PPV) but low specificity and negative predictive value (NPV). Thus, a positive result may be quite useful in guiding treatment, but a negative result does not rule out infection.[37]

Cultures from aspiration need to be held for at least 14 days on aerobic, anaerobic, and broth media.[35] Recent investigations into IL-6 and leukocyte esterase for synovial samples have yet to yield readily available reliable testing.[38,39] Alpha defensin measurement (Synovasure—Zimmer/Biomet, Warsaw IN) is commercially available but has been met with mixed literature reviews.[40]

Next-generation sequencing (NGS), in which the bacterial genome is identified, has been reported for diagnostic use in periprosthetic joint infection (PJI).[41-44] While this technique is intellectually appealing, its clinical use is still evolving. When NGS is performed in native shoulders during arthroplasty, more bacteria are identified compared to culture results.[45] This may be due to dead bacteria, or there may be a normal bacterial load in synovial joints that is yet to be understood. The study of the microbiome of specific parts of the body, including synovial joints, has demonstrated that few places in the body are truly sterile. Some investigators believe that there may be a role of bacteria as a causative agent in arthritis.[46]

INFECTION (ALSO ADDRESSED IN CHAPTERS 32 AND 49)

The first concern to address if one is considering arthroplasty for PFS reconstruction is that of infection. When surgical treatment of proximal humeral fractures fails, one must always consider the possibility of an underlying infection. If infection has been ruled out, or infection has been treated as outlined below, then one can proceed to reconstruction based on the structural pathology, with specific attention to the soft tissue envelope of the proximal humerus.

Many postoperative infections about the shoulder are clinically clear, especially when they occur early.

Indolent infections are much more difficult to diagnose. Therefore, it is important to have a high index of suspicion when evaluating failed proximal humerus fracture treatments. The rate of low-grade infection after fracture fixation in the shoulder may be higher than after fracture fixation of hips and knees.[47]

A painful or dysfunctional shoulder after treatment for fracture which is obviously infected needs to be aggressively treated. The more common and difficult presentation is the failed fracture fixation or primary arthroplasty for fracture with an indolent infection.

The shoulder which is clearly infected will typically have pain, erythema, swelling, and induration. The laboratory workup will often be notable for increased CRP, ESR, and a high WBC count with increased neutrophils. Drainage and/or sinus tracts may be present. Aspiration will usually yield grossly purulent fluid that can be analyzed for cell count and differential. Clinical scenarios like this are often infected with a staph species or a gram-negative bacterium.

An obvious infection in a posttraumatic proximal humerus fracture which will undergo eventual arthroplasty must first undergo aggressive debridement including hardware removal. A decision has to be made as to a single-stage reconstruction with immediate implantation or a multistage reconstruction with delayed final implantation.[36,47-50] When delayed implantation is chosen, a polymethyl methacrylate (PMMA) spacer is placed to maintain the resection space, afford some support/stability, and provide antibiotics via elution.

The more common clinical situation in a posttraumatic shoulder is one of an indolent infection. The shoulder surgeon should have a high index of suspicion for infection when evaluating failed proximal humeral fracture fixation. This is not typically a clear clinical presentation as laboratory studies (CBC, ESR, CRP) are typically negative, nuclear medicine studies such as Indium labeled WBC scans are negative, and joint aspirations have negative gram stains and cultures. As noted, newer tests, including interleukin six (IL-6), alpha defensin, leukocyte esterase, and NGS, are evolving as methods of diagnosing infection. In these situations, the surgeon can consider attempting to answer the infection question with a less invasive approach such as joint aspiration or arthroscopic evaluation.[37] If a less invasive approach could change the treatment plan, it should be considered. Typically, it is useful if one can prove that a painful shoulder is not infected, then a progression to reconstruction based on the pathology can be performed in a single stage. The concern with this approach is the potential for false negatives from a joint aspiration or arthroscopic tissue acquisition. If the diagnostic workup demonstrates absence of infection and a reconstruction is undertaken only to have positive intraoperative cultures from deeper tissue, a dilemma is created. The possibility of a false negative leading to a reconstruction in

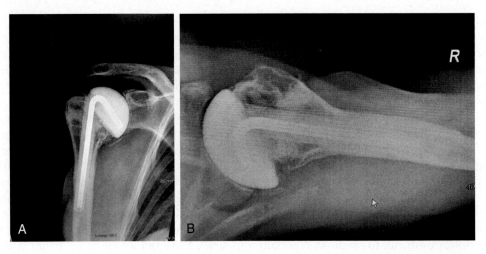

FIGURE 31.3 This patient presented with a draining wound and failed open reduction and internal fixation (ORIF) of a proximal humerus fracture. Despite removal of hardware and debridement, she required humeral head excision and polymethyl methacrylate (PMMA) spacer. She recovered well and decided not to proceed with a second-stage procedure. 5.5 years after placement of the PMMA spacer anteroposterior (AP) (**A**) and axillary (**B**) radiographs demonstrate a commercially made PMMA spacer. It is centrally reduced on the glenoid.

the face of an indolent infection supports the logic of treating any possible infection with an interval PMMA spacer.

Single-stage treatment of a known infection, utilizing complete component removal, debridement, and reimplantation is an emerging concept with some recent literature supporting its practice. Stone et al showed similar low reinfection rates with a single-stage procedure. However, reinfection rates were higher in those with *Staphylococcus aureus* or coagulase-negative *Staphylococcus* species, suggesting additional procedures may be required in these patients.[48,49,51]

Single-stage treatment of an uncertain or suspected infection consists of removal of any hardware, aggressive debridement, and final arthroplasty reconstruction. Postoperative antibiotics should be administered until final cultures are obtained, which is at 2 to 3 weeks.[48] This approach probably has a higher risk of failure. Therefore, it is helpful in these situations to discuss preoperatively with the patient and infectious disease specialist as to what the plan will be if the intraoperative cultures are positive for infection. Will the debridement and short course of antibiotics be considered sufficient and the patient then be followed off antibiotics, or will the patient be treated for a full course and then followed closely, or will lifetime suppression be utilized? Having a plan defined preoperatively will help patient compliance with treatment and avoids disappointment that they are not finished with treatment following the surgery.

Multistage treatment of infections is preferred by most surgeons.[50] We typically proceed with a multistage option when the goal is complete eradication of the infection, a long-life expectancy for the patient, and a desire to eventually discontinue all antibiotics. A multistage operation will allow for antibiotic treatment to be tailored to a defined organism for the appropriate

duration, and clearance of the infection can be confirmed either at the time of final implantation or during an intermediary stage.

The first-stage of a multistage revision for infection includes aggressive debridement with hardware removal. A PMMA HA spacer is placed with a broad-spectrum antibiotic delivered from the device via elution. Antibiotics placed in the device are typically gentamycin, tobramycin, or vancomycin; or some combination of the three. Infectious disease consultation is typically obtained to determine the best choice. These antibiotic PMMA hemiarthroplasties can be made in the operating room from molds and are also commercially manufactured. We prefer the commercially manufactured because of time saved, increased strength, and better elution of antibiotics.[52,53]

The PMMA spacer maintains the resection gap, preventing contraction of tissues, keeps the tissue planes defined, all of which will ease the second-stage dissection and implantation. While the spacers can enhance stability and function, some are surprisingly pain free and functional. There are some patients, typically those with long and protracted previous courses, who experience enough pain relief and improved function with a PMMA spacer in place that they choose to accept the spacer as definitive treatment. While this is an off-label use of any commercial device and neither the commercially available or back table assembled devices are designed for long-term use, this approach is reasonable and has shown good longevity in some patients[53] **(FIGURE 31.3)**.

The standard treatment after stage one is to change from the broad-spectrum antibiotic that was started immediately postoperatively to a more tailored approach, based on the data from the operating room and culture results. The majority of infections are from *C. acnes*, which typically does not grow in cultures until 11 days or more after surgery.[34,37,42] This requires that all cultures should be held for 2 to 3 weeks. Sonication of the implant has been demonstrated to improve culture results, although this technology is not universally available.[54,55] The postoperative delay until culture results are available has led to interest in deoxyribonucleic acid (DNA) analysis of tissue from revisions to more quickly identify the pathogens and allow for earlier specific and directed antibiotic therapy. Polymerase chain reaction (PCR) results are typically returned in 48 hours, with next-generation sequencing (NGS) results obtained in approximately 1 week.[41-45]

Oral antibiotics are administered after a predefined intravenous (IV) regimen. There is divergence of opinion on when to proceed with the second stage. Some surgeons wait for a specific time off all antibiotics, allow the ESR and CRP to normalize, and then proceed with final implantation as a second and final stage. Some surgeons aspirate the joint off antibiotics to assess for persistent infection. The more cautious approach is to carry out a PMMA spacer exchange off antibiotics, obtaining deep tissue cultures, and/or DNA analysis to confirm the infection is eradicated before proceeding to the third and final stage.[50] If there is still infection at this intermediary second-stage, then the process of antibiotic treatment can be repeated, until the infection is eradicated allowing reimplantation to proceed. After an infection has been treated, whether in a single or multistage process, the final arthroplasty reconstruction will be determined by the remaining bony and soft tissue status.

DYSFUNCTION AFTER FRACTURE FROM NONSKELETAL ISSUES

Arthroplasty for PFS requires the surgeon to carefully assess the bony and soft tissue anatomy of the glenohumeral joint and the surrounding tissues. ATSA requires a well-functioning rotator cuff and deltoid, while RTSA requires only a well-functioning deltoid to work. A complete absence of the rotator cuff may limit rotation, although the deltoid may provide some compensation. The role of tendon transfers to restore external rotation following RTSA is evolving.[56] The needed muscle-tendon units must have intact innervation, intact or reconstructable insertions, and functional excursion. Soft tissue pathologies that will affect proximal humeral fracture recovery and function include nerve injuries, primary tendon dysfunction, and joint stiffness.

Neurologic

Nerve injuries can occur primarily from fractures and secondarily after surgical intervention. A history of a fracture-dislocation, especially one with prolonged pressure on the axillary nerve from a dislocated humeral head or difficult extraction of a humeral head incarcerated in the axilla should alert the surgeon to the possibility of an axillary nerve abnormality. Lateral deltopectoral approaches, long deltoid splitting approaches, and anterior deltoid atrophy anterior to surgical approaches should alert one to the possibility of denervation of part of the deltoid.

If there is dysfunction of the axillary nerve and all three heads of the deltoid are not functioning adequately, no type of shoulder arthroplasty will be successful. The options for treatment of an axillary nerve injury in the setting of PFS include waiting for recovery and proceeding with "standard" reconstruction, exploration, and neurolysis/repair of the axillary nerve, transferring a branch of the radial nerve and tendon/muscle transfers. If the axillary nerve and/or deltoid cannot be restored or the function replaced, an arthroplasty should not be performed. Options would include nonoperative management, resection arthroplasty, or glenohumeral arthrodesis. Neurological injuries around the shoulder are discussed in Chapter 39.

Rotator Cuff Dysfunction

If one is considering an ATSA, the rotator cuff should be near normal in its function. If this is not the case, RTSA is the preferred option. Rotator cuff dysfunction may occur from pathologies other than nerve injury. There may be loss of the rotator cuff tendon insertions due to tuberosity malunion or osteolysis. The rotator cuff may have been torn as a result of the injury that caused the initial fracture, or there may have been an acute on chronic rotator cuff injury, such that a well-compensated proximal humerus becomes dysfunctional after a fracture.

Evaluation should examine for rotator cuff dysfunction, especially loss of active external rotation. If this exists, one can consider a latissimus dorsi tendon transfer, although due to the changes in mechanics of a reverse shoulder arthroplasty, this may not be needed.[56]

Severe Stiffness, Contracture, and Loss of Motion

If a surgeon is considering reconstruction with an ATSA, not only will a functional rotator cuff be needed but also the proximal humerus and rotator cuff will need to move independently of the deltoid. When there is severe loss of motion and no apparent independent motion of the rotator cuff and deltoid, one has to consider if surgical dissection of the pathology will result in recovery of this independent motion and recovery of function of the rotator cuff. In these situations, MRI examination of the rotator cuff is helpful to ensure that a potential tissue plane exists between a functional rotator cuff and the deltoid. If the surgeon finds that a release of a severely contracted shoulder can only be done by releasing the rotator cuff, then an RTSA will be necessary.

NONUNION AND MALUNION

Malunion of the proximal humerus may be tolerated when not severe or if functional demands are limited.[3,4] A nonunion may be asymptomatic and well tolerated, but

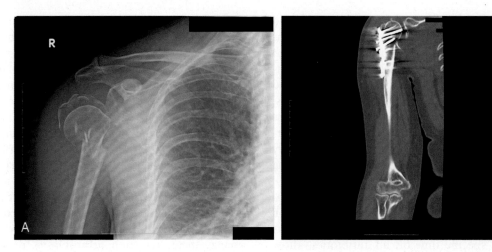

FIGURE 31.4 This 55-year-old woman fell while hiking. **A,** Imaging revealed a head-splitting proximal humerus fracture with vagus impaction of the majority of the head, displacement of the tuberosities, and comminution at the surgical neck. Open reduction and internal fixation (ORIF) was performed emergently. **B,** Follow-up upon her return home prompted a computed tomography (CT) scan, which demonstrated loss of fixation with backing out of the locking screws and penetration of the fixation through the humeral head.

this is uncommon. Fracture malunion and nonunions can occur at different sites including the tuberosities, surgical neck, anatomic neck, or a combination of these.[22,57] The head fragment may be in a single piece, fractured at the anatomic neck level, or have intra-articular components. Nonunion also will typically have pain generated from motion of the ununited fragment. Pain and dysfunction can be from rotator cuff dysfunction, mechanical impingement of the tuberosities, altered mechanics of the shoulder, and soft tissue scaring and contracture (both intrinsic and extrinsic). There are no absolute indicators of significance: a malunion or nonunion are significant when there is dysfunction that the patient finds meaningful.

Isolated osteotomy for malunited proximal humeral fractures can result in improvements in both pain and function when performed in the proper setting, with attention to soft tissue as well as the bony deformity.[20,58] Surgical neck nonunions (Boileau type 3) in patients with adequate bone should be treated with bone grafting and rigid fixation.[21] For complex clinical situations with nonunion or malunion of the proximal humerus, especially in the lower demand patient, arthroplasty is often the preferred solution. When considering arthroplasty for the treatment of proximal humeral nonunion or malunion, a key factor is the status of the rotator cuff and the tuberosities. Osteotomy of the tuberosity combined with arthroplasty has been unsuccessful in all but one study in which no impact was noted.[21,22,57,59-62] When the decision is made to proceed with arthroplasty of the shoulder, the surgeon must decide between an anatomic or reverse prosthesis.

HA AND ATSA

Intracapsular PFS in Boileau classification (types 1 and 2) carry the treatment recommendation of ATSA. Further studies have refined these recommendations to consider the use of RTSA when there is rotator cuff

atrophy and when there is varus malalignment of the proximal humerus, which would require placing the humeral implant in varus position.[26,27,61]

Normal or near-normal rotator cuff tissue and function, in addition to normal, or well-aligned tuberosities are necessary for a successful HA or ATSA. In the rare situation in which the malunion or nonunion is limited to the articular surface and the glenoid anatomy is normal, an HA can provide a successful outcome as long as the rotator cuff is functional. A proximal humeral nonunion/malunion that is amenable to a humeral prosthesis may also have posttraumatic glenoid changes. This clinical situation is most likely encountered after failed ORIF in which protruding screws have damaged the glenoid. In this situation, an ATSA can be considered **(FIGURE 31.4)**.

If the posttraumatic process involves a tuberosity malunion/nonunion that is reconstructable, an ATSA can be considered. While restoring anatomy to normal is typically the goal for a posttraumatic reconstruction, one has to be cognizant that tuberosity osteotomy to correct a malunion or tuberosity repair to correct a nonunion is generally not as reliable with either HA or ATSA.[21,22,57,59-61] One reconstructive solution for tuberosity malunion is to position the humeral head component in a "best fit" position, keeping the head centered in the glenoid and 5 to 10 mm above the greater tuberosity.[26,59-62] Early prosthetic designs required alteration in the entry point of the stem, into the canal, downsizing the stem, and/or utilizing cement. Modern modular components with variable offset from the stem now make this technique more reproducible and avoid the need to cement a downsized stem.

REVERSE TOTAL SHOULDER ARTHROPLASTY

RTSA does not require normal tuberosities or an intact and functional rotator cuff. Deltoid function must be present or restored for an RTSA to function. Due to

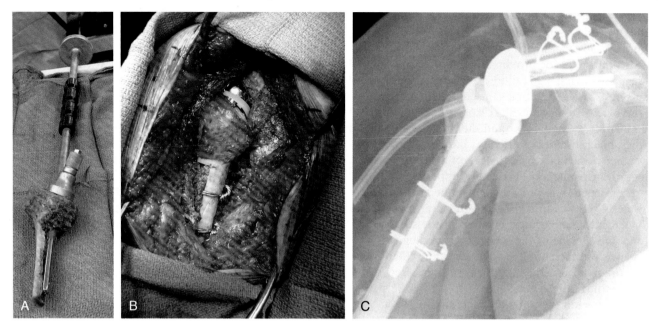

FIGURE 31.5 Allograft prosthetic component (APC) reconstruction of the proximal humerus. **A**, A proximal humeral allograft is prepared with the final humeral stem cemented in place on the back table. Cancellous or morselized cortical allograft bone is placed at the interface prior to insertion. A flange of cortical bone projects beyond the circumferential bone and the tuberosities are left intact. **B**, The APC construct is cemented into host bone, and bone graft is placed under and around the flange, in addition to the interface. The flange of bone is secured with cerclage fixation, and if possible, with a plate (this construct was short, and good proximal fixation would not be obtained, so a plate was used). **C**, Postoperative radiograph shows the well-approximated interface. There are more than two shaft diameters of flange overlapping host humerus.

extrinsic contractures between the deltoid and rotator cuff in PFS, extensive releases are often required. If the rotator cuff is not functional or is heavily scared with extensive adhesions, the proximal humerus may need to be skeletonized to allow for reconstruction with maximized range of motion. Aggressive release must be balanced with tendon retention as the more functional rotator cuff that remains attached to an RTSA, the more active range of motion expected from the reconstruction. Releasing all the soft tissue attachments to the proximal humerus will increase the risk of instability. However, even if all of the soft tissue is released, normal or near-normal tuberosities should contribute to stability due to the "deltoid wrap" effect.[63]

Raiss et al have shown an unacceptably high rate of dislocation when the tuberosities are resected. Thus, the tuberosities and rotator cuff should be preserved whenever possible to improve outcomes and decrease complications.[28]

If the deformity from the posttraumatic process is not severe, an RTSA can be performed without addressing the tuberosities.[27,61] Severe deformity of the tuberosities as seen in Boileau type 4 fractures have been treated with osteotomy with some success.[30] But, as in ATSA, most studies demonstrate high rates of complications such as nonunion and dislocation when tuberosity osteotomy is combined with RTSA.[23,25,28,64] Boileau initially recommended RTSA for category 2—ie, extracapsular pathology.[22] This included both

surgical neck nonunions and extracapsular fractures, which would also require tuberosity osteotomy. Later recommendations were altered to recommend fixation with bone grafting for type 3 pathology (surgical neck nonunions), leaving RTSA for extracapsular fractures with severe tuberosity displacement.[21] Resorption and nonunion of the tuberosities in type 3 PFS are problematic because it increases the risk of instability following RTSA.[23,28] While Boileau eventually recommended RTSA only for type 4 pathology, other authors have reported good results when RTSA is for type 1 and type 2 pathology.[27,61] Type 1 fractures with varus deformity have been shown to do poorly following ATSA and, as a result, RTSA should also be considered for these intracapsular injuries.[26]

Depending on the soft tissue envelope, the tuberosity malunion, and the overall deformity of the shoulder, it is possible, although uncommon, that the entire proximal humerus, with tuberosities, will need to be resected. This is especially true in varus deformity, as any "head cut" of substance will remove at least a portion of the tuberosities. It is also possible that even if the tuberosities remain that the posttraumatic deformity is significant enough to preclude a useful deltoid wrap. In this situation, there are two options for tuberosity reconstruction. An allograft prosthetic composite (APC) will not only support the prosthesis but will also provide the important "deltoid wrap" from the tuberosities, which improves stability and function **(FIGURE 31.5)**. Although

APCs provide the required anatomy of the proximal humerus, the results have been marginal. Martinez reported a 50% failure rate in six APCs combined with RTSA performed for proximal humeral nonunion.[65] In addition to having high failure rates due to infection and resorption, APCs are time-consuming procedures due to the extensive amount of "carpentry" required to fit the allograft to the patient and the prosthesis. Fixation of the humeral stem typically has little to no rotational resistance, which increases the risk of a nonunion at the allograft-host junction. The other option for tuberosity reconstruction is prosthetic. A humeral replacement prosthesis (HRP) utilizes the prosthetic proximal body to replace the tuberosities. Fixation of the stem is both within and outside of the humerus, providing torsional resistance and increasing angular strength **(VIDEO 31.1)**. The proximal humeral body has variably sized tuberosities, which allows the surgeon to create the proper amount of deltoid wrap and attach any functional soft tissue for additional stability **(FIGURE 31.6)**.

OSTEONECROSIS AND POSTTRAUMATIC ARTHRITIS

Patients who sustain a proximal humerus fracture may initially have a period of healing and improved function. Some eventually develop changes affecting the articular surface, which results in increased pain and loss of function. Osteonecrosis (ON) is a complication resulting from damage to the blood supply to the humeral head. Reports in the literature suggest this may occur in up to 75% of displaced 4-part fractures, with other studies reporting much lower incidences in the 15% to 30% range. There is likely a lower incidence in less complex fracture patterns, and the differences may also reflect how fractures are classified.[66,67] Recent literature has suggested that the posterior humeral circumflex artery is the dominant blood supply representing 64% of the blood supply to the humeral head.[68] Fracture patterns with long medial metaphyseal fragments greater than 8 mm are associated with a lower incidence of ON. Additionally, simple fracture patterns, an intact medial hinge, angular displacement less than 45°, absence of a dislocation or head-split, and tuberosity displacement less than 10 mm have also been shown to be protective against ON.[69]

Early diagnosis of humeral head ON may present options to preserve the articular surface,[70] but this is less likely to be possible when the etiology is posttraumatic. If the area of ON is significant and progresses to collapse, it will eventually lead to glenohumeral arthritis. Arthroplasty treatment prior to involvement of the glenoid can involve just the humeral head, with partial or total resurfacing, stemless humeral devices, or stemmed HA, depending on the proximal humerus anatomy, the extent of the ON, and the implants available. While literature has demonstrated that in glenohumeral arthritis, an ATSA is more reliable than an HA, ON may present a unique indication where HA can be considered if the glenoid is completely uninvolved.[71] When reconstructing with a HA, if a stemmed device is used, it should be a platform stem, such that conversion to an ATSA or RTSA can be done if glenoid degeneration develops. In addition, preoperative discussion with the patient should include the possibility of an ATSA if significant glenoid involvement is encountered. Just as in ATSA for glenohumeral arthritis, resurfacing the glenoid when there are glenoid degenerative changes from ON results in better outcomes than HA.[71]

When ON occurs following ORIF, screw protrusion often results in damage to the glenoid necessitating resurfacing of the humeral head and the glenoid. ATSA can be considered if the tuberosities are well-aligned and the rotator cuff functions well. However, ON with collapse in the presence of tuberosity malalignment, proximal humeral deformity, and compromised rotator cuff function is best treated by RTSA **(FIGURE 31.7)**.

AUTHORS' RECOMMENDATIONS AND TECHNIQUES

After a thorough history and physical examination as detailed above, any decision to proceed with arthroplasty for PFS is made jointly with the patient. Expected as well as contingency operative plans are outlined, and expectations for surgery, recovery, and outcomes are discussed. The possibility of infection is always considered and worked through as described above.

When deciding on treatment options, it is helpful to consider the status of the rotator cuff, tuberosities, and deltoid. These findings, combined with the presence or absence of scarring, will direct the selection of the preferred treatment from the options of HA, ATSA, RTSA, or HRP RTSA **(TABLE 31.1)**.

Tuberosity Osteotomy

It is our preference to avoid tuberosity osteotomy in PFS treated by arthroplasty. In younger patients with higher functional demands, if the prosthetic humeral head cannot be adjusted to a tuberosity malunion as described above, tuberosity osteotomy can be considered **(FIGURE 31.8)**. However, these situations are uncommon. If indicated, the patient should have an understanding of the required postoperative management and the anticipated outcomes. Tuberosity repair is performed using the techniques described by Boileau for tuberosity fixation in acute fractures with fixation of the tuberosities around the stem.[72] Tuberosity osteotomy is performed using the bicipital groove as a guide between the greater and lesser tuberosity. After osteotomy, soft tissue releases should be performed, including the rotator interval, middle glenohumeral ligament, and the inferior glenohumeral ligament. Four horizontal mattress nonabsorbable doubled/looped sutures are placed around the greater tuberosity at the bone/

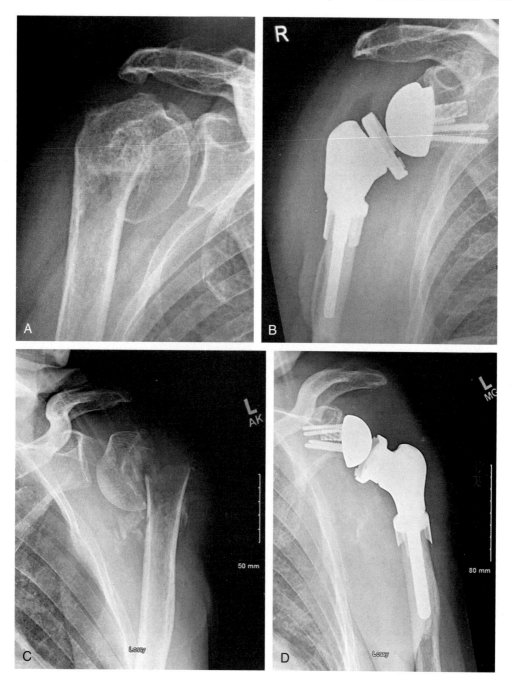

FIGURE 31.6 This woman sustained a proximal humeral fracture from a ground-level fall. After 8 months of nonoperative treatment, she had continued pain and limited motion. Active forward flexion was to 75°, with active external rotation of zero. **A,** Preoperative radiograph demonstrates what is best described as a Boileau type 1 injury, as it was intracapsular without a dislocation component. The head is in severe varus with an intra-articular split. **B,** Postoperative radiograph after humeral reconstruction prosthesis (HRP). This reconstruction was chosen to avoid tuberosity osteotomy/fixation but still provides deltoid wrap. Four months after reconstruction, her pain was minimal, active forward flexion was 100° and external rotation was 20°. This 76-year-old male presented 6 months following left proximal humerus fracture that was treated nonoperatively, 6 months prior. Examination showed a flail shoulder, with elevation of the arm only through scapular motion. His axillary nerve function was intact. **C,** Preoperative radiographs showing two-part, surgical neck nonunion with complete discontinuity. **D,** Postoperative radiographs showing HRP. Consideration was given to surgical fixation of the nonunion with plating and bone graft. However, given his age and activity level, reverse shoulder replacement with humeral reconstruction prosthesis was elected.

tendon interface, two superiorly and two inferiorly. These sutures must freely slide. Two vertical cerclage sutures are then placed into bone tunnels on either side of the bicipital groove and into the humeral canal. The

humeral implant is then placed in proper position, with 5 to 6 cm between the superior portion of the humeral head and the upper border of the pectoralis tendon insertion.[73] After proper placement, the four doubled/

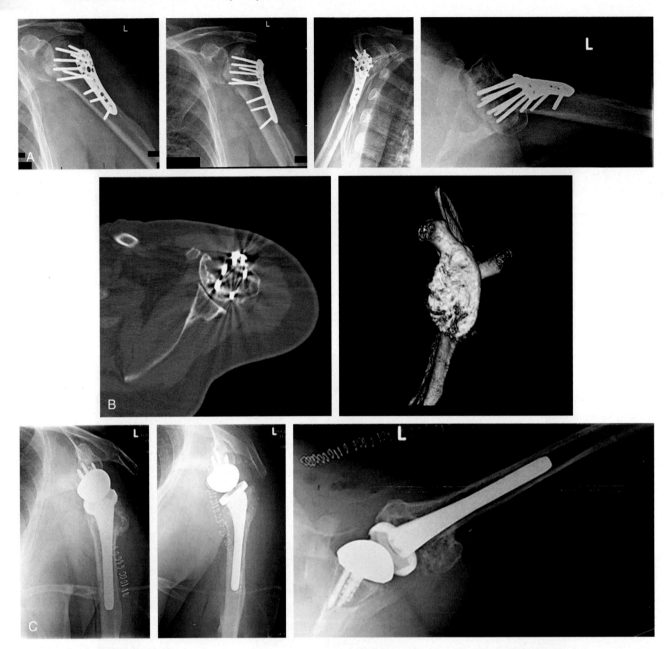

FIGURE 31.7 A, A 69-year-old male 2 years after open reduction and internal fixation (ORIF) of the proximal humerus. **B**, Osteonecrosis (ON) developed with flattening of the head and secondary glenoid changes. **C**, The combination of posttraumatic arthritis and tuberosity malunion made reverse total shoulder arthroplasty (RTSA) the preferred procedure.

TABLE 31.1 Arthroplasty Requirements for Postfracture Sequelae (PFS)

	Functional RTC Necessary	Normal or Near-Normal Tuberosity Profile	Severe Preoperative Scarring and/or Stiffness	Deltoid Function Needed
Hemiarthroplasty	✔	✔		✔
Anatomic total shoulder arthroplasty (ATSA)	✔	✔		✔
Reverse total shoulder arthroplasty (RTSA)		✔	✔	✔
Humeral replacement prosthetic (HRP) reverse total shoulder arthroplasty			✔	✔

The options for arthroplasty are dependent on the function of the rotator cuff and deltoid, the presence or absence of severe stiffness/scaring and tuberosity anatomy.

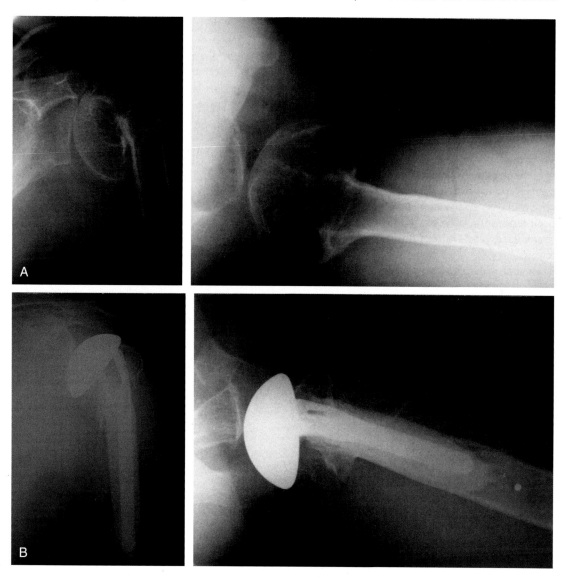

FIGURE 31.8 This 52-year-old woman was 2 years after this proximal humerus fracture treated nonoperatively. **A**, With varus malunion, she was very active and desired to return to swimming. The glenoid was not involved. **B**, Corrective osteotomy was performed to restore alignment with a cemented hemiarthroplasty. Varus malunion after a proximal humerus fracture with glenohumeral arthritis cannot be treated with a standard arthroplasty unless the tuberosities are osteotomized.

looped horizontal cerclage sutures are wrapped around the humeral implant, and the joint is reduced. Two of the horizontal cerclage sutures are then tightened and tied, positioning the greater tuberosity 5 mm below the superior surface of the humeral head. A racking hitch knot is tied.[74] The remaining double/looped cerclage sutures are then passed through the lesser tuberosity bone/tendon interface (superiorly and inferiorly) and then tied with the same racking hitch knot, pulling the lesser tuberosity to the humeral stem (**VIDEO 31.2**). Lastly, the vertical cerclage sutures from the humeral shaft are passed through the greater and lesser tuberosity bone/tendon interface and tied, further securing the fragments around the stem. After these steps, the tuberosities, stem, and shaft should all move as a continuous unit.

Anatomic Total Shoulder Arthroplasty

PFS with nondisplaced or minimally displaced tuberosities can be considered for ATSA. We consider minimally displaced tuberosities as those which will allow the prosthetic humeral head to be placed 5 to 10 mm above the greater tuberosity. The rotator cuff must have reasonably normal musculature, tendon insertions and excursion. Deformity is accommodated with a modular, stemmed device, with variable offset, or with a stemless device, which can be placed centered on the tuberosities, without concern for the relationship to the intramedullary canal. If there is slightly greater tuberosity malunion, but the construct otherwise looks functional, a concomitant acromioplasty can be considered.[20] Varus deformity is carefully evaluated, as stems placed in varus for type 1 patterns have demonstrated poor outcomes.[26] If the glenoid articular cartilage is intact, then an HA can be performed, but in most situations, glenoid replacement is necessary and preferred. If intraoperative findings show significant rotator cuff deficiency, then RTSA should be performed.

Pearls for ATSA

- Use a platform stem
- Consider a stemless device to accommodate malunion of tuberosities or surgical neck
- Plan subscapularis approach based on tuberosity shape: peel, tenotomy, osteotomy
- Evaluate any hardware's impact on rotator cuff status and function
- Varus deformity warrants consideration for reverse (see case 3a)
- Every planned ATSA for PFS should have an RTSA plan as backup
- Use offset head to adjust head 5 to 10 mm above tuberosity
- Consider acromioplasty if there is slightly more tuberosity malunion
- Tuberosity osteotomy should be done only in very selected situations and when the patient recognizes the difficulty in achieving a successful outcome

Reverse Total Shoulder Arthroplasty

Currently, our indications for a standard RTSA for PFS include any anatomy where a standard or short stem can be placed and achieve good fixation and when there is sufficient tuberosity anatomy to allow for deltoid wrap. Every attempt is made to maintain functional rotator cuff tissue attached, but often with complex fracture patterns or failed previous surgery, the rotator cuff is scarred and dysfunctional and must be released.

HRP stems are used when there is not a good deltoid wrap and in situations when the proximal humeral anatomy will not allow stem implantation without tuberosity osteotomy. It is not unusual for impacted, displaced three- and four-part malunions to have such scarring and deformity that a proximal humeral replacement is necessary due to both loss of proximal bone and severely displaced tuberosities. Surgical neck nonunions, as well as some malunions (especially those in varus), are also often treated with HRP. The availability of HRP implants has replaced the use of APCs in our practice. The additional time in the operating room for reconstruction with allograft, combined with the possibility of allograft resorption no longer makes this a preferred option.

Pearls for RTSA

- Variable offset glenospheres are beneficial to provide tension without lengthening

- Consider an HRP when tuberosities are deficient or osteotomy would be required
- Maintain functional rotator cuff when possible for stability and function but release as necessary for exposure and reduction
- A 4- to 6-week delay for any formal postoperative therapy may decrease the risk of stress fracture
- Altering the stem position as a result of the proximal humeral deformity may be acceptable

VIDEO 31.3: 5.5-year follow-up demonstrates functional motion with forward flexion of 145°, external rotation of 50°, and internal rotation of T12.

REFERENCES

1. Lopiz Y, Alcobía-Díaz B, Galán-Olleros M, García-Fernández C, Picado AL, Marco F. Reverse shoulder arthroplasty versus nonoperative treatment for 3- or 4-part proximal humeral fractures in elderly patients: a prospective randomized controlled trial. *J Shoulder Elbow Surg.* 2019;28(12):2259-2271.
2. Pinkas D, Wanich TS, DePalma AA, Gruson KI. Management of malunion of the proximal humerus: current concepts. *J Am Acad Orthop Surg.* 2014;22(8):491-502.
3. Rangan A, Handoll H, Brealey S, et al. Surgical vs nonsurgical treatment of adults with displaced fractures of the proximal humerus: the PROFHER randomized clinical trial. *J Am Med Assoc.* 2015;313(10):1037-1047.
4. Roberson TA, Granade CM, Hunt Q, et al. Nonoperative management versus reverse shoulder arthroplasty for treatment of 3- and 4-part proximal humeral fractures in older adults. *J Shoulder Elbow Surg.* 2017;26(6):1017-1022.
5. Chalmers PN, Slikker W, Mall NA, et al. Reverse total shoulder arthroplasty for acute proximal humeral fracture: comparison to open reduction-internal fixation and hemiarthroplasty. *J Shoulder Elbow Surg.* 2014;23(2):197-204.
6. Gallinet D, Clappaz P, Garbuio P, Tropet Y, Obert L. Three or four parts complex proximal humerus fractures: hemiarthroplasty versus reverse prosthesis. A comparative study of 40 cases. *Orthop Traumatol Surg Res.* 2009;95(1):48-55.
7. Garrigues GE, Johnston PS, Pepe MD, Tucker BS, Ramsey ML, Austin LS. Hemiarthroplasty versus reverse total shoulder arthroplasty for acute proximal humerus fractures in elderly patients. *Orthopedics.* 2012;35(5):e703-e708.
8. Boyle MJ, Youn SM, Frampton CMA, Ball CM. Functional outcomes of reverse shoulder arthroplasty compared with hemiarthroplasty for acute proximal humeral fractures. *J Shoulder Elbow Surg.* 2013;22(1):32-37.
9. Cuff DJ, Pupello DR. Comparison of hemiarthroplasty and reverse shoulder arthroplasty for the treatment of proximal humeral fractures in elderly patients. *J Bone Joint Surg Am.* 2013;95(22):2050-2055.
10. Sebastia-Forcada E, Cebrián-Gómez R, Lizaur-Utrilla A, Gil-Guillén V. Reverse shoulder arthroplasty versus hemiarthroplasty for acute proximal humeral fractures. A blinded, randomized, controlled, prospective study. *J Shoulder Elbow Surg.* 2014;23(10):1419-1426.
11. Olerud P, Ahrengart L, Ponzer S, Saving J, Tidermark J. Hemiarthroplasty versus nonoperative treatment of displaced 4-part proximal humeral fractures in elderly patients: a randomized controlled trial. *J Shoulder Elbow Surg.* 2011;20(7):1025-1033.
12. Boons HW, Goosen JH, van Grinsven S, van Susante JL, van Loon CJ. Hemiarthroplasty for humeral four-part fractures for patients 65 years and older: a randomized controlled trial. *Clin Orthop Relat Res.* 2012;470(12):3483-3491.
13. Norris TR, Green A, McGuigan FX. Late prosthetic shoulder arthroplasty for displaced proximal humerus fractures. *J Shoulder Elbow Surg.* 1995;4(4):271-280.
14. Torchia MT, Austin DC., Cozzolino N, Jacobowitz L, Bell JE. Acute versus delayed reverse total shoulder arthroplasty for the

treatment of proximal humeral fractures in the elderly population: a systematic review and meta-analysis. *J Shoulder Elbow Surg.* 2019;28(4):765-773.

15. Siegel JA, Dines DM. Techniques in managing proximal humeral malunions. *J Shoulder Elbow Surg.* 2003;12(1):69-78.

16. Hanson B, Neidenbach P, de Boer P, Stengel D. Functional outcomes after nonoperative management of fractures of the proximal humerus. *J Shoulder Elbow Surg.* 2009;18(4):612-621.

17. Torrens C, Corrales M, Vilà G, Santana F, Cáceres E. Functional and quality-of-life results of displaced and nondisplaced proximal humeral fractures treated conservatively. *J Orthop Trauma.* 2011;25(10):581-587.

18. Shannon SF, Wagner ER, Houdek MT, Cross WW, Sánchez-Sotelo J. Reverse shoulder arthroplasty for proximal humeral fractures: outcomes comparing primary reverse arthroplasty for fracture versus reverse arthroplasty after failed osteosynthesis. *J Shoulder Elbow Surg.* 2016;25(10):1655-1660.

19. Kristensen MR, Rasmussen JV, Elmengaard B, Jensen SL, Olsen BS, Brorson S. High risk for revision after shoulder arthroplasty for failed osteosynthesis of proximal humeral fractures. *Acta Orthop.* 2018;89(3):345-350.

20. Beredjiklian PK, Iannotti JP, Norris TR., Williams GR. Operative treatment of malunion of a fracture of the proximal aspect of the humerus. *J Bone Joint Surg Am.* 1998;80(10):1484-1497.

21. Boileau P, Trojani C, Chuinard C, Lehuec JC, Walch G. Proximal humerus fracture sequelae: impact of a new radiographic classification on arthroplasty. *Clin Orthop Relat Res.* 2006;442:121-130.

22. Boileau P, Trojani C, Walch G, Krishnan SG, Romeo A, Sinnerton R. Shoulder arthroplasty for the treatment of the sequelae of fractures of the proximal humerus. *J Shoulder Elbow Surg.* 2001;10(4):299-308.

23. Zafra M, Uceda P, Flores M, Carpintero P. Reverse total shoulder replacement for nonunion of a fracture of the proximal humerus. *Bone Joint J.* 2014;96(9):1239-1243.

24. Kilic M, Berth A, Blatter G, et al. Anatomic and reverse shoulder prostheses in fracture sequelae of the humeral head. *Acta Orthop Traumatol Turc.* 2010;44(6):417-425.

25. Martinez AA, Calvo A, Bejarano C, Carbonel I, Herrera A. The use of the Lima reverse shoulder arthroplasty for the treatment of fracture sequelae of the proximal humerus. *J Orthop Sci.* 2012;17(2):141-147.

26. Moineau G, McClelland WB, Trojani C, Rumian A, Walch G, Boileau P. Prognostic factors and limitations of anatomic shoulder arthroplasty for the treatment of posttraumatic cephalic collapse or necrosis (type-1 proximal humeral fracture sequelae). *J Bone Joint Surg Am.* 2012;94(23):2186-2194.

27. Alentorn-Geli E, Guirro P, Santana F, Torrens C. Treatment of fracture sequelae of the proximal humerus: comparison of hemiarthroplasty and reverse total shoulder arthroplasty. *Arch Orthop Trauma Surg.* 2014;134(11):1545-1550.

28. Raiss P, Edwards TB, da Silva MR, Bruckner T, Loew M, Walch G. Reverse shoulder arthroplasty for the treatment of nonunions of the surgical neck of the proximal part of the humerus (type-3 fracture sequelae). *J Bone Joint Surg Am.* 2014;96(24):2070-2076.

29. Mansat P, Bonnevialle N. Treatment of fracture sequelae of the proximal humerus: anatomical vs reverse shoulder prosthesis. *Int Orthop.* 2015;39(2):349-354.

30. Grubhofer F, Wieser K, Meyer DC, Catanzaro S, Schürholz K, Gerber C. Reverse total shoulder arthroplasty for failed open reduction and internal fixation of fractures of the proximal humerus. *J Shoulder Elbow Surg.* 2017;26(1):92-100.

31. Wagner ER, McLaughlin R, Sarfani S, Cofield RH, Sperling JW, Sanchez-Sotelo J, Elhassan BT. Long-term outcomes of glenohumeral arthrodesis. *J Bone Joint Surg Am.* 2018;100(7):598-604.

32. Smet LD. Bipolar latissimus dorsi flap transfer for reconstruction of the deltoid. *Acta Orthop Belg.* 2009;75(1):32-36.

33. Kotwal PP, Mittal R, Malhotra R. Trapezius transfer for deltoid paralysis. *J Bone Joint Surg Br.* 1998;80(1):114-116.

34. Paxton ES, Green A, Krueger VS. Periprosthetic infections of the shoulder: diagnosis and management. *J Am Acad Orthop Surg.* 2019;27(21):e935-e944.

35. Matsen FA III, Butler-Wu S, Carofino BC, Jette JL, Bertelsen A, Bumgarner R. Origin of propionibacterium in surgical wounds and evidence-based approach for culturing propionibacterium from surgical sites. *J Bone Joint Surg Am.* 2013;95(23):e1811-7.

36. Nelson GN, Davis DE, Namdari S. Outcomes in the treatment of periprosthetic joint infection after shoulder arthroplasty: a systematic review. *J Shoulder Elbow Surg.* 2016;25(8):1337-1345.

37. Dilisio MF, Miller LR, Warner JJP, Higgins LD. Arthroscopic tissue culture for the evaluation of periprosthetic shoulder infection. *J Bone Joint Surg Am.* 2014;96(23):1952-1958.

38. Villacis D, Merriman JA, Yalamanchili R, Omid R, Itamura J, Rick Hatch GF. Serum interleukin-6 as a marker of periprosthetic shoulder infection. *J Bone Joint Surg Am.* 2014;96(1):41-45.

39. Nelson GN, Paxton ES, Narzikul A, Williams G, Lazarus MD, Abboud JA. Leukocyte esterase in the diagnosis of shoulder periprosthetic joint infection. *J Shoulder Elbow Surg.* 2015;24(9):1421-1426.

40. Han X, Xie K, Jiang X, et al. Synovial fluid alpha-defensin in the diagnosis of periprosthetic joint infection: the lateral flow test is an effective intraoperative detection method. *J Orthop Surg Res.* 2019;14(1):274.

41. Tarabichi M, Alvand A, Shohat N, Goswami K, Parvizi J. Diagnosis of Streptococcus canis periprosthetic joint infection: the utility of next-generation sequencing. *Arthroplast Today.* 2018;4(1):20-23.

42. Namdari S, Nicholson T, Abboud J, et al. Comparative study of cultures and next-generation sequencing in the diagnosis of shoulder prosthetic joint infections. *J Shoulder Elbow Surg.* 2019;28(1):1-8.

43. Goswami K, Tarabichi M, Tan T, Shohat N, Alvand A, Parvizi J. Utility of next generation sequencing in the diagnosis of periprosthetic joint infection. *Orthop Proc.* 2019;101-B(4).

44. Goswami K, Parvizi J. Culture-negative periprosthetic joint infection: is there a diagnostic role for next-generation sequencing? *Expert Rev Mol Diagn.* 2020;20(3):269-272.

45. Rao AJ, MacLean IS, Naylor AJ, Garrigues GE, Verma NN, Nicholson GP. Next-generation sequencing for diagnosis of infection: is more sensitive really better? *J Shoulder Elbow Surg.* 2020;29(1):20-26.

46. Berthelot JM, Sellam J, Maugars Y, Berenbaum F. Cartilage-gut-microbiome axis: a new paradigm for novel therapeutic opportunities in osteoarthritis. *RMD Open.* 2019;5(2):e001037.

47. Klatte TO, Sabihi R, Guenther D, Kamath AF, Rueger JM, Gehrke T, Kendoff D. High rates of occult infection after shoulder fracture fixation: considerations for conversion shoulder arthroplasty. *HSS J.* 2015;11(3):198-203.

48. Hsu JE, Gorbaty JD, Whitney IJ, Matsen FA. Single-stage revision is effective for failed shoulder arthroplasty with positive cultures for propionibacterium. *J Bone Joint Surg Am.* 2016;98(24):2047-2051.

49. Stone GP, Clark RE, O'Brien KC, Vaccaro L, Simon P, Lorenzetti AJ, Stephens BC, Frankle MA. Surgical management of periprosthetic shoulder infections. *J Shoulder Elbow Surg.* 2017;26(7):1222-1229.

50. Tseng WJ, Lansdown DA, Grace T, Zhang AL, Feeley BT, Hung LW, Ma CB. Outcomes of revision arthroplasty for shoulder periprosthetic joint infection: a three-stage revision protocol. *J Shoulder Elbow Surg.* 2019;28(2):268-275.

51. Garrigues GE, Zmistowski B, Cooper AM, Green A; ICM Shoulder Group. Proceedings from the 2018 International Consensus Meeting on Orthopedic Infections: management of periprosthetic shoulder infection. *J Shoulder Elbow Surg.* 2019;28(6S):S67-S99.

52. Coffey MJ, Ely EE, Crosby LA. Treatment of glenohumeral sepsis with a commercially produced antibiotic-impregnated cement spacer. *J Shoulder Elbow Surg.* 2010;19(6):868-873.

53. Cronin KJ, Hayes CB, Sajadi KR. Antibiotic cement spacer retention for chronic shoulder infection after minimum 2-year follow-up. *J Shoulder Elbow Surg.* 2020;29(9):e325-e329.

54. Kobayashi N, Bauer TW, Tuohy MJ, Fujishiro T, Procop GW. Brief ultrasonication improves detection of biofilm-formative bacteria around a metal implant. *Clin Orthop Relat Res.* 2007;457:210-213.

55. Esteban J, Gomez-Barrena E, Cordero J, Martin-de-Hijas NZ, Kinnari TJ, Fernandez-Roblas R. Evaluation of quantitative analysis of cultures from sonicated retrieved orthopedic implants in diagnosis of orthopedic infection. *J Clin Microbiol.* 2008;46(2):488-492.

56. Young BL, Connor PM, Schiffern SC, Roberts KM, Hamid N. Reverse shoulder arthroplasty with and without latissimus and teres major

transfer for patients with combined loss of elevation and external rotation: a prospective, randomized investigation. *J Shoulder Elbow Surg.* 2020;29(5):874-881.

57. Dines DM, Warren RF, Altchek DW, Moeckel B. Posttraumatic changes of the proximal humerus: malunion, nonunion, and osteonecrosis. Treatment with modular hemiarthroplasty or total shoulder arthroplasty. *J Shoulder Elbow Surg.* 1993;2(1):11-21.

58. Benegas E, Zoppi Filho A, Ferreira Filho AA, et al.. Surgical treatment of varus malunion of the proximal humerus with valgus osteotomy. *J Shoulder Elbow Surg.* 2007;16(1):55-59.

59. Antuna SA, Sperling JW, Sánchez-Sotelo J, Cofield RH. Shoulder arthroplasty for proximal humeral malunions: long-term results. *J Shoulder Elbow Surg.* 2002;11(2):122-129.

60. Mansat P, Guity MR, Bellumore Y, Mansat M. Shoulder arthroplasty for late sequelae of proximal humeral fractures. *J Shoulder Elbow Surg.* 2004;13(3):305-312.

61. Willis M, Min W, Brooks JP, et al. Proximal humeral malunion treated with reverse shoulder arthroplasty. *J Shoulder Elbow Surg.* 2012;21(4):507-513.

62. Jacobson JA, Duquin TR, Sanchez-Sotelo J, Schleck CD, Sperling JW, Cofield RH. Anatomic shoulder arthroplasty for treatment of proximal humerus malunions. *J Shoulder Elbow Surg.* 2014;23(8):1232-1239.

63. Hamilton MA, Diep P, Roche C, et al. Effect of reverse shoulder design philosophy on muscle moment arms. *J Orthop Res.* 2015;33(4):605-613.

64. Raiss P, Edwards TB, Collin P, et al. Reverse shoulder arthroplasty for malunions of the proximal part of the humerus (Type-4 fracture sequelae). *J Bone Joint Surg Am.* 2016;98(11):893-899.

65. Martinez AA, Bejarano C, Carbonel I, Iglesias D, Gil-Albarova J, Herrera A. The treatment of proximal humerus nonunions in older patients with reverse shoulder arthroplasty. *Injury.* 2012;43(suppl 2):S3-S6.

66. Schai P, Imhoff A, Preiss S. Comminuted humeral head fractures: a multicenter analysis. *J Shoulder Elbow Surg.* 1995;4(5):319-330.

67. Sarris I, Weiser R, Sotereanos DG. Pathogenesis and treatment of osteonecrosis of the shoulder. *Orthop Clin North Am.* 2004;35(3):397-404.

68. Hettrich CM, Boraiah S, Dyke JP, Neviaser A, Helfet DL, Lorich DG. Quantitative assessment of the vascularity of the proximal part of the humerus. *J Bone Joint Surg Am.* 2010;92(4):943-948.

69. Hertel R, Hempfing A, Stiehler M, Leunig M. Predictors of humeral head ischemia after intracapsular fracture of the proximal humerus. *J Shoulder Elbow Surg.* 2004;13(4):427-433.

70. Mont MA, Maar D, Urquhart M, Lennox D, Hungerford D. Avascular necrosis of the humeral head treated by core decompression. A retrospective review. *J Bone Joint Surg Br.* 1993;75(5):785-788.

71. Schoch BS, Barlow JD, Schleck C, Cofield RH, Sperling JW. Shoulder arthroplasty for post-traumatic osteonecrosis of the humeral head. *J Shoulder Elbow Surg.* 2016;25(3):406-412.

72. Boileau P, Walch G, Krishnan SG. Tuberosity osteosynthesis and hemiarthroplasty for four-part fractures of the proximal humerus. *Tech Shoulder Elb Surg.* 2000;1(2):96-109.

73. Murachovsky J, Ikemoto RY, Nascimento LGP, Fujiki EN, Milani C, Warner JJP. Pectoralis major tendon reference (PMT): a new method for accurate restoration of humeral length with hemiarthroplasty for fracture. *J Shoulder Elbow Surg.* 2006;15(6):675-678.

74. Boileau P, Alami G, Rumian A, Schwartz DG, Trojani C, Seidl AJ. The doubled-suture Nice knot. *Orthopedics.* 2017;40(2): e382-e386.

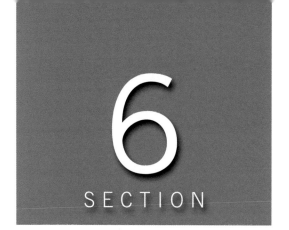

Complications

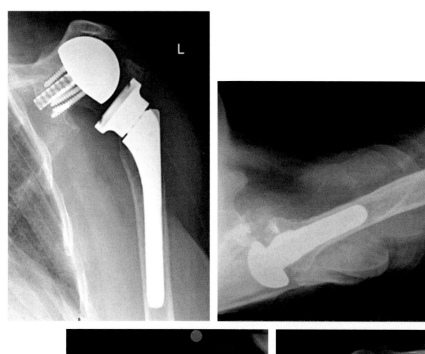

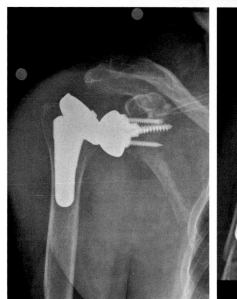

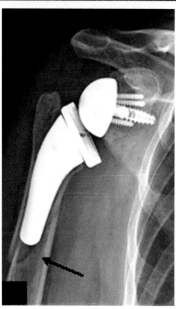

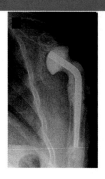

32

Infection (Anatomical Total Shoulder Arthroplasty and Reverse Total Shoulder Arthroplasty)

Stephen A. Parada, MD, Daniel B. Buchalter, MD, and Lynn A Crosby, MD

INTRODUCTION

The 2018 International Consensus Meeting (ICM) on Orthopaedic Infections provided important guidelines to define a periprosthetic joint infection (PJI) of the shoulder as characterized by either one definite criteria **(TABLE 32.1)**[1] or by six or more points derived from minor criteria **(TABLE 32.2)**.

While infection after anatomical total shoulder arthroplasty (ATSA) continues to be an uncommon, although potentially devastating, complication, early reports of reverse total shoulder arthroplasty (RTSA) demonstrated higher rates of overall complications, including infection.[2,3] These series reported an infection rate of up to 6.7%. As implant designs and surgeon experience increased, these infection rates have decreased substantially and are now reported as less than 3% in systematic review articles.[4,5] While the reasons are not completely clear, infection rate following ATSA is consistently lower than that following RTSA. Increased surface area of the implanted devices and larger dead space are thought to be the possible reasons which may explain this difference.[6]

RISK FACTORS

Risk factors for PJI following shoulder arthroplasty include younger age, male sex, obesity, immunodeficiency, nutritional deficiency, diabetes mellitus, traumatic arthroplasty, and revision procedures for prior failed arthroplasty.[7-18]

Younger age and male gender are theorized to be risk factors for PJI because these populations are more likely to have had trauma, rheumatoid arthritis, or *Cutibacterium acnes* (*C. acnes*, formerly *Propionibacterium acnes*), an increasingly common organism in PJI.[10,19] Class 3 obesity (BMI ≥40 kg/m²), poor glycemic control (hemoglobin A1c > 8.0 mg/dL), and malnutrition (preoperative albumin <3.5 g/dL) are all associated with an increased risk of PJI.[7,8,13]

Several types of immunodeficiency are suggested to increase the risk of PJI. Rheumatoid arthritis has previously been associated with an increased risk of PJI,[9] though newer research suggests it poses no greater risk.[14] Additionally, the use of intra-articular corticosteroid injections within 3 months of surgery has been implicated in recent literature.[15] Lastly, systemic lupus erythematosus, systemic corticosteroid therapy, and chemotherapy have all been implicated, but data suggesting they lead to increased risk are over 20 years old.[16,17]

Revision arthroplasty has been found to have an infection rate twice that of primary shoulder arthroplasty in some reviews (5.8% compared with 2.9%).[4] Alternatively, data are mixed on whether previous nonarthroplasty shoulder surgery increases PJI risk, though any prior shoulder surgery may increase the risk of subdermal *C. acnes* inoculation.[14,18,20]

MICROBIOLOGY

Although *Staphylococcus* has historically been the most commonly isolated PJI bacteria, now the low-virulent *C. acnes* predominates.[10] *C. acnes* is a gram-positive anaerobic bacillus that was once thought to be a contaminant, but is now known to be a pathologic organism.[21] Other commonly reported bacteria responsible for PJI include coagulase-negative *Staphylococcus*, *Klebsiella*, and *Escherichia coli*.[22] *C. acnes* is normal skin flora and is found frequently in the epidermal and subdermal layers of the shoulder at the regular incision site, especially in male patients.[20,23] Presence of sebaceous follicle glands also contributes to a 2.5 times increase in relative risk of *C. acnes* PJI in male patients compared with women.[24]

DIAGNOSIS

Clinical presentation of a patient with PJI can occur at any time following shoulder arthroplasty. Patients can present acutely **(FIGURE 32.1)** or even years after surgery. Clinical examination may have limited value in the majority of cases, as PJI findings that are typical in other joints are not as common in the shoulder.[25] Fever, surrounding erythema, palpable joint effusions, and sinus tracts communicating with the glenohumeral joint are rare. Physical examination can be characterized by pain, both with active motion and strength testing. History typically reveals aching pain in the joint or soreness that can be worse at night. Patients do not commonly report an acute onset of pain but rather an insidious onset.

TABLE 32.1 The 2018 International Consensus Meeting Definition of Periprosthetic Shoulder Infection—Definite Criteria

Presence of sinus tract from skin to prosthesis
Gross intra-articular pus
Two positive tissue cultures with phenotypically identical virulent organisms

Diagnostic Studies

Imaging studies are important components of the diagnostic evaluation of a patient with a suspected PJI. These generally start with standard radiographs which may demonstrate soft tissue swelling or even an effusion in the setting of an acute PJI **(FIGURE 32.2)**. In cases of chronic PJI, component loosening or hardware failure may be visible **(FIGURE 32.3)**. Scapular notching in the setting of an RTSA that is associated with lucency behind the baseplate should also raise concerns for a potential PJI. Other chronic changes that can be visualized on standard radiographs in the setting of PJI are endosteal scalloping, bone resorption

TABLE 32.2 The 2018 International Consensus Meeting Definition of Periprosthetic Shoulder Infection—Minor Criteria

Finding	Points
Unexpected wound drainage	4
Single positive tissue culture with virulent organism	3
Single positive tissue culture with low-virulence organism	1
Second positive tissue culture (identical low-virulence organism)	3
Humeral loosening	3
Positive frozen section (5 PMNs in ≥5 high-power fields)	3
Positive preoperative aspirate culture (low or high virulence)	3
Elevated synovial neutrophil percentage (>80%)[a]	2
Elevated synovial WBC count (>3000 cells/μL)[a]	2
Elevated ESR (>30 mm/h)[a]	2
Elevated CRP level (>10 mg/L)[a]	2
Elevated synovial α-defensin level	2
Cloudy fluid	2

CRP, C-reactive protein; ESR, erythrocyte sedimentation rate; PMN, polymorphonuclear leukocyte; WBC, white blood cell.
[a]Beyond 6 weeks from recent surgery.

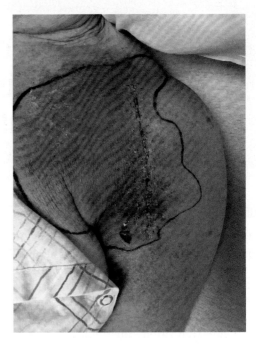

FIGURE 32.1 Photograph depicting an acute infection in the left shoulder of a patient 2 weeks after shoulder arthroplasty. The area of erythema has been outlined with a marker.

of the proximal humerus or glenoid, periosteal reaction, and lucency around the humeral or glenoid implants.[25]

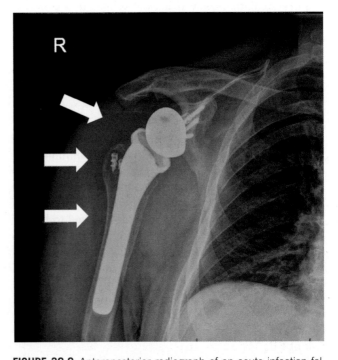

FIGURE 32.2 Anteroposterior radiograph of an acute infection following reverse total shoulder arthroplasty that had been performed over 6.5 years ago. The patient presented with fever and acute pain after suspected hematologic seeding. Arrows outline the large effusion. Metallic anchors from a previous rotator cuff repair are present in the proximal humerus.

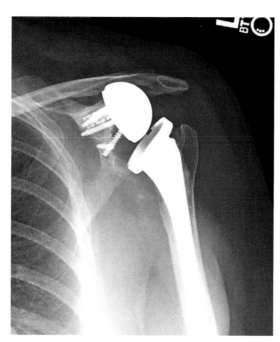

FIGURE 32.3 Anteroposterior radiograph of a reverse total shoulder arthroplasty demonstrating severe notching and hardware failure consisting of baseplate loosening and a broken screw consistent with a chronic infection.

Advanced imaging studies may be indicated for the patient where the diagnosis is uncertain. Computed tomography (CT) is particularly useful to evaluate for lucency around the glenoid implant in both ATSA and RTSA. CT arthrogram may be utilized to further evaluate a loose glenoid component in ATSA while also evaluating the integrity of the rotator cuff as this may be a factor in surgical planning.[26] Magnetic resonance imaging can be performed with metal artifact reduction techniques and may be useful to assess the soft tissue structures around the shoulder as well as to evaluate for osteolysis and component loosening, although these have not been fully explored to assess their utility in confirming a diagnosis of PJI.[27] A technetium-99m three-phase bone scan is another useful imaging modality because of its sensitivity for detecting loosening. However, the lack of specificity makes it difficult to differentiate aseptic from septic loosening, especially in recently implanted prostheses that experience remodeling-related increased uptake for up to 1 year after surgery.[28] Some findings that may be more associated with infection as opposed to loosening are irregular contiguous bone activity extending laterally with mild activity at the pedestal **(FIGURE 32.4)**. Further confirmation could be obtained with radiolabeled leukocyte imaging, but this is not considered a routine component of testing for PJI.

Laboratory Studies

Laboratory studies are a key component of the evaluation of a patient with a suspected PJI. Common laboratory studies are serum white blood cell (WBC) count with differential, erythrocyte sedimentation rate (ESR), and C-reactive protein (CRP). These studies have a high specificity but a low sensitivity and can often be within normal limits especially with low-virulent organisms such as *C. acnes*.[25] Overall sensitivities of ESR and CRP in the diagnosis of PJI of the shoulder are less than 50% and are much lower than the sensitivities for diagnosing PJI in the knee or hip.[29] Serum interleukin 6 (IL-6) can be ordered in many institutions, although depending on availability, it may have to be calculated at an outside institution and take several days for results to return. IL-6 has been found to have a lower sensitivity compared with ESR and CRP for predicting indolent PJI in the shoulder.[30]

Shoulder Aspiration-Based Studies

Along with serologic testing, synovial fluid analysis is a critically important step in the diagnosis of shoulder PJI. The presence of gross intra-articular purulence identified during aspiration, arthroscopy, or open surgery is one of the definite 2018 ICM criteria for shoulder PJI. Additionally, cloudy synovial fluid, positive cultures obtained during aspiration, an elevated synovial neutrophil percentage (>80%), synovial WBC count (>3000 cells/μL), and α-defensin level (an antimicrobial peptide) are all 2018 ICM minor criteria for shoulder PJI. Importantly, lower neutrophil percentage and WBC count thresholds do not necessarily rule out infection, especially in lower inflammatory response infections such as *C. acnes*. In the knee arthroplasty literature, cut-off values as low as neutrophil percentage >64% and WBC >1100 cells/10^{-3} cm^3 have been used to diagnose PJI,[31] though similarly low thresholds have not been proposed for shoulder PJI.

Recently, several other synovial fluid biomarkers have been used to assist in the diagnosis of shoulder PJI, but validation with larger cohorts is required to determine their value. Specifically, synovial IL-6, granulocyte-macrophage colony-stimulating factor, interferon-γ, IL-1β, IL-2, IL-8, and IL-10 were found to be significantly elevated in cases of revision shoulder arthroplasty that were found to be infected.[32] A combined model of IL-6, tumor necrosis factor-α (TNF-α), and IL-2 had a sensitivity of 0.80, specificity of 0.93, and positive and negative predict values of 0.87 and 0.89, respectively. This combined synovial fluid cytokine analysis is more effective than standard serum ESR and CRP in diagnosing PJI of the shoulder. A unique advantage of synovial α-defensin is that it can be analyzed within hours and rapid testing kits are available for analysis within minutes. This study has also been shown to be more effective than serum ESR and CRP for diagnosing shoulder PJI.[33]

Compared with the hip and knee, shoulder PJIs generally produce a lower synovial inflammatory

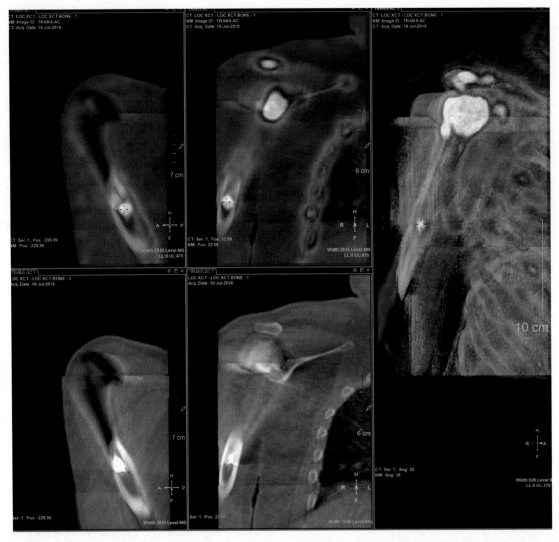

FIGURE 32.4 Images from a bone scan three-phase limited area study with single photon emission computed tomography. Bone flow phase images demonstrate irregular contiguous bone activity extending laterally with activity at the pedestal as well. These findings are associated with infection more than for aseptic loosening.

response, resulting in lower synovial fluid production and more difficulty in obtaining fluid during aspiration. Preoperative shoulder aspiration for the diagnosis of PJI is reported to be possible in only 39% to 56% of patients, with 29% to 78% of these aspirations producing positive cultures,[34,35] and a 34% false negative culture rate.[36] Despite its shortcomings, preoperative shoulder aspiration can be a useful tool in the diagnosis of shoulder PJI. If aspiration is going to be performed as part of the PJI workup, we recommend that it be performed with a sterility protocol that exceeds the standard protocol utilized for shoulder injections. This will maximize the value of the aspiration. Furthermore, if image guidance (fluoroscopy or ultrasound) is readily available, we recommend its use to lower the chance of a false negative based on a dry aspiration.

Tissue Biopsy

Often, laboratory analysis and imaging studies will still not be confirmatory for the presence of a PJI, and surgeons must decide whether or not to proceed with a revision surgery even though the possibility of a PJI remains a possibility. In this setting, a surgical biopsy can be helpful. The specimens obtained are cultured for an extended period of time, up to 18 days for *C. acnes*,[37] to allow sufficient time for culture results to be definitive prior to any type of revision procedure. These biopsies can be performed as either an open or arthroscopic procedure. Obtaining tissue for culture is preferred over the use of swabs. As *C. acnes* is an anaerobic bacteria, it must quickly be transferred to a sterile container and not remain exposed to air. Our preferred method for tissue culture is to use sterile instruments that have not yet been utilized during the case to remove tissue and then have the operating room nurse open a sterile container. The nurse passes the sterile container to the assistant who uses another unused sterile instrument to sweep the tissue into the container. This is preferred over multiple sterile containers left open throughout the case prior to the harvesting of tissue. At least five cultures should be sent and each one should be obtained from different anatomic areas of the shoulder. Dilisio et al studied the utility of arthroscopic biopsy in 19 patients who had suspected PJI. In their study, they found a 100% sensitivity and specificity compared to cultures obtained from joint aspirate which had a sensitivity of only 16.7%.[38] Tashjian et al also evaluated open and arthroscopy prerevision tissue biopsy and found a sensitivity of 0.75 with a specificity of 0.60.[39] It is our preference to perform an arthroscopic biopsy on potential PJI cases in which the diagnosis remains uncertain despite imaging and laboratory analysis. Any subsequent case is planned at least 21 days after the arthroscopy to allow for final cultures to return.

TREATMENT

The goal of treatment procedures for an infected shoulder arthroplasty patient is to eradicate the infection and preserve as much function as possible. In most cases, the soft tissue supporting the shoulder joint, specifically the rotator cuff, may not be fully functional as a result of the infectious process and the treatment needed to eliminate the infection. The availability of RTSA as a revision procedure has had a major impact on regaining function when revision surgery is necessary as part of the overall treatment for the infected arthroplasty.

In this section, the treatment options of debridement with preservation of the implant, one-stage revision, and two-stage revision will be discussed. These are presented as treatment options as are the guidelines for their utilization. It is essential that the treating surgeons rely on their own judgment to determine what procedure is in the patient's best interest for eradicating the infection and preserving postoperative function.

Irrigation and Debridement and Preservation of the Implant

An acute PJI, defined as an infection that occurs within 6 weeks of the shoulder arthroplasty procedure, is a rare event. An infection that is apparent this early is most likely related to a superficial wound cellulitis or a suture-related abscess. Deep infections after shoulder arthroplasty are rarely diagnosed in this early stage. However, when one does occur, it can present with pain out of proportion to what would be expected during the early recovery and rehabilitation period. If the diagnosis can be made, early irrigation and debridement (I&D) may be

a successful treatment approach with the goal of retaining the implants.[10,34,40-42] However, only limited data are available regarding outcomes after I&D and retention of the prosthesis in the acute setting. In a series of 10 shoulder arthroplasties with PJI, Dennison et al reported that 30% (3/10) of patients who underwent I&D required revision for persistent infection, 60% (6/10) of patients required chronic antibiotic suppression, and 57% (4/7) of patients who did not require revision for persistent infection reported satisfactory or excellent outcomes.[43] Of note, 6 of the 10 patients underwent I&D greater than 6 weeks after index arthroplasty. Coste et al reported on 8 patients treated with I&D, finding a 12% persistent infection rate, a 62.5% reoperation rate, and overall unsatisfactory results.[44] Again, only two of the eight patients had acute infections, though these two patients had the best outcomes.

For all arthroplasty cases we routinely use endotracheal intubation so that muscle paralysis can be achieved intraoperatively. Additionally, patients receive a single-shot, ultrasound-guided interscalene block for pain control unless contraindicated by gross purulence or a large effusion that obscures the neurovascular anatomy. We then wash the skin with a 4% chlorhexidine gluconate solution followed by a 3% hydrogen peroxide rinse before a standard surgical preparation. All scrubbed personnel wear body exhaust suits (sterile hoods) during primary and revision cases.

When performing an I&D procedure for acute infection in an ATSA, the modular humeral head is removed to allow for as extensive a debridement as possible. The glenoid component is most often cemented into place and is nonmodular and cannot be exchanged in this setting. When an RTSA is in place, the polyethylene liner can be removed along with the glenosphere to allow for a more complete I&D. Some systems have additional modular components which can also be removed to gain a more extensive exposure for debridement. When the I&D is completed, all modular components are replaced. Alternatively, in an RTSA we have also soaked the glenosphere in antibiotic fluid irrigation, scrubbed with a brush, and then reinserted. Obtaining proper cultures is an essential part of this procedure. Our protocol is to obtain cultures from the subcutaneous tissue and also when entering the glenohumeral joint. It has been recommended that at least five different biopsy specimens should be collected from different areas of the shoulder joint and that is the protocol we follow. Positive results are considered if on frozen section there are five or more leukocytes on five or more high-powered fields (HPFs).[1] All cultures should be monitored for 18 days for the diagnosis of *C. acnes* to be ruled out. After cultures are taken and tissue has been debrided, we irrigate with an antibiotic solution of at least 3 L by gravity irrigation using cystoscopy tubing, followed by 3 L of normal saline

(NS). The antibiotic irrigation solution is 3 L of NS with additional bacitracin (150,000 units), Neosporin irrigant (9 mL), and vancomycin (3 g). An additional 1 g of vancomycin powder is placed into the deep layer of the wound. We close the wound over a suction drain, which in most cases can be removed after 24 hours or when the fluid output is minimal. The deltopectoral interval is closed with a monofilament suture and the skin is closed with a monofilament layer in the subcutaneous tissue followed by skin staples. No braided sutures are utilized. Since *Staphylococcus aureus (S. aureus)* is expected to grow in culture within the first 48 hours, patients remain hospitalized for this time period to rule out *S. aureus* as a source if there is sufficient suspicion. This allows us to optimize antibiotic coverage before discharge.

One-Stage Revision

Very few reports exist regarding the outcomes following a one-stage revision for a deep infection following shoulder arthroplasty. Most are small case reports with no long-term follow-up, making it difficult to define the indications for a one-stage revision and to recommend when it should be utilized. Despite this, Kunutsor et al recently performed a systematic review and meta-analysis of 147 one-stage revisions at an average of 3-year follow-up, finding an overall success rate for elimination infection of 94.7%, a noninfectious complication rate of 12.1%, and acceptable functional outcomes.[45] The most important determination regarding one-stage revision is the necessity of identifying the causative organism before the revision procedure is performed. The methods described earlier can be utilized. If the organism identified is sensitive to appropriate antibiotic treatment, then a single-stage revision can be considered and may be preferable since patients do not necessarily require a second operation. However, if the organism cannot be identified prior to revision, then a two-stage revision is the preferred procedure. Certain organisms, even if identified prior to revision, may be best treated by a two-stage procedure. These include gram-negative organisms, multiple organisms, or when cultures identify more than one organism at the time of aspiration or arthroscopy.[42,46,47]

For one-stage revisions, we again use endotracheal intubation and muscle relaxation, a single-shot interscalene block, a 4% chlorhexidine gluconate solution wash followed by a 3% hydrogen peroxide rinse prior to standard surgical preparation, and body exhaust suits. When performing a one-stage revision, it is important to remove all implants, including all retained cement and any rotator cuff anchors left in the greater tuberosity from the index procedure. We recommend a biopsy and culture of the tissue at the bone interface as this tissue can have a large concentration of the organism. After an aggressive I&D procedure as described in the section above, we recommend cementing the revision humeral stem in place during this revision setting. Antibiotic-impregnated cement is utilized and is specific to the known organism when possible. If the soft tissue envelope (eg, rotator cuff) is at all in question, an RTSA should be utilized as the revision implant, though patient age must be considered.[46,48,49] While primary RTSA in younger patients leads to substantial functional improvement without clinical deterioration at 10 years, it can be associated with a nearly 40% complication rate that is likely even higher if used in the setting of PJI.[50] When performing a revision on a prior ATSA in the setting of a competent rotator cuff, we remove all cement from the glenoid and cement a new glenoid component in place in a physiological young patient. In a younger patient with a deficient cuff, the decision must be made to either proceed with a hemiarthroplasty or conversion to an RTSA. In elderly patients where glenoid bone stock is insufficient to allow for conversion to an RTSA, a hemiarthroplasty can also be considered **(FIGURE 32.5)**. The wound should be closed over a drain and an appropriate antibiotic regimen followed based upon the recommendation of the infectious disease (ID) specialist. This is usually 2 to 4 weeks of intravenous antibiotics depending on the organism involved. The IL-6 should be monitored as well as the CRP and ESR levels. If these levels stay elevated, a prolonged course of oral antibiotics may be required. While Kunutsor et al reported that one-stage revisions for PJI do well up to 3 years,[45] no longer term outcomes are available to recommend one-stage revision at this time.

Two-Stage Revision

In multiple studies evaluating the two-stage approach for treatment of deep infection following shoulder arthroplasty, the overall success rate for eliminating infection was 91%, the noninfectious complication rate was 18.9%, and there were acceptable functional outcomes.[36,45,48,51-57] Notably, the meta-analysis by Kunutsor et al suggests that one-stage revision is at least equally effective as two-stage revision in controlling infection, improving function, and limiting noninfectious complication.[45] Nonetheless, our recommended procedure in most cases is to perform a two-stage revision and we would counsel surgeons to carefully consider the indications for I&D with retention of implants and one-stage revisions. Most failures following two-stage revision are felt to be secondary to failure to identify the organism, inadequate I&D, and/or failure to utilize antibiotics postoperatively for an appropriate amount of time.

When performing a two-stage procedure, if the organism has not been identified, we recommend holding the antibiotics until adequate cultures have been obtained during the procedure. Endotracheal intubation, muscle relaxation, a single-shot interscalene block, a 4%

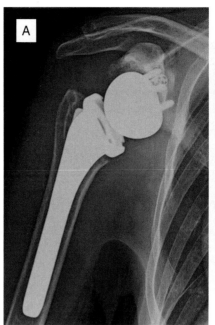
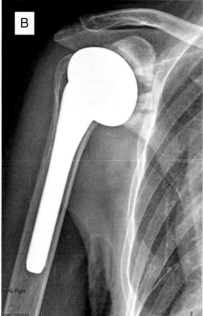
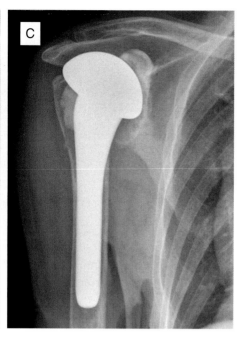

FIGURE 32.5 Anteroposterior radiograph of a reverse total shoulder arthroplasty in a 78-year-old woman who had gross purulence on aspiration (**A**). Due to the patient's poor general health, the decision was made to perform a one-stage irrigation and debridement and conversion to a hemiarthroplasty to avoid any future surgery if possible (**B**). At 4 years postoperatively, there was no recurrence of infection. Radiograph demonstrates moderate glenoid erosion; however, no loosening of the prosthesis was found (**C**).

chlorhexidine gluconate solution wash followed by a 3% hydrogen peroxide rinse prior to standard surgical preparation, and body exhaust suits are again utilized. If there is a sinus tract present, it is important to excise this tissue during the initial debridement. There may be extensive scarring in the subdeltoid space, and care should be taken to preserve deltoid function with careful dissection. Removal of all bursal tissues and release of all adhesions is important. The axillary nerve is at risk in any revision surgery, and it must be identified and protected before proceeding with an aggressive I&D. The subscapularis is released and tagged if felt that it can be preserved. However, in most cases, RTSA will be the implant of choice for the second-stage procedure (**FIGURE 32.6**). It is the surgeon's choice whether to preserve the subscapularis or simply debride it if there is extensive necrosis from the infection. All previous deep suture materials and capsular tissues must be removed. If previous rotator cuff anchors were left in place in the greater tuberosity at the time of the index surgery, they are removed at the first stage of the revision. Cultures are taken from the subcutaneous and deep tissues. Biopsies are obtained from at least five different sites as described previously. Releases are performed to obtain adequate external rotation before attempting to dislocate the implants.[49,51]

After the initial dissection and dislocation of the humeral implant, the humeral head can be removed which allows visualization of the glenoid implant. In most cases, the glenoid component is easily removed with a rongeur or osteotome. All cement must be removed from the glenoid vault, and a small handheld burr can aid in this removal. It is important to preserve as much glenoid bone stock as possible during this debridement and removal of the cement. Whenever removing an implant, the tissue from the bone-implant interface must be biopsied and cultured as this tissue can have a high yield for the organism. The humeral stem can usually be removed by utilizing the specific implant manufacturer's extraction instruments. However, if these tools are not available, using standard revision instrumentation is recommended. If the implant is cemented or well-fixed, the use of a needle-tipped burr around the proximal aspect of the implant to loosen it has been found to be very helpful. A bone tamp can then be used to back out the implant after it has been released. On rare occasions, an osteotomy may be necessary to release a well-fixed or cemented implant. A bone window can be made distally leaving a large enough bridge of proximal bone to prevent the tuberosities from splitting and separating when the implant is removed. An ultrasonic cement removal device, burrs, and osteotomes can then be used to remove any remaining cement from the humeral canal. These ultrasonic devices utilize high heat, and great care must be taken to prevent bone penetration to limit any risk of radial nerve injury. Additional detailed descriptions of stem removal techniques are included in Chapter 41. Cultures and biopsies should also be obtained from the bone-implant interface around the humeral component. The entire humeral canal, glenoid vault, and soft tissue

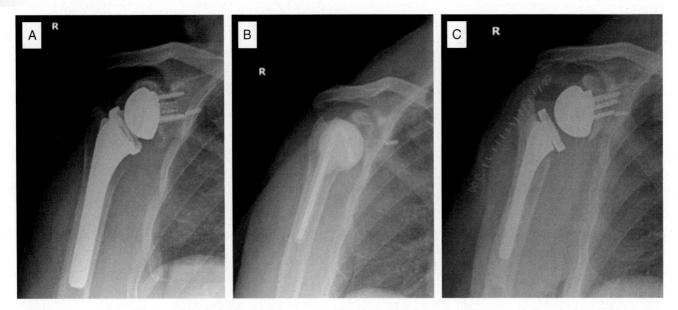

FIGURE 32.6 Anteroposterior radiograph of a reverse total shoulder arthroplasty (RTSA) demonstrating hardware failure and a broken screw consistent with a chronic infection (**A**). After staged procedure consisting of extensive debridement, removal of hardware with the exception of the broken screw deep in the glenoid vault and placement of an antibiotic spacer with a cuff of antibiotic cement (**B**). Following revision, RTSA with a cemented humeral component was performed after 6 weeks of antibiotic treatment and normalization of infection labs (**C**).

are now irrigated with a pulse lavage utilizing the antibiotic solution described above. If an osteotomy was performed, the bone window is now replaced and secured with polydioxanone suture or cerclage wire if required.

Placement of an antibiotic-impregnated cement spacer is recommended, which can either be made from a mold at the time of surgery or a commercially produced

cement spacer can be used (**FIGURE 32.7**). It is recommended that a small amount of antibiotic-impregnated cement be used to form a collar around the implant to help secure the spacer in place and prevent rotation. A small amount of antibiotic cement can be placed into the glenoid vault to help protect it from further damage that may be caused by contact with the humeral cement

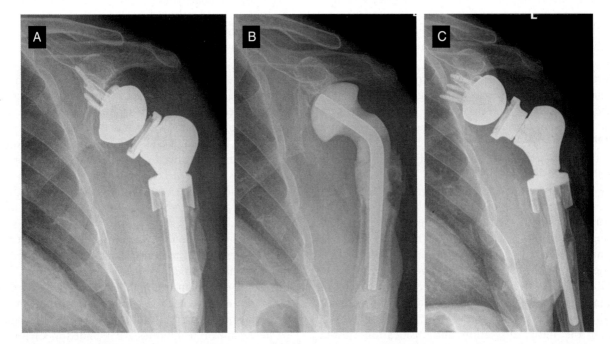

FIGURE 32.7 Anteroposterior radiograph of a revision proximal humerus replacement reverse total shoulder arthroplasty (RTSA) demonstrating lucencies about the glenoid and humerus prostheses (**A**) in a 67-year-old man. Because of the bone loss due to the resection of the proximal humerus, an antibiotic spacer for the hip was placed (**B**). After 6 weeks of treatment with antibiotics for *Cutibacterium acnes*, he had normalization of infection labs and a revision proximal humerus replacement RTSA was performed (**C**).

spacer. A deep drain is placed, and the wound is closed. If the rotator cuff tissue is salvable, it can be repaired with a monofilament suture. The skin can be closed with either monofilament suture or staples.

The parameters used to determine when it is appropriate to proceed with the second stage of the revision have not been clearly defined. Serum IL-6 shows promise as a marker to follow to assist in making this determination, though care must be taken as it may not reliably identify indolent infections like *C. acnes*.[58] However, no long-term controlled studies have been performed to date to make a firm recommendation. CRP and ESR are inflammatory markers that can also be followed but these markers can take many months to return to normal while IL-6 can be one of the first inflammatory markers to return to normal. We feel that the sooner a revision can be performed in these infected cases, the better a functional result will be obtained.[48] As such, following 6 weeks of antibiotic treatment, if IL-6 is normal or trending downward, we proceed to the second stage of the revision. However, even in this context, the second stage needs to be done safely and the infection fully eradicated in order to obtain a satisfactory long-term outcome.

During the second stage of the revision procedure, the same skin incision is utilized and again all nonviable tissues are removed as part of a complete debridement. Biopsies are taken and if the WBC per HPF is >5, then a repeat I&D with placement of new antibiotic spacer is performed. If biopsies are negative, then cultures are again taken; however, empiric antibiotic treatment is not routinely utilized. In most cases, the rotator cuff tissue, even if tagged or repaired in the first stage, is not viable at this point and should be debrided. Therefore, RTSA is often the preferred implant. The antibiotic spacer is removed using a bone tamp, rongeurs, and/or osteotomes. An extensive I&D is now carried out to eliminate any remaining cement debris or nonviable tissue. The humeral canal and glenoid vault are dried with sponge packing and long suction tips. The glenoid may require bone grafting before placement of the baseplate. Given the infected milieu, autograft is theoretically preferable to allograft but comes with significant donor site morbidity if structural support is needed.[59] Therefore, we often use femoral head allograft. A cement restrictor is placed in the humeral canal and then filled with specific antibiotic-impregnated cement according to the organism that was cultured if possible. Cementing the implant is recommended as it will give immediate stability and allow for secondary protection from the antibiotic. A drain is placed and the wound closed in the standard fashion. Postoperatively, cultures are closely monitored, and in the case that they are positive after the second stage, then a treatment course with antibiotics is discussed with ID. Importantly, urgent return to the operating room is not planned.

Antibiotic Therapy

When evaluating a suspected PJI that requires arthroscopic biopsy due to inconclusive laboratory results, we recommend holding antibiotics at the time of the biopsy and monitoring cultures to determine if a PJI is present. If the cultures are positive, then a two-stage procedure is generally recommended **(FIGURE 32.8)**. In the case that the cultures do not return positive, but there remains a high suspicion of infection due to other signs such as hardware failure or loosening, a thorough discussion needs to occur with the patient to discuss treatment options and potential risks and complications of each possible treatment course.

Regardless of which treatment course is chosen, consultation with a musculoskeletal ID specialist is performed preoperatively and further discussion follows after surgery. We recommend meeting frequently with your hospital's ID department to find a willing partner to consult with, rather than consulting with the member of the department who happens to be on-call on the day that you require assistance. We consider musculoskeletal ID to be a subspecialty area that ideally should be developed in every institution that provides both ID consultations and orthopedic care. Continued follow-up with ID during the postoperative period can result in early identification of a situation in which antibiotic coverage does not seem to be effective, indicating the possibility of a gram-negative rod (GNR) being the causative organism. Although rare, it is possible for a PJI to be due to a GNR such a *Klebsiella* or *E. coli*.[22]

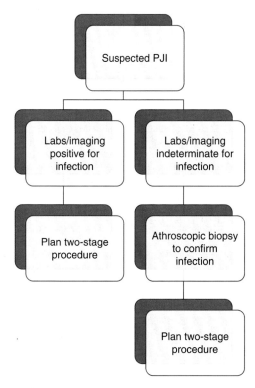

FIGURE 32.8 Algorithm for suspected periprosthetic joint infection (PJI).

CONCLUSION

One of the most important aspects of the evaluation and treatment of PJI following shoulder arthroplasty is maintaining a high index of suspicion for infection when patients report continued pain and are not progressing as anticipated. We have also encountered acute infection presenting several years after the index surgery in patients who were previously doing well. In true acute infections, I&D with replacement of all modular components followed by a course of intravenous antibiotics can be considered. The use of single-stage revisions has, as of yet, an undefined role in our treatment armamentarium given the limited long-term data, though it may be preferable when the organism has been preoperatively identified. Two-stage revisions have had a high success rate, are the gold standard for the treatment of hip and knee PJI, and should be considered the procedure of choice for PJI following shoulder arthroplasty except for in selected circumstances.

REFERENCES

1. Garrigues GE, Zmistowski B, Cooper AM, et al. Proceedings from the 2018 International Consensus Meeting on Orthopedic Infections: the definition of periprosthetic shoulder infection. *J Shoulder Elbow Surg.* 2019;28(suppl 6):S8-S12.
2. Boileau P, Watkinson D, Hatzidakis AM, Hovorka I. Neer Award 2005: the Grammont reverse shoulder prosthesis. Results in cuff tear arthritis, fracture sequelae, and revision arthroplasty. *J Shoulder Elbow Surg.* 2006;15(5):527-540.
3. Wall B, Nove-Josserand L, O'Connor DP, Edwards TB, Walch G. Reverse total shoulder arthroplasty: a review of results according to etiology. *J Bone Joint Surg Am.* 2007;89(7):1476-1485.
4. Zumstein MA, Pinedo M, Old J, Boileau P. Problems, complications, reoperations, and revisions in reverse total shoulder arthroplasty: a systematic review. *J Shoulder Elbow Surg.* 2011;20(1):146-157.
5. Bohsali KI, Bois AJ, Wirth MA. Complications of shoulder arthroplasty. *J Bone Joint Surg Am.* 2017;99(3):256-269.
6. Cheung E, Willis M, Walker M, Clark R, Frankle MA. Complications in reverse total shoulder arthroplasty. *J Am Acad Orthop Surg.* 2011;19(7):439-449.
7. Garcia GH, Fu MC, Webb ML, Dines DM, Craig EV, Gulotta LV. Effect of metabolic syndrome and obesity on complications after shoulder arthroplasty. *Orthopedics.* 2016;39(5):309-316.
8. Garcia GH, Fu MC, Dines DM, Craig EV, Gulotta LV. Malnutrition: a marker for increased complications, mortality, and length of stay after total shoulder arthroplasty. *J Shoulder Elbow Surg.* 2016;25(2):193-200.
9. Holcomb JO, Hebert DJ, Mighell MA, et al. Reverse shoulder arthroplasty in patients with rheumatoid arthritis. *J Shoulder Elbow Surg.* 2010;19(7):1076-1084.
10. Singh JA, Sperling JW, Schleck C, Harmsen WS, Cofield RH. Periprosthetic infections after total shoulder arthroplasty: a 33-year perspective. *J Shoulder Elbow Surg.* 2012;21(11):1534-1541.
11. Richards J, Inacio MC, Beckett M, et al. Patient and procedure-specific risk factors for deep infection after primary shoulder arthroplasty. *Clin Orthop Relat Res.* 2014;472(9):2809-2815.
12. Wagner ER, Houdek MT, Schleck CD, et al. The role age plays in the outcomes and complications of shoulder arthroplasty. *J Shoulder Elbow Surg.* 2017;26(9):1573-1580.
13. Cancienne JM, Brockmeier SF, Werner BC. Association of perioperative glycemic control with deep postoperative infection after shoulder arthroplasty in patients with diabetes. *J Am Acad Orthop Surg.* 2018;26(11):e238-e245.
14. Morris BJ, O'Connor DP, Torres D, Elkousy HA, Gartsman GM, Edwards TB. Risk factors for periprosthetic infection after reverse shoulder arthroplasty. *J Shoulder Elbow Surg.* 2015;24(2):161-166.
15. Werner BC, Cancienne JM, Burrus MT, Griffin JW, Gwathmey FW, Brockmeier SF. The timing of elective shoulder surgery after shoulder injection affects postoperative infection risk in Medicare patients. *J Shoulder Elbow Surg.* 2016;25(3):390-397.
16. Wirth MA, Rockwood CA Jr. Current concepts review-complications of total shoulder-replacement arthroplasty. *J Bone Joint Surg Am.* 1996;78(4):603-616.
17. Wirth MA, Rockwood CA Jr. Complications of shoulder arthroplasty. *Clin Orthop Relat Res.* 1994;307:47-69.
18. Werthel JD, Hatta T, Schoch B, Cofield R, Sperling JW, Elhassan BT. Is previous nonarthroplasty surgery a risk factor for periprosthetic infection in primary shoulder arthroplasty? *J Shoulder Elbow Surg.* 2017;26(4):635-640.
19. Koh CK, Marsh JP, Drinkovic D, Walker CG, Poon PC. Propionibacterium acnes in primary shoulder arthroplasty: rates of colonization, patient risk factors, and efficacy of perioperative prophylaxis. *J Shoulder Elbow Surg.* 2016;25(5):846-852.
20. Falconer TM, Baba M, Kruse LM, et al. Contamination of the surgical field with propionibacterium acnes in primary shoulder arthroplasty. *J Bone Joint Surg Am.* 2016;98(20):1722-1728.
21. Patel A, Calfee RP, Plante M, Fischer SA, Green A. Propionibacterium acnes colonization of the human shoulder. *J Shoulder Elbow Surg.* 2009;18(6):897-902.
22. Parada SA, Shaw KA, Eichinger JK, Stadecker MJ, Higgins LD, Warner JJP. Survey of shoulder arthroplasty surgeons' methods for infection avoidance of *Propionibacterium. J Orthop.* 2018;15(1):177-180.
23. Matsen FA III, Butler-Wu S, Carofino BC, Jette JL, Bertelsen A, Bumgarner R. Origin of propionibacterium in surgical wounds and evidence-based approach for culturing propionibacterium from surgical sites. *J Bone Joint Surg Am.* 2013;95(23):e1811-e1817.
24. Hou C, Gupta A, Chen M, Matsen FA III. How do revised shoulders that are culture positive for *Propionibacterium* differ from those that are not? *J Shoulder Elbow Surg.* 2015;24(9):1427-1432.
25. Mook WR, Garrigues GE. Diagnosis and management of periprosthetic shoulder infections. *J Bone Joint Surg Am.* 2014;96(11):956-965.
26. Paxton ES, Green A, Krueger VS. Periprosthetic infections of the shoulder: diagnosis and management. *J Am Acad Orthop Surg.* 2019;27(21):e935-e944.
27. Nwawka OK, Konin GP, Sneag DB, Gulotta LV, Potter HG. Magnetic resonance imaging of shoulder arthroplasty: review article. *HSS J.* 2014;10(3):213-224.
28. Gyftopoulos S, Rosenberg ZS, Roberts CC, et al. ACR appropriateness criteria imaging after shoulder arthroplasty. *J Am Coll Radiol.* 2016;13(11):1324-1336.
29. Piper KE, Fernandez-Sampedro M, Steckelberg KE, et al. C-reactive protein, erythrocyte sedimentation rate and orthopedic implant infection. *PLoS One.* 2010;5(2):e9358.
30. Grosso MJ, Frangiamore SJ, Saleh A, et al. Poor utility of serum interleukin-6 levels to predict indolent periprosthetic shoulder infections. *J Shoulder Elbow Surg.* 2014;23(9):1277-1281.
31. Parvizi J, Zmistowski B, Berbari EF, et al. New definition for periprosthetic joint infection: from the workgroup of the Musculoskeletal Infection Society. *Clin Orthop Relat Res.* 2011;469(11):2992-2994.
32. Frangiamore SJ, Saleh A, Grosso MJ, et al. Neer Award 2015: analysis of cytokine profiles in the diagnosis of periprosthetic joint infections of the shoulder. *J Shoulder Elbow Surg.* 2017;26(2):186-196.
33. Frangiamore SJ, Saleh A, Grosso MJ, et al. α-Defensin as a predictor of periprosthetic shoulder infection. *J Shoulder Elbow Surg.* 2015;24(7):1021-1027.
34. Sperling JW, Kozak TK, Hanssen AD, Cofield RH. Infection after shoulder arthroplasty. *Clin Orthop Relat Res.* 2001;382:206-216.
35. Codd TP, Yamaguchi K, Pollock RG, Flatow EL, Bigliani LU. Infected shoulder arthroplasties: treatment with staged reimplantations vs. resection arthroplasty. *J Shoulder Elbow Surg.* 1996;5(2):S5.
36. Strickland J, Sperling J, Cofield R. The results of two-stage reimplantation for infected shoulder replacement. *J Bone Joint Surg Br.* 2008;90(4):460-465.

37. Pottinger P, Butler-Wu S, Neradilek MB, et al. Prognostic factors for bacterial cultures positive for Propionibacterium acnes and other organisms in a large series of revision shoulder arthroplasties performed for stiffness, pain, or loosening. *J Bone Joint Surg Am.* 2012;94(22):2075-2083.

38. Dilisio MF, Miller LR, Warner JJ, Higgins LD. Arthroscopic tissue culture for the evaluation of periprosthetic shoulder infection. *J Bone Joint Surg Am.* 2014;96(23):1952-1958.

39. Tashjian RZ, Granger EK, Zhang Y. Utility of prerevision tissue biopsy sample to predict revision shoulder arthroplasty culture results in at-risk patients. *J Shoulder Elbow Surg.* 2017;26(2):197-203.

40. Crosby LA. Complications. In: Crosby LA, ed. *Total Shoulder Arthroplasty.* American Academy of Orthopaedic Surgeons; 2000:39-46.

41. Romano CL, Borens O, Monti L, Meani E, Stuyck J. What treatment for periprosthetic shoulder infection? Results from a multicentre retrospective series. *Int Orthop.* 2012;36(5):1011-1017.

42. Weber P, Utzschneider S, Sadoghi P, Andress HJ, Jansson V, Muller PE. Management of the infected shoulder prosthesis: a retrospective analysis and review of the literature. *Int Orthop.* 2011;35(3):365-373.

43. Dennison T, Alentorn-Geli E, Assenmacher AT, Sperling JW, Sanchez-Sotelo J, Cofield RH. Management of acute or late hematogenous infection after shoulder arthroplasty with irrigation, debridement, and component retention. *J Shoulder Elbow Surg.* 2017;26(1):73-78.

44. Coste JS, Reig S, Trojani C, Berg M, Walch G, Boileau P. The management of infection in arthroplasty of the shoulder. *J Bone Joint Surg Br.* 2004;86(1):65-69.

45. Kunutsor SK, Wylde V, Beswick AD, Whitehouse MR, Blom AW. One- and two-stage surgical revision of infected shoulder prostheses following arthroplasty surgery: a systematic review and meta-analysis. *Sci Rep.* 2019;9(1):232.

46. Cuff DJ, Virani NA, Levy J, et al. The treatment of deep shoulder infection and glenohumeral instability with debridement, reverse shoulder arthroplasty and postoperative antibiotics. *J Bone Joint Surg Br.* 2008;90(3):336-342.

47. Hackett DJJ, Crosby LA. Evaluation and treatment of the infected shoulder arthroplasty. *Bull Hosp Jt Dis.* 2013;71:88-93.

48. Coffey MJ, Ely EE, Crosby LA. Treatment of glenohumeral sepsis with a commercially produced antibiotic-impregnated cement spacer. *J Shoulder Elbow Surg.* 2010;19(6):868-873.

49. Crosby LA. Two stage revision of infected total shoulder arthroplasty. In: Abrams JS, Bell RH, Tokish JM, eds. *Advanced Reconstruction Shoulder 2.* 2nd ed. American Academy of Orthopaedic Surgeons; 2016:479-485.

50. Ernstbrunner L, Suter A, Catanzaro S, Rahm S, Gerber C. Reverse total shoulder arthroplasty for massive, irreparable rotator cuff tears before the age of 60 years: long-term results. *J Bone Joint Surg Am.* 2017;99(20):1721-1729.

51. Crosby LA. Infected total shoulder arthroplasty: two stage revision. In: Zuckerman JD, ed. *Advanced Reconstruction Shoulder.* American Academy of Orthopaedic Surgeons; 2007:605-612.

52. Florschutz AV, Lane PD, Crosby LA. Infection after primary anatomic versus primary reverse total shoulder arthroplasty. *J Shoulder Elbow Surg.* 2015;24(8):1296-1301.

53. Gorman MT, Crosby LA. Treatment of deep infection after total shoulder arthroplasty with an antibiotic-impregnated cement spacer. *Tech Shoulder Elbow Surg.* 2006;7(2):82-85.

54. Jawa A, Shi L, O'Brien T, et al. Prosthesis of antibiotic-loaded acrylic cement (PROSTALAC) use for the treatment of infection after shoulder arthroplasty. *J Bone Joint Surg Am.* 2011;93(21):2001-2009.

55. Mileti J, Sperling JW, Cofield RH. Reimplantation of a shoulder arthroplasty after a previous infected arthroplasty. *J Shoulder Elbow Surg.* 2004;13(5):528-531.

56. Sabesan VJ, Ho JC, Kovacevic D, Iannotti JP. Two-stage reimplantation for treating prosthetic shoulder infections. *Clin Orthop Relat Res.* 2011;469(9):2538-2543.

57. Seitz WH Jr, Damacen H. Staged exchange arthroplasty for shoulder sepsis. *J Arthroplasty.* 2002;17(4 suppl 1):36-40.

58. Villacis D, Merriman JA, Yalamanchili R, Omid R, Itamura J, Rick Hatch GF III. Serum interleukin-6 as a marker of periprosthetic shoulder infection. *J Bone Joint Surg Am.* 2014;96(1):41-45.

59. Ammon P, Stockley I. Allograft bone in two-stage revision of the hip for infection. Is it safe? *J Bone Joint Surg Br.* 2004;86(7):962-965.

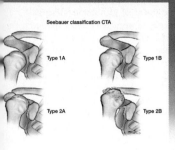

33 Component Loosening and Scapular Notching

Diego Lima, MD and Gregory J. Gilot, MD

INTRODUCTION

Component loosening remains one of the central concerns following total shoulder arthroplasty (TSA) and, in this context, the glenoid component is more of a concern than the humeral component.[1] Both symptomatic and asymptomatic loosening of the glenoid and/or humeral components following TSA have been reported to account for approximately one-third of all complications associated with anatomic total shoulder arthroplasty (ATSA) and reverse total shoulder arthroplasty (RTSA).[2]

Aseptic glenoid component loosening after ATSA occurs more frequently than aseptic humeral component loosening. Radiographic evidence of loosening often occurs in the absence of clinical symptoms. Therefore, it is essential to confirm that pain in association with radiographic evidence of loosening is secondary to loosening and not another cause. The presence of component migration is a very reliable sign that the component is loose and the cause of symptoms.[3]

CLINICAL AND RADIOGRAPHIC EVALUATION

The literature reports an incidence of radiographic glenoid component loosening from 12% to 94%.[3] Early glenoid loosening can be the result of eccentric stress distribution because of excessive humeral component translation as occurs with rotator cuff deficiency or instability. Other possible causes for early loosening include inadequate initial fixation, poor bony support, and infection. A thorough physical exam must be performed on any patient with persistent shoulder pain following shoulder arthroplasty to identify the potential etiology. In addition to range of motion, rotator cuff function and glenohumeral stability should be assessed and correlated with associated discomfort.[3,4]

Immediate postoperative radiolucent lines around the glenoid component (up to 94%) may represent inadequate immediate fixation resulting from the surgical technique or suboptimal cementing technique. Although several studies have reported a high incidence of radiolucent lines, direct correlation to symptomatic loosening has not been identified. Furthermore, the exact significance of the size and location of the radiolucent lines has not been clearly established. A lucent line that is progressive around the perimeter of the component or one that widens on serial radiographs should raise concern for true loosening. Lucent lines that progress or exceed 1.5 to 2 mm in width are more suggestive of true, symptomatic loosening (**FIGURE 33.1**).[5] Of course, any translation of the component (ie, shifting or tilting) or overall displacement of the component is a clear indication of loosening.[3] Much less information is available on the significance of humeral radiolucent lines. Radiographic findings consistent with humeral loosening include component subsidence or migration into varus, progressive radiolucent line formation, cortical scalloping, and distal pedestal formation (**FIGURE 33.2**).[6] Radiolucent lines have been reported more frequently around uncemented humeral components. In a recent study, Sanchez-Sotelo et al defined the "at risk" humeral component to be a component in which two of three observers identify tilt or subsidence or a radiolucent line 2 mm or greater in width present in three or more zones (**FIGURE 33.3**). In general, any component with subsidence or shift in position is typically deemed to be loose.[3]

Shoulder radiographs can be difficult to interpret with respect to component loosening. If there is metal backing to the glenoid component, only a slight change in angle of the x-ray beam will obscure interface changes. The 40-degree posterior oblique view is an improvement over the standard anterior-posterior view in assessing the interface between the glenoid implant and the bone. We have found fluoroscopically positioned views to be most consistent for evaluating not only the glenoid component, but also the humeral component. It is also useful to have a series of radiographs taken over time to identify progressive changes that would not be evident on a single radiograph.[1]

By recognizing the characteristic patient presentation and having high-quality serial radiographs, it is usually possible to diagnose component loosening without needing more complex studies. However, occasionally they are needed. Arthrography, in addition to outlining the rotator cuff tendons, will display synovitis, which is often present in situations where component loosening occurs. Also, dye can track between the bone-cement interface. However, the accuracy of this test for the diagnosis

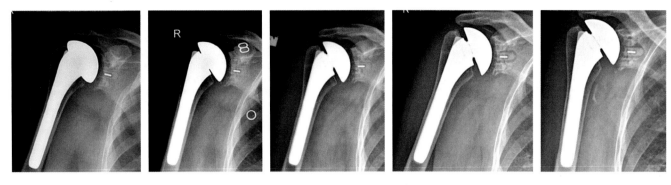

FIGURE 33.1 Postoperative radiographic series showing progression of radiolucency lines after an anatomic total shoulder arthroplasty in the same patient. Time from surgery, starting on the left: 1 year, 3 years, 5 years, 7 years, and 9 years.

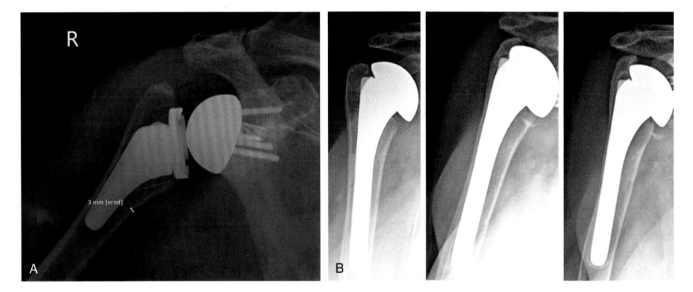

FIGURE 33.2 (A) Radiographic evidence of stress shielding exhibiting thinning of the medial cortex after a reverse total shoulder arthroplasty; **(B)** sequential postoperative films after 1 year, 4 years, and 7 years with evidence of scalloping around the stem, pedestal formation at the tip of the stem, and complete loosening and subsidence of the stem.

of component loosening has not been fully assessed. Shoulder arthroscopy has been suggested as one means to diagnose glenoid loosening in cases where a diagnosis cannot be established by less invasive means.[1]

ANATOMIC TOTAL SHOULDER ARTHROPLASTY

Aseptic Glenoid Loosening in TSA

The most common long-term complication following TSA is glenoid loosening, which accounts for approximately 24% of all complications. A recent systematic review reported that asymptomatic radiolucent lines occurred at a rate of 7.3% per year after primary ATSA, with symptomatic glenoid loosening and surgical revision occurring at rates of 1.2% and 0.8% annually, respectively. Radiolucent lines around glenoid components are common; however, they do not necessarily precede symptomatic loosening or indicate a need for revision **(FIGURE 33.4)**. The etiology of glenoid loosening is likely multifactorial and may be related to implant

design, surgical technique, patient characteristics, and the integrity of the rotator cuff. Knowledge of the native glenoid anatomy and pathology, indications and techniques for implantation, mechanisms of failure, and the rationale behind various implant designs allows the surgeon to minimize complications and maximize outcomes following ATSA. Franklin et al developed a system for classifying radiolucency around keeled glenoid components that was later adapted by Lazarus et al to classify loosening around pegged components **(FIGURE 33.5)**. These classification systems are frequently utilized and have become the standard; however, the interobserver and intraobserver reliability of each has not been established.[5]

The classic mechanism by which anatomic glenoid components loosen over time is the "rocking-horse" phenomenon **(FIGURE 33.6)**. When the component is edge-loaded, it is compressed at one side, resulting in tensile forces on the opposite side. The resulting micromotion or rocking eventually results in compromise

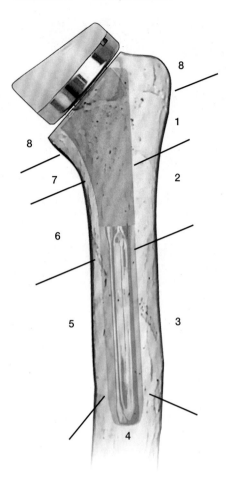

FIGURE 33.3 Humeral stem divided into thirds. Bone adjacent to the stem is divided into eight zones: Zones 1, 2, and 3 represent the lateral aspect of the stem at the proximal, middle, and distal thirds, respectively. Zone 4 is the area around the distal stem tip. Zones 5, 6, 7, and 8 denote the medial portion of the stem from the distal middle, proximal thirds, and base, respectively.

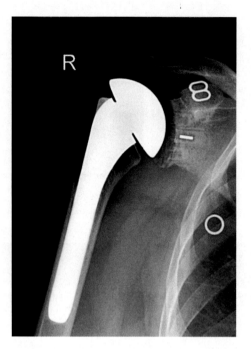

FIGURE 33.4 Radiolucent lines around the glenoid component on an anatomic total shoulder arthroplasty 3 years following surgery.

at the bone-cement interface. Although this theory has not been proven conclusively in clinical or laboratory studies, it is supported by clinical experience. Edge-loading can be worsened by glenohumeral instability and rotator cuff dysfunction, ultimately leading to a rapid progression of glenoid loosening. Similar edge-loading effects and excessive implant micromotion are thought to occur when glenoid components are implanted in retroversion or superior inclination. Eccentric implant wear patterns and implant micromotion likely exacerbate the process of loosening through generation of polyethylene wear debris and particle-induced osteolysis. Another factor that contributes to loosening is potential compromise of the bone-cement interface as a result of thermal necrosis during the cementing process. Stress-shielding of bone adjacent to a rigid cement mantle or adjacent to an uncemented metal-backed component has also been implicated as a cause of radiolucent lines and clinical loosening. The influence of inflammation and biologic factors is

likely of great importance, although it remains poorly understood. Inflammatory cytokines can be part of the arthritic disease process leading to shoulder arthritis and can also be increased as a response to foreign body wear particles from metal or polyethylene. These cytokines may share a role in the development of glenoid component loosening over time.[5]

Glenoid Implant Designs

Efforts to decrease glenoid loosening have resulted in changes to prosthetic design and implantation techniques. Currently, a wide variety of glenoid component options are available, including metal-backed, all-polyethylene, hybrid, bone ingrowth or ongrowth, inset, and augmented designs **(FIGURE 33.7)**. Many recent clinical and biomechanical studies have examined these implant options. A thorough knowledge of glenoid anatomy, pathology, implant options, indications, and principles of implantation is necessary to optimize the outcome following ATSA and ultimately, to decrease the incidence of glenoid component loosening.[5]

Glenoid Component Shape

Modern glenoid components are available in several shapes and sizes. Some implants are pear-shaped to mimic the shape of the normal glenoid, whereas others are elliptical. An anatomic pear shape offers the potential for less implant overhang superiorly and less uncovered bone inferiorly, but this shape has not been shown to be superior to elliptical designs. This may be because the arthritic glenoid is not often pear-shaped, and properly

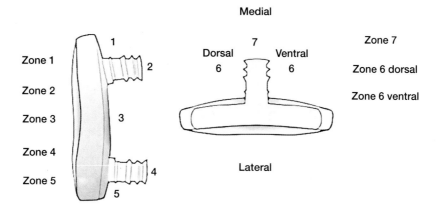

FIGURE 33.5 This drawing represents the zoning and grading systems to determine the risk of loosening on an anatomic glenoid implant. They are measured for width and scored according to Lazarus and Molé, adapted to two-pegged design. Zones 1 to 5 are evaluated on AP view. Zone 1: area under the superior portion; zone 3: area under the implant in between the two pegs; zone 5: area under the inferior portion of the implant. Zones 2 and 4: areas around the superior and inferior pegs. Zones 6 and 7 are evaluated on axial view. Zone 6 ventral: area under the ventral or anterior part of the implant and correspondingly zone 6 dorsal as the area under the dorsal or posterior part of it; zone 7: area around the two pegs in line on axial view. Radiolucent line thickness scoring system: <1 mm = 1 point; 1 to 2 mm = 2 points; >2 mm = 3 points. Score of 6 points or less is classified as having no loosening; 7 to 12 points as risk for loosening; and 13 and above to be loose, according to a previously published study.

sized elliptical implants often fit well after reaming. The backside of the components may be flat or curved. Curved designs have the potential advantage of resisting micromotion more effectively than flat designs. Curved implants theoretically convert shear stresses to compressive stresses to improve the stability of the implant. In a radiographic comparison of flat and convex components, Szabo et al reported that, at 2 years, glenoid designs with

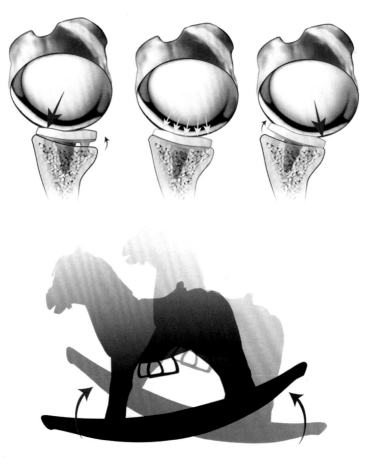

FIGURE 33.6 Rocking-horse phenomenon experienced by an edge-loaded anatomic glenoid implant.

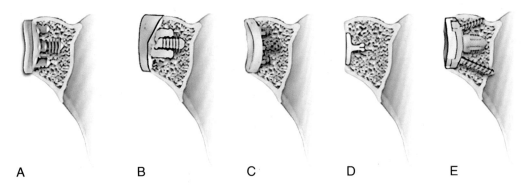

FIGURE 33.7 Different designs of glenoid implants: **(A)** all-polyethylene; **(B)** all-poly with augment; **(C)** hybrid with cage; **(D)** inset; **(E)** metal back.

a curved back had better seating and significantly better radiolucency scores than flat back components. In a follow-up study, however, the same patients showed no difference in progression of radiolucent lines at 10 years. Recently, inset glenoid designs have been developed to aid implant stability. By maintaining a peripheral rim of bone, displacement and micromotion can be minimized by preventing edge-loading.[5] It provides a partial resurfacing while preserving the glenoid rim, capsule, and labrum. To date, only limited data are available to document the outcomes with this component design. Davis reported seven patients who underwent TSA with an inset glenoid component for severe glenoid bone loss. At a mean follow-up of 34 months, there were significant improvements in range of motion, pain, and Single Assessment Numeric Evaluation scores with no complications or revisions. Gunther and Lynch reported on seven patients who underwent TSA with an inset glenoid component for severe glenoid bone stock deficiency with an average 4 years of follow-up. All radiographs were classified as "low risk" for glenoid loosening. Although more research is necessary, this may be a future option in severe glenoid deformity and deficiency.[7] The development of augmented glenoid implants has introduced another design parameter that may impact the risk of loosening.[5] A finite element analysis comparing two different all-polyethylene anatomic glenoid designs showed that a wedge-type of augmented glenoid provided better implant fixation and stress profiles with less micromotion than a step-type design. Longer-term clinical outcome studies are needed to determine the impact of these design modifications on radiolucencies and loosening **(FIGURE 33.8).**[8]

Glenohumeral Radial Mismatch

The ideal conformity between the humeral and glenoid implant has not yet been determined. A fully conformed articulation, such as the original Neer prosthesis, may uniformly distribute stress at the implant-bone interface **(FIGURE 33.9)**. However, normal glenohumeral translation can then occur only with articular separation and edge-loading. Translation can occur more freely with less conformity between the implants, but then contact pressures are not uniform.[5] A biomechanical study looking at different radial mismatches (RMs) demonstrated that greater than 10 mm of RM resulted in loosening of the glenoid component.[9] Another biomechanical and finite element analysis showed that greater RM has the advantage of providing greater glenohumeral stability but with higher implant and cement mantle stress levels and micromotion, which was worse when using a step-cut than a full-wedge design for augmented glenoids.[10]

Walch et al reported that there were fewer radiolucent lines at 2-year follow-up when the RM was at least 6 mm. However, they did not establish an upper limit for the mismatch. Schoch et al evaluated 451 TSAs at a mean follow-up of 5.4 years using a variation of RM between 3.4 and 7.7 mm and showed no statistically significant difference between the groups with respect to the incidence of glenoid radiolucent lines or Lazarus

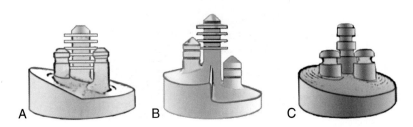

FIGURE 33.8 Current options available for augmented anatomic glenoid implants: **(A)** half-wedge; **(B)** step; **(C)** full-wedge.

Original Neer design

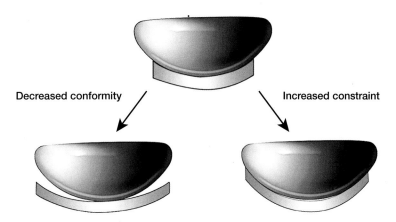

FIGURE 33.9 Conformity refers to the difference between the humeral head radius and the glenoid radius. Constraint is determined by glenoid wall height and is independent of conformity. Two articulations may have identical conformity and different constraints.

score. This finding suggests that optimal RM may extend below 6.0 mm, as previously recommended by Walch et al, without affecting the incidence and grade of glenoid radiolucencies. However, in a more recent study, an RM of the less than 4.5 mm was associated with an increased incidence of radiolucent lines and decreased patient-reported outcome scores at a mean follow-up of 41 months.[11]

Optimal RM in ATSA remains an unanswered question. A complete understanding of optimal RM will require consideration of other factors including implant position and rotator cuff function.[5]

Glenoid Metal-Backed Components

Early efforts to improve the stability of glenoid components and reduce the incidence of loosening led to the development of metal-backed implants. Most of these implants were uncemented and fixed to the glenoid with screws. These designs had a high failure rate, with early loosening, screw breakage, polyethylene dissociation, and the need for revision. Later efforts improved this design with the incorporation of a bony ingrowth material on the metal backing. Taunton et al examined the results of TSA with one such implant, reporting a 31% revision rate associated with loosening and an implant survival rate of 52% at 10 years. Porous ingrowth was improved and screw fixation was eliminated from the design. The metal backing was changed to a monoblock polyethylene platform with a central bony ingrowth attachment. However, these components fractured at the keel-glenoid junction or through the bone ingrowth platform, resulting in an unacceptably high failure rate. These implants were redesigned yet again, and the bony ingrowth platform and its connection to the polyethylene have been solidified to resist fracture. Modern metal-backed implants may hold promise; however, because of the history of loosening and catastrophic failure of early

components, judicious use and close monitoring of these implants are recommended.[5]

Glenoid Polyethylene Components

All-polyethylene implants have proved to be a more durable option than metal-backed implants. This may be related in part to the favorable mechanical properties of all-polyethylene implants that result in decreased stress at the implant-bone interface. This is the reason why most glenoid implants used today are all polyethylene. Many of the advances in polyethylene processing and manufacturing associated with hip and knee arthroplasty have been applied to glenoid components. Cross-linked, ultrahigh-molecular-weight polyethylene has been shown to have favorable wear properties and a low incidence of wear-induced osteolysis. Backside texture of all-polyethylene cemented implants has also been examined, and rough texture and threading of pegs have been shown to improve implant pull-out strength. Most all-polyethylene components are designed for cemented fixation around three or four pegs or a central keel. Several comparative studies have examined pegged and keeled implants and most have shown no significant difference in implant survival or clinical outcome despite a reported higher rate of radiolucent lines with keeled implants.[5] In a biomechanical study, Roche et al reported the results of eccentric loading with similar RMs using a peg and keel glenoid and found no difference in edge displacement between the two designs.[12] In a prospective randomized trial comparing pegged and keeled components, Edwards et al showed that, even with the careful application of modern cementing technique, pegged components were radiographically superior to keeled glenoid components. At present the use of both keeled and pegged components can be supported based upon the clinical data reported.

Hybrid Glenoid Designs

In recent years, several variations to the traditional all-polyethylene pegged implants have been introduced all with the goal of improving implant stability. Divergent pegs have been used to provide additional stability against micromotion. All-polyethylene components that allow for bone ongrowth onto an interference-fit central peg provide the possibility of long-term biologic fixation. These "hybrid" components are characterized by central noncemented fixation and peripheral cemented fixation. Promising clinical results have been reported particularly when radiographic density is observed between the flutes of the central peg, indicating bone ingrowth. Other newer implants have been designed to take advantage of the bone ingrowth potential of porous-coated metal and the favorable mechanical properties of polyethylene by adding an optional porous-coated metal central post to a polyethylene-pegged component.[5]

Clinical and biomechanical studies have demonstrated excellent bone ingrowth but have also reported problems with metal debris formation, fracture, and/or dissociation at the metal-polyethylene interface. These complications have been accompanied by early revisions for aseptic loosening.[13] Nelson et al. have reported a 36% rate of radiolucency lines at a minimum 5-year follow up on radiographic evaluation, when used exclusively hybrid glenoids after TSA. Nonetheless, they presented no cases with aseptic loosening.[14] It has been also reported as little as less than 2% revision rates due to aseptic loosening when a hybrid glenoid is used.[15] However, a recent matched cohort comparison, including same humerus component, reported a lower incidence of loosening compared to all-polyethylene glenoids (1.3% vs 3.8%) and lower revision rates with a minimum of 2 years of follow-up.[13]

Aseptic Humeral Loosening

In ATSA, the humeral component is responsible for a small number of complications and revision surgeries. In a study of 1423 patients who underwent ATSA from 1984 to 2004, Cil et al reported an 83% humeral component survival at 20 years.[16] The early-design Neer II humeral component had a 98% survival rate. In a series of 1112 TSAs, isolated humeral loosening occurred in only 0.3% of cases. Given the relative rarity of isolated humeral loosening, if encountered, the surgeon must suspect and carefully evaluate for the possibility of a low-grade infection and potential other sources of the reported symptoms.[7,16,17] The micromotion associated with humeral component loosening results in progressive endosteal bone erosion. The cortices become thinner; subsidence and progressive varus can result, ultimately leading to shaft fracture or perforation.

Cemented Versus Press-Fit Stems

Cemented humeral stems used to be the preferred method for fixation in ATSA patients, with long-term studies reporting excellent results and durability. Cemented fixation became popular because of concerns about aseptic loosening of smooth, diaphyseal humeral components and the decreased risk of intra-operative periprosthetic fracture when used in patients with poor bone quality. Uncemented (press-fit) fixation has become increasingly popular because of concerns for bone stock preservation, surgical time, complications associated with cement pressurization, and the difficulty of removing a well-cemented humeral component during revision surgery. Early studies on press-fit humeral stems reported concerns for loosening primarily because of the use a smooth stem designed for cemented fixation. Matsen et al in a study of 131 patients, who underwent ATSA with a press-fit metaphyseal taper stem design, reported a lower rate of humeral component loosening compared with patients who underwent ATSA with a press-fit diaphyseal cylindrical humeral component. In other series, the rates of aseptic humeral component loosening have ranged from 0.0% to 1.6%. Analysis of pooled data from the series with the largest numbers of patients showed that revision for humeral loosening remained uncommon at 2.6% for cemented implants and 7.47% for uncemented implants—thereby providing further evidence that aseptic loosening is an infrequent occurrence.[18]

However, osteolysis of the proximal humerus has been reported in ATSA patients with either cemented or uncemented humeral components. In a study of 395 TSA patients, Raiss et al reported osteolysis of the proximal humerus in a high percentage of the patients with a well-fixed humeral component. Although osteolysis of the proximal humerus occurred secondary to glenoid wear in many of these patients, the authors also reported stress shielding in 63% of the patients with a long stem, press-fit, uncemented humeral component. Stress shielding has also been reported in ATSA patients with a short stem humeral component. Theoretically, the incidence of stress shielding should increase with increased humeral stem length because the probability of diaphyseal loading increases with increased humeral stem length. In a review of the radiographs of 64 ATSA patients, Nagels et al reported a direct relationship between stress shielding about the humeral component and diaphyseal contact—the greater the diaphyseal fill, the higher the incidence of stress shielding—, suggesting lower stress shielding and loosening rates with properly designed and implanted short stems.[18]

Patient age, bone quality, humeral component design, and surgeon preference are the most important factors to consider in the selection of a cemented or press-fit humeral component. However, the rate of humeral

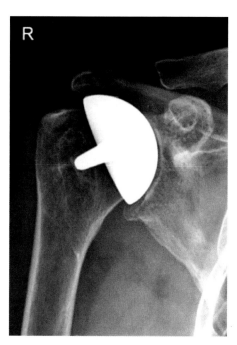

FIGURE 33.10 A 78-year-old patient with radiographic evidence of proximal migration and loosening of a stemless humeral component.

component complications is relatively low compared to glenoid component complications in patients who undergo ATSA using a variety of humeral stem and fixation options.[16]

Stemless Components

Stemless shoulder arthroplasty is a new and emerging surgical procedure and, as such, no long-term clinical and radiographic studies have been published. In a study of 91 patients who underwent placement of a stemless ongrowth humeral implant with a 2-year follow-up, no loosening, complications, or revisions specific to the humeral implant were noted. In a quasi-randomized clinical trial comparing that same implant with a standard cemented, stemmed ATSA implant, no differences were found in regard to clinical outcomes, implant survival, or radiolucent lines.[8] Another study of 61 patients with osteoarthritis, posttraumatic arthritis, or osteonecrosis who underwent stemless shoulder arthroplasty (44 hemiarthroplasties and 19 ATSAs), Huguet et al reported intraoperative lateral humeral cortical fracture in 5 patients, all of which healed uneventfully. With a mean follow-up of 3.5 years (range 36-51 months), the authors reported humeral component revision in four patients all of which were unrelated to the humeral component. The authors also reported no evidence of subsidence, loosening, osteolysis, stress shielding, or radiolucent lines on radiographs obtained at final follow-up **(FIGURE 33.10)**. In a study of 78 patients (mean age, 58 years) who underwent stemless shoulder arthroplasty (39 hemiarthroplasties and 39 ATSAs), Habermeyer et al reported partial osteolysis under the cranial part of the humeral component without loosening in 3 of the patients (3.8%); in 2 of these 3 patients, the partial osteolysis was observed in combination with glenoid component loosening. The rates of radiolucent lines and glenoid component loosening observed were similar to those in patients who underwent shoulder arthroplasty with a stemmed humeral component. An area of lower density cancellous bone in the proximal humerus was observed in 41.3% of the patients, which did not appear to affect clinical outcome. The overall complication rate was 12.8%, and the overall revision surgery rate was 9%; however, none of the patients underwent revision surgery for component loosening.[16] These early overall results suggest that, at this point in time, stemless humeral components are a reasonable option in shoulder arthroplasty.

REVERSE TOTAL SHOULDER ARTHROPLASTY

Baseplate Loosening and Scapular Notching

Although glenoid component loosening is common in ATSA, it is uncommon following RTSA. When loosening does develop, it often results in proximal migration and tipping of the component into superior inclination. Unless significant trauma occurs, which could lead to catastrophic failure, component migration can be a relatively subtle process because the locking screws create a fixated construct that must cut through the vault to completely compromise baseplate stability, even in the absence of central post incorporation. The major challenge created by baseplate loosening is the associated loss of glenoid bone stock. Removal of a loose component can leave a substantial osseous defect making reconstruction challenging. These reconstructive techniques are discussed in Chapter 43.[6]

Favard reported an incidence of glenoid component migration of 28.5% of patients after a minimum follow-up of 8 years.[19] Another study with long-term outcomes, reported a 6.25% rate of loosening on the glenoid side after an RTSA with a mean follow-up of 44 months.[20] A 15-year follow-up study by Gerber et al in 2018 reported a 2% incidence of aseptic glenoid loosening following RTSA performed for irreparable rotator cuff tears.[21] There have been rare reports of complete baseplate loosening as a result of progressive scapular notching (SN). The clinical effects and mechanisms of notching will be discussed.

SCAPULAR NOTCHING

Pathogenesis

Scapular notching (SN) is a radiographic finding, which may occur following RTSA. The term is used to describe an erosive lesion at the axillary border of the scapular neck that occurs when the medial rim of the humeral liner abuts against the scapular neck with the arm in adduction. It can cause an osteolytic process as

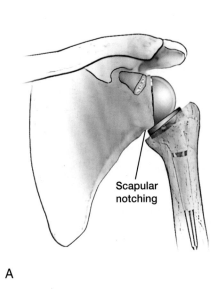

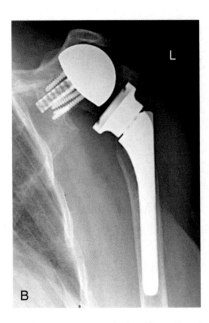

FIGURE 33.11 Illustration **(A)** and radiograph **(B)** depicting scapular notching after a reverse total shoulder arthroplasty. Observe a broken screw on the baseplate.

a result of wear debris from the polyethylene liner. The clinical effect of notching was uncertain until recently **(FIGURE 33.11)**. However, several reports suggest a correlation between the presence of SN and functional outcomes.[22-24] The radiographic incidence increases with increasing follow-up and has been reported in up to 70% of patients.[22,25-27] Factors that contribute to SN include prosthetic design, scapular anatomy, and implant position.[25,27] Notching can be progressive and extend beyond the most inferior screw, suggesting that an osteolytic response does occur in addition to the mechanical impingement.[26,27]

In 1985, Grammont introduced the first successful RTSA. One of the distinguishing biomechanical characteristics of Grammont's design included medialization of the center of rotation (CoR) of the glenoid implant. This decreased the shear force and lever arm across the glenoid bone-implant interface. Distalization of the glenoid implant served to tension the deltoid. The combination of these factors resulted in a lower rate of glenoid implant failure that was characteristic of previous designs. However, this design frequently resulted in contact between the inferior-medial rim of the humeral implant polyethylene and the scapular neck with the arm in adduction. Mechanical engagement of the humeral cup with the scapular neck has been linked to the development of bone loss, polyethylene wear, osteolysis, glenoid implant loosening, and failure associated with compromise of clinical outcomes.[23] While studies have utilized cadaveric models, finite element analysis, computational modeling, and retrospective radiographic review to examine factors related to an impingement-free shoulder range of motion following RTSA as well as factors associated with notching as seen

on postoperative radiographs, the relationship between dynamic osseous impingement and subsequent development of notching as visualized on radiographs in a clinical population has not been clearly defined. The ability to position the glenosphere or humeral component to avoid osseous impingement along the scapular neck may prevent the development of notching.[25] Previous studies have demonstrated that prosthesis design parameters, patient attributes, diagnosis, and surgical technique predispose to SN **(FIGURE 33.12)**.[28] As a result, surgeons often use specific implantation methods, even employing glenoid bone grafting techniques to minimize notching in designs that are prone to the development of this problem.[26]

The factors causing SN are now better understood. Lateralization of the CoR and a decrease in the humeral component neck-shaft angle are probably the most relevant modifications to minimize the risk of notching. Along with those changes, the surgical technique has also evolved to position the glenoid baseplate at least flush with the inferior glenoid rim so that some amount of glenosphere overhang is present **(FIGURE 33.13)**. Glenosphere overhang has been identified as one of the most important factors to prevent the development of SN.[29] SN was described by Sirveaux et al in their analysis of the midterm results of the Delta (DePuy, Warsaw, IN, USA) shoulder prosthesis, which was a Grammont-style reverse design.[24,27] When investigators compared pre- to postoperative radiographs of 80 Grammont-style RTSAs, they identified the phenomenon as "a defect of the bone in the inferior part of the glenoid component." It was eventually recognized that the symmetric geometry of the polyethylene humeral component and drastically medialized CoR also contributed to this phenomenon.

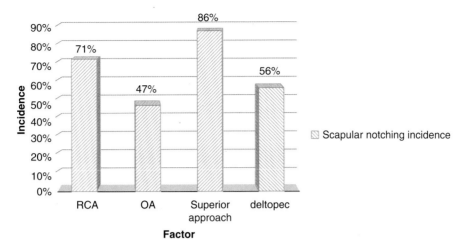

FIGURE 33.12 Graph showing different factors that influence the risk of scapular notching. deltopec, deltopectoralis approach; OA, osteoarthritis; RCA, rotator cuff arthropathy.

Sirveaux et al developed a classification system for SN at the same time Nerot's group reported a very similar classification system, hence the designation of the Nerot-Sirveaux classification system for SN.[27]

INCIDENCE

The reported incidence of SN varies widely (0%-96%) and can be explained by the different implant design characteristics, variation in placement of the glenoid component, surgical approach used, and patient's anatomy, among other reasons.[23,24,29] A 2015 systematic review of 37 studies and 3150 patients revealed notching rates between 4.6% and 50.8%. Recent studies evaluating the effect of implant design and position report notching rates as low as 10% to 30%, indicating that these two factors play an important role. By contrast, other studies have found notching rates in excess of 50% and reaching as high as 80% to 96%. Some of the variability in reported incidence is attributable to the length of follow-up since higher grades have been associated

with longer follow-up. For example, in 2008, Cuff and colleagues reported that zero out of 96 patients showed radiographic signs of notching at 2 years, but a subsequent follow-up of the same cohort at 5 years reported an increase in SN to 9% **(FIGURE 33.14)**.[23,30-35]

Anatomic Considerations

Several studies have demonstrated that decreased scapular neck length (SNL) leads to increased rates of notching. In general, SNL is measured as the distance between the lateral column of the scapula and the articular surface of the glenoid on a Grashey AP radiograph. A cadaver study of 442 scapulae from 221 cadavers showed a mean SNL of 10.6 ± 3.3 mm **(FIGURE 33.15)**. Male specimens trended toward a longer SNL than female specimens, and Caucasians had significantly longer SNLs compared to African Americans. In a 2014 analysis of 50 RTSA patients, those with notching were found to have a mean SNL of 8.9 mm as compared with those without notching who had a mean SNL of 12.1 mm ($P = 0.0012$). This

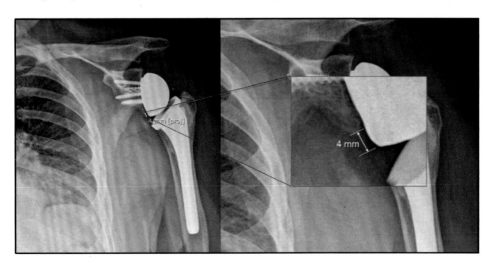

FIGURE 33.13 Glenosphere overhang (4 mm) in relation to the inferior rim of the glenoid used to increase impingement-free range of motion.

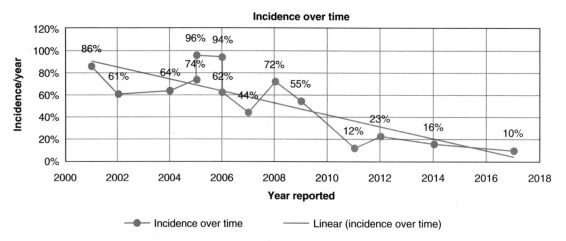

FIGURE 33.14 Graph showing variation in incidence of scapular notching over time. From 2001 to 2009, all implants used were Grammont style. From 2010 to 2018, all implants used were lateralized style.

suggested that those with smaller than average SNL are at an increased risk of notching. Shorter neck lengths result in a smaller adduction arc, increasing the likelihood of impingement between the humeral implant and the inferior scapular neck. When performing an RTSA on patients with an SNL less than 9.0 mm, glenoid augmentation should be considered, or an implant with increased lateral offset used. Patients with rotator cuff arthropathy or inflammatory arthropathy often have superior-medial migration of the humeral head against the glenoid, leading to glenoid bone loss and a shorter SNL. Significant glenoid deformity and malpositioning of the glenoid baseplate into a superior or superior tilt position may increase the risk of notching.[23]

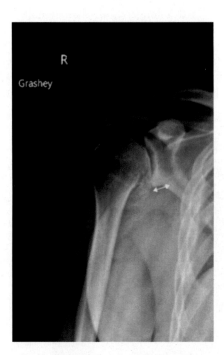

FIGURE 33.15 Measurement of scapular neck length on anterior-posterior radiographic view.

RADIOGRAPHIC ANALYSIS

Presurgical Imaging

The prevention of SN starts with adequate presurgical imaging Typically, standard Grashey anterior-posterior (AP) views in external and internal rotation and an axillary lateral view are obtained.[22] A computed tomography (CT) study with 3D reconstruction scan is recommended when abnormal glenoid anatomy is suspected. Although two-dimensional CT scans are helpful in identifying lesions of the glenoid, angles on a given CT image are influenced by the gantry angle, or angle of the x-ray beam relative to the patient, which may vary considerably with changes in patient position inside the CT scanner.[23]

Postsurgical Imaging

As noted, the Nerot-Sirveaux classification system for SN is a radiographically based tool that describes the amount and extent of bone loss in patients with notching after RTSA.[22-24] Sirveaux et al utilized an AP radiograph tangential to the baseplate (a true AP of the shoulder in the scapular plane), because this view permits visualization of the glenosphere and scapular neck without superimposition of the humeral component. Sirveaux et al and Nerot's group both classified the scapular notch as grades 1 to 4 based on the size of the defect visualized on the AP radiograph. Grade 1 describes a defect confined to the pillar; grade 2 represents a defect confluent with the inferior-most screw; grade 3 represents a defect extending above the inferior-most screw; and grade 4 represents a defect that involves the central post **(FIGURE 33.16)**. Grades 1 and 2 are considered to be the limit by which purely mechanical erosion may occur. Grades 3 and 4 are likely the result of a biologic response to polyethylene particles resulting in osteolysis. Radiographic evaluation of SN is performed using standard radiographs. A

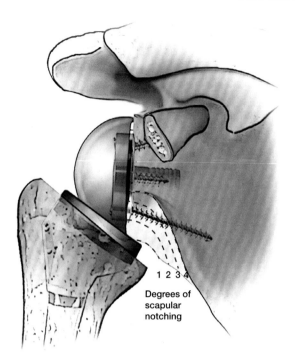

FIGURE 33.16 Sirveaux-Nerot classification for scapular notching: grade 1: defect contained within the pillar; grade 2: notch with the lower screw; grade 3: notch is localized over the lower screw; and grade 4: notch extends under the baseplate.

true Grashey AP view is obtained with the x-ray beam tangential to the glenoid baseplate to view it in profile. Scapular lateral and axillary views should also be obtained.[23,24,27] The accuracy of this grading system has been evaluated to a limited degree. In a series of 60 shoulders, Sadoghi et al reported excellent interobserver reliability between two observers using the Sirveaux classification system.[24] In another study of 190 cases, utilizing three observers, the interobserver reliability was low with an overall κ value of 0.43.[24] However, in another study the interobserver and intraobserver reliability of the Sirveaux classification was "almost perfect" with a κ coefficient value of >0.86.[27] These variable results, though interesting, have not changed the preference for use of the Nerot-Sirveaux classification system.

SURGICAL TECHNIQUES TO MINIMIZE NOTCHING

Surgical Approach

Surgical approach may also play a role in the development of SN. The anterosuperior approach (or deltoid splitting approach) has been associated with an increased risk of notching. In one series of 337 shoulders undergoing RTSA by either an anterosuperior or deltopectoral approach, the incidence of SN was 86% when an anterosuperior approach was used, compared with only 56% when a deltopectoral approach was used (P < 0.0001). Another study reported an SN incidence of

74% using the anterosuperior approach and 63% with the deltopectoral approach (P > 0.05). During an anterosuperior approach, one may misjudge the true inferior border of the glenoid. This situation may result in superior placement or superior tilt of the glenosphere or both, which is known to increase the risk of notching and would explain the increased rates of notching reported. Currently, the most common approach for RTSA is deltopectoral. Regardless of the approach utilized, it is important to fully expose the inferior glenoid to minimize the risk of inadvertent superior placement or tilt of the glenoid component. This may be more easily accomplished with the deltopectoral approach. However, the choice of surgical approach is multifactorial of which surgeon's preference is an important consideration.[23]

Glenosphere Tilt

In biomechanical models, inferior glenoid tilt affords a greater arc of impingement-free motion with a more even distribution of force at the bone-glenoid implant interface. However, optimal glenoid tilt is dependent on other design and anatomic factors, such as lateralization of the glenosphere and humeral prosthesis neck-shaft angle. Therefore, achieving inferior glenoid tilt is more important in a standard Grammont-style prosthesis with a nonlateralized glenosphere and a 155° neck-shaft angle.[23,25]

Glenosphere Placement

Placing the glenosphere with inferior overhang and less medialization of the baseplate appears to be very effective in reducing the incidence of SN with the least adverse consequences.[23,24] Nyffeler et al performed an in vitro study of cadaver scapulae to determine optimal glenosphere placement. They measured adduction angles in the scapular plane in four scenarios as follows: (1) superior placement with exposed inferior glenoid[23]; (2) neutral placement with the glenosphere flush with the inferior glenoid rim[24]; (3) glenosphere extending below the inferior glenoid rim; and (4) the glenosphere tilted inferiorly 15° and flush with the inferior scapular neck.[25] Scenario 3 provided the greatest impingement-free adduction angle (P < 0.001), which was confirmed in different clinical studies (Simovitch et al in 2007 and de Wilde et al in 2010). Limitations exist on the amount of overhang that is possible with concentric designs before fixation in glenoid bone may be compromised. Eccentric glenospheres have been designed in an effort to increase inferior overhang while maintaining fixation within the glenoid. In 2014, Poon et al compared notching rates between concentric and eccentric implants. Notching was not observed in either group when the overhang was at least 3.5 mm. In addition, there was no difference in clinical outcomes with a minimum of 3.5 mm overhang. Consequences of excessive inferior placement of the glenosphere include overtensioning of the deltoid, the need for increased humeral resection, compromised glenoid fixation, and a potential increase in acromial stress fractures.[23,25] Richetti et al, using multivariate modeling, demonstrated that the combination of inferior and lateral or posterior and lateral glenosphere placement was strongly predictive of the absence of notching, confirming the importance of lateralization. In both univariate and multivariate analyses, posterior glenosphere position was strongly predictive of the absence of notching. Posterior glenosphere position has been less commonly discussed, compared with inferior and lateral placement, as being important in avoiding notching. Translational changes (lateral, posterior, and inferior) to the glenosphere position have been shown to be more effective in avoiding impingement than changes in version and inclination.[25] This suggests that preoperative planning of the preferred implant position based on the osseous anatomy and kinematic range-of-motion criteria may help to avoid notching postoperatively. These authors further suggest that for implant systems with a medialized CoR, placing the glenosphere in a maximally inferior position while maximizing posterior and lateral placement as allowed by the osseous anatomy is an important guideline to minimize notching. This approach may be generalizable to any RTSA system, although the appropriate amount of inferior, lateral, or posterior glenosphere placement is likely implant design-specific.[25]

Glenosphere Design

Similar to glenospheres with an inferior overhang, those with a lateralized offset appear to protect against SN. Standard Grammont glenospheres have a medialized CoR at the glenoid border and a predisposition toward notching. A lateralized CoR more closely replicates the physiologic COR and is associated with a decreased risk of notching. Lateral offset can be achieved in different ways, including by intrinsic design or with bone or metal augmentation of the glenoid. Autograft or allograft bone augmentation effectively increases the SNL **(FIGURE 33.17)**. The advantage of lateralization with a bone graft is that the CoR is maintained at the bone-implant interface while simultaneously restoring offset. Concerns exist regarding incorporation of the intercalary bone graft positioned between the native glenoid and the baseplate prosthesis. The use of large diameter glenospheres provides a more stable, impingement-free ROM and decreases notching. These benefits need to be balanced against the potential increased tension on the construct.[23,29]

Humeral Implant Design

As the prosthesis neck-shaft angle decreases, the humeral articulating surface becomes more vertical and positioned in more abduction relative to the shaft. In a cadaver model, this has been shown to improve impingement-free adduction while also providing more lateral offset. However, as the neck-shaft angle is decreased, contact stresses are increased and tend to shift inferiorly along the onlay polyethylene. This situation could potentially lead to edge-loading with increased generation of polyethylene wear particles, which theoretically could result in glenoid osteolysis and contribute to notching in the absence of mechanical impingement. Similarly, decreased polyethylene depth appears to improve the adduction angle. However, this decreases the contact area and resistance to shear forces. The reduced constraint and decreased "jump distance" may increase the risk of instability. A recent systematic review of 38 studies including more than 2000 RTSAs performed with either 155° or 135° of humeral neck-shaft inclination found that implants with 155° of inclination produced significantly higher rates of SN. SN was found in only 2.8% in the 135° group versus 16.8% in the 155° group ($P < 0.0001$). No difference in the dislocation rate was observed between the two groups. Each of the individual parameters discussed with regard to glenoid and humeral prosthesis design, offset, and placement can contribute to notching. Ultimately, it is the combination of these parameters that will have the greatest effect on notching rates and clinical outcomes.[23]

Clinical Outcomes

Mechanical impingement along the scapular pillar has the potential to result in increased discomfort, reduced active ROM, and compromised outcomes. Despite several early studies which did not describe any negative clinical effects, more recent studies have demonstrated that SN, and specifically higher grades of notching, is associated with worse clinical outcomes.[22-24,26,27] A study by Mollon et al demonstrated that the majority of previous studies were insufficiently powered to detect the clinical impact. Their series of 464 patients with a minimum of 2 years follow-up demonstrated that RTSA provided significant mean improvements compared to preoperative data for all active ROM measurements and functional outcome score, in all patients. However, at latest follow-up, patients with SN had significantly worse outcomes in 4 of 6 outcomes scores and significantly less active abduction, forward flexion, and strength compared with patients without SN. The SN group also had significantly less mean improvement in preoperative to postoperative outcomes in the Constant score and strength as well a significantly higher complication rate (23.4% vs 9.4%; $P = 0.0051$) and revision rate (10.6% vs 1.4%; $P = 0.0004$) **(FIGURE 33.18)**. They also noted that the SN group had a significantly higher incidence of humeral radiolucent lines (27.7% vs 13.8%; $P = 0.0157$).[26,32]

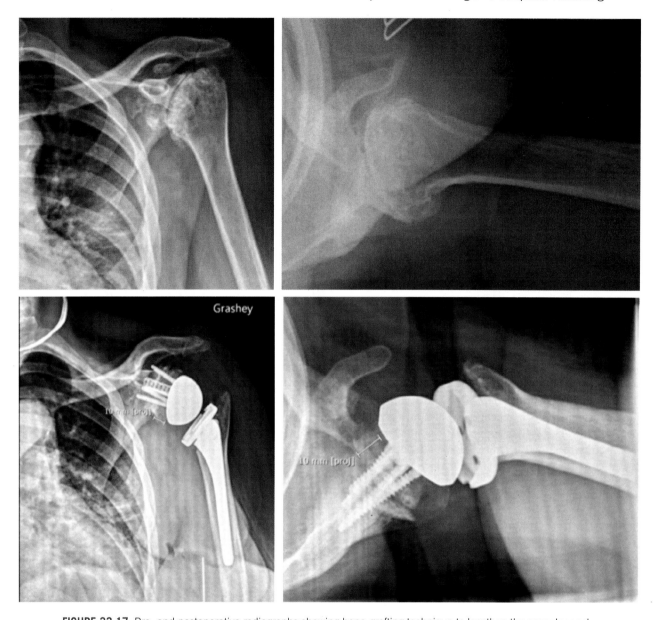

FIGURE 33.17 Pre- and postoperative radiographs showing bone-grafting technique to lengthen the scapular neck.

ASEPTIC HUMERAL LOOSENING IN RTSA

Aseptic loosening of the humeral stem in RTSA generally occurs in less than 2% of cases with previous reports ranging from 0% to 5.8%.[36] Radiographic changes include the presence of osteolysis, radiolucent lines, and stress shielding. Osteolysis was defined as endosteal scalloping, scalloping at the bone-implant junction, or presence of cystic changes within the humeral metaphyseal bone. Stress shielding was defined as uniform regional decrease in bone density. This finding has been proposed to occur through two mechanisms. First, the solid implants used during shoulder arthroplasty have a lower modulus of elasticity than the hollow cortical bone,

making them a stiffer construct. This causes a reduction in stress transfer in the proximal portion of the bone. The second mechanism relates to the rigid distal fixation of the stem in the diaphysis, which results in decreased load in the metaphyseal area.[37]

Gilot et al performed a multicenter, retrospective, blinded, case-control radiographic study of aseptic humeral stem loosening in RTSA. They evaluated 177 cemented and 115 press-fit humeral stems after RTSA for rotator cuff arthropathy. At mean follow-up of 39 months, the overall loosening rate was 0.74%, with no significant difference between the cemented and press-fit groups.[38]

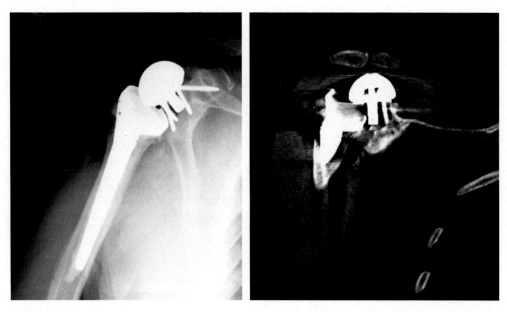

FIGURE 33.18 Radiographic and CT images showing catastrophic loosening and notching after reverse total shoulder arthroplasty.

In a study of 98 shoulders with uncemented trabecular stems, 9 (9.2%) showed subsidence of 2 mm or less at 1 year and none showed subsidence of more than 2 mm. Subsidence did not progress the interval from 1 to 2 years nor did any stems appear at risk for loosening based upon criteria published in previous reports assessing radiographic stability.[39]

There is an expectation, like in any form of arthroplasty, that the rate of implant loosening will increase over time. In a group of studies with longer follow-up time, there has been a higher rate of loosening (2% vs 0.8%, $P \leq 0.01$). The accuracy of reporting true humeral radiolucent lines from loosening can be questioned because stress-shielding can mimic humeral radiolucent lines. The stress transfer that occurs through the implant rather than the adjacent bone can result in resorption of the cortices and tuberosities. With cortical resorption a radiolucency can appear between the implant and the cortex, which may mimic the radiolucency of loosening. Stress-shielding may explain why humeral radiolucent lines around uncemented stems appear to become more frequent in cohorts with longer follow-up.[40]

Stemless RTSA

Stemless shoulder arthroplasty was developed to alleviate the stem-associated intraoperative and postoperative complications and the difficulties of revisions. Early results with respect to the humeral component have been encouraging. Moroder et al reported that the clinical and radiographic outcomes of stemless RTSA in their cohort was not inferior to conventional RTSA.[41] Levy et al reported excellent results in 102 consecutive patients with follow-up of 2 to 7 years who underwent stemless RTSA. Radiographic analysis showed no radiolucencies around either the humeral or glenoid components at latest follow-up. Ballas and Beguin reported the results of a prospective, single-surgeon series of 56 TESS stemless implants with a mean follow-up of 58 months. At the latest follow-up, there were no periprosthetic humeral radiolucencies, migration, or loosening of the humeral component. Teissier et al[30] reported on 101 patients with 105 stemless TESS implants, with a minimum follow-up period of 24 months. Radiographically, inferior SN occurred in 17 cases (19%). The notching rate was higher when the glenometaphyseal angle increased, the inferior tilt decreased ($P = 0.003$), and when the neck-shaft angle increased. There was no evidence of component loosening. Overall, these results support the continued use and development of stemless RTSA. However, longer-term follow-up is needed to determine true implant survival rates.

CONCLUSION

Although the vast majority of patients have excellent pain relief and functional outcomes following ATSA and RTSA, component loosening will continue to be a focus for all shoulder arthroplasty surgeons. Glenoid component loosening following ATSA is the most significant issue. Humeral component loosening following ATSA and RTSA is a much less significant issue. Future areas that may improve implant survival include advances in surgical approach, such as computer-assisted surgical planning and intra-operative navigation; advances in humeral component geometry and fixation, such as stemless, short-stem, and convertible implants; advances in bearing surfaces, such as pyrocarbon, ceramic, and metal-on-metal; and advances in glenoid component geometry and fixation, such as augmented components, in-growth pegs, and inlay glenoid components.[7,42]

Despite the fact the SN is much better understood now and its incidence has been decreasing over time as a result of new implant designs, improved insertion techniques, and a better understanding of the biomechanics of the RTSA, more work needs to be done to understand the contributions of SN to loosening or component failure.

REFERENCES

1. Iannotti JP, Williams GR. *Disorders of the Shoulder: Diagnosis & Management.* 2nd ed. Lippincott Williams & Wilkins; 2007.
2. Favard L. Revision of total shoulder arthroplasty. *Orthop Traumatol Surg Res.* 2013;99(1 suppl):S12-S21.
3. Warner JJPI, Joseph P, Flatow EL. *Complex and Revision Problems in Shoulder Surgery.* 2nd ed. Lippincott Williams & Wilkins (LWW); 2005:608.
4. Bonnevialle N, Melis B, Neyton L, et al. Aseptic glenoid loosening or failure in total shoulder arthroplasty: revision with glenoid reimplantation. *J Shoulder Elbow Surg.* 2013;22(6):745-751.
5. Pinkas D, Wiater B, Wiater JM. The glenoid component in anatomic shoulder arthroplasty. *J Am Acad Orthop Surg.* 2015;23(5):317-326.
6. Chalmers PN, Boileau P, Romeo AA, Tashjian RZ. Revision reverse shoulder arthroplasty. *J Am Acad Orthop Surg.* 2019;27(12):426-436.
7. Tashjian RZ, Chalmers PN. Future frontiers in shoulder arthroplasty and the management of shoulder osteoarthritis. *Clin Sports Med.* 2018;37(4):609-630.
8. Sabesan VJ, Lima DJL, Whaley JD, Pathak V, Zhang L. Biomechanical comparison of 2 augmented glenoid designs: an integrated kinematic finite element analysis. *J Shoulder Elbow Surg.* 2019;28(6):1166-1174.
9. Sabesan VJ, Ackerman J, Sharma V, Baker KC, Kurdziel MD, Wiater JM. Glenohumeral mismatch affects micromotion of cemented glenoid components in total shoulder arthroplasty. *J Shoulder Elbow Surg.* 2015;24(5):814-822.
10. Sabesan VJ, Lima DJL, Whaley JD, Pathak V, Zhang L. The effect of glenohumeral radial mismatch on different augmented total shoulder arthroplasty glenoid designs: a finite element analysis. *J Shoulder Elbow Surg.* 2019;28(6):1146-1153.
11. Hasler A, Meyer DC, Tondelli T, Dietrich T, Gerber C. Radiographic performance depends on the radial glenohumeral mismatch in total shoulder arthroplasty. *BMC Musculoskelet Disord.* 2020;21(1):206.
12. Roche C, Angibaud L, Flurin PH, Wright T, Zuckerman J. Glenoid loosening in response to dynamic multi-axis eccentric loading: a comparison between keeled and pegged designs with an equivalent radial mismatch. *Bull Hosp Jt Dis.* 2006;63(3-4):88-92.
13. Friedman RJ, Cheung E, Grey SG, et al. Clinical and radiographic comparison of a hybrid cage glenoid to a cemented polyethylene glenoid in anatomic total shoulder arthroplasty. *J Shoulder Elbow Surg.* 2019;28(12):2308-2316.
14. Nelson CG, Brolin TJ, Ford MC, Smith RA, Azar FM, Throckmorton TW. Five-year minimum clinical and radiographic outcomes of total shoulder arthroplasty using a hybrid glenoid component with a central porous titanium post. *J Shoulder Elbow Surg.* 2018;27(8):1462-1467.
15. Levy DM, Metzl JA, Vorys GC, Levine WN, Ahmad CS, Bigliani LU. Clinical and radiographic outcomes of total shoulder arthroplasty with a hybrid dual-radii glenoid component. *Am J Orthop (Belle Mead NJ).* 2017;46(6):E366-E373.
16. Lazarus MD, Cox RM, Murthi AM, Levy O, Abboud JA. Stemless prosthesis for total shoulder arthroplasty. *J Am Acad Orthop Surg.* 2017;25(12):e291-e300.
17. Gartsman GE, Edwards TB. *Shoulder Arthroplasty.* 1st ed. Saunders; 2008:1-544.
18. Keener JD, Chalmers PN, Yamaguchi K. The humeral implant in shoulder arthroplasty. *J Am Acad Orthop Surg.* 2017;25(6):427-438.
19. Favard L, Katz D, Colmar M, Benkalfate T, Thomazeau H, Emily S. Total shoulder arthroplasty—arthroplasty for glenohumeral arthropathies: results and complications after a minimum follow-up of 8 years according to the type of arthroplasty and etiology. *Orthop Traumatol Surg Res.* 2012;98(4 suppl):S41-S47.
20. Sirveaux F, Favard L, Oudet D, Huquet D, Walch G, Molé D. Grammont inverted total shoulder arthroplasty in the treatment of glenohumeral osteoarthritis with massive rupture of the cuff. Results of a multicentre study of 80 shoulders. *J Bone Joint Surg Br.* 2004;86(3):388-395.
21. Gerber C, Canonica S, Catanzaro S, Ernstbrunner L. Longitudinal observational study of reverse total shoulder arthroplasty for irreparable rotator cuff dysfunction: results after 15 years. *J Shoulder Elbow Surg.* 2018;27(5):831-838.
22. Beltrame A, Di Benedetto P, Cicuto C, Cainero V, Chisoni R, Causero A. Onlay versus Inlay humeral steam in Reverse Shoulder Arthroplasty (RSA): clinical and biomechanical study. *Acta Biomed.* 2019;90(12 suppl):54-63.
23. Friedman RJ, Barcel DA, Eichinger JK. Scapular notching in reverse total shoulder arthroplasty. *J Am Acad Orthop Surg.* 2019;27(6):200-209.
24. Schneider MM, Toft F, Kolling C, et al. Limited reliability of grading scapular notching according to Nerot-Sirveaux on anteroposterior radiographs. *Arch Orthop Trauma Surg.* 2019;139(1):7-13.
25. Kolmodin J, Davidson IU, Jun BJ, et al. Scapular notching after reverse total shoulder arthroplasty: prediction using patient-specific osseous anatomy, implant location, and shoulder motion. *J Bone Joint Surg Am.* 2018;100(13):1095-1103.
26. Simovitch R, Flurin PH, Wright TW, Zuckerman JD, Roche C. Impact of scapular notching on reverse total shoulder arthroplasty midterm outcomes: 5-year minimum follow-up. *J Shoulder Elbow Surg.* 2019;28(12):2301-2307.
27. Young BL, Cantrell CK, Hamid N. Classifications in brief: the Nerot-Sirveaux classification for scapular notching. *Clin Orthop Relat Res.* 2018;476(12):2454-2457.
28. Lévigne C, Garret J, Boileau P, Alami G, Favard L, Walch G. Scapular notching in reverse shoulder arthroplasty: is it important to avoid it and how? *Clin Orthop Relat Res.* 2011;469(9):2512-2520.
29. Torrens C, Miquel J, Martinez R, Santana F. Can small glenospheres with eccentricity reduce scapular notching as effectively as large glenospheres without eccentricity? A prospective randomized study. *J Shoulder Elbow Surg.* 2020;29(2):217-224.
30. Feeley BT, Zhang AL, Barry JJ, et al. Decreased scapular notching with lateralization and inferior baseplate placement in reverse shoulder arthroplasty with high humeral inclination. *Int J Shoulder Surg.* 2014;8(3):65-71.
31. Huri G, Familiari F, Salari N, Petersen SA, Doral MN, McFarland EG. Prosthetic design of reverse shoulder arthroplasty contributes to scapular notching and instability. *World J Orthop.* 2016;7(11):738-745.
32. Mollon B, Mahure SA, Roche CP, Zuckerman JD. Impact of scapular notching on clinical outcomes after reverse total shoulder arthroplasty: an analysis of 476 shoulders. *J Shoulder Elbow Surg.* 2017;26(7):1253-1261.
33. Nicholson GP, Strauss EJ, Sherman SL. Scapular notching: recognition and strategies to minimize clinical impact. *Clin Orthop Relat Res.* 2011;469(9):2521-2530.
34. Sadoghi P, Leithner A, Vavken P, et al. Infraglenoidal scapular notching in reverse total shoulder replacement: a prospective series of 60 cases and systematic review of the literature. *BMC Musculoskelet Disord.* 2011;12:101.
35. Wierks C, Skolasky RL, Ji JH, McFarland EG. Reverse total shoulder replacement: intraoperative and early postoperative complications. *Clin Orthop Relat Res.* 2009;467(1):225-234.
36. Brolin TJ, Cox RM, Horneff JG III, et al. Humeral-sided radiographic changes following reverse total shoulder arthroplasty. *Arch Bone Jt Surg.* 2020;8(1):50-57.
37. Bulhoff M, Spranz D, Maier M, Raiss P, Bruckner T, Zeifang F. Mid-term results with an anatomic stemless shoulder prosthesis in patients with primary osteoarthritis. *Acta Orthop Traumatol Turc.* 2019;53(3):170-174.

38. Gilot G, Alvarez-Pinzon AM, Wright TW, et al. The incidence of radiographic aseptic loosening of the humeral component in reverse total shoulder arthroplasty. *J Shoulder Elbow Surg.* 2015;24(10):1555-1559.

39. Bogle A, Budge M, Richman A, Miller RJ, Wiater JM, Voloshin I. Radiographic results of fully uncemented trabecular metal reverse shoulder system at 1 and 2 years' follow-up. *J Shoulder Elbow Surg.* 2013;22(4):e20-e25.

40. Grey B, Rodseth RN, Roche SJ. Humeral stem loosening following reverse shoulder arthroplasty: a systematic review and meta-analysis. *JBJS Rev.* 2018;6(5):e5.

41. Moroder P, Ernstbrunner L, Zweiger C, et al. Short to mid-term results of stemless reverse shoulder arthroplasty in a selected patient population compared to a matched control group with stem. *Int Orthop.* 2016;40(10):2115-2120.

42. Petkovic D, Kovacevic D, Levine WN, Jobin CM. Management of the failed arthroplasty for proximal humerus fracture. *J Am Acad Orthop Surg.* 2019;27(2):39-49.

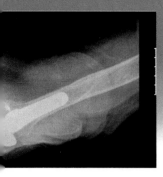

34 The Unstable Anatomic Total Shoulder Arthroplasty

Sri Pinnamaneni, MD and Lawrence Gulotta, MD

INTRODUCTION

Stability in the normal native glenohumeral joint is maintained by the interaction of multiple static and dynamic stabilizers. The bony articulation plays a minor role in providing stability. Dynamic stabilizers, including the deltoid and rotator cuff, contribute significantly to the stability of the glenohumeral joint by providing active compression of the humeral head against the glenoid and within the coracoacromial arch during shoulder range of motion (ROM).

When performing an anatomic total shoulder arthroplasty (ATSA), many of the static and dynamic stabilizers of the native shoulder are altered. These include extensive capsular releases and often resections. In addition, the subscapularis tendon is generally taken down and then repaired at the end of the operation. With these alterations, successfully assessing and maintaining adequate stability of the implant can be challenging. In an ATSA, minimal stability is provided by the implanted metal on polyethylene bearing surface; therefore, implant size, position, and soft-tissue balancing are of paramount importance.

The number of ATSAs has increased significantly over the last decade and is projected to continue to increase. While ATSA shows excellent long-term outcomes and 10-year survivorship, the complication rates can be as high as 14.7%.[1,2] With increasing numbers of ATSAs being performed around the world, surgeons performing this procedure should be well versed in the diagnosis and management of instability following ATSA. The purpose of this chapter is to provide an overview of the diagnosis and management of instability after ATSA.

EPIDEMIOLOGY AND CLASSIFICATION

Instability following ATSA is a common cause of persistent pain and dysfunction and represents a relatively frequent indication for revision surgery. The rate of shoulder instability in the literature after ATSA has ranged from 1.0% to 31%.[1-4] While the reported rate of instability after shoulder arthroplasty has decreased over the last decade, instability after ATSA still represents the third most common complication (after glenoid loosening and glenoid wear).[2] Instability after shoulder arthroplasty is a challenging problem to treat and can result from a combination of soft-tissue insufficiency and implant malpositioning.[5,6] Despite revision surgery for instability, over two-thirds of patients can have recurrent symptoms.[5]

Instability following ATSA is generally classified by the direction of displacement—anterior, posterior, superior, or inferior. It is further characterized based on chronicity (early vs late) and the cause of instability. When assessing and addressing instability following ATSA, it is essential to understand the direction, chronicity, and cause of the instability to determine an appropriate treatment plan.

DIAGNOSTIC EVALUATION

History

Evaluation of instability of any prosthetic joint should always include a comprehensive history and physical examination. Instability should be considered with any patient with a history of pain and dysfunction after ATSA.[7] In more subtle cases of instability and subluxation, the patient's primary complaint may only be pain with little, if any, suggestion of mechanical symptoms.[5,8]

The onset of symptoms and its relationship to the time from surgery is crucial information to obtain. Patients present with instability at an average of 2.1 years following ATSA.[9] Certain causes of instability can present in the immediate postoperative period, including malpositioned implants and acute subscapularis failure. Conversely, implant oversizing or excess lateral offset may lead to attritional wear of the rotator cuff resulting in late instability.

It is essential to identify any history of recent trauma. For example, patients with acute trauma would raise suspicion for a rotator cuff tear. Understanding the patient-specific patterns of symptoms and dysfunction can provide clues to the diagnosis and direction of instability. For example, patients with anterior instability often complain of symptoms with the arm in abduction and external rotation. Alternatively, patients with posterior instability can have worsening symptoms when the arm is in flexion and adduction.

The initial indication for arthroplasty should be carefully reviewed. For example, patients who had significant posterior glenoid wear before the index ATSA can be predisposed to placement of the glenoid component in a retroverted position.[10] These patients are more likely to have posterior instability. Patients with rheumatoid arthritis frequently have deficient soft tissues as a result of the nature of the underlying disease process and can present with rotator cuff insufficiency following ATSA.[11] Patients with limited external rotation or a preoperative history of multiple prior anterior shoulder surgeries are at an increased risk for postoperative subscapularis rupture or insufficiency and anterior instability.[12]

Physical Examination

A careful physical examination is important to establish the diagnosis and direction of instability. Inspection for deltoid and rotator cuff atrophy is important. Location of previous incisions and status of the surrounding skin should be evaluated, especially if there is a suggestion of infection. Any concern for infection should prompt the clinician to proceed with further diagnostic workup as described in Chapter 32.

Passive and active ROM should be evaluated, with particular attention to deltoid and rotator cuff function. Deficits of passive and active ROM should be noted. In the early postoperative setting, increased passive external rotation can point toward possible subscapularis failure.[12] The operative shoulder should also be assessed for anterosuperior escape with active forward elevation.

The positions of apprehension should be assessed. A comprehensive motor and sensory examination should be performed with specific attention to axillary nerve and brachial plexus. Postoperative axillary nerve palsy is a known complication of ATSA. Focused special testing should also be completed. The lift-off and belly-press test should be performed to assess the subscapularis. However, these tests are often difficult to perform in the setting of an ATSA. The sulcus test can reveal inferior laxity, and the load and shift test can assess for increased anterior and posterior translation.[5,8]

Standard Radiographs

Standard radiographs are an essential component of the initial evaluation. Radiographic studies should include a true anteroposterior image (Grashey) of the glenohumeral joint, a scapular Y view, and an axillary view. The true anteroposterior radiograph shows implant position, fixation, and the relationship between the humeral and glenoid components. The scapular Y lateral view can show the anterior to posterior position of the implant in relation to the glenoid. Additionally, an axillary view is essential to evaluate the glenoid component position, fixation, glenoid bone stock, version, and the relative position of the humeral component in relation to the glenoid. Comparison to previous radiographs can identify progressive changes, including osteolysis, implant loosening, eccentric glenoid wear, and superior migration. Anterior translation can indicate subscapularis insufficiency. Superior translation is consistent with superior rotator cuff insufficiency.

Advanced Imaging

While standard radiographs can provide useful information, the utility of the radiographs can be impacted by the patient's positioning and by the imaging technique.[13,14] In this context, a computed tomography (CT) scan can help evaluate the glenoid component position, fixation, glenoid bone stock, glenoid version, and the position of the humeral component in relation to the glenoid.[13,14] It is essential to utilize metal artifact reduction techniques to enhance visualization. An ultrasound can evaluate the rotator cuff without metallic artifact. However, an ultrasound cannot evaluate for implant loosening and position.[15] Magnetic resonance imaging (MRI) is oftentimes not helpful because of the associated artifact. An MRI with multiacquisition with variable-resonance image combination (MAVRIC) sequencing may be useful to identify the soft-tissue integrity, including fatty infiltration of the muscle bellies.[16] Alternatively, a CT arthrogram can evaluate the rotator cuff and assess glenoid bone stock, version, implant position, and fixation. If a CT arthrogram is planned, it can be used as an opportunity for aspiration if there is concern about infection.

Anterior Instability

Etiology

The incidence of anterior instability is approximately 0.9%[1,2] and represents 16% of all instability after ATSA.[1,2] The most common cause of anterior instability is disruption or insufficiency of the subscapularis tendon.[1,2,12] After ATSA, the subscapularis tendon acts as a primary anterior compressor and serves to balance the posterior rotator cuff. Additionally, it also acts as a static soft-tissue restraint to anterior subluxation. Subscapularis function can be variable in patients following ATSA.[17] In a retrospective study of 41 patients, Miller et al showed that the lift-off test and belly-press test was abnormal in the majority of patients.[17]

Subscapularis tendon failure after ATSA is a potentially devastating complication that can result in significant pain, disability, and even implant failure.[6,8,12,17] Most cases of subscapularis failures are related to soft-tissue integrity and implant positioning, but can be multifactorial **(TABLE 34.1)**. Soft-tissue integrity risk factors for subscapularis failures include a history of prior anterior shoulder surgeries that violate the subscapularis, including prior lengthening procedures for internal rotation contractures and previous open anterior stabilization procedures.[12] Aggressive physical therapy,

TABLE 34.1 Anterior Instability

Causes	Treatment Options
Subscapularis rupture/insufficiency	Primary Repair
Humeral component anteversion	± Component revision
Overstuffed humeral component	± Augmentation
Glenoid component anteversion	
Excessive lateralization of the joint line	Conversion to RTSA
Anterior deltoid dysfunction	

RTSA, reverse total shoulder arthroplasty.

early return to increased activity, or acute trauma in the early postoperative period can place excessive stress on the subscapularis repair and result in a subscapularis compromise.

Authors have proposed different techniques of subscapularis management during ATSA to optimize postoperative healing, including tendon-to-tendon repair, tendon-to-bone repair, and lesser tuberosity osteotomy.[18-22] The reported failure rate of primary subscapularis repairs and reattachments has been reported to be as high as 44%.[19] A compilation of the current literature is inconclusive whether one technique is clearly superior to another to prevent postoperative subscapularis failure.[18-22] Any technique that optimizes subscapularis healing will help improve clinical outcomes after ATSA.

Implant malpositioning in the form of excessive combined humeral or glenoid component anteversion can cause unexpected stress on the anterior structures and the subscapularis repair resulting in anterior instability.[7,23] Considering there is a wide variation in the normal humeral head retroversion and glenoid version, an anatomic humeral head osteotomy to re-create the anatomic retroversion and treating anterior glenoid bone loss is essential during the index ATSA.[24] Excessive lateralization by overstuffing the joint with a large humeral head, large glenoid component, or placing the humeral component in varus can place undue stress on the subscapularis repair and result in failure.[6,8,12,19]

The diagnosis of chronic anterior instability can be subtle. Subscapularis failure can present with progressive development of internal rotation weakness or a sense of apprehension with the arm in abduction and external rotation. Symptoms may present more acutely after a traumatic event. Increased external rotation on the operative side compared to the contralateral side or a significant change from earlier examinations can point to a subscapularis tear. Special testing, including belly-press and the lift-off test for subscapularis testing, is not highly reliable in the setting of ATSA.[17] In cases of apparent anterior instability or subluxation, standard radiographs can be diagnostic **(FIGURE 34.1)**. If the subscapularis was managed with a lesser tuberosity osteotomy during the index surgery, it is very important to evaluate radiographs for displacement of the reattached lesser tuberosity. In subtle cases of anterior

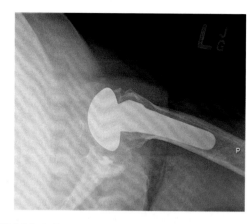

FIGURE 34.1 Axillary radiograph demonstrating anterior instability.

instability, MRI, CT arthrograms, and ultrasound may be helpful in the diagnosis of rotator cuff tears, tendon quality, retraction, and associated muscle atrophy **(FIGURES 34.2 and 34.3)**. CT scan can also help identify the version and positioning of the humeral and glenoid components.

Treatment

If the patient is diagnosed with a subscapularis tear or insufficiency, the clinical decision-making relies on multiple important variables, including age, time from index ATSA, and quality of the tissue **(TABLE 34.1)**. In the setting of acute subscapularis tear (<12 weeks from index ATSA) in a young patient with healthy tissue, acute primary repair of the subscapularis should be attempted.

In most cases, the prior deltopectoral interval is used. Oftentimes, the subscapularis tear retracts into the subcoracoid space. The subscapularis tendon should be identified carefully and all subdeltoid, subacromial,

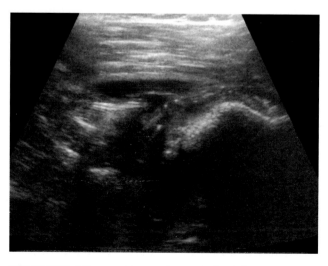

FIGURE 34.2 Ultrasound image demonstrating failure and retraction of the subscapularis repair after acute trauma.

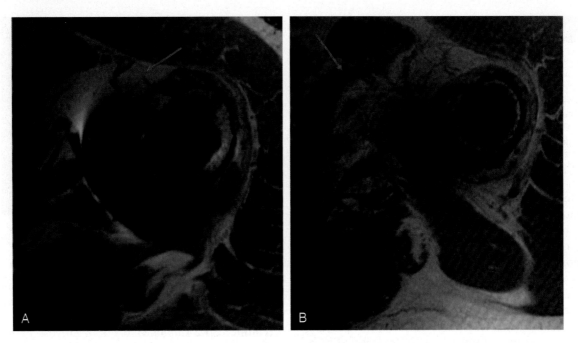

FIGURE 34.3 Coronal magnetic resonance images (MRIs) with arrows demonstrating (**A**) failure of lesser tuberosity osteotomy repair and (**B**) loss of reduction with retraction of the boney lesser tuberosity osteotomy fragment after acute trauma.

and subcoracoid adhesions should be released. Circumferential releases must be completed, including mobilization along the rotator interval and anterior glenoid. Care should be taken when dissecting in the subcoracoid space. The goal of these releases is to maximize tendon mobilization. Next, the tendon edge should be debrided to healthy tissue. The tendon excursion can be checked using a blunt Allis clamp or a separate traction stitch. At this point, the surgeon should check the position and sizing of the humeral and glenoid components. If the humeral head component is oversized, revision to a smaller humeral head should be considered. If there is excessive anteversion of the humeral and glenoid components, component revision and repositioning should be considered. The surgeon can use a combination of suture anchors and suture augmentation to repair the subscapularis tendon to the lateral stump and lesser tuberosity. It is important to carefully plan the placement of suture anchors around the humeral stem. If a tension-free subscapularis tendon repair cannot be completed or the tendon is of poor quality, an allograft augmentation can be considered using an Achilles tendon or iliotibial band (ITB). There are limited outcome data on allograft augmentation for subscapularis repairs.[8,25] Alternatively, with poor tissue quality in an older patient, a revision to reverse total shoulder arthroplasty (RTSA) should be considered.

Primary repair of late-onset subscapularis tear (>12 weeks from index ATSA) is less predictable. In these patients, it is essential to understand the patient's complaints and review patient expectations. The first mode of treatment in chronic subscapularis insufficiency

is nonoperative conservative care with physical therapy, activity modification, nonsteroidal anti-inflammatory medications. If the patient has continued pain and dysfunction despite treatment with conservative measures, revision surgery can be considered.

Pectoralis major tendon transfers and Achilles tendon allograft reconstructive procedures have been reported with limited and unreliable results for subscapularis tears following ATSA.[26-28] For this reason, our opinion is that these techniques should rarely be considered. In the setting of late-onset subscapularis tear (>12 weeks from index ATSA) in an older patient with inadequate tissue who has failed nonoperative treatment, conversion to RTSA should be considered and can be successful (**FIGURE 34.4**). Conversion to an RTSA provides a more constrained implant that does not rely on the rotator cuff for stability.

Outcomes

There have been few studies reporting on treatment outcomes after acute and chronic subscapularis failure following ATSA. In a cohort of 51 patients with anterior instability, Ahers et al reported an 87% incidence of subscapularis tear and reported success in restoring stability in only 40% of the patients using a variety of techniques.[28] Miller et al reported that outcomes were better if the subscapularis repair was performed early versus late.[12] We reviewed the results at our institution of 15 patients who underwent a revision procedure to treat subscapularis failure after ATSA. Seven patients underwent a primary repair and four had successful outcomes. The three patients who had poor outcomes underwent a

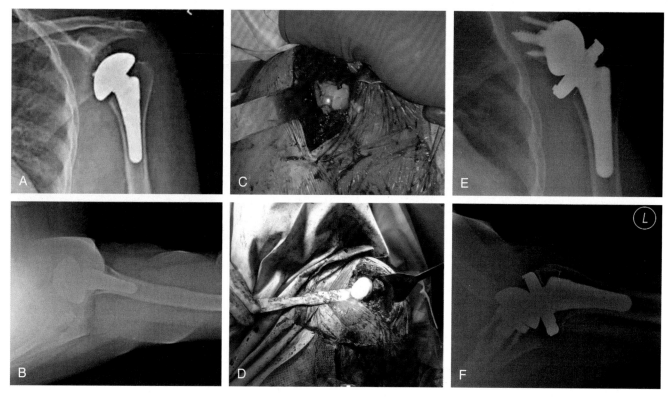

FIGURE 34.4 Anteroposterior (**A**) and axillary (**B**) radiographs in a patient with anterior shoulder instability secondary to a late subscapularis failure. Conversion to reverse total shoulder arthroplasty (RTSA) was performed using convertible humeral stem. **C**, Glenoid component is removed using a combination of flexible osteotomes, rongeur, needle-tip burr, and trephine. **D**, Modular humeral head is removed, and a humeral tray with polyethylene socket is implanted with retention of the well-fixed humeral stem. Postoperative anteroposterior (**E**) and axillary (**F**) radiographs after conversion to RTSA.

subsequent conversion to RTSA. When primary repair was attempted in cases >12 weeks after index ATSA, patients were more likely to have worse outcomes. In the 10 patients who ultimately underwent revision to RTSA, the average University of California Los Angeles (UCLA) score was 24.6/30, and the Simple Shoulder Test (SST) score was 8.9/12. In our cohort, younger patients with early subscapularis failures had the best outcomes after primary repairs. Older patients and those with late-onset subscapularis failures with muscle atrophy did best with conversion to RTSA.

Posterior Instability

Etiology

The incidence of posterior instability is approximately 1%[1,2] and represents 20% of all instability following ATSA.[1,2] Causes of posterior instability include implant malpositioning and soft-tissue imbalance, with most cases being multifactorial **(TABLE 34.2)**. The most common cause of posterior instability is implant malpositioning in the form of excessive humeral, glenoid, or combined component retroversion.[8] In patients with glenohumeral osteoarthritis, it is common to have posterior glenoid bone loss with associated posterior subluxation, posterior capsular laxity, and tight anterior structures.

These factors should be recognized and corrected during the index ATSA.

Posterior glenoid bone erosion (Walch B and C glenoid deformities) are risk factors for placement of excessively retroverted implants leading to postoperative posterior instability.[5,29-31] Excessive humeral retroversion (>45°) with associated glenoid retroversion (>20°) has been associated with posterior instability.[23,32] Additionally, the rate of posterior humeral head subluxation is 85% when glenoid retroversion is >20°.[32] Prior to the index ATSA, CT scan should be used to understand the glenoid bone stock, version, and humeral head subluxation.[13,30,33] Restoration of glenoid version to between 0° and 10° can potentially correct preoperative posterior subluxation and center the humeral

TABLE 34.2 Posterior Instability

Causes	Treatment Options
Glenoid component retroversion	Revision of glenoid component
Humeral component retroversion	± Revision of humeral component
Tight subscapularis	± Posterior capsular plication
Posterior capsular laxity	± Subscapularis lengthening
	Conversion to RTSA

RTSA, reverse total shoulder arthroplasty.

head on the glenoid component.[32] Techniques to treat posterior glenoid version include eccentric reaming, use of augmented glenoid implants, and use of bone grafts. Additionally, other authors have described using intraoperative computer-assisted navigation to optimize glenoid component placement.[34]

Inadequate soft-tissue balancing can also contribute to posterior instability. Tight anterior structures (subscapularis and capsule), posterior capsular laxity, and posterior rotator cuff dysfunction are predisposing factors if not corrected during the index ATSA.[5,8] Excessive resection and releases of the posterior capsule can increase the risk for posterior instability. Additionally, multiple previous anterior instability surgeries can lead to tight anterior structures and subsequently cause posterior instability.[10]

The diagnosis of posterior subluxation can be subtle and definitive diagnosis can be difficult. Symptoms may present more acutely as instability after a traumatic event. In subtle cases of posterior instability, the patient may only complain of pain and apprehension, with the arm forward flexed and adducted with a posteriorly directed force. The load and shift test may show increased anterior to posterior translation.[5,8] Radiographs should be carefully assessed for implant malpositioning **(FIGURE 34.5)**. In cases of chronic posterior instability, radiographs of the glenoid should be carefully evaluated for eccentric polyethylene wear, osteolysis, and loosening. Advanced imaging with a CT scan and MRI can be helpful for identifying humeral and glenoid component malposition, loosening, eccentric glenoid polyethylene wear, posterior subluxation, and integrity of the rotator cuff. In addition to current imaging, the imaging before the index ATSA should also be evaluated for posterior glenoid deformity and humeral head subluxation.

Treatment

If the patient is diagnosed with posterior instability secondary to implant positioning, the clinical decision-making relies on multiple important variables including age, time from index ATSA, preoperative ROM, status of the rotator cuff, glenoid bone stock, and position of the implants **(TABLE 34.2)**. Advanced imaging should be reviewed and assessed for implant position and integrity of the rotator cuff. In young patients with implant malpositioning in the early postoperative setting with good ROM, an intact rotator cuff and good glenoid bone stock, revision ATSA surgery with correction of the malpositioned implants should be considered.

The goals of revision ATSA for posterior instability are (1) correction and restoration of the glenoid version; (2) to balance the soft tissues appropriately; and (3) to center the humeral head. When considering revision of the glenoid component, it is important to preoperatively plan for the anticipated bone loss during the explantation of the glenoid component. The surgical approach

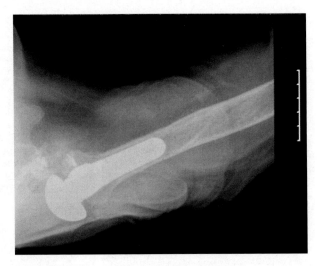

FIGURE 34.5 .Axillary radiograph demonstrating posterior instability.

will usually utilize the prior deltopectoral interval. For subscapularis management, the tendon length can be maintained with a subscapularis peel. A 360° release, including mobilization of the subscapularis along the rotator interval and the anterior glenoid, should be completed. A Z-lengthening of the subscapularis tendon can be considered, although lengthening procedures of the subscapularis have been shown to increase the risk of postoperative rupture and insufficiency.[12] Alternatively, the subscapularis can be reattached more medially to achieve the desired lengthening without compromise of tissue quality. A partial release of the pectoralis major tendon may also be required to increase external rotation motion and improve exposure and mobilization.

For revision of an excessively retroverted glenoid component, correction can be obtained by eccentric anterior reaming, use of an augmented glenoid component, or use of bone graft.[35-38] The use of patient-specific guides or intraoperative computer-assisted navigation can be considered to help optimize accurate placement of the glenoid component.[34] For the humeral component, it is important to assess the humeral component retroversion because excessive retroversion can also contribute to posterior instability. Studies have shown that placing the stem in increased anteversion is an ineffective technique to improve posterior instability.[24,39] The humeral head can be placed with increased anterior offset to help center the humeral head component on the glenoid.[40] The humeral head can also be revised to a larger size to improve stability, but care should be taken to avoid overstuffing. For soft-tissue balancing, a posterior capsular plication can be a helpful technique to decrease persistent posterior laxity and translation. With the humeral head component removed, placing purse-string sutures or figure-of-eight stitches medially and laterally in the posterior capsule can help restore stability for persistent intraoperative posterior instability.[41] Before final implantation, stability and soft-tissue tensioning of the shoulder with the trial components in place should be assessed. Anterior to posterior translation of the humeral head should not exceed 30% to 50% of the glenoid diameter, and the humeral head should spontaneously recenter on the glenoid implant after the translational force is released.[8] If posterior translation exceeds 50% or if the head does not self-reduce, then additional techniques, as described above, should be utilized. If these techniques do not provide intraoperative stability, then the use of an RTSA should be considered even in a young patient.

In the setting of chronic posterior instability in older patients, with poor ROM, rotator cuff insufficiency, or inadequate glenoid bone stock, it is essential to understand the patient's specific complaints and the factors causing the instability. It is also essential to carefully review patient expectations. The first mode of treatment is nonoperative care with physical therapy, activity modification, and nonsteroidal anti-inflammatory medications. If the patient has continued pain and dysfunction despite treatment with these measures, revision surgery with conversion from ATSA to RTSA can be considered.

Outcomes

There are limited studies looking at the results of patients undergoing revision for posterior instability following ATSA. Persistent instability can persist in 36% of patients despite revision surgery.[5] Moeckel et al reported on the treatment of three cases of posterior instability from their cohort of 236 total shoulder arthroplasties. Two patients were successfully treated nonoperatively, and one failed multiple revision surgeries and eventually underwent implant removal.[8] Ahrens et al reported on a cohort of 29 cases of posterior instability following ATSA, reporting success in restoring stability in 53% of patients after revision surgery.[28] These studies demonstrate the difficulty of successfully treating posterior instability after ATSA. Patients should be counseled carefully that the risk of complications, recurrence, and reoperation is high. In patients with early-onset instability with malpositioned implants, revision ATSA with implant revision should be considered. However, in the vast majority of patients, given its increased durability and predictable outcomes, RTSA should be considered in older patients and appropriately indicated younger patients.

Superior Instability

Etiology

The incidence of superior instability is approximately 3%[1,2] and represents 61% of all instability following ATSA.[1,2] The most common cause of proximal migration and anterosuperior instability is progressive rotator cuff insufficiency leading to tearing and dysfunction

TABLE 34.3 Superior Instability

Causes	Treatment Options
Rotator cuff insufficiency	Rotator Cuff Repair
Overstuffed humeral component	
Excessive lateralization of the joint line	Conversion to RTSA
Superior inclination of the glenoid component	
Coracoacromial arch insufficiency	
Anterior deltoid dysfunction	

RTSA, reverse total shoulder arthroplasty.

(TABLE 34.3).[1,2,11,23,42] Failure of the subscapularis or posterior-superior rotator cuff leads to an imbalance in the concavity-compression mechanism of the glenohumeral joint. This rotator cuff dysfunction, in addition to the shear force produced by the deltoid muscle, subluxates the humeral head superiorly. Superior migration can cause the "rocking horse" glenoid phenomenon, resulting in eccentric loading of the glenoid component, leading to early glenoid loosening and failure.[24]

Approximately, 55% of patients have rotator cuff insufficiency or dysfunction 15 years after ATSA.[42] The size of the rotator cuff tear is correlated with the risk of proximal migration.[43] The rate of rotator cuff tears following ATSA is approximately 11% to 17% and increases as the length of follow-up increases.[44] Risk factors for progressive rotator cuff insufficiency include patients with a history of inflammatory arthropathy like rheumatoid arthritis or multiple previous operations.

Humeral components placed with excessive height can increase the stress on the rotator cuff and lead to decreased motion, increased pain, and eventual rotator cuff tendon failure **(FIGURES 34.6** and **34.7)**. The humeral component articular surface should be between 5 and 8 mm above the greater tuberosity.[24] Alternatively, a best-fit circle technique can be used to assess the humeral height on postoperative radiographs.[45] Placing a humeral component higher than 5 to 10 mm places increased stress on the inferior ligaments in abduction, increases the stress on the rotator cuff, raises the joint center of rotation, and decreases the moment arms of the infraspinatus and subscapularis.[46] Increased superior glenoid component inclination can result in superior shear forces and also contribute to superior subluxation.

Anterior deltoid insufficiency and coracoacromial arch insufficiency can contribute to anterosuperior escape. The coracoacromial arch includes the coracoid, acromion, and coracoacromial ligament. In conjunction with a rotator cuff tear, disruption of any part of the arch may result in an inability to counteract the compressive forces of the deltoid and result in anterosuperior instability.[47] The coracoacromial arch can be disrupted during the surgical approach or as a result of prior surgeries.

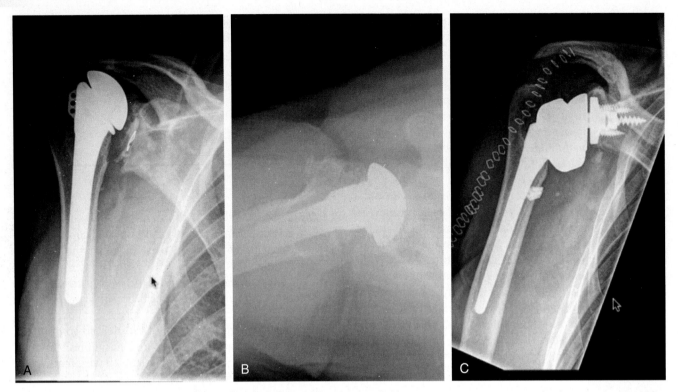

FIGURE 34.6 Anteroposterior **(A)** and axillary **(B)** radiographs in a patient with superior migration of the humeral implant secondary to chronic rotator cuff insufficiency. Postoperative anteroposterior **(C)** radiographs after conversion to reverse total shoulder arthroplasty (RTSA) and revision of the humeral stem.

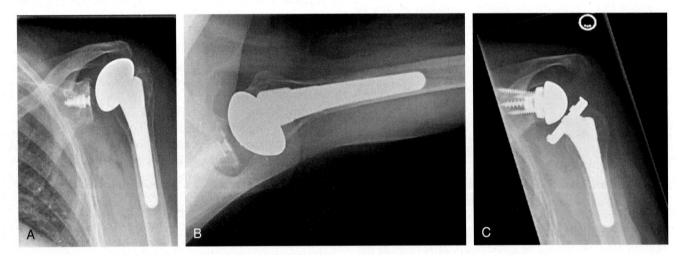

FIGURE 34.7 Anteroposterior **(A)** and axillary **(B)** radiographs in a patient with superior migration of the humeral implant secondary to rotator cuff insufficiency. Postoperative anteroposterior **(C)** radiographs after conversion to reverse total shoulder arthroplasty (RTSA) with convertible humeral stem.

The diagnosis of superior instability can often be made based on history and physical examination. Symptoms are usually gradual in onset and progressively worsening. Patients describe decreased ROM and functional limitations. Physical examination findings include loss of active ROM and rotator cuff weakness and pseudoparalysis. In chronic cases, radiographs should be evaluated for superior migration **(FIGURES 34.6** and **34.7)**. In patients with pain and early finding, MRI can be helpful to assess the integrity of the rotator cuff and identify fatty infiltration.

Treatment

In the setting of chronic superior migration or instability after ATSA, it is essential to understand the patient's specific complaints, cause of instability, and carefully review patient expectations. The first mode of treatment in chronic superior migration may be nonoperative care with physical therapy, activity modification, an anterior deltoid strengthening exercise program, and nonsteroidal anti-inflammatory medications. Despite having superior migration on radiographs, the patient might have minimal symptoms because rotator cuff disease in the setting of ATSA can be well tolerated.[44] If the patient has continued pain and dysfunction despite treatment with these measures, revision surgery can be considered **(TABLE 34.3)**.

In a young patient, who has primary complaints of pain but can elevate their arm and has a repairable rotator cuff tear, rotator cuff repair can be considered. However, rotator cuff repairs in the setting after ATSA have been shown to have poor clinical results.[48] Additionally, soft-tissue reconstruction procedures including coracoacromial arch reconstructions procedures have limited outcome data and have generally not been successful.[31]

In most patients with superior instability who have failed nonoperative treatment, the most predictable revision surgery is conversion to RTSA **(FIGURES 34.6 and 34.7)**.[49] During conversion from ATSA to RTSA, standard revision principles should be used by the surgeon, including proper knowledge of revision instruments based upon the implants in place and the implants to be utilized. In most cases, the prior deltopectoral interval is used and exposure and mobilization should be maximized to avoid excessive stress. The choice of implants during the index ATSA can have a significant effect on the revision technique. Many contemporary implants utilize a platform convertible implant system (Chapter 44) that allows for conversion to RTSA without removal of a well-fixed humeral stem and can result in shorter operating room (OR) times and less blood loss **(FIGURES 34.4 and 34.7)**. In patients with significant superior migration, it can sometimes be challenging to reduce the components and achieve the proper balance. In this setting, the remaining portion of the superior rotator cuff should be released. If the shoulder is still irreducible or too tight, revision of the humeral stem should be performed. Convertible humeral components are only beneficial if they are in proper position and a stable, balanced construct can be achieved.

Outcomes

Hattrup et al showed that repair of the rotator cuff in the setting of ATSA has poor clinical outcomes with 14 of the 18 patients in their cohort having poor outcomes.[48] Revision from ATSA to RTSA has generally predictable results with 78% excellent or good results and consistent improvements in forward elevation from 50° to 130°.[50] Abdel et al reported good short-term results in a cohort of 33 unstable ATSA patients who underwent conversion to RTSA with 31/33 maintaining stability at 3.5 years after surgery.[51] Additionally, Hernandez et al

reported 87% and 79% survivorship at 2 and 5 years, respectively, in their series of revisions of ATSA to RTSA for instability.[49]

CONCLUSION

While the incidence of instability after shoulder arthroplasty has decreased over time, instability is the third most common complication following ATSA. Comprehensive preoperative planning and meticulous surgical technique are crucial to preventing postoperative instability. A careful history and physical evaluation provide important information about the direction and cause of instability. Radiographs and advanced imaging are essential to arrive at an accurate identification of the underlying factors causing instability. Accurate diagnosis allows the surgeon to develop an appropriate treatment plan for the patient. Anterior instability is primarily caused by acute or chronic subscapularis insufficiency. Posterior instability is most likely caused by implant malpositioning and inadequate soft-tissue balancing. Superior instability is primarily caused by progressive rotator cuff insufficiency. In most cases of instability in the early postoperative period, revision surgery with component revision can be considered. In most cases of late-onset instability, nonoperative care should be the first line of treatment. If nonoperative treatment fails, a revision to RTSA should be considered. The reported clinical results after revision surgery for instability following ATSA are somewhat limited and variable, so preoperative patient counseling is crucial. However, given its increased durability and predictable outcomes, RTSA can be considered even in appropriately indicated younger patients.

REFERENCES

1. Bohsali KI, Wirth MA, Rockwood CA. Complications of total shoulder arthroplasty. *J Bone Joint Surg.* 2006;88(10):2279-2292. doi:10.2106/JBJS.F.00125
2. Bohsali KI, Bois AJ, Wirth MA. Complications of shoulder arthroplasty. *J Bone Joint Surg Am.* 2017;99(3):256-269. doi:10.2106/JBJS.16.00935
3. Cofield RH, Edgerton BC. Total shoulder arthroplasty: complications and revision surgery. *Instr Course Lect.* 1990;39:449-462.
4. Chin PYK, Sperling JW, Cofield RH, Schleck C. Complications of total shoulder arthroplasty: are they fewer or different? *J Shoulder Elbow Surg.* 2006;15(1):19-22. doi:10.1016/j.jse.2005.05.005
5. Sanchez-Sotelo J, Sperling JW, Rowland CM, Cofield RH. Instability after shoulder arthroplasty: results of surgical treatment. *J Bone Joint Surg.* 2003;85(4):622-631. doi:10.2106/00004623-200304000-00006
6. Kany J, Jose J, Katz D, et al. The main cause of instability after unconstrained shoulder prosthesis is soft tissue deficiency. *J Shoulder Elbow Surg.* 2017;26(8):e243-e251. doi:10.1016/j.jse.2017.01.019
7. Hasan SS, Leith JM, Campbell B, Kapil R, Smith KL, Matsen FA. Characteristics of unsatisfactory shoulder arthroplasties. *J Shoulder Elbow Surg.* 2002;11(5):431-441. doi:10.1067/mse.2002.125806
8. Moeckel BH, Altchek DW, Warren RF, Wickiewicz TL, Dines DM. Instability of the shoulder after arthroplasty. *J Bone Joint Surg.* 1993;75(4):492-497. doi:10.2106/00004623-199304000-00003
9. Deshmukh AV, Koris M, Zurakowski D, Thornhill TS. Total shoulder arthroplasty: long-term survivorship, functional outcome, and quality

of life. *J Shoulder Elbow Surg*. 2005;14(5):471-479. doi:10.1016/j.jse.2005.02.009

10. Sperling JW, Antuna SA, Sanchez-Sotelo J, Schleck C, Cofield RH. Shoulder arthroplasty for arthritis after instability surgery. *J Bone Joint Surg*. 2002;84(10):1775-1781. doi:10.2106/00004623-200210000-00006

11. Trail IA, Nuttall D. The results of shoulder arthroplasty in patients with rheumatoid arthritis. *J Bone Joint Surg*. 2002;84(8):1121-1125. doi:10.1302/0301-620X.84B8.12695

12. Miller BS, Joseph TA, Noonan TJ, Horan MP, Hawkins RJ. Rupture of the subscapularis tendon after shoulder arthroplasty: diagnosis, treatment, and outcome. *J Shoulder Elbow Surg*. 2005;14(5):492-496. doi:10.1016/j.jse.2005.02.013

13. Nyffeler RW, Jost B, Pfirrmann CWA, Gerber C. Measurement of glenoid version: conventional radiographs versus computed tomography scans. *J Shoulder Elbow Surg*. 2003;12(5):493-496. doi:10.1016/S1058-2746(03)00181-2

14. Friedman RJ, Hawthorne KB, Genez BM. The use of computerized tomography in the measurement of glenoid version. *J Bone Joint Surg*. 1992;74(7):1032-1037. doi:10.2106/00004623-199274070-00009

15. Sofka CM, Adler RS. Sonographic evaluation of shoulder arthroplasty. *Am J Roentgenol*. 2003;180(4):1117-1120. doi:10.2214/ajr.180.4.1801117

16. Sperling JW, Potter HG, Craig EV, Flatow E, Warren RF. Magnetic resonance imaging of painful shoulder arthroplasty. *J Shoulder Elbow Surg*. 2002;11(4):315-321. doi:10.1067/mse.2002.124426

17. Miller SL, Hazrati Y, Klepps S, Chiang A, Flatow EL. Loss of subscapularis function after total shoulder replacement: a seldom recognized problem. *J Shoulder Elbow Surg*. 2003;12(1):29-34. doi:10.1067/mse.2003.128195

18. Caplan JL, Whitfield B, Neviaser RJ. Subscapularis function after primary tendon to tendon repair in patients after replacement arthroplasty of the shoulder. *J Shoulder Elbow Surg*. 2009;18(2):193-196. doi:10.1016/j.jse.2008.10.019

19. Gerber C, Yian EH, Pfirrmann CAW, Zumstein MA, Werner CML. Subscapularis muscle function and structure after total shoulder replacement with lesser tuberosity osteotomy and repair. *J Bone Joint Surg*. 2005;87(8):1739-1745. doi:10.2106/JBJS.D.02788

20. Scalise JJ, Ciccone J, Iannotti JP. Clinical, radiographic, and ultrasonographic comparison of subscapularis tenotomy and lesser tuberosity osteotomy for total shoulder arthroplasty. *J Bone Joint Surg*. 2010;92(7):1627-1634. doi:10.2106/JBJS.G.01461

21. Giuseffi SA, Wongtriratanachai P, Omae H, et al. Biomechanical comparison of lesser tuberosity osteotomy versus subscapularis tenotomy in total shoulder arthroplasty. *J Shoulder Elbow Surg*. 2012;21(8):1087-1095. doi:10.1016/j.jse.2011.07.008

22. Lapner PLC, Sabri E, Rakhra K, Bell K, Athwal GS. Comparison of lesser tuberosity osteotomy to subscapularis peel in shoulder arthroplasty: a randomized controlled trial. *J Bone Joint Surg*. 2012;94(24):2239-2246. doi:10.2106/JBJS.K.01365

23. Wirth MA, Rockwood CA. Complications of total shoulder-replacement arthroplasty. *J Bone Joint Surg*. 1996;78(4):603-616. doi:10.2106/00004623-199604000-00018

24. Iannotti JP, Spencer EE, Winter U, Deffenbaugh D, Williams G. Prosthetic positioning in total shoulder arthroplasty. *J Shoulder Elbow Surg*. 2005;14(1 suppl):111S-121S. doi:10.1016/j.jse.2004.09.026

25. Iannotti JP, Antoniou J, Williams GR, Ramsey ML. Iliotibial band reconstruction for treatment of glenohumeral instability associated with irreparable capsular deficiency. *J Shoulder Elbow Surg*. 2002;11(6):618-623. doi:10.1067/mse.2002.126763

26. Konrad GG, Sudkamp NP, Kreuz PC, Jolly JT, McMahon PJ, Debski RE. Pectoralis major tendon transfers above or underneath the conjoint tendon in subscapularis-deficient shoulders: an in vitro biomechanical analysis. *J Bone Joint Surg*. 2007;89(11):2477-2484. doi:10.2106/JBJS.F.00811

27. Burnier M, Elhassan BT, Sanchez-Sotelo J. Surgical management of irreparable rotator cuff tears: what works, what does not, and what is coming. *J Bone Joint Surg Am*. 2019;101(17):1603-1612. doi:10.2106/JBJS.18.01392

28. Ahrens P, Boileau P, Walch G. Anterior and posterior instability after unconstrained shoulder arthroplasty. In: Walch G, Boileau P, Molé

D, eds. *Shoulder Prostheses: Two to Ten Year Follow-up*. Montpellier Sauramps Medical; 2001:359-393.

29. Godenèche A, Boileau P, Favard L, et al. Prosthetic replacement in the treatment of osteoarthritis of the shoulder: early results of 208 cases. *J Shoulder Elbow Surg*. 2002;11(1):11-18. doi:10.1067/mse.2002.120140

30. Klepps S, Hazrati Y, Flatow E, May L, May PW. Management of glenoid bone deficiency during shoulder replacement. *Tech Shoulder Elbow Surg*. 2003;4(1):4-17. doi:10.1097/00132589-200303000-00002

31. Warren RF, Coleman SH, Dines JS. Instability after arthroplasty: the shoulder. *J Arthroplasty*. 2002;17(4 suppl 1):28-31. doi:10.1054/arth.2002.32543

32. Habermeyer P, Magosch P, Lichtenberg S. Recentering the humeral head for glenoid deficiency in total shoulder arthroplasty. *Clin Orthop Relat Res*. 2007;457:124-132. doi:10.1097/BLO.0b013e31802ff03c

33. Kwon YW, Powell KA, Yum JK, Brems JJ, Iannotti JP. Use of three-dimensional computed tomography for the analysis of the glenoid anatomy. *J Shoulder Elbow Surg*. 2005;14(1):85-90. doi:10.1016/j.jse.2004.04.011

34. Stanley RJ, Edwards TB, Sarin VK, Gartsman GM. Computer-aided navigation for correction of glenoid deformity in total shoulder arthroplasty. *Tech Shoulder Elbow Surg*. 2007;8(1):23-28. doi:10.1097/BTE.0b013e31802ca571

35. Gerber A, Warner JJP. Management of glenoid bone loss in shoulder arthroplasty. *Tech Shoulder Elbow Surg*. 2001;2(4):255-266. doi:10.1097/00132589-200112000-00005

36. Neer CS II, Morrison DS. Glenoid bone-grafting in total shoulder arthroplasty. *J Bone Joint Surg*. 1988;70(8):1154-1162. doi:10.2106/00004623-198870080-00006

37. Hill JM, Norris TR. Long-term results of total shoulder arthroplasty following bone-grafting of the glenoid. *J Bone Joint Surg*. 2001;83(6):877-883. doi:10.2106/00004623-200106000-00009

38. Antuna SA, Sperling JW, Cofield RH, Rowland CM. Glenoid revision surgery after total shoulder arthroplasty. *J Shoulder Elbow Surg*. 2001;10(3):217-224. doi:10.1067/mse.2001.113961

39. Spencer EE, Valdevit A, Kambic H, Brems JJ, Iannotti JP. The effect of humeral component anteversion on shoulder stability with glenoid component retroversion. *J Bone Joint Surg*. 2005;87(4):808-814. doi:10.2106/JBJS.C.00770

40. Kim HMM, Chacon AC, Andrews SH, et al. Biomechanical benefits of anterior offsetting of humeral head component in posteriorly unstable total shoulder arthroplasty: a cadaveric study. *J Orthop Res*. 2016;34(4):666-674. doi:10.1002/jor.23048

41. Alentorn-Geli E, Assenmacher AT, Sperling JW, Cofield RH, Sánchez-Sotelo J. Plication of the posterior capsule for intraoperative posterior instability during anatomic total shoulder arthroplasty. *J Shoulder Elbow Surg*. 2017;26(6):982-989. doi:10.1016/j.jse.2016.10.008

42. Young AA, Walch G, Pape G, Gohlke F, Favard L. Secondary rotator cuff dysfunction following total shoulder arthroplasty for primary glenohumeral osteoarthritis: results of a multicenter study with more than five years of follow-up. *J Bone Joint Surg*. 2012;94(8):685-693. doi:10.2106/JBJS.J.00727

43. Haines IA, Trail IA, Nuttall D, Birch A, Barrow A. The results of arthroplasty in osteoarthritis of the shoulder. *J Bone Joint Surg*. 2006;88(4):496-501. doi:10.1302/0301-620X.88B4.16604

44. Levy D, Abrams G, Harris J, Bach B, Nicholson G, Romeo A. Rotator cuff tears after total shoulder arthroplasty in primary osteoarthritis: a systematic review. *Int J Shoulder Surg*. 2016;10(2):78-84. doi:10.4103/0973-6042.180720

45. Alolabi B, Youderian AR, Napolitano L, et al. Radiographic assessment of prosthetic humeral head size after anatomic shoulder arthroplasty. *J Shoulder Elbow Surg*. 2014;23(11):1740-1746. doi:10.1016/j.jse.2014.02.013

46. Nyffeler RW, Sheikh R, Jacob HAC, Gerber C. Influence of humeral prosthesis height on biomechanics of glenohumeral abduction: an in vitro study. *J Bone Joint Surg*. 2004;86(3):575-580. doi:10.2106/00004623-200403000-00017

47. Fagelman M, Sartori M, Freedman KB, Patwardhan AG, Carandang G, Marra G. Biomechanics of coracoacromial arch modification. *J Shoulder Elbow Surg*. 2007;16(1):101-106. doi:10.1016/j.jse.2006.01.010

48. Hattrup SJ, Cofield RH, Cha SS. Rotator cuff repair after shoulder replacement. *J Shoulder Elbow Surg.* 2006;15(1):78-83. doi:10.1016/j.jse.2005.06.002

49. Hernandez NM, Chalmers BP, Wagner ER, Sperling JW, Cofield RH, Sanchez-Sotelo J. Revision to reverse total shoulder arthroplasty restores stability for patients with unstable shoulder prostheses. *Clin Orthop Relat Res.* 2017;475(11):2716-2722. doi:10.1007/s11999-017-5429-z

50. Walker M, Willis MP, Brooks JP, Pupello D, Mulieri PJ, Frankle MA. The use of the reverse shoulder arthroplasty for treatment of failed total shoulder arthroplasty. *J Shoulder Elbow Surg.* 2012;21(4):514-522. doi:10.1016/j.jse.2011.03.006

51. Abdel MP, Hattrup SJ, Sperling JW, Cofield RH, Kreofsky CR, Sanchez-Sotelo J. Revision of an unstable hemiarthroplasty or anatomical total shoulder replacement using a reverse design prosthesis. *Bone Joint J.* 2013;95-B(5):668-672. doi:10.1302/0301-620X.95B5.30964

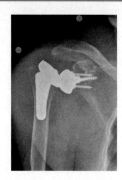

35 The Unstable Reverse Shoulder Arthroplasty

Joaquin Sanchez-Sotelo, MD, PhD

Reverse total shoulder arthroplasty (RTSA) is a very successful procedure. However, complications do occur after RTSA. Dislocation is one of the most common complications leading to revision surgery after RTSA.[1-3] In this chapter, we will review the epidemiology and risk factors for instability after RTSA as well as evaluation and management strategies when this complication occurs.

EPIDEMIOLOGY AND RISK FACTORS FOR INSTABILITY AFTER REVERSE TOTAL SHOULDER ARTHROPLASTY

Multiple factors may contribute to instability following RTSA, either in isolation or combined. In essence, for an RTSA not to dislocate, the components have to be properly oriented in space, the tension of the surrounding soft-tissues needs to be sufficient, and all sources of impingement with the potential to lever out and dislocate the arthroplasty must be eliminated.

Frankle et al have categorized the factors that contribute to dislocation after RTSA into three groups: loss of compression, impingement, and loss of containment **(TABLE 35.1)**.[4] *Loss of compression* describes laxity between the humeral and glenoid components, and it can be secondary to insufficient deltoid and/or rotator cuff tension. *Loss of containment* is secondary to gross implant failure (component disassociation or fracture) or advanced polyethylene wear. *Impingement* between the humerus and scapula, the implant and the scapula, or with fibrotic soft tissues may also lead to dislocation. Obese patients with a large body habitus may experience dislocation secondary to abutment of the upper arm with the trunk, combined with traction secondary to the heavy weight of their arm.

Reported rates of dislocation after RTSA have varied widely, and at least in primary RTSA, they seem to have decreased over time. At the Hospital for Special Surgery, the dislocation rate after the first 57 RTSAs performed was 16%.[5] At Stanford University, the reported rate of dislocation was 9.2%.[6] Zumstein et al performed a meta-analysis of studies published between 1995 and 2008 and reported a mean dislocation incidence of 4.7%.[7] A similar dislocation rate of 4% was reported by the Hawkins group.[8] The Rothman and Rush groups have reported identical dislocation rates of 2.9%.[9,10] However, Dr Zuckerman's group has reported a dislocation rate of 0.5% in a study on 591 primary RTSA,[11] and similarly, in a study from the Mayo Clinic on 1649 primary RTSA implanted between 2009 and 2015, the rate of reoperation for dislocation after reverse shoulder arthroplasty (RSA) was under 0.5%.[12]

The dislocation rate reported by different studies have been influenced likely by the type of implants used, performing the procedure during the learning curve, the underlying diagnosis, and the mix of primary and revision procedures. For example, when assessing the outcome of RTSA for proximal humerus nonunion, Raiss et al reported a very high dislocation rate of 34%, but many of the shoulders that dislocated had been managed with resection of the tuberosities.[13] Interestingly, in one small series, RTSA performed specifically for treatment of glenohumeral instability was not reported to have a higher instability rate than when performed for cuff tear arthropathy, with only one subluxation leading to revision surgery in each group.[14]

Several studies have tried to identify risk factors for dislocation following RTSA. These can be divided into patient-related factors and procedure-related factors **(TABLE 35.2)**. *Patient-related factors* identified in the peer-reviewed literature include male gender, obesity, RTSA for proximal humerus nonunion or other fracture sequelae, axillary nerve injury, prior (open) surgery, and revision shoulder arthroplasty,[3,4,6,9,10,13,15] although one study did not find a correlation between body mass index (BMI) and RTSA dislocation.[16] Similarly, *procedure-related factors* associated with a higher dislocation rate have included inadequate soft-tissue tension, impinging heterotopic ossification, polyethylene disassociation or wear, resection of the tuberosities at the time of the procedure, and superior baseplate inclination.[13,17-19] However, in one study, cuff tear arthropathy was found to be protective against dislocation.[9]

The relationship between subscapularis repair or integrity and dislocation rates after RTSA continues to be a matter of debate. Scientific analysis of the studies focused on this issue is complicated by the wide range of implants used in various publications as well as little information on the rate of subscapularis healing when repaired.

TABLE 35.1 Frankle Classification of Instability After RTSA

I	Loss of compression	a	Undersized Implants
		b	Loss of deltoid contour
		c	Humeral height loss
		d	Subscapularis deficiency
		e	Acromion/scapular fracture
		f	Deltoid dysfunction
II	Loss of containment	a	Mechanical failure
		b	Alteration of D/R ratio (humerosocket depth)
III	Impingement	a	Soft-tissue or bony impingement
		b	Prosthetic malalignment
		c	Body habitus

D/R, depth/radius; RTSA, reverse total shoulder arthroplasty. (Used with permission from Abdelfattah A, Otto RJ, Simon P, et al. Classification of instability after reverse shoulder arthroplasty guides surgical management and outcomes. *J Shoulder Elbow Surg.* 2018;27(4):e107-e118.)

TABLE 35.2 Risk Factors for Dislocation After RTSA Reported in the Literature

Patient-related factors

- Male gender
- Obesity and large body habitus
- RTSA for proximal humerus nonunion and other traumatic sequelae
- Prior (open) surgery
- Revision surgery
- Axillary or brachial plexus palsy
- Severe cuff insufficiency
- Deltoid insufficiency

Procedure-related factors

- Inadequate soft-tissue tension
- Impinging heterotopic ossification
- Polyethylene dissociation or wear
- Tuberosity resection

RTSA, reverse total shoulder arthroplasty.

Chalmers et al[10] and Cheung et al[6] reported lower rates of dislocation when the subscapularis was repaired, whereas Vourazeris et al[20] and Roberson et al[21] found no differences in dislocation rates when the subscapularis was repaired or not. A meta-analysis published in 2019 indicated that repair of the subscapularis at the time of RTSA leads to lower dislocation rates for both medialized and lateralized designs (pooled dislocation rates were 4.1% in the nonrepair group and 0.7% in the repair group).[22] In addition, when subscapularis repair cannot be performed, or it is not performed intentionally, use of a lateralized implant seems to decrease the dislocation rate.

EVALUATION OF THE UNSTABLE REVERSE SHOULDER ARTHROPLASTY

History and Physical Examination

As with other shoulder conditions, evaluation of patients presenting with instability following RTSA requires a careful history and physical examination. Not uncommonly, patients presenting with dislocation early after surgery are not aware that the prosthesis is dislocated, since many do not experience major pain due to the dislocation episode.[10] The main complaint of patients who develop a late dislocation is a sudden loss of motion and function in association with pain.

It is important to determine whether the dislocation has occurred after a primary or a revision RTSA, as well as to record a number of other important details, including the patient's BMI, the indication for the index surgery, prior surgeries, the chronology of the dislocation, and any indication of possible deep infection or neurological dysfunction after surgery. Careful review of prior operative reports cannot be overemphasized: What implants were used? What was the condition of the rotator cuff? Was the subscapularis intact at the time of exposure? Was the subscapularis repaired? Were any unexpected intraoperative difficulties noted?

Physical examination should be directed to evaluate the patient's body habitus, assess the condition and status of the skin incision, identify tenderness or deformity along the acromion or spine of the scapula (indicative of a fracture or nonunion) that might contribute to instability, carefully assess the deltoid for integrity and contraction, and perform a detailed neurovascular examination to identify any evidence of injury to the axillary nerve, suprascapular nerve, or brachial plexopathy. Measuring range of motion is typically impractical in the setting of a dislocated RSA. Little attention is paid to the position of the scapula in space; however, it is our opinion that scapular malposition, oftentimes secondary to kyphosis of the thoracic spine, may also contribute to RTSA instability.

Radiographs

Anteroposterior and axillary radiographs will confirm the dislocation and show its direction, with anterior being most common **(FIGURE 35.1)**.[6,10] Whenever possible, it is important to review radiographs obtained prior to dislocation to measure global lateral offset and arm lengthening. Obtaining full-length radiographs of both humeri with magnifier markers is particularly important when evaluating these patients **(FIGURE 35.2)**.[23]

Any available radiographs should be assessed for component position and fixation, as well as any indication of component fracture or dissociation. On the humeral side, alignment of the humeral component in excessive varus or valgus will have a direct impact on the polyethylene opening angle. This problem seems to

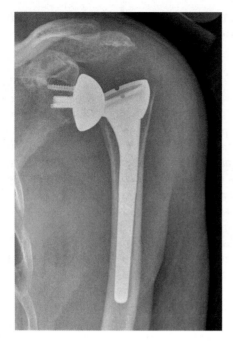

FIGURE 35.1 Dislocated reverse shoulder arthroplasty.

insufficiency? Is the greater tuberosity nonunited or malunited in a position where it may create levering impingement? Radiographs should also be scrutinized for heterotopic bone formation, deformity of the acromion or spine with or without fracture or nonunion, notching indicative of impingement between the humeral component and the medial scapular pillar, and humeral or glenoid osteolysis possibly indicative of polyethylene wear.[4,17]

Advanced Imaging Studies

Computed tomography (CT) is often useful in the evaluation of patients with a dislocated RTSA. CT allows more accurate evaluation of component position (especially on the glenoid side) and may also reveal occult notching or ectopic bone formation. In addition, CT scans are useful to assess the acromion and spine of the scapula for fracture and the possibility of associated nonunion or malunion. Greater tuberosity resorption, nonunion, or malunion is also best assessed on a CT scan. Finally, the degree of atrophy and fatty infiltration of the rotator cuff and deltoid can be assessed. We have not found MRI or bone scan particularly useful for the evaluation of the dislocated RTSA.

Electromyogram and Nerve Conduction Studies

Any abnormality in the motor or sensory examination of the brachial plexus and its branches should prompt obtaining an electromyogram with nerve conduction studies. We have a low threshold to order this test when the physical examination findings are inconclusive, since occult axillary nerve or brachial plexus dysfunction may play a major role in instability after RTSA.

be much more prevalent now that ultrashort stems are being widely used.[24] On the glenoid side, gross malposition in version or inclination may facilitate instability. Inclination can be assessed using the radiographic projection of the floor of the supraspinatus fossa as a reference.[25]

It is particularly important to assess the condition of the greater tuberosity, especially when RTSA was performed for acute trauma or sequelae of trauma: Is the greater tuberosity resorbed, indicative of cuff

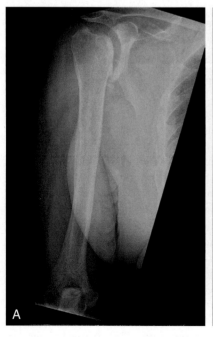
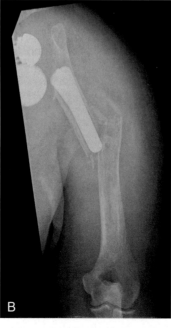

FIGURE 35.2 A and **B**, Radiographs of both humeri with magnifier markers may be used to determine relative changes in humeral length (markers not shown here).

Additional Evaluation

Although the value of preoperative evaluation of the failed shoulder arthroplasty for infection may have a low diagnostic yield, in my practice, I have decided to evaluate every failed shoulder arthroplasty with laboratory studies that include a complete cell count, erythrocyte sedimentation rate, and C-reactive protein, as well as an aspiration of intra-articular fluid for cell count, differential cell count, and cultures. In addition, one sample of tissue for pathologic assessment and five samples of tissue for culture are obtained at the time of revision of every failed shoulder arthroplasty.

THE ROLE OF CLOSED REDUCTION

Closed reduction is the standard initial treatment for dislocation after total hip arthroplasty and can be expected to be successful in the vast majority of situations.[26] For the dislocated RTSA, several studies mention closed reduction as a possible treatment option.[9] Some authors have reported attempted closed reduction,[27] whereas others recommend proceeding directly to revision surgery.[5]

Closed reduction may be attempted in the office, or it may require regional or general anesthesia with or without muscle relaxation. Fluoroscopy is useful to guide and confirm closed reduction. The reduction maneuver usually involves placing the humerus in neutral rotation and combining axial traction with direct translation of the humeral metaphysis into the reduction position, typically by applying a posteriorly directed force.[28] After closed reduction, the shoulder is immobilized in abduction and neutral rotation for 6 weeks to maximize congruency between the glenosphere and humeral bearing.

The reported success of closed reduction has varied. Edwards et al reported a successful closed reduction in two of seven shoulders.[27] Chalmers et al treated nine shoulders with closed reduction, and four of the nine remained stable.[10] Teusink et al reported a 62% success rate (13 of 21 shoulders) for shoulders that could be closed reduced in the office. Kusin et al reported a 30% success rate (10 of 22 shoulders) with closed reduction after RTSA dislocation in a study using the National Surgical Quality Improvement Program (NSQIP) database.[16] Several other authors have reported that in their studies, none of the dislocations were treated successfully with closed reduction.[6,8,9,17]

SURGICAL MANAGEMENT OF THE UNSTABLE REVERSE SHOULDER ARTHROPLASTY

Revision Strategies to Maximize Stability

The reported failure rate of surgical management for the unstable RTSA continues to be unacceptably high.[1,4-6,10,17] This may be related, at least in part, to difficulties in identifying and addressing all factors contributing to instability in each individual shoulder. The goals of surgical management include the following: (1) eliminating all sources of impingement that may lever the arthroplasty causing the dislocation; (2) optimizing component sizing and position; and (3) adjusting soft-tissue tension. Rarely, isolated removal of bone or scar tissue may render the RTSA stable. In most situations, surgeons exchange the glenosphere and polyethylene as well. More extensive component revision is frequently needed to implant new components in a position that restores stability. Severe cuff and deltoid deficiency may contribute to instability in some shoulders and can be addressed with muscle and tendon transfers. Rarely, instability cannot be solved unless the nonunited spine of the scapula is stabilized. Some unstable RTSAs fail multiple attempts to correct instability and require one of various salvage procedures.

Impingement: Identification and Management

When evaluating the dislocated RTSA prior to surgical management, radiographs and CT should be carefully scrutinized to identify any areas of potential impingement as the etiology of the instability. Common sources of bony impingement include *osteophytes* of the glenoid or proximal humerus that were not removed at the time of the original RTSA surgery, *ectopic bone*, and the superior aspect of the *medial scapular pillar* in RTSA using a medialized glenoid and a horizontal polyethylene opening angle. Impingement with the medial scapular pillar may be particularly relevant in shoulders with a short glenoid neck, such as those with glenohumeral dysplasia. A burr may be used around the perimeter of the implanted glenoid component to remove any scapular bone that might contribute to impingement causing instability. A retained, malpositioned, or malunited *greater tuberosity* after RSA for trauma or its sequelae may contribute to dislocation. The greater tuberosity may also need to be trimmed down when prominent in shoulders with supraspinatus and infraspinatus disruption. Finally, thick inferior *pseudocapsule* contributes to instability in many dislocated RTSA, especially chronic situations that have been dislocated for a few weeks. Complete excision of this tissue is necessary in almost every shoulder to minimize recurrence of instability.

Glenosphere and Polyethylene Exchange

Exchange of the glenosphere may improve stability through several mechanisms. Similar to the hip joint,[29] a larger glenosphere will provide a greater arc of motion before impingement and also a larger jump distance. In addition, a glenosphere providing more lateral offset will add tension to the soft tissues and decrease the chances of impingement between the humeral component and the scapula. As such, our strategy when dealing with the unstable RTSA is to implant a larger glenosphere with lateralization and posteroinferior eccentricity. However, exchange to a much larger glenosphere may be limited by the surrounding soft-tissue envelope (**FIGURE 35.3**).

Exchange of the polyethylene bearing is performed almost routinely in order to (1) implant a new liner that

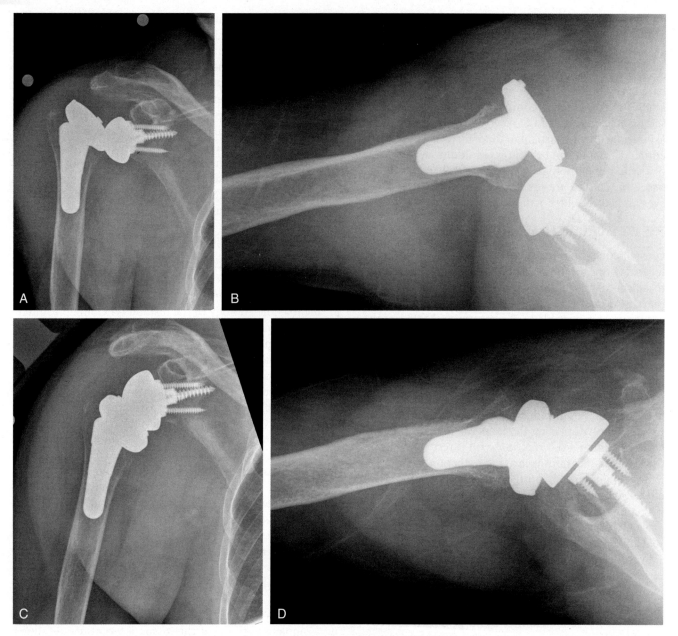

FIGURE 35.3 Successful management of dislocation after reverse total shoulder arthroplasty with exchange of the glenosphere and humeral bearing. **A and B,** Preoperative anteroposterior and axillary radiographs. **C and D,** Anteroposterior and axillary radiographs after revision for glenosphere and polyethylene exchange.

has not been subjected to wear; (2) facilitate exposure to the inferior pseudocapsule, ectopic bone, and the glenoid; and (3) match the diameter of the newly implanted glenosphere. A new polyethylene may be all that is needed for a late dislocation attributed solely to polyethylene disassociation or severe polyethylene wear, although that circumstance is uncommon. Polyethylene liners with greater constraint are also available. They provide a larger jump distance, but they may also lead to earlier impingement. As such, careful trialing of constrained liners is mandatory, and we tend to use them only as a last resort. Very often, the thickness of the humeral bearing is increased at the time of revision surgery to

optimize soft-tissue tension. However, in shoulders with a shortened humerus, the available thicknesses for the humeral bearing may be insufficient. In addition, care must be taken when using very thick bearings to avoid lengthening the arm to the point of overstretching the brachial plexus, deltoid, and any remaining rotator cuff.

Component Revision

Revision of the glenoid and/or humeral component becomes necessary in a number of circumstances, including loosening, gross malposition, component fracture, and severe humeral bone loss. Revision of a well-fixed baseplate must be considered with caution since removal of the baseplate may lead to catastrophic bone loss that might compromise the entire reconstruction.

Similarly, revision of a well-fixed humeral component should only be performed when absolutely needed. However, poor version, incorrect height, varus/valgus malalignment of the humeral component, and severe bone loss may require correction in order to achieve a stable RTSA. Shortening of the humerus can be confirmed with comparative right and left humeri radiographs and will lead to insufficient soft-tissue tension.[4] A humeral component implanted in varus may lead to an excessively vertical polyethylene (**FIGURE 35.4**), whereas excessive valgus may lead to impingement between the polyethylene and scapula.[24] Version abnormalities may facilitate dislocation through loss of containment and/or impingement. Finally, in the presence of substantial humeral bone loss, the absence of the greater tuberosity may decrease deltoid tension (loss of "deltoid wrapping" around the tuberosity[30]), and the attachment sites for the subscapularis, posterosuperior cuff, and, in larger defects, the deltoid are compromised, leading to loss of soft-tissue restraints.

When component revision is performed for dislocation after RTSA, the reconstruction should be planned with sufficient global lateralization so that the lateral aspect of the greater tuberosity extends close to the anatomic position in the native shoulder. The glenoid component should be implanted in adequate version and inferior tilt. As noted, implantation of a larger glenosphere with posteroinferior eccentricity and some degree of glenoid lateralization obtained using bone graft, a thicker baseplate, or a glenosphere with built-in lateralization are recommended.

On the humeral side, every effort should be made to implant the new humeral component in adequate alignment, version, and height. Although a moderate amount of bone loss may be addressed by implanting the component "proud," substantial bone loss requires consideration of either an allograft-prosthetic composite or a modular segmental replacement.[31,32] Modular segmental prostheses are extremely versatile and useful. However, the main complication reported after revision to a reverse modular segmental replacement is precisely dislocation. As such, our preference has been to use allograft-prosthetic composites and order the bone allograft with soft-tissue attachments so that any remaining rotator cuff and the deltoid, if needed, can be repaired to the allograft tendon stumps (**FIGURE 35.5**).[32] This is particularly useful when muscle and tendon transfers are recommended in the setting of revision RTSA for shoulders with substantial proximal humerus bone loss.

The Role of Muscle and Tendon Transfers

Adequate tension of the deltoid and any rotator cuff that remains contributes to the stability of RTSA. As mentioned previously, the effect of an intact subscapularis on RSA stability remains controversial. In the native shoulder, an intact posterosuperior rotator cuff functions as a posterior restraint to anterior translation and, as such, an intact cuff contributes to RTSA stability. When the posterior cuff is completely absent, including the teres minor, tendon transfers may be useful not only

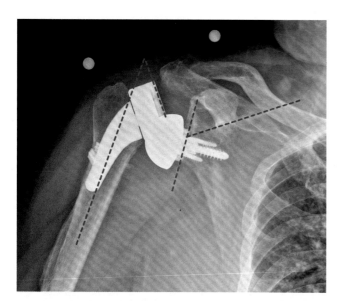

FIGURE 35.4 Varus malalignment of short humeral components may lead to an excessively vertical polyethylene angle that may contribute to instability. Superior tilt of the glenoid component may contribute to instability as well. Blue lines indicate the effective opening angle of the humeral bearing. Red lines indicate superior tilt of the baseplate in reference to the floor of the supraspinatus fossa.

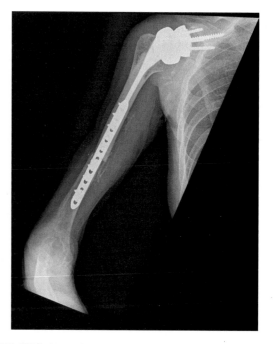

FIGURE 35.5 Allograft-prosthetic composite has the potential to improve stability by restoring humeral length, tensioning the deltoid muscle through the so-called wrapping effect, and providing an opportunity for secure soft-tissue reattachment.

to restore active external rotation but also to increase joint stability.

Transfer of the latissimus dorsi with or without the teres major in the setting of RTSA has been reported to provide good outcomes in terms of motion and strength.[33] However, its potential role as a soft-tissue stabilizer to prevent instability after RTSA has not been investigated. When the latissimus dorsi and teres major have been compromised by prior surgeries, we have considered transfer of the lower trapezius in the setting of RTSA, a well-established technique of surgical management of irreparable rotator cuff tears.[34] Regarding unstable RTSAs with subscapularis deficiency, we have occasionally transferred the insertion of the pectoralis major proximally to the lesser tuberosity in an effort to create one more soft-tissue constraint against anterior dislocation.

Deltoid dysfunction is the main factor contributing to RTSA dislocation in many shoulders.[4,17] It may be secondary to a neurological deficit—ie, axillary nerve, brachial plexus palsy, or cervical radiculopathy—or a postsurgical deltoid deficiency or tear. Neurological reasons for deltoid dysfunction may recover spontaneously or require specific treatment (transfer of branches of the radial nerve to the axillary nerve,[35] cervical spine decompression). Rarely, a severely stretched or detached deltoid may be successfully imbricated or repaired to the acromion and scapular spine. Deltoid deficiency may also be addressed with a pedicled transfer of the pectoralis major. Although this procedure has been reported mostly to improve function,[36] it may also be effective in restoring RTSA stability.

The Role of Internal Fixation for Acromion or Spine Fractures

Fractures of the acromion and scapular spine are known complications of RTSA. These fractures have been reported with increase in frequency for certain RTSA designs.[37] Pain and loss of motion and strength are the most commonly reported symptoms after these fractures.[38] However, at least theoretically, these fractures could also contribute to instability. Not uncommonly the lateral fractured fragment angles inferiorly, effectively shortening the deltoid muscle. The resultant insufficient deltoid tension could allow dislocation to occur. However, the outcome of internal fixation for scapular spine fractures in the setting of RTSA has been reported to be unpredictable.[38,39] The potential value of open reduction and internal fixation of scapular spine fractures to restore stability after RTSA remains undetermined.

Salvage Solutions

Certain shoulders continue to dislocate after RTSA despite multiple reoperation attempts. There may be times when further revision to another RTSA incorporating many of the elements described above remains unsuccessful. In those circumstances, salvage solutions may need to be considered.

Glenohumeral Cerclage

Tashjian et al have reported use of a glenohumeral cerclage for salvage of recalcitrant instability after RTSA.[40] Heavy caliber nonabsorbable suture or tape is passed behind the glenoid and tied either around the humeral prosthesis in the presence of proximal humerus bone loss or after passage through humeral bone tunnels. All three shoulders included in their report remained stable at 6 months, 10 months, and 18 months, respectively. From my own experience, I have used this cerclage technique successfully in one case **(FIGURE 35.6)**.

Revision to Humeral Hemiarthroplasty or Hemi-Reverse

Another salvage procedure is to revise the failed RTSA to a hemiarthroplasty. This procedure may be planned as a permanent solution or as a temporary method to allow the soft tissues to contract once the relative lengthening of the RTSA has been eliminated in hopes that after soft-tissue shortening, a stable RTSA could be implanted. Classically, revision involves removal of the reverse glenoid component and revision to a humeral head hemiarthroplasty. Reported functional outcomes after conversion of RTSA to a humeral hemiarthroplasty are relatively poor, and hemiarthroplasty instability can occur, but further surgery can typically be avoided.[41] Since glenoid bone stock is more limited than humeral bone stock, some authors recommend revising the failed RTSA to a "hemi-reverse," removing the humeral component and leaving the glenosphere to articulate with the remaining proximal humerus bone. This may allow for a more constrained articulation with better stability and motion and may also facilitate RTSA reimplantation since the glenoid remains undisturbed.

Arthrodesis

Glenohumeral fusion is frequently mentioned in academic discussions on salvage options for the failed

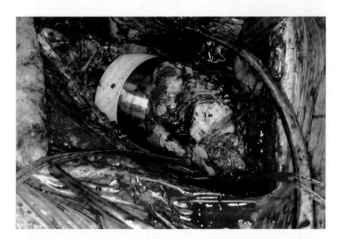

FIGURE 35.6 Recalcitrant instability after reverse shoulder arthroplasty has been reported to be successfully managed with glenohumeral cerclage.

shoulder arthroplasty. However, the ability to achieve a solid fusion mass is compromised by the magnitude of the bone defect present after removal of the unstable RTSA. Scalise and Iannotti reported successful fusion in five of the seven shoulders included in their study, but several shoulders required more than one grafting and fixation procedure to achieve union. In addition, a vascularized fibular autograft was used in some shoulders.[42]

Resection Arthroplasty

For patients with recalcitrant RTSA instability despite multiple reoperation attempts, resection arthroplasty with removal of all components may need to be considered. Severe deltoid insufficiency, associated periprosthetic joint infection, and severe glenoid bone loss are frequently present in those shoulders considered for resection arthroplasty. Similar to what has been reported for revision of RTSA to hemiarthroplasty, the functional outcome is typically poor.[43]

Reported Outcomes

Reported outcomes after surgical management of the unstable RTSA have not been particularly promising. In the study by Gallo et al, only three of the nine shoulders included were stable at most recent follow-up, with two shoulders persistently dislocated and two shoulders resected.[5] Chalmers et al reported persistent instability requiring conversion to hemiarthroplasty in 2 of the 11 shoulders included in their study.[10] Kohan et al reported recurrent instability after revision surgery in 29% of the dislocations that had occurred early (within 3 months after the index procedure) and 40% of their late dislocations.[17] In the study by Abdelfattah et al, 5 of the 26 shoulders (19%) followed up for a minimum of 2 years after revision surgery remained unstable.[4] Cheung et al reported recurrent instability in 5 of the 11 shoulders (45%) treated surgically by placement of a thicker polyethylene insert. Clearly, further advances are needed to improve the outcome of surgical management for the unstable RTSA.

CONCLUSION

Dislocation following RTSA remains a challenging complication to treat. Although the rate of dislocation has continued to decrease to under 1% after primary contemporary RTSA, rates are still high after revision and for certain patients and conditions. Main risk factors for dislocation after RTSA include male gender, obesity, axillary or brachial plexus injury, prior open surgery, revision surgery, RTSA for sequelae of trauma, inadequate soft-tissue tension, deltoid insufficiency, superior baseplate inclination, tuberosity resection at the time of arthroplasty, implant disassociation, and polyethylene wear. Controversy remains regarding the relationship between subscapularis integrity and risk of dislocation.

The evaluation of patients presenting with an unstable RTSA must include a thorough history and physical examination to understand the chronology of the dislocation, the nature of the index procedure, as well as the condition of the deltoid, acromion, scapular spine, axillary nerve, and brachial plexus. Shoulder radiographs are often complemented with radiographs of both humeri with magnifier markers to measure relative humeral length as well as CT. Electromyography and nerve conduction studies and a workup for infection may also be indicated based upon the findings at the time of evaluation.

The success of closed reduction followed by shoulder immobilization has been reported to range between 0% and 60%. The success of surgical management for the dislocated RTSA has been reported to range between 55% and 82% **(TABLE 35.3)**. Conceptually, instability after RTSA may be classified as secondary to loss of compression, loss of containment, and impingement. However, frequently there are several contributing

TABLE 35.3 Common Strategies for Surgical Management of Dislocation After RTSA	
Eliminate sources of impingement	• Osteophytes • Ectopic bone • Medial scapular pillar • Greater tuberosity • Pseudocapsule
Optimize glenosphere size and position	• Larger diameter • Lateral offset (lateralized) • Posteroinferior eccentricity
Humeral bearing exchange	• Larger diameter • Thicker • Constrained (selective)
Baseplate revision	• Adequate tilt and version
Humeral component revision	• Adequate height, version and alignment • Consider reconstruction using a modular segmental prosthesis or an allograft-prosthesis composite in shoulders with severe proximal humerus bone loss
Muscle and tendon transfers	• Transfer of the latissimus dorsi, teres major, or lower trapezius to the greater tuberosity or proximal humeral shaft may act as posterior restraints against anterior dislocation • Transfer of the pectoralis major to the lesser tuberosity may create one more layer of soft-tissue constraint against anterior dislocation • Pedicled pectoralis major transfer to replace deltoid function.
Internal fixation of fractures of the acromion or spine	• Theoretically should contribute to stability; role largely unknown

RTSA, reverse total shoulder arthroplasty.

factors that need to be addressed to render the arthroplasty stable. When surgical management is considered, exchange of the glenosphere and humeral components combined with removal of sources of impingement may be sufficient in selected cases. However, complex shoulders may require revision of one or both components, tendon transfers, or internal fixation of a scapular spine fracture or nonunion. There are some unstable RTSAs that cannot be stabilized despite one or more reoperation procedures. In these situations, salvage with glenohumeral cerclage, conversion to humeral hemiarthroplasty or hemi-reverse, arthrodesis, or resection arthroplasty may all need to be considered.

A careful review of the literature on this topic really highlights the need to ensure stability at the time of primary RTSA. If dislocation occurs, a detailed analysis of all possible contributing factors needs to be performed before reoperation is considered. The relatively high rate of failure after reoperation likely reflects failure to recognize and address the several factors that may not be obvious but may have contributed to the instability.

REFERENCES

1. Markes AR, Cheung E, Ma CB. Failed reverse shoulder arthroplasty and recommendations for revision. *Curr Rev Musculoskelet Med.* 2020;13(1):1-10.
2. Barco R, Savvidou OD, Sperling JW, Sanchez-Sotelo J, Cofield RH. Complications in reverse shoulder arthroplasty. *EFORT Open Rev.* 2016;1(3):72-80.
3. Werner BC, Burrus MT, Begho I, Gwathmey FW, Brockmeier SF. Early revision within 1 year after shoulder arthroplasty: patient factors and etiology. *J Shoulder Elbow Surg.* 2015;24(12):e323-e330.
4. Abdelfattah A, Otto RJ, Simon P, et al. Classification of instability after reverse shoulder arthroplasty guides surgical management and outcomes. *J Shoulder Elbow Surg.* 2018;27(4):e107-e118.
5. Gallo RA, Gamradt SC, Mattern CJ, et al. Instability after reverse total shoulder replacement. *J Shoulder Elbow Surg.* 2011;20(4):584-590.
6. Cheung EV, Sarkissian EJ, Sox-Harris A, et al. Instability after reverse total shoulder arthroplasty. *J Shoulder Elbow Surg.* 2018;27(11):1946-1952.
7. Zumstein MA, Pinedo M, Old J, Boileau P. Problems, complications, reoperations, and revisions in reverse total shoulder arthroplasty: a systematic review. *J Shoulder Elbow Surg.* 2011;20(1):146-157.
8. Clark JC, Ritchie J, Song FS, et al. Complication rates, dislocation, pain, and postoperative range of motion after reverse shoulder arthroplasty in patients with and without repair of the subscapularis. *J Shoulder Elbow Surg.* 2012;21(1):36-41.
9. Padegimas EM, Zmistowski BM, Restrepo C, et al. Instability after reverse total shoulder arthroplasty: which patients dislocate? *Am J Orthop (Belle Mead NJ).* 2016;45(7):E444-E450.
10. Chalmers PN, Rahman Z, Romeo AA, Nicholson GP. Early dislocation after reverse total shoulder arthroplasty. *J Shoulder Elbow Surg.* 2014;23(5):737-744.
11. Friedman RJ, Flurin P-H, Wright TW, Zuckerman JD, Roche CP. Comparison of reverse total shoulder arthroplasty outcomes with and without subscapularis repair. *J Shoulder Elbow Surg.* 2017;26(4):662-668.
12. Kang JR, Dubiel MJ, Cofield RH, et al. Primary reverse shoulder arthroplasty using contemporary implants is associated with very low reoperation rates. *J Shoulder Elbow Surg.* 2019;28(6 suppl):S175-S180.
13. Raiss P, Edwards TB, da Silva MR, Bruckner T, Loew M, Walch G. Reverse shoulder arthroplasty for the treatment of nonunions of the surgical neck of the proximal part of the humerus (type-3 fracture sequelae). *J Bone Joint Surg Am.* 2014;96(24):2070-2076.
14. Hasler A, Fornaciari P, Jungwirth-Weinberger A, Jentzsch T, Wieser K, Gerber C. Reverse shoulder arthroplasty in the treatment of glenohumeral instability. *J Shoulder Elbow Surg.* 2019;28(8):1587-1594.
15. Theodoulou A, Krishnan J, Aromataris E. Risk of poor outcomes in patients who are obese following total shoulder arthroplasty and reverse total shoulder arthroplasty: a systematic review and meta-analysis. *J Shoulder Elbow Surg.* 2019;28(11):e359-e376.
16. Kusin DJ, Ungar JA, Samson KK, Teusink MJ. Body mass index as a risk factor for dislocation of total shoulder arthroplasty in the first 30 days. *JSES Open Access.* 2019;3(3):179-182.
17. Kohan EM, Chalmers PN, Salazar D, Keener JD, Yamaguchi K, Chamberlain AM. Dislocation following reverse total shoulder arthroplasty. *J Shoulder Elbow Surg.* 2017;26(7):1238-1245.
18. Wren ER, Noud P. Polyethylene dislocation after a reverse total shoulder arthroplasty with an intact glenohumeral joint. *JSES Int.* 2020;4(1):169-173.
19. Tashjian RZ, Martin BI, Ricketts CA, Henninger HB, Granger EK, Chalmers PN. Superior baseplate inclination is associated with instability after reverse total shoulder arthroplasty. *Clin Orthop Relat Res.* 2018;476(8):1622-1629.
20. Vourazeris JD, Wright TW, Struk AM, King JJ, Farmer KW. Primary reverse total shoulder arthroplasty outcomes in patients with subscapularis repair versus tenotomy. *J Shoulder Elbow Surg.* 2017;26(3):450-457.
21. Roberson TA, Shanley E, Griscom JT, et al. Subscapularis repair is unnecessary after lateralized reverse shoulder arthroplasty. *JB JS Open Access.* 2018;3(3):e0056.
22. Matthewson G, Kooner S, Kwapisz A, Leiter J, Old J, MacDonald P. The effect of subscapularis repair on dislocation rates in reverse shoulder arthroplasty: a meta-analysis and systematic review. *J Shoulder Elbow Surg.* 2019;28(5):989-997.
23. Lädermann A, Walch G, Lubbeke A, et al. Influence of arm lengthening in reverse shoulder arthroplasty. *J Shoulder Elbow Surg.* 2012;21(3):336-341.
24. Lädermann A, Chiu JC-H, Cunningham G, et al. Do short stems influence the cervico-diaphyseal angle and the medullary filling after reverse shoulder arthroplasties? *Orthop Traumatol Surg Res.* 2020;106(2):241-246.
25. Boileau P, Gauci M-O, Wagner ER, et al. The reverse shoulder arthroplasty angle: a new measurement of glenoid inclination for reverse shoulder arthroplasty. *J Shoulder Elbow Surg.* 2019;28(7):1281-1290.
26. Sanchez-Sotelo J, Haidukewych GJ, Boberg CJ. Hospital cost of dislocation after primary total hip arthroplasty. *J Bone Joint Surg Am.* 2006;88(2):290-294.
27. Edwards TB, Williams MD, Labriola JE, Elkousy HA, Gartsman GM, O'Connor DP. Subscapularis insufficiency and the risk of shoulder dislocation after reverse shoulder arthroplasty. *J Shoulder Elbow Surg.* 2009;18(6):892-896.
28. Teusink MJ, Pappou IP, Schwartz DG, Cottrell BJ, Frankle MA. Results of closed management of acute dislocation after reverse shoulder arthroplasty. *J Shoulder Elbow Surg.* 2015;24(4):621-627.
29. Sanchez-Sotelo J, Berry DJ. Epidemiology of instability after total hip replacement. *Orthop Clin North Am.* 2001;32(4):543-552, vii.
30. Roche CP, Diep P, Hamilton M, et al. Impact of inferior glenoid tilt, humeral retroversion, bone grafting, and design parameters on muscle length and deltoid wrapping in reverse shoulder arthroplasty. *Bull Hosp Jt Dis.* 2013;71(4):284-293.
31. Guven MF, Aslan L, Botanlioglu H, Kaynak G, Kesmezacar H, Babacan M. Functional outcome of reverse shoulder tumor prosthesis in the treatment of proximal humerus tumors. *J Shoulder Elbow Surg.* 2016;25(1):e1-e6.
32. Sanchez-Sotelo J, Wagner ER, Sim FH, Houdek MT. Allograft-prosthetic composite reconstruction for massive proximal humeral bone loss in reverse shoulder arthroplasty. *J Bone Joint Surg Am.* 2017;99(24):2069-2076.
33. Puskas GJ, Catanzaro S, Gerber C. Clinical outcome of reverse total shoulder arthroplasty combined with latissimus dorsi transfer for the treatment of chronic combined pseudoparesis of elevation and external rotation of the shoulder. *J Shoulder Elbow Surg.* 2014;23(1):49-57.

34. Elhassan BT, Sanchez-Sotelo J, Wagner ER. Outcome of arthroscopically assisted lower trapezius transfer to reconstruct massive irreparable posterior-superior rotator cuff tears. *J Shoulder Elbow Surg.* 2020;29(10):2135-2142.

35. Salazar DH, Chalmers PN, Mackinnon SE, Keener JD. Reverse shoulder arthroplasty after radial-to-axillary nerve transfer for axillary nerve palsy with concomitant irreparable rotator cuff tear. *J Shoulder Elbow Surg.* 2017;26(1):e23-e28.

36. Elhassan BT, Wagner ER, Werthel J-D, Lehanneur M, Lee J. Outcome of reverse shoulder arthroplasty with pedicled pectoralis transfer in patients with deltoid paralysis. *J Shoulder Elbow Surg.* 2018;27(1):96-103.

37. Ascione F, Kilian CM, Laughlin MS, et al. Increased scapular spine fractures after reverse shoulder arthroplasty with a humeral onlay short stem: an analysis of 485 consecutive cases. *J Shoulder Elbow Surg.* 2018;27(12):2183-2190.

38. Patterson DC, Chi D, Parsons BO, Cagle PJ. Acromial spine fracture after reverse total shoulder arthroplasty: a systematic review. *J Shoulder Elbow Surg.* 2019;28(4):792-801.

39. Toft F, Moro F. Does ORIF of rare scapular spine fractures sustained after reverse shoulder arthroplasty benefit elderly patients? A case-series appraisal. *Orthop Traumatol Surg Res.* 2019;105(8):1521-1528.

40. Tashjian RZ, Broschinsky K, Chalmers PN. Glenohumeral cerclage for salvage of recalcitrant instability after reverse total shoulder arthroplasty. *J Shoulder Elbow Surg.* 2018;27(8):e259-e263.

41. Glanzmann MC, Kolling C, Schwyzer H-K, Audigé L. Conversion to hemiarthroplasty as a salvage procedure for failed reverse shoulder arthroplasty. *J Shoulder Elbow Surg.* 2016;25(11):1795-1802.

42. Scalise JJ, Iannotti JP. Glenohumeral arthrodesis after failed prosthetic shoulder arthroplasty. *J Bone Joint Surg Am.* 2008;90(1):70-77.

43. Muh SJ, Streit JJ, Lenarz CJ, et al. Resection arthroplasty for failed shoulder arthroplasty. *J Shoulder Elbow Surg.* 2013;22(2):247-252.

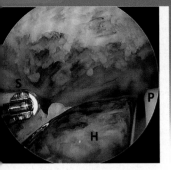

36 Stiffness After Arthroplasty

Robert M. Zbeda, MD and Peter D. McCann, MD

INTRODUCTION

Stiffness of the shoulder following primary anatomic total shoulder arthroplasty (ATSA) and reverse total shoulder arthroplasty (RTSA) is poorly defined and often underreported as a unique surgical complication but is a common reason for dissatisfaction in patient-reported outcome studies.[1-11] In a comprehensive review of complications of shoulder arthroplasty in 19,000 cases, stiffness was not listed as a unique complication.[12] Further confusing this issue, shoulder stiffness is often merely one of several factors accounting for failure following shoulder arthroplasty.

The purpose of this chapter is to define shoulder stiffness as a unique complication following shoulder arthroplasty; review the preoperative, intraoperative, and postoperative causes of stiffness; and provide an overview of the various treatments of shoulder stiffness based on etiology.

DEFINITION OF SHOULDER STIFFNESS

Stiffness as a unique complication following total shoulder arthroplasty may be defined as severe limitation of passive range of motion sufficient to compromise the basic activities of daily living necessary for independent self-care. A 2012 study quantified the range of motion required to perform the activities assessed by three validated shoulder patient-reported outcome measures: American Shoulder and Elbow Surgeons Score, the Simple Shoulder Test, and the University of Pennsylvania Shoulder Score.[13] The average motion required to perform 10 functional activities were flexion, 121°; extension, 46°; abduction, 128°; cross body adduction, 116°; external rotation at 90° abduction, 59°; and internal rotation with the arm at the side, 102°. External rotation with the arm at the side was not recorded, nor was the correlation of humeral internal rotation with the common clinical measurement of internal rotation, ie, posterior reach (the highest midline spinal segment reached by the tip of the hitch-hiking thumb). The authors concluded that full range of motion of the shoulder is not required to perform the routine activities of daily living as defined in these three shoulder-specific patient-reported outcome measures. Hence, one could define

shoulder stiffness as a complication following shoulder arthroplasty as range of motion less than the functional range of motion reported in the study.

Another definition of shoulder stiffness is the range of motion accounting for failure following total shoulder arthroplasty as reported by various investigators. In his 1982 report, Neer defined an unsatisfactory result following ATSA as <90° elevation and <25° external rotation,[14] although the basis for these parameters was not discussed. Reporting on the characteristics of 139 failed shoulder arthroplasties, Hasan et al defined stiffness as the inability to perform activities relating to shoulder mobility as components of the Simple Shoulder Test: tuck in shirt, place hand behind head, place coin on shelf, and wash opposite shoulder.[5]

Another definition of shoulder stiffness to consider is the degree of limitation of motion that would indicate surgical intervention. Thorsness and Romeo recommended arthroscopic release for postarthroplasty patients with less than 90° forward flexion and less than 20° external rotation in the absence of component malposition or infection.[15] Finally, in a study investigating severe preoperative external rotation deficits and RTSA outcomes, Carafino and coauthors defined stiffness as external rotation <20°.[16]

The lack of consensus on the definition of stiffness following shoulder arthroplasty contributes to its underreporting in the orthopedic literature. There are no accepted criteria for the degree of limitation of motion following shoulder arthroplasty that would qualify as a unique complication. Numerous reports of complications of shoulder arthroplasty either have not even included stiffness as a reason for failure or, when listed as a complication requiring revision surgery, have reported stiffness at a very low rate of 0.3% to 1%.[1,16] On the other hand, reporting on the reasons for patient dissatisfaction following shoulder arthroplasty, Franta and colleagues have stated that stiffness of the shoulder is the most common complaint, occurring in up to 74% of patients.[3]

For the purpose of this discussion, the degree of limitation of passive range of motion to define stiffness as a unique complication and a cause for a poor outcome following shoulder arthroplasty should be less than the range of motion required for functional use as described in the report of Namdari et al and, based on the several studies cited above, may reasonably be defined as forward elevation less than 90°, external rotation less than 20°, and internal rotation to the gluteal region ("unable to tuck in shirt" in the Simple Shoulder Test), consistent with the range of motion Neer considered "unsatisfactory," Thorsness and Romeo considered as an indication for arthroscopic release, Carofino et al considered "stiff," and Franta et al reported as "unsatisfactory shoulder arthroplasties"[3,13-15,17] **(TABLE 36.1)**.

ETIOLOGY OF STIFFNESS

Identification of the etiology of stiffness following shoulder arthroplasty will both direct current treatment and, through better understanding of the causes of stiffness, prevent stiffness in subsequent cases. Analysis of shoulder stiffness following arthroplasty can be divided into preoperative, intraoperative, and postoperative factors.

Preoperative Factors

Preoperative limited range of motion is the most common cause of stiffness following shoulder arthroplasty.[14,17,18] Patients with fracture sequelae, failed open reduction internal fixation (ORIF) or hemiarthroplasty for proximal humerus fracture, failed shoulder arthroplasty, and advanced glenohumeral osteoarthritis with severe limitation of motion (less than 90° forward elevation, less than 0° external rotation, and internal rotation to the gluteal region) are especially at risk for postoperative stiffness.[7,8,16,19-28] Such patients must be counseled preoperatively of the risk of postoperative stiffness in an effort to appropriately manage postoperative clinical expectations.

Patient motivation and engagement are other important preoperative factors that will influence shoulder stiffness postoperatively. Appropriate selection of patients who understand the importance of postoperative rehabilitation and commit to its duration of up to 12 months following surgery will also help prevent postoperative stiffness.

Finally, prosthetic design can be considered a preoperative factor that influences stiffness postoperatively. Many patients undergoing RTSA fail to regain internal rotation, regardless of the particular design of the replacement. There is no consensus on the reason for limited internal rotation in some patients, but it may be related to body habitus, design characteristics of the prosthesis, as well as variations in size and version of the individual components. Limited internal rotation does not appear to be related to repair of the subscapularis tendon or to the constraint inherent to the RTSA design since impingement-free range of motion would allow for adequate internal rotation for activities of daily living.[29-34] Consequently, patients considering RTSA should be counseled preoperatively regarding the possibility of limited internal rotation postoperatively.

Intraoperative Factors

Intraoperative factors contributing to stiffness following arthroplasty can be divided into soft tissue– and implant-related issues. Operative techniques addressing these factors will be discussed in other chapters. In general, soft tissue management includes extensive lysis of adhesions in the subacromial and subdeltoid spaces, anterior and inferior capsular resection, as well as biceps tenotomy or tenodesis. In ATSA, component size and

TABLE 36.1 Definitions of Shoulder Stiffness Following Arthroplasty

Quantitative Assessment

Author	Year	Flexion	Extension	Abduction	Cross-Body Adduction	External Rotation at 90° Abduction	External Rotation at 0° Abduction
Carofino[17]	2020	–	–	–	–	–	20°
Thorsness[15]	2016	90°	–	–	–	–	20°
Namdari[13]	2012	121°	46°	128°	116°	59°	–
Neer[14]	1982	90°	–	–	–	–	25°

Qualitative Assessment

Author	Y	Definition
Hasan[5]	2002	• Tuck in shirt • Place hand behind head • Place coin on shelf • Wash opposite shoulder

Proposed Definition

- Flexion: <90°
- External rotation: <20°
- Internal rotation: gluteal region
- Compromise of basic activities of daily living

position should permit 50% translation of the humeral component on the glenoid, as well as sufficient adduction, and internal rotation for the operative hand to touch the opposite shoulder. An oversized humeral component will not permit the desired translation intraoperatively (overstuffing) and will account for stiffness and pain postoperatively **(FIGURE 36.1)**.

In RTSA, implant size and orientation should allow for reduction under appropriate soft tissue tension to ensure stability. Superior glenosphere placement will limit forward elevation due to impingement of the humerus on the acromion and should be avoided. Finally, excessive force to achieve reduction, due to inadequate soft tissue releases, insufficient proximal humeral resection, or an excessively large glenosphere or humeral polyethylene liner, will increase tension on the deltoid and limit elevation as well.[10]

Postoperative Factors

In the absence of infection, component malposition, and certain preoperative factors predisposing to postoperative limitation of motion, inadequate rehabilitation is the most important postoperative factor accounting for stiffness following shoulder arthroplasty.[35] Patient motivation and commitment are key to achieve the desired range of motion and strength postoperatively, preferably with a surgeon-directed home-based program that may be supplemented by traditional physical therapy supervised by a therapist knowledgeable in shoulder

rehabilitation. Heterotopic ossification has been reported as a cause of shoulder stiffness following both anatomic and reverse TSA, more commonly when shoulder replacement is performed for the treatment of proximal humerus fractures or fracture sequelae.[10] However, in the senior author's (PDM) experience, heterotopic ossification is an extremely uncommon cause of stiffness following shoulder arthroplasty for nonfracture cases. Finally, delayed onset of shoulder stiffness and pain without a traumatic history, following a period of having achieved satisfactory range of motion postoperatively, is a sign of a postoperative periprosthetic joint infection until proven otherwise. The diagnosis and treatment of infection following shoulder arthroplasty are discussed in Chapter 32.

TREATMENT OF SHOULDER STIFFNESS

The treatment of shoulder stiffness following both ATSA and RTSA is based on etiology and may be considered in three broad categories:

1. periprosthetic joint infection
2. component malposition (height, version, size)
3. soft tissue adhesions and contractures; no infection, no component malposition

Management of infection is reviewed in Chapter 32, and component malposition as a cause of shoulder stiffness managed by revision surgery is discussed in Chapters 41 to 44.

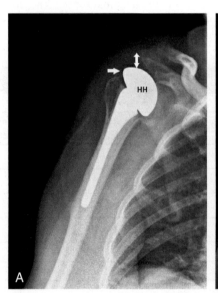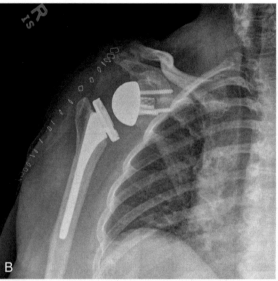

FIGURE 36.1 A, Radiograph of a 72-year-old patient who presented at 16 months following hemiarthroplasty of the right shoulder for osteoarthritis. She had severe pain, limited range of motion, and weakness unresponsive to over 12 months of physical therapy. Passive forward elevation 90°, active elevation 45°, passive external rotation 60°, active 30°. She had never achieved satisfactory range of motion following surgery, and evaluation for periprosthetic joint infection was negative. Cause of failure was implant malposition with an oversized humeral component (HH) placed superiorly (single arrow) accounting for stiffness and rotator cuff insufficiency as evidenced by weakness and a high riding humerus (double arrow). **B,** Radiograph of revision of case in **A** to a reverse total shoulder arthroplasty demonstrating the value of a platform system. The extended central peg of the glenoid baseplate was placed into the central hole of the anatomic glenoid component in an appropriate position thereby preserving glenoid bone stock. Conversion of the humeral component was easily achieved by simple exchange of the anatomic head with a reverse component, obviating the need to remove a well-fixed cemented humeral stem.

The mainstay of managing stiffness following arthroplasty with well-positioned components and no evidence of infection is a comprehensive rehabilitation program. In rare circumstances, arthroscopic lysis of adhesions and capsular release may be considered. It is worth repeating that the best treatment of stiffness following shoulder arthroplasty is prevention. Preoperative education should include not only the importance of postoperative rehabilitation but also the fact that, although the majority of improvement in function following shoulder arthroplasty will be achieved by 6 months postoperatively, improvement in motion and strength will continue for as long as 24 months following surgery.[35,36] Patients frustrated by limited range of motion during the early and midterm recovery less than 6 months following surgery should be encouraged to stay with the program.

Managing patient expectations preoperatively is equally important. As previously mentioned, patients with pain and severe limitation of motion preoperatively should be advised that relief of pain following shoulder arthroplasty is predictable and achieved consistently in the vast majority of cases but that dramatic improvement in range of motion is less predictable and inferior to the motion achieved by patients without severe preoperative restriction of motion.[2,27]

A surgeon-directed home exercise program should be the fundamental basis of postoperative rehabilitation and is the most effective way to both prevent and treat stiffness following shoulder arthroplasty.[14,35] The program should be reviewed with the patient as part of presurgical education, and handouts illustrating the various exercises are a helpful resource for patients performing the exercises at home (**FIGURE 36.2**). This program emphasizes active-assisted stretching exercises performed independently by the patient briefly (1-2 minutes per session) and frequently (3-5 sessions daily) at home. Patients should be instructed to range the shoulder to the limit of motion and then to push additional motion another inch and hold the stretch for 5 seconds. It is appropriate to experience soreness during the stretch, but the maneuver should not be so aggressive as to lead to pain that persists for more than 2 minutes after the stretching session. Overly aggressive stretching causing pain may further injure healing soft tissues, increase swelling, and limit range of motion.[37] Nonnarcotic medications and icing may be recommended to address soreness following the exercises, but opioids must be avoided. The common concept of "no pain, no gain" is discouraged. This home-based program for stretching should be continued for up to 9 to 12 months following surgery since late gains in range of motion can be achieved. However, as previously mentioned, the majority of motion is typically regained by 6 months postoperatively. Supplementation of this home exercise program with a formal program supervised by a physical therapist experienced in shoulder therapy is helpful for many

patients but should be considered as a complement, not a substitute, for a home-based program.

Arthroscopic releases for stiffness may be considered following shoulder arthroplasty in shoulders with no evidence of infection and with well-positioned components refractory to a rehabilitation program for 1 year following shoulder arthroplasty. However, there is no consensus on specific indications for arthroscopy in the painful and stiff shoulder following ATSA, and the procedure is infrequently reported.[38-40] Vezeridis and coworkers considered 50% loss of external rotation compared with the opposite shoulder, refractory to physical therapy for a minimum of 4 months as an indication for arthroscopic release.[41] Thorsness and Romeo recommended arthroscopic release following ATSA for patients with well-positioned components, no signs of infection, and less than 90° forward elevation and less than 20° external rotation unresponsive to physical therapy.[15]

Hersch and Dines reported on 13 shoulder arthroscopies performed on patients with painful and stiff arthroplasties in whom infection and malaligned components had been ruled out at an average 33 months following the index arthroplasty. Multiple procedures were performed including mini-open rotator cuff repair, distal clavicle excision, subacromial decompression, capsular releases, and biceps tenotomy. Average preoperative forward elevation was 76°, and at an average of 22 months' follow-up, forward elevation improved to 126° as did functional outcome scores. The authors concluded that arthroscopy of the shoulder for patients with painful arthroplasty should be considered in select patients as an alternative to revision arthroplasty.[42]

Doherty et al reported on 14 patients who underwent shoulder arthroscopy at an average 65 months' following the index arthroplasty for stiff and painful shoulders with normal implant alignment, normal C-reactive protein and white blood cell counts, and no clinical evidence of infection. The primary indication for arthroscopy was to obtain biopsy for culture, given the low accuracy of shoulder aspiration to diagnose periprosthetic joint infection. Preoperative range of motion was not described, and only 2 of the 12 shoulders underwent capsular release. Three shoulder biopsies (21%) were positive, all for *Cutibacterium acnes*. The authors concluded that diagnostic arthroscopy was a helpful adjunct in managing these select patients, especially the ability to obtain biopsies for culture to rule out occult infection.[43]

Tytherleigh-Strong et al reported on 29 patients who underwent arthroscopy for a painful and stiff shoulder at an average of 38 months following shoulder arthroplasty. All components were well aligned, and one patient had a known acute infection that was treated successfully with an arthroscopic washout and intravenous antibiotics for 6 weeks. Multiple procedures were performed including subacromial decompression,

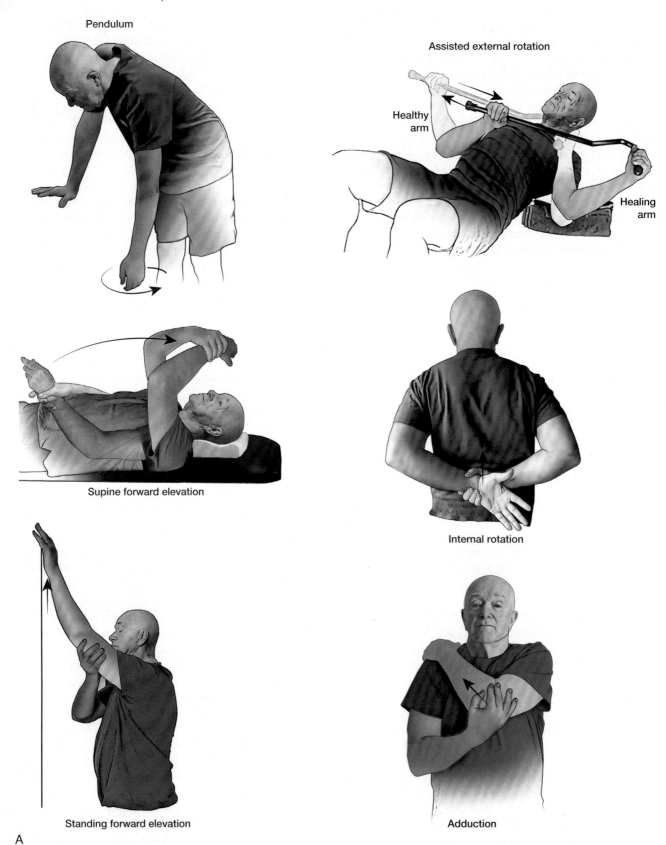

Pendulum

Assisted external rotation

Healthy arm

Healing arm

Supine forward elevation

Internal rotation

Standing forward elevation

Adduction

A

FIGURE 36.2 Simple home exercise instructions for patients demonstrating active assisted stretching **(A)** and strengthening exercises **(B)** as recommended by Neer.

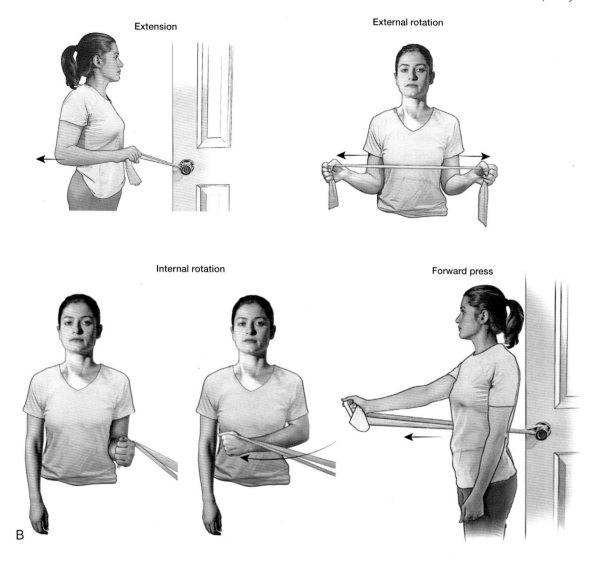

Extension

External rotation

Internal rotation

Forward press

B

FIGURE 36.2 cont'd

removal of a loose body, and capsular release, and at an average of 13 months following arthroscopy, the average Constant-Murley score improved significantly from a preoperative score of 23 to 63 postoperatively. The authors concluded that arthroscopy of the "problem shoulder arthroplasty," ie, the stiff and painful shoulder without a diagnosis following a standard investigation to rule out infection and component malalignment, is beneficial in selected patients with subacromial impingement or capsular fibrosis.[44]

These studies suggest that, in the rare patient with severe stiffness (forward elevation <90° and external rotation <20°) following ATSA that compromises activities of daily living and has not improved following a 12-month rehabilitation program, with no evidence of infection or malaligned components, arthroscopic lysis of adhesions and capsular release may be considered.

The principles of arthroscopic release of the stiff ASTA are the same as those guiding releases in the nonarthroplasty shoulder: capsular release and resection of all interarticular

adhesions, bursectomy, and extensive release of scar and adhesions in the subacromial space and lateral gutter. However, several unique aspects of arthroscopic release of the stiff ASTA warrant special mention **(VIDEO 36.1)**.

The posterior capsule is often quite thickened in the stiff arthroplasty shoulder, thereby obliterating the usual "soft spot" commonly palpable as a landmark for the routine posterior portal. Careful but firm pressure, using a blunt trocar, should be used to enter the glenohumeral joint in an effort to avoid damage to the glenoid and humeral components. Once intra-articular, the reflection of the humeral head distorts the anatomy, disorienting the surgeon who may be unable to distinguish the real from the mirror images of tissues and instruments **(FIGURE 36.3)**.

Thickened and contracted anterior capsule and rotator interval tissue may preclude the usual percutaneous method of establishing the anterior portal and necessitate an inside-out technique using a switching stick from the posterior portal. Once the anterior portal is established, an electrocautery device is used to sequentially divide the rotator interval scar and superior capsule with care not to violate the more superficial subscapularis tendon. As the tight anterosuperior tissue is divided, gentle external rotation and abduction of the shoulder will improve access to release the inferior capsule. If present, the biceps tendon should be divided, and the intra-articular portion resected. Even if suspicion for infection is low, multiple biopsies should be obtained for culture. The arthroscope is then transferred to the anterior portal, and release of the posterior contracted tissue is performed using electrocautery via the posterior portal.

The arthroscope is then introduced into the subacromial space through the posterior portal, and adhesions in the subacromial and, especially, the lateral and anterior subdeltoid gutters, are lysed with electrocautery via a lateral portal. If there is a prominent anterior acromion impinging on the underlying rotator cuff tendons, an anterior acromioplasty can be considered, but in the senior author's experience, this is rarely required. Finally, and only following a complete arthroscopic release of all accessible intra- and extra-articular soft tissue contractures, a gentle manipulation of the shoulder can be considered to regain additional terminal range of motion. Only minimal force should be used to minimize the risk of humeral shaft or tuberosity fracture.

Shoulder stiffness following RTSA is much less common than that following ATSA. However, similar principles mentioned above for ATSA apply. Patients with stiffness prior to RTSA (fracture sequelae, failed ORIF, failed arthroplasty) have a greater risk of postoperative stiffness. Rehabilitation exercises remain the mainstay of treatment of stiffness following RTSA as for ATSA.

Most improvement in range of motion is achieved within 6 months of the index arthroplasty but may continue for up to 2 years following surgery.[36]

Arthroscopic release for stiffness following RTSA is rare, and, as such, the indications have not been well delineated. Only 2 of the 14 cases reported by Doherty et al were performed in patients with RTSA.[43] From the senior author's perspective, the indications should be similar to those described for stiffness following ATSA. However, the significant preoperative rotator cuff compromise that is often present in patients undergoing RTSA presents a confounding variable that must be considered in the evaluation of postoperative stiffness. Technically, arthroscopy of the RTSA shoulder is less disorienting than that following ATSA since, in the absence of the superior rotator cuff, the glenohumeral joint and subacromial space are continuous, thereby widening the field of view (**FIGURE 36.4; VIDEO 36.2**).

In patients with RTSA who have been unable to regain active range of motion after 1 year of a proper exercise program further assessment may be needed. Limited active range of motion in the presence of much better passive range of motion is not an indication for arthroscopic releases. There must be the combination of limited active and passive range of motion for arthroscopic release to be considered. It is also important to recognize that as of this writing the limited experience with arthroscopic release for stiffness following RTSA makes this somewhat "uncharted territory." An

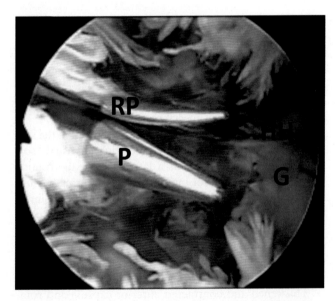

FIGURE 36.3 Posterior arthroscopic view of a right ATSA in the lateral decubitus position. A blunt probe (P) is placed in the anterior portal and its reflection (RP) mirrored on the humeral head (HH). There is marked synovitis within the joint, and the glenoid component (G) seen in the inferior aspect of the field. ATSA, anatomic total shoulder arthroplasty.

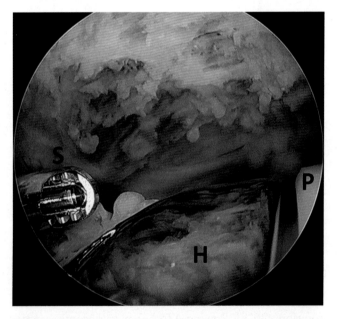

FIGURE 36.4 Posterior arthroscopic view of a left RTSA in the beach chair position. A shaver (S) is placed in the lateral portal and reflected on the proximal aspect of the humeral component (H). The polyethylene insert (P) is seen to the right of the field. Arthroscopic view of an RTSA is less disorienting than that of an ATSA owing to the fact that, in the absence of the superior rotator cuff, the glenohumeral joint is continuous with the subacromial space thereby widening the field of view. ATSA, anatomic total shoulder arthroplasty; RTSA, reverse total shoulder arthroplasty.

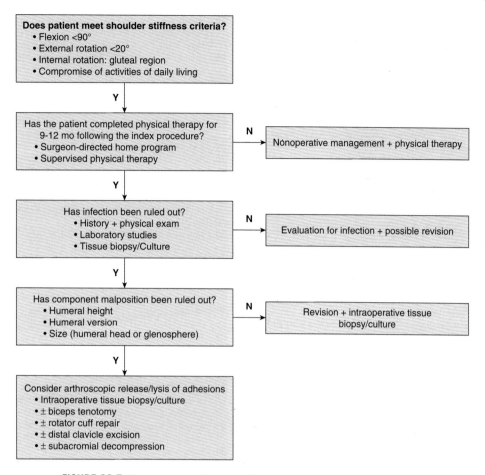

FIGURE 36.5 Treatment algorithm for stiffness following shoulder arthroplasty.

algorithmic approach to shoulder stiffness following arthroplasty is summarized in **FIGURE 36.5**.

CONCLUSION

Stiffness following total shoulder arthroplasty is infrequently cited in the literature as an isolated surgical complication. However, in reports of patient-reported outcomes, shoulder stiffness was the most common cause of patient dissatisfaction. Limited range of motion of the shoulder is often associated with other more commonly recognized complications of both anatomic and reverse shoulder arthroplasty, further complicating the role of stiffness alone as a unique complication.

A definition of stiffness of the shoulder following arthroplasty that may be considered as an isolated complication has been proposed: passive forward elevation <90°, external rotation <20°, and internal rotation limited to the gluteal region, sufficient to compromise the basic activities of daily living. Appreciation of this definition as well as an understanding of the etiology of stiffness will help guide appropriate management.

The majority of stiff shoulders following arthroplasty is successfully managed with rehabilitation exercises, preferably a surgeon-directed home program supplemented by supervised physical therapy, for 9 to 12 months following the index procedure. Arthroscopic release for those selected patients who have failed a comprehensive rehabilitation program, in the absence of infection or component malalignment, is beneficial. Revision arthroplasty is reserved for those stiff shoulders caused by infection or malpositioned components. An understanding of all the factors predisposing the shoulder to severe limitation of motion following surgery, and addressing these factors preoperatively, intraoperatively, and postoperatively will help minimize shoulder stiffness after arthroplasty.

REFERENCES

1. Aldinger PR, Raiss P, Rickert M, Loew M. Complications in shoulder arthroplasty: an analysis of 485 cases. *Int Orthop.* 2010;34(4):517-524. doi:10.1007/s00264-009-0780-7
2. Bacle G, Nove-Josserand L, Garaud P, Walch G. Long-term outcomes of reverse total shoulder arthroplasty: a follow-up of a previous study. *J Bone Joint Surg Am.* 2017;99(6):454-461. doi:10.2106/JBJS.16.00223
3. Franta AK, Lenters TR, Mounce D, Neradilek B, Matsen FA. The complex characteristics of 282 unsatisfactory shoulder arthroplasties. *J Shoulder Elbow Surg.* 2007;16(5):555-562. doi:S1058-2746(07)00215-7
4. Gauci MO, Cavalier M, Gonzalez JF, et al. Revision of failed shoulder arthroplasty: epidemiology, etiology, and surgical options. *J Shoulder Elbow Surg.* 2020;29(3):541-549. doi:S1058-2746(19)30531-2

5. Hasan SS, Leith JM, Campbell B, Kapil R, Smith KL, Matsen FA. Characteristics of unsatisfactory shoulder arthroplasties. *J Shoulder Elbow Surg.* 2002;11(5):431-441. doi:S1058274602000599

6. Luedke C, Kissenberth MJ, Tolan SJ, Hawkins RJ, Tokish JM. Outcomes of anatomic total shoulder arthroplasty with B2 glenoids: a systematic review. *JBJS Rev.* 2018;6(4):e7. doi:10.2106/JBJS.RVW.17.00112

7. Neyton L, Kirsch JM, Collotte P, et al. Mid- to long-term follow-up of shoulder arthroplasty for primary glenohumeral osteoarthritis in patients aged 60 or under. *J Shoulder Elbow Surg.* 2019;28(9):1666-1673. doi:S1058-2746(19)30182-X

8. Saltzman BM, Chalmers PN, Gupta AK, Romeo AA, Nicholson GP. Complication rates comparing primary with revision reverse total shoulder arthroplasty. *J Shoulder Elbow Surg.* 2014;23(11):1647-1654. doi:10.1016/j.jse.2014.04.015

9. Simovitch R, Flurin PH, Wright TW, Zuckerman JD, Roche C. Impact of scapular notching on reverse total shoulder arthroplasty midterm outcomes: 5-year minimum follow-up. *J Shoulder Elbow Surg.* 2019;28(12):2301-2307. doi:S1058-2746(19)30292-7

10. Wiater BP, Moravek JE, Wiater JM. The evaluation of the failed shoulder arthroplasty. *J Shoulder Elbow Surg.* 2014;23(5):745-758. doi:10.1016/j.jse.2013.12.003

11. Wierks C, Skolasky RL, Ji JH, McFarland EG. Reverse total shoulder replacement: intraoperative and early postoperative complications. *Clin Orthop Relat Res.* 2009;467(1):225-234. doi:10.1007/s11999-008-0406-1

12. Bohsali KI, Bois AJ, Wirth MA. Complications of shoulder arthroplasty. *J Bone Joint Surg Am.* 2017;99(3):256-269. doi:10.2106/JBJS.16.00935

13. Namdari S, Yagnik G, Ebaugh DD, et al. Defining functional shoulder range of motion for activities of daily living. *J Shoulder Elbow Surg.* 2012;21(9):1177-1183. doi:10.1016/j.jse.2011.07.032

14. Neer CS, Kirby RM. Revision of humeral head and total shoulder arthroplasties. *Clin Orthop Relat Res.* 1982;170(170):189-195.

15. Thorsness RJ, Romeo AA. Stiffness following shoulder arthroplasty: to manipulate or not. *Semin Arthroplasty: JSES.* 2016;27(2):104-107. doi:10.1053/j.sart.2016.08.006

16. Petkovic D, Kovacevic D, Levine WN, Jobin CM. Management of the failed arthroplasty for proximal humerus fracture. *J Am Acad Orthop Surg.* 2019;27(2):39-49. doi:10.5435/JAAOS-D-17-00051

17. Carofino B, Routman H, Roche C. The influence of pre-operative external rotation weakness or stiffness on reverse total shoulder arthroplasty outcomes. *JSES Open Access.* 2020;4:382-387.

18. Abboud JA, Anakwenze OA, Hsu JE. Soft-tissue management in revision total shoulder arthroplasty. *J Am Acad Orthop Surg.* 2013;21(1):23-31. doi:10.5435/JAAOS-21-01-23

19. Raiss P, Edwards TB, Collin P, et al. Reverse shoulder arthroplasty for malunions of the proximal part of the humerus (type-4 fracture sequelae). *J Bone Joint Surg Am.* 2016;98(11):893-899. doi:10.2106/JBJS.15.00506

20. Crosby LA, Wright TW, Yu S, Zuckerman JD. Conversion to reverse total shoulder arthroplasty with and without humeral stem retention: the role of a convertible-platform stem. *J Bone Joint Surg Am.* 2017;99(9):736-742. doi:10.2106/JBJS.16.00683

21. Friedman RJ, Eichinger J, Schoch B, et al. Preoperative parameters that predict postoperative patient-reported outcome measures and range of motion with anatomic and reverse total shoulder arthroplasty. *JSES Open Access.* 2019;3(4):266-272. doi:10.1016/j.jses.2019.09.010

22. Jobin CM, Galdi B, Anakwenze OA, Ahmad CS, Levine WN. Reverse shoulder arthroplasty for the management of proximal humerus fractures. *J Am Acad Orthop Surg.* 2015;23(3):190-201. doi:10.5435/JAAOS-D-13-00190

23. Lindbloom BJ, Christmas KN, Downes K, et al. Is there a relationship between preoperative diagnosis and clinical outcomes in reverse shoulder arthroplasty? An experience in 699 shoulders. *J Shoulder Elbow Surg.* 2019;28(6S):S110-S117. doi:S1058-2746(19)30257-5

24. Raiss P, Alami G, Bruckner T, et al. Reverse shoulder arthroplasty for type 1 sequelae of a fracture of the proximal humerus. *Bone Joint J.* 2018;100-B(3):318-323. doi:10.1302/0301-620X.100B3.BJJ-2017-0947.R1

25. Sajadi KR, Kwon YW, Zuckerman JD. Revision shoulder arthroplasty: an analysis of indications and outcomes. *J Shoulder Elbow Surg.* 2010;19(2):308-313. doi:10.1016/j.jse.2009.05.016

26. Shields E, Wiater JM. Patient outcomes after revision of anatomic total shoulder arthroplasty to reverse shoulder arthroplasty for rotator cuff failure or component loosening: a matched cohort study. *J Am Acad Orthop Surg.* 2019;27(4):e193-e198. doi:10.5435/JAAOS-D-17-00350

27. Chalmers PN, Boileau P, Romeo AA, Tashjian RZ. Revision reverse shoulder arthroplasty. *J Am Acad Orthop Surg.* 2019;27(12):426-436. doi:10.5435/JAAOS-D-17-00535

28. Boileau P. Complications and revision of reverse total shoulder arthroplasty. *Orthop Traumatol Surg Res.* 2016;102(1 suppl):S33-S43. doi:10.1016/j.otsr.2015.06.031

29. Hamilton MA, Diep P, Roche C, et al. Effect of reverse shoulder design philosophy on muscle moment arms. *J Orthop Res.* 2015;33(4):605-613. doi:10.1002/jor.22803

30. Kim MS, Jeong HY, Kim JD, Ro KH, Rhee SM, Rhee YG. Difficulty in performing activities of daily living associated with internal rotation after reverse total shoulder arthroplasty. *J Shoulder Elbow Surg.* 2020;29(1):86-94. doi:S1058-2746(19)30394-5

31. Kontaxis A, Chen X, Berhouet J, et al. Humeral version in reverse shoulder arthroplasty affects impingement in activities of daily living. *J Shoulder Elbow Surg.* 2017;26(6):1073-1082. doi:S1058-2746(16)30625-5

32. Werner BS, Chaoui J, Walch G. The influence of humeral neck shaft angle and glenoid lateralization on range of motion in reverse shoulder arthroplasty. *J Shoulder Elbow Surg.* 2017;26(10):1726-1731. doi:S1058-2746(17)30212-4

33. Wright MA, Keener JD, Chamberlain AM. Comparison of clinical outcomes after anatomic total shoulder arthroplasty and reverse shoulder arthroplasty in patients 70 years and older with glenohumeral osteoarthritis and an intact rotator cuff. *J Am Acad Orthop Surg.* 2020;28(5):e222-e229. doi:10.5435/JAAOS-D-19-00166

34. Friedman RJ, Flurin PH, Wright TW, Zuckerman JD, Roche CP. Comparison of reverse total shoulder arthroplasty outcomes with and without subscapularis repair. *J Shoulder Elbow Surg.* 2017;26(4):662-668. doi:S1058-2746(16)30448-7

35. Neer CS. *Shoulder Reconstruction.* 1st ed. WB Saunders; 1990:487-535.

36. Simovitch RW, Friedman RJ, Cheung EV, et al. Rate of improvement in clinical outcomes with anatomic and reverse total shoulder arthroplasty. *J Bone Joint Surg Am.* 2017;99(21):1801-1811. doi:10.2106/JBJS.16.01387

37. Tauro JC, Paulson M. Shoulder stiffness. *Arthroscopy.* 2008;24(8):949-955. doi:10.1016/j.arthro.2008.03.014

38. Itoi E, Arce G, Bain GI, et al. Shoulder stiffness: current concepts and concerns. *Arthroscopy.* 2016;32(7):1402-1414. doi:10.1016/j.arthro.2016.03.024

39. Elhassan B, Ozbaydar M, Massimini D, Higgins L, Warner JJ. Arthroscopic capsular release for refractory shoulder stiffness: a critical analysis of effectiveness in specific etiologies. *J Shoulder Elbow Surg.* 2010;19(4):580-587. doi:10.1016/j.jse.2009.08.004

40. Parker DB, Smith AC, Flekenstein CM, Hasan SS. Arthroscopic Evaluation and treatment of complications that arise following prosthetic shoulder Arthroplasty. *JBJS Rev.* 2020;8(8):e20.00020-e20.00028. doi:10.2106/JBJS.RVW.20.00020

41. Vezeridis PS, Goel DP, Shah AA, Sung SY, Warner JJ. Postarthroscopic arthrofibrosis of the shoulder. *Sports Med Arthrosc Rev.* 2010;18(3):198-206. doi:10.1097/JSA.0b013e3181ec84a5

42. Hersch JC, Dines DM. Arthroscopy for failed shoulder arthroplasty. *Arthroscopy.* 2000;16(6):606-612. doi:S0749-8063(00)83174-6

43. Doherty C, Furness ND, Batten T, White WJ, Kitson J, Smith CD. Arthroscopy of the symptomatic shoulder arthroplasty. *J Shoulder Elbow Surg.* 2019;28(10):1971-1976. doi:S1058-2746(19)30173-9

44. Tytherleigh-Strong GM, Levy O, Sforza G, Copeland SA. The role of arthroscopy for the problem shoulder arthroplasty. *J Shoulder Elbow Surg.* 2002;11(3):230-234. doi:10.1067/mse.2002.122257

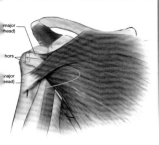
Rotator Cuff Failure:
Early and Late

Ian R. Byram, MD and Joseph T. Labrum IV, MD

INTRODUCTION

Anatomic total shoulder arthroplasty (ATSA) has proven to be effective in alleviating pain and restoring function in the setting of severe glenohumeral osteoarthritis. Although this procedure provides reliable, positive outcomes for most patients, complications can be encountered in the early and late postoperative course. The most common complication of ATSA is rotator cuff dysfunction.[1,2] The dynamic stability provided to the shoulder by the rotator cuff is pivotal for proper function of the native glenohumeral joint, and its importance is magnified in the reconstructed shoulder after removal of osteophytes and capsular releases. Unlike reverse total shoulder arthroplasty, ATSA recreates the native unconstrained glenohumeral joint and requires a functional rotator cuff for stability. Rotator cuff pathology in the setting of total shoulder arthroplasty can lead to increased pain, instability, arthroplasty component loosening or failure, need for revision surgery, and poor clinical outcomes. This chapter reviews the epidemiology, etiology, prevention, diagnosis, and management of rotator cuff failure in the setting of ATSA.

EPIDEMIOLOGY AND ETIOLOGY

Rotator cuff failure is a recognized complication following ATSA. It can present in both the early postoperative period as well as long after successful ATSA. Rotator cuff pathology can arise as a result of multiple biologic and biomechanical processes, with the majority of cases representing degenerative rotator cuff failure, traumatic rotator cuff injury, infectious etiology, and technique-related implant and soft tissue complications.

Frequency

Rotator cuff failure represents the most common complication following ATSA. Young et al observed rotator cuff dysfunction to be the most common complication in their cohort of 518 ATSAs, reporting an incidence of 16.8% at an average follow-up of 8.6 years. In addition, they found that the incidence of rotator cuff dysfunction following total shoulder arthroplasty increased with increasing postoperative follow-up.[1] They estimated total shoulder arthroplasty (TSA) survivorship free of secondary rotator cuff dysfunction to be 100% at 5-year follow-up, 84% at 10-year follow-up, and 45% at 15-year follow-up.[1] Chin et al similarly observed rotator cuff failure to be the most common complication following ATSA.[2] They observed a total of 53 complications in a cohort of 421 ATSAs at an average follow-up of 4.2 years, with 32% (17/53) of complications resulting from rotator cuff tears.[2] Chin et al noted only four cases of acute rotator cuff failure within the 90-day postoperative period, all of which were due to subscapularis repair failure.[2] Deshmukh et al carried out a retrospective review of 320 consecutive ATSAs and observed instability and secondary traumatic rotator cuff injury in approximately 1% of cases.[3]

Biomechanical and Biologic Etiology

Degenerative

The most common etiology of rotator cuff insufficiency following ATSA is degenerative rotator cuff dysfunction. As degenerative rotator cuff disease progresses, the dynamic stability provided to the prosthetic glenohumeral articulation is compromised. This lack of stability results in altered joint reactive forces, thereby subjecting the glenoid and humeral components to abnormal stresses and loads. Mechanically, this results in humeral component translation and eccentric loading of the glenoid component, leading to the "rocking horse phenomenon."[1,4] Secondary rotator cuff dysfunction is a chronic process encountered in long-term ATSA follow-up. In a review of 596 cases, Young et al noted that secondary rotator cuff dysfunction occurred only after the 5-year follow-up interval.[1] Preoperative magnetic resonance imaging (MRI) finding of fatty infiltration of the infraspinatus has been noted to be a statistically significant predictor for development of secondary rotator cuff dysfunction following ATSA.[1] Fatty degeneration of the rotator cuff has been associated with poor clinical outcomes following ATSA.[5]

Traumatic

Traumatic rotator cuff failure can occur following injury to the shoulder that results in a sudden contracture of the rotator cuff. This complication can present with or without concurrent glenohumeral dislocation and can occur at any point postoperatively. However, the subscapularis is most vulnerable to failure in the acute postoperative period following ATSA, because of the time required for healing of the subscapularis tenotomy (SST), lesser tuberosity osteotomy (LTO), or subscapularis tendon reattachment. Subscapularis failure commonly takes place following a sudden active internal rotation moment or forced external rotation moment in the setting of an incompletely healed subscapularis. Similar to degenerative rotator cuff pathology, traumatic rotator cuff insufficiency results in uncoupling of the balanced rotator cuff forces that function to stabilize the glenohumeral articulation, resulting in ATSA instability.

Infection-Related Rotator Cuff Failure

Periprosthetic joint infection (PJI) in the setting of ATSA is an uncommon yet devastating complication. Total shoulder replacement complicated by PJI can result in chronic inflammation and degeneration of the rotator cuff, resulting in subsequent rotator cuff failure. PJI following total shoulder arthroplasty has an estimated incidence of 0.7% to 4.0%.[4,6] A retrospective review of 2588 primary ATSAs by Singh et al observed the 5-, 10-, and 20-year prosthetic infection–free rates to be 99.3%, 98.5%, and 97.2%, respectively.[7] The authors found that male sex and younger age were significant risk factors for the development of PJI.[7] The prevention, evaluation, diagnosis, and management of PJI following total shoulder replacement, which will be covered extensively in Chapters 32 and 49, can be challenging and should be considered in presentations of rotator cuff dysfunction following TSA.

Technique-Related Rotator Cuff Failure and Prevention in ATSA

Although rotator cuff deficiency following TSA is in many cases unavoidable, there are several iatrogenic, technique-related errors that can also result in this complication. Surgeons should be aware of these potential pitfalls in order to minimize the risk of future rotator cuff failure.

Superior inclination of the glenoid component on immediate postoperative radiographs following ATSA has been noted as a significant risk factor for the development of secondary cuff dysfunction.[1] As such, surgeons should remove all inferior glenoid osteophytes and critically evaluate inclination prior to glenoid reaming and preparation.

Studies evaluating LTO, SST, and subscapularis peel have shown excellent clinical results with all techniques.[8] The literature on the recovery of subscapularis strength following these techniques remains mixed.[8] Lapner et al found no clinical differences at 2-year follow-up in TSA patients randomized to subscapularis peel versus LTO,[9] but others have shown improved subscapularis function and healing rates with ATSA performed using a LTO.[10-12] Scalise et al reported a prospective evaluation of 35 TSAs comparing SST and LTO, noting higher clinical outcome scores, superior subscapularis tendon retear rates, and universal osteotomy healing in the LTO cohort.[10] Similarly, Jandhyala et al noted improved subscapularis function following anatomic TSA with LTO when compared with SST as assessed with the graded belly press test in a consecutive cohort of 36 TSAs.[11] A recent biomechanical analysis by Terrier et al evaluating subscapularis function in the setting of ATSA observed that a dysfunctional subscapularis disrupts the mechanical force coupling of the rotator cuff, resulting in a decrease in infraspinatus force.[13] This imbalance results in a compensatory increase in force on the supraspinatus and middle deltoid, inducing upward migration of the humeral head and eccentric contact and stress patterns across the glenoid component.[13] Subscapularis deficiency can disrupt the mechanical equilibrium of the glenohumeral joint and may play a role in the development of secondary rotator cuff dysfunction. As such, surgeons should utilize meticulous surgical technique regardless of which technique is utilized to maintain proper subscapularis healing and function following ATSA.

Failure to restore native glenoid version during ATSA in cases with excessive pathologic glenoid retroversion (Walch B2 and B3 glenoids) may also play a role in rotator cuff–related failure. Donohue et al observed a significant and direct association between fatty infiltration of the infraspinatus, teres minor, and combined posterior rotator cuff muscles and increasing glenoid retroversion in glenohumeral arthritis.[14] Given these findings, failure to address pathologic glenoid retroversion may further predispose patients to secondary rotator cuff dysfunction following ATSA.

Glenoid and humeral component size mismatch and failure to completely remove humeral neck osteophytes are theorized to contribute to suboptimal ATSA outcome by resulting in improperly tensioned soft tissues and altered joint kinematics, which may lead to secondary rotator cuff dysfunction. "Overstuffing" the joint with a large humeral head may increase stress on the rotator cuff leading to progressive dysfunction.[4,15,16]

Aggressive physical therapy regimens with excessive external rotation exercises have been cited as a source of acute subscapularis failure postoperatively.[4] An intraoperative assessment of the subscapularis repair is necessary to establish postoperative range-of-motion parameters for the rehabilitation program. Surgeons should utilize a standardized physical therapy protocol and clearly communicate the goals of this regimen to their patients and physical therapist colleagues. Postoperative ATSA rehabilitation protocols will be reviewed in depth in Chapter 15.

DIAGNOSIS

Diagnosis of rotator cuff failure following ATSA is challenging and requires a multifaceted approach owing to its variable presentation. In a retrospective review of 18 rotator cuff failures following ATSA, Hattrup et al observed that presentation typically included complaints of continued pain, lack of motion, instability, and weakness but was not uniform in nature.[17] Given this variability, surgeons should be prepared to utilize multiple diagnostic tools to determine the etiology of shoulder complaints in patients following total shoulder arthroplasty. These tools include history, physical examination, radiographs, ultrasonography, MRI, arthrography, and diagnostic arthroscopy.

History and Physical Examination

History and physical examination are the mainstays of rotator cuff evaluation following ATSA. Hattrup et al observed that history and physical examination were sufficient to identify two-thirds of cases of rotator cuff failures, with the remaining one-third of cases requiring additional diagnostic modalities.[17]

Information obtained from a complete history should include onset, location, character, and severity of symptoms as well as exacerbating activities or actions. A thorough past surgical history regarding the affected shoulder should also be obtained. History should also include medical comorbidities, tobacco use, and a review of constitutional symptoms including fevers, chills, and recent illnesses. Rotator cuff failure following ATSA can occur in both the early and late postoperative period. Any history of shoulder trauma accompanied by subsequent shoulder dysfunction should raise concern for acute rotator cuff failure. A history of sudden functional decline, pain, or instability following total shoulder replacement should raise concern for subscapularis failure. In contrast, a history of more gradual weakness, pain, or instability long after successful shoulder replacement surgery should raise concern for secondary rotator cuff dysfunction.

Physical examination is an important tool in assessing total shoulder dysfunction postoperatively. Rotator cuff strength testing should be performed on all patients who present with shoulder pain in the setting of a previous total shoulder replacement. Basic inspection, palpation, range of motion (ROM), and neurovascular assessment should be performed. Rotator cuff strength testing maneuvers can be utilized to assess the integrity of the subscapularis, supraspinatus, infraspinatus, and teres minor. These maneuvers include the empty can test and drop arm test (supraspinatus), external rotation lag sign (supraspinatus, infraspinatus), Hornblower test (teres minor), and lift off test and belly press test (subscapularis).[4] Although these tests are clinically useful, the presence or absence of abnormalities on rotator cuff strength

testing alone can be unreliable. A retrospective review of rotator cuff strength testing following successful ATSA observed that 67.5% of patients had abnormalities on lift off testing and 66.6% of patients had abnormalities on belly press testing.[18] The abdominal compression test is reported to have a sensitivity of 25% and a specificity of 73% in diagnosing subscapularis failure following ATSA when compared with ultrasound evaluation as the gold standard.[19] Armstrong et al observed the positive and negative predictive values of the abdominal compression test to be 13% and 86%, respectively, in the diagnosis of postarthroplasty subscapularis failure.[19] In instances where patient history, physical examination, and radiographs are indicative of rotator cuff failure, further imaging modalities can be deferred. Conversely, in cases with ambiguous physical examination findings and normal radiographs, further work-up is indicated. In these situations, additional imaging modalities should be utilized to determine the origin of shoulder dysfunction.

Laboratory Evaluation

PJI should be included in the differential for every patient who presents with shoulder complaints in the setting of a total shoulder replacement. The presentation of PJI may be atypical given the indolent nature of *Cutibacterium acnes*, the most common causal organism in TSA PJI.[4] Workup should include C-reactive protein, erythrocyte sedimentation rate, and complete blood count with differential on all patients as well as a joint aspiration when indicated. If an aspiration is obtained, it should be assessed for a minimum of 2 weeks.[4] Normal laboratory values unfortunately do not rule out the diagnosis of PJI. The evaluation and management of periprosthetic joint infection in the setting of TSA, covered in depth in Chapter 32, is highly pertinent to the workup of the painful total shoulder replacement with suspected rotator cuff failure.

Diagnostic Imaging

Radiographs

Standard radiographs should be obtained in all patients presenting with ATSA dysfunction,[4] including true anteroposterior (AP) radiographs of the shoulder with the humerus in internal and external rotation in addition to an axillary view.[1,20] Proximal humeral subluxation can be appreciated on the true AP shoulder, or Grashley view, by evaluating the acromiohumeral interval as well as the relative center of the glenoid and humeral components.[1] An acromiohumeral interval of less than 6 mm is considered pathognomonic for rotator cuff pathology.[20,21] Superior migration of the humeral component with respect to the glenoid component, ie, anterosuperior escape, can be categorized according to the classification system developed by Torchia et al.[22] Anterosuperior escape is often the result of failure of the subscapularis and/or supraspinatus, also referred to as a "rotator interval lesion."[4,22] When present in the setting of ATSA, these radiographic findings are highly concerning for secondary rotator cuff failure.

Ultrasonography

Ultrasound imaging is an extremely useful adjunct in the diagnosis of rotator cuff dysfunction following ATSA.[19,23] It is sensitive and specific in the diagnosis of rotator cuff pathology.[23,24] Although this technique is less comprehensive than MRI and arthrography, it does offer a noninvasive, cost-effective, and efficient method of evaluating the rotator cuff in the setting of a painful shoulder arthroplasty.[23] In addition, ultrasound evaluation allows localization of secondary rotator cuff failure and is less susceptible to interfering signal artifact in the setting of prosthetic components than MRI.[23] When clinical suspicion of secondary rotator cuff dysfunction is high and ultrasonography results are equivocal, advanced imaging should be considered.

Magnetic Resonance Imaging

MRI has historically had limited value in the workup of dysfunction following TSA as a result of the substantial metal artifact that obscures radiographic evaluation. Metal artifact reduction sequence (MARS) MRI can optimize radiographic evaluation of the TSA by suppressing this artifact.[25] This imaging modality can provide a more thorough assessment of the size and location of secondary rotator cuff failure as well as degree of tendon retraction when compared with arthrography.[26] MARS MRI has been successfully utilized to diagnose rotator cuff failure following TSA.[25,26]

Computed Tomography Arthrography

Computed tomography (CT) arthrography is also highly sensitive and specific in detecting full-thickness rotator cuff tears. This imaging modality can also elucidate other sources of TSA dysfunction including osteolysis and humeral or glenoid implant loosening or failure, although its accuracy in these applications remains limited.[27] Although arthrography is highly accurate in diagnosing full-thickness rotator cuff tears, it provides limited evaluation of the location of rotator cuff failure and degree of tendon retraction.[26] Both CT arthrography and MRI can shed light on the acuity or chronicity of rotator cuff compromise by evaluating fatty degeneration of the rotator cuff muscles.

Arthroscopic Evaluation

If clinical suspicion for secondary cuff failure or other TSA complications is high and the diagnostic evaluation is inconclusive, diagnostic arthroscopy can be considered.[4,28,29] Hersch et al reported on 13 arthroscopies performed in patients with both early and late

TSA dysfunction of unclear etiology and found it to be a reliable diagnostic tool.[29] Diagnoses included secondary rotator cuff failure, biceps pathology, and capsular contracture.[29] Guild et al performed 13 arthroscopies in 7 ATSAs and 6 reverse TSAs with post-arthroplasty dysfunction and were able to successfully treat 46% (6/13) of their cohort with arthroscopic procedures, avoiding the need for further revision surgery.[28] Arthroscopic evaluation is often a last resort in the evaluation of dysfunction following ATSA, as it is technically demanding, invasive, and a potential cause of novel complications.[29] Despite these drawbacks, it does provide an effective means of evaluating component loosening, rotator cuff integrity, and the presence of infection by synovial biopsy.[28,29]

Arthroscopic Evaluation Case Example

A 70-year-old man with persistent pain and weakness approximately 1 year following ATSA. Radiologic, electromyography, and laboratory workup was nondiagnostic. Arthroscopic evaluation was performed, revealing an intact rotator cuff but loose glenoid component (**VIDEO 37.1**). The glenoid component was removed arthroscopically, and thorough debridement was performed. Despite a negative fluid aspiration, multiple synovial biopsies revealed *C. acnes* infection. This patient was subsequently treated with resection of the humeral implant, placement of antibiotic spacer, and intravenous antibiotics before reimplantation with reverse TSA.

TREATMENT

Nonoperative

Treatment of pain or instability secondary to rotator cuff failure after ATSA remains challenging. To date, the literature on primary rotator cuff repair in the setting of ATSA has shown poor clinical outcomes.[17] As a result, nonoperative management has become the mainstay of treatment for asymptomatic or minimally symptomatic rotator cuff failure following ATSA.[4,17] This commonly includes activity modification, physical therapy, and analgesics. Nonoperative management is typically avoided in cases of acute postoperative rotator cuff failure or posttraumatic rotator cuff failure with pseudoparalysis or instability. When contemplating operative versus nonoperative treatment, surgeons should consider patient age, activity level, rotator cuff viability, chronicity and degree of rotator cuff failure, and, most importantly, severity of shoulder dysfunction in order to determine a unique, patient-based approach.

Rotator Cuff Repair

Rotator cuff repair in the setting of ATSA with secondary rotator cuff failure can be performed, but results are unpredictable at best.[4,17] Hattrup et al experienced a 20% success rate in 20 patients with ATSA complicated by rotator cuff failure. Attempts at repair failed in 14 patients, with the majority requiring further revision surgery.[17] Given the unsatisfactory outcomes that have been reported to date, many surgeons recommend nonoperative management of rotator cuff failure in the setting of ATSA except in cases of acute traumatic tears that result in profound dysfunction or instability.[17] In this clinical situation, rotator cuff repair should be performed as soon as possible in order to minimize tendon retraction and maximize the potential for success.[17] Standard techniques including tissue mobilization, tuberosity preparation, and adequate fixation should be used when performing rotator cuff repair following ATSA.

Reconstruction and Augmentation Procedures

Capsular reconstruction and augmentation of rotator cuff repair can be utilized in the setting of massive cuff tears or chronic tears that may be irreparable with standard techniques. Successful anterior capsular reconstruction using dermal allograft for the treatment of an irreparable subscapularis tear in the setting of ATSA has been reported.[30] Additional experience is needed to determine the role of this intervention in the treatment of rotator cuff failure following ATSA. In our practice, we choose to utilize dynamic tendon transfers to restore anterior stability and internal rotation.

Tendon Transfer for Subscapularis Failure

Tendon transfer can be utilized in cases of ATSA subscapularis failure where direct subscapularis repair is not possible. Options for tendon transfer include both the pectoralis major and latissimus dorsi (LD) tendons.[31,32] These interventions should be considered ATSA salvage procedures.[4] Surgeons should closely evaluate the viability of the rotator cuff as well as the degree of TSA instability resulting from secondary rotator cuff failure. Tendon transfers for subscapularis failure should be avoided in cases with static subluxation of the humeral head.[32]

Pectoralis Major Transfer: Operative Technique

Pectoralis major transfer has been described to augment or replace a deficient subscapularis **(FIGURE 37.1)**.[33-36] Techniques involving transfer of the entire pectoralis insertion,[36] the upper half of the pectoralis,[33,34] and the sternal head of the pectoralis have been employed based on surgeon preference.[35] In all techniques, the pectoralis insertion is identified along the lateral border of the humerus, lateral to the long head of the biceps. The desired portion for transfer is then sharply released and mobilized with traction sutures. Care must be taken to avoid an overly aggressive release, as the lateral pectoral nerve is at risk with releases greater than 8 cm medially.[36] A bone trough is made on the superolateral aspect of the greater tuberosity for attachment of the transferred

tendon. In the technique described by Warner, the sternal head of the pectoralis is transferred deep to the clavicular head to the lesser tuberosity, allowing the clavicular head to serve as a pulley and recreate the more native line of pull of the subscapularis.[35] Attachment may be performed with either sutures through bone tunnels or suture anchors.

Passage of the transferred pectoralis deep to the conjoined tendon is also described in some techniques as this route minimizes the anterior vector and maximizes the inferior vector of the pectoralis on the humeral head by allowing the conjoined tendon to serve as a pulley.[34,36] However, transfer of the tendon behind the conjoined tendon places the musculocutaneous nerve at risk and must be performed with caution after visualizing the nerve. In our practice, we have abandoned transfer under the coracoid owing to the potential risk of injury to the musculocutaneous nerve.

Pectoralis Major Transfer: Outcomes

Resch et al described the technique of transferring the clavicular portion of the pectoralis under the conjoined tendon in 12 patients with subscapularis deficiency, 4 of whom demonstrated instability prior to transfer. With mean follow-up of 28 months, 9 of 12 patients demonstrated good or excellent outcomes with no recurrent instability in any of the 4 patients at final follow-up.[34] Galatz et al also demonstrated satisfactory results in 11 of 14 patients with mean follow-up of 17 months utilizing a transfer of the entire pectoralis behind the conjoined tendon.[36] However, in the setting of anterior glenohumeral subluxation with subscapularis insufficiency following ATSA, pectoralis transfer has not been as successful.[32] Elhassan et al reported improvement in the shoulder subjective score and pain in only one of eight patients undergoing pectoralis transfer following ATSA, demonstrating generally poor outcomes in this setting.[32]

Latissimus Dorsi Transfer: Operative Technique

Owing to the inability of the pectoralis to recreate the vector angle of the subscapularis, the LD transfer has been described as an alternative for treatment of the subscapularis deficient shoulder **(FIGURE 37.2; VIDEO 37.2)**.[31,37,38] Originating posterior to the chest wall, the LD has a vector more similar to the subscapularis than the pectoralis, capable of recreating an inferior and posterior directed force on the humeral head. Its potential in reproducing the function of the subscapularis has been demonstrated in a cadaveric study, both in isolation as well as in conjunction with the teres major (TM). Although the risk of nerve injury is low with isolated transfers of the LD and TM to the lesser tuberosity, axillary and radial nerve compression can occur with a combined transfer to the upper portion of the lesser tuberosity.[37]

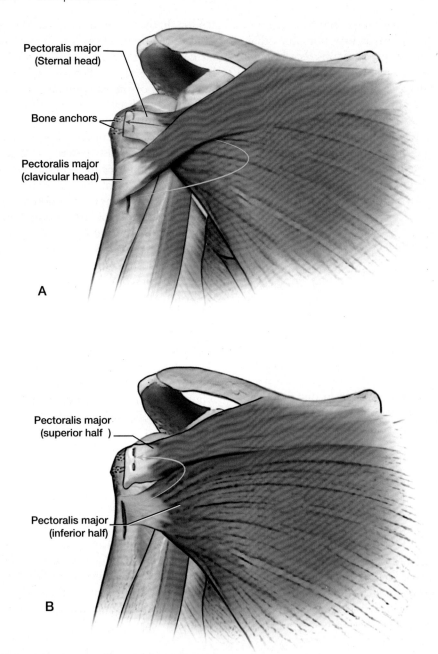

Pectoralis major
(Sternal head)

Bone anchors

Pectoralis major
(clavicular head)

A

Pectoralis major
(superior half)

Pectoralis major
(inferior half)

B

FIGURE 37.1 An illustration depicting a pectoralis major transfer in the treatment of subscapularis deficiency. **A,** Transfer of the sternal head of the pectoralis under the clavicular head for the treatment of subscapularis deficiency.[35] **B,** Transfer of the superior half of the pectoralis tendon for the treatment of subscapularis deficiency.[33]

The LD tendon insertion on the humerus is identified and is sharply released preserving as much of the tendinous insertion as possible. It is then dissected free from the TM insertion located deep and distal to the LD. Traction sutures are placed in the tendon using a locking whipstitch technique, and it is mobilized **(FIGURE 37.3A)**. The lesser tuberosity is then prepared with a rasp and rongeur to create a bleeding surface for healing. Two anchors are utilized on the upper portion of the lesser tuberosity, and sutures are passed in horizontal mattress fashion through the LD tendon and tied **(FIGURE 37.3B)**. The remaining strands of suture are then combined with the initial traction sutures

and loaded into a lateral row knotless anchor placed adjacent to the greater tuberosity to create a double row construct. When substantial tissue exists, sutures can be placed between the upper portion of the transferred LD tendon and the leading edge of the supraspinatus with the arm in 30° external rotation to simulate a rotator interval closure.

Latissimus Dorsi Transfer: Case Example

A 57-year-old woman 7 months following ATSA developed dynamic anterior instability after a motor vehicle accident. CT arthrogram revealed complete rupture of the subscapularis with fatty degeneration of the muscle

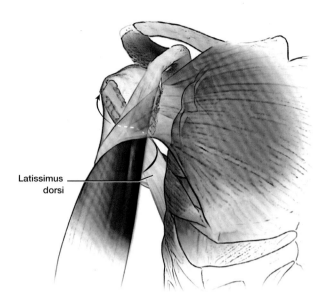

Latissimus
dorsi

FIGURE 37.2 An illustration depicting a latissimus dorsi transfer in the treatment of subscapularis deficiency.

belly. Physical examination revealed limited active forward elevation to 130° and a positive belly press test. We elected to perform latissimus transfer to the lesser tuberosity with the technique described above to restore active internal rotation and stability. At 4-month follow-up, the patient had 160° of forward elevation with improvement in belly press testing.

Latissimus Dorsi Transfer: Outcomes

There is experience reported on the use of LD transfers in patients with subscapularis failure without previous ATSA. Elhassan reported on 56 patients who underwent LD transfer for irreparable subscapularis tears, showing improvements in pain, motion, subjective shoulder score,

and Constant scores at mean follow-up of 13 months. At final follow-up, however, 10 of 38 patients had continued proximal humeral migration.[39] In a series of 24 patients with irreparable subscapularis tears who underwent LD transfer with mean follow-up of 27 months, Mun et al reported improvements in American Shoulder and Elbow Surgeons (ASES), Constant, and visual analog scale scores. Positive belly press test results were reversed in 18/24 (75%) patients at final follow-up.[31] Utilizing an arthroscopic technique for LD transfer in a small case series, Kany et al showed improvement in subjective shoulder score, Constant score, and belly press testing in four of five patients with minimum 12-month follow-up.[38] Although these reports show promising results for LD transfer in the treatment of irreparable subscapularis tear, there are no studies analyzing LD transfer as treatment for subscapularis insufficiency in the setting of ATSA.

Postoperative Management

LD transfer and pectoralis major transfer are managed in a similar fashion postoperatively. The patient is placed in a shoulder abduction brace for 6 weeks. Passive ROM and pendulum exercises are initiated 1 week postoperatively, limiting external rotation to 30° and avoiding active internal rotation and extension. Active-assisted ROM is initiated at 6 weeks postoperative and active ROM at 8 weeks. Gentle strengthening is begun at 3 months with restrictions lifted at 4 months.

Revision to Reverse TSA

In patients with irreparable rotator cuff failure with static subluxation of the humeral head and advanced age, revision of ATSA to reverse TSA can be achieved with satisfactory results. Conversion of ATSA to reverse TSA is covered in depth in Chapters 41 to 44.

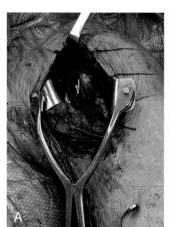
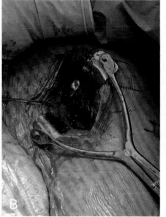
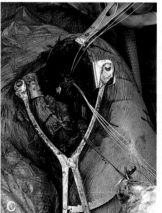
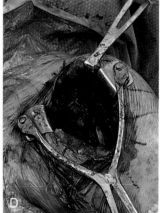

FIGURE 37.3 Intraoperative images of a latissimus dorsi transfer utilized for the treatment of an ATSA complicated by dynamic anterior instability secondary to complete rupture of the subscapularis. **A**, illustrates the exposed humeral head secondary to late subscapularis failure following anatomic TSA. **B**, illustrates mobilization of the latissimus tendon with traction sutures prior to transfer. **C**, depicts suture anchor placement on the lesser tuberosity for transfer of the latissimus tendon. **D**, shows the transferred latissimus dorsi tendon covering the humeral head.

CONCLUSION

Rotator cuff failure following total shoulder arthroplasty remains a significant complication that is commonly encountered by shoulder arthroplasty surgeons. Rotator cuff pathology can present both in the early postoperative period as well as long after successful anatomic TSA. This diagnosis can have negative effects on clinical outcomes and patient satisfaction and requires careful evaluation so that an effective patient-specific treatment plan can be determined using the techniques described.

REFERENCES

1. Young AA, Walch G, Pape G, et al. Secondary rotator cuff dysfunction following total shoulder arthroplasty for primary glenohumeral osteoarthritis: results of a multicenter study with more than five years of follow-up. *J Shoulder Elbow Surg.* 2012;94(8):685-693.
2. Chin PY, Sperling JW, Cofield RH, et al. Complications of total shoulder arthroplasty: are they fewer or different? *J Shoulder Elbow Surg.* 2006;15(1):19-22.
3. Deshmukh AV, Koris M, Zurakowski D, et al. Total shoulder arthroplasty: long-term survivorship, functional outcome, and quality of life. *J Shoulder Elbow Surg.* 2005;14(5):471-479.
4. Eichinger JK, Galvin JW. Management of complications after total shoulder arthroplasty. *Curr Rev Musculoskelet Med.* 2015;8(1):83-91.
5. Edwards TB, Boulahia A, Kempf JF, et al. The influence of rotator cuff disease on the results of shoulder arthroplasty for primary osteoarthritis: results of a multicenter study. *J Bone Joint Surg Am.* 2002;84(12):2240-2248.
6. Coste JS, Reig S, Trojani C, et al. The management of infection in arthroplasty of the shoulder. *J Bone Joint Surg Br.* 2004;86(1):65-69.
7. Singh JA, Sperling JW, Schleck C, et al. Periprosthetic infections after total shoulder arthroplasty: a 33-year perspective. *J Shoulder Elbow Surg.* 2012;21(11):1534-1541.
8. Bornes TD, Rollins MD, Lapner PL, et al. Subscapularis management in total shoulder arthroplasty: current evidence comparing peel, osteotomy, and tenotomy. *J Shoulder Elbow Arthroplasty.* 2018;2:1-10.
9. Lapner PL, Wood KS, Zhang T, et al. The return of subscapularis strength after shoulder arthroplasty. *J Shoulder Elbow Surg.* 2015;24(2):223-228.
10. Scalise JJ, Ciccone J, Iannotti JP. Clinical, radiographic, and ultrasonographic comparison of subscapularis tenotomy and lesser tuberosity osteotomy for total shoulder arthroplasty. *J Bone Joint Surg Am.* 2010;92(7):1627-1634.
11. Jandhyala S, Unnithan A, Hughes S, et al. Subscapularis tenotomy versus lesser tuberosity osteotomy during total shoulder replacement: a comparison of patient outcomes. *J Shoulder Elbow Surg.* 2011;20(7):1102-1107.
12. Levine WN, Munoz J, Hsu S, et al. Subscapularis tenotomy versus lesser tuberosity osteotomy during total shoulder arthroplasty for primary osteoarthritis: a prospective, randomized controlled trial. *J Shoulder Elbow Surg.* 2019;28(3):407-414.
13. Terrier A, Larrea X, Malfroy Camine V, et al. Importance of the subscapularis muscle after total shoulder arthroplasty. *Clin Biomech (Bristol, Avon).* 2013;28(2):146-150.
14. Donohue KW, Ricchetti ET, Ho JC, et al. The association between rotator cuff muscle fatty infiltration and glenoid morphology in glenohumeral arthritis. *J Bone Joint Surg Am.* 2018;100(5):381-387.
15. Ding DY, Mahure SA, Akuoko JA, et al. Total shoulder arthroplasty using a subscapularis-sparing approach: a radiographic analysis. *J Shoulder Elbow Surg.* 2015;24(6):831-837.
16. Schoch B, Abboud J, Namdari S, et al. Glenohumeral mismatch in anatomic total shoulder arthroplasty. *JBJS Rev.* 2017;5(9):e1.
17. Hattrup SJ, Cofield RH, Cha SS. Rotator cuff repair after total shoulder replacement. *J Shoulder Elbow Surg.* 2006;15(1):78-83.
18. Miller SL, Hazrati Y, Klepps S, et al. Loss of subscapularis function after total shoulder arthroplasty: a seldom recognized problem. *J Shoulder Elbow Surg.* 2003;12(1):29-34.
19. Armstrong AD, Southam JD, Horne AH, et al. Subscapularis function after total shoulder arthroplasty: electromyography, ultrasound, and clinical correlation. *J Shoulder Elbow Surg.* 2016;25(10):1674-1680.
20. Merolla G, Di Pietto D, Romano S, et al. Radiographic analysis of shoulder anatomical arthroplasty. *Eur J Radiol.* 2008;68(1):159-169.
21. Gruber G, Bernhardt GA, Clar H, et al. Measurement of the acromiohumeral interval on standardized anteroposterior radiographs: a prospective study of observer variability. *J Shoulder Elbow Surg.* 2010;19(1):10-13.
22. Torchia ME, Cofield RH, Settergren CR. Total shoulder arthroplasty with the Neer prosthesis: long-term results. *J Shoulder Elbow Surg.* 1997;6(6):495-505.
23. Prickett WD, Teefey SA, Galatz LM, et al. Accuracy of ultrasound imaging of the rotator cuff in shoulders that are painful postoperatively. *J Bone Joint Surg Am.* 2003;85(6):1084-1089.
24. Al-Shawi A, Badge R, Bunker T. The detection of full thickness rotator cuff tears using ultrasound. *J Bone Joint Surg Br.* 2008;90(7):889-892.
25. Talbot BS, Weinberg EP. MR imaging with metal-suppression sequences for evaluation of total joint arthroplasty. *Radiographics.* 2016;36(1):209-225.
26. Sperling JW, Potter HG, Craig EV, et al. Magnetic resonance imaging of the painful shoulder arthroplasty. *J Shoulder Elbow Surg.* 2002;11(4):315-321.
27. Mallo GC, Burton L, Coats-Thomas M, et al. Assessment of painful total shoulder arthroplasty using computed tomography arthrography. *J Shoulder Elbow Surg.* 2015;24(10):1507-1511.
28. Guild T, Kuhn G, Rivers M, et al. The role of arthroscopy in painful total shoulder arthroplasty: is revision always necessary? *Arthroscopy.* 2020;36(6):1508-1514.
29. Hersch JC, Dines DM. Arthroscopy for failed shoulder arthroplasty. *Arthroscopy.* 2000;16(6):606-612.
30. Myers D, Triplet JJ, Johnson DB, et al. Anterior capsular reconstruction using dermal allograft for an irreparable subscapularis tear after shoulder arthroplasty: a case report. *JBJS Case Connect.* 2020;10(1):e0468.
31. Mun SW, Kim JY, Yi SH, et al. Latissimus dorsi transfer for irreparable subscapularis tendon tears. *J Shoulder Elbow Surg.* 2018;27(6):1057-1064.
32. Elhassan B, Ozbaydar M, Massimini D, et al. Transfer of pectoralis major for the treatment of irreparable tears of subscapularis: does it work? *J Bone Joint Surg Br.* 2008;90(8):1059-1065.
33. Wirth MA, Rockwood Jr CA. Operative treatment of irreparable rupture of the subscapularis. *J Bone Joint Am.* 1997;79(5):722-731.
34. Resch H, Povacz P, Ritter E, et al. Transfer of the pectoralis major muscle for the treatment of irreparable rupture of the subscapularis tendon. *J Bone Joint Surg Am.* 2000;82(3):372-382.
35. Warner J. Management of massive irreparable rotator cuff tears: the role of tendon transfer. *Instr Course Lect.* 2001;50:63-71.
36. Galatz L, Conner P, Calfee R, et al. Pectoralis major transfer for anterior-superior subluxation in massive rotator cuff tear. *J Shoulder Elbow Surg.* 2003;12(1):1-5.
37. Elhassan B, Christensen TJ, Wagner ER. Feasibility of latissimus and teres major transfer to reconstruct irreparable subscapularis tendon tear: an anatomic study. *J Shoulder Elbow Surg.* 2015;23(4):492-499.
38. Kany J, Guinand R, Croutzet P, et al. Arthroscopic-assisted latissimus dorsi transfer for subscapularis deficiency. *Eur J Orthop Surg Traumatol.* 2016;26(3):329-334.
39. Elhassan B, Wagner E, Kany J. Latissimus dorsi transfer for irreparable subscapularis tear. *JSES Int Open Access.* 2019;3(4):248-249.

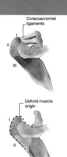

38 Acromion and Scapula Fractures After Reverse Total Shoulder Arthroplasty

Ryan Colley, DO and Jonathan C. Levy, MD

INTRODUCTION

Reverse total shoulder arthroplasty (RTSA) continues to have expanded indications for various shoulder pathology. Although originally RTSA was intended for rotator cuff arthropathy, it is now commonly used for acute fractures, massive irreparable rotator cuff tears without arthritis, severe arthritis with glenoid bone loss, and revision shoulder arthroplasty.[1,2] In fact, RTSA is now being performed on younger patients with greater confidence.[3,4] The increased utilization of RTSA has brought about a greater appreciation of complications and a focused effort to define strategies for prevention and management.[5-12] Postoperative fractures of the acromion and scapula have surfaced as a complication uniquely more common to RTSA than other forms of shoulder arthroplasty.[13] One of the difficulties with these fractures involves the seemingly elusive diagnosis. Although often times they are associated with sudden and dramatic impacts on pain and function, the presentation may be more subtle. Acromion fractures in the setting of RTSA have traditionally been treated without surgery as operative management is unpredictable. In this chapter, we hope to guide the shoulder surgeon to have a better understanding of how to identify and manage acromial and scapula fractures after RTSA.

ANATOMY

Deltoid activity is critical to functional recovery following RTSA. The deltoid muscle has a broad origin across the lateral third of the clavicle, acromion, and scapular spine.[11] It consists of three heads: anterior, middle, and posterior, which function as a shoulder flexor, abductor, and extensor, respectively. Following RTSA, the deltoid has a critical role in restoration of shoulder elevation[14] and likely plays an impactful role in restoration of external rotation especially with increasing lateralization of the humerus.[14-18] With all RTSA systems, the arm is typically lengthened,[7,11,19] which increases the abductor moment arm of the deltoid,[11,20] as the center of rotation of the shoulder is moved medially. The increased abductor moment improves the mechanical advantage of the deltoid to facilitate shoulder function. In addition, the increased

arm length and deltoid tension provide a compression between the components enhancing stability of the semi-constrained RTSA prosthesis.[11,21] When postoperative acromion fractures occur, the length-tension relationship of the deltoid is altered, as the acromion often tilts inferiorly (FIGURE 38.1). This displaces the deltoid origin, which will not only impact strength but also may create impingement between the acromion and greater tuberosity during attempted elevation. In addition, the loss of deltoid tension (and associated compression) has been reported to be associated with prosthetic instability (FIGURE 38.2).[22] With acromion fractures being observed in various areas along the length of the acromion, the impact on function seems to be related to the amount of deltoid origin involved, with more medial fractures demonstrating worse functional outcomes.[19]

CLASSIFICATION

In order to have a better understanding of postoperative acromion fractures following RTSA, two classification systems have been described (FIGURE 38.3). Both of these classification systems are descriptive and based on anatomic location of the fracture. Crosby et al[23] performed a retrospective review of 22 postoperative fractures and developed a system based on location of the fracture relative to the acromioclavicular (AC) joint. Type I fractures were described as small fractures along the anterior acromion, which includes the origin of the coracoacromial ligament. Type II fractures occur posterior to the AC joint. Finally, type III fractures are considered posterior acromion or base of the scapular spine. The hypothesis behind type III fractures involved a stress reaction from the tip of superior metaglene screw. The reproducibility of the Crosby classification has not been evaluated.

Levy et al[19] described postoperative acromion fractures based on the location of the fracture relative to the deltoid origin (see FIGURE 38.3). This classification system was based on the principle that greater amounts of deltoid origin are impacted by more medial acromion fractures, with the greatest involvement of deltoid origin being involved in the base of the acromion fractures. Thus, the more medial the acromion fracture, the

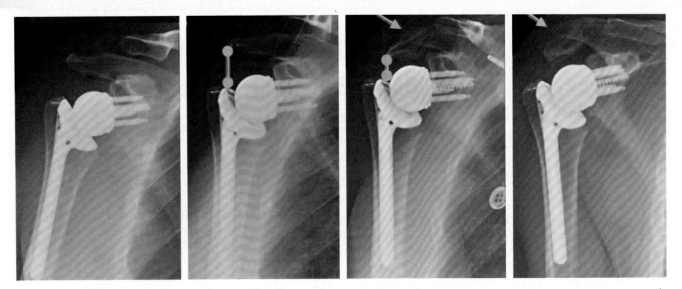

FIGURE 38.1 Postoperative acromion fracture resulting in inferior tilt of acromion. Notice the decreased acromial to greater tuberosity distance. This fracture resulted in pain from impingement and ultimately decreased function.

higher the fracture type; the higher the fracture type, the more the deltoid origin was involved, resulting in worse outcomes. In the study that defined the classification system, a consecutive series of 18 patients with postoperative acromion or scapular spine pain was evaluated. Of the 18 patients, 7 had negative results on radiographs and required a computed tomography (CT) scan for further evaluation. Type I fractures were described as those through the midpart of the acromion involving the acromion origin of the anterior deltoid and a portion of the middle deltoid. Type II fractures involve the entire

origin of the middle deltoid together with the acromion origin of the anterior deltoid. Type III fractures involve the anterior, middle, and posterior deltoid origin. The interobserver reliability and agreement were excellent in this study, helping to validate this classification system.

Despite the availability of two classification systems, many articles simply describe fracture location and determine whether it is related to trauma, stress fatigue, or spontaneous. Mayne et al[24] rationalized that the bony pathology comprises a spectrum for which the earliest presentation is a stress reaction. If the process is able to

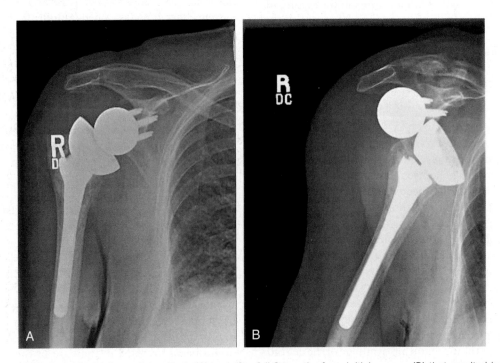

FIGURE 38.2 Anteroposterior radiographs postoperatively (**A**) and after fall 9 months from initial surgery (**B**) that resulted in type III scapular spine fracture and dislocated RTSA. The scapular spine fracture is still visible.

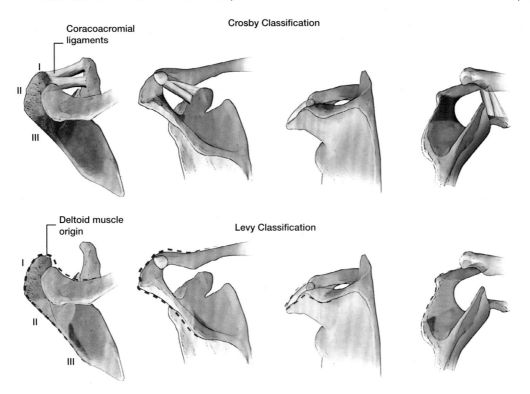

FIGURE 38.3 Acromion fracture classification.

continue, a nondisplaced fracture may occur. Finally, in the worst situation, a complete displaced fracture may result. Clinical results deteriorate based on the location and displacement of the fracture.

ETIOLOGY

Acromion fractures are often seen in patients prior to RTSA. With rotator cuff dysfunction, the superior directed forces created by the unopposed deltoid create stress across the acromion, often creating erosive changes, fractures, and fragmentation of the acromion. Preoperative acromion fractures have been reported in patients treated with RTSA.[25] Among 457 consecutive patients treated with RTSA, Walch et al. reported a 9% incidence (41/457 patients) of preoperative acromion fractures, with 23 patients having an os acromiale, 17 with fragmentation of the acromion, and 1 having a nonunion of the scapular spine. Of interest, the impact on postoperative outcomes was minimal as Constant scores and subjective results were no different from those of patients without acromion pathology. Similar findings were reported by Aibinder et al[26] who reported no impact on postoperative outcomes in patients with preoperative os acromiale. Although postoperative radiographs demonstrated acromion tilt, this did not have an impact on outcome when compared with patients without inferior tilt of the os acromiale. Thus, it is commonly accepted that preoperative acromion

fractures can essentially be ignored and no change in operative planning is necessary when performing RTSA in these patients.

The true etiology of postoperative acromion or scapular spine fractures is not known. A multitude of factors have been implicated as contributing factors including age, osteoporosis, acromion wear, previous acromioplasty, humeral lengthening, glenoid component screw location and trajectory, retractor placement, release of the coracoacromial ligament, acromion length, delta angle, preoperative glenoid inclination, and greater tuberosity impingement. However, to date, few definitive risk factors have been identified. In a case-control study comparing patients with postoperative acromion fractures with controls, Otto et al[27] examined the clinical risk factors in 53 patients with postoperative scapular fractures. The only significant risk factor identified was osteoporosis, which was present in 30.8% of patients with an acromion fracture. Screw position, smoking, body mass index, endocrine disease, chronic steroids, excessive alcohol use, and autoimmune disease were found to be no different between control and fracture cohorts. This observation was subsequently confirmed in a more recent study.[28]

Surgical indication also likely plays a role, especially considering that patients with rotator cuff tear arthropathy often have acromion wear and fragmentation. In a systematic review of the RTSA literature, acromion fractures were reported to be most common after RTSA for inflammatory arthritis (10.9%) and massive rotator cuff tears (3.8%) and lowest for degenerative joint disease (2.7%), posttraumatic arthritis (2.1%), and acute fractures.[29]

Excessive humeral lengthening has been implicated as a potential contributor to acromial stress. Although evidence suggests that lengthening of the humerus is associated with neurologic symptoms following RTSA,[30] it would make sense that excessive lengthening could contribute to postoperative acromion fractures as stress is transmitted to the acromion.[7,9,19,24,27] Humeral lengthening is compounded by inferiorly translating the glenosphere, utilizing humeral components with valgus neck-shaft angles, and adding additional humeral-sided augmentations to the polyethylene insert. Furthermore, in an on-lay design implant when the polyethylene is placed on top of the anatomic neck osteotomy, higher rates of fractures of the base of the acromion spine were reported.[31] In contrast, when the humeral shell was placed within the metaphysis of the proximal humerus (in-lay), the incidence of acromion fractures decreased by more than 50% (11%-4%) when compared with previously published work using an earlier-generation implant system **(FIGURE 38.4)**.[32]

Use of a lateralized center of rotation has been thought to play a role in acromial stress fractures as well. Wong et al[33] were the first to suggest this theory utilizing a fine element analysis (FEA) of 10 RTSA reconstructed cadaveric shoulders with a 38-mm glenosphere and a 155° neck-shaft angle. By varying glenoid inferior translation, lateral offset, and humeral lateralization at a 155° angle, this FEA model suggested that glenosphere lateralization increased stress by 17.2%, whereas humeral lateralization increased stress by only 1.7%. Conversely, humeral medialization decreased stress by 1.4%. The concentration of this stress occurred along the lateral aspect of the acromion in this FEA model. A recent systematic review of 90 articles noted that lateralized glenosphere designs had a significantly higher rate of acromion fractures when compared with medial glenosphere designs.[23]

The position, length, and trajectory of glenoid component screws have also been implicated in contributing to acromion fractures.[23,27,34] Crosby et al[23] initially described three patients with fractures of the base of the scapular spine associated with a superior fixation screw. The concern was that the superior screw functioned as a stress riser. Subsequently, the authors modified their technique in an effort to prevent this complication, completely eliminating the use of screws placed above the glenoid midpoint. In a clinical series of 318 patients, Kennon et al[34] compared the incidence of postoperative acromial and scapular spine fractures among patients treated with and without superior screws. There was a significantly higher rate of base of the acromial fractures among patients with screws placed superior to the glenoid midpoint (4.4%) when compared with patients treated after the modification in surgical technique (0%). This clinical series was supported by a cadaveric mechanical testing model of this surgical technique

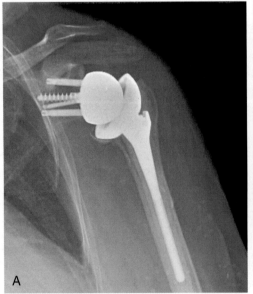 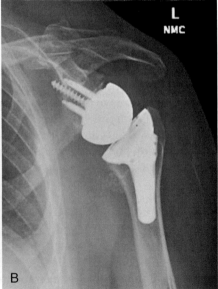

FIGURE 38.4 A, Demonstrating reverse shoulder arthroplasty with a more onlay humeral design with bottom of humeral polyethylene at or above the humeral cut surface. **B,** Inlay humeral design with bottom of the humeral polyethylene below the cut surface.

modification, as superior screw constructs demonstrated a lower load to failure (1077 vs 1970 N). With virtual planning, the trajectory of superior screws used for glenoid component fixation can be better appreciated. Those that are directed toward the base of the scapular spine can be shortened to avoid becoming a potential stress riser. The treating surgeon should be well aware of the screw trajectories and modify the length if necessary. However, there is no consensus on the optimal number, length, or trajectory of screws.

The role of the coracoacromial ligament has been thought to be a soft-tissue stabilizer for the acromion and lessen the stress transmitted to the acromion following RTSA. Taylor et al[16] reported an increase in scapular spine strain following transection of the coracoacromial ligament. Preservation of the coracoacromial ligament during RTSA exposure should thus be considered as a potential method of lowering the stress transmitted to the acromion.

Recently, Schenk et al[28] investigated multiple preoperative and postoperative factors associated with acromion fractures. Specifically, they focused on the delta angle. The delta angle is defined by a line connecting the superior and the inferior border of the glenoid fossa and a second line from the lateral acromial border through the center of rotation of the glenohumeral joint measured on anteroposterior radiographs. The preoperative angle is called delta 1, and the postoperative angle is called delta 2. The difference between these two angles from pre- to postoperatively was defined as the delta angle **(FIGURE 38.5)**.

They found a significantly larger delta angle in the fracture group (29.4° ± 8.1° vs 19.5° ± 9.7°). They also found greater lateralization of the humerus to be protective of acromion fractures. Humeral lateralization may result in a more horizontal pull of the deltoid and decrease the stress across the acromion.

Using a multicenter database, Routman et al[35] performed a retrospective review of 4125 reverse total shoulder arthroplasties (RTSAs) with a medialized glenosphere/lateralized humeral implant and reported a 1.77% incidence of acromial/scapular fractures. Risk factors for developing an acromion or scapula fracture were female sex, rheumatoid arthritis, cuff tear arthropathy, and an increased number of baseplate screws.

INCIDENCE AND DIAGNOSIS

The incidence of acromial and scapular fractures has been reported to be between 0% and 11%.[2,7,19] In a recent systematic review by Patterson et al,[36] a 4.14% incidence of fractures was observed. In another systematic review by King et al,[29] the incidence was slightly lower at 2.8%. In a large recent study by Zuckerman et al, the overall incidence was 1.77%.[35] What confounds the actual incidence is the difficulty identifying and diagnosing a postoperative fracture. Often, patients present with acute pain along the acromion or scapular spine. However, standard radiographs are often negative.[19,27] Although fractures typically present early in the postoperative recovery, they have been observed many years

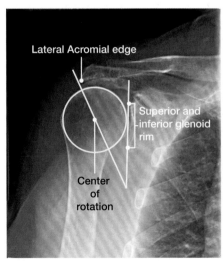
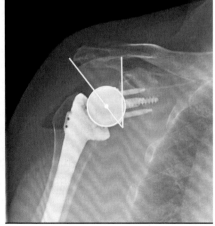

Delta 1   Delta 2

FIGURE 38.5 Delta angle is defined by a line connecting the superior and inferior borders of the glenoid fossa and a second line from the lateral acromial border through the center of rotation of the glenohumeral joint measured on the anteroposterior radiographs. The preoperative angle is delta 1, and the postoperative angle is delta 2. The difference between these two angles is the delta angle.

following surgery,[9,19,22,24,27,37] as Teusink et al[38] reported a fracture more than 8 years following RTSA. In addition to acute pain, patients typically display an abrupt change in function. In fact, when patients present with an acute episode of pain associated with a sudden loss of function and tenderness following RTSA, the diagnosis of a postoperative acromion fracture should be strongly considered. Although postoperative acromion fractures are typically attributed to a stress reaction, cases of traumatic fractures have also been reported.

As with any shoulder evaluation, a thorough examination of the entire shoulder girdle should be performed. One of the key findings is point tenderness along the acromion or spine of the scapula. If the fracture is displaced a gross deformity may be present, as the lateral acromion is often tilted inferiorly. Stressing the lateral acromion may elicit pain and detectable motion at the fracture site, especially when a displaced fracture is present. Rarely, ecchymosis occurs without acute trauma. Active and passive range-of-motion measurements should be performed and compared with previous postoperative values. Often times the patient's functional status exhibits a significant decline from prior postoperative evaluations.

Standard radiographs should be performed as part of the initial evaluation. A quality axillary lateral image is important and should include the entire scapula, as Levy type III fractures can often be missed if the field of view of the radiograph is too focused. On anteroposterior radiographs, assessment for a change in the acromion to greater tuberosity distance and tilt of the acromion can be observed (see **FIGURE 38.1**).[27] Once again, comparisons with previous radiographs are important to help recognize these often-subtle changes. Unfortunately, despite clinical signs and symptoms of an acromion fracture, radiographs commonly do not identify the fracture.[19,23,24,27,38,39] Otto et al[27] reported an accuracy of radiographs at detecting acromion fractures to be 78.8%. Levy et al[19] also demonstrated that interobserver reliability was poor for diagnosis of fractures with radiographs and similarly noted that 39% of patients ultimately diagnosed with acromion fractures were found to have negative radiographs based on the blinded review of three fellowship-trained shoulder surgeons. If clinical suspicion is high for an acromion or spine fracture, CT scan of the shoulder girdle is often utilized for diagnosis. Alternatively, Nicolay et al[40] described the use of single-photon emission computerized tomography/CT for the diagnosis of atraumatic scapular spine fracture.

OUTCOMES

Although postoperative acromion or scapular fracture following RTSA is a rarely reported complication, patients who sustain this complication report inferior function compared with initial recovery following the procedure. As outlined in a systematic review by Patterson et al,

these fractures result in lower average postoperative outcome scores, loss of range of motion, persistent pain, and dissatisfaction.[36] Measured outcome scores (ASES [American Shoulder & Elbow Society], Constant, VAS [Visual Analog Scale] pain, SANE [Single Assessment Numeric Evaluation], SST [Simple Shoulder Test]) all decreased in patients with fractures when compared with those who did not sustain a fracture.[2,22,25,28,35,39]

Teusink et al[38] performed a case-control study of 25 patients who sustained postoperative acromion and scapular spine fractures, comparing these patients with matched controls (n = 100) based on age, sex, follow-up, indication, and primary versus revision surgery. Patients with acromion fractures improved the ASES score by an average of 21 but were significantly worse than the comparison group. Range of motion was also less in the fracture cohort. In this series, outcomes were not impacted by the location of the fracture.

Although functional outcomes can be impacted by postoperative acromion and scapular spine fractures, the subtype of fracture has the greatest impact on ultimate functional recovery. Those patients with Levy type I or type II fractures often recover a substantial degree of function and remain typically satisfied with the outcome.[19,38] However, this is not the case for type III base of the acromion fractures, as functional recovery is rare. Levy et al[19] reported that 50% of patients with type III fractures were unsatisfied at the most recent follow-up, with significant improvements observed only in the postoperative SANE score, which improved from an average score of 5 to 49. Crosby et al[23] recognized the dramatic impact that the base of the acromion fractures can have on functional recovery and recommended surgical fixation of these fractures (**FIGURE 38.6**).

TREATMENT OPTIONS

The mainstay of treatment for postoperative acromion and scapular spine fractures has been nonoperative management. Nonsurgical treatment options include immobilization (typically using an abduction pillow) for 4 to 6 weeks or until tenderness over the acromion resolves. The analgesic effect of nasal calcitonin, which can follow vertebral compression fractures[41] and distal radius fractures,[10] has potential as a treatment option. As soon as pain over the fracture has resolved or healing is visible on radiographs, a focused rehabilitation program directed at restoration of motion and function can be initiated.

Neyton et al[11] reported outcomes of patients with postoperative acromion fractures following a Grammont-based RTSA design. Among the 19 patients, nonoperative treatment resulted in inferior results when compared with patients with non-acromion fracture RTSA, with base of the acromion fractures having the worst impact on function. Teusink et al[38] reported outcomes of patients with postoperative acromion fractures

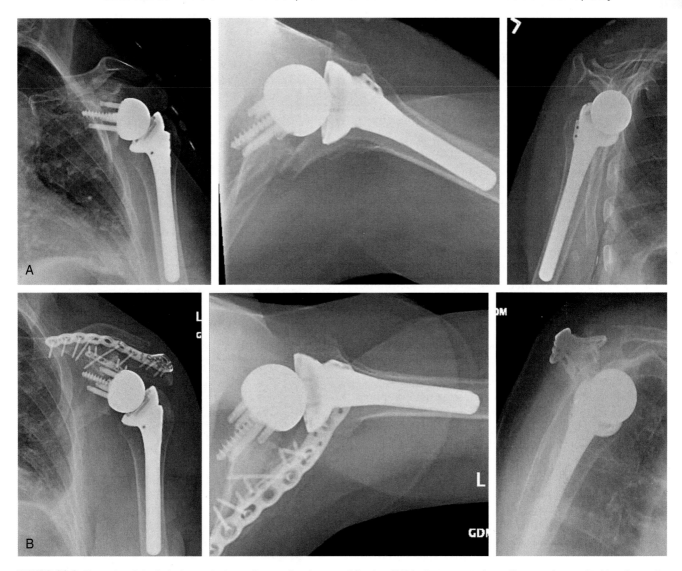

FIGURE 38.6 Example of dual plating technique of acromion fracture following RTSA. Anteroposterior, axillary, and scapular Y radiographs showing type III scapular spine fracture with tilt of the acromion (**A**). Postoperative images showing dual plate fixation (**B**).

following RTSA utilizing a lateralized center of rotation design. Among the 25 patients with fractures, nonoperative treatment once again resulted in inferior results when compared with matched controls, with a higher revision rate in patients who sustained acromion fractures. In a series of patients reported by the Mayo Clinic using a variety of RTSA designs, outcomes of 12 postoperative acromion fractures were compared with a 4:1 matched cohort of patients who underwent RTSA without acromion fractures. In this series, which contained patients with only type I and type II fractures, no difference was found in motion or ASES scores between those with and without acromion fractures.[12] These studies give support to management of type I and type II fractures with nonoperative measures. However, the negative impact of type III acromion base fractures on outcomes is significant and justifies consideration of surgical intervention.

Unfortunately, operative fixation of acromion fractures can be challenging owing to poor bone quality and the inferior-directed stress of the deltoid in the setting of RTSA. Nonetheless, there are several reports that describe successful fixation of these fractures. Neyton et al[11] reported a nonunion of one of two patients treated with surgical fixation of postoperative acromion fractures. Crosby et al[23] reported surgical fixation of four type 2 fractures and four type 3 base of the acromion fractures. With only one of four type 3 fractures developing into a nonunion, the series reported by Crosby represents the highest union rate in the literature. Similar to Crosby, Rouleau et al[42] recommended surgical fixation of type 3 base of the acromion fractures. In this series, seven patients with type 3 fractures were treated using a dual plating technique with three developing nonunions (43%) of which two were treated with revision surgical fixation. Further investigations to identify the optimal method of fracture fixation is needed to help define optimal surgical methods for treating these difficult fractures, as reported nonunion rates remain excessively high.

CASE #1

A 64-year-old man with history of failed prior rotator cuff surgery underwent an uncomplicated RTSA. At the patient's initial postoperative appointment, he was doing well with no pain. At 6 weeks, his forward flexion improved to 120° without pain. However, 3 months following the operation, he returned to the office with increasing pain and diminished function. Forward flexion became limited to 35°, abduction to 40°, and external rotation to 50°. He had significant pain with abduction, and there was point tenderness along the acromion. X-ray and CT evaluation identified a type II acromion fracture. Initial treatment was nonoperative, utilizing an abduction orthosis for 4 weeks, until pain resolved. Following pain resolution with direct palpation over the acromion, the patient was still unsatisfied with his function and persistent discomfort and crepitus would occur with abduction. Radiographs demonstrated a nonunited type 2 acromial fracture with associated decreased space between the acromion and humeral RTSA component. A shared decision was made for operative fixation. The patient underwent an open acromioplasty and tuberoplasty. In addition, a larger glenosphere was utilized (32-36 N, DJO) to distalize the glenosphere by 2 mm and medialize the center of rotation. The polyethylene was also switched from standard size to +4 to further distalize the humeral component from the acromion. The goal was to maximize impingement-free range of motion **(FIGURE 38.7)**. The surgery was uneventful. At 6 months following the revision procedure, the patient demonstrated a VAS pain score 0, ASES 70, SST 8, and SANE 64. Despite improvements in active motion with forward elevation to 160°, the patient remained dissatisfied.

CASE #2

An 84-year-old left hand dominant woman with history of bilateral reverse shoulder arthroplasties presented to the office after sustaining a fall on to her left shoulder. The patient was 6 months following a left RTSA. After the fall, the patient noted a significant decline in function. On examination, she had point tenderness and crepitus along the scapular spine. The left shoulder demonstrated pseudoparalysis with active forward elevation of 10°, abduction 0°, external rotation 0°, and internal rotation to the side. Standard radiographs demonstrated well-positioned reverse shoulder replacement with an acute type 3 fracture, not originating at any glenoid baseplate screw **(FIGURE 38.8)**. Owing to the acute nature and significant decline in patient's function,

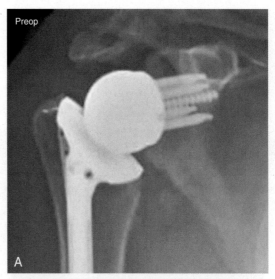

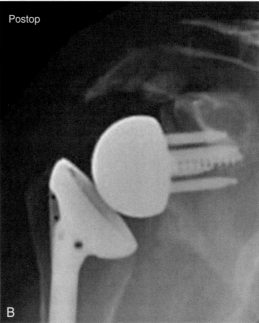

FIGURE 38.7 Preoperative (**A**) and postoperative (**B**) radiographs following revision arthroplasty for acromion fracture. The patient underwent an open acromioplasty and tuberoplasty. In addition, the glenosphere and polyethylene were exchanged to larger sizes to maximize impingement-free range of motion.

decision was made to proceed with operative intervention. The patient underwent a dual plating technique with Superior Lateral Clavicle plate (Stryker, Mahwah, NY) and additional orthogonal Utility Plate (Stryker) with additional suture fixation using figure-of-8 suture orientation across the fracture **(FIGURE 38.9)**. She was placed in a postoperative shoulder abduction orthosis for 6 weeks. At the 6-week postoperative appointment, the patient was doing well with no pain. Her range of motion demonstrates forward flexion to 105°, abduction 85°, and external rotation 35°.

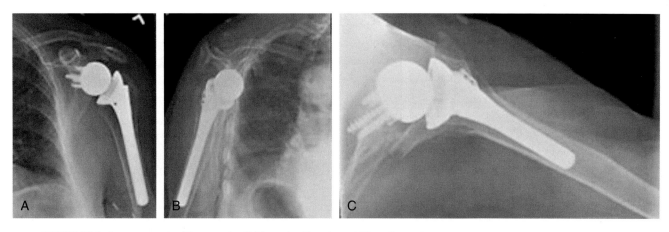

FIGURE 38.8 Anteroposterior (**A**), scapular Y (**B**), and axillary lateral (**C**) radiographs demonstrating a type III acromion fracture.

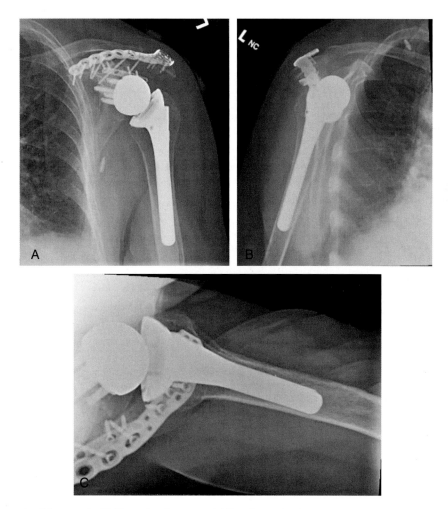

FIGURE 38.9 Anteroposterior (**A**), scapular Y (**B**), and axillary lateral (**C**) radiographs demonstrating open reduction internal fixation of type 3 acromion fracture with the dual plating technique.

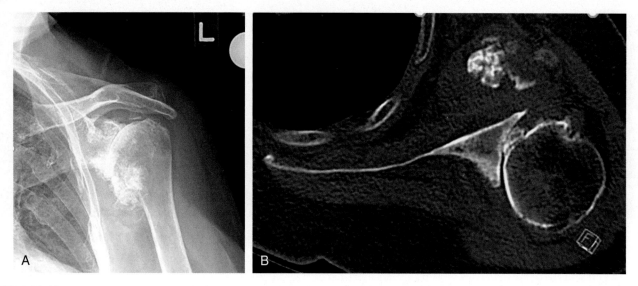

FIGURE 38.10 Preoperative imaging showing advanced glenohumeral osteoarthritis with severe retroversion (**A**) and posterior humeral head subluxation (**B**).

CASE #3

An 81-year-old woman with a history of glenohumeral osteoarthritis with severe retroversion and subluxation **(FIGURE 38.10)** underwent uncomplicated RTSA **(FIGURE 38.11)**. She was progressing until she returned for her 6-week postoperative visit with increasing shoulder pain and difficulty lifting the arm. On examination the shoulder demonstrated 40° of active forward elevation, 40° of abduction, and 15° of external rotation all with significant pain. The patient was exquisitely tender to palpation posteriorly along the scapula. Radiographs show a type II acromion fracture with tilt of the acromion **(FIGURE 38.12)**. Decision was made to perform dual plate fixation (Acumed, Inc) **(FIGURE 38.13)**. Two weeks postoperatively the patient noted increased pain and hardware prominence. Radiographs showed loss of fixation, and the decision was made to remove the hardware **(FIGURE 38.14)**. At final follow-up, the patient has mild pain with active forward elevation to 90°.

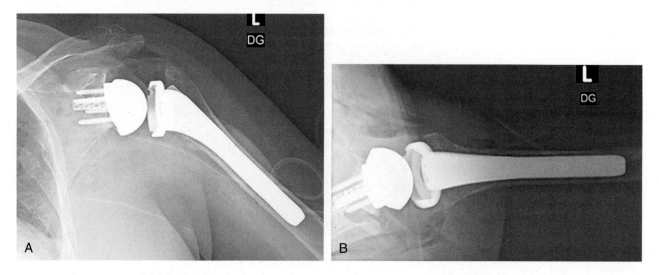

FIGURE 38.11 A and **B**, Initial postoperative radiographs of uncomplicated RTSA.

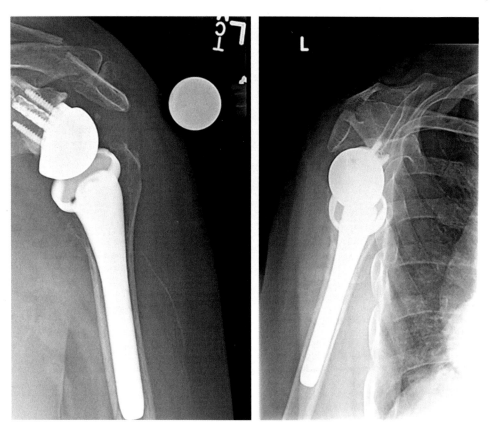

FIGURE 38.12 Anteroposterior and scapular Y radiographs showing type II acromion fracture with inferior tilt of the acromion.

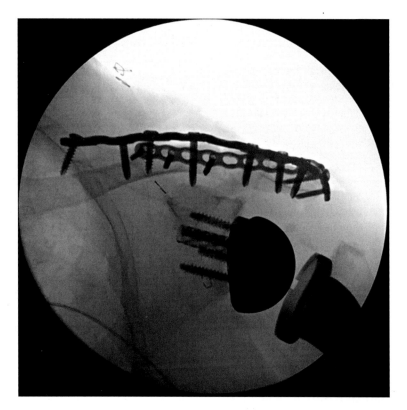

FIGURE 38.13 Intraoperative fluoroscopy demonstrating reduction and dual plate fixation of acromion fracture.

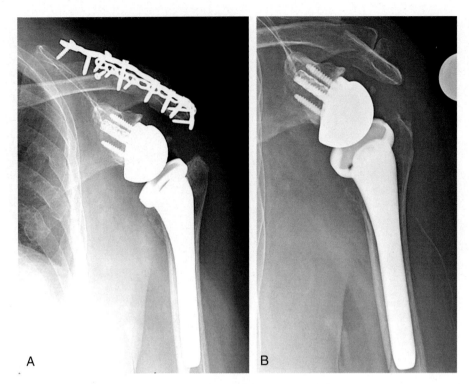

FIGURE 38.14 A and **B**, Anteroposterior radiographs demonstrating loss of fixation followed by removal of hardware.

AUTHOR'S TIPS TO AVOID ACROMION AND SCAPULAR SPINE FRACTURES

Given the concern for postoperative acromion fractures following RTSA, a number of modifications to surgical technique are now being utilized. When utilizing a lateralized center of rotation glenosphere, lengthening of the humerus is minimized. This is accomplished through the use of an inlay humeral component and avoiding any glenosphere overhang inferior to the glenoid. Posterior-superior screws are avoided, and the preferred orientation of the glenoid baseplate places the superior screw directly superior. A shorter superior screw is typically utilized unless it is clear from surgical planning that the screw exits more anteriorly away from the base of the scapular spine. During exposure, the coracoacromial ligament is preserved to unload stress on the acromion. Finally, efforts are made to avoid impingement of the greater tuberosity on the acromion during abduction, and assessment is made by elevating the arm to 90° and rotating the arm through full internal and external rotation. In cases where impingement occurs, use of a tuberoplasty from the greater tuberosity or the use of a semiconstrained polyethylene, which allows for further inset of the humerus, can be utilized.

CONCLUSION

Postoperative acromion and scapular spine fractures represent an infrequent but impactful complication following RTSA. Patients with risk factors such as osteoporosis should be counseled regarding the elevated risk of fracture. Despite preventive efforts, these fractures will likely continue to be observed following RTSA. Further innovations into management of type 3 fractures are needed to provide patients with reduced pain and improved functional recovery.

REFERENCES

1. Dubrow S, Streit JJ, Muh S, Shishani Y, Gobezie R. Acromial stress fractures: correlation with acromioclavicular osteoarthritis and acromiohumeral distance. *Orthopedics.* 2014;37:e1074-e1079. doi:10.3928/01477447-20141124-54

2. Jiang JJ, Toor AS, Shi LL, Koh JL. Analysis of perioperative complications in patients after total shoulder arthroplasty and reverse total shoulder arthroplasty. *J Shoulder Elbow Surg.* 2014;23:1852-1859. doi:10.1016/j.jse.2014.04.008

3. Bachman D, Nyland J, Krupp R. Reverse-total shoulder arthroplasty cost-effectiveness: a quality-adjusted life years comparison with total hip arthroplasty. *World J Orthop.* 2016;7:123-127. doi:10.5312/wjo.v7.i2.123

4. Wahlquist TC, Hunt AF, Braman JP. Acromial base fractures after reverse total shoulder arthroplasty: report of five cases. *J Shoulder Elbow Surg.* 2011;20:1178-1183. doi:10.1016/j.jse.2011.01.029

5. Barco R, Savvidou OD, Sperling JW, Sanchez-Sotelo J, Cofield RH. Complications in reverse shoulder arthroplasty. *EFORT Open Rev.* 2016;1:72-80. doi:10.1302/2058-5241.1.160003

6. Cheung E, Willis M, Walker M, Clark R, Frankle MA. Complications in reverse total shoulder arthroplasty. *J Am Acad Orthop Surg.* 2011;19:439-449.

7. Frankle M, Siegal S, Pupello D, Saleem A, Mighell M, Vasey M. The reverse shoulder prosthesis for glenohumeral arthritis associated with severe rotator cuff deficiency. A minimum two-year follow-up study of sixty patients. *J Bone Joint Surg Am.* 2005;87:1697-1705. doi:10.2106/jbjs.D.02813

8. Hamid N, Connor PM, Fleischli JF, D'Alessandro DF. Acromial fracture after reverse shoulder arthroplasty. *Am J Orthop (Belle Mead NJ).* 2011;40:E125-E129.

9. Hattrup SJ. The influence of postoperative acromial and scapular spine fractures on the results of reverse shoulder arthroplasty. *Orthopedics*. 2010;33:302. doi:10.3928/01477447-20100329-04

10. Karponis A, Rizou S, Pallis D, et al. Analgesic effect of nasal salmon calcitonin during the early post-fracture period of the distal radius fracture. *J Musculoskelet Neuronal Interact*. 2015;15(2):186-189.

11. Neyton L, Erickson J, Ascione F, Bugelli G, Lunini E, Walch G. Grammont Award 2018: scapular fractures in reverse shoulder arthroplasty (Grammont style). Prevalence, functional, and radiographic results with minimum 5-year follow-up. *J Shoulder Elbow Surg*. 2019;28(2):260-267. doi:10.1016/j.jse.2018.07.004

12. Werthel JD, Schoch BS, van Veen SC, et al. Acromial fractures in reverse shoulder arthroplasty: a clinical and radiographic analysis. *JSEA*. 2018;2:2471549218777628.

13. Farshad M, Gerber C. Reverse total shoulder arthroplasty—from the most to the least common complication. *Int Orthop*. 2010;34:1075-1082. doi:10.1007/s00264-010-1125-2 http://dx.doi.org/10.1007/s00264-010-1125-2

14. Gagey O, Hue E. Mechanics of the deltoid muscle. A new approach. *Clin Orthop*. 2000;375:250-257.

15. Groh GI, Groh GM. Complications rates, reoperation rates, and the learning curve in reverse shoulder arthroplasty. *J Shoulder Elbow Surg*. 2014;23:388-394. doi:10.1016/j.jse.2013.06.002

16. Taylor S, Kontaxis A, Chen X, et al. *Coracoacromial Ligament Transection Increases Scapular Spine Strains Following Reverse Total Shoulder Arthroplasty*. Paper 386, AAOS; 2019, Las Vegas, Nevada.

17. Virani NA, Cabezas A, Gutiérrez S, Santoni BG, Otto R, Frankle M. Reverse shoulder arthroplasty components and surgical techniques that restore glenohumeral motion. *J Shoulder Elbow Surg*. 2013;22(2):179-187. doi:10.1016/j.jse.2012.02.004

18. Virani NA, Williams CD, Clark R, Polikandriotis J, Downes KL, Frankle MA. Preparing for the bundled-payment initiative: the cost and clinical outcomes of reverse shoulder arthroplasty for the surgical treatment of advanced rotator cuff deficiency at an average 4-year follow-up. *J Shoulder Elbow Surg*. 2013;22:1612-1622. doi:10.1016/j.jse.2013.01.003

19. Levy JC, Anderson C, Samson A. Classification of postoperative acromial fractures following reverse shoulder arthroplasty. *J Bone Joint Surg Am*. 2013;95:e104. doi:10.2106/jbjs.K.01516

20. Berliner JL, Regalado-Magdos A, Ma CB, et al. Biomechanics of reverse total shoulder arthroplasty. *J Shoulder Elbow Surg*. 2015;24:150-160.

21. Greiner S, Schmidt C, Herrmann S, Pauly S, Perka C. Clinical performance of lateralized versus non-lateralized reverse shoulder arthroplasty: a prospective randomized study. *J Shoulder Elbow Surg*. 2015;24(9):1397-1404. doi:10.1016/j.jse.2015.05.041

22. Lópiz Y, Rodríguez-González A, García-Fernández C, et al. Scapula insufficiency fractures after reverse total shoulder arthroplasty in rotator cuff arthropathy: what is their functional impact? *Rev Esp Cir Ortop Traumatol*. 2015;59:318-325.

23. Crosby LA, Hamilton A, Twiss T. Scapula fractures after reverse total shoulder arthroplasty: classification and treatment. *Clin Orthop Relat Res*. 2011;469:2544-2549.

24. Mayne IP, Bell SN, Wright W, Coghlan JA. Acromial and scapular spine fractures after reverse total shoulder arthroplasty. *Shoulder Elbow*. 2016;8:90-100. doi:10.1177/1758573216628783

25. Walch G, Mottier F, Wall B, Boileau P, Molé D, Favard L. Acromial insufficiency in reverse shoulder arthroplasties. *J Shoulder Elbow Surg*. 2009;18:495-502. doi:10.1016/j.jse.2008.12.002

26. Aibinder WR, Schoch BS, Cofield RH, Sperling JW, Sánchez-Sotelo J. Reverse shoulder arthroplasty in patients with os acromiale. *J Shoulder Elbow Surg*. 2017;26(9):1598-1602. doi:10.1016/j.jse.2017.02.012

27. Otto RJ, Virani NA, Levy JC, et al. Scapular fractures after reverse shoulder arthroplasty: evaluation of risk factors and the reliability of a proposed classification. *J Shoulder Elbow Surg*. 2013;22:1514-1521.

28. Schenk P, Aichmair A, Beeler S, Ernstbrunner L, Meyer DC, Gerber C. Acromial fractures following reverse total shoulder arthroplasty: a cohort controlled analysis. *Orthopedics*. 2020;43(1):15-22

29. King JJ, Dalton SS, Gulotta LV, Wright TW, Schoch BS. How common are acromial and scapular spine fractures after reverse shoulder arthroplasty?: a systematic review. *Bone Joint J*. 2019;101-B(6):627-634. doi:10.1302/0301-620X.101B6.BJJ-2018-1187.R1

30. Lädermann A, Lübbeke A, Mélis B, et al. Prevalence of neurologic lesions after total shoulder arthroplasty. *J Bone Joint Surg Am*. 2011;93(14):1288-1293. doi:10.2106/JBJS.J.00369

31. Ascione F, Kilian CM, Laughlin MS, et al. Increased scapular spine fractures after reverse shoulder arthroplasty with a humeral onlay short stem: an analysis of 485 consecutive cases. *J Shoulder Elbow Surg*. 2018;27(12):2183-2190. doi:10.1016/j.jse.2018.06.007

32. Levy JC, Berglund D, Vakharia R, et al. Primary monoblock inset reverse shoulder arthroplasty resulted in decreased pain and improved function. *Clin Orthop Relat Res*. 2019;477(9):2097-2108. doi:10.1097/CORR.0000000000000761

33. Wong MT, Langohr GDG, Athwal GS, Johnson JA. Implant positioning in reverse shoulder arthroplasty has an impact on acromial stresses. *J Shoulder Elbow Surg*. 2016;25(11):1889-1895. doi:10.1016/j.jse.2016.04.011

34. Kennon JC, Lu C, McGee-Lawrence ME, Crosby LA. Scapula fracture incidence in reverse total shoulder arthroplasty using screws above or below metaglene central cage: clinical and biomechanical outcomes. *J Shoulder Elbow Surg*. 2017;26(6):1023-1030. doi:10.1016/j.jse.2016.10.018

35. Routman HD, Simovitch RW, Wright TW, Flurin PH, Zuckerman JD, Roche CP. Outcomes of and risk factors for acromial or scapular fractures after reverse shoulder arthroplasty with a medialized glenoid/lateralized humeral implant. *J Bone Joint Surg*. 2020;102(19):1724-1733.

36. Patterson DC, Chi D, Parsons BO, Cagle PJ Jr. Acromial spine fracture after reverse total shoulder arthroplasty: a systematic review. *J Shoulder Elbow Surg*. 2019;28(4):792-801. doi:10.1016/j.jse.2018.08.033

37. Camarada L, Phadnis J, Clitherow HD, et al. Mesh plates for scapula fixation. *Tech Shoulder Elbow Surg*. 2015;16:79-84.

38. Teusink MJ, Otto RJ, Cottrell BJ, Frankle MA. What is the effect of postoperative scapular fracture on outcomes of reverse shoulder arthroplasty? *J Shoulder Elbow Surg*. 2014;23:782-790. doi:10.1016/j.jse.2013.09.010

39. Levy JC, Blum S. Postoperative acromion base fracture resulting in subsequent instability of reverse shoulder replacement. *J Shoulder Elbow Surg*. 2012;21:e14-e18. doi:10.1016/j.jse.2011.09.018

40. Nicolay S, De Beuckeleer L, Stoffelen D, et al. Atraumatic bilateral scapular spine fracture several months after bilateral reverse total shoulder arthroplasty. *Skeletal Radiol*. 2014;43:699-702.

41. Knopp-Sihota JA, Newburn-Cook CV, Homik J, Cummings GG, Voaklander D. Calcitonin for treating acute and chronic pain of recent and remote osteoporotic vertebral compression fractures: a systematic review and meta-analysis. *Osteoporos Int*. 2012;23(1):17-38. doi:10.1007/s00198-011-1676-0

42. Rouleau DM, Gaudelli C. Successful treatment of fractures of the base of the acromion after reverse shoulder arthroplasty: case report and review of the literature. *Int J Shoulder Surg*. 2013;7:149-152.

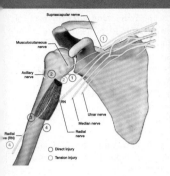

39 Neurological Complications and Shoulder Arthroplasty

Bertrand Coulet, MD, PhD, Geert Alexander Buijze, MD, PhD, FEBHS, and Pierre-Henri Flurin, MD

INTRODUCTION

Neurological complications following shoulder arthroplasty are not frequent, with a reported incidence of less than 5%, but are probably underestimated since a majority spontaneously recover.[1] Nevertheless, in unfavorable cases, often affecting elderly patients with reduced neurological regeneration potential, their management is not straightforward. For the purpose of this chapter, we have designed a decision-making algorithm for the treatment of neurological complications after shoulder arthroplasty, based on a review of the neuroanatomy of the shoulder, the pathophysiology of these complications, and their neurological and palliative management.

SHOULDER NEUROANATOMY

The shoulder has two articular systems, *scapulothoracic* and *glenohumeral* (*GH*), each consisting of two muscle groups with their own innervation (**FIGURE 39.1**). The *scapulothoracic* system has a posterior group, whose main motor is the *trapezius*, innervated very proximally by the eleventh paired cranial nerve (*accessory nerve*), and an anterior one, the most important of which is the *serratus anterior* innervated by the *long thoracic nerve*, originating from the C5-C7 nerve roots of the brachial plexus. The GH joint also has two muscle groups. The first includes the rotator cuff muscles, including the *supra-* and *infraspinatus*, which are innervated by the suprascapular nerve arising from the *superior trunk of the brachial plexus*, as well as the *teres minor* innervated by a branch of the *axillary nerve* (*AN*) and the *subscapularis* innervated by two individual branches. The second muscle group includes the *deltoid* innervated by the terminal branch of the *AN* arising from the *posterior cord*.

This double innervation pattern and the presence of these two systems imply that complete paralysis of the shoulder is exceptional, except in the case of very proximal lesions, and that there is important potential for compensation, within the same system and also between the two systems. This important concept explains the delays in the diagnosis of certain deficits that can be perfectly compensated for.

The proximity of the brachial plexus and its terminal branches is one of the causes of neurological complications during arthroplasty, through direct injuries (blunt or compression) and especially through stretching (**FIGURE 39.2**).

The *suprascapular nerve* has a short trajectory after its emergence from the *superior trunk* and presents several points of vulnerability. The first point is at the *suprascapular notch* before entering the *supraspinatus fossa*, where it constitutes a fixed point making it particularly vulnerable to traction. The second is located in the *spinoglenoid notch*, a crossing point between *supra-* and *infraspinatus fossae*. These two zones are in direct contact with the glenoid, where the center of the articular surface is located at 28 and 12 mm, respectively, in the anterosuperior and posterosuperior planes.[2]

The *axillary nerve*, upon emergence, has a posterior trajectory less than 11 mm from the lower capsule of the GH joint.[3] Its exit from the *quadrilateral space* as it winds around the humerus constitutes a point of fixation and, above all, a zone of close contact with the humeral metaphysis (5-8 mm).[1,4] The *AN* will therefore be vulnerable during any procedure involving the lower part of the capsule, and also by traction when the internally rotated humerus is translated posteriorly. An anterosuperior approach is not without risk. As Burkhead et al[5] have shown, the classic mean safety distance for the AN of 50 mm below the acromion is reduced to 30 mm in abduction.

After its emergence, the *radial nerve* has a more direct path but several points of vulnerability. The first is the passage under the *latissimus dorsi* tendon and its insertion zone, the proximity of which varies greatly depending on the position of the arm, as shown by Gates et al.[6] In adduction-internal rotation, this distance is minimal (15 mm), whereas it is maximal in abduction-external rotation (52 mm). The second is the area where the radial nerve wraps around the humerus, constituting a point of fixation, but, above all, an area of close contact with its gutter, making it particularly vulnerable in the event of fracture or cement extravasation.[7,8]

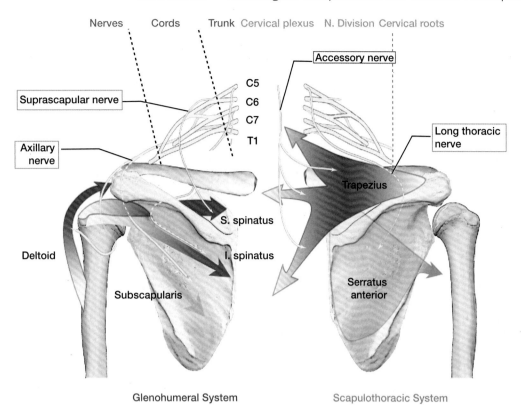

FIGURE 39.1 Schematic presentation of the neuroanatomy of the shoulder with the two-joint systems represented. The scapulothoracic system with its two main motors and their proximal innervation, the trapezius innervated by the accessory nerve (eleventh cranial nerve) and the serratus anterior innervated by the long thoracic nerve. The glenohumeral system with the rotator cuff innervated by the suprascapular nerve and the deltoid innervated by the axillary nerve.

More medially, the area where the *musculocutaneous nerve* crosses the coracobrachialis muscle represents an area of potential direct trauma by a retractor and also of point of fixation subject to stretching injury. The other nerves of the brachial plexus are more distant but can be damaged indirectly by a traction mechanism. As in obstetric lesions, it is the upper roots and trunks that will be most vulnerable because of a vertical traction vector.

CLASSIFICATION OF NERVE INJURIES AND GENERAL CONSIDERATIONS

Pathophysiology and Classification

There are two types of nerve lesions: (1) the frank disruption without any possible spontaneous recovery, and more frequent in the shoulder; (2) continuous lesions as a result of traction or crushing, whose prognosis of spontaneous recovery is very variable depending on the extent of the trauma.

Seddon,[9] followed by Sunderland[10] **(TABLE 39.1),** classified these nerve injuries according to the nature of the lesion and prognosis. The importance of the axonal trauma was emphasized, from a simple injury (neurapraxia) recovering spontaneously in a few weeks to a more important injury with distal Wallerian degeneration, the recovery of which is conditioned by the integrity of the nerve sheaths. If the basal lamina of the Schwann cell is intact, the nerve sheath guides the regeneration of axons (axonotmesis) and recovery is possible but takes longer and is often incomplete. This regrowth depends on the patient's capacity for axonal regeneration (important factors include age and tobacco use) and the type of nerve involved. Conversely, if the nerve sheath for axonal regrowth is destroyed (neurotmesis), although the nerve is in continuity, axonal regeneration is impossible.

Mackinnon described an additional type[11] in which these different stages exist in the same nerve for different fascicles and at several levels, constituting mosaic lesions at the origin of an early recovery whose progression stagnates rapidly.

Mechanisms of Injury

Several mechanisms can cause nerve damage in the shoulder with varying consequences:

- A **nerve section** is the most obvious, the deficit is complete without spontaneous recovery.
- A **stretching mechanism** is by far the most common. It will be more severe with greater displacement and occurs along the axis of the nerve over a short

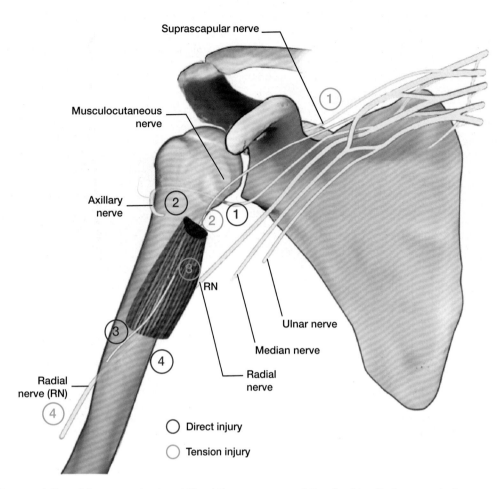

FIGURE 39.2 Representation of the areas of vulnerability of the nerves around the shoulder. Red represents the areas of potential direct trauma, and blue represents the points of nerve fixation that could cause traction injuries. AN, axillary nerve; CBM, coracobrachialis muscle; MCN, musculocutaneous nerve; MN, median nerve; RN, radial nerve; SScN, suprascapular nerve; UN, ulnar nerve.

segment. This mechanism can affect several nerves at the same time.

- A **crushing mechanism** by a retractor or a blunt instrument.

Nagda et al[12] performed intraoperative nerve monitoring during total shoulder arthroplasty (TSA). They showed signs of nerve alertness in 57% of the shoulders, regressive after neutralization or removal of the retractor, but almost half retained postoperative disturbances based on electroneuromyography (ENMG). They observed diffuse involvement of the brachial plexus in 50% of cases and of the musculocutaneous nerve and AN in a comparable manner in 20%. Shinagawa et al, [13] with a similar monitoring method during reverse TSA (RTSA), showed that the AN is the most vulnerable, especially during the preparation of the humerus and the glenoid. Lenoir et al[14] reported an anatomical study of the tension (stress) on the nerves during the insertion of an RTSA. They observed significant increases in tension on the axillary and radial nerves during exposure of the humerus when it is in a position of internal rotation and

extension. External rotation becomes potentially hazardous beyond 45° except for the AN and above 60° for all nerves when associated with extension. Furthermore, exposure of the glenoid increases the tension on the axillary, radial, and musculocutaneous nerves, especially during posterior translation of the head. A polyethylene insert greater than 3 mm also potentially increases tension on the axillary, radial, and musculocutaneous nerves. Inserts larger than 9 mm can impact all the nerve structures.

Epidemiology

Neurological complications after shoulder arthroplasty are underestimated, with an incidence reported to be less than 1% in the overall literature.[15-18] However, this complication when actively sought, is more common, as Lynch et al[1] observed it in 4.3% of shoulder arthroplasties. The incidence is increased in women without any association to the patient's morphology and also in cases of revision, rheumatoid arthritis, or osteoarthritis and in those with significant limitation of preoperative

TABLE 39.1 Different Types of Neurological Lesions According to the Seddon and Sunderland Classifications Including Their Clinical and ENMG Presentations and Prognosis

| Nerve Injury | Histopathologic Changes | Degree of Nerve Injury | | Prognostic | ENMG |
		Seddon Classification	Sunderland Classification	Recovery	Fibrillations
	Axon: nerve conduction bloc No Wallerian degeneration Muscle: no denervation	Neurapraxia	Type I	Spontaneous, fast (few weeks)	None
	Axon: stop of nerve conduction Wallerian degeneration Intact basal membrane Axonal regeneration Muscle: denervation	Axonotmesis	Type II	Spontaneous, slow, complete	Present
	Axon: stop of nerve conduction Wallerian degeneration Intact basal membrane but injured myelin sheath Axonal regeneration Muscle: denervation		Type III	Spontaneous, slow, incomplete like "perfect nerve repair"	Present
	Axon: stop of nerve conduction Wallerian degeneration Injuries of all nerve sheaths—nerve appearing macroscopically in continuity No axonal regeneration Muscle: denervation	Neurotmesis	Type IV	No recovery	Present
	Complete nerve section		Type V	No recovery	Present
	Mixed injury (Mackinnon)		Type VI	Variable	Present

external rotation. The diagnosis is delayed in the majority of cases. Two-thirds can be expected to recover within 6 months. More than half of the cases that do not recover have an AN paralysis. Injury to the radial nerve is mainly related to cement extravasation or fractures of the humerus. More recently, Kim et al[19] and Ball et al[15] showed that RTSAs resulted in a 20% incidence of neurological deficit due, in part, to the distalization of the construct. The AN was affected in almost 50% of cases, followed by the radial nerve in 20%, the musculocutaneous nerve in 10%, and the median nerve in 10%. In these series of RTSAs, the suprascapular nerve was injured by protruding glenoid screws.

RTSAs are particularly at risk for several reasons including the more extensive mobilization of the humerus due to the frequent absence of the rotator cuff and the inherent distalization of the humerus.[4-16,20]

The prognosis for these lesions is generally good with almost 90% being neurapraxias and an average recovery time of 7 months for the AN and 5 to 6 months for the other nerves. Finally, the deltopectoral approach seems to place the nerves at greater risk, especially in the absence of release of the anterior fibers of the deltoid, perhaps as a result of excessive stress on retractors.

TOWARD A SURGICAL STRATEGY

When faced with a neurological complication following TSA, it is possible to adopt a standard approach that is applicable to all lesions **(TABLE 39.2)**.

The **first stage (initial phase)** consists of establishing the precise identification of the lesion, topography, mechanism, and the impact of the neurological deficit

TABLE 39.2 Management of a Neurological Complication After Shoulder Arthroplasty From the Initial Phase to the Sequelae Stage

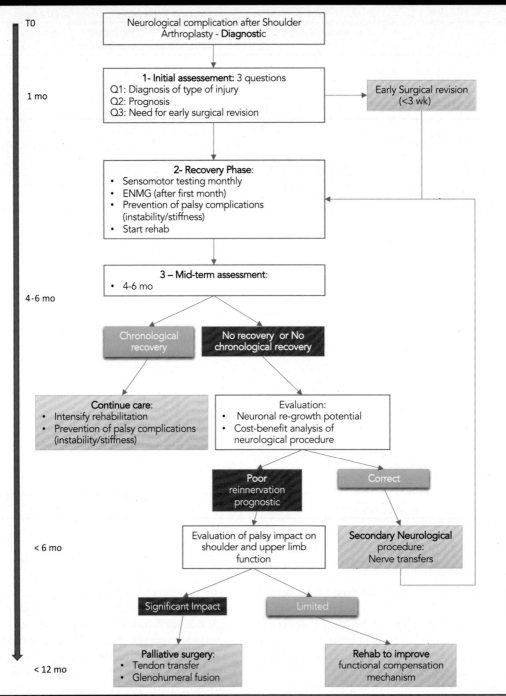

on the outcome of the arthroplasty. This analysis should make it possible to answer three questions that will determine management:

- Should immediate surgical intervention be considered?
- What impact will this paralysis have on the short- and long-term function of the arthroplasty?
- What is the prognosis of the lesion in this patient, and is spontaneous recovery possible?

The **second stage** is a **recovery and follow-up phase.** Regardless of whether or not revision surgery has been performed, specific clinical and paraclinical evaluation criteria are established, with a time limit beyond which the absence of recovery must prompt reconsideration of the treatment plan.

The **third stage** occurs 4 to 6 months after the initial operation (or revision surgery if it was necessary) with a careful evaluation of the initial strategy and the results with the goal of determining a definitive treatment plan:

- If the patient is recovering, the plan should continue with an increased emphasis on rehabilitation.
- If there are no clinical and paraclinical signs of recovery, management should be redirected based upon axonal regeneration capacity and the functional impact of the paralysis. If the patient has some potential for axonal regrowth, a neurological intervention may be considered; otherwise, the patient will be directed toward the final phase which is neurological consolidation.

The **phase of neurological consolidation** corresponds to the stabilization of the neurological status when recovery is no longer progressing. At this point recovery may be significant or minimal to none. The recovery and the impact of the residual motor deficit on function are assessed followed by discussion, if necessary, of tendon transfers or joint stabilization procedures.

Initial Evaluation—Diagnostic Circumstances

The immediate postoperative diagnosis is not always obvious, as the neurological examination of the shoulder is often masked by pain or impossible in the case of analgesic peripheral nerve catheters or prolonged regional anesthetic blocks.

Overall, three main circumstances may be encountered:

- **Concern about a technical (iatrogenic) intraoperative complication or maneuver** (aggressive periarticular release, diaphyseal fracture of the humerus): In this situation, a careful assessment of the deficit is needed (excluding local analgesia). Once the diagnosis is established a decision concerning immediate operative intervention is made.
- **Complete or partial (distal) upper limb deficit involving the hand or elbow in the immediate postoperative phase:** In the absence of any obvious intraoperative incident or difficulty, this probably represents a traction injury or compression without nerve interruption. Spontaneous recovery is considered possible.
- **Discovery of a secondary deficit during the recovery phase** that does not follow the usual chronology: This is usually an observation made during rehabilitation and should be assessed in the context of the two previous situations described.

Nerve Injury Analysis

The evaluation of the neurological deficit is based upon clinical findings utilizing reference sensory-motor tests to locate the neurological lesion. A distinction is made between truncular lesions in which deficits are limited to the territory of a nerve (axillary, radial, musculocutaneous) and more extensive plexus lesions corresponding to the root level. Truncular lesions may result from all mechanisms of injury, whereas plexus or pluritruncular lesions are most often the result of stretching or compression mechanisms with intact neural continuity resulting in a better prognosis. In the initial phase, the ENMG is of little additional value, but radiographs and advanced imaging (computed tomography scan, ultrasound) are often necessary to search for a skeletal, hardware/implant, cement extrusion, or hematoma as a cause of the deficit.

Prognostic Factors for Neurologic Recovery

There are two prognostic factors that impact neurological recovery and determine therapeutic strategy and the potential need for an eventual neurological procedure.

The first is the **capacity for axonal regeneration**, which is directly related to the age of the patient. In the specific case of complications of TSA, especially RTSA, patients are almost exclusively elderly. Very few authors have reported on nerve transfer results after the age of 60 years. Although the procedure is often inferior, it can be useful in producing a contraction of the deltoid at M3 following AN transfer on the five-point scale of the British Medical Research Council (BMRC). This corresponds to an active abduction of the shoulder against gravity without any form of resistance by the examiner.[21-24] In this age group a minimal delay in management is essential.

The second prognostic factor is **receptiveness of the muscle to innervation. For adequate receptiveness to muscle innervation** the classic 6-month delay should be respected. Ideally, surgery is planned no later than 4 months knowing that beyond 9 months the results are much less successful and that no useful results have been obtained after 12 months.[10,24,25] Indeed, beyond this period, muscle atrophy is extensive and the motor endplates have degenerated to irreversible fibrosis. This period includes the time of management and the time of axonal regrowth.

The work of Gillis et al[26] is most relevant as they reported a series of 50 shoulders in a population aged between 50 and 77 years who were reinnervated following brachial plexus paralysis. Only 35% obtained a useful BMRC result >3 without a correlation between age and the outcome, although the initiation of treatment before the 6-month deadline was clearly highlighted.

Short-Term Outcome of Shoulder Arthroplasty

The primary complications that result from neurological deficits after shoulder arthroplasty are stiffness and especially instability. The risk of instability is considerable both in cases of extensive (plexus) palsy and also in the relatively frequent situation of AN paralysis following RTSA. Close monitoring is essential, because shoulders that have lost sensitivity subluxation may go unnoticed.

At the end of this assessment, four questions should be answered:

- What is the topography, nature, and prognosis of the neurological injury?
- Does the lesion require suturing or immediate nerve release? In this situation, this procedure should be performed as soon as possible (ideally within 3 weeks).
- What is the patient's axonal regeneration potential?
- What is the impact of short-term paralysis on the arthroplasty?

Phase of Recovery Follow-up

Postoperative rehabilitation should continue uninterrupted to avoid the additional complications of stiffness and instability. This phase is marked by sensation and motor testing to monitor for the first signs of reinnervation. ENMG becomes relevant from the third week onward. From this stage on it confirms the neurological deficit by the denervation potentials (fibrillations) in the paralyzed muscles. Thereafter, its major benefit is that it can show very early the first signs of reinnervation even before a voluntary clinical contraction. Furthermore, ENMG can also highlight ductal syndromes of the ulnar or median nerves.

The recovery chronology is very important and specific to each nerve. In the case of plexus injury, recovery proceeds proximal to distal and is then called synchronous. Asynchronous recovery is indicative of polymorphic neurological injury. In fact, a distal-first type of recovery indicates a more severe proximal injury.

Each nerve follows a recovery specific to its anatomy. For the AN, the posterior bundle is innervated first, followed by the middle and anterior bundles. For the radial nerve, the brachioradialis muscle is innervated first, followed by the extensors of the wrist and fingers. The suprascapular nerve first reinnervates the supraspinatus and then the infraspinatus. When the first signs of recovery are observed, rehabilitation should be intensified. During the recovery phase, the following question should guide the decision-making process:

- Is the recovery chronological? If so, follow-up should be continued. If the patient's recovery does not follow the chronology expected, several questions should be asked and management adapted:
  - What is the nerve regeneration potential of this type of lesion in this patient?
  - What is the functional tolerance of the deficit?

At this stage, operative management may include nerve repair with or without a graft in the case of a localized lesion or, more commonly, a nerve transfer.

Neurological Consolidation Phase

This period of variable duration is characterized by the recognition that the patient will no longer improve neurologically and that he or she has completed any compensatory mechanisms. If the functional deficit is too great, palliative procedures such as tendon transfer or osteoarticular fusion should be considered.

SURGICAL PRINCIPLES: WHEN AND HOW

The surgical management of nerve injuries is not systematic. The mechanism of injury, being most often stretching or compression, indicates that the vast majority of these complications recover spontaneously, and moreover, compensatory mechanisms are often effective. Before deciding if surgery is indicated, it is essential to assess the impact of the palsy and the possible benefits of the proposed treatment on the functional outcome of the arthroplasty. One needs to bear in mind that spontaneous recovery, when possible, provides the best outcome and that, after nerve surgery or tendon transfer, the outcome of arthroplasty is altered. There are two categories of surgical options that should be considered successively.

Restorative procedures are dependent on the patient's axonal regeneration potential; always limited in older patients, offering a result that is often modest but useful; and also inferior to spontaneous recovery. These procedures must be proposed early to be effective, but not too early to avoid hindering spontaneous recovery that would provide a better outcome.

Palliative procedures are considered later in the process when the patient has completed neurological recovery based on the compensatory mechanisms and tolerance of the deficit. These include tendon transfers or GH arthrodesis.

Neurological Procedures

Restorative neurological procedures have limitations. The neurological lesion must be identified and surgically accessible. Beyond these technical challenges, these procedures have two limiting factors previously considered[27,28]: first, **the capacity for axonal regeneration** directly linked to the age of the patient, and second, the **receptiveness of the muscle to innervation**, directly linked to the timing of management (ideally before 6 months).

Neurolysis, Nerve Repair, and Grafting

By releasing compression on the nerve, neurolysis promotes axonal flow, limiting Wallerian degeneration and promoting axonal regeneration in the event of neurotmesis. Direct nerve repair, which in theory is the most suitable, requires precise knowledge of the area of injury and whether it is surgically accessible. Ideally, it is performed within 3 weeks in order to avoid nerve retraction as well as an intercalated nerve graft, which would compromise the outcome.[21,28] Repair is reserved for intraoperative iatrogenic events with a clear corresponding deficit, the mechanism of injury being direct (eg, frank nerve section or severe crushing injury). At the slightest suspicion about the quality of the proximal nerve segment and if the patient has the correct axonal regeneration potential, it will be more reproducible to proceed directly with nerve transfer.

Nerve Transfer

Nerve transfers utilize the motor innervation of a healthy muscle to reinnervate another paralyzed muscle. They have been developed in recent years,[29] initially for proximal palsies, particularly of the brachial plexus. This technique has several advantages: it uses donor nerves of known quality, can compensate for the loss of nerve substance, and allows the neurotization to be as close as possible to the effector, optimizing the capacity for muscle reinnervation.[30] Garg et al[18] have very clearly shown the superiority of nerve transfers over grafts for shoulder reanimation with 74% successful results (BMRC > 4) compared with 46%, respectively. These techniques do not exclude the potential for axonal regeneration and muscle receptiveness. These techniques can be used for palsies after shoulder arthroplasty with certain restrictions[31] based on the reduced axonal regeneration capacity of this population and the local surgical conditions complicating the procedure. In summary, it seems desirable in our opinion to consider the transfers according to their targets.

Nerve Transfer for Rotator Cuff Reinnervation

These transfers are rarely used in this clinical setting since most of the time following arthroplasty neurological lesions of the suprascapular nerve are extremely distal and not amenable to nerve transfer. In fact, the suprascapular nerve can be identified only after its emergence from the superior trunk. Its distal segment will be intact only in very proximal lesions of the brachial plexus. Finally, the indications for neurotization of the suprascapular nerve will only be in those plexus injuries that have not recovered. The only nerve transfer that can actually be used is the accessory nerve to the suprascapular nerve. However, the results are still limited, potentially providing only GH stabilization.

Nerve Transfer for Deltoid Reinnervation

Nerve transfers to reinnervate the deltoid are more commonly utilized because, in the absence of deltoid, the function of the shoulder is compromised and the restoration of even slight muscle contraction improves the functional outcome considerably. The main nerve transfer applicable for this deficit is that of the branches of the radial nerve destined for the triceps (medial, lateral, or long head) to the AN. This transfer is all the more interesting as it allows neurotization on the AN very close to the effector. Moreover, it has a very limited impact on the donor site, as the extension of the elbow is only

very partially weakened, and is of little use in the case of shoulder paralysis. This transfer is performed through a posterior approach, which is devoid of any previous surgical procedure. The only prerequisite is the integrity of the innervation of the triceps, which must be confirmed. This transfer can therefore only be considered in cases of isolated shoulder palsy (**FIGURE 39.3**). Injury to the brachial plexus affecting C7 or the posterior trunk, which in turn affects the radial nerve, is a contraindication.

Other nerve transfers can be used to reinnervate the deltoid such as the medial nerve of pectoralis major or the intercostal nerves, but they have almost no indication in this context. Apart from being technically challenging to perform on a previously operated shoulder, they require an intact AN as soon as it emerges from the posterior trunk and are very distant from the deltoid target to be performed without an intercalary graft.

Tendon Transfers

The principle of tendon transfers is to use a functional muscle to restore deficient function. Widely used in the hand and the elbow, tendon transfers are utilized less commonly in the shoulder because function is reserved not only for a muscle but rather to a group. Morphologically, the shoulder muscles have tendon blades rather than true tendons, which makes transfer more difficult. Finally, as shown in **FIGURE 39.4** is the mechanical performance (force and course) of the various shoulder muscles proposed by Herzberg et al,[32] the deltoid muscle performs much better than any other muscle that can be transferred to replace it. Furthermore, normal shoulder function requires the coordinated activation of muscles that will be difficult to replace by a single transfer. For this reason, tendon transfers will only be indicated following RTSA in which the main objective of the treatment of a neurological complication is to restore a deficient basic function. This may involve external rotation or abduction or more simply stabilization of the GH joint to allow some scapulothoracic compensation. In some cases, tendon transfers will have more limited objectives such as avoiding implant dislocation.

Unlike nerve transfers, tendon transfers are not dependent on the time of treatment, but they must comply with certain rules. The transferred muscle must be at least rated at 4 according to the BMRC rating, the axis of its fibers must be parallel to that of the function to be restored, and the passive range of motion of the joint must be sufficient. There is a paucity of the literature on the subject, which is explained by the fact that motor deficits in the shoulder after arthroplasty are relatively well tolerated and compensated for. Moreover, a weak deltoid is not always incompatible with the functioning of an RTSA. Lädermann et al[33] reported a series of 50

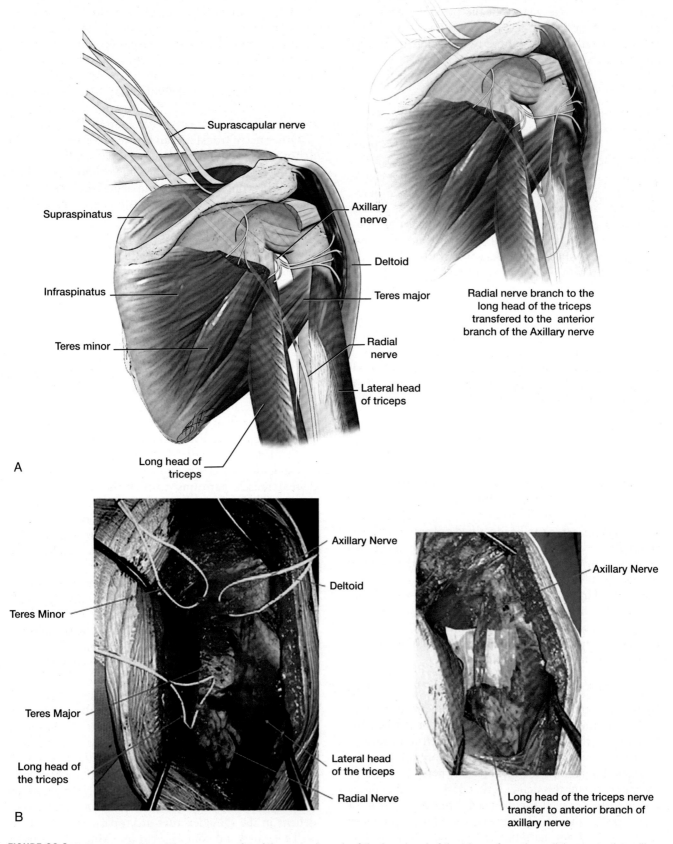

FIGURE 39.3 A, Representation of the nerve transfer of the motor branch of the long head of the triceps from the radial nerve to the axillary nerve. This is a posterior approach to a right shoulder with a schematic representation and intraoperative views (**B**) before and after the transfer with the long and lateral heads of the triceps having been separated.

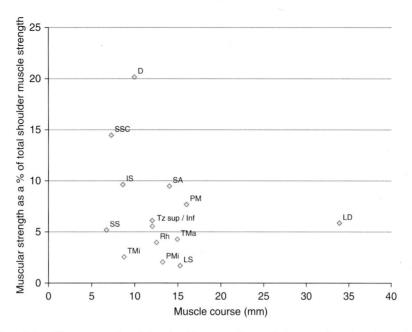

FIGURE 39.4 Representation of the different muscles of the shoulder according to their strength and stroke as described by Herzberg. The deltoid is the most powerful muscle and is difficult to substitute for by the transfer of another muscle. D, deltoid; IS, infraspinatus; LD, latissimus dorsi; LS, levator scapula; PM, pectoralis major; PMi, pectoralis minor; Rh, rhomboid; SA, serratus anterior; SSC, subscapularis; SS, supraspinatus; TMi, teres minor; Tz, trapezius.

RTSAs with a deficient deltoid whose results were satisfactory (mean flexion of more than 120° and mean Constant score of 58). These results demonstrate that a weak deltoid is compatible with reasonable function after RTSA.

Arthrodesis

The final option is to stabilize the GH joint by arthrodesis to allow some compensation by scapulothoracic mobility. It is unusual to consider this option since the joint is usually stiff and arthrodesis is necessary only when the prosthesis is unstable and painful. Beyond the shoulder, arthrodesis allows the elbow to be flexed more, making it easier to position the hand in space. Technically, this procedure is challenging, as it must compensate for a significant loss of bone after the implant has been removed. We use, in addition to a corticocancellous graft, a fibular strut graft embedded in the humeral diaphysis and passed through the acromioglenoid space (**FIGURE 39.5**). The fibular strut graft provides primary stability and fills the loss of substance and provides a rigid fixation point for osteosynthesis. The fibular embedding facilitates the positioning of the arthrodesis with 30° of flexion and abduction and 20° to 30° of internal rotation. Osteosynthesis is performed with plate and screw fixation. The construct must be protected for several months, as achieving a fusion requires a long time. The results are comparable with those obtained with primary arthrodesis.

CLINICAL SUBTYPES AND THEIR MANAGEMENT

Generally, there are two main clinical subtypes, plexus and truncal paralysis, the most problematic being that of the AN.

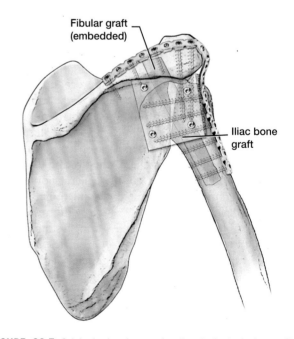

FIGURE 39.5 Original glenohumeral arthrodesis technique after shoulder arthroplasty. Use of a fibula embedded in the space between the acromion, scapula, glenoid, clavicle, and the humeral shaft. Addition of a corticocancellous graft posteriorly with screw fixation. Osteosynthesis of the construct with plate and screws.

Brachial Plexus Palsy

The incidence of brachial plexus injuries varies greatly across studies, depending on whether one considers immediate postoperative deficits that often rapidly recover or only those that persist. This is evident in two publications on the subject. Lynch et al[1] reported an incidence of almost 70%, whereas more recently, Kim et al[19] reported only 6%, when considering persistent deficits only. These palsies result in a sensory-motor deficit involving the roots or truncular system. Secondary to a traction mechanism, it is generally a neurapraxia, rarely an axonotmesis, and is generally of good prognosis.

Persistent deficits usually involve the most proximal C5, C6, or even C7 nerve roots or trunks, as they are more vertical. The distinction between a combined plexus and truncular nerve injury is important, because in the latter a direct nerve injury is possible. A plexus injury is often characterized in the initial phase by a deficit of the whole upper limb with dysesthesias in the hand and asynchronous recovery.

The protocol for monitoring recovery should be structured. It requires thorough monthly comparative sensitivity-motor testing and, at the slightest doubt, an ENMG to assess the first signs of reinnervation. The recovery phase must be followed closely so as not to miss the opportunity for successful nerve restorative surgery. With regard to proximal injuries, various authors[15] report recovery within 6 months in more than 90% of cases. The absence of signs of reinnervation within 6 months is a poor prognosis and should be discussed if the patient's age supports consideration of a nerve transfer procedure. In these patients there may be an associated elbow flexion deficit, the management of which is prioritized over that of the shoulder because in the absence of elbow flexion, the upper limb is dysfunctional. For plexus palsy, neurological procedures include double transfers of the accessory nerve to the suprascapular nerve and the branch to the long or lateral head of the triceps to the AN. For elbow flexion, if necessary, some fascicles of the ulnar nerve can be transferred to the musculocutaneous nerve according to the technique described by Oberlin et al.[34] In the general population, these transfers provide almost 70% functionally satisfactory results.[24,35-37] In elderly patients, the results are less predictable,[25,38-40] with most requiring a simple stabilization of the shoulder, which is often sufficient.

In the rare situation when the deficits of the shoulder are major and particularly disabling, GH arthrodesis becomes essential to allow for scapulothoracic compensation. In case of failure of a nerve transfer, and in the presence of an unstable painful shoulder, tendon transfers are generally impossible owing to the lack of transferable muscles. It will then be necessary to opt for a procedure to stabilize the GH joint by arthrodesis or, as proposed by Elkwood et al,[41] a stabilizing transfer from the upper and middle trapezius to the deltoid using the technique described by Bateman et al.[42]

Axillary Nerve Palsy

The AN is involved in almost 50% of neurological complications, and more than 40% are isolated deficits.[19] Paralysis of the deltoid has a considerable impact on shoulder function, particularly following RTSA. The consequences of this deficit are less serious following anatomical total shoulder arthroplasty (ATSA) with an intact rotator cuff. The injury mechanism is highly variable, ranging from simple traction causing a neurapraxia to more significant direct intraoperative injuries that do not recover.

Diagnosis may be delayed owing to postoperative muscle injury and the use of analgesic anesthetic blocks. The initial injury assessment based on sensory-motor testing is fundamental to distinguishing between isolated forms of AN deficit and combined forms with brachial plexus injury.

In the case of isolated AN, an intraoperative event or a postoperative compression factor (eg, hematoma) requiring rapid surgical treatment must be eliminated. Acute measures to prevent additional sequelae including dislocation and stiffness should be initiated.

The structured monthly follow-up protocol is started. At 1 month, the ENMG should confirm the isolated nature of the AN paralysis and provide an early indication of prognosis. At 4 months, a precise ENMG evaluation is considered important, because in the absence of signs of reinnervation a neurological procedure must be performed before the sixth month.

In general, AN paralysis due to reasons other than an iatrogenic section recovers spontaneously in more than 80% of cases within 2 to 8 months, depending on the type of injury.[14,19] These are also the injuries for which neurological procedures, particularly nerve transfers, are the most effective. Moreover, compensation mechanisms are important since even a weak deltoid is not strictly incompatible with the limited function of an RTSA, as well as an ATSA.[43] Therefore, in this type of lesion it is essential to closely monitor neurological recovery and, in the absence of signs of recovery at 4 to 6 months, propose a nerve transfer procedure, specifically a branch of the radial nerve to the AN, because even in elderly patients this technique allows a useful result to be obtained (BMRC > 3) provided it is performed early when the muscle is still very receptive.[26] A tendon transfer will only be considered as a second step in case of failure of recovery and in the absence of adequate compensation.

Radial to Axillary Nerve Transfer

This transfer was described by Leechavengvongs et al[24,37] for use in cases of brachial plexus paralysis and has been shown to provide better results than conventional grafts,[21,30,44] because the transferred nerve fascicles are mainly motor and healthy and the neurotization is performed as close as possible to the effector. In the literature, there have been no reports describing neurological procedures performed following AN paralysis after TSA, but in the context of isolated AN paralysis in over 50 subjects, nerve transfers seem to be superior.[45] The approach required for TSA is not difficult because the transfer approach is posterior in a surgically healthy area. The nerve branch to the long head of the triceps, or even the medial or lateral head, may be used depending on local conditions.

After protective immobilization for 3 weeks, rehabilitation can be resumed while waiting for the first signs of clinical reinnervation (muscle contraction BMRC > 2), which begins on average between 6 and 8 months[24] and marks the beginning of its intensification.

Tendon Transfer

Tendon transfers are considered only after at least 8 months and only as a remedy in cases of contraindications or failure of a neurological procedure. Three main situations may be encountered: (1) inefficiency of compensatory mechanisms, (2) implant instability often with permanent inferior subluxation, and (3) a deficit in a particular component of mobility of the shoulder such as external rotation. Several tendon transfers have been described to address these issues.

Deltoid Reanimation Transfer

Transfer of the latissimus dorsi entirely in place of the deltoid as described by Itoh et al[46] is a very theoretical indication, but no cases have been reported following arthroplasty. The transfer of the upper trapezius to the deltoid described by Bateman et al[42] **(FIGURE 39.6)** is effective because of the direction of its fibers in the event of inferior shoulder subluxation,[41] but this procedure also has not been reported for use in the context of shoulder arthroplasty. Only the pedicled pectoralis major transfer has been used following arthroplasty. Elhassan et al[47,48] reported a large series of pectoralis major transfers performed in one stage for arthroplasty in association with deltoid paralysis with satisfactory results. In their series, they sometimes combined this transfer with that of the latissimus dorsi or lower trapezius to restore external rotation. However, no cases have been reported following arthroplasty complicated by deltoid palsy. This transfer performed secondarily appears to be technically more difficult, since the muscle is transferred in its entirety with a reversal on its pedicle.

Glenohumeral Fusion

The principle is to stabilize the GH joint to allow compensation by the intact scapulothoracic musculature. A GH arthrodesis enhances the mobility and strength of the scapulothoracic articulation and also of the elbow, allowing better positioning of the hand in space. Fusion will be indicated in the case of very deficient shoulder function without effective compensation, and especially in the case of severe pain or associated instability. This is a demanding procedure with a lengthy rehabilitation; hence, the indication will have to be carefully considered and thoroughly discussed with the patient.

Radial Nerve

Isolated paralysis of the radial nerve accounts for 15% of nerve complications.[19] It is often linked to an injury along the humeral groove during an intraoperative fracture or cement extravasation in revision cases.[8] When this deficit is identified in the immediate postoperative period, it is important to explore the nerve to increase the chance of recovery.[20] In the case of confirmed radial nerve palsy and a nonrepairable injury in this elderly population, in the absence of recovery, one must not delay too long before proceeding with palliative procedures. It is recommended to perform tendon transfers within the first year after the injury. Tendon transfer procedures will restore extension of the wrist and fingers. Extension of the elbow is often preserved because the branches to the triceps are proximal to the point of entry into the humeral sulcus.

Suprascapular Nerve Palsy

Accounting for approximately 5% of cases, isolated lesions of the suprascapular nerve are rare.[19] They are most often related to material protrusion into the suprascapular notch or, more frequently, into the spinoglenoid notch, usually as a result of the fixation screws of the RTSA glenoid base plate. This injury could explain certain deficits in external rotation and residual posterior pain phenomena. There are only a few indications for surgical exploration, as these areas are difficult to access. Exceptions are the need for surgical revision of the implant based on malposition or excessive screw length, which should be documented radiographically before proceeding. In theory, a secondary transfer of the lower trapezius or latissimus dorsi to restore external rotation could be discussed, but to our knowledge, no cases have been reported on this subject. Sometimes the deficit of the suprascapular nerve coexists in more proximal plexus involvement reaching the C5C6 roots, as described above.

Musculocutaneous Nerve Palsy

Injury to the musculocutaneous nerve is relatively infrequent and has two subtypes. The first is a global injury of plexus origin with a generally good prognosis for recovery. The second is a localized injury linked to compression from retraction of the coracobrachialis. The distinction between the two clinical subtypes is quite

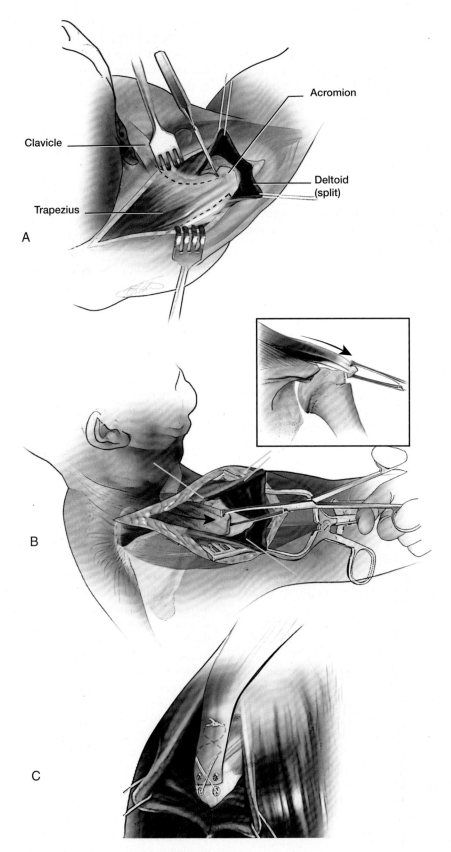

FIGURE 39.6 A-C, Transfer of the upper trapezius to the humerus for the treatment of deltoid paralysis.

straightforward with careful motor-sensory testing. The procedure for monitoring recovery is the same as described above. The 6-month period without signs of recovery is applicable as for all other plexus or truncal injuries. For plexus injury, the procedure to follow is the same as described above. For localized isolated injury to the musculocutaneous nerve, a nerve transfer using a few ulnar nerve fascicles has been described by Oberlin et al.[49] This unique nerve transfer procedure could be considered after having carefully evaluated the potential for compensation. In fact, in these isolated deficits, the brachioradialis remains functional and often allows sufficient compensatory elbow flexion in an elderly patient.

In the absence of recovery, a tendon transfer may be considered to restore elbow flexion. In the case of a C5C6-type deficit, a Steindler-type procedure with osteotomy of the medial epicondyle and fixation to the anterior surface of the humerus will optimize the compensation mechanisms. Alternatively, a transfer from the triceps to the biceps will restore flexion of the elbow.

HOW TO AVOID NEUROLOGICAL COMPLICATIONS?

The adage "prevention is better than cure" absolutely applies to neurological complications after arthroplasty because the results to be expected after nerve repair, transfer, or palliative treatment are satisfactory but not excellent. All procedures discussed in this chapter can be avoided primarily by identifying high-risk situations. There is no single preventive practice, but rather there is a succession of precautions and practices that should be applied when performing shoulder arthroplasty, especially in at-risk patients (**FIGURE 39.7**). Certain preoperative situations increase the risk, such as female patients independent of body habitus, inflammatory pathologies such as juvenile polyarthritis, and ongoing methotrexate therapy. Arthroplasty performed for osteoarthritis with significant limitation of external rotation also presents a higher risk.

The risk is clearly increased in revision and primary RTSA, particularly if the humerus is lengthened by more than 2 cm. During the operation, certain parts of the procedure are particularly at risk for jeopardizing neurological structures. For example, exposure using a short deltopectoral approach will require more forceful retraction. Bladed retractors on the coracobrachialis may cause compression of the musculocutaneous nerve. During preparation of the humerus, the position of extension and external rotation stretches the nerves, especially when the patient is in a very supine position. Before sectioning the subscapularis muscle, it is important to identify the location of the AN by palpation (the only exception to the no touch rule for nerves), and some even suggest visualizing it during revisions.

Exposure of the glenoid is also a critical step for the AN, especially if the humerus is contracted in an adduction-internal rotation position. This brings the nerve and the capsule closer together and increases the tension on the nerve. This position also places the radial nerve at risk. It is crucial to be mindful of any hazardous movements beyond 45° of external rotation that may jeopardize nerve structures, particularly when combined with extension. From a technical perspective, excessive length of the glenoid baseplate screws can be problematic, especially in the anterior and posterior superior quadrants.

SUMMARY

With an incidence of less than 5%, neurological complications following shoulder arthroplasty are probably underestimated, as the vast majority recover spontaneously. The primary mechanism of injury is stretching and rarely that of direct neurological injury. A distinction is made between global forms of injury—brachial plexus palsies, which generally have a good prognosis—and truncular forms mainly affecting the axillary nerve. Management of the latter is generally more complex owing to the older age of most patients resulting in poorer prognosis for nerve regeneration.

The goal of this chapter is to review the various nerve injury subtypes, evaluate their severity and prognosis, and, above all, propose a therapeutic strategy applicable to the patients, who are most commonly older, in the specific context of shoulder arthroplasty. Faced with this type of complication, a relatively standardized decision-making algorithm can be followed.

Initially, a precise injury assessment is essential to establish a prognosis for recovery. Apart from the obvious direct surgical events requiring a rapid reintervention, the first few months require a precise diagnostic evaluation and, above all, close monitoring for possible spontaneous recovery. In the absence of signs of recovery after 4 to 6 months, the shared decision-making process should not be delayed as early reinnervation is key to avoid muscle atrophy and loss of reinnervation potential. Nerve transfers using healthy motor fascicles close to the muscle effector are generally preferred, depending largely on the nerve regeneration potential related to the patient's age and nicotine dependence.

Beyond this period or after failure of neurological procedures, the extent of the functional deficit and the compensation mechanisms will be reevaluated. In the absence of compensatory recovery, palliative procedures such as tendon transfer or glenohumeral arthrodesis will be considered. Prevention of this complication is essential and requires an up-to-date knowledge of the procedure and the situations that place the neurological structures at risk.

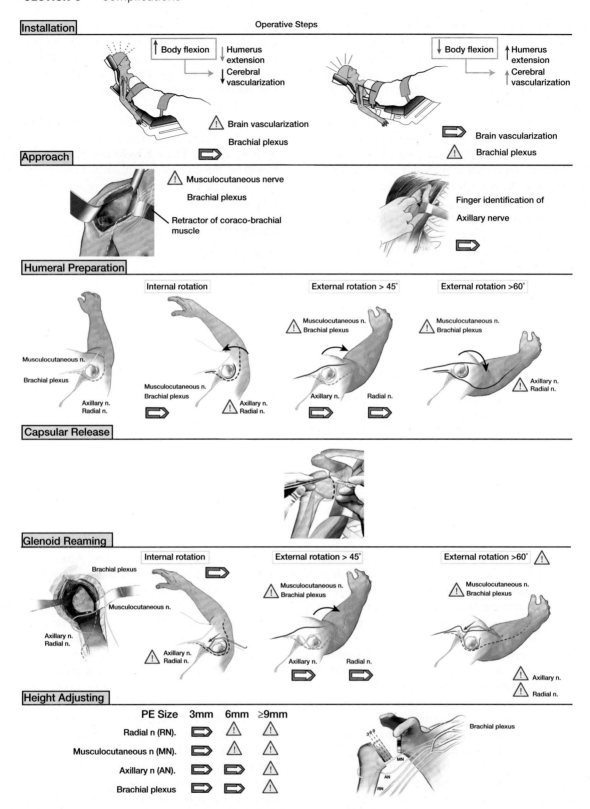

FIGURE 39.7 This illustration shows the different stages of a shoulder arthroplasty and the specific risk factors for nerve damage at each stage of the procedure. When a nerve is at risk it is represented by the sign indicating danger (triangle and exclamation mark); the use of the horizontal arrow indicates that the structure is not particularly at risk. When positioning the patient, a more upright body position decreases cerebral vascularization but protects the neurological structures, especially the brachial plexus, by reducing the amount of extension of the humerus necessary for exposure. During the approach, identifying the axillary nerve by palpation seems to be a prudent option. This nerve is also at risk during capsular release. During exposure of the humerus and during glenoid exposure, significant internal rotation increases tension on the axillary and radial nerves, while external rotation beyond 45° places tension on the brachial plexus and the musculocutaneous nerve and external rotation beyond 60° places all the neurological structures under tension. Finally, the distalization of the humerus also presents a situation that influences the tension of the neurological structures based on the amount of displacement.

REFERENCES

1. Lynch NM, Cofield RH, Silbert PL, Hermann RC. Neurologic complications after total shoulder arthroplasty. *J Shoulder Elbow Surg.* 1996;5(1):53-61.
2. Leschinger T, Hackl M, Buess E, et al. The risk of suprascapular and axillary nerve injury in reverse total shoulder arthroplasty: an anatomic study. *Injury.* 2017;48(10):2042-2049.
3. Apaydin N, Uz A, Bozkurt M, Elhan A. The anatomic relationships of the axillary nerve and surgical landmarks for its localization from the anterior aspect of the shoulder: axillary nerve and surgical landmarks. *Clin Anat.* 2007;20(3):273-277.
4. Lädermann A, Stimec BV, Denard PJ, Cunningham G, Collin P, Fasel JHD. Injury to the axillary nerve after reverse shoulder arthroplasty: an anatomical study. *Orthop Traumatol Surg Res.* 2014;100(1):105-108.
5. Burkhead WZ, Scheinberg RR, Box G. Surgical anatomy of the axillary nerve. *J Shoulder Elbow Surg.* 1992;1(1):31-36.
6. Gates S, Sager B, Collett G, Chhabra A, Khazzam M. Surgically relevant anatomy of the axillary and radial nerves in relation to the latissimus dorsi tendon in variable shoulder positions: a cadaveric study. *Shoulder Elbow.* 2020;12(1):24-30.
7. Fu MC, Hendel MD, Chen X, Warren RF, Dines DM, Gulotta LV. Surgical anatomy of the radial nerve in the deltopectoral approach for revision shoulder arthroplasty and periprosthetic fracture fixation: a cadaveric study. *J Shoulder Elbow Surg.* 2017;26(12):2173-2176.
8. Bassora R, Namdari S, Beharrie AW, Inzerillo VC, Abboud JA. Late-onset radial nerve palsy after closed treatment of a periprosthetic humerus fracture: a case report. *JBJS Case Connect.* 2020;10(1):e0510.
9. Seddon HJ. Classification of nerve injuries. *Br Med J.* 1942;2:237-239.
10. Sunderland S. *Nerves and Nerve Injuries.* 2nd ed. Churchill Livingstone; 1978.
11. Wood MD, Johnson PH, Myckatyn TM. Anatomy and physiology for the peripheral nerve surgeon. In: Mackinnon SE, ed. *Nerve Surgery.* Thieme Medical; 2015.
12. Nagda SH, Rogers KJ, Sestokas AK, et al. Neer Award 2005: peripheral nerve function during shoulder arthroplasty using intraoperative nerve monitoring. *J Shoulder Elbow Surg.* 2007;16(3):S2-S8.
13. Shinagawa S, Shitara H, Yamamoto A, et al. Intraoperative neuromonitoring during reverse shoulder arthroplasty. *J Shoulder Elbow Surg.* 2019;28(8):1617-1625.
14. Lenoir H, Dagneaux L, Canovas F, Waitzenegger T, Pham TT, Chammas M. Nerve stress during reverse total shoulder arthroplasty: a cadaveric study. *J Shoulder Elbow Surg.* 2017;26(2):323-330.
15. Ball CM. Neurologic complications of shoulder joint replacement. *J Shoulder Elbow Surg.* 2017;26(12):2125-2132.
16. Bois AJ, Knight P, Alhojailan K, Bohsali KI. Clinical outcomes and complications of reverse shoulder arthroplasty used for failed prior shoulder surgery: a systematic review and meta-analysis. *JSES Int.* 2020;4(1):156-168.
17. Lädermann A, Lübbeke A, Mélis B, et al. Prevalence of neurologic lesions after total shoulder arthroplasty. *J Bone Joint Surg Am.* 2011;93(14):1288-1293.
18. Walton M, Makki D, Brookes-Fazakerley S. Complications of shoulder arthroplasty. In: Trail IA, Funk L, Rangan A, Nixon M, eds. *Textbook of Shoulder Surgery.* [Internet]. Springer International Publishing; 2019:367-381. http://link.springer.com/10.1007/978-3-319-70099-1_23
19. Kim HJ, Kwon TY, Jeon YS, Kang SG, Rhee YG, Rhee S-M. Neurologic deficit after reverse total shoulder arthroplasty: correlation with distalization. *J Shoulder Elbow Surg.* 2020;29:1096-1103.
20. Lee JS, Kim JY, Jung H-J, Jung H-S, Baek J-H. Radial nerve recovery after thermal injury due to extruded cement during humeral revision in total elbow arthroplasty. *J Shoulder Elbow Surg.* 2013;22(12):e23-e25.
21. Wolfe SW, Johnsen PH, Lee SK, Feinberg JH. Long-nerve grafts and nerve transfers demonstrate comparable outcomes for axillary nerve injuries. *J Hand Surg.* 2014;39(7):1351-1357.
22. Desai MJ, Daly CA, Seiler JG, Wray WH, Ruch DS, Leversedge FJ. Radial to axillary nerve transfers: a combined case series. *J Hand Surg.* 2016;41(12):1128-1134.
23. Miyamoto H, Leechavengvongs S, Atik T, Facca S, Liverneaux P. Nerve transfer to the deltoid muscle using the nerve to the long head of the triceps with the da Vinci Robot: six cases. *J Reconstr Microsurg.* 2014;30(06):375-380.
24. Leechavengvongs S, Witoonchart K, Uerpairojkit C, Thuvasethakul P. Nerve transfer to deltoid muscle using the nerve to the long head of the triceps, part II: a report of 7 cases. *J Hand Surg.* 2003;28(4):633-638.
25. Bertelli JA, Ghizoni MF. Reconstruction of C5 and C6 brachial plexus avulsion injury by multiple nerve transfers: spinal accessory to suprascapular, ulnar fascicles to biceps branch, and triceps long or lateral head branch to axillary nerve. *J Hand Surg.* 2004;29(1):131-139.
26. Gillis JA, Khouri JS, Kircher MF, Spinner RJ, Bishop AT, Shin AY. Outcomes of shoulder abduction after nerve surgery in patients over 50 years following traumatic brachial plexus injury. *J Plast Reconstr Aesthet Surg.* 2019;72(1):12-19.
27. Terzis JK, Barmpitsioti A. Axillary nerve reconstruction in 176 posttraumatic plexopathy patients. *Plast Reconstr Surg.* 2010;125(1):233-247.
28. Bonnard C, Anastakis D, Van Melle G, Narakas A. Isolated and combined lesions of the axillary nerve. A review of 146 cases. *J Bone Joint Surg Br.* 1999;81(2):212-217.
29. Garg R, Merrell GA, Hillstrom HJ, Wolfe SW. Comparison of nerve transfers and nerve grafting for traumatic upper plexus palsy: a systematic review and analysis. *J Bone Joint Surg Am.* 2011;93(9):819-829.
30. Koshy JC, Agrawal NA, Seruya M. Nerve transfer versus interpositional nerve graft reconstruction for posttraumatic, isolated axillary nerve injuries: a systematic review. *Plast Reconstr Surg.* 2017;140(5):953-960.
31. Salazar DH, Chalmers PN, Mackinnon SE, Keener JD. Reverse shoulder arthroplasty after radial-to-axillary nerve transfer for axillary nerve palsy with concomitant irreparable rotator cuff tear. *J Shoulder Elbow Surg.* 2017;26(1):e23-e28.
32. Herzberg G, Urien JP, Dimnet J. Potential excursion and relative tension of muscles in the shoulder girdle: relevance to tendon transfers. *J Shoulder Elbow Surg.* 1999;8(5):430-437.
33. Lädermann A, Walch G, Denard PJ, et al. Reverse shoulder arthroplasty in patients with pre-operative impairment of the deltoid muscle. *Bone Joint J.* 2013;95-B(8):1106-1113.
34. Oberlin C, Béal D, Leechavengvongs S, Salon A, Dauge MC, Sarcy JJ. Nerve transfer to biceps muscle using a part of ulnar nerve for C5-C6 avulsion of the brachial plexus: anatomical study and report of four cases. *J Hand Surg.* 1994;19(2):232-237.
35. Teboul F, Kakkar R, Ameur N, Beaulieu J-Y, Oberlin C. Transfer of fascicles from the ulnar nerve to the nerve to the biceps in the treatment of upper brachial plexus palsy. *J Bone Joint Surg Am.* 2004;86(7):1485-1490.
36. Bertelli JA, Ghizoni MF. Results of spinal accessory to suprascapular nerve transfer in 110 patients with complete palsy of the brachial plexus. *J Neurosurg Spine.* 2016;24(6):990-995.
37. Leechavengvongs S, Malungpaishorpe K, Uerpairojkit C, Ng CY, Witoonchart K. Nerve transfers to restore shoulder function. *Hand Clin.* 2016;32(2):153-164.
38. Xiao F, Zhao X, Lao J. Comparative study of single and dual nerve transfers for repairing shoulder abduction. *Acta Neurochir (Wien).* 2019;161(4):673-678.
39. Texakalidis P, Tora MS, Lamanna JJ, Wetzel J, Boulis NM. Combined radial to axillary and spinal accessory nerve (SAN) to suprascapular nerve (SSN) transfers may confer superior shoulder abduction compared with single SA to SSN transfer. *World Neurosurg.* 2019;126:e1251-e1256.
40. Leechavengvongs S, Witoonchart K, Uerpairojkit C, Thuvasethakul P, Malungpaishrope K. Combined nerve transfers for C5 and C6 brachial plexus avulsion injury. *J Hand Surg.* 2006;31(2):183-189.
41. Elkwood A, Rose M, Kaufman M, et al. Shoulder subluxation pain as a secondary indication for trapezius to deltoid transfer. *J Brachial Plex Peripher Nerve Inj.* 2018;13(01):e20-e23.

42. Bateman JE. Transplant of the trapezius for aductor paralysis of the shoulder. *J Bone Joint Surg Br.* 1948;30B(1):221.

43. Kermarrec G, Werthel JD, Canales P, Valenti P. Review and clinical presentation in reverse shoulder arthroplasty in deltoid palsy. *Eur J Orthop Surg Traumatol.* 2018;28(4):747-751.

44. Hardcastle N, Texakalidis P, Nagarajan P, Tora MS, Boulis NM. Recovery of shoulder abduction in traumatic brachial plexus palsy: a systematic review and meta-analysis of nerve transfer versus nerve graft. *Neurosurg Rev.* 2019;43:951-956. http://link.springer.com/10.1007/s10143-019-01100-9

45. Willis CB, Ahmadi S. Radial-to-axillary nerve transfer resolves symptoms of axillary nerve injury due to proximal humerus fracture-dislocation in an elderly patient treated with hemiarthroplasty. *Orthopedics.* 2019;42(4):e395-e398.

46. Itoh Y, Sasaki T, Ishiguro T, Uchinishi K, Yabe Y, Fukuda H. Transfer of latissimus dorsi to replace a paralyzed anterior deltoid. A new technique using an inverted pedicled graft. *J Bone Joint Surg Br.* 1987;69(4):647-651.

47. Elhassan BT, Wagner ER, Werthel J-D, Lehanneur M, Lee J. Outcome of reverse shoulder arthroplasty with pedicled pectoralis transfer in patients with deltoid paralysis. *J Shoulder Elbow Surg.* 2018;27(1):96-103.

48. Le Hanneur M, Lee J, Wagner ER, Elhassan BT. Options of bipolar muscle transfers to restore deltoid function: an anatomical study. *Surg Radiol Anat.* 2019;41(8):911-919.

49. Oberlin C, Ameur NE, Teboul F, Beaulieu J-Y, Vacher C. Restoration of elbow flexion in brachial plexus injury by transfer of ulnar nerve fascicles to the nerve to the biceps muscle. *Tech Hand Up Extrem Surg.* 2002;6(2):86-90.

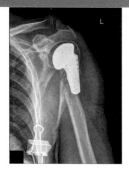

40 Treatment of Periprosthetic Fractures

Leesa M. Galatz, MD, Alexander J. Vervaecke, MD, and Brad Parsons, MD

INTRODUCTION

Periprosthetic shoulder fractures are potentially devastating complications and can present substantial challenges for the treating orthopedic surgeon. Currently considered relatively rare, the increasing use of shoulder arthroplasty in general will ensure a similar rise in the absolute number of complications, making them more common.[1] The periprosthetic fractures may be anatomically located at the humerus or scapula (glenoid, acromion, or coracoid), and a clear distinction is made between an intra- and postoperative occurrence. The scope of this chapter will mainly be focused on periprosthetic humerus fractures and to a lesser extent on periprosthetic glenoid fractures. While the incidences vary widely in the literature, intraoperative humerus fractures are most frequently reported and occur in 1.2% to 6.5% of primary shoulder arthroplasties. Postoperative humerus fractures most often originate from traumatic events, and an incidence between 0.2% and 12.9% is reported.[2] The majority of modifiable risk factors for fractures are directly related to technical errors during surgery such as poor exposure, endosteal notching, and cortical perforation and can therefore potentially be avoided. While multiple classifications systems are present, they are mostly based upon small unvalidated series that somewhat limits their transferability to relevant treatment algorithms. Higher nonunion rates are reported for periprosthetic fractures in comparison to native fractures, and most individuals undergoing shoulder arthroplasty tend to belong to an older and more osteopenic population. Considering the already limited bone stock of the proximal humerus and glenoid vault, these factors further increase treatment difficulties. Intraoperative fractures should be stabilized at the time of the index procedure. Postoperative fractures may require revision surgery but can often be treated nonoperatively. Two important factors have to be assessed when determining optimal treatment: (1) implant stability and (2) fracture stability. Generally, with a stable implant and a stable fracture, nonoperative treatment can be utilized. Unstable fractures at the tip or below the stem will often need to be reduced and fixated as typical diaphyseal humerus fractures. Unstable implants

in combination with periprosthetic fractures warrant implant revision and fracture fixation.

INTRAOPERATIVE INCIDENCE

Fractures are the most frequent intraoperative complications during primary and revision shoulder arthroplasties.[3,4] A single-center retrospective analysis of 2588 total shoulder arthroplasties (TSAs) and 1431 hemiarthroplasties (HAs) performed over 32 years reported intraoperative fractures in 47 (40 humerus, 5 glenoid, 2 unspecified) and 15 (8 humerus, 7 glenoid) cases, respectively.[5] Furthermore, an analysis of the National Joint Registry of England, Wales, Northern Ireland and the Isle of Man (NJR) between 2011 and 2015 reported 315 intraoperative complications in 12,559 primary shoulder arthroplasties, of which the majority were humeral fractures (110 humerus fractures, 87 glenoid fractures).[3] While these results are consistent with other published reports, the incidence is most likely underestimated due to the inherent limitation of database studies that rely on surgeons reporting their complications. Higher incidences are reported in revision arthroplasty procedures. Athwal et al retrospectively analyzed all primary and revision shoulder arthroplasties performed in their center between 1980 and 2002 and found that fractures were more than twice as likely to occur in revision surgery (14 of 422, 3.3%) compared to those in primary arthroplasty (31 of 2666, 1.2%).[6] Additionally, Wagner et al evaluated the medical records of 230 revision procedures performed between 2005 and 2012 and found an incidence of 15.7%.[7] Utilizing the same aforementioned NJR database, Ingoe et al further confirmed this increased risk as fractures occurred in 50 revision cases.[4] Summarized, the intraoperative incidence varies between 1.2% and 15.7% for both primary and revision shoulder arthroplasty **(TABLE 40.1)**.

POSTOPERATIVE INCIDENCE

The incidence of postoperative periprosthetic humeral fractures as reported in the literature is quite variable. Boyd et al identified seven cases with postoperative periprosthetic humeral fractures between 1974 and 1988 resulting in an incidence of 1.6%.[9] Similar results

TABLE 40.1 Summary of Reported Intraoperative Incidences of Periprosthetic Fractures in Both Primary and Revision Shoulder Arthroplasty

Study	Procedure	No. of Arthroplasties	Incidence	Anatomical Location			
				Tuberosities	Metaphysis	Shaft	Multi
1. Athwal et al (2009)[6]	Primary	2666	31 (1.2%)	19	6	16	3
	Revision	422	14 (3.3%)				1
2. Singh et al (2012)[5]	Primary	4019	62 (1.5%)	Unspecified			
	ATSA	2588	47 (1.8%)				
	HA	1431	15 (1.0%)				
3. Atoun et al (2014)[8]	Primary	31	2 (6.5%)	–	2	–	–
4. Wagner et al (2015)[7]	Revision	230	36 (15.7%)	30	3	3	–
5. García-Fernández et al (2015)[14]	Primary	163	2 (1.2%)	–	2	1	–
	Revision	40	1 (2.5%)				
6. Ingoe et al (2017)[4]	Revision	1455	35 (2.4%)	Unspecified			
7. Cowling et al (2017)[3]	Primary	12,599	202 (1.6%)	Unspecified			
	ATSA	3712	52 (1.4%)				
	HA	1928	45 (2.3%)				
	RTSA	4590	103 (2.2%)				
	SL	2329	2 (0.1%)				

Incidence is given as the total number with percentage between parentheses. *ATSA*, anatomic total shoulder arthroplasty; *HA*, hemiarthroplasty; *RTSA*, reverse total shoulder arthroplasty; *SL*, stemless hemiarthroplasty.

were found by Wright et al (1.8%) and Worland et al (2.38%).[10,11] In the study by Singh et al, 43 (36 humerus, 5 glenoid, 2 unspecified) postoperative humeral fractures occurred in 4019 primary shoulder arthroplasties (0.9%).[5] Chin et al reported on only 1 postoperative fracture in 431 patients (0.2%) with a mean follow-up of 4.2 years, whereas Atoun et al reported four fractures in a series of 31 short-stemmed reverse total shoulder arthroplasty (RTSA) implants (12.9%).[8,12] In summary, the postoperative incidence varies between 0.2% and 12.9% **(TABLE 40.2)**.

RISK FACTORS

Intraoperative Risk Factors

Considering that patient characteristics often cannot be altered or modified, identification of the primary risk factors associated with periprosthetic fractures allows the surgeon to apply extra care and consider alternative technical approaches in those patients at high risk. Established unmodifiable risk factors for intraoperative periprosthetic humerus fractures are female gender, a preoperative diagnosis of posttraumatic arthritis or osteonecrosis, and revision arthroplasty. Although no studies were able to directly attribute a higher incidence of intraoperative periprosthetic fractures to osteopenia and osteoporosis, these conditions will certainly

be a factor in the higher relative risk in female patients. Modifiable risk factors are strongly related to the choice of implant, surgical technique, and potential technical errors. The use of press-fit humeral stems showed a relative risk of 2.9× greater than the use of cemented implants **(TABLE 40.3)**.[6] As the endosteal surface at the level of the diaphysis is asymmetrical and elliptical in cross sections, endosteal notching can result from using cylindrical intramedullary reamers and can potentially increase the risk of fractures when inserting the broach or final press-fit implant.[15,16] Cementing the humeral component allows the use of a smaller size implant, and therefore over-reaming can be avoided, thereby reducing the risk of fracture. These results, however, are based on a historical cohort. Between 1980 and 2002, press-fit humeral stems relying on diaphyseal fixation predominated. The introduction of newer stems with metaphyseal fixation and "bony ingrowth" coating potentially mitigating the increased fracture risk associated with the use of press-fit stems.[17] Werthel et al found no difference in both intra- and postoperative fractures between cemented and cementless stems in 4636 primary arthroplasties performed between 1970 up to 2012.[18]

One study reported a lower relative fracture risk with the superior approach compared to that with the deltopectoral approach.[3] The authors hypothesized that this difference was more likely attributable

TABLE 40.2 Summary of Reported Postoperative Incidences of Periprosthetic Fractures in Both Primary and Revision Shoulder Arthroplasty

Study	Procedure	No of Athroplasties	Incidence	Wright and Cofield		
				A	B	C
1. Boyd et al (1992)[9]	Primary	436	7 (1.6%)	Unspecified		
2. Wright et al (1995)[10]	Primary	499	9 (1.8%)	1	5	3
3. Worland et al (1999)[11]	Primary	256	6 (2.3%)	2	3	1
4. Kumar et al (2004)[13]	Primary	3091	19 (0.6%)	6	6	3
5. Chin et al (2006)[12]	Primary	431	1 (0.2%)	Unspecified		
6. Singh et al (2012)[5]	Primary	4019	43 (1.1%)	20 shaft fractures further unspecified		
	ATSA	2588	23 (0.9%)	15 shaft fractures further unspecified		
	HA	1431	18 (1.3%)			
7. Atoun et al (2014)[8]	Primary RTSA	31	4 (12.9%)	4 metaphyseal fractures		
8. García-Fernández et al (2015)[14]	Primary RTSA	203	4 (2.0%)	1	3	–

Incidence is given as the total number with percentage between parentheses. *ATSA*, anatomic total shoulder arthroplasty; *HA*, hemiarthroplasty; *RTSA*, reverse total shoulder arthroplasty.

TABLE 40.3 Summary of Literature on Risk Factors for Intraoperative Periprosthetic Fractures in Both Primary and Revision Shoulder Arthroplasty

Study	Risk Factors	Reference	Quantification of Risk	
			Relative Risk	*P-Value*
1. Athwal et al (2009)[6]	Female	Male	3.3×	0.0006
	Revision	Primary	2.8×	0.003
	Press-fit stem	Cemented	2.9×	0.046
Study	**Risk Factors**	**Reference**	**Quantification of Risk**	
			Odds Ratio and 95% CI	*P-Value*
2. Singh et al (2012)[5]	Female	Male	4.19 (1.82-9.62)	<0.001
	Posttraumatic osteoarthritis	Rheumatoid arthritis	2.55 (0.92-7.12)	0.04
3. Wagner et al (2015)[7]	Female	Male	2.41 (1.11-5.68)	0.03
	Prior instability	No instability	2.65 (1.18-5.93)	0.02
	Prior HA	ATSA	2.34 (1.13-4.84)	0.03

ATSA, anatomic total shoulder arthroplasty; *CI*, confidence interval; *HA*, hemiarthroplasty.

to surgeon differences and the rationale of using the superior approach in less-complicated cases than to the approach itself. Higher incidences of intraoperative fractures were also found for RTSA and stemmed HAs compared to those for anatomical and resurfacing arthroplasties. This trend correlated to a relative risk of 1.4 for RTSA and 1.9 for HA compared to TSA in a multivariable analysis adjusting for age, sex, indication for surgery, and American Society of Anesthesiologists grade. Taking into consideration that the former two implant types will more often be utilized in acute or trauma settings and for patients with a larger inherent risk for fractures, it remains difficult to directly attribute the higher risk solely to the implant type when different implants would have been selected based upon the operative indications.[3] While revision arthroplasty itself is a significant risk factor for intraoperative periprosthetic humeral fractures, subgroup analysis of revision cases showed that female sex, history of prior instability, and prior HA are also risk factors with an odds ratio of 2.41 ($P = 0.03$), 2.65 ($P = 0.02$), and 2.34 ($P = 0.03$), respectively.[7] Interestingly, a history of a prior cemented primary arthroplasty did not significantly increase the risk of intraoperative fractures in this study.

Intraoperative glenoid fractures are related to excessive retraction, reaming, or the glenoid fixation technique. A higher risk is reported in cases with a preexisting unloaded glenoid. This may be the case with rotator cuff–deficient shoulders with superior humeral head migration or after prolonged periods of immobilization. Patients with rheumatoid arthritis, osteoporosis, or rotator cuff arthropathy have relatively soft glenoids in contrast to the sclerotic changes associated with osteoarthritis, and the risk of fracture may be higher in these subgroups.[19]

Postoperative Risk Factors

The comorbidity burden of a patient is a determining factor when assessing for postoperative periprosthetic fracture risk. A strong association has been identified between patients having multiple comorbidities and an increased risk of postoperative fractures.[5] This can be explained due to older, frail patients being at risk of falling, even more so when they undergo polypharmaceutical treatment, which is often present postoperatively. Preexisting osteopenia and rheumatoid arthritis lead to significant bone loss and increase the likelihood of fractures. Burrus et al showed a clear increased fracture risk in shoulder arthroplasties performed in patients for steroid-associated and posttraumatic osteonecrosis.[20] Similar to the intraoperative risk factors, both female gender and endosteal notching are also significant in the postoperative setting. Endosteal notching or asymmetrical intramedullary reaming leads to a cortical thickness mismatch that acts as a "stress riser" with increased susceptibility to fracture after even minor trauma. Of course, cortical perforation or gross shaft compromise during the index procedure also increases the subsequent fracture risk.

Patients with combined ipsilateral elbow and shoulder arthroplasties are of significant concern. The stress riser between the tips of both humeral implants potentially increases the risk of fractures even with minimal trauma.[21,22] Inglis et al hypothesized that in those patients, short-stemmed humeral components should be utilized to preserve a sufficient bony bridge between both the proximal and distal cement mantles or that the bony bridge should be filled with cement to decrease stress concentrations between the ends of the humeral components. Biomechanical modeling, however, showed only a minimal benefit when filling the canal with cement, and no significant correlation was found regarding the length of the bone bridge and stress concentrations.[23] On balance, ipsilateral shoulder and elbow arthroplasties

should avoid the stress riser effect of having two humeral stems that end in close proximity.

MECHANISM OF INJURY

Most intraoperative periprosthetic humeral fractures in primary arthroplasties are the result of technical errors. Achieving adequate exposure can be challenging, and care has to be taken to avoid forceful rotation (especially external rotation) and excessive soft-tissue retraction or generally while applying too much force or torque to the humerus as these are known to increase the risk of fractures.[24] Obtaining adequate soft-tissue releases especially in stiff posttraumatic shoulders or in revision arthroplasty will facilitate exposure and reduce fracture risk. Other possible mechanisms causing fractures are related to canal preparation and implantation. As described, endosteal notching should be avoided when reaming the canal as this can increase the susceptibility for fractures taking place by adding a stress riser. Over-reaming can weaken the endosteal cortex, and inadequate reaming before broaching can cause cortical notching or a diaphyseal fracture especially in patients with weakened osteopenic bone.[25] In addition, using an oversized trial or final implant or performing a reduction in an excessively tight shoulder (primarily with RTSA) can also cause an intraoperative fracture. During revision arthroplasty, most fractures occur during humeral stem removal.[7] Therefore, utilizing a systematic approach with implant specific extraction instruments is required when trying to minimize the fracture risk. Performing a controlled cortical window or a longitudinal osteotomy also facilitates the removal of a well-fixed humeral stem when other implant-bone interface separation methods pose a high fracture risk.[26,27] Intraoperative glenoid fractures may result from retraction, reaming, or the baseplate fixation technique. Similarly to the prevention of periprosthetic humerus fractures, obtaining optimal soft-tissue releases in stiff shoulders is crucial to avoid glenoid injury. The correction of retroversion or inclination of highly deformed glenoids with eccentric reaming may reduce overall glenoid bone stock and lead to glenoid peg perforation or gross fracturing. Furthermore, uncareful removal of glenoid osteophytes can also cause intraoperative glenoid fractures. It is important to identify patients who have an increased risk for glenoid fractures due to soft bone or a reduced bone mineral density and for whom the use of a hand reamer might be preferential to machined reaming.

Postoperative fractures seem to most frequently occur subsequent to a fall on the outstretched upper limb or due to other traumatic events.[24] In select cases, preexisting implant loosening or periprosthetic osteolysis resulting in cortical weakening can be responsible for periprosthetic fractures in the absence of notable trauma.[13,28]

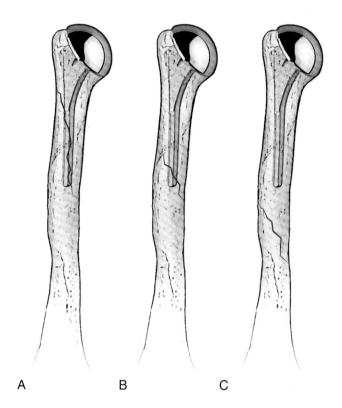

A   B   C

FIGURE 40.1 Wright and Cofield classification for periprosthetic humerus fractures. **A**, Fractures centered at the tip of the stem with proximal extension greater than one-third of the length of the stem. **B**, Fractures centered at the tip of the stem with proximal extension less than one-third of the length of the stem. **C**, Fractures located distal to the tip of the stem.

CLASSIFICATIONS

The first classification of periprosthetic humerus fractures was published in 1995 by Wright and Cofield.[10] In their series of nine patients, they found that the outcome of treatment was related to the fracture configuration and fracture location relative to the tip of the humeral stem. They classified fractures as follows: type A fractures are centered at the tip of the humeral implant and extend proximally (extension greater than one-third of the length the stem); type B fractures remain centered at the tip of the stem; and type C fractures are located distal to the prosthesis (**FIGURE 40.1**). Validation of the classification by Andersen et al showed acceptable intraobserver agreement (mean κ 0.69). However, the interobserver agreement was poor (mean κ 0.37). The Campbell classification, described in 1998, was similarly based upon the most distal extent of the fracture.[29] Region 1 fractures involved the greater or lesser tuberosity; region 2 fractures are located in the metaphyseal region of the proximal humerus; region 3 fractures extend to the proximal diaphysis; and region 4 fractures involve the mid- and distal humeral diaphysis.

In 1999, Worland et al proposed an alternative classification system that utilized the fracture anatomy combined with implant stability.[11] Type A fractures were limited to the region of the tuberosities; type B fractures represent fractures around the stem and are divided as spiral fractures with a stable stem (B1), transverse or short oblique fractures and stable stem (B2), and the presence of an unstable stem (B3); and type C fractures are fractures distal to the implant. Groh also developed a classification system that was very similar to the system described by Wright and Cofield.[30]

The latest and most extensive classification system was developed by Kirchhoff in 2016 and retrospectively validated using the data from 19 patients.[31] Six patients, implant, and fracture factors are utilized to develop a treatment algorithm. First, a distinction is made between stemless (A), anatomic (B), and RTSA (C). Second, the general anatomical location of the fracture is used to differentiate between acromion (A), glenoid (G), and humerus (H) periprosthetic fractures. Third, the stemless and anatomical shoulder arthroplasties are divided into HAs (H) and TSAs (T). Fourth, the functional status of the rotator cuff is described as intact (I) or defective/torn (T). Fifth, the exact humeral fracture location relative to the stem is outlined as being in the region of the tuberosities (1), as a spiral (2) or oblique (3) diaphyseal fracture, or as a fracture distal to the stem (4). For stemless humeral implants, this division is limited to fractures at the tuberosities (1) or distal to the tuberosities (4). Finally, the implant stability is evaluated and noted as stable (S) or loose (L) (**FIGURE 40.2**). In the attempted validation, prior medical records, imaging (CT scans and metal artifact reduction sequence protocol MRI scans), and anatomic and clinical signs of rotator cuff deficiency were assessed to evaluate and score the rotator cuff function. Fracture patterns and radiolucency at the bone-implant interface on standard radiographs and CT scans were used to assess prosthesis stability and loosening. The retrospective analysis of 19 cases by two surgeons showed discrepancies in the scoring of one patient (interrater variability, κ = 0.94). In addition, a poor clinical outcome occurred in only one patient, in which the treatment algorithm was applied.

The available fracture classification systems should be utilized to understand the fracture pattern and the stability of the implant with the goal of developing a treatment plan. These classification systems provide a mechanism for investigators to compare treatment outcomes. The relative limited number of periprosthetic humeral fractures that occur has limited the ability to assess the advantages of one classification system over another. Most important is for each treating orthopedic surgeon to utilize a system they are comfortable with and that provides a basis for treatment.

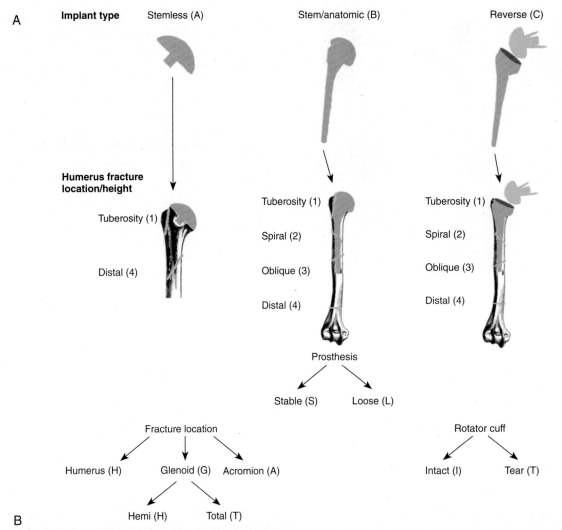

Type	Treatment	Type	Treatment	Type	Treatment
A-A-X-X-X-X	Conservative vs ORIF	B-A-X-X-X-X	Conservative vs ORIF	C-A-X-X	Conservative vs ORIF
A-G-H-I-X-X	Conservative vs ORIF vs TEP	B-G-H-I-X-X	Conservative vs ORIF vs TEP	C-G-X-L	Revision glenoid
A-G-H-T-X-X	Convert to reversed	B-G-H-T-X-X	Convert to reversed	C-H-1-S	Conservative vs ORIF
A-G-T-I-X-S	Conservative	B-G-T-I-X-S	Conservative	C-H-2-S	ORIF
A-G-T-I-X-L	Revise glenoid	B-G-T-I-X-L	Revision glenoid	C-H-3-S	ORIF
A-G-T-T-X-X	Convert to reversed	B-G-T-T-X-X	Convert to reversed	C-H-X-L	Convert to reversed long stem +/- ORIF
A-H-H-I-1-S	ORIF	B-H-H-I-X-S	ORIF		
A-H-H-I-1-L	Convert to anatomic stem	B-H-H-I-X-L	Revise to TEP + new stem		
A-H-H-T-1-L	Convert to reversed	B-H-H-T-X-S	Convert to reversed		
A-H-H-T-4-L	Convert to reversed + ORIF vs reversed long stem	B-H-H-T-1-L	Convert to reversed		
		B-H-H-T-2-L	Convert to reversed + ORIF		
		B-H-H-T-3-L	Convert to reversed + long stem		
		B-H-H-T-4-L	Convert to reversed long stem + ORIF		

FIGURE 40.2 Kirchhoff classification for periprosthetic shoulder fractures.

Type	Localisation	Glenoid	Cuff	Height		Prosthesis	Therapy	
A Stemless	A acromial	H Hemi	I Intact	1 Tuberosities		S stable	A-A-X-X-X-X →	conservative vs. ORIF
	G glenoidal	T Total	T Tear			L loose	A-G-H-I-X-X →	conservative vs. ORIF vs. TEP
	H humeral						A-G-H-T-X-X →	convert to reversed
							A-G-T-I-X-S →	conservative
				4 Distal			A-G-T-I-X-L →	revision glenoid
							A-G-T-T-X-X →	convert to reversed
							A-H-H-I-1-S →	ORIF
							A-H-H-I-1-L →	convert to anatomic stem
							A-H-H-T-1-L →	convert to reversed
							A-H-H-T-4-L →	convert to reversed + ORIF vs. reversed long stem
B Anatomic	A acromial	H Hemi	I Intact	1 Tuberosities		S stable	B-A-X-X-X-X →	conservative vs. ORIF
	G glenoidal	T Total	T Tear	2 Spiral		L loose	B-G-H-I-X-X →	conservative vs. ORIF vs. TEP
	H humeral			3 Oblique			B-G-H-T-X-X →	convert to reversed
				4 Distal			B-G-T-I-X-S →	conservative
							B-G-T-I-X-L →	revision glenoid
							B-G-T-T-X-X →	convert to reversed
							B-H-H-I-X-S →	ORIF
							B-H-H-I-X-L →	revise to TEP + new stem
							B-H-H-T-X-S →	convert to reversed
							B-H-H-T-1-L →	convert to reversed
							B-H-H-T-2-L →	convert to reversed + ORIF
							B-H-H-T-3-L →	convert to reversed + long stem
							B-H-H-T-4-L →	convert to reversed long stem + ORIF
C Reversed	A acromial			1 Tuberosities		S stable	C-A-X-X →	conservative vs. ORIF
	G glenoidal			2 Spiral		L loose	C-G-X-L →	revision glenoid
	H humeral			3 Oblique			C-H-1-S →	conservative vs. ORIF
				4 Distal			C-H-2-S →	ORIF
							C-H-3-S →	ORIF
							C-H-X-L →	convert to reversed long stem vs. convert to reversed long stem + ORIF

FIGURE 40.2, cont'd

TREATMENT

When determining treatment, the main two questions that need to be asked are (1) is the implant stable and (2) is the fracture stable. In addition, the fracture displacement, location, timing (intra- or postoperative), and general alignment as well as patient characteristics such as age, activity level, comorbidities, and bone quality also need to be considered before selecting the optimal treatment strategy.[24,32] Overall goals include achieving fracture union with a stable implant with acceptable recovery of range of motion and function. For intraoperative fractures specifically, preserving the original rehabilitation plan and obtaining a stable construct that allows for immediate motion should be regarded as the main objective whenever possible. Additional treatment for intraoperative fractures is generally not needed for minimally displaced or nondisplaced fractures in satisfactory alignment with a stable implant. Diaphyseal fractures can be treated utilizing the same fixation principles for humeral shaft fractures that occur without the presence of an implant. Periprosthetic humerus fractures in association with a loose humeral stem will often require revision arthroplasty to optimize patient outcomes. In addition, fractures treated nonoperatively with subsequent nonunion or failure of reduction should also be treated operatively if the general health and comorbidity status of the patients allows for a procedure of such magnitude (**FIGURE 40.3**).[32]

Intraoperative Humerus Fractures

Accurate characterization of the location and the extent of the intraoperative fracture is necessary to apply correct treatment principles. Identification and visualization of the fracture can be achieved by using direct exposure after extending the deltopectoral approach or by using intraoperative fluoroscopy.[6] Undisplaced and stable fractures limited to the greater tuberosity can be managed without a significant change of the initial operative plan and without additional specific fixation, provided that the implant is stable and the fracture is not at risk for displacement.[6] Postoperatively, standard rehabilitation programs can be utilized in these cases. However, if any fracture motion or displacement is present, transosseous suture fixation of the fractured tuberosity with nonabsorbable sutures around the humeral implant or cerclage wiring is strongly advisable to prevent the rotator cuff from further displacing the fracture (**FIGURE 40.4**).[33] If an anatomic reduction cannot be achieved or maintained with suture fixation alone, a conversion to a fracture type stem with a metaphyseal porous coating that increases the bony ingrowth potential and that has specific suture fixation

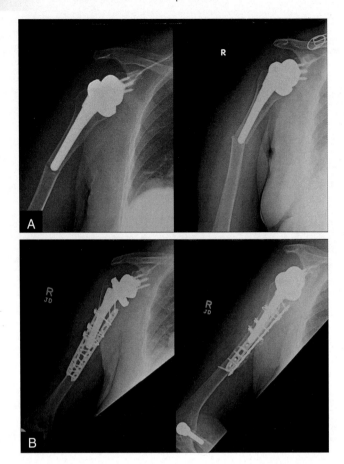

FIGURE 40.3 A 68-year-old woman with postoperative periprosthetic humerus fracture sustained after fall. Nonoperative treatment was initially attempted; however, sequential follow-up revealed worsening of alignment in both the coronal and sagittal plane. On preoperative CT imaging, no signs of stem loosening were present. **A,** Anteroposterior (AP) and lateral views after injury showed a transverse mid-diaphyseal humerus fracture located at the tip of the stem. **B,** AP and lateral views after open reduction and double plate fixation; a combination of both screws and cable constructs was utilized to obtain fracture stability.

sites should be considered. In some cases, with insufficient rigid fixation of the tuberosities and rotator cuff attachment sites, conversion to reverse arthroplasty is also an option depending on the clinical circumstances **(FIGURE 40.5).** Autologous or allograft bone augmentation can be necessary in revision cases with prior tuberosity resorption or in patients with a severely deficient proximal humeral bone stock.

Whenever the tuberosity fracture extends more distally to the proximal humeral shaft, it is recommended to exchange the stem to a long-stemmed humeral implant that extends at least two to three times the length of the cortical diameter past the fracture site.[13,29] In addition, supplemental rigid fixation devices such as cerclage wires, cables, rigid tapes, and/or plate fixation should be used to augment the stability of the construct. Cortical strut allografts are an additional option for providing much-needed construct rigidity in patients with severe osteopenia or bone deficiency.[34] The same principles of bridging the fracture site with the humeral stem and adding supplemental fixation apply to humeral shaft fractures centered at the tip of the stem without involvement of the tuberosities. When deciding on augmenting the construct by cementing the humeral component, care has to be taken to avoid extrusion of the cement through the fracture site.[24,32] The heat generated by the exothermic polymerization of the cement can cause significant nerve injury, and the cement itself will hinder bone healing when situated between the fracture lines. Intraoperative fractures that are located distal to the tip of the stem can also be treated with long-stem humeral implants in combination with additional fixation. However, cases in which the fracture extends into the distal humerus can make it impossible to adequately bridge or span the fracture site with the implant by the recommended two to three cortical diameters. In these

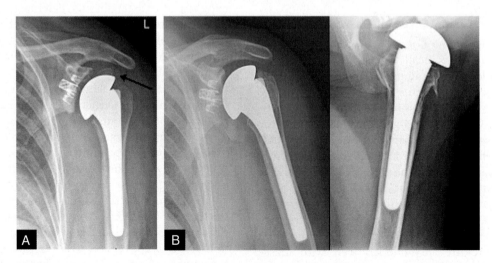

FIGURE 40.4 A 65-year-old woman presented with greater tuberosity fracture at 2 weeks postoperatively. **A,** Anteroposterior (AP) view of the greater tuberosity fracture with mediosuperior migration of the fragment due to the rotator cuff. **B,** Postoperative AP and lateral views after open reduction and suture fixation of the tuberosity fragment.

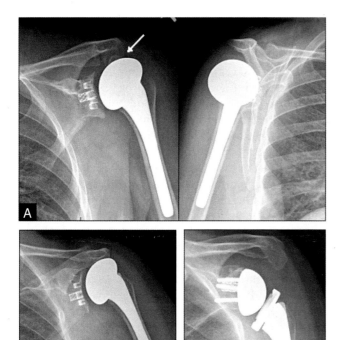

FIGURE 40.5 A 67-year-old woman with unrecognized greater tuberosity fracture at 2 weeks postoperatively. **A**, Anteroposterior (AP) and lateral views at 2 weeks postoperatively show migrated greater tuberosity fracture, which was not recognized. **B**, AP view at 6 months postoperatively shows superior migration. Clinical findings were consistent with severe rotator cuff dysfunction. **C**, AP view after conversion to reverse total shoulder arthroplasty.

Postoperative Humerus Fractures

Verifying the stability of the implant in place—that is, is it loose or not?—is an important factor to consider when deciding on the treatment of postoperative periprosthetic humeral fractures. Specific fracture patterns or preexisting radiolucency at the bone-implant interface can be indicative of humeral implant loosening. Sanchez-Sotelo et al noted that the presence of a radiolucent line measuring ≥2 mm in more than three of the eight zones around the stem correlates with clinical loosening of the humeral component in the absence of fractures.[35] Additionally, previously obtained sequential radiographs can be analyzed to identify subtle changes in implant positioning. CT imaging will provide more detailed information on radiolucency surrounding the uncemented stem and can also be helpful to evaluate the remaining bone stock. Steinman reported that some Wright and Cofield type A fractures (fractures located at the tip of the stem and extending proximally) are at risk of being associated with a loose implant, especially if the fracture line is oblique and extends proximally over the full length of the stem.[32] When there is significant overlap between the fracture pattern and the stem in addition to >2 mm displacement and >20° angulation, they recommended stem revision and fracture fixation.[32] While all these measures will aid the preoperative preparation and planning, the intraoperative assessment of the actual fixation of the implant will ultimately determine the treatment strategy. In humeral shaft fractures, implant stability can be assessed when the implant is exposed by applying direct pressure to determine if motion is present. If the implant is loose, then proximal exposure can proceed; if the implant is not loose, then the procedure can focus on fracture stabilization.[36]

cases, with very distal humeral shaft extension, plate and screw or cable fixation should be expanded to the distal humerus to improve the rigidity of the construct **(FIGURES 40.6 and 40.7)**.

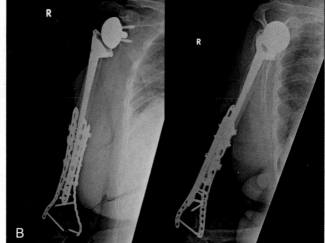

FIGURE 40.6 An 82-year-old woman with postoperative periprosthetic humerus fracture at the tip of a long-stem reverse total shoulder arthroplasty implant. **A**, Anteroposterior (AP) and lateral views postinjury. **B**, AP and lateral views after triple plate fixation with screw and cable constructs.

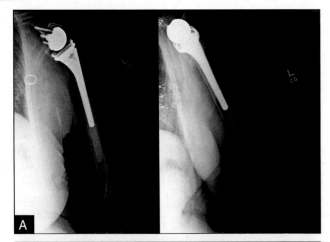

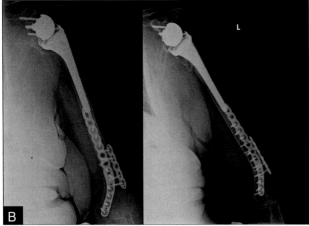

FIGURE 40.7 An 84-year-old woman with a postoperative periprosthetic humerus fracture distal to the stem of the cemented reverse total shoulder arthroplasty. **A**, Anteroposterior (AP) and lateral views postinjury. **B**, AP and lateral views after treatment with dual-plate and screw fixation.

In the absence of implant instability, minimally displaced or minimally angulated fractures can be treated with the use of a fracture brace **(FIGURES 40.8** and

40.9). However, the rate of union with nonoperative treatment is relatively low, and subsequent operative measures are often necessary. When combining the union rates of several case series, only 16 of 37 patients (43%) treated nonoperatively progressed to union. Disruption of the endosteal blood supply as a result of implant placement and potential distraction of the fracture due to the exposed end of the implant may be contributing factors to these low healing rates.[9,37] A trial of nonoperative treatment with sequential clinical and radiographic follow-up may be utilized, and surgery can be deferred as long as the alignment is maintained and the patient shows progressive clinical signs of union.

In general, displaced tuberosity fractures that occur postoperatively in patients undergoing anatomic total shoulder arthroplasty (ATSA) or HA require open reduction and internal fixation to preserve rotator cuff function and clinical outcomes. Similar to the intraoperative repair technique, transosseous nonabsorbable sutures or cerclage wires can be used. If an anatomical reduction of the tuberosity cannot be maintained with the fixation options available or if significant compromise/degeneration of the rotator cuff is identified, then conversion to RTSA should be performed. This includes compromise of the posterosuperior rotator cuff (supraspinatus and infraspinatus) or the subscapularis. Humeral shaft fractures with a loose humeral component require revision and fracture fixation. Comparable to the treatment of intraoperative fractures, replacement of the humeral component with a long-stem implant that bridges the fracture site by at least two to three cortical diameters is necessary combined with additional rigid fixation. The choice of plate and screw or cable constructs, cerclage wires, and/or strut allografts should depend on the fracture pattern, location, and bone quality **(FIGURE 40.10)**.

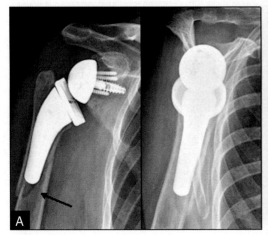

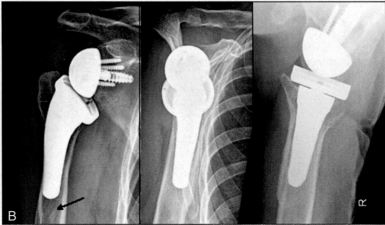

FIGURE 40.8 A 73-year-old woman with postoperative periprosthetic humerus fracture at the tip of short-stem reverse total shoulder arthroplasty implant. **A**, Anteroposterior (AP) and lateral views show acceptable alignment and minimal displacement of the fracture (black arrow) **B**, AP, lateral, and axillary views 6 months posttrauma following nonoperative treatment (6 weeks of sling immobilization) show fracture healing (black arrow).

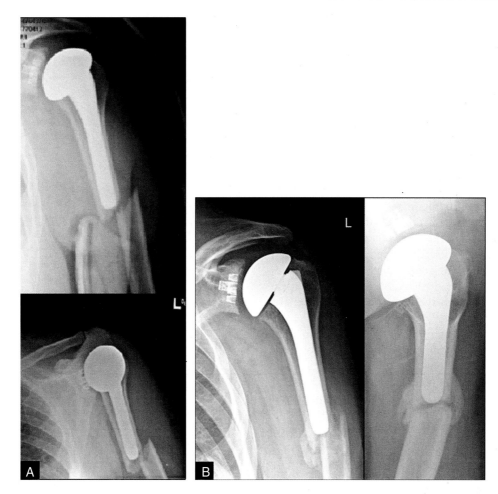

FIGURE 40.9 A 67-year-old man with postoperative periprosthetic humerus fracture 5 years after anatomic total shoulder arthroplasty. Patient did not want to consider surgery and insisted on nonoperative treatment. **A**, Anteroposterior (AP) and lateral views after trauma. **B**, AP and axillary views at 3 months posttrauma. Patient was treated with a coaptation splint for 2 weeks followed with a fracture brace for 3 months.

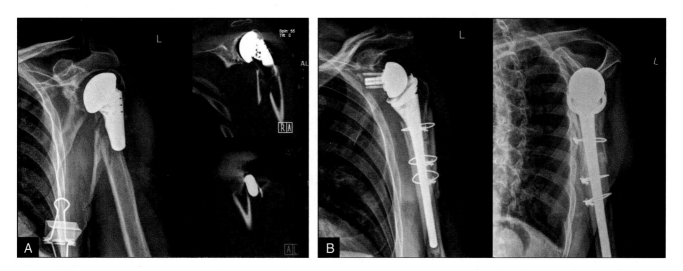

FIGURE 40.10 A 77-year-old man with postoperative comminuted periprosthetic humerus fracture at the tip of a short-stem anatomic total shoulder arthroplasty implant. **A**, Anteroposterior (AP) view and coronal and sagittal CT imaging postinjury. **B**, AP and scapular Y views after conversion arthroplasty to long-stem reverse total shoulder arthroplasty with struts and cables.

Intra- and Postoperative Glenoid Fractures

When an intraoperative glenoid fracture occurs, the amount of bone stock available to support the glenoid baseplate needs to be assessed. Small or partial fractures may not necessitate a change in intraoperative care. If adequate support of the baseplate cannot be guaranteed, however, it is advisable to not proceed with glenoid resurfacing and rather perform a "ream and run" or not ream the glenoid at all and convert to a HA procedure.[38] If the glenoid fracture fragments are large enough, screw fixation may be attempted, possibly in combination with a bone graft. Transitioning from an all-polyethylene cemented baseplate to a metal-backed glenoid component may also form an alternative method as this allows for the use of additional screws. Specifically for RTSA, a metaglenoid with a long central peg and baseplate fixation screws may be used to reduce smaller or partial glenoid fractures and achieve both fracture and implant stability.[19]

Similarly to intraoperatively, the degree of baseplate support and glenoid component stability or loosening needs to be considered in postoperative glenoid fractures. Glenoid component loosening may require revision of the glenoid component (all-polyethylene component to metal-backed glenoid) or conversion to another shoulder implant design (ATSA to RTSA or RTSA to HA) **(FIGURE 40.11)**.

COMPLICATIONS

Both intra- and postoperative fractures present an increased risk for other complications as a result of prolonged operative time, the need for additional dissection and exposure, and the placement of internal fixation devices. Nerve injuries can be potentially devastating complications and are described in several case series. Athwal et al described 6 associated nerve injuries (three partial brachial plexus, two radial nerve, one isolated ulnar nerve) in a series of 45 intraoperative fractures.[6] Andersen et al noted two radial nerve injures in their series of 36 postoperative fractures. Wolf et al also described two radial nerve injuries in their smaller series of eight postoperative fractures. Fortunately, most palsies were transient and recovered between 5 days and 12 months postoperatively. When extending the deltopectoral approach to an anterior approach for periprosthetic humeral shaft fractures, it is advisable to split the brachialis muscle in its midline so that the lateral part of the muscle can function as soft-tissue protection between the radial nerve and the retractors.[32] In addition, the position of the radial nerve in the spiral groove on the posterior aspect of the humerus has to be carefully considered when using fixation devices such as cables, cerclage wires, or anterior to posterior screws to minimize the risk of iatrogenic nerve injury. Cadaveric studies have shown that the radial nerve enters the spiral

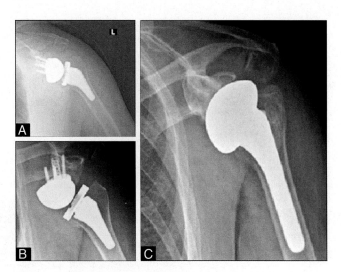

FIGURE 40.11 A 79-year-old woman with postoperative glenoid fracture. **A,** Anteroposterior (AP) view of short-stemmed reverse total shoulder arthroplasty performed for osteoarthritis. **B,** Fall 6 weeks postoperatively caused glenoid fracture with significant loosening and displacement of the metaglenoid. **C,** AP view after conversion to hemiarthroplasty.

groove at an average distance of 4 cm distal to the inferior facet of the latissimus dorsi tendon insertion, which can function as reference point. Dissection and use of hardware distal or in proximity to this point should be performed carefully if it is necessary.[39]

CONCLUSION

With the significant overall rise in shoulder arthroplasties performed, periprosthetic shoulder fractures are bound to become more common. As most fractures occur intraoperatively, employing preventive procedural measures is of great importance to prevent the associated technical challenges. These measures consist of identifying the patients who are at risk, considering alternative surgical approaches, and avoiding surgical errors such as forceful rotation, excessive retraction, inadequate soft-tissue releases, or over-reaming. Treatment principles rely on the assessment of both the fracture and implant stability, and treatment should be individually decided on for each patient based upon the fracture configuration, alignment, and overall patient factors.

REFERENCES

1. Day JS, Paxton ES, Lau E, Gordon VA, Abboud JA, Williams GR. Use of reverse total shoulder arthroplasty in the Medicare population. *J Shoulder Elbow Surg.* 2015;24(5):766-772.
2. Bohsali KI, Bois AJ, Wirth MA. Complications of shoulder arthroplasty. *J Bone Joint Surg Am.* 2017;99:256-269.
3. Cowling PD, Holland P, Kottam L, Baker P, Rangan A. Risk factors associated with intraoperative complications in primary shoulder arthroplasty. *Acta Orthop.* 2017;88:587-591.
4. Ingoe HM, Holland P, Cowling P, Kottam L, Baker PN, Rangan A. Intraoperative complications during revision shoulder arthroplasty: a study using the National Joint Registry dataset. *Shoulder Elbow.* 2017;9:92-99.

5. Singh JA, Sperling J, Schleck C, Harmsen W, Cofield R. Periprosthetic fractures associated with primary total shoulder arthroplasty and primary humeral head replacement: a thirty-three-year study. *J Bone Joint Surg Am*. 2012;94:1777-1785.

6. Athwal GS, Sperling JW, Rispoli DM, Cofield RH. Periprosthetic humeral fractures during shoulder arthroplasty. *J Bone Joint Surg Am*. 2009;91:594-603.

7. Wagner ER, Houdek MT, Elhassan BT, Sanchez-Sotelo J, Cofield RH, Sperling JW. What are risk factors for intraoperative humerus fractures during revision reverse shoulder arthroplasty and do they influence outcomes? *Clin Orthop Relat Res*. 2015;473:3228-3234.

8. Atoun E, Van Tongel A, Hous N, et al. Reverse shoulder arthroplasty with a short metaphyseal humeral stem. *Int Orthop*. 2014;38(6):1213-1218. doi:10.1007/s00264-014-2328-8

9. Boyd AD Jr, Thornhill TS, Barnes CL. Fractures adjacent to humeral prostheses. *J Bone Joint Surg Am*. 1992;74:1498-1504.

10. Wright TW, Cofield RH. Humeral fractures after shoulder arthroplasty. *J Bone Joint Surg Am*. 1995;77:1340-1346.

11. Worland RL, Kim DY, Arredondo J. Periprosthetic humeral fractures: management and classification. *J Shoulder Elbow Surg*. 1999;8:590-594.

12. Chin PY, Sperling JW, Cofield RH, Schleck C. Complications of total shoulder arthroplasty: are they fewer or different? *J Shoulder Elbow Surg*. 2006;15:19-22.

13. Kumar S, Sperling JW, Haidukewych GH, Cofield RH. Periprosthetic humeral fractures after shoulder arthroplasty. *J Bone Joint Surg Am*. 2004;86(4):680-689.

14. García-Fernández C, López-Morales Y, Rodríguez A, López-Durán L, Marco Martínez F. Periprosthetic humeral fractures associated with reverse total shoulder arthroplasty: incidence and management. *Int Orthop*. 2015;39(10):1965-1969.

15. Lee M, Chebli C, Mounce D, Bertelsen A, Richardson M, Matsen F. Intramedullary reaming for press-fit fixation of a humeral component removes cortical bone asymmetrically. *J Shoulder Elbow Surg*. 2008;17(1):150-155.

16. Choo AM, Hawkins RH, Kwon BK, Oxland TR. The effect of shoulder arthroplasty on humeral strength: an in vitro biomechanical investigation. *Clin Biomech (Bristol, Avon)*. 2005;20(10):1064-1071.

17. Keener JD, Chalmers PN, Yamaguchi K. The humeral implant in shoulder arthroplasty. *J Am Acad Orthop Surg*. 2017;25(6):427-438.

18. Werthel JD, Lonjon G, Jo S, Cofield R, Sperling JW, Elhassan BT. Long-term outcomes of cemented versus cementless humeral components in arthroplasty of the shoulder: a propensity score-matched analysis. *Bone Joint J*. 2018;100-B(9):1260.

19. Melis B, Marongiu G. *Intraoperative fracture in reverse shoulder arthroplasty*. In: *Reverse Shoulder Arthroplasty. Current Techniques and Complications*. Springer Nature Switzerland AG; 2019:333-339.

20. Burrus MT, Cancienne JM, Boatright JD, Yang S, Brockmeier SF, Werner BC. Shoulder arthroplasty for humeral head avascular necrosis is associated with increased postoperative complications. *HSS J*. 2018;14(1):2-8.

21. Inglis AE, Inglis AE Jr. Ipsilateral total shoulder arthroplasty and total elbow replacement arthroplasty: a caveat. *J Arthroplasty*. 2000;15(1):123-125. doi:10.1016/s0883-5403(00)91441-4

22. Gill DR, Cofield RH, Morrey BF. Ipsilateral total shoulder and elbow arthroplasties in patients who have rheumatoid arthritis. *J Bone Joint Surg Am*. 1999;81(8):1128-1137.

23. Plausinis D, Greaves C, Regan WD, Oxland TR. Ipsilateral shoulder and elbow replacements: on the risk of periprosthetic fracture. *Clin Biomech (Bristol, Avon)*. 2005;20(10):1055-1063.

24. Fram B, Elder A, Namdari S. Periprosthetic humeral fractures in shoulder arthroplasty. *JBJS Rev*. 2019;7(11):e6.

25. Gonzalez JF, Alami GB, Baque F, Walch G, Boileau P. Complications of unconstrained shoulder prostheses. *J Shoulder Elbow Surg*. 2011;20(4):666-682.

26. Sahota S, Sperling JW, Cofield RH. Humeral windows and longitudinal splits for component removal in revision shoulder arthroplasty. *J Shoulder Elbow Surg*. 2014;23(10):1485-1491.

27. Van Thiel GS, Halloran JP, Twigg S, Romeo AA, Nicholson GP. The vertical humeral osteotomy for stem removal in revision shoulder arthroplasty: results and technique. *J Shoulder Elbow Surg*. 2011;20(8):1248-1254.

28. Greiner S, Stein V, Scheibel M. Periprosthetic humeral fractures after shoulder and elbow arthroplasty. *Acta Chir Orthop Traumatol Cech*. 2011;78(6):490-500.

29. Campbell JT, Moore RS, Iannotti JP, Norris TR, Williams GR. Periprosthetic humeral fractures: mechanisms of fracture and treatment options. *J Shoulder Elbow Surg*. 1998;7:406-413.

30. Groh GI, Heckman MM, Wirth MA, Curtis RJ, Rockwood CA Jr. Treatment of fractures adjacent to humeral prostheses. *J Shoulder Elbow Surg*. 2008;17(1):85-89.

31. Kirchhoff C, Beirer M, Brunner U, Buchholz A, Biberthaler P, Crönlein M. Validation of a new classification for periprosthetic shoulder fractures. *Int Orthop*. 2018;42(6):1371-1377.

32. Steinmann SP, Cheung EV. Treatment of periprosthetic humerus fractures associated with shoulder arthroplasty. *J Am Acad Orthop Surg*. 2008;16(4):199-207.

33. Gebrelul A, Green A, Schacherer T, Khazzam M. Periprosthetic humerus fractures: classification, management, and review of the literature. *Ann Joint*. 2018;3:49.

34. Thés A, Klouche S, de Tienda M, Bauer T, Hardy P. Cortical onlay strut allograft with cerclage wiring of periprosthetic fractures of the humerus without stem loosening: technique and preliminary results. *Eur J Orthop Surg Traumatol*. 2017;27(4):553-557.

35. Sanchez-Sotelo J, Wright TW, O'Driscoll SW, Cofield RH, Rowland CM. Radiographic assessment of uncemented humeral components in total shoulder arthroplasty. *J Arthroplasty*. 2001;16(2):180-187.

36. Andersen JR, Williams CD, Cain R, Mighell M, Frankle M. Surgically treated humeral shaft fractures following shoulder arthroplasty. *J Bone Joint Surg Am*. 2013;95(1):9-18.

37. Cameron B, Iannotti J. Periprosthetic fractures of the humerus and scapula: management and prevention. *Orthop Clin North Am*. 1999;30:305-318.

38. Boyle S, Watts A, Trail I. Periprosthetic fractures around the shoulder. *Shoulder Elbow* 2012;4(1):1-10.

39. Fu MC, Hendel MD, Chen X, Warren RF, Dines DM, Gulotta LV. Surgical anatomy of the radial nerve in the deltopectoral approach for revision shoulder arthroplasty and periprosthetic fracture fixation: a cadaveric study. *J Shoulder Elbow Surg*. 2017;26(12):2173-2176.

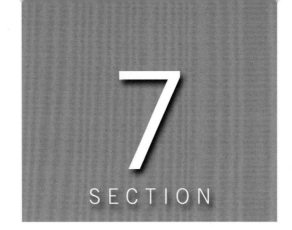

Revision Shoulder Arthroplasty: Techniques

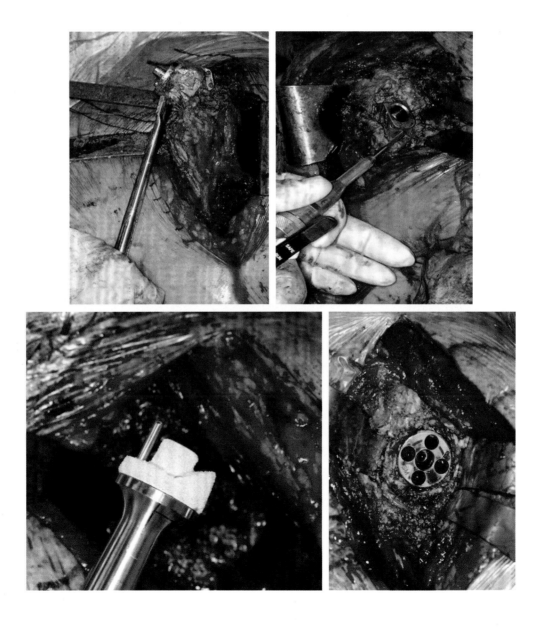

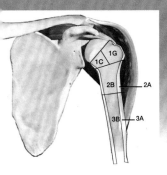

41 The Humeral Component

Jennifer Tangtiphaiboontana, MD and John W. Sperling, MD, MBA

INTRODUCTION

Revision of the humeral component may be necessary for various reasons including aseptic loosening, infection, periprosthetic fracture, revision from hemiarthroplasty or anatomic to a reverse in nonconvertible implants, or for increased exposure of the glenoid. Removal of a well-fixed humeral component is fraught with challenges and may result in significant bone loss and fracture.

PREOPERATIVE EVALUATION

In preparation for revision surgery, a careful and thorough preoperative evaluation must be performed. This includes a detailed history and physical examination, close attention to signs or symptoms suggestive of infection, standard radiographs, and copies of the prior operative reports as needed. If there is clinical concern for infection, further testing is obtained including a complete blood cell count with differential, C-reactive protein level, erythrocyte sedimentation rate, and ultrasound- or fluoroscopic-guided shoulder aspiration.

Preoperative imaging of the shoulder should include a complete series of shoulder x-rays including Grashey, anterior-posterior (AP) with the arm in internal and external rotation, and axillary views. If there is notable bone loss of the proximal humerus, additional humeral x-rays (AP and lateral views) of bilateral arms are obtained to allow for proper assessment of humeral length. Thorough evaluation of shoulder radiographs is crucial and can help surgeons anticipate intraoperative challenges and the potential for bone loss with stem extraction.[1]

The rate of humeral loosening ranges from 0% to 7% and is often associated with glenoid component issues.[2-9] The presence of humeral loosening, in the absence of other mechanical reasons for arthroplasty failure, should also raise suspicion for an occult infection.[10] The humeral component is closely scrutinized on radiographs for evidence of subsidence, change in alignment, osteolysis, and radiolucent lines (RLLs). The stem is considered loose if there are circumferential RLLs or if a shift in stem position has occurred on successive radiographs. A stem is considered to be "at risk" of loosening if RLLs of 2 mm or more are present in three or more zones.[11-13] Although the use of bone scans to evaluate for loosening or infection has been well described in the hip and knee arthroplasty literature, it is not commonly used for shoulder arthroplasty. If loosening is not readily apparent on routine radiographs, further evaluation with a computed tomography (CT) scan may be helpful; however, metal artifact from the implant may limit the ability to assess for loosening. Metal artifact reduction techniques can increase the information obtained from the CT scan.

Metaphyseal bone loss of the proximal humerus may be a result of acute or chronic trauma, infection, sequelae of tumor resection, or revision surgery arthroplasty. When proximal bone loss is ≥4 cm, revision shoulder arthroplasty with structural allograft or a tumor prosthesis may be necessary. Evaluation for proximal humeral bone loss has recently been described by the Proximal Humeral Arthroplasty Revision Osseous in Sufficiency (PHAROS) classification system (**FIGURE 41.1**).[14] The authors propose three types of bone loss with alphanumeric subtypes. Type 1 describes epiphyseal bone loss and is subdivided into Type 1C for calcar bone loss and Type 1G for greater tuberosity loss. Type 2 describes metadiaphyseal bone loss, defined as the bone proximal to the deltoid attachment. Subtype 2A includes cortical thinning >50% of the expected cortical thickness with associated epiphyseal bone loss. Subtype 2B describes bone loss of the metadiaphyseal and epiphyseal regions. Type 3 is diaphyseal bone loss extending below the deltoid with subtypes 3A for those with cortical thinning >50% of the expected cortical thickness and subtype 3B for patients with compromise of the diaphysis with loss of the epiphysis and metadiaphysis. Types 2 and 3 were more likely to need structural bone grafting or proximal humeral or total humeral replacements. Intraoperative greater tuberosity fixation was encountered primarily in Types 1 and 2. Proximal humeral bone loss has important implications in revision shoulder arthroplasty as these patients often have associated rotator cuff insufficiency. The loss of the proximal humeral contour will also alter the lateral tension on the deltoid and result in increased rates of instability if not recognized and addressed during revision surgery.

PHAROS Classification

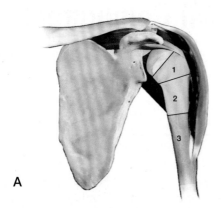 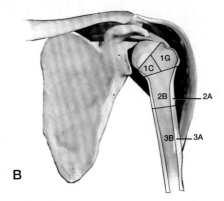

A   B

FIGURE 41.1 This schematic demonstrates the Proximal Humeral Arthroplasty Revision Osseous in Sufficiency (PHAROS) classification system for humeral bone loss in revision shoulder arthroplasty. Numeric (**A**) types include Type 1 with epiphyseal bone loss, Type 2 with metadiaphyseal bone loss above with deltoid attachment, and Type 3 with diaphyseal bone loss extending below the deltoid attachment. Alphanumeric (**B**) subtypes include Type 1C with calcar compromise, Type 1G with greater tuberosity compromise, Type 2A with cortical thinning of the metadiaphysis >50% of the expected cortical thickness based on the noninstrumented portion of the humerus with associated epiphyseal loss or cortical thinning, Type 2B with bone loss above the deltoid of some metadiaphysis and the epiphysis, Type 3A with diaphyseal cortical thinning, and Type 3B with compromise of the majority of the diaphysis with loss of the epiphysis, metadiaphysis, and part of the diaphysis below the deltoid insertion.

Other radiographic findings around a humeral component include stress shielding of the calcar that can occur with press-fit implants or osteolysis. While the clinical relevance of stress shielding remains unknown, humeral osteolysis has been associated with worse outcomes, glenoid component loosening, and polyethylene wear.[15]

EXPOSURE

Patients are placed in the beach chair position and the operative arm rests on a sterile Mayo stand. The deltopectoral approach is preferred in revision shoulder arthroplasty because of the ability to extend distally into an anterolateral approach. This allows for a more extensile approach for complex reconstructions. The cephalic vein marks the interval between the deltoid and pectoralis major. However, it may have been ligated in prior surgeries. When the interval is difficult to identify because of scarring or lack of a cephalic vein, an interval can be created proximally starting 1 cm lateral to the coracoid and continuing distally toward the humerus. The upper border of the pectoralis major tendon insertion on the humerus is released for further exposure. Once the conjoined tendon is identified, careful blunt dissection underneath the tendon develops the subcoracoid space. A blunt retractor is placed underneath the conjoined tendon to expose the subscapularis tendon. Next, the arm is placed in slight forward flexion and abduction to facilitate release of adhesions in the subacromial and subdeltoid space. An arthrotomy is performed by releasing the rotator interval and continuing distally into a subscapularis tenotomy or peel with the

arm in slight external rotation and adduction to relax the axillary nerve. With gentle external rotation of the arm, a generous inferior capsular release is performed around the humeral neck and continued distally on the humerus as needed to allow for dislocation of the shoulder with minimal force. Adequate soft-tissue release is required to reduce the risk of iatrogenic fractures of the humerus. The superior rotator cuff and posterior capsule may also need to be released for additional exposure. Once the humeral component is dislocated, additional retractors are placed between the glenoid and humeral component, and the humeral head or tray is removed using a low-profile removal fork. Scar tissue overlying the humeral stem is removed to expose the interface between the stem and the bone or cement mantle.

HUMERAL STEM REMOVAL

Loose humeral stems are easily removed using a needle-nose rongeur or implant-specific extraction device. Removal of a well-fixed humeral stem can be challenging and potentially destructive to the native bone stock. Various techniques have been described to minimize bone loss and morbidity during revision surgery.

Router Bit Technique

The router bit technique was described by Sperling et al and uses a handheld high-speed motorized device with a router bit attachment (Stryker Total Performance System, 2.3 × 15.9 mm² tapered router bit, reference #5120-071-023, Stryker Instruments, Kalamazoo, Michigan) **(FIGURE 41.2A)** to circumferentially break the implant-bone or implant-cement interface of a well-fixed implant

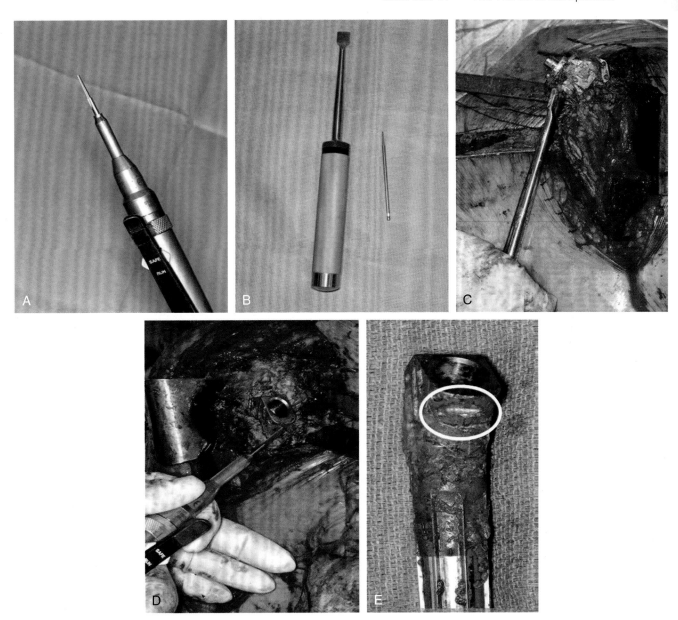

FIGURE 41.2 Router bit technique for humeral component removal. **A**, Router bit device. **B**, Narrow square tip impactor. **C**, Placement of the impactor along the medial collar of the humeral component to remove the implant in a retrograde fashion using a mallet. **D and E**, Creation of a groove (indicated by the oval) in the medial aspect of the humeral component to facilitate removal with the impactor.

proximally **(VIDEO 41.1)**.[16] The router bit is buried as far in as possible without violating the cortex. If the implant has a medial collar, a needle-nosed rongeur can be used to remove the minimal amount of bone needed to gain access to the ingrowth surface underneath the collar. A narrow square tip impactor **(FIGURE 41.2B)** is placed on the undersurface of the medial collar, and the mallet is used to strike the impactor to remove the stem in a retrograde fashion **(FIGURE 41.2C)**. If the humeral stem does not have a collar, a metal cutting helicoidal burr attachment (3.2 × 18.3 mm², reference #5120-080-020; Stryker Instruments, Kalamazoo, Michigan) can be used with the handheld device to create a groove in the proximal, medial aspect of the stem **(FIGURE 41.2D and E)**. The

square tip impactor can then be placed in the groove to remove the stem.

The router bit extraction technique is successful in removing 98.6% of humeral stems while minimizing the amount of proximal bone loss.[16] Only four stems in this study required the addition of a cortical window for extraction. All cases that required a cortical window had standard length stems. Two patients had dense cement mantles with thin humeral cortices, and two patients had stems with proximal ingrowth coating and was fully textured and fluted distally. This technique offers several advantages over an osteotomy. It maintains an intact column of bone to allow for revision to a press-fit stem and preserves the various tendon attachments to the proximal humerus. It can also be used to remove any type of humeral stem and does not require the use of a manufacturer-specific extraction device. The disadvantage of this technique is the limited exposure of the intramedullary canal, which may be needed to remove the distal cement mantle, especially in the setting of an infection.

Humeral Osteotomy

Longitudinal osteotomies of the humerus can also be used to extract well-fixed stems or facilitate cement removal from the canal (**FIGURE 41.3A**). Prior to creating the osteotomy, a narrow osteotome is used around the top of the implant to break the interface between the implant and the tuberosities. Van Thiel et al described a vertical humeral osteotomy (VHO) technique in which a 10 cm unicortical osteotomy is created with a micro oscillating saw lateral to the bicipital groove extending distally between the pectoralis tendon and deltoid insertion.[17] The distal extent of the osteotomy is just below the deltoid insertion and does not go beyond the tip of the implant. A series of osteotomes are placed vertically in the osteotomy and gently twisted to open the humerus and create visible gaps between the bone or cement and the stem. The humeral component is removed in a retrograde fashion with an impactor and mallet. Johnston et al described a variation of the humeral osteotomy in which an osteotomy is created in the center of the bicipital groove, and a 2.5 mm drill hole is made at the distal end of the osteotomy to prevent split propagation of the distal cortex.[18] After removal of the stem and cement mantle, the osteotomy is repaired by placing two 18-gauge Luque wires circumferentially around the proximal humerus followed by canal preparation and placement of a trial stem. Care must be taken to avoid iatrogenic injury to the radial nerve while repairing the osteotomy. The inferior border of the latissimus dorsi serves as a reliable landmark for passing the distal cerclage wires as the radial nerve is located approximately 2.7 cm medial and 4 cm distal to the inferior aspect of the tendon insertion.[19,20]

Humeral Window

An anterior humeral window can be used to remove a well-fixed humeral component, especially those with distal fixation or a fully textured stem (**FIGURE 41.3B**).[21,22] Alternatively, a medial metaphyseal window may be used to expose the cement mantle and porous on-growth or in-growth region of a proximally textured or cemented implant (**FIGURE 41.3C**). Advantages of the window are that it grants more access to the implant and exposes a greater surface area for the surgeon with a reliable healing rate. Disadvantages of this technique include a higher rate of intraoperative fracture when compared to the longitudinal osteotomy.[22]

The size of the humeral window varies and is dependent on several factors: cement distribution, regions of

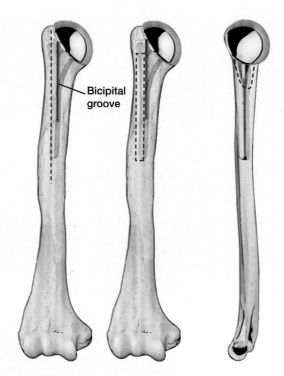

FIGURE 41.3 Examples of osteotomies to assist with removal of a well-fixed humeral component. **A**, Longitudinal osteotomy positioned lateral to the bicipital groove. **B**, Anterior humeral window made 3 cm distal to the humeral cut and approximately 1 cm wide. **C**, Medial window used to facilitate removal of bone or cement around the proximal aspect of the implant.

bone deficiency, and anticipated length of the revision stem. The anterior window is created with a micro oscillating saw beginning 3 cm distal to the humeral cut to preserve the strength of the tuberosities, including the attachment site for the subscapularis. The two vertical osteotomies for the window are approximately 1 cm apart, allowing access to the anterior, medial, and lateral aspects of the prosthetic humeral stem. These vertical osteotomies extend 1 cm distal to the end of the implant being removed. The superior and inferior aspects of the pectoralis major insertion are released, leaving the central portion of the tendon attached to the window. The window is completed with a horizontal osteotomy with a saw or osteotome. A series of flexible osteotomes can be used to break the bone-implant or bone-cement interface around the component prior to removal. The window is repaired with No. 5 circumferential sutures, Luque wires, or cables. The upper portion of the pectoralis major is repaired to the humerus with two drill holes slightly medial to the window, and the lower aspect of the pectoralis major is sutured to deltoid insertion.

Cemented Stems

Removal of a stable cemented stem presents another set of challenges and is often more difficult to remove and results in greater humeral bone loss than removal of an uncemented stem.[1] After successful removal of the implant, removing the remaining cement mantle can also be a challenge. Several techniques have been described to assist with removing the cement mantle when exposure of the intramedullary canal is limited. Levy et al described a technique to sequentially remove the cement mantle by using a cannulated screw system.[23] First, a threaded guidewire is advanced through the cement under fluoroscopic guidance. Next, a cannulated drill bit is passed over the wire followed by a cannulated tap or screw, which is advanced approximately 2 to 3 cm into the cement mantle. A vise grip is connected to the proximal end of the tap or screw, and a mallet is used to strike the vise grip to remove the cement. Loose fragments of cement can be removed with a pituitary rongeur or long forceps. An endoscope may also be used to assess for residual cement within the canal.[24,25] An ultrasonic device is another technique for cement removal; however, this has largely fallen out of use due to the risk of thermal injury to the bone and surrounding soft tissues and neurovascular structures.[26]

Complete cement removal from the canal may be desirable, especially in cases of infection. However, it may not be possible in certain cases, and efforts to do so may result in further bone loss and fracture. Currently, there is no literature available that describes the effects of retained cement on the successful treatment of prosthetic joint infections of the shoulder.[27] Therefore, we favor preserving bone over complete removal of the cement mantle.

IMPLANT SELECTION AND FIXATION

The decision of stem length and method of fixation is dependent on the amount of bone remaining after removal of the humeral component. If an osteotomy or cortical window is used, a longer stem implant should be used to bypass the defect. Impaction bone grafting, with cancellous allograft, of osteolytic lesions in the tuberosity or metaphysis can be used to increase the fixation if a press-fit stem is selected.

When the proximal humeral bone is well preserved, conversion to a longer humeral stem may not always be necessary. Wagner et al reported good short-to-intermediate-term results with a low complication rate in 39 patients who were revised from a long humeral component to a short bone-preserving implant **(FIGURE 41.4)**.[28] The use of a short-stemmed implant for revision arthroplasty offers several advantages including continued preservation of the metaphyseal bone and avoids the need to remove distal cement. A short stem component also reduces implant interference in cases where patients have an ipsilateral total elbow arthroplasty (TEA) or may need a TEA in the future.

Cement within cement technique may be used when revising a previously cemented stem **(FIGURE 41.5)**.

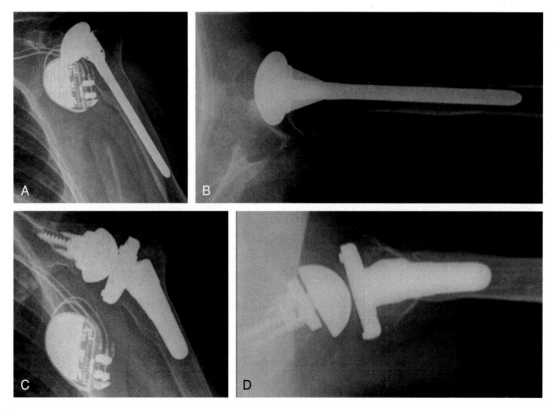

FIGURE 41.4 Revision of a well-fixed hemiarthroplasty stem (**A and B**) to a short-stemmed reverse shoulder arthroplasty (**C and D**). The humeral stem was removed using the router bit technique and x-rays demonstrate preservation of the proximal humeral bone.

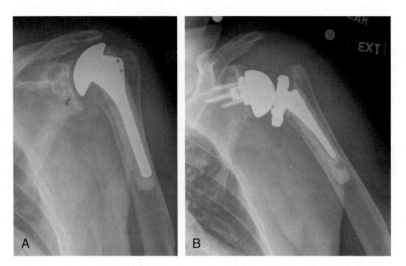

FIGURE 41.5 A and B, Revision of previously cemented humeral component to a reverse prothesis using the cement-within-cement technique with a stable humeral component at 5-year follow-up.

After removing the humeral component, the cement mantle should be carefully evaluated for stability and loose fragments removed. The remaining cement is roughened with a burr to allow for improved interdigitation prior to cementing in the new stem. A narrower and shorter stem is preferred to allow for an adequate cement mantle. This technique results in significant improvement in pain and shoulder motion and an overall implant revision-free survival of 95% and 91% at 2 and 5 years, respectively.[29] Of the 38 shoulders included in the study, seven nondisplaced fractures of the greater tuberosity occurred intraoperatively during implant removal. Only three fractures required suture stabilization, and all fractures healed radiographically. Three shoulders (8%) had radiographic lucency around the humeral component, but only one was determined to be at risk.

Management of Proximal Bone Loss

Marked proximal humeral bone loss, typically defects of ≥4 cm, may be reconstructed with the use of a proximal humeral replacement or allograft-prosthetic composites (APCs). Failure to address proximal bone loss results in problems of instability, weakness, and stem loosening due to lack of metaphyseal fixation to support the humeral component, risk of humeral shortening, rotator cuff insufficiency, and inadequate lateral tensioning of the deltoid.

The benefits of reconstruction with an APC include the potential for repair of the patient's remaining rotator cuff to the allograft, restoration of the proximal humeral anatomy, and increased fixation of the humeral component. The downsides of this technique include the possibility of nonunion, graft resorption, infection, prolonged operative times, increased costs, and graft availability. Despite these concerns, the current literature demonstrates encouraging results. Chacon et al reported the

outcomes of 25 patients who underwent revision shoulder arthroplasty with an APC with an average bone loss of 53.6 mm and found significant improvements in functional outcomes and motion.[30] Graft resorption or fragmentation occurred in 4 (17%) patients. Sanchez-Sotelo et al reported similar improvements in pain and functional outcomes in 26 patients with 2- and 5-year revision-free survival rates of 96%.[31] A long-term follow-up study by Cox et al demonstrated 10-year and beyond 10-year revision-free survival rates of 78% and 67%, respectively.[32]

Revision with a proximal humeral replacement or tumor prosthesis has several advantages over APCs as the operation can be completed in a more efficient manner and eliminates the concerns with graft availability, healing, or resorption. Good clinical outcomes have been reported with the use of proximal humeral replacement in revision shoulder arthroplasty with a low dislocation rate of 3% and humeral loosening rate of 13% **(VIDEO 41.2)**.[33] Cement fixation of the stem is recommended as current implant designs do not allow for adequate resistance against rotational forces and may reduce the rate of humeral loosening.

MANAGEMENT OF INTRAOPERATIVE COMPLICATIONS

Iatrogenic fractures of the humerus are the most common intraoperative complication in revision shoulder arthroplasty and rates vary from 3.3% to 16%.[34,35] A majority of fractures occur during implant removal. Risk factors associated with intraoperative fracture include female sex ratio, history of instability, and prior hemiarthroplasty.[35] Extensive scaring and inadequate exposure may also increase the risk of fracture due to aggressive retraction and increase torque across the humerus. Humeral stems with proximal fins also place the greater tuberosity at increase risk for fracture during removal. Other patient characteristics that place the humerus at risk for fracture include osteopenia, rheumatoid arthritis, and shoulder stiffness due to posttraumatic arthritis.

Treatment of intraoperative fractures is based on the location of the fracture, available bone stock, prosthesis type, and stability. Nondisplaced tuberosity fractures that maintain a large soft tissue sleeve and are stable after placement and reduction of the components may successfully be treated without further fixation.[29] Displaced tuberosity fractures are fixed with suture or cerclage wiring. Metaphyseal or calcar fractures can also be stabilized using suture or wire cerclage. Fractures of the humeral shaft may be treated with a long stem prosthesis with supplement fixation using cable or suture cerclage, plate fixation, or strut allograft. If the stem requires cement fixation, care must be taken to avoid cement extrusion through the fracture site as it may impair fracture healing and result in injury to the radial nerve.

The occurrence of an intraoperative fracture does not appear to have negative effects on the overall outcome. Wagner et al reported the outcomes of 36 shoulders that sustained a fracture during revision surgery and found no difference in pain relief, shoulder motion, patient-reported outcomes, and revision-free survival rates when compared to a revision shoulder arthroplasty cohort without intraoperative fracture.[35]

CONCLUSION

Successful revision of the humeral component requires careful preoperative planning and adequate soft-tissue releases to reduce the risk of fracture. Removal of the component should begin with the most bone-preserving technique, such as the router bit technique, and progress to an osteotomy or humeral window as needed. Implant options largely depend on the amount of bone remaining after removal of the humeral component, and those with a significant amount of bone loss should be addressed with a tumor prosthesis or APC.

REFERENCES

1. O'Briain DE, Simon P, Christmas KN, et al. Do preoperative radiographs help predict intraoperative challenges in revision surgery after previous shoulder hemiarthroplasty? *J Shoulder Elbow Surg.* 2019;28(6): S161-S167. http://www.ncbi.nlm.nih.gov/pubmed/31196511
2. Raiss P, Schmitt M, Bruckner T, et al. Results of cemented total shoulder replacement with a minimum follow-up of ten years. *J Bone Joint Surg Am.* 2012;94(23):e1711-10. http://www.ncbi.nlm.nih.gov/pubmed/23224391
3. Gonzalez JF, Alami GB, Baque F, Walch G, Boileau P. Complications of unconstrained shoulder prostheses. *J Shoulder Elbow Surg.* 2011;20:666-682. http://www.ncbi.nlm.nih.gov/pubmed/21419661
4. Bohsali KI, Wirth MA, Rockwood CA. Complications of total shoulder arthroplasty. *J Bone Joint Surg Am.* 2006;88(10):2279. http://www.ncbi.nlm.nih.gov/pubmed/17015609
5. Wiater BP, Moravek JE, Wiater JM. The evaluation of the failed shoulder arthroplasty. *J Shoulder Elbow Surg.* 2014;23:745-758.
6. Cil A, Veillette CJH, Sanchez-Sotelo J, Sperling JW, Schleck CD, Cofield RH. Survivorship of the humeral component in shoulder arthroplasty. *J Shoulder Elbow Surg.* 2010;19(1):143-150.
7. Keener JD, Chalmers PN, Yamaguchi K. The humeral implant in shoulder arthroplasty. *J Am Acad Orthop Surg.* 2017;25:427-438.
8. Gilot G, Alvarez-Pinzon AM, Wright TW, et al. The incidence of radiographic aseptic loosening of the humeral component in reverse total shoulder arthroplasty. *J Shoulder Elbow Surg.* 2015;24(10):1555-1559.
9. Grey B, Rodseth RN, Roche SJ. Humeral stem loosening following reverse shoulder arthroplasty: a systematic review and meta-analysis. *JBJS Rev.* 2018;6(5):e5.
10. Pottinger P, Butler-Wu S, Neradilek MB, et al. Prognostic factors for bacterial cultures positive for Propionibacterium acnes and other organisms in a large series of revision shoulder arthroplasties performed for stiffness, pain, or loosening. *J Bone Joint Surg Am.* 2012;94(22):2075-2083.
11. Sperling JW, Cofield RH, O'Driscoll SW, Torchia ME, Rowland CM. Radiographic assessment of ingrowth total shoulder arthroplasty. *J Shoulder Elbow Surg.* 2000;9(6):507-513.
12. Sanchez-Sotelo J, O'Driscoll SW, Torchia ME, Cofield RH, Rowland CM. Radiographic assessment of cemented humeral components in shoulder arthroplasty. *J Shoulder Elbow Surg.* 2001;10(6):526-531.
13. Matsen FA, Iannotti JP, Rockwood CA. Humeral fixation by press-fitting of a tapered metaphyseal stem. A prospective radiographic study. *J Bone Joint Surg Am.* 2003;85(2):304-308.
14. Chalmers PN, Romeo AA, Nicholson GP, et al. Humeral bone loss in revision total shoulder arthroplasty: the proximal humeral arthroplasty revision osseous insufficiency (PHAROS) classification system. *Clin Orthop Relat Res.* 2019;477(2):432-441.
15. Raiss P, Edwards TB, Deutsch A, et al. Radiographic changes around humeral components in shoulder arthroplasty. *J Bone Joint Surg Am.* 2014;96(7):e54. http://www.ncbi.nlm.nih.gov/pubmed/24695931
16. Kang JR, Logli AL, Tagliero AJ, Sperling JW. The router bit extraction technique for removing a well-fixed humeral stem in revision shoulder arthroplasty. *Bone Joint Lett J.* 2019;101-B(10):1280-1284.
17. Van Thiel GS, Halloran JP, Twigg S, Romeo AA, Nicholson GP. The vertical humeral osteotomy for stem removal in revision shoulder arthroplasty: results and technique. *J Shoulder Elbow Surg.* 2011;20(8): 1248-1254. http://www.ncbi.nlm.nih.gov/pubmed/21420326
18. Johnston PS, Creighton RA, Romeo AA. Humeral component revision arthroplasty: outcomes of a split osteotomy technique. *J Shoulder Elbow Surg.* 2012;21(4):502-506.
19. Fu MC, Hendel MD, Chen X, Warren RF, Dines DM, Gulotta LV. Surgical anatomy of the radial nerve in the deltopectoral approach for revision shoulder arthroplasty and periprosthetic fracture fixation: a cadaveric study. *J Shoulder Elbow Surg.* 2017;26(12): 2173-2176.
20. Pearle AD, Kelly BT, Voos JE, Chehab EL, Warren RF. Surgical technique and anatomic study of latissimus dorsi and teres major transfers. *J Bone Joint Surg Am.* 2006;88(7):1524-1531.
21. Sperling JW, Cofield RH. Humeral windows in revision shoulder arthroplasty. *J Shoulder Elbow Surg.* 2005;14(3):258-263.
22. Sahota S, Sperling JW, Cofield RH. Humeral windows and longitudinal splits for component removal in revision shoulder arthroplasty. *J Shoulder Elbow Surg.* 2014;23(10):1485-1491.
23. Berglund DD, Kurowicki J, Rosas S, et al. Cannulated system for sequential intramedullary cement extraction from humerus during revision shoulder arthroplasty. *Tech Orthop.* 2019;34(1):50-52. http://insights.ovid.com/crossref?an=00013611-201903000-00012
24. Takagi M, Tamaki Y, Kobayashi S, Sasaki K, Takakubo Y, Ishii M. Cement removal and bone bed preparation of the femoral medullary canal assisted by flexible endoscope in total hip revision arthroplasty. *J Orthop Sci.* 2009;14(6):719-726.
25. Reilly P, Rees J, Carr A. Technical notes and tips: an aid to removal of cement during revision elbow replacement. *Ann R Coll Surg Engl.* 2006;88(2):231.
26. Goldberg SH, Cohen MS, Young M, Bradnock B. Thermal tissue damage caused by ultrasonic cement removal from the humerus. *J Bone Joint Surg Am.* 2005;87(3):583-591.
27. Garrigues GE, Zmistowski B, Cooper AM, et al. Proceedings from the 2018 International Consensus Meeting on Orthopedic Infections: management of periprosthetic shoulder infection. *J Shoulder Elbow Surg.* 2019;28(6):S67-S99.

28. Wagner ER, Statz JM, Houdek MT, Cofield RH, Sánchez-Sotelo J, Sperling JW. Use of a shorter humeral stem in revision reverse shoulder arthroplasty. *J Shoulder Elbow Surg.* 2017;26(8):1454-1461.

29. Wagner ER, Houdek MT, Hernandez NM, Cofield RH, Sanchez-Sotelo J, Sperling JW. Cement-within-cement technique in revision reverse shoulder arthroplasty. *J Shoulder Elbow Surg.* 2017;26(8):1448-1453.

30. Chacon A, Virani N, Shannon R, Levy JC, Pupello D, Frankle M. Revision arthroplasty with use of a reverse shoulder prosthesis-allograft composite. *J Bone Joint Surg Am.* 2009;91(1):119-127.

31. Sanchez-Sotelo J, Wagner ER, Sim FH, Houdek MT. Allograft-prosthetic composite reconstruction for massive proximal humeral bone loss in reverse shoulder arthroplasty. *J Bone Joint Surg Am.* 2017;99(24):2069-2076.

32. Cox JL, McLendon PB, Christmas KN, Simon P, Mighell MA, Frankle MA. Clinical outcomes following reverse shoulder arthroplasty–allograft composite for revision of failed arthroplasty associated with proximal humeral bone deficiency: 2- to 15-year follow-up. *J Shoulder Elbow Surg.* 2019;28(5):900-907.

33. Shukla DR, Lee J, Mangold D, Cofield RH, Sanchez-Sotelo J, Sperling JW. Reverse shoulder arthroplasty with proximal humeral replacement for the management of massive proximal humeral bone loss. *J Shoulder Elbow Arthroplast.* 2018;2:247154921877984. http://journals.sagepub.com/doi/10.1177/2471549218779845

34. Athwal GS, Sperling JW, Rispoli DM, Cofield RH. Periprosthetic humeral fractures during shoulder arthroplasty. *J Bone Joint Surg Am.* 2009;91(3):594-603.

35. Wagner ER, Houdek MT, Elhassan BT, Sanchez-Sotelo J, Cofield RH, Sperling JW. What are risk factors for intraoperative humerus fractures during revision reverse shoulder arthroplasty and do they influence outcomes? *Clin Orthop Relat Res.* 2015;473(10):3228-3234.

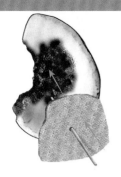

CHAPTER

42

The Glenoid Component in Anatomic Total Shoulder Arthroplasty

Thomas W. Wright, MD and Joseph J. King, MD

INTRODUCTION

The need for glenoid revision in anatomic total shoulder arthroplasty (ATSA) is unfortunately a relatively common indication for revision shoulder arthroplasty. Glenoid loosening is one of the leading reasons for ATSA revision reported in the literature.[1-10] Glenoid loosening can be due to rotator cuff failure or soft tissue imbalance leading to eccentric glenoid loading, infection, poor implantation technique, osteolysis, or mechanical failure of the glenoid component over time.[6,9,11] Multiple types of ATSA glenoid components exist and the surgeon revising the implants should be familiar with the different implants that may be encountered including all-polyethylene, metal-backed, augmented, hybrid with a metal ongrowth surface and inlay designs. The rate of clinical glenoid loosening in all-polyethylene ATSA components ranges from 0% to 48%,[2,7,10,12-17] with one large recent meta-analysis reporting a mean of 15% in 25 studies.[2] Glenoid loosening in metal-backed implants has been reported in 0% to 29% of cases,[2,8,12,18-21] with a recent meta-analysis reporting a mean of 5% in 10 studies.[2] Lower rates of glenoid loosening have been reported for hybrid glenoid[16,22-24] and inlay glenoid components[25,26]; however, these studies generally have short-term follow-up. In addition, hybrid components may be more difficult to revise due to bone ingrowth (but easier than metal-backed components), and inlay glenoids leave a large glenoid defect due to the initial removal of subchondral bone. However, careful removal of a hybrid glenoid may preserve more bone for subsequent reconstruction than an entirely loose all-polyethylene glenoid. Rates of asymptomatic glenoid loosening or glenoid loosening not needing revision have been reported as high as 48% in ATSAs at long-term follow-up,[7] but little is known about the percentage of these cases that may become symptomatic in the future. However, the rate of glenoid lucent lines and glenoid loosening has been shown to increase over time,[2,7,16,27,28] which means shoulder surgeons will be seeing many more revisions in the future. Generally, a loose glenoid component is easy to remove. The challenge and technical difficulty comes in the subsequent reconstruction.

Revision of a well-fixed glenoid component is a less common scenario compared with revision of a loose glenoid component, but presents a greater challenge compared with loose glenoids. Revision of a well-fixed ATSA glenoid can be encountered in cases of rotator cuff failure requiring revision to reverse total shoulder arthroplasty (RTSA), treatment of periprosthetic infection, and humeral component failure or periprosthetic fracture needing revision to RTSA. When removing a well-fixed glenoid, the goal is to remove the implant with the loss of as little glenoid bone as possible. This is more difficult in metal-backed ingrowth implants due to a strong bone-implant interface. With removal of a well-fixed component, native glenoid bone may be sacrificed. It is important to plan for implant removal, so the surgeon has the appropriate tools to effectively and efficiently remove the implant. This will be discussed later in this chapter.

EVALUATION

As in the evaluation of all patients with shoulder pain, a comprehensive history and physical examination is critical for assessment of patients who may require ATSA glenoid revision. In patients with glenoid loosening, start-up pain is common, which can decrease with light use and increase with heavy use of the extremity. Generally, rest pain is absent in aseptic glenoid loosening. Evaluation for other etiologies of pain is critical as radiographs may show glenoid loosening, but this loosening can be asymptomatic and pain may be coming from other causes. Patients that have night pain and pain at rest should raise the surgeon's suspicion of deep infection. A history of shoulder warmth, redness, or persistent postoperative drainage or swelling should increase this suspicion. Limited passive range of motion associated with constant pain is frequently encountered when a periprosthetic infection is present. Range of motion and strength should be assessed during the physical examination to determine if the rotator cuff is functional. A decrease in range of motion over time is frequently encountered in patients with glenoid loosening or rotator cuff tear. In addition, a complete neurologic examination of the affected extremity will help exclude neurologic causes of shoulder dysfunction.

High-quality radiographs are an important and essential part of the diagnostic evaluation.[29] An adequate Grashey radiograph is helpful to confirm glenoid loosening and glenoid component medialization, as well as whether the humeral component is high-riding.[11] An adequate axillary view is helpful to determine if there is loss of anterior or posterior glenoid bone due to component subsidence and will also identify anterior or posterior humeral translation suggesting subscapularis or posterior rotator cuff insufficiency.[6,29] Comparison of previous radiographs will identify how the appearance of the glenoid component has changed over time and can confirm glenoid migration in cases of subtle loosening. Computed tomography (CT) scans are helpful for diagnosis in cases where subtle glenoid loosening is not obvious on radiographs and also in the evaluation of glenoid bone stock and version. They also provide additional information about rotator cuff muscle atrophy and the acromiohumeral interval,[6] as well as the visualization of periprosthetic fractures. One study showed that a CT scan with the patient in the lateral decubitus position and maximum shoulder forward flexion nearly eliminated metal artifact from ATSAs, which may be useful when evaluating subtle glenoid lucencies.[30] We recommend a preoperative CT scan on all patients undergoing revision for a loose glenoid component to better evaluate the glenoid bone stock. We frequently use three-dimensional CT reconstructions to help assess the amount and location of glenoid bone loss. The Antuña classification, first described in 2001, characterized lesions as central, peripheral, or combined and graded the extent of the bone loss as mild, moderate, or severe **(TABLE 42.1)**. Subsequently, Williams and Iannotti expanded Antuña classification—taking into account the glenoid subchondral bone, vault, and rim—to assist in determining glenoid component fixation options in the setting of revision TSA.[31] Gupta and colleagues described an expanded classification scheme to guide surgical management which was focused on revision RTSA with glenoid bone loss.[32] This will be discussed further in Chapter 43.

Preoperative serum inflammatory markers (white blood cell [WBC], erythrocyte sedimentation rate, and C-reactive protein) are recommended[6] and can be useful if they are elevated without another explanation. However, low-virulent organism infections such as *Cutibacterium acnes* and *Staphylococcus epidermidis* are common in the shoulder and are frequently associated with normal values for the inflammatory markers.[33,34] Preoperative aspiration should be performed when there is high suspicion of infection. However, one intra-articular sample is really only helpful if bacteria grows from the culture or has a highly elevated WBC count.[33] In addition, the threshold for white blood cell count in aspirated fluid to confirm infection has not

TABLE 42.1 Antuña Classification

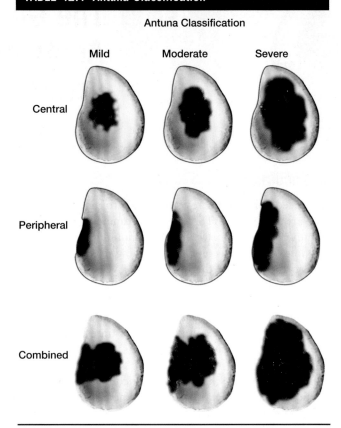

Antuna Classification

been studied extensively in shoulder arthroplasty,[33,34] partly because the exact definition of a shoulder periprosthetic infection is unclear.[35] Arthroscopic evaluation may be a useful adjunct especially in cases where there is concern for glenoid loosening without definitive radiographic evidence.[36] During arthroscopy, biopsies of the synovium can be obtained (dry scope) for both culture and pathology and the glenoid component and glenoid bone interface can be evaluated for glenoid component loosening. If there is definite glenoid loosening on arthroscopic evaluation and the infection concern is low, arthroscopic-assisted removal of the glenoid component is an option for possible definitive treatment of a painful ATSA.[37,38] While no gold standard algorithm exists for preoperative workup for a patient with glenoid loosening, the options discussed should be considered based on the patient's age, probability of infection, and possible etiologies of glenoid loosening based on history, physical examination, and imaging.

REMOVING THE GLENOID COMPONENT

The glenoid component in ATSA will require revision in cases of symptomatic loosening, cuff failure, infection, and whenever the shoulder is being converted to RTSA. Adequate glenoid exposure is paramount for glenoid component removal and subsequent reconstruction, especially in cases of significant glenoid bone loss. Glenoid removal can be easy in cases of a loose all-polyethylene glenoid and can be extremely onerous with some ingrowth implants. This step is very important in order to minimize the amount of native glenoid bone loss. The amount of remaining native glenoid bone stock following glenoid removal is critical in determining the type of reconstruction that can be performed.

Prior to surgery, the initial plan and backup plan for reconstruction must be clearly understood and articulated to the patient. If the goal is glenoid removal only with conversion to hemiarthroplasty, there are two options if the all-polyethylene glenoid is loose. One option is removing it arthroscopically and the other is open removal.

Arthroscopic removal has the advantage of not violating the subscapularis again. Frozen section biopsies and cultures can be obtained. These should be done with a dry scope if possible to increase the positive yield. Arthroscopically, the bone-polyethylene glenoid interface is cleared of all fibrous tissues. The viewing portal is posterior and the working portal is anterior, but additional portals can be added as needed. Generally, the portal in the rotator cuff interval is used for removal of the implant. The glenoid implant is then sectioned with an osteotome or burr and each section is removed through the anterior portal using a grasper. Loose cement can also be excised following implant removal and bone grafting of any glenoid defects can be performed.

When performing open glenoid implant removal, it is important to obtain excellent exposure, which requires removing the humeral head on a modular implant and releasing all subacromial and subdeltoid adhesions. Frozen section biopsies are always obtained from multiple locations targeting the biofilm areas especially where granulation tissue or synovitis is observed. All fibrous tissue is then removed circumferentially from around the glenoid component. If the glenoid component is a cemented all-polyethylene or poly-ingrowth implant, a curved narrow osteotome is placed at the anterior interface of the glenoid component with the native glenoid and another at the posterior interface. Gentle pressure is applied to both, and in the majority of the cases, the implant is easily removed using lateral traction with minimal bone compromise. If this is not successful, then working completely around the implant with the osteotomes (narrow flexible osteotomes) in different directions will usually be successful. If the implant is not loose and removal is becoming difficult, a sharp osteotome can be placed at the anterior glenoid polyethylene interface and carefully driven posteriorly to separate the pegs or keel from the glenoid implant articular face, thereby leaving the cemented/ingrowth pegs/keel in the native bone. In this manner, the native glenoid bone stock is not disrupted. At this point, if the implant is not infected, the revision to RTSA can be performed

with no attempt to remove the well-fixed polyethylene and cement. The placement of the reverse baseplate on a stable cement/polyethylene platform gives excellent fixation with no further damage to glenoid bone (**FIGURE 42.1A-G**). However, in implants that use a central hole for the baseplate, this area needs to be prepared with a high-speed pencil tip burr. It is important not to use the burr as a drill as it will deflect off the remaining cement and create additional bone destruction. If the implant is infected, then the polyethylene and cement should be removed with a high-speed pencil tip burr. This process can be destructive to the native glenoid and should be performed in a controlled and careful manner. Drill bits can be used to remove the polyethylene components, but a burr is better for the cemented areas. Having the appropriate equipment available is essential for successful removal of an ATSA glenoid.

Metal composite polyethylene glenoids, if not loose, can pose an additional challenge as they are often well fixed. The manner of removal depends on the type of implant. If a hybrid caged implant is present, drilling out the bone inside the cage and then tapping the cage removes the central fixation with minimal bony destruction (**FIGURE 42.2A-G**). Other metal composite glenoids may require using a high-speed pencil tip burr around the outside and then removing the peg. Unfortunately, this results in greater bone loss. In some cases, it might be possible to move the central fixation of the reverse baseplate to a different area on the glenoid, leaving the well-fixed peg in place. However, often there is insufficient available area to permit this technique. It is also important to not accept a suboptimal placement of the glenoid baseplate to avoid removing the central peg. Metal-backed glenoids can be particularly challenging if they have significant ingrowth. Some of these are convertible to RTSA, and if infection is not present, then conversion to RTSA can be performed relatively easily. However, if not convertible and/or infected, removing these implants can be very destructive to the native glenoid. If the ingrowth material is tantalum and there is no infection present, it might be wise to fix the baseplate directly through the tantalum and into the host bone. Sterile petroleum jelly can be used to collect the metallic debris as you drill through this implant to avoid accumulation in the joint space.

RECONSTRUCTING THE GLENOID

The plan for reconstructing the glenoid after removing the glenoid implant must be carefully thought out and discussed with the patient prior to surgery. Contingency plans also need to be discussed as the initial plan may need to change once the glenoid is inspected after component removal. The Antuña classification is helpful with planning (**TABLE 42.1**).[39] As noted, there are three classes of glenoid deficiencies: central, peripheral, and combined, each being further divided into mild, moderate,

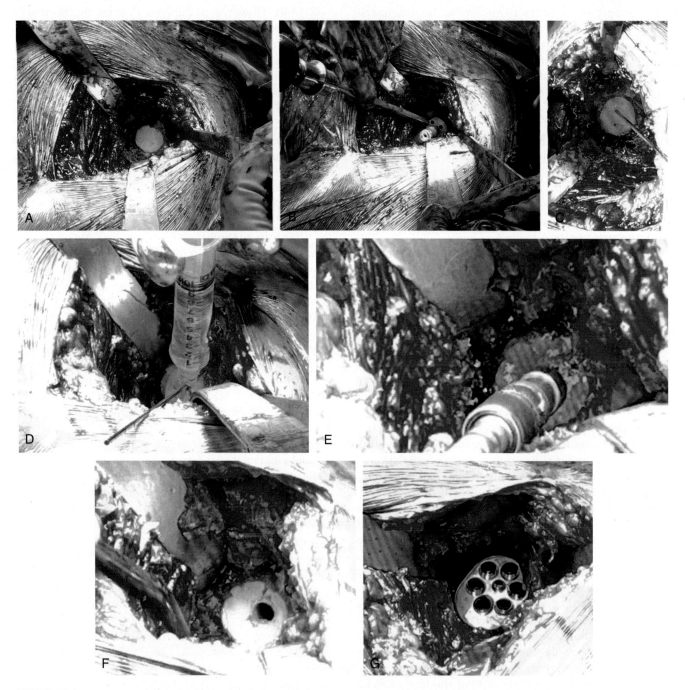

FIGURE 42.1 Inset glenoid. **A,** Glenoid is exposed noting a well-fixed inset all-poly implant. Implant was not removed in order to minimize destruction to glenoid bone stock. **B,** Kirschner wire (K-wire guide) placed to obtain starting point. K-wire drilled with inferior tilt parallel to the anterior glenoid neck. **C,** K-wire placed through the poly in the correct orientation. **D,** Sterile K-Y jelly placed to capture drilling debris. **E,** Cannulated drill placed over K-wire and poly cement and bone drilled for the central hole. **F,** Picture of hole through the poly. **G,** Baseplate placed in central hole.

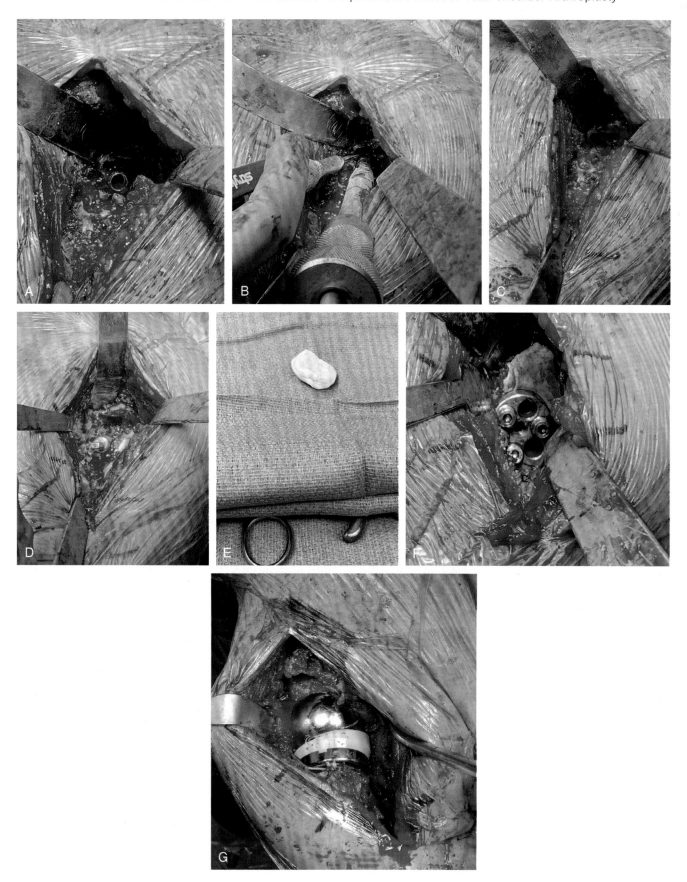

FIGURE 42.2 Intraoperative photographs. **A**, Composite failed glenoid with polyarticular face removed—note well-healed cage in the bone. **B**, Cage removal by drilling out center and using tap to remove. **C**, Remaining glenoid defect, which is severe. **D**, Center drill hole made and kept open while using impaction grafting around it. **E**, Montage graft used to repair posterior superior glenoid wall. This graft has been mixed and now has a uniform light tan color and is ready for implantation. **F**, Baseplate in place graft noted superior. **G**, Implant assembled.

or severe. In general, central contained defects, once they have been fully debrided and irrigated, are relatively easy to manage. Our protocol for debridement and irrigation includes use of dilute betadine, followed by dilute hydrogen peroxide and finally dilute chlorhexidine as lavages. We then change gloves and proceed with the reconstruction.

ATSA is an option when there is minimal bone loss and an adequate rotator cuff. This can be performed by repreparing the glenoid in the standard fashion after impaction bone grafting of small defects if necessary. If there is any remaining cement, a burr should be used for removal followed by glenoid preparation. Reaming of the glenoid surface should be performed to assure adequate backside contact for the new ATSA glenoid. When necessary, eccentric reaming can be performed to correct excessive version. It is important to emphasize that revision to ATSA should only be reserved for cases with little to no bone loss, in cases where adequate peg or keel fixation can be achieved and when adequate rotator cuff is present. In reality, this set of conditions rarely presents itself in the revision setting. We rarely revise an ATSA to an ATSA: the revision is almost always to a RTSA, which is far more forgiving ad has a more predictable outcome.

For RTSA with a contained defect, our approach is to drill the central post screw hole and leave the drill in place. Allograft cubes are then crushed and impacted into the defect, followed by removing the drill and placing the baseplate **(FIGURE 42.3A-I)**.

When a wall of the glenoid is missing—ie., an uncontained defect—the revision procedure becomes much more complicated. The deficient wall needs to be reconstructed before performing the impaction grafting. If the defect is small, a small piece of structural allograft can be placed to fill the defect followed by impaction grafting. Alternatively, Montage (Abyrx, Irvington NY), a calcium phosphate putty that gets very hard, sticks to bone, and does not wash away with blood, can be used to fix small- to moderate-sized wall defects followed by impaction grafting. Montage graft is prepared by opening the two foil packages just before use and kneading the two components together for 45 seconds or until the components are uniformly mixed creating a light tan color. The graft is then molded and placed into the defect.

For massive wall and vault defects or Antuña-combined defects, the decision of what needs to be done depends on the state of the host and their willingness to accept a baseplate failure or a staged procedure. If the host has had multiple operations and is physically frail, it might be best to convert to a hemiarthroplasty **(FIGURE 42.4A-E)** or antibiotic spacer **(FIGURE 42.5A-D)** as the definitive treatment. Similarly, if there is a high index of suspicion that the

joint might be infected, then removing all components and all cement followed by a two-stage procedure is advisable rather than using allograft in a possibly infected wound. Assuming the host is willing to possibly undergo a staged procedure, a structural allograft is obtained (humeral head, femoral head, or proximal femur—the neck is an excellent graft source). If autograft is preferred, then the iliac crest is the donor site of choice for large defects. The distal clavicle can be used for small defects. Preoperative planning software can be helpful for planning these revisions. Unfortunately, intraoperative navigation is often impossible to utilize due to metallic artifact.

The allograft or autograft is fashioned to fit the vault defect. The glenoid neck is fully exposed anteriorly to help place the guide wire for central fixation of the baseplate. Unfortunately, there is little to guide the surgery as to inclination, but in our experience it is difficult to inferiorly incline the baseplate (favorable) and easy to superiorly incline the baseplate (can lead to failure). The central guide pin is placed without graft in the way as this is the most important step for success. The allograft is prepared, and a hole is drilled in it to accept the guide pin. The graft is placed over the guide wire. It can be preliminarily held in place by Kirschner wires (K-wires) directed through the deltoid so as to be out of the way. A reamer is placed over the guide pin and reaming is performed to smooth the graft so it is contiguous with the remaining glenoid bone. Drilling for the central post is performed with a cannulated drill. A baseplate with an extended cage, post, or screw is placed so as to maximize fixation into the host bone. Peripheral screws are then placed **(FIGURE 42.6A-I)**. If baseplate fixation is secure, then a one-stage reconstruction is performed **(FIGURE 42.7A-D** RTSA revision bone graft). When medial bone loss is present and the grafting did not reapproximate the native joint line, a lateralized glenosphere should be used to enhance stability and create an appropriate deltoid wrap and compression vector. If the allograft or autograft has sufficiently lateralized the bone, a standard glenosphere can be used. If baseplate fixation is not secure, a two-stage procedure is preferred. There are two options: the baseplate can be left in place without a glenosphere **(FIGURE 42.8A-C)** or a glenosphere can be placed but the humeral construct is not mated with the glenosphere **(FIGURE 42.9A-D)** so as to minimize shear forces and allow incorporation of the graft. A second procedure completing the RTSA will then be performed at least 6 months in the later to allow graft incorporation.

Another option in cases with severe bone loss is to use a custom baseplate created after an appropriate CT has been performed. Unfortunately, due to the presence of metal, this may require a two-stage procedure to remove the humeral and glenoid implant and

Contained Central Defect

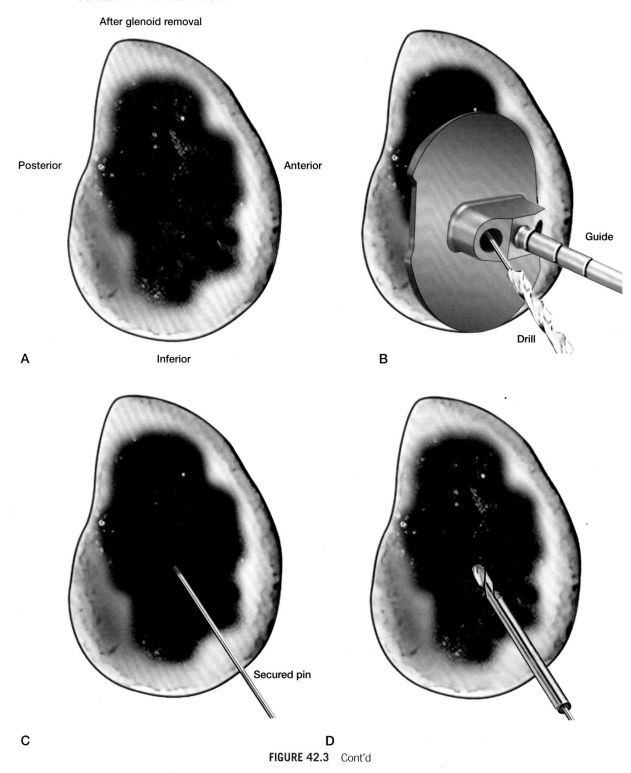

FIGURE 42.3 Cont'd

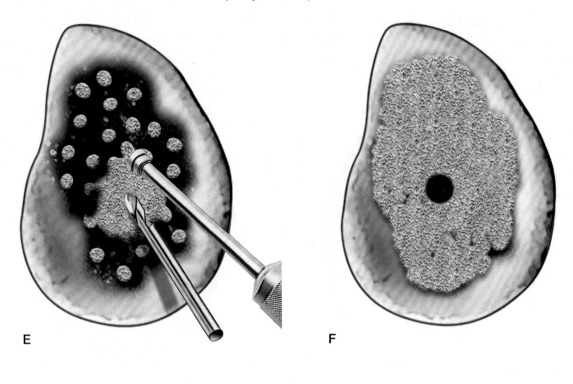

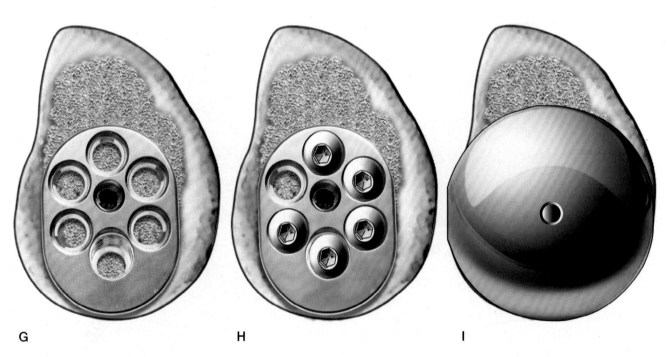

FIGURE 42.3 Impaction grafting. **A,** Schematic drawing of a glenoid with a large contained central defect after glenoid implant has been removed. **B,** Drill guide placed to determine the appropriate location for the central drill hole. **C,** Kirschner wire (K-wire) placed parallel to the anterior neck and with inferior tilt. Ideally want greater than 20 mm of bone. **D,** Cannulated drill drills central hole. **E,** Drill left in place and allograft croutons are crushed in the defect. **F,** Entire defect is now filled with allograft by impaction grafting leaving the central hole open. **G,** Extended post or screw baseplate placed. **H,** Four to six peripheral multiaxial compression screws are placed and then locked via locking caps. **I,** Glenosphere is now placed on stable baseplate.

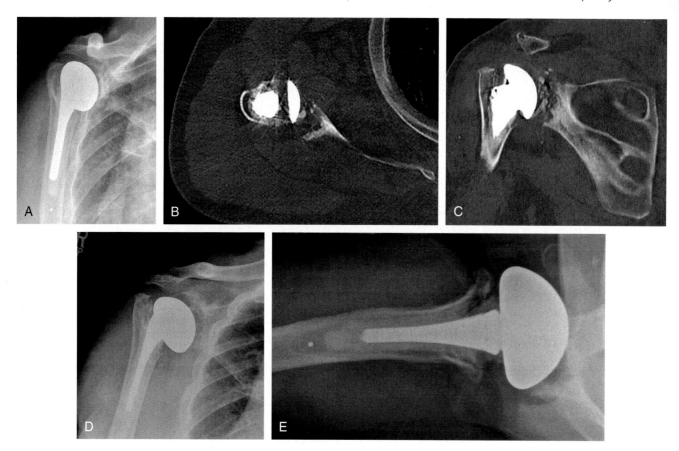

FIGURE 42.4 Total shoulder arthroplasty revised to hemiarthroplasty. **A,** Grashey view preoperatively—note medial migration of the glenoid as shown by the relationship between the lateral edge of the tuberosity and the lateral acromion. **B,** Axillary computed tomography (CT) showing significant loss of bone with minimal remaining glenoid for reverse total shoulder arthroplasty baseplate fixation. **C,** Coronal oblique CT demonstrating extreme glenoid bone loss due to loose glenoid. **D,** Grashey view of hemiarthroplasty cemented into old cement mantle. Note the oversized head that fits into the glenoid defect restoring some lateralization of the humerus. **E,** Axillary lateral view of hemiarthroplasty sitting in the glenoid defect but centered.

permit a high-quality CT to be obtained. The CT is used to make the custom implant. A polymethyl methacrylate (PMMA) antibiotic spacer can be placed in the interim as it will not interfere with the CT scan for preoperative planning. This solution, while available, is currently very expensive **(FIGURE 42.10).**

REVISION FOR INFECTION

Shoulder arthroplasty infection is discussed extensively in Chapter 32. When infection is present, our approach is to remove all foreign materials, including suture, metal, polyethylene, and cement. Complete debridement is followed sequentially by soaking with dilute betadine, dilute hydrogen peroxide, and dilute chlorhexidine. If the host is healthy and not immunocompromised and no structural graft is needed, a primary exchange arthroplasty is performed. If the host is not healthy or

a structural allograft/autograft is required, then a two-stage procedure will be performed. All infected patients require 6 weeks of intravenous antibiotics based on the intraoperative cultures.

DECISION ON TYPE OF RECONSTRUCTION

The decision to revise an anatomic shoulder arthroplasty to an RTSA, ATSA, or hemiarthroplasty is predicated on the quality of the rotator cuff and the remaining glenoid bone stock. If the quality of the glenoid and rotator cuff is good (rarely occurs but most often will be encountered with a painful hemiarthroplasty), then conversion to an ATSA can be performed. If either the glenoid or the rotator cuff is of poor quality or the host is elderly, then conversion to an RTSA is the treatment of choice. In cases of severe bone loss in a poor host, a hemiarthroplasty may be the optimal solution.

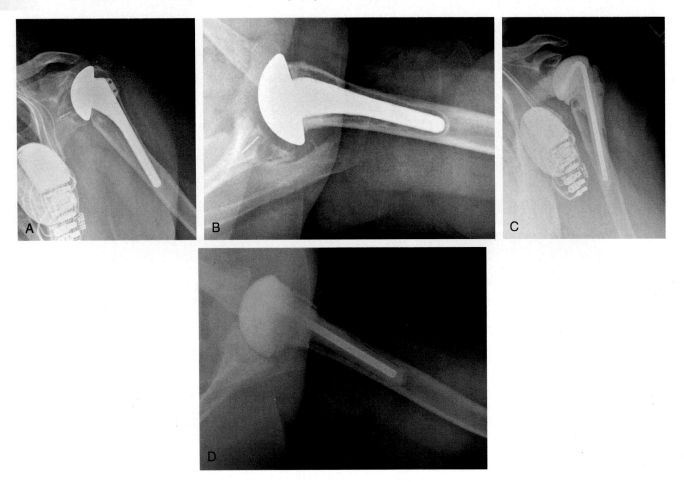

FIGURE 42.5 Total shoulder arthroplasty revised to an antibiotic spacer used as definitive treatment. **A**, Grashey view preoperatively. **B**, Axillary lateral preoperative view of an infected anatomic total shoulder arthroplasty. **C**, Grashey view of the antibiotic spacer. Glenoid has been allograft impaction grafted. **D**, Axillary lateral view of the antibiotic spacer.

RESULTS

The outcomes of revision surgery are not nearly as good as after primary surgery. The reason for this difference is likely multifactorial and due to soft tissue compromise as a result of multiple procedures, weakness of surrounding musculature, and deficiency of native bone following removal of prior implants.

A preliminary study from our institution of 64 revision shoulder arthroplasties followed for more than 2 years showed that hemiarthroplasties had an average Constant score of 48, RTSA of 58, and TSA of 64.[a] This same study noted that ASES scores reached minimal clinically important difference for ATSA[24] and RTSA[22] but not for hemiarthroplasty.[17] This is a somewhat unfair comparison as the ATSAs were performed in optimal revision patients, the RTSAs in less optimal

[a]We thank Atsushi Endo for unpublished data.

patients, and the hemiarthroplasties in the most severe cases. Raphael et al[40] showed that ATSAs revised to ATSAs had mildly improved UCLA and Constant scores compared to patients converted to hemiarthroplasty, although the arthroscopic glenoid excision cases had similar outcomes to the ATSAs. One study reported that revision of ATSA as a result of glenoid loosening or failure to another ATSA had a complication rate of 17% and a radiographic loosening rate of 67% in 42 cases.[41] However, there was a 16-point improvement in the Constant score to 57.[41] Sheth et al[42] reported that 20 revision ATSAs performed *for* all failure mechanisms revised to another ATSA resulted in a revision rate of 35%. Those patients who did not undergo revision had good outcome scores (ASES score 70, SANE 66). Of note, these 20 revision ATSAs to ATSA comprised only 4% of all the revision shoulder surgeries performed during the study period.[42] The same authors reported that 40 ATSAs revised to RTSA had an average ASES

Combined Defect

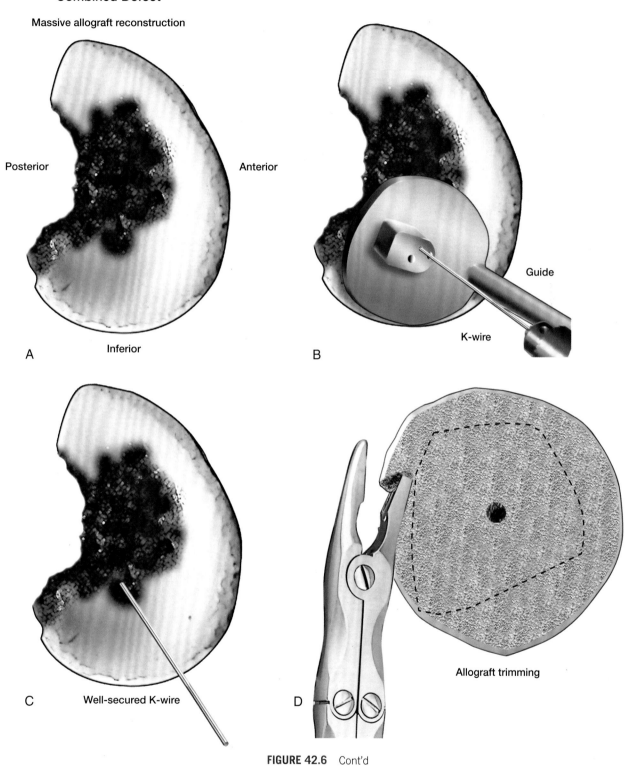

Massive allograft reconstruction

Posterior

Anterior

A   Inferior

Guide

K-wire

B

C   Well-secured K-wire

Allograft trimming

D

FIGURE 42.6 Cont'd

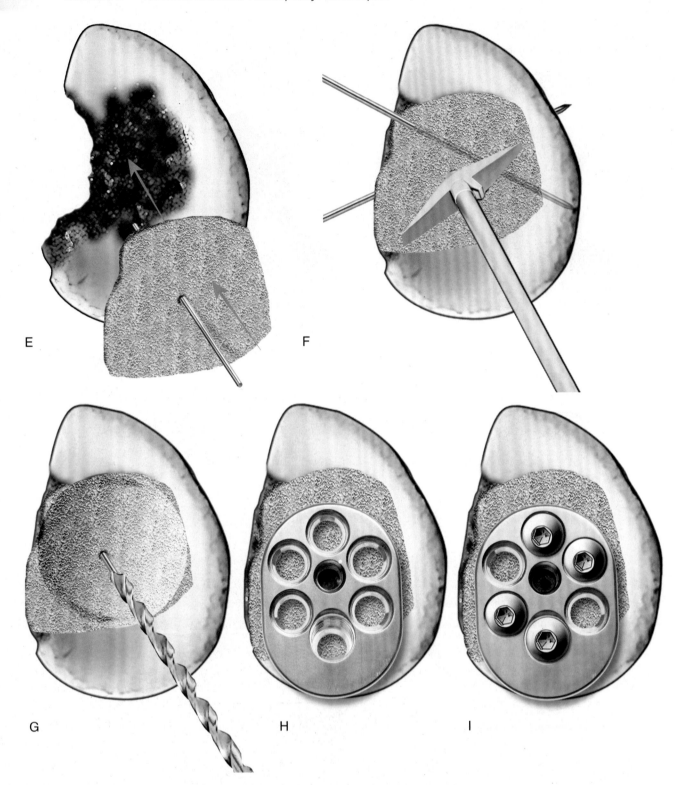

FIGURE 42.6 Massive allograft reconstruction for combined glenoid defect. **A**, Schematic drawing of a combined central and peripheral glenoid defect after removal of implant. **B**, Guide to determine appropriate Kirschner wire (K-wire) starting position. **C**, K-wire placed with inferior tilt and parallel to anterior glenoid neck with goal to obtain at least 20 mm of bone purchase. **D**, Allograft trimmed and oriented prior to K-wire placement. A 4.5 drill hole is placed through the center of the allograft. **E**, Allograft is placed over the K-wire. **F**, Allograft is secured in place by two K-wires placed through the posterior deltoid into the graft and then the host. They are placed in such a manner as to be out of the way of the cannulated reamer. **G**, Cannulated drill drills through the allograft and host bone. **H**, Baseplate with extended post is placed. **I**, Four to six peripheral compression screws are placed through graft and host and then locked with locking caps. The glenosphere can now be placed on this stable baseplate.

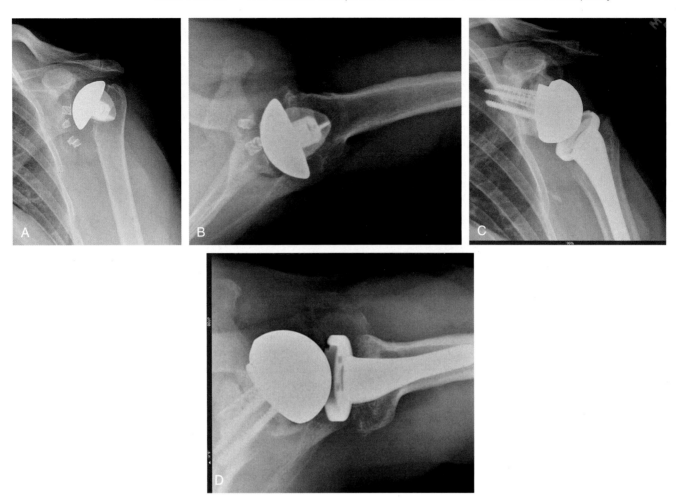

FIGURE 42.7 Loose glenoid revision to reverse total shoulder arthroplasty (RTSA). **A**, Grashey view of loose glenoid in anatomic total shoulder arthroplasty (ATSA). The majority of the loose glenoid is in the axillary recess. **B**, Axillary lateral preoperative view of failed ATSA. **C**, Grashey view of postoperative reconstruction with an RTSA using a combination bone grafting technique of impaction grafting and superior glenoid wall reconstruction with Montage. **D**, Axillary lateral of the RTSA reconstruction.

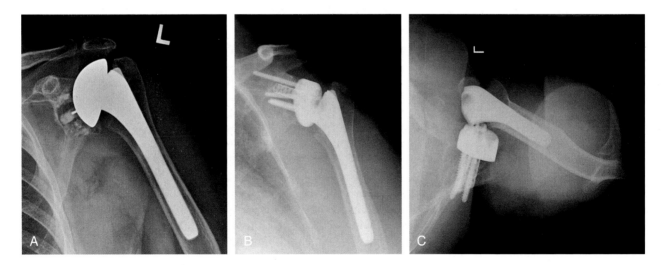

FIGURE 42.8 Two-stage reconstruction with inadequate glenoid support bone graft compressed in the place with the baseplate and platform stem left in place. This is not the desirable technique. Soft tissue is placed between the humerus and baseplate. **A**, Grashey view of an anatomic total shoulder arthroplasty with a loose glenoid. **B**, Grashey radiograph of the baseplate and humerus in place but not coupled after grafting. Allograft soft tissue is interposed. The stem was a platform stem and not pulled. This is not the preferred technique for two-stage bone grafting. **C**, Axillary lateral view postreconstruction.

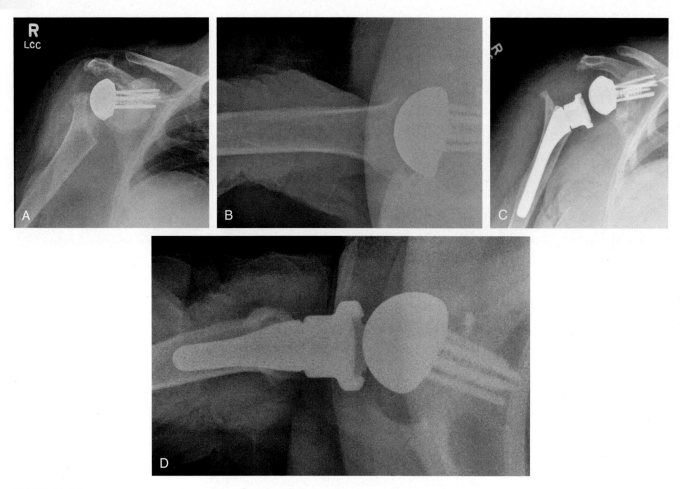

FIGURE 42.9 Two-stage reconstruction with bone grafting of glenoid and no humeral stem (recommended technique). **A**, Grashey first stage; some frail patients will stop at this phase as moderate stability can occur if the glenosphere gets inset into the humerus. **B**, Axillary lateral view of stage 1. **C**, Grashey view after coupling stage 2. The second stage procedure is performed at 6 months or longer after the first stage. **D**, Axillary lateral view of stage 2.

score of 59, but this included some patients with multiple revisions.[5] Shields et al[43] showed that 35 patients who underwent revision of an ATSA to RTSA had similar ASES scores (68) compared to a matched cohort of primary RTSAs, although patient satisfaction and Simple Shoulder Test scores were worse. Another study of ATSAs revised to RTSAs showed a 31-point improvement in the Constant score to 55.[44]

Complications following revision shoulder arthroplasty for glenoid loosening are common. The most common complications following revision of an ATSA to another ATSA are glenoid loosening, instability, and rotator cuff failure.[1,41,42,45] Complications encountered in revision to RTSA are glenoid loosening, instability, periprosthetic fracture (including scapular spine fractures), and infection.[1,5,44,46] One large recent database study

found that of ATSAs that were revised, the re-revision rate was much lower after revision to RTSA (7.5%) versus hemiarthroplasty (19%) or ATSA (22.7%).[1] This is contrary to a nondatabase study that showed a high revision rate in ATSAs revised to RTSA (31%), which was higher compared with a matched comparison group of primary RTSAs (13%).[43] Another study reported a 21% revision rate of ATSAs revised to RTSA in 37 patients.[44] One study noted a significant increase in the number of revisions to RSTAs compared with hemiarthroplasty or ATSA between 2005 and 2016.[47] In this study, RTSA was used more commonly in patients with glenoid loosening, indicating that RTSA use in revision situations has increased possibly due to better outcomes and decreased complications in the revision shoulder arthroplasty setting.

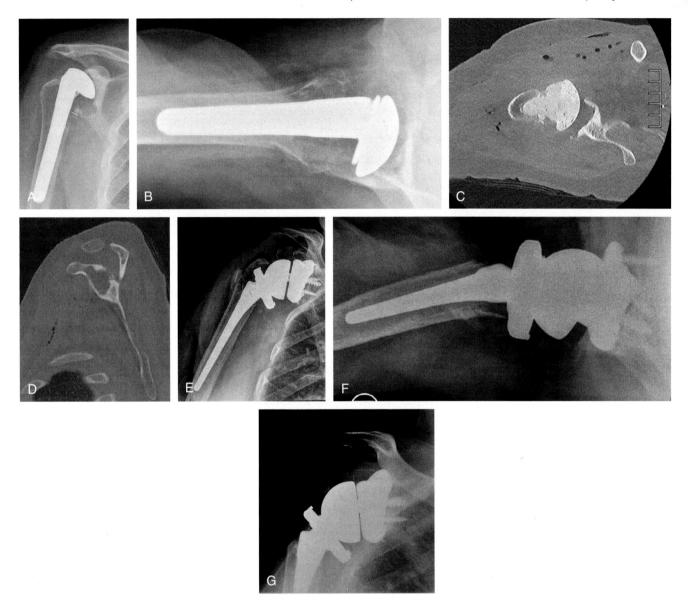

FIGURE 42.10 Two-stage reconstruction with a custom baseplate. **A**, Poorly placed total shoulder arthroplasty with loose glenoid and cuff failure Grashey view. **B**, Axillary lateral of the same patient. **C**, Implants were removed and a cement spacer was placed so a good computed tomography (CT) could be performed and used for the custom implant. **D**, CT showing the glenoid defect. **E**, Grashey view of the custom reconstruction. **F**, Axillary lateral of the custom implant. **G**, Grashey 2.5 years s/p placement of custom implant. (Courtesy of Brad Schoch.)

CONCLUSION

Revision shoulder arthroplasty is a salvage procedure requiring carful preoperative planning and shared decision-making with the patient. The need for massive allograft or autograft as well as the possibility of a two-staged procedure should be discussed with every patient undergoing a revision shoulder arthroplasty. The outcomes, particularly following revision to RTSA, are fair and not comparable to a primary procedure. Similarly, complications are more common and more significant than in a well-executed primary shoulder arthroplasty. As our ATSA implants, preoperative planning, intraoperative tools, and experience improve, the percentage of revision shoulder arthroplasties will decrease; however, with revisions, the outcomes currently remain somewhat unpredictable.

REFERENCES

1. Dillon MT, Prentice HA, Burfeind WE, Singh A. Risk factors for re-revision surgery in shoulder arthroplasty. *J Am Acad Orthop Surg.* 2020. doi:10.5435/JAAOS-D-19-00635
2. Kim DM, Aldeghaither M, Alabdullatif F, et al. Loosening and revision rates after total shoulder arthroplasty: a systematic review of cemented all-polyethylene glenoid and three modern designs of metal-backed glenoid. *BMC Musculoskelet Disord.* 2020;21(1):1-16.

3. Brown JS, Gordon RJ, Peng Y, Hatton A, Page RS, Macgroarty KA. Lower operating volume in shoulder arthroplasty is associated with increased revision rates in the early postoperative period: long-term analysis from the Australian Orthopaedic Association National Joint Replacement Registry. *J Shoulder Elbow Surg*. 2020;29:1104-1114.

4. Gauci M-O, Cavalier M, Gonzalez J-F, et al. Revision of failed shoulder arthroplasty: epidemiology, etiology, and surgical options. *J Shoulder Elbow Surg*. 2020;29(3):541-549.

5. Sheth MM, Sholder D, Getz CL, Williams GR, Namdari S. Revision of failed hemiarthroplasty and anatomic total shoulder arthroplasty to reverse total shoulder arthroplasty. *J Shoulder Elbow Surg*. 2019;28(6):1074-1081.

6. Pinkas D, Wiater B, Wiater JM. The glenoid component in anatomic shoulder arthroplasty. *J Am Acad Orthop Surg*. 2015;23(5):317-326.

7. Raiss P, Schmitt M, Bruckner T, et al. Results of cemented total shoulder replacement with a minimum follow-up of ten years. *J Bone Joint Surg Am*. 2012;94(23):e1711-10.

8. Taunton MJ, McIntosh AL, Sperling JW, Cofield RH. Total shoulder arthroplasty with a metal-backed, bone-ingrowth glenoid component: medium to long-term results. *J Bone Joint Surg Am*. 2008;90(10):2180-2188.

9. Matsen FA III, Clinton J, Lynch J, Bertelsen A, Richardson ML. Glenoid component failure in total shoulder arthroplasty. *J Bone Joint Surg Am*. 2008;90(4):885-896.

10. Page RS, Pai V, Eng K, Bain G, Graves S, Lorimer M. Cementless versus cemented glenoid components in conventional total shoulder joint arthroplasty: analysis from the Australian Orthopaedic Association National Joint Replacement Registry. *J Shoulder Elbow Surg*. 2018;27(10):1859-1865.

11. Flurin PH, Marczuk Y, Janout M, Wright TW, Zuckerman J, Roche CP. Comparison of outcomes using anatomic and reverse total shoulder arthroplasty. *Bull Hosp Jt Dis (2013)*. 2013;71(suppl 2):101-107.

12. Gauci MO, Bonnevialle N, Moineau G, Baba M, Walch G, Boileau P. Anatomical total shoulder arthroplasty in young patients with osteoarthritis: all-polyethylene versus metal-backed glenoid. *Bone Joint J*. 2018;100(4):485-492.

13. Merolla G, Ciaramella G, Fabbri E, Walch G, Paladini P, Porcellini G. Total shoulder replacement using a bone ingrowth central peg polyethylene glenoid component: a prospective clinical and computed tomography study with short- to mid-term follow-up. *Int Orthop*. 2016;40(11):2355-2363.

14. Gazielly DF, Scarlat MM, Verborgt O. Long-term survival of the glenoid components in total shoulder replacement for arthritis. *Int Orthop*. 2015;39(2):285-289.

15. Vavken P, Sadoghi P, von Keudell A, Rosso C, Valderrabano V, Müller AM. Rates of radiolucency and loosening after total shoulder arthroplasty with pegged or keeled glenoid components. *J Bone Joint Surg Am*. 2013;95(3):215-221.

16. Friedman RJ, Cheung E, Grey SG, et al. Clinical and radiographic comparison of a hybrid cage glenoid to a cemented polyethylene glenoid in anatomic total shoulder arthroplasty. *J Shoulder Elbow Surg*. 2019;28(12):2308-2316.

17. Parks DL, Casagrande DJ, Schrumpf MA, Harmsen SM, Norris TR, Kelly JD II. Radiographic and clinical outcomes of total shoulder arthroplasty with an all-polyethylene pegged bone ingrowth glenoid component: prospective short-to medium-term follow-up. *J Shoulder Elbow Surg*. 2016;25(2):246-255.

18. Panti JP, Tan S, Kuo W, Fung S, Walker K, Duff J. Clinical and radiologic outcomes of the second-generation Trabecular Metal™ glenoid for total shoulder replacements after 2–6 years follow-up. *Arch Orthop Trauma Surg*. 2016;136(12):1637-1645.

19. Styron JF, Marinello PG, Peers S, Seitz WH. Survivorship of trabecular metal anchored glenoid total shoulder arthroplasties. *Tech Hand Up Extrem Surg*. 2016;20(3):113-116.

20. Vuillermin CB, Trump ME, Barwood SA, Hoy GA. Catastrophic failure of a low profile metal-backed glenoid component after total shoulder arthroplasty. *Int J Shoulder Surg*. 2015;9(4):121.

21. Budge MD, Nolan EM, Heisey MH, Baker K, Wiater JM. Results of total shoulder arthroplasty with a monoblock porous tantalum glenoid component: a prospective minimum 2-year follow-up study. *J Shoulder Elbow Surg*. 2013;22(4):535-541.

22. Nelson CG, Brolin TJ, Ford MC, Smith RA, Azar FM, Throckmorton TW. Five-year minimum clinical and radiographic outcomes of total shoulder arthroplasty using a hybrid glenoid component with a central porous titanium post. *J Shoulder Elbow Surg*. 2018;27(8):1462-1467.

23. Metzl JA, Vorys GC, Levine WN, Ahmad CS, Bigliani LU. Clinical and radiographic outcomes of total shoulder arthroplasty with a hybrid dual-radii glenoid component. *Am J Orthop*. 2017;46(6):E366-E373.

24. Schoch BS, Zarezadeh A, Priddy M, King JJ, Wright TW. Uncemented fixation of a monoblock ingrowth polyethylene glenoid: early follow-up. *J Shoulder Elbow Surg*. 2020;29:968-975.

25. Gunther SB, Tran SK. Long-term follow-up of total shoulder replacement surgery with inset glenoid implants for arthritis with deficient bone. *J Shoulder Elbow Surg*. 2019;28(9):1728-1736.

26. Cvetanovich GL, Naylor AJ, O'Brien MC, Waterman BR, Garcia GH, Nicholson GP. Anatomic total shoulder arthroplasty with an inlay glenoid component: clinical outcomes and return to activity. *J Shoulder Elbow Surg*. 2020;29:1188-1196.

27. Schoch B, Schleck C, Cofield RH, Sperling JW. Shoulder arthroplasty in patients younger than 50 years: minimum 20-year follow-up. *J Shoulder Elbow Surg*. 2015;24(5):705-710.

28. Papadonikolakis A, Neradilek MB, Matsen FA III. Failure of the glenoid component in anatomic total shoulder arthroplasty: a systematic review of the English-language literature between 2006 and 2012. *J Bone Joint Surg Am*. 2013;95(24):2205-2212.

29. Hernandez-Ortiz EG, Christmas KN, Simon P, et al. Improving preoperative planning of revision surgery after previous anatomic total shoulder arthroplasty. *J Shoulder Elbow Surg*. 2019;28(6):S168-S174.

30. Gregory T, Hansen U, Khanna M, et al. A CT scan protocol for the detection of radiographic loosening of the glenoid component after total shoulder arthroplasty. *Acta Orthop*. 2014;85:91-96.

31. Williams GR Jr, Iannotti JP. Options for glenoid bone loss: composites of prosthetics and biologics. *J Shoulder Elbow Surg*. 2007;16(5 suppl):S267-S272.

32. Gupta A, Thussbas C, Koch M, et al. Management of glenoid bone defects with reverse shoulder arthroplasty-surgical technique and clinical outcomes. *J Shoulder Elbow Surg*. 2018;27(5):853-862.

33. Garrigues GE, Zmistowski B, Cooper AM, Green A. Proceedings from the 2018 International Consensus Meeting on Orthopedic Infections: evaluation of periprosthetic shoulder infection. *J Shoulder Elbow Surg*. 2019;28(6s):S32-S66.

34. Ahmadi S, Lawrence TM, Sahota S, et al. Significance of perioperative tests to diagnose the infection in revision total shoulder arthroplasty. *Arch Bone Jt Surg*. 2018;6(5):359.

35. Garrigues GE, Zmistowski B, Cooper AM, Green A. Proceedings from the 2018 International Consensus Meeting on Orthopedic Infections: the definition of periprosthetic shoulder infection. *J Shoulder Elbow Surg*. 2019;28(6s):S8-S12.

36. Guild T, Kuhn G, Rivers M, Cheski R, Trenhaile S, Izquierdo R. The role of arthroscopy in painful shoulder arthroplasty: is revision always necessary? *Arthroscopy*. 2020;36:1508-1514.

37. Venjakob AJ, Reichwein F, Nebelung W. Arthroscopic removal of a polyethylene glenoid component in total shoulder arthroplasty. *Arthrosc Tech*. 2015;4(2):e149-e152.

38. O'Driscoll SW, Petrie RS, Torchia ME. Arthroscopic removal of the glenoid component for failed total shoulder arthroplasty: a report of five cases. *J Bone Joint Surg Am*. 2005;87(4):858-863.

39. Antuna SA, Sperling JW, Cofield RH, Rowland CM. Glenoid revision surgery after total shoulder arthroplasty. *J Shoulder Elbow Surg*. 2001;10(3):217-224.

40. Raphael BS, Dines JS, Warren RF, et al. Symptomatic glenoid loosening complicating total shoulder arthroplasty. *HSS J*. 2010;6(1):52-56.

41. Bonnevialle N, Melis B, Neyton L, et al. Aseptic glenoid loosening or failure in total shoulder arthroplasty: revision with glenoid reimplantation. *J Shoulder Elbow Surg*. 2013;22(6):745-751.

42. Sheth M, Sholder D, Padegimas EM, et al. Failure of anatomic total shoulder arthroplasty with revision to another anatomic total shoulder arthroplasty. *Arch Bone Jt Surg*. 2019;7(1):19.

43. Shields E, Wiater JM. Patient outcomes after revision of anatomic total shoulder arthroplasty to reverse shoulder arthroplasty for rotator cuff failure or component loosening: a matched cohort study. *J Am Acad Orthop Surg*. 2019;27(4):e193-e198.

44. Melis B, Bonnevialle N, Neyton L, et al. Glenoid loosening and failure in anatomical total shoulder arthroplasty: is revision with a reverse shoulder arthroplasty a reliable option? *J Shoulder Elbow Surg*. 2012;21(3):342-349.

45. Aibinder WR, Schoch B, Schleck C, Sperling JW, Cofield RH. Revisions for aseptic glenoid component loosening after anatomic shoulder arthroplasty. *J Shoulder Elbow Surg*. 2017;26(3):443-449.

46. Bois AJ, Knight P, Alhojailan K, Bohsali KI. Clinical outcomes and complications of reverse shoulder arthroplasty used for failed prior shoulder surgery: a systematic review and meta-analysis. *JSES Int*. 2020;4(1):156-168.

47. Wagner ER, Chang MJ, Welp KM, et al. The impact of the reverse prosthesis on revision shoulder arthroplasty: analysis of a high-volume shoulder practice. *J Shoulder Elbow Surg*. 2019;28(2):e49-e56.

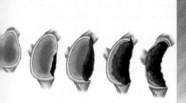

43 The Glenoid Component in Reverse Total Shoulder Arthroplasty

Andrew R. Jensen, MD, MBE, Samuel Antuña, MD, PhD, and John W. Sperling, MD, MBA

INTRODUCTION

As the incidence of primary anatomic total shoulder arthroplasty (ATSA) and reverse total shoulder arthroplasty (RTSA) continue to rise, there will be a greater need for revision shoulder arthroplasty procedures. Often, these revision procedures are complicated by a loss of glenoid bone stock that leads to tenuous fixation of the glenoid component. At times, surgical techniques to restore, augment, or circumvent glenoid bone loss are required to obtain stable and durable glenoid component fixation during revision RTSA. These techniques will be the focus of this chapter.

EPIDEMIOLOGY AND RISK FACTORS

Severe glenoid bone loss is often due to aseptic loosening of a preexisting ATSA or RTSA glenoid implant. Aseptic loosening of the glenoid component in ATSA is one of the most common modes of total shoulder arthroplasty (TSA) failure and, when the glenoid component becomes loose due to the "rocking horse phenomenon," can leave a cavitary defect in the remaining glenoid.[1] Additionally, when, otherwise, well-fixed glenoid components are removed during a revision procedure, the remaining glenoid can have significant bony defects that require consideration.

Unlike in the case of ATSA, the rates of aseptic loosening of primary RTSA glenoid components are relatively low. Bitzer and colleagues reviewed 202 patients who had undergone RTSA and found that there was a 3% incidence of glenoid component aseptic loosening.[2] The rate of RTSA glenoid component loosening is higher in certain situations, such as following revision surgery, when glenoid bone graft is used and in female patients. In the same aforementioned study, Bitzer and colleagues found that the rate of aseptic loosening of the glenoid was 10% following revision surgery.[2] A meta-analysis of 6583 RTSA surgeries from 2019 found that there was a baseplate loosening rate of 0.90% for primary and 3.64% for revision RTSA.[3] Therefore, rerevision of RTSA with glenoid bone loss can pose a significant technical challenge.

Frequently, glenoid augmentation is required during revision RTSA. One study from the Mayo Clinic reported that 29% of 143 consecutive revision RTSA procedures over a 5-year period required glenoid augmentation for bone loss. Because of this, surgeons who perform revision shoulder arthroplasty should be prepared to address various types and severities of glenoid defects intraoperatively with an assortment of techniques which will be discussed in this chapter.

EVALUATION OF GLENOID BONE LOSS

Clinical History and Physical Examination

Following RTSA, baseplate loosening may present early after initial fixation or late, related to baseplate malposition or bone graft resorption. Traumatic etiologies must be excluded. Patients with loose glenoid components after shoulder arthroplasty may have no clinical symptoms, with the diagnosis being made on routine postoperative imaging. In fact, patients may not develop symptoms until years after the glenoid component is first noted to be loose. Unfortunately, this symptomatic delay can actually exacerbate glenoid defect severity if and when revision surgery is ultimately required.

When these patients are symptomatic, they often report pain deep in the shoulder that is worse with activity. A thorough physical examination should include visualization of the shoulder girdle for muscle atrophy and previous incisions, evaluation of deltoid integrity and scapular motion, measurement of active and passive shoulder range of motion, as well as rotator cuff strength and performance of a thorough neurovascular examination.

In any failed shoulder arthroplasty, infection must be ruled out with inflammatory laboratory tests and possibly shoulder aspiration or surgical biopsies.[4] Additionally, for patients requiring revision surgery, the identity of previous implants should be confirmed on radiographs and from the operative note, if available.

Radiographic Analysis

Routine standard radiographs should be obtained for all patients. Our standard series includes Grashey anteroposterior (AP) radiographs in internal and external rotation as well as an axillary view. It is best to compare with previous radiographs, if available, to assess for interval bone loss. One can consider using fluoroscopic guidance for proper positioning to obtain adequate imaging.[4]

Advanced imaging with computed tomography (CT) and three-dimensional (3D) reconstruction is recommended for all patients. If ATSA glenoid component loosening is in question, a CT arthrogram can delineate lucent lines around the polyethylene component. Use of metal artifact reduction software for CT scans may improve glenoid vault visualization in cases of metal burden around the glenoid vault.

Advanced imaging can also be processed through preoperative planning software to help the surgeon optimize baseplate fixation and glenosphere orientation.[5] These software programs utilize CT data to calculate baseplate contact area, screw lengths, and glenosphere version and inclination and allow the surgeon to change these virtual surgical variables. This planning process can be particularly helpful in cases with glenoid bone loss in which surface anatomy is distorted. Studies have shown that the use of preoperative planning software can improve glenoid baseplate guide pin accuracy in terms of version, inclination, and location.[5] A further extension of preoperative planning software utility is the creation and use of patient-specific instrumentation (PSI) guides and/or intraoperative navigation. Custom PSI guides that conform to patient anatomy and allow for optimal glenoid guide pin placement can be created from preoperative planning software data, while intraoperative navigation systems use optical tracking after anatomic registration in conjunction with preoperative CT data to direct the surgeon in accurate glenoid component placement.[5] While both PSI and intraoperative navigation are exciting technologies, their clinical utility remains to be proven, and currently, they require specialized surgical equipment and are associated with additional operating room time and cost.[5]

Characterization of Glenoid Bone Defects

Antuña and colleagues were the first to classify glenoid bone loss in revision shoulder arthroplasty **(FIGURE 43.1)**.[6] Their classification, which was published in 2001, characterized lesions as central, peripheral, or combined and graded the extent of each as mild, moderate, or severe. Subsequently, Williams and Iannotti expanded Antuña's classification—taking into account the glenoid subchondral bone, vault, and rim—to assist in determining glenoid component fixation options in the setting of revision TSA.[7]

As the Antuña classification predated RTSA availability in the United States, Gupta and colleagues described a classification scheme to guide surgical management during revision RTSA with glenoid bone loss **(FIGURE 43.2)**.[8] They similarly classified glenoid bone loss as centric or eccentric and graded the severity one through four. With this classification scheme, they recommended that centric defects be treated with impaction grafting, eccentric

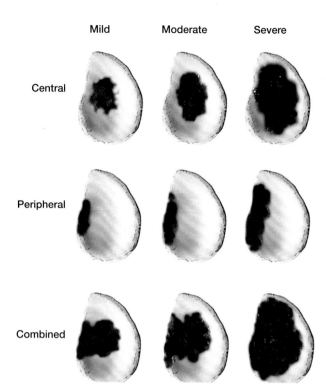

FIGURE 43.1 Antuña Classification of glenoid bone loss. Bone loss is classified according to location (central, peripheral, or combined) and severity.

defects with corticocancellous structural bone grafting, and that severe defects of either nature be staged.[8]

Although preoperative glenoid bone defect evaluation and classification is important, intraoperative reassessment of the remnant glenoid morphology prior to definitive baseplate fixation is critical. Preoperative radiographic evaluation of glenoid bone, particularly in the setting of retained implants, can be inaccurate.[8] Also, the process of implant removal can worsen glenoid defects despite best efforts to preserve bone stock. As part of the reconstructive surgical procedure, we recommend full assessment of the glenoid bone stock after all hardware and overlying soft tissues have been removed from the native glenoid prior to proceeding with reconstruction.

TREATMENT OPTIONS

Many treatment options exist for patients who present with glenoid bone loss, ranging from nonoperative measures to salvage surgeries **(TABLE 43.1)**.

Nonoperative Treatment

While surgical intervention is indicated for the majority of patients with failed shoulder arthroplasties and glenoid bone loss, there are a few categories of patients for whom nonoperative treatment, including activity modifications and anti-inflammatory medications, is

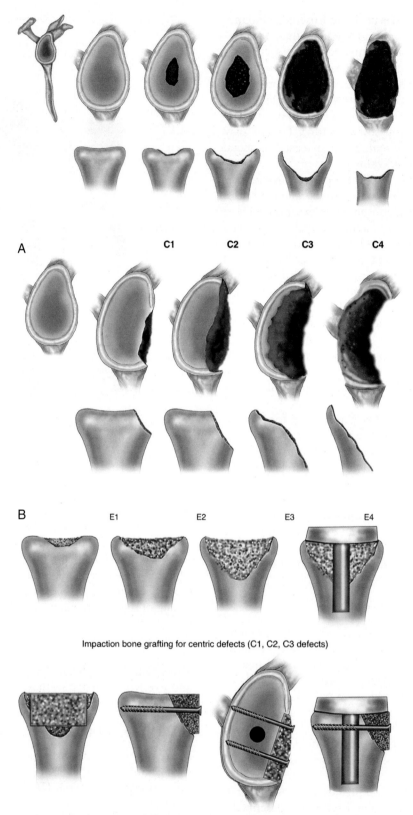

FIGURE 43.2 Gupta Classification of glenoid bone loss. Bone loss is classified as concentric (**A**) or eccentric (**B**). Glenoid reconstruction during shoulder arthroplasty is dictated by the nature and severity of the bone loss (**C**).

TABLE 43.1 Treatment Options for Failed Shoulder Arthroplasty in the Setting of Glenoid Bone Loss

Nonoperative	Revision RTSA Options		Salvage
Conservative management	Standard RTSA	RTSA with augmented baseplate	Two-stage glenoid bony reconstruction
	RTSA with nonstructural bone graft	RTSA with metallic glenoid reconstruction	Conversion to hemiarthroplasty
	RTSA with structural autograft	RTSA using the alternate scapular spine centerline	Resection arthroplasty
	RTSA with structural allograft		Glenohumeral arthrodesis

RTSA, reverse total shoulder arthroplasty.

an acceptable option. Currently, it is standard of care to treat asymptomatic ATSA patients who have radiographic evidence of glenoid component loosening nonoperatively.[4] As mentioned, these patients can remain asymptomatic for years despite a loose glenoid component. Some mildly symptomatic patients may refuse further surgical intervention due to adequate upper extremity function. Secondary stabilization of loose or even displaced RTSA glenoid components has been described that may result in acceptable shoulder function after a trial of nonoperative management.[9] Additionally, patients who are medically unfit for revision surgery or participation in the required postoperative rehabilitation should be managed nonoperatively. Patients with glenoid component loosening treated nonoperatively, however, may have progressive symptoms and worsening glenoid bone loss **(FIGURE 43.3)**. Therefore, it is essential to follow these patients at regular intervals.

Conversion to Hemiarthroplasty

In the case of a failed shoulder arthroplasty, one surgical option is to remove the glenoid component and convert the RTSA to a hemiarthroplasty. Downsides of conversion to hemiarthroplasty, as opposed to revision to another RTSA, include worse biomechanical function

of the shoulder due to medialization of the humerus and the potential for subsequent rapid glenoid bone loss.[4] Accordingly, in a study of 79 patients with glenoid aseptic loosening following RTSA, Ladermann and colleagues found that revision RTSA significantly improved range of motion, function score, and pain scores, whereas revision hemiarthroplasty did not improve any of these outcomes.[10] In this study, 70% of patients revised to RTSA were satisfied or very satisfied, compared with just 31% of those revised to hemiarthroplasty.[9] Therefore, we only recommend conversion to hemiarthroplasty as a viable surgical option in extenuating circumstances **(FIGURE 43.4)**.

Revision RTSA With Glenoid Augmentation

For patients with failed shoulder arthroplasties and glenoid bone defects, regardless of the etiology, often the best surgical treatment option is revision to RTSA. At times, the glenoid bone loss may be sufficiently limited that standard reaming and glenoid preparation will address the defect. When defects are larger and potentially compromise baseplate stability, the glenoid should be augmented to achieve baseplate stability. Options for glenoid augmentation include the use of bone graft, metal, or a salvage reconstructive procedure.

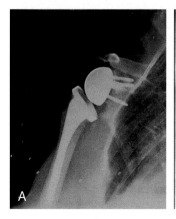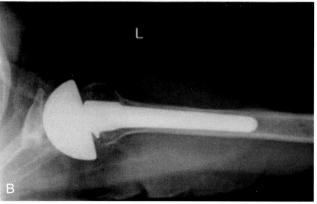

FIGURE 43.3 Nonoperative management of reverse total shoulder arthroplasty (RTSA) with scapular notching. A patient with inferior scapular notching following RTSA (**A**). Note the loose glenoid component. The patient was treated nonoperatively. Glenoid component loosening progressed, resulting in severe glenoid bone loss, gross component displacement, and broken hardware (**B**).

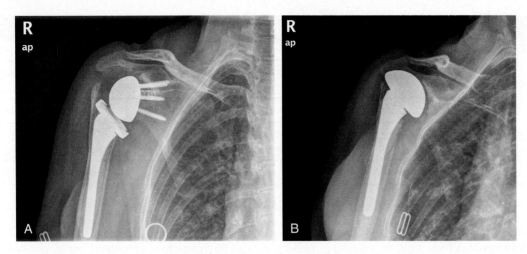

FIGURE 43.4 Conversion of failed reverse total shoulder arthroplasty (RTSA) to hemiarthroplasty. A failed RTSA demonstrating humeral component subsidence and bone loss (**A**). After glenoid component removal during the revision surgery, there was insufficient bone stock for revision to RTSA, and so the patient was converted to a hemiarthroplasty (**B**) with successful pain relief but poor function.

Bone Grafts

There are a variety of bone graft options for glenoid defects that have been described, with a variety of unique biologic and mechanical properties (**TABLE 43.2**). Generally speaking, these bone graft options can be divided into autograft versus allograft options.

Autograft can be cancellous or structural in nature. Local cancellous bone, such as that from the humeral metaphysis, can be used to augment small- or medium-sized glenoid defects that do not compromise the cortical rim. Often, in revision surgery, humeral cancellous autograft may not be readily available. However, if the humeral component needs to be revised in a revision RTSA, some metaphyseal cancellous bone graft can often be obtained. In these situations, bone graft can be impacted into the glenoid defects with the use of bone

tamps and a mallet. Care should be taken to not fracture an intact glenoid cortical rim.

Structural autograft options include humeral cortical bone, tricortical iliac crest, and distal clavicle. Humeral cortical autograft is only readily available during revision RTSA when the humeral component also requires revision, similar to humeral cancellous bone. The rim of cortical bone, if sufficiently large to address the glenoid defect, can be saved from the revision humeral cut to reconstruct the glenoid by placing it into the glenoid defect while seating the baseplate (**FIGURE 43.5**).

Tricortical iliac crest is the most commonly reported structural autograft option for revision RTSA with significant glenoid defects. Its use was pioneered by Norris.[11] Tricortical iliac crest autograft is a versatile option because of its large size that can be adjusted based on intraoperative assessment of the glenoid defect.

TABLE 43.2 Glenoid Bone Graft Options

	Bone Graft	Structure	Comments
Autograft	Humeral cancellous bone	Cancellous only	Impaction grafting for contained defects, if available
	Humeral cortical bone	Corticocancellous	If humeral stem requires revision with a deeper humeral cut
	Tricortical iliac crest	Corticocancellous	Large structural glenoid defects
	Distal clavicle	Corticocancellous	Patients with AC arthritis; may aid in glenoid component removal
Allograft	Cancellous bone	Cancellous only	Impaction grafting for contained defects
	Tricortical iliac crest	Corticocancellous or cancellous	Large structural glenoid defects
	Femoral head or neck	Corticocancellous or cancellous	Large structural glenoid defects
	Femoral cortex	Corticocancellous	Do not use

AC, acromioclavicular.

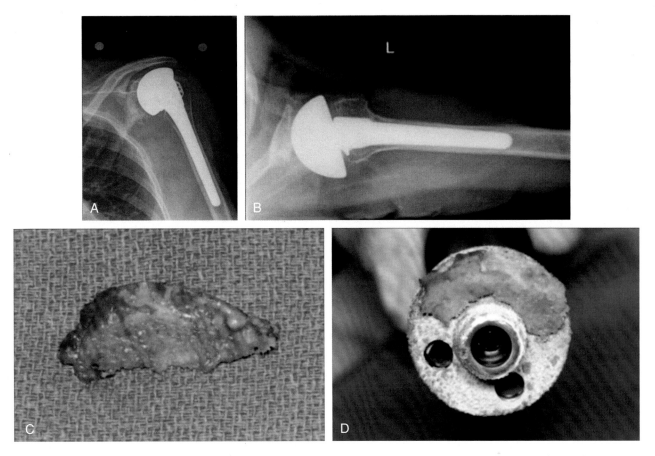

FIGURE 43.5 Humeral autograft for posterior glenoid bone loss during revision of hemiarthroplasty to reverse total shoulder arthroplasty (RTSA). A prior hemiarthroplasty with glenoid cartilage loss (**A**) and posterior glenoid bone loss (**B**) was revised for pain and loss of function. The humeral stem required removal and, therefore, a wedge of structural humeral corticocancellous autograft (**C**) was able to be harvested from the revision humeral neck cut. This structural autograft wedge was applied to the posterior aspect of the glenoid baseplate (**D**) to account for the posterior glenoid bone loss.

Also, additional cancellous bone can be harvested from the graft site as needed. The disadvantages of this option include the additional incision and donor site pain, which is often significant. Patients must have their iliac crests prepped and draped preoperatively.

To perform tricortical iliac crest grafting, the glenoid bone defect is first assessed for size and shape. Then a standard approach to the iliac crest is undertaken. After measuring the required bone graft length, one technique is to osteotomize the bone, fashion the graft to the glenoid defect, provisionally fix the graft to the glenoid with Kirschner wires (K-wires), and then insert the glenoid baseplate on top of the construct. Alternatively, the technique as described by Norris can be utilized, wherein the iliac crest is reamed and the baseplate is inserted in situ, after which the baseplate with the iliac crest is osteotomized as a unit and transferred to the glenoid for the final implantation. The osteotomized baseplate/bone graft unit must be fashioned with a rongeur to fit the remnant glenoid contour. One peripheral locking screw can be inserted into the iliac crest while in situ to prevent the graft from spinning during final insertion.

Distal clavicle autograft has been described in the treatment of shoulder instability with glenoid bone loss.[12] Similarly, the distal clavicle can be resected and used for central or peripheral glenoid bone loss during revision RTSA. This technique has a few notable benefits. First, it only requires extending the deltopectoral incision slightly proximally, as opposed to creating an entirely new incision with the resulting morbidity of other structural autograft options. Second, it can treat concomitant acromioclavicular (AC) osteoarthritis if present. Third, resection of the distal clavicle provides an advantageous exposure of the glenoid implant/bone interface for implant removal. A small osteotome can be inserted from superior to inferior through the inferior AC joint capsule to aid in implant removal.

Allograft options also can be cancellous or structural. Allograft cancellous bone chips are commonly used to fill nonstructural contained defects when cancellous autograft is not available, as is often the case in revision surgery.

Many structural allograft options have been described in the literature, including femoral head, neck, shaft, and iliac crest. The technique described by Tashjian and

TABLE 43.3 Augmented Glenoid Baseplates Available in the United States

Company	RTSA System	Type of Wedge Augment
Zimmer-Biomet	Comprehensive reverse shoulder system	Half-wedge
Tornier	Aequalis perform reversed	Half- or full-wedge
Exactech	Equinoxe	Full-wedge

colleagues utilizes a wedge of femoral head allograft that is shaped to the contour of the glenoid bone defect.[13] Allograft cancellous bone chips can also be harvested from the remaining femoral head after the wedge is created. Of note, femoral shaft allograft should not be used for revision RTSA. A study that compared the use of femoral shaft allograft to femoral neck allograft found that all femoral shaft grafts failed to incorporate, while 78% of femoral neck allografts successfully incorporated.[14]

Metal Augments

As an alternative to bony options, metal augments can be used to reconstruct glenoid defects during revision RTSA. Generally speaking, there are two metal reconstructive options available—the use of glenoid baseplates that are augmented on the backside to account for partial glenoid bone loss and custom metallic implants that reconstruct the entire glenoid with fixation to an individual's remaining scapula.

Augmented baseplates have additional metal on the backside, either a half- or full-wedge for eccentric wear or a flat back for centric wear to compensate for glenoid bone loss. Though newer than the use of bone graft for these situations, a number of augmented baseplates now exist in the US market for RTSA in the setting of bone loss **(TABLE 43.3)**. The augmented baseplate can be rotated to match the glenoid defect, for example, to account for superior **(FIGURE 43.6)** or posterior **(FIGURE 43.7)** bone loss. The porous metal on the backside of the baseplate allows for bony ingrowth and a stable construct by contacting native bone. Relative to structural bone grafting options, the use of augmented metal baseplates is also time efficient and does not include the concerns of donor site morbidity.

If insufficient glenoid exists to implant a standard glenoid baseplate, either with the use of bone grafts or metal augments, the options are to perform a two-staged bony glenoid reconstruction or to reconstruct the glenoid with a custom metallic implant called the Vault Reconstruction System (VRS; Zimmer Biomet, Warsaw, IN, USA).[15] The benefit of using VRS for these salvage situations is that severe glenoid deformities can be addressed in a single surgery and without the concern for potential nonunion. However, these custom implants are expensive and require weeks to create. The VRS implant is fixed to the remaining scapular bone through patient-specific drill guides and screws to reconstruct the missing glenoid vault, and a glenosphere is attached to the fixed VRS implant onto its morse taper **(FIGURE 43.8)**.

Implant Fixation

It is not currently known how much contact must exist between native glenoid and the baseplate to obtain adequate time-zero fixation and stability that results in a durable glenoid construct. Formaini and colleagues performed a biomechanical study to assess this question, in which they fixed an RTSA baseplate with peripheral locking screws onto a bone surrogate and measured the resulting amount of micromotion during shear and compressive forces with decreasing amounts of bone contact.[16] They found that there was no difference in fixation with 100%, 75%, or 50% contact but that at 25% contact there was significantly greater micromotion above a critical threshold.[16] However, in a clinical study, Lorenzetti and colleagues reviewed 57 patients with glenoid bone loss who had undergone primary RTSA with bone grafting and found a low glenoid loosening rate even though there was an average of just 17% contact between the glenoid baseplate and native bone.[17] In this study, there was no significant association between host bone contact and functional outcomes at mean of 46 months.[17] Therefore, it is currently unclear just how much native glenoid is required for adequate baseplate stability.

Another option for obtaining adequate baseplate fixation in cases of significant glenoid bone loss has been described by Frankle and colleagues using a corridor of preserved bone from the glenoid to the base of the scapular spine called the alternate scapular spine centerline.[18] In this technique, the baseplate's central screw is directed toward the base of the scapular spine instead of toward the glenoid vault base by adjusting the guide pin's angulation approximately 30° posteriorly and 15° superiorly. Benefits of this approach include easier instrumentation and avoiding a two-staged approach. However, the resulting glenosphere position is by design anteverted, which may affect range of motion or anterior impingement on the coracoid and conjoint tendon.

Lastly, if the surgeon is unable to obtain adequate baseplate fixation despite these techniques, salvage surgical options include staging an RTSA, resection arthroplasty, and glenohumeral arthrodesis. In a two-stage glenoid reconstruction for failed RTSA, the glenoid bone stock is first replenished via bone grafting, and then, after bone graft healing is confirmed radiographically, a second procedure is performed at a later date to complete the RTSA implantation. This two-staged option is rarely needed. Gupta and colleagues evaluated 94 patients with preoperative bone loss who underwent RTSA and found that there were able to obtain adequate

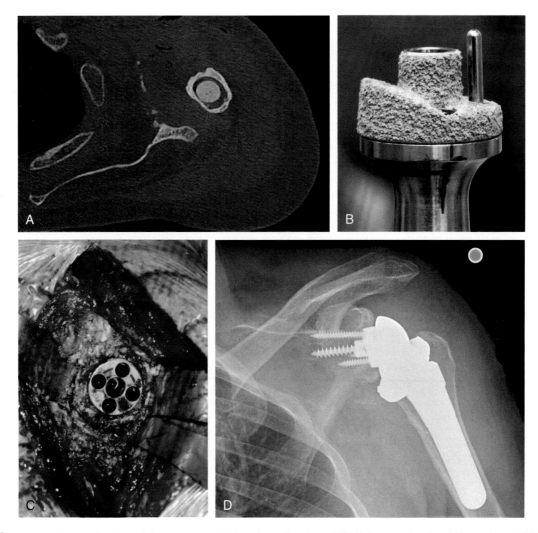

FIGURE 43.6 Augmented baseplate in revision reverse total shoulder arthroplasty (RTSA) for superior glenoid bone loss. A failed ATSA with stemless humeral component resulting in central and superior glenoid bone defect (**A**). A half-wedged augmented glenoid baseplate was used to account for the superior bone defect (**B**). The augmented glenoid component is inserted onto the glenoid (**C**) resulting in a stable glenoid implant with the appropriate restoration of offset and tilt (**D**).

single-stage fixation in 92.5% of cases.[8] Other salvage options include resection arthroplasty, which can alleviate pain but also results in limited function, and glenohumeral arthrodesis, which is a complex reconstruction in which consolidation can be difficult to achieve.

REPORTED OUTCOMES

One complicating factor when reviewing the outcomes of RTSA with glenoid bone loss is that many studies have combined primary and revision surgeries into the same cohort.[19-21] It is important, however, to separate the two groups, as revision RTSA cases have much worse outcomes at baseline, regardless of the type of glenoid augmentation. Malahias and colleagues performed a systematic review of studies reporting the outcomes of bone grafting for RTSA and found that the revision surgery rate was just 3% for primary RTSA but 21% for revision RTSA.[22] Therefore, the nature of the RTSA

(revision or primary) is critical to account for before applying the findings of outcome studies broadly.[3]

In regard to the success of bone grafting for glenoid bone loss in RTSA, the reported radiographic incorporation rates have varied from 75% to 95%.[19-21,23] There are two caveats to be aware of regarding these data. First, many studies included both primary and revision RTSA surgeries, as mentioned above. Second, postoperative radiographs and CT scans likely underrepresent bone nonunion rates. In a cadaver study assessing the ability of CT scan to demonstrate bone gaps after RTSA, Ferreria and colleagues showed that the sensitivity of CT to identify bone graft resorption was just 38%.[24] Bone grafting in revision RTSA may have lower union rates than is reported in the literature.

In the few studies that have evaluated clinical outcomes in patients with structural glenoid bone graft during revision RTSA, the early and mid-term results

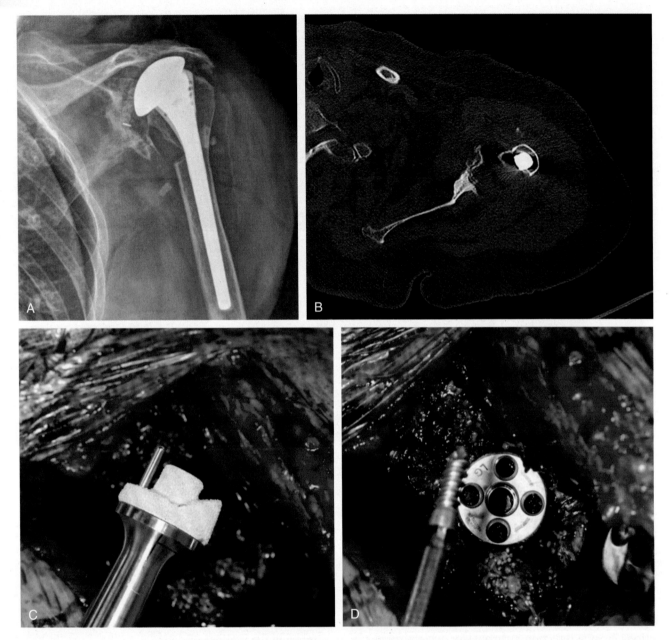

FIGURE 43.7 Augmented baseplate in revision reverse total shoulder arthroplasty (RTSA) for posterior glenoid bone loss. A failed anatomic total shoulder arthroplasty (ATSA) (**A**) resulting in severe posterior glenoid bone defect (**B**). A large half-wedged augmented glenoid baseplate was used to account for the posterior bone loss (**C**). After implantation (**D**), glenoid implant stability was achieved with the appropriate offset and tilt.

have been disappointing. Wagner and colleagues evaluated 40 such patients and found that the 5-year implant revision-free survival was just 76%.[25] In their study of RTSAs with structural bone graft, when just the revision RTSA cases are considered, Ho and colleagues found a 50% radiographic failure rate and 38% revision rate at 2 years.[20] Mahylis and colleagues evaluated 15 patients who underwent revision RTSA with structural tricortical iliac crest autograft and found that 40% of patients had some degree of bone graft resorption at 2 years.[26] In a recent systematic review, the reoperation rate for revision RTSAs augmented with glenoid bone graft was found to be 24.4% at 2- to 4-year follow-up.[22] Because of these

data, we are guarded with respect to the long-term success of structural bone graft in revision RTSA cases.

There are few studies that have reported the outcomes of augmented baseplates in RTSA with glenoid bone loss. One that retrospectively compared augmented glenoid baseplates to structural bone graft in primary RTSA found that there were no complications in the 39 patients treated with augmented baseplates while 15% of the 41 patients who received structural bone graft had a complication, including two loose glenoid components.[27] Although this study did not include revision RTSA cases, the fact that the authors compared augmented baseplates to structural bone graft and found lower complication

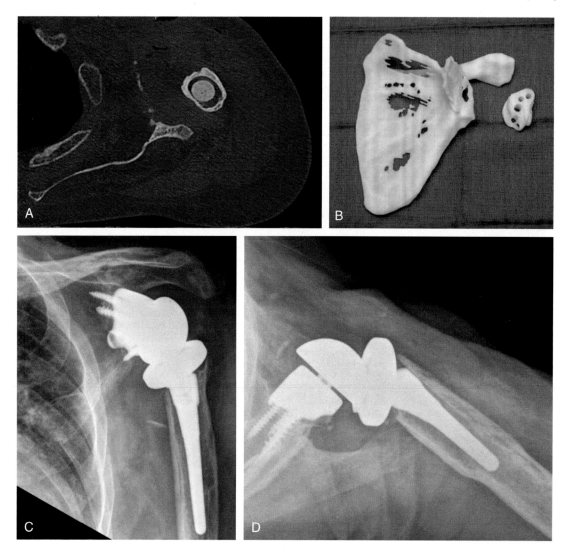

FIGURE 43.8 Vault reconstruction system (VRS) for catastrophic glenoid bone loss in revision reverse total shoulder arthroplasty (RTSA). A patient who had undergone multiple revision shoulder arthroplasties for infection had severe glenoid bone erosion (**A**) that precluded the use of a standard baseplate with bone graft or an augmented baseplate. A custom VRS was created along with three-dimensional (3D) printed model scapula and implant (**B**). At 6 weeks postoperatively, the anteroposterior (AP) (**C**) and axillary (**D**) radiographs demonstrate excellent restoration of glenoid stability, offset, and tilt.

rates in the former gives us preliminary confidence in the use of augmented glenoid baseplates in place of structural bone graft for revision RTSA cases.

CONCLUSION

Glenoid bone loss is a not infrequent complicating factor in patients undergoing revision RTSA. For small contained defects, local cancellous autograft or cancellous allograft bone chips can be used to fill in nonstructural voids. For structural glenoid defects that would otherwise render the glenoid baseplate unstable, options include structural auto- or allograft or augmented glenoid baseplates. In these circumstances, our preference is to use augmented baseplates due to the high rates of clinical failure with structural bone graft in revision RTSA procedures. For catastrophic glenoid bone loss, options include metallic

glenoid reconstruction, two-stage bony reconstruction, and use of the alternate scapular spine centerline.

The long-term outcomes of revision RTSA with the various glenoid augmentation options are not currently known. Future studies should compare the outcomes of glenoid-augmenting modalities for these complex revision procedures.

REFERENCES

1. Karelse A, Van Tongel A, Verstraeten T, et al. Rocking-horse phenomenon of the glenoid component: the importance of inclination. *J Shoulder Elbow Surg.* 2015;24(7):1142-1148.
2. Bitzer A, Rojas J, Patten IS, et al. Incidence and risk factors for aseptic baseplate loosening of reverse total shoulder arthroplasty. *J Shoulder Elbow Surg.* 2018;27(12):2145-2152.
3. Rojas J, Choi K, Joseph J, et al. Aseptic glenoid baseplate loosening after reverse total shoulder arthroplasty: a systematic review and meta-analysis. *JBJS Rev.* 2019;7(5):e7.

4. Walch G, Boileau P, Neyton L. Revision of the glenoid component. In: Cofield RH, Sperling JW, eds. *Revision and Complex Shoulder Arthroplasty*. Lippincott Williams & Wilkins; 2010:105-113.

5. Rodriguez JA, Entezari V, Iannotti J, et al. Pre-operative planning for reverse shoulder replacement: the surgical benefits and their clinical translation. *Ann Jt*. 2019;4(1):1-15.

6. Antuna SA, Sperling JW, Cofield RH, et al. Glenoid revision surgery after total shoulder arthroplasty. *J Shoulder Elbow Surg*. 2001;10(3):217-224.

7. Williams GR Jr, Iannotti JP. Options for glenoid bone loss: composites of prosthetics and biologics. *J Shoulder Elbow Surg*. 2007;16(5 suppl):S267-S272.

8. Gupta A, Thussbas C, Koch M, et al. Management of glenoid bone defects with reverse shoulder arthroplasty-surgical technique and clinical outcomes. *J Shoulder Elbow Surg*. 2018;27(5):853-862.

9. Ladermann A, Schwitzguebel AJ, Edwards TB, et al. Glenoid loosening and migration in reverse shoulder arthroplasty. *Bone Joint Lett J*. 2019;101-b(4):461-469.

10. Ladermann A, Denard PJ, Collin P. Massive rotator cuff tears: definition and treatment. *Int Orthop*. 2015;39(12):2403-2414.

11. Norris TR, Iannotti JP. Functional outcome after shoulder arthroplasty for primary osteoarthritis: a multicenter study. *J Shoulder Elbow Surg*. 2002;11(2):130-135.

12. Kwapisz A, Fitzpatrick K, Cook JB, et al. Distal clavicular osteochondral autograft augmentation for glenoid bone loss: a comparison of radius of restoration versus Latarjet graft. *Am J Sports Med*. 2018;46(5):1046-1052.

13. Tashjian RZ, Broschinsky K, Stertz I, et al. Structural glenoid allograft reconstruction during reverse total shoulder arthroplasty. *J Shoulder Elbow Surg*. 2020;29(3):534-540.

14. Ozgur SE, Sadeghpour R, Norris TR. Revision shoulder arthroplasty with a reverse shoulder prosthesis: use of structural allograft for glenoid bone loss. *Orthopade*. 2017;46(12):1055-1062.

15. Dines DM, Gulotta L, Craig EV, et al. Novel solution for massive glenoid defects in shoulder arthroplasty: a patient-specific glenoid vault reconstruction system. *Am J Orthop (Belle Mead NJ)*. 2017;46(2):104-108.

16. Formaini NT, Everding NG, Levy JC, et al. The effect of glenoid bone loss on reverse shoulder arthroplasty baseplate fixation. *J Shoulder Elbow Surg*. 2015;24(11):e312-e319.

17. Lorenzetti A, Streit JJ, Cabezas AF, et al. Bone graft augmentation for severe glenoid bone loss in primary reverse total shoulder arthroplasty: outcomes and evaluation of host bone contact by 2D-3D image registration. *JB JS Open Access*. 2017;2(3):e0015.

18. Klein SM, Dunning P, Mulieri P, et al. Effects of acquired glenoid bone defects on surgical technique and clinical outcomes in reverse shoulder arthroplasty. *J Bone Joint Surg Am*. 2010;92(5):1144-1154.

19. Jones RB, Wright TW, Zuckerman JD. Reverse total shoulder arthroplasty with structural bone grafting of large glenoid defects. *J Shoulder Elbow Surg*. 2016;25(9):1425-1432.

20. Ho JC, Thakar O, Chan WW, et al. Early radiographic failure of reverse total shoulder arthroplasty with structural bone graft for glenoid bone loss. *J Shoulder Elbow Surg*. 2020;29(3):550-560.

21. Lopiz Y, Garcia-Fernandez C, Arriaza A, et al. Midterm outcomes of bone grafting in glenoid defects treated with reverse shoulder arthroplasty. *J Shoulder Elbow Surg*. 2017;26(9):1581-1588.

22. Malahias MA, Chytas D, Kostretzis L, et al. Bone grafting in primary and revision reverse total shoulder arthroplasty for the management of glenoid bone loss: a systematic review. *J Orthop*. 2020;20:78-86.

23. Paul RA, Maldonado-Rodriguez N, Docter S, et al. Glenoid bone grafting in primary reverse total shoulder arthroplasty: a systematic review. *J Shoulder Elbow Surg*. 2019;28(12):2447-2456.

24. Ferreira LM, Knowles NK, Richmond DN, et al. Effectiveness of CT for the detection of glenoid bone graft resorption following reverse shoulder arthroplasty. *Orthop Traumatol Surg Res*. 2015;101(4):427-430.

25. Wagner E, Houdek MT, Griffith T, et al. Glenoid bone-grafting in revision to a reverse total shoulder arthroplasty. *J Bone Joint Surg Am*. 2015;97(20):1653-1660.

26. Mahylis JM, Puzzitiello RN, Ho JC, et al. Comparison of radiographic and clinical outcomes of revision reverse total shoulder arthroplasty with structural versus nonstructural bone graft. *J Shoulder Elbow Surg*. 2019;28(1):e1-e9.

27. Jones RB, Wright TW, Roche CP. Bone grafting the glenoid versus use of augmented glenoid baseplates with reverse shoulder arthroplasty. *Bull Hosp Jt Dis (2013)*. 2015;73(suppl 1):S129-S135.

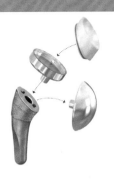

44 Conversion of an Anatomic Total Shoulder Arthroplasty or Hemiarthroplasty to Reverse Total Shoulder Arthroplasty:
The Use of a Platform System

Stephen Yu, MD and Joseph D. Zuckerman, MD

INTRODUCTION

Shoulder arthroplasty is now an increasingly common surgery based upon the significant growth over the past decade. Anatomic total shoulder arthroplasty (ATSA) remains the gold standard for the treatment of glenohumeral arthritis with an intact rotator cuff. Hemiarthroplasty (HA) remains a widely utilized procedure that produces favorable outcomes when it is used in patients with primarily humeral-sided degenerative conditions. It had been used extensively for the treatment of proximal humeral fractures and in cuff tear arthropathy. More recently, HA has been replaced by the reverse total shoulder arthroplasty (RTSA) as the preferred procedure for these conditions. RTSA is now used extensively for revision of HA and ATSA. This will become increasingly important because as the number of shoulder arthroplasties increases, there will be an inevitable increase in the number of revisions performed. Although the outcomes of shoulder arthroplasty have been improving over the years, the longer-term implant survival remains approximately 80% at 15 years.[1] Revisions of HA and ATSA are challenging procedures both for the patients and the surgeons.

Glenoid component loosening and rotator cuff failure are among the most common indications for revision. It has been reported that up to 55% of patients have some degree of rotator cuff dysfunction following ATSA.[2] Sperling et al reported a rate of 28% of anterior-superior escape secondary to severe rotator cuff dysfunction in patients with HA and ATSA at 15 years' follow-up, necessitating revision to RTSA.[3] A recent systematic review, Knowles et al, reported that the primary indication for shoulder arthroplasty revision in 26% of cases was rotator cuff tear or deficiency; glenoid-sided indications for revision, which included glenoid component loosening and bone loss/erosion, accounted for 22% of the indications. A humeral-sided indication, such as humeral loosening, only accounted for 7%.[4] It has been consistently demonstrated that the indications for revision do not commonly involve the humeral component, and that conversion from HA or ATSA to RTSA is most commonly secondary to rotator cuff dysfunction.

Conversion of HA or ATSA to RTSA has become increasingly common, particularly as the indications for primary RTSA have expanded. Although patients largely benefit from these procedures, some early studies demonstrated a high complication rate ranging from 22% to 43%.[5] Certainly, overall risk is higher in the revision setting in comparison to index procedures. However, in these early published reports, the complications were primarily humeral sided and were frequently related to the morbidity of extracting the humeral stem. Extracting a well-fixed stem often requires the use of a humeral osteotomy or cortical window. These additional procedures significantly contribute to increased operative time, blood loss, cost, and, most importantly, the overall risk of the procedure.

Extraction of humeral stems can result in complications, such as intraoperative humeral shaft fracture or damage to adjacent structures. Current designs have incorporated a modular, convertible humeral component that can be retained to reduce the need for stem removal and potentially mitigate these complications. Crosby et al reported on the utility of a convertible platform system and demonstrated that the stem was able to be retained in up to 78% of cases being revised to RTSA.[6] Similarly, Kany et al reported that 72% were able to be retained in their series.[7] These reports support the potential benefits of a convertible humeral stem when revision to RTSA is necessary.

DESIGN RATIONALE AND ADVANTAGES OF A CONVERTIBLE PLATFORM SYSTEM

Prior to the development of the modular platform humeral stem, every procedure necessitated the removal of an otherwise well-fixed and well-positioned humeral component in order to convert from HA or ATSA to an RTSA. Revising the humeral component in many situations was considered unnecessary and was only performed so it could be converted to an RTSA system. With a convertible platform humeral stem, additional surgery could be avoided by replacing the modular humeral component and either inserting the glenoid component (for revisions of HA) or revising the glenoid component (for revisions of ATSA). However, it is important to emphasize that retention of the stem requires it to be both well fixed and well positioned in order to achieve the goals of the revision procedure.

Most convertible platform systems offer the same modular features found in many of the nonconvertible shoulder arthroplasty systems. Newer designs have only expanded the modularity available for convertible stems **(FIGURES 44.1 and 44.2)**. This offers more options at the humeral head-neck junction, thereby allowing greater modularity for humeral component version; varying degrees of length and offset, neck angle, center of rotation; inlay versus onlay designs, and humeral head eccentricity. These characteristics can be adjusted intraoperatively to "fine-tune" the final position, balance, and stability of the construct to potentially enhance the clinical outcomes.

CONSIDERATIONS IN THE UTILITY OF A PLATFORM SYSTEM

It is always important to be careful when adopting new technology and implant designs and this is also true for convertible stems. Regardless of the potential advantages of a convertible stem, it is also important to consider new modes of failure that may be introduced. Increasing modularity can be associated with unique modes of failure such as increased wear, failure at the modular junctions, and the potential for implant dissociation.

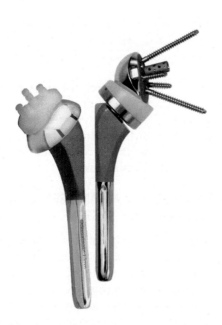

FIGURE 44.1 Convertible platform shoulder arthroplasty system Used with permission from © Exactech, Inc.)

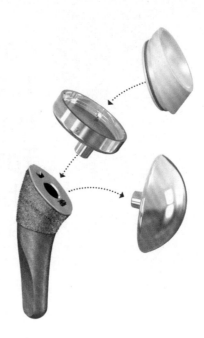

FIGURE 44.2 Convertible platform shoulder arthroplasty system Image reprinted with permission from Stryker Corporation. © 2021 Stryker Corporation. All rights reserved.)

Fortunately, early and midterm results have been promising, but long-term outcomes are still needed. Currently, no unique modes of failure have been reported with the use of convertible stems, but ongoing evaluation is certainly required.

Retaining a convertible humeral stem may present itself as an advantage, but should not be taken for granted. The position and fixation of the existing humeral stem should be critically evaluated, and if it is anything less than acceptable, the stem should be extracted and revised. In all cases where a convertible stem is in place, it is essential that the preoperative plan includes the necessary equipment and implants for stem removal if it becomes necessary. The final decision about stem "convertibility" cannot be made until the glenoid component is in place and trial reductions have been performed and found to be satisfactory.

CLINICAL EVALUATION

As with any potential revision, a careful and comprehensive preoperative evaluation is required. This includes history and physical examination, appropriate laboratory studies, and imaging studies. The symptoms should be carefully evaluated for indications of potential humeral component loosening. The indications for revision procedure should be clearly identified. Revision shoulder arthroplasty is extensively discussed in Section 7 and will not be reviewed here; however, we would emphasize the importance of obtaining previous operative reports and specific information about the implants in place to confirm whether or not the humeral stem is convertible. This will have important implications for the planning of the revision procedure. All implant-specific instruments should be available for modular head removal as well as stem extraction if this becomes necessary.

SURGICAL TECHNIQUE

Revision of a convertible stem to RTSA follows the important principles that are addressed in detail in Chapters 41, 42, and 43. In this chapter, we will focus on the surgical steps that are unique to this specific procedure. The most important first step is complete exposure of the proximal humerus and the humeral component. This will require release of the subscapularis (if intact) as well as release of the capsule so that the humerus can be externally rotated to 90°. Once the modular humeral head is exposed, it should be removed with the extraction device specific for the system in place. At this point, careful evaluation of the humeral stem is essential. Soft tissue surrounding the proximal portion of the stem should be removed so that the bone-prosthesis interface or the bone-cement interface is exposed. Confirmation that the component is well fixed should be obtained. Visualization of the upper portion of the stem is most easily accomplished by placing humerus in extension, adduction, and external rotation. Additional soft tissue releases about the proximal humerus may be necessary for proper immobilization and should be performed at this stage. In addition, the soft tissue overlying the proximal portion of the stem may be better visualized with the arm in this position and should be removed. Any bony prominences about the proximal humerus that overlie the proximal portion of the stem should be evaluated and removed if problematic.

The humeral component should also be carefully evaluated to confirm the appropriate position. If the stem is excessively proud, reduction and soft tissue tension may be problematic. A recessed stem is usually less problematic as long as any bony prominences are removed. The version of the component should also be carefully assessed. Retroversion in the range of 20° to 40° is acceptable. Conversion to an RTSA does provide some latitude with respect to version but significant malrotation can predispose to instability and is an indication for stem removal and revision.

At this point with the humeral stem completely exposed, attention can be turned to the glenoid. Retraction of the proximal humerus posteriorly with the stem in place does provide some degree of protection from the stresses that may be applied during retraction and manipulation. This lessens the chance of iatrogenic fracture. Insertion of the glenoid component should then proceed according to the steps for the specific implant system being utilized. Once the glenoid baseplate is secured in position, we utilize trial glenosphere components and do not place the final glenosphere until trial reductions are completed and final components are determined.

Attention is then directed back to the humeral component and the very important trialling process to assess the construct. Trial reductions are performed with humeral base plates and polyethylene inserts to determine if appropriate soft tissue tensioning and stability can be achieved. Intraoperative decision-making proceeds according to the same principles utilized for primary RTSA with the goal of achieving a stable construct that is neither excessively tight nor loose and provides the stability needed for range of motion and function. Range of motion should be assessed in the operating room and includes maximum forward elevation, abduction to 90° with internal and external rotation, and adduction combined with extension and external rotation. Traction should be applied to the arm to determine the separation between the humeral and glenoid components. Ease of trial reduction is an important factor in determining whether the appropriate size components are in place. If the soft tissue tension and stability parameters are acceptable, then trial components could be removed and final components placed. If there is concern about excessive tension, then additional soft tissue releases can be performed. However, if there is difficulty obtaining a trial reduction or there are concerns about stability after utilization of all modular component options, then revision of the humeral stem will be necessary and should be performed. It is essential to complete the procedure with a stable construct in place that achieved the goals of the procedure. If this cannot be achieved with the convertible humeral stem, then revision of all components should be performed.

ILLUSTRATIVE CASES

Case 1: Conversion of Well-Positioned Platform Stem

A 73-year-old, right-hand-dominant man presents with a history of bilateral anatomic shoulder replacements. The right side was performed 8 years ago **(FIGURE 44.3A and B)** and the left 7 years ago. He was doing well until 1 year prior to presentation. For the past 1 year, he has had increasing pain and limitation in range of motion of the right shoulder. On physical examination, forward elevation is to 60°, external rotation to 40°, and internal rotation to the posterior. Strength testing revealed 4/5 strength in the supraspinatus with pain, otherwise he is 5/5 in all other muscle groups.

X-rays showed superior migration of the humeral head consistent with rotator cuff compromise. There was also lucency about the glenoid keel suggestive of component loosening **(FIGURE 44.3C and D)**.

Based upon the rotator cuff failure and glenoid radiolucency, revision to RTSA was performed. Intraoperatively, the rotator cuff was found to be deficient and the glenoid was grossly loose. The humeral component was found to be well fixed and well positioned. Decision was made to retain the humeral component.

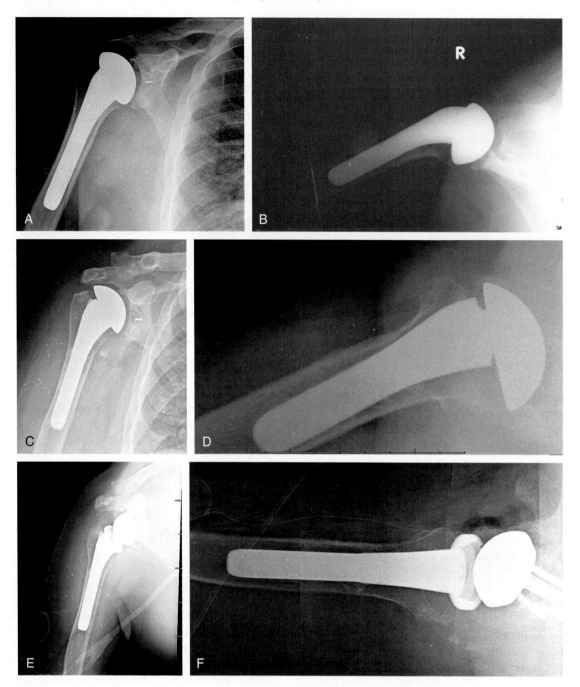

FIGURE 44.3 A and **B**, Early postoperative radiographs. **C** and **D**, Current radiographs with superior migration of the humeral component and glenoid radiolucency. **E** and **F**, Immediate postoperative radiographs of the conversion reverse total shoulder arthroplasty with the humeral stem retained.

The modular components were removed. The glenoid was revised to RTSA components with femoral head allograft used to fill the contained glenoid defect. Trial reductions demonstrated a stable construct and the final components were implanted (**FIGURE 44.3E** and **F**).

Postoperatively, the patient did well reporting satisfactory pain relief and improved function. One year following surgery, active forward elevation was to 135°, external rotation to 30°, and internal rotation to the posterior ilium.

Case 2: Revision of Poorly Positioned Platform Humeral Stem

A 61-year-old man underwent right anatomic total shoulder replacement approximately 3 years previously. He always felt the shoulder was "not right" because of discomfort and limited range of motion. Over the past year, he experienced increasing pain about the right shoulder with *greater functional limitations*. Physical examination showed forward elevation is to 75°, external rotation to 20°, and internal rotation to his lumbar spine.

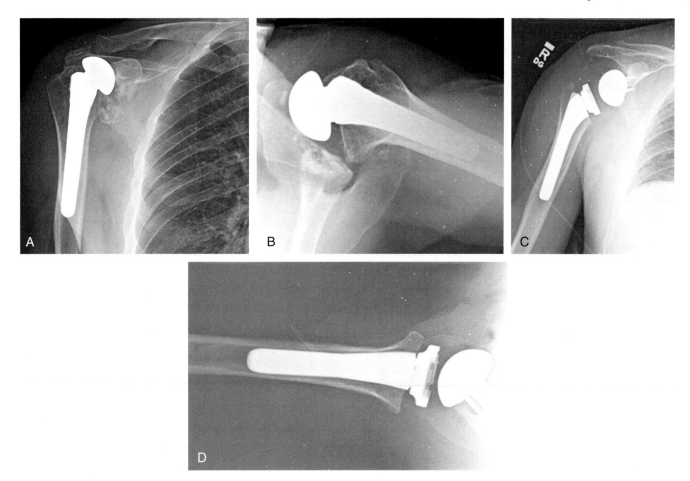

FIGURE 44.4 A and **B**, Preoperative radiographs showing superior migration, anterior instability, inadequate proximal humeral resection, and varus stem position. **C** and **D**, Immediate postoperative radiographs.

Serial radiographs demonstrated progressive superior migration of the humeral head and anterior dislocation of the humeral head, consistent with subscapularis and superior rotator cuff failure. Although a convertible humeral stem was in place, it was malpositioned in varus with an inadequate proximal humeral resection (**FIGURE 44.4A** and **B**). Conversion to RTSA was recommended.

Intraoperatively, the rotator cuff was found to be deficient. The humeral component was evaluated and was confirmed to be proud and malpositioned, and it was removed using thin osteotomes and an extraction device. Removal of the well-fixed glenoid could be performed without significant compromise of the bone. Conversion to RTSA was performed (**FIGURE 44.4C** and **D**).

The patient did very well postoperatively and was satisfied with his outcome. Range of motion was significantly improved with forward elevation to 150°, external rotation to 30°, and internal rotation to the lumbosacral area.

Case 3: Conversion of Modular Platform Humeral Stem

This patient is a 74-year-old woman with a history of bilateral shoulder replacements. She underwent left shoulder HA 1.5 years prior to initial presentation for treatment of osteonecrosis of the humeral head. She also previously underwent right anatomic shoulder replacement for glenohumeral arthritis.

She initially presented with left shoulder complaints, with increasing pain secondary to rotator cuff compromise and glenoid erosion (**FIGURE 44.5A** and **B**). On examination, she had 80° of forward elevation, 30° of external rotation, and internal rotation to the posterior ilium. Conversion to RTSA was recommended.

Intraoperatively, her humeral stem was found to be well fixed and well positioned. Her index left shoulder HA was a convertible humeral stem, so decision was made to retain the stem and utilize the convertible adapter tray and the glenoid component for this system (**FIGURE 44.5B** and **C**).

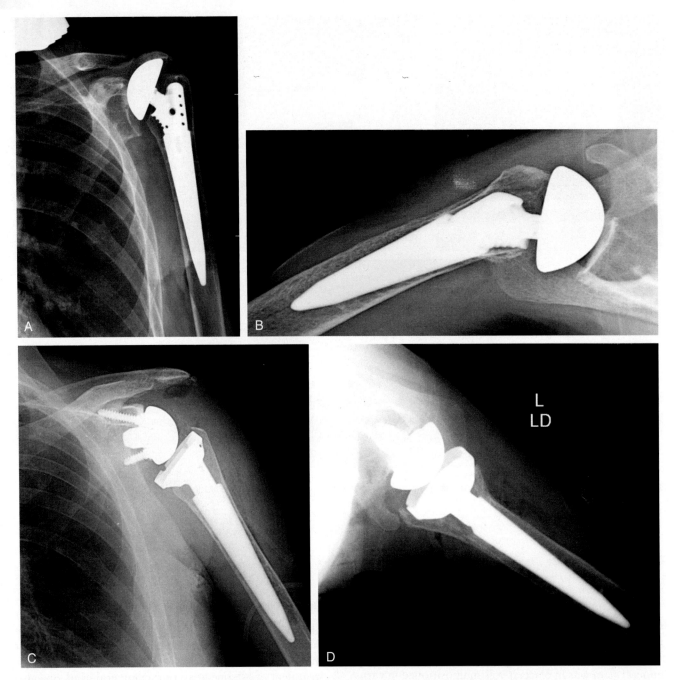

FIGURE 44.5 A 74-year-old female who underwent left proximal humeral replacement for treatment of osteonecrosis. 18 months following surgery she complains of pain and loss of motion. Radiographs (**A** and **B**) show glenoid erosion and superior migration consistent with rotator cuff compromise. The modular, platform stem allowed conversion to RTSA while retaining the diaphyseal portion of the stem and replacing the metaphyseal modular component (**C** and **D**).

Postoperatively, the patient did very well at 9 years of follow-up reporting excellent functional scores and significant improvements in range of motion with 160° of forward elevation, 45° of external rotation, and internal rotation to the lumbar spine.

Case 4: Conversion of Well-Fixed Nonplatform Stem

This patient is a 73-year-old man who was presented 3 years following right ATSA. He did well for approximately 1 year after surgery but has had progressively worsening pain and loss of motion since that time. An

arthroscopic lysis of adhesions and manipulation had been performed without improvement. Active range of motion showed forward elevation of 60°, external rotation with the arm at the side to 30°, and internal rotation to the lumbar spine.

Radiographs demonstrated significant superior migration consistent with rotator cuff failure (**FIGURE 44.6A** and **B**). Revision to RTSA was recommended.

At the time of surgery, the components were found to be well fixed. The nonplatform humeral component was well positioned and could be removed with minimal

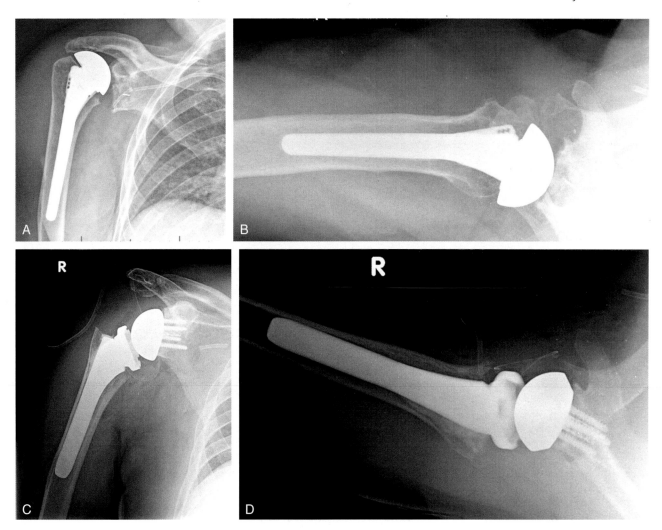

FIGURE 44.6 A 73-year-old male who presents three years after right ATSA with continuing pain and loss of motion (**A** and **B**). Findings were consistent with rotator cuff compromise. The well positioned, nonplatform stem required removal and conversion to RTSA was performed (**C** and **D**).

bone loss. Femoral head allograft was used to fill the contained glenoid defect after implant removal. RTSA was performed (**FIGURE 44.6C** and **D**).

Postoperatively, the patient did very well. He reported excellent pain relief and improvement in shoulder function with forward elevation to 140°, external rotation to 30°, and internal rotation to the posterior ilium.

Case 5: Conversion of Poorly Positioned Nonplatform Stem

This patient is an 81-year-old man who previously underwent a right proximal humeral replacement for treatment of degenerative arthritis. He reported that he was "never satisfied with the result." For 3 years he had experienced increasing pain and loss of range of motion. Examination showed painful, limited range of motion. Radiographs showed an inferiorly malpositioned humeral stem in varus. There was loss of glenoid articular cartilage and erosion (**FIGURE 44.7A** and **B**).

Revision to RTSA was recommended. The stem was malpositioned and required revision. Even if it had

been a platform stem, it could not have been used for conversion because of the malposition. The stem could be removed with minimal bone loss and the humeral neck resection was revised. RTSA was performed (**FIGURE 44.7C** and **D**).

Postoperatively, this patient did very well. Two years after revision, he reported minimal discomfort. Active forward elevation was 140°, external rotation was to 25°, and internal rotation to the posterior ilium.

CLINICAL OUTCOMES AND COMPLICATIONS

Most convertible systems have been introduced within the past decade. Initially, there were only a few select systems available. However, as the benefits of convertible systems became evident, more of the orthopedic implant companies began to design and produce convertible stems for their shoulder arthroplasty systems. Going forward, we anticipate that the majority of, if not all, humeral components will eventually be convertible. Currently, there are many different convertible systems available (**TABLE 44.1**).

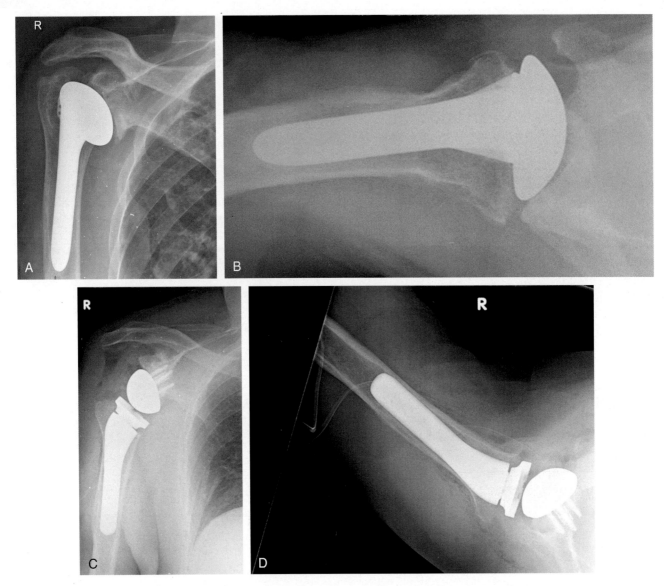

FIGURE 44.7 An 81-year-old male who presents 3 years following right proximal humeral replacement for glenohumeral arthritis describing continued pain since the procedure. Radiographs (**A** and **B**) showed the humeral component malpositioned in varus and inferior to the greater tuberosity. Revision to RTSA was performed with removal of the nonplatform stem (**C** and **D**). The malposition of the stem would have precluded stem retention even if it had been a platform system.

In the evaluation of convertible platform systems, there are two specific areas of outcomes that should be evaluated. First should be clinical outcomes of the system when it is utilized for primary cases. This data is necessary to confirm that the new design did not

TABLE 44.1 Convertible Systems

Exactech—Equinoxe
DePuy Synthes—GLOBAL UNITE
Stryker—ReUnion
DJO—Altivate
Smith and Nephew—PROMOS
Zimmer Biomet—Comprehensive
Wright Medical/Tornier—Aequalis
Arthrex—Univers
Integra—Titan

provide any negative outcomes compared with nonconvertible stems. Second is the evaluation of convertible stems during revision procedures. We will address both of these areas. Currently, only short- to midterm, level 4 data is available for convertible shoulder arthroplasty systems utilized in the primary setting. Clinical outcome data of these systems have been overall acceptable and comparable with nonconvertible systems.[8-10] Updegrove et al reported substantial increases in two clinical outcome scores at 2 years which were similar to the nonconvertible counterpart of the same manufacturer.[8] Another short-term study by Goetzmann et al demonstrated similar findings with a different system. They reported significant increases in Constant shoulder scores and range of motion, similar to published data of standard nonconvertible implants. No mechanical complications were reported that could be considered unique to the convertible system.[9] In a registry study by Audige et al, several convertible stem systems were used for fracture sequelae indications. At 5 years postoperatively, good results were experienced for range of motion and outcome scores.[10] Although longer term studies and survival analyses of these systems are needed, there is no current evidence that suggests the expected longevity of convertible stems to be less than the nonconvertible counterparts in the primary setting.

There are considerable data available on the use of convertible stems during revisions to RTSA. A meta-analysis by Kirsch et al included seven studies with 236 revisions of which 113 shoulders underwent humeral stem revision and 123 utilized a convertible platform stem that was retained. Both HA and ATSA underwent conversion to RTSA. Overall complications were significantly higher in the patients requiring humeral stem revision (42%) compared with those that did not require stem revision (7%).[5] Flury et al reported a 38% overall complication rate in their series of revisions of ATSA to RTSA conversions. Every patient underwent exchange of all components as none of the systems were convertible platforms.[11] In a study by Weber-Spickschen et al in which all revisions to RTSA utilized platform stems, the complication rate was reported to be 7%.[12] Dilisio et al reported similar results in a small series comparing retained stems in convertible platform systems with exchanged stems in nonconvertible systems.[13]

Complication rates represent a combination of a variety of events that can occur intraoperatively and postoperatively. To determine the impact of the use of a platform stem it is important to assess both complications and the impact on intraoperative surgical variables, specifically blood loss and duration of the procedure. The use of a convertible platform stem and the ability to retain the implanted stem has the potential to positively impact both parameters.

The primary advantage of convertible humeral stems is the ability to avoid the need for stem removal and thereby minimize the risk of intraoperative humeral fracture. In the systematic review performed by Kirsch et al, intraoperative humeral shaft fractures occurred in 16% of the stem exchange group compared with 2% in the stem retention group. Also, humeral osteotomies were necessary in the exchange group while none were required in the retention group. These results are consistently echoed in other case series, with studies reporting minimal to zero rates of humeral-sided complications for retained stems.[6,13,14]

Additional procedures like humeral osteotomies and cortical windows are not reported as complications since they are performed in order to facilitate stem removal. They represent "planned" intraoperative fractures to avoid an "unplanned" one. These procedures add complexity, morbidity, and cost to each case and result in some degree of bone loss **(FIGURE 44.8)**. Therefore, potentially avoiding the need for these procedures would be expected to have a positive impact.

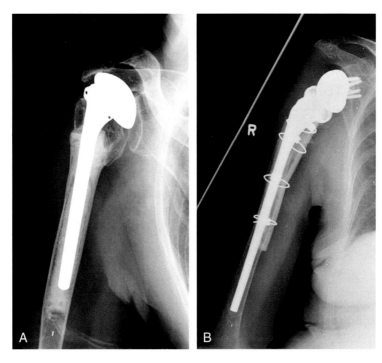

FIGURE 44.8 Conversion of nonplatform stems (**A**) can often require humeral osteotomy for stem removal and necessitate reconstruction using strut grafts (**B**) which is associated with increased operative time, blood loss, and potential for complications.

Intraoperative Blood Loss and Operative Time

It is intuitive that there would be reduced intraoperative blood loss in stem retention cases and this finding has consistently been reported. Kirsch et al found a decrease in blood loss by a mean difference of 260 mL when the surgeon was able to retain the humeral stem. They also found that with stem retention rather than exchange, there was a mean difference of 62 minutes in surgical time.[5]

Crosby et al reported similar results for both estimated blood loss and operative time in the stem retention group, with a mean difference of 200 mL and 65 minutes, respectively.[6] Although these comparative studies have not focused on cost, it is reasonable to conclude that with stem retention, there would be significant cost savings versus stem exchange. These cost savings would include not only the cost of the new stem but also the additional cost associated with increased operative time and management of complications.

Revision of HA and ATSA to RTSA using convertible stems has been shown to achieve results at least as satisfactory as revisions requiring stem exchange.[6,9,12] Dilisio et al did not identify a difference in patient outcomes between retained and extracted humeral stems based upon the Subjective Shoulder Value, ASES, and Simple Shoulder Test scores at 2 years postoperatively.[13] Crosby et al reported similar results for Constant and ASES scores were not statistically different between the two groups at 2 years.[6]

CONCLUSION

Conversion of HA and ATSA to RTSA can be a technically demanding procedure. Modular platform shoulder arthroplasty systems have the potential for this procedure to be performed without removal of the humeral stem. If the humeral stem is to be retained, it must be well fixed and well positioned. The advantages of stem retention and conversion to RTSA include a reduction of intraoperative fractures, humeral bone preservation, decreased intraoperative blood loss, reduced operative time, and fewer overall complications. These results support the use of convertible platform systems in the performance of primary shoulder arthroplasty.

REFERENCES

1. Torchia ME, Cofield RH, Settergren CR. Total shoulder arthroplasty with the Neer prosthesis: long-term results. *J Shoulder Elbow Surg.* 1997;6:495-505.
2. Young AA, Walch G, Pape G, Gohlke F, Favard L. Secondary rotator cuff dysfunction following total shoulder arthroplasty for primary glenohumeral osteoarthritis: results of a multicenter study with more than five years of follow-up. *J Bone Joint Surg Am.* 2012;94:685-693. doi:10.2106/JBJS.J.00727
3. Sperling JW, Cofield RH, Rowland CM. Minimum fifteen year follow-up of Neer hemiarthroplasty and total shoulder arthroplasty in patients aged fifty years or younger. *J Shoulder Elbow Surg.* 2004;13:604-613. doi:10.1016/j.jse.2004.03.013
4. Knowles NK, Columbus MP, Wegmann K, Ferreira LM, Athwal GS. Revision shoulder arthroplasty: a systematic review and comparison of North American vs. European outcomes and complications. *J Shoulder Elbow Surg.* 2020;29(5):1071-1082. doi:10.1016/j.jse.2019.12.015
5. Kirsch JM, Khan M, Thornley P, et al. Platform shoulder arthroplasty: a systematic review. *J Shoulder Elbow Surg.* 2018;27(4):756-763. doi:10.1016/j.jse.2017.08.020
6. Crosby LA, Wright TW, Yu S, Zuckerman JD. Conversion to reverse total shoulder arthroplasty with and without humeral stem retention: the role of a convertible-platform stem. *J Bone Joint Surg Am.* 2017;99(9):736-742. doi:10.2106/JBJS.16.00683
7. Kany J, Amouyel T, Flamand O, Katz D, Valenti P. A convertible shoulder system: is it useful in total shoulder arthroplasty revisions? *Int Orthop.* 2015;39(2):299-304. doi:10.1007/s00264-014-2563-z
8. Updegrove GF, Nicholson TA, Namdari S, Williams GR, Abboud JA. Short-term results of the DePuy global unite platform shoulder system: a two-year outcome study. *Arch Bone Jt Surg.* 2018;6(5):353-358.
9. Goetzmann T, Molé D, Aisene B, et al. A short and convertible humeral stem for shoulder arthroplasty: preliminary results. *J Shoulder Elb Arthroplast.* 2017;1(1):1-9. doi:10.1177/2471549217722723
10. Audigé L, Graf L, Flury M, Schneider MM, Müller AM. Functional improvement is sustained following anatomical and reverse shoulder arthroplasty for fracture sequelae: a registry-based analysis. *Arch Orthop Trauma Surg.* 2019;139(11):1561-1569. doi:10.1007/s00402-019-03224-5
11. Flury MP, Frey P, Goldhahn J, Schwyzer HK, Simmen BR. Reverse shoulder arthroplasty as a salvage procedure for failed conventional shoulder replacement due to cuff failure – Midterm results. *Int Orthop.* 2011;35:53-60.
12. Weber-Spickschen TS, Alfke D, Agneskirchner JD. The use of a modular system to convert an anatomical total shoulder arthroplasty to a reverse shoulder arthroplasty. *Bone Joint J.* 2015;97-B(12):1662-1667. doi:10.1302/0301-620X.97B12.35176
13. Dilisio MF, Miller LR, Siegel EJ, Higgins LD. Conversion to reverse shoulder arthroplasty: humeral stem retention versus revision. *Orthopedics.* 2015;38(9):e773-e779.
14. Castagna A, Delcogliano M, de Caro F, et al. Conversion of shoulder arthroplasty to reverse implants:clinical and radiological results using a modular system. *Int Orthop.* 2013;37(7):1297-1305.

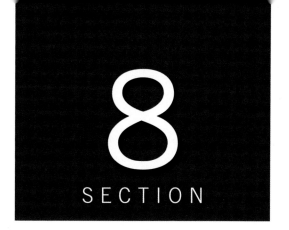

SECTION

Special Situations

PHAROS Classification

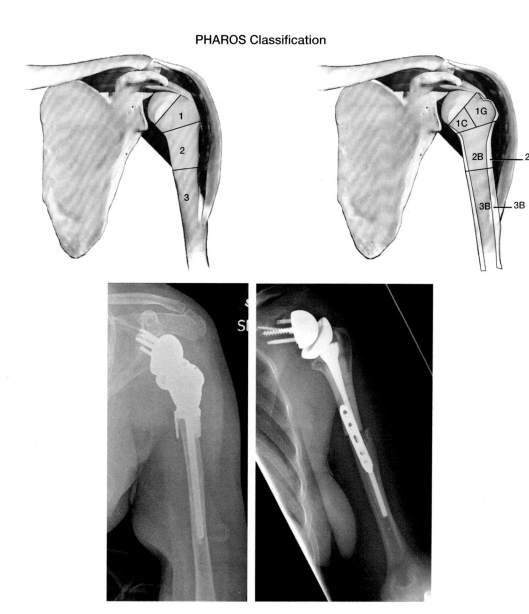

8

Special Situations

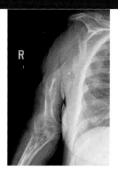

45 Massive Humeral Bone Loss

Bradley S. Schoch, MD and Jean-David Werthel, MD

INTRODUCTION

Humeral bone loss represents a challenging problem for shoulder surgeons, especially in the setting of arthroplasty reconstruction. Bone loss can occur secondary to trauma, prior surgery, infection, osteolysis, or oncologic destruction. Newer humeral implants for shoulder arthroplasty have trended toward uncemented humeral fixation with certain stem designs causing stress shielding and loss of lateral humeral or calcar bone. Removal of these well-fixed uncemented stems can lead to iatrogenic humeral bone loss with the associated destruction of both cortical and cancellous bone. In rare cases, a humeral osteotomy may even be required.[1] Loss of the proximal humerus architecture can then lead to loss of function and glenohumeral instability.

There are many techniques available to help restore or replace humeral bone stock and restore shoulder function for patients who present with massive humeral bone loss. However, understanding the pattern of bone loss and treatment options available are vital to being adequately prepared for this complex revision surgery. This chapter is designed to describe the classification of humeral bone loss, review the reconstructive treatment options for shoulder arthroplasty in the setting of massive humeral bone loss, and outline tendon transfer techniques that may assist in improving functional outcomes.

CLASSIFICATION

Historically, classification of proximal humeral bone loss has been described in the setting on oncologic resection. Multiple systems have been described, often in relation to sacrificed anatomic structures and the type of oncologic resection performed. In the setting of the shoulder girdle, Malawer et al[2] proposed a classification system for shoulder-girdle resections in patients undergoing limb-sparing procedures. Bone loss following oncologic resections can be very similar to the bone loss encountered in patients undergoing revision arthroplasty. However, of the six resection types described, only one involves the humerus in isolation (Type I). It is then subdivided into Type 1A (preservation of the deltoid insertion and/or rotator cuff) and Type 2B (resection of the deltoid tuberosity or rotator cuff). With this classification system, it is difficult to describe the variations of proximal humeral bone loss which can be treated with humeral implants ranging from standard primary components to a total humerus.

Furthermore, in the setting of revision arthroplasty, oncologic classification systems fail to take into account the quality of remaining bone, which has significant clinical implications when considering reconstructive techniques. Given the limitations with previous classification systems, Chalmers et al[3] proposed a classification system for humeral bone loss in the setting of revision shoulder arthroplasty **(FIGURE 45.1)**. This has been termed the Proximal Humeral Arthroplasty Revision Osseous inSufficiency (PHAROS) classification. The authors designed this system around both the presence and absence of critical bony structures (greater tuberosity, calcar, deltoid insertion) as well as the quality of the remaining cortical bone. The proximal humerus was then divided into three sections: epiphysis (tuberosities and calcar bone), metadiaphyseal bone (between the epiphysis and deltoid insertion), diaphysis (below the deltoid insertion). Type 1 epiphyseal lesions were subdivided into deficiencies at the calcar (Type 1C) and greater tuberosity (Type 1G). The clinical photo in **FIGURE 45.2** is an example of a Type 1C defect. Both metadiaphyseal (Type 2) and diaphyseal (Type 3) compromise was further classified as thinning of greater than 50% of the cortex (Type 2A or 3A) or frank loss of cortical bone (Type 2B or 3B).

IMPLANT OPTIONS

When performing revision shoulder arthroplasty, surgeons must be aware of both existing and potential iatrogenic bone loss, which can occur at the time of surgery. Prior to revision surgery, surgeons should consider the level of cementation (when present), the on-growth properties and metaphyseal filling of the humeral stem to be removed, and cortical bone quality. During extraction, metaphyseal bone loss can be anticipated. Iatrogenic bone loss patterns differ based on both the implanted stem and extraction techniques. Depending on the quality of cortical bone, surgeons may be able to anticipate potential cortical bone loss at the time of stem extraction. Prior to stem

PHAROS Classification

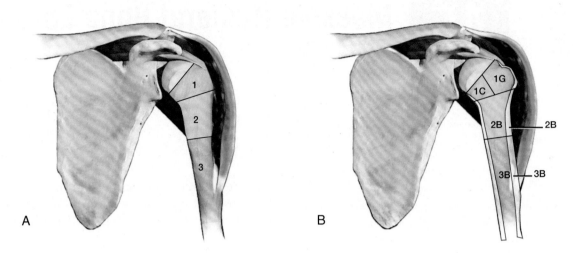

FIGURE 45.1 Illustration demonstrating the Proximal Humeral Arthroplasty Revision Osseous inSufficiency (PHAROS) classification as described by Chalmers et al.

extraction, it is important to measure the length of the humerus by measuring from the humeral calcar to a structure which is likely to be preserved after humeral component explant or bone resection. This measurement can then be used during the reconstruction to ensure restoration of appropriate humeral length. Depending on the extent of anticipated bone loss, surgeons must be adequately prepared at the time of surgery, which often may involve having multiple implant options available.

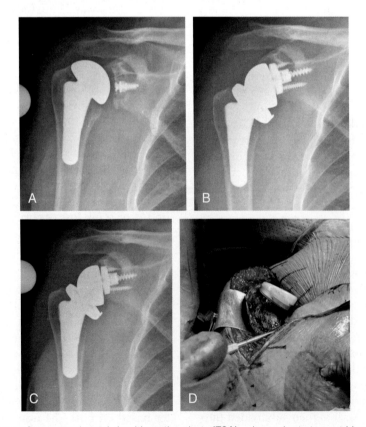

FIGURE 45.2 Postoperative x-rays after anatomic total shoulder arthroplasty (TSA) using a short-stemmed humeral component (**A**), 9 months post–stem implantation x-rays (**B**) (after conversion to reverse shoulder arthroplasty [RSA] for subscapularis failure) showing early calcar osteolysis, and 14 months post–stem implantation x-rays showing progressive stress shielding along the humeral calcar (**C**). Intraoperative photo from revision surgery (**D**) showing bone loss of the humeral calcar proximal to the ongrown junction of the stem.

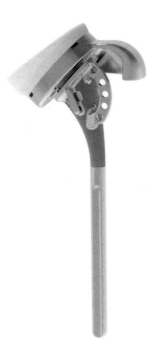

FIGURE 45.3 Fracture humeral stem with metallic greater tuberosity augment designed to restore the deltoid wrapping angle Image reprinted with permission from Exactech, Inc. © Exactech, Inc. All rights reserved.)

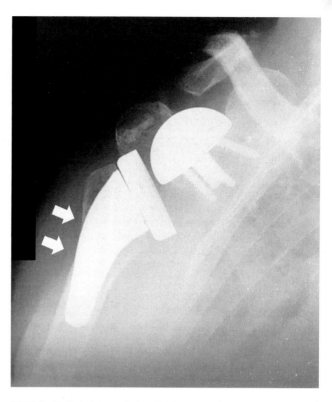

FIGURE 45.4 Anteroposterior (AP) x-rays show an uncemented humeral stem with a large metaphyseal filling ratio with lateral stress shielding (arrows) leading to complete lateral humeral cortex defect.

Primary Arthroplasty Stems

Primary arthroplasty has historically been performed with humeral stems that require both canal reaming and metaphyseal broaching to achieve rotational stability. However, new generations of humeral implants have employed shorter stems and broach-only techniques in an effort to preserve humeral bone stock and prevent stress shielding.[4]

The use of primary implants at the time of revision surgery is possible in the setting of Type 1 deficits, where the metadiaphyseal bone remains intact.

Caution should be taken when using these techniques with significant Type 1G defects, where the greater tuberosity is absent. In a study of 420 patients undergoing reverse total shoulder arthroplasty (RTSA) for proximal humerus fractures, Ohl et al compared a group of patients with iatrogenic bone loss (tuberosity excision) to a group with healed or malunited/resorbed/nonunited greater tuberosities. Postoperative instability was significantly higher in shoulders with resected tuberosities (12.5%).[5] This is likely due to loss of the deltoid wrapping angle and the rotator cuff deficiency, which both provide a compressive force across the glenohumeral joint and reduce postoperative instability.[6] Therefore, surgeons should be cautious when using standard medialized glenoid/medialized humerus[7] RTSA implants in the setting of greater tuberosity bone loss. In the future, metal augmentation of the greater tuberosity will be available in conjunction with standard stem fixation options **(FIGURE 45.3)**.

Fixation of standard stems in proximal humeri with Type 1 bony deficits can be performed in both uncemented and cemented fashion, depending on the system selected.[8] It is important to achieve rotational stability regardless of fixation type. When using cement, this can be performed using traditional techniques or cementing into a previous cement mantle at the time of revision when no infection is suspected (cement-within-cement technique).[9] When cancellous bone is compromised in the metaphyseal region, rotational stability can also be obtained with impaction grafting of auto- or allograft bone.[10] This technique has been used successfully in the setting of revision surgery, where bone loss is isolated to the epiphyseal/metaphyseal cancellous bone. Lastly, rotational stability can be achieved by simply increasing the size of the humeral stem until adequate cortical contact is achieved at the metaphyseal portion of the implant. However, fixation using this technique has led to significant stress shielding and longer term loss of humeral bone in the area of cortical contact.[11] **(FIGURE 45.4)**.

Some surgeons have also attempted to treat Type 2a bone defects with standard stems. In a study of 32 revision RTSA with (16) and without (16) proximal humeral bone loss, Stephens et al[12] documented similar improvements in pain and patient-reported outcome measures. However, in those with proximal humeral bone loss, patients demonstrated significantly less forward elevation ($100°$ vs $135°$, $P = 0.022$) and external rotation ($19°$ vs $34°$, $P = 0.009$). Furthermore, the authors noted

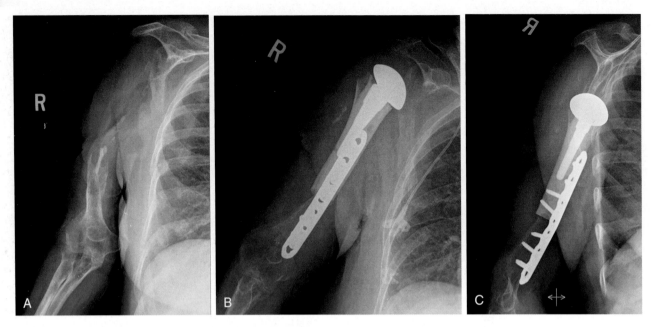

FIGURE 45.5 A, Preoperative anteroposterior (AP) x-ray showing a 57-year-old female with massive humeral bone loss (Type 3B) following treatment of a periprosthetic humerus fracture which became infected with methicillin-resistant *Staphylococcus aureus* (MRSA). She had a document axillary nerve injury on the same side with disruption of the deltoid insertion. **B** and **C,** She was treated with an allograft prosthetic composite (APC) reconstruction using compression plating.

higher rates of aseptic humeral loosening in shoulders with proximal humeral bone loss (19% vs 0).[12]

Long-Stem Monoblock

In the setting of bone loss proximal to the deltoid insertion (Type 1 and Type 2) or with smaller defects distally, arthroplasty can be performed with long-stemmed monoblock humeral components. Similar to reconstruction with standard stems, consideration should be given to greater tuberosity bone loss and the deltoid wrapping angle. When reconstructing with long-stemmed humeral components, these are often cemented into the remaining diaphyseal bone. Cementing can be performed the entire length of the stem or only at the most proximal aspect of the bone-implant interface. During preparation, care must be taken to avoid a distal cortical perforation.[13] It is important to remember that these long-stemmed components are straight and do not accommodate for the natural bow of the humerus. Intraoperative fluoroscopy may be useful during humeral preparation for these implants to ensure that diaphyseal reaming remains within the intramedullary canal.

In addition to intraoperative complications, previous reports on these prostheses have raised concern about high rates of aseptic humeral loosening. In a study of 124 revision shoulder arthroplasties performed with long-stem cemented humeral components, the authors noted a 10% rate of aseptic humeral loosening.[14] The failure rates with this prosthesis are likely related to the high torsional loads, which occur with use of the forearm during daily activity. Following reconstruction

in the setting of humeral bone loss, humeral implants experience increased rotational micromotion, which may lead to failure at the bone cement interface.[15] This method of failure likely explains the higher rates of aseptic loosening when standard humeral stems are used to treated proximal humeral bone loss in revision RTSA.[12] For these reasons, we prefer not to use long-stemmed components in isolation in the setting of proximal humeral bone loss, which involves complete loss of the greater tuberosity.

Allograft Prosthetic Composite

In cases of proximal humeral bone loss exceeding 5 cm, reconstruction using standard or long-stem implants is not possible even with the use of eccentric glenospheres or augmented humeral trays. One option for this more distal bone loss is reconstruction with an allograft prosthetic composite (APC). This has historically been used for Type 2 and Type 3 bone loss **(FIGURE 45.5).** This procedure involves removing proximal poor quality bone and replacing the bony defect with a frozen allograft. Our general preference is to use a size-matched proximal humerus allograft, but when unavailable, alternative grafts such as a distal tibia can be utilized. A standard or long-stemmed humeral component is then placed into/through the allograft bone and then mated with the remaining native bone. Fixation into the host bone has been described using both cemented and uncemented techniques. The junction between the allograft and native bone can be supplemented with plate fixation and local bone grafting.

Previous authors have recommended reconstruction with an APC when bone loss exceeds 5 cm from the native humeral calcar. However, this remains as level 5 evidence (expert opinion) based on surgical experience.[16,17] Advantages of APC reconstruction include restoration of bone stock, reproduction of the deltoid wrapping angle, and ability to repair soft tissues to the allograft with the potential for biologic healing. In a study of 14 APCs undergoing revision surgery, all or a portion of the allograft was able to be retained in 64% of cases.[18]

Multiple studies have reported clinical success with APCs used in both the hemiarthroplasty and RTSA configurations. However, long-term success of shoulder reconstruction with an APC hemiarthroplasty remains unclear. In a study of 21 APC hemiarthroplasties following tumor resection, El Beaino et al reported 48% of patients showed evidence of superior subluxation (>1 cm) at 1-year follow-up despite reattachment of the rotator cuff musculature.[19] The authors do not report functional outcomes, but the presence of superior subluxation is concerning for failure of the rotator cuff repair, which would place the patient at high risk for meaningful loss of shoulder function.[20] In addition to rotator cuff failure, resections that sacrifice the deltoid insertion have also been shown to have poorer range of motion and function following APC reconstruction with a hemiarthroplasty.[21]

Because of concern about the long-term function of hemiarthroplasty with rotator cuff repair, APC reconstruction with a reverse shoulder configuration has become increasingly popular.[22,23] Sanchez-Sotelo et al[24] reported on 26 patients treated with reverse APC reconstructions for massive proximal humeral bone loss. At a mean follow-up of 4 years, mean forward elevation had improved from 41° to 98° ($P < 0.0001$). Patients also demonstrated acceptable function, with a mean American Shoulder and Elbow Surgeons (ASES) functional score of 66.1. Implant survivorship at 5 years was 92%.

Despite successes described with APC reconstruction, surgeons should expect a higher level of complications following these surgeries compared to primary arthroplasty. Long-term success of this construct depends on the junction of the host bone to the humeral allograft. Compression plating has become increasingly popular to secure the APC construct to host bone to improve healing rates.[19,24] Described techniques to increase bony union include transverse cuts with compression plating, step-cut mating with cable and/or plate fixation, and dome osteotomy with compression plating.[24-26] However, nonunion at the junction of the host/allograft remains the most common complication.[21] Other complications include aseptic loosening, instability, periprosthetic fracture, graft osteolysis, and infection.

Modular Reconstruction Prostheses

As humeral bone loss progresses to involve the deltoid insertion, substantial structural loss of the proximal humerus architecture is present. As bone loss increases, reconstruction with standard components becomes impossible, and long-stem components are at increased risk of mechanical failure. Based on the concern with traditional components, modular reconstruction prostheses have been developed, which allow for replacement of humeral bone stock with metallic components. These devices traditionally involve fixation of a humeral stem into the remaining diaphysis, with multiple-sized proximal body attachments, which can be used to reconstruct the proximal humeral bone loss. Attachment sites for soft tissues are often incorporated into the design in an attempt to restore function. However, long-term stability of the remaining repaired soft tissues to hydroxyapatite-coated metal components remains in question. Early reports on the use of these types of prosthesis have shown encouraging results.[27,28]

Similar to APC reconstruction, modular reconstruction prostheses can be implemented in both a hemiarthroplasty or RTSA configuration. When used for tumor surgery, these are often used as an RTSA, as long as the deltoid remains intact and functional.[27] In the setting of revision surgery, the amount of remaining glenoid bone stock may dictate whether or not a glenosphere can be securely placed. Strategies to restore humeral length and offset are important. Soft tissue repairs and/or transfers may also help to minimize postoperative dead space.

Restoration of stability following RTSA reconstruction using a modular reconstruction prosthesis is critical to restoring function following surgery. For cases in which the deltoid insertion or conjoint tendon origin is disrupted, longitudinal tension may be difficult to obtain without overlengthening the arm. Humeral lateralization and restoration of the deltoid wrapping angle with the use of a modular reconstruction prosthesis also imparts secondary stability. The availability of multiple proximal body size diameters is important to filling the soft tissue envelope and restoring the deltoid wrapping angle. These implants can take the place of the missing tuberosities as well as restore the metaphyseal flare (FIGURE 45.6). Soft tissues can also be attached to the prosthesis, but in our experience, soft tissue integration to the metal components remains poor.

In addition to stability, long-term secure fixation of the implant is also a serious concern because of the large rotational forces that develop at the humeral bone/implant interface. Rotational stability can be achieved using cement fixation. However, this is susceptible to rotational stress fatigue over time and delated aseptic loosening, which has been observed in traditional long-stemmed prostheses.[15]

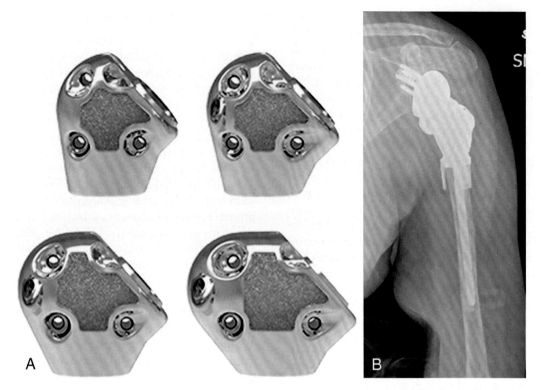

FIGURE 45.6 The humeral reconstruction prosthesis (Exactech, Gainesville FL) (**A**) has multiple proximal body options which come in varying sizes to replicate the shape of the tuberosities and metaphyseal flare. **B**, The size options allow for appropriate restoration of the missing humeral tuberosities and restoration of the deltoid wrapping angle. (Used with permission from © Exactech, Inc.)

Newer modular humeral prostheses have been designed to restore long-term rotational stability following reconstruction in the setting of massive humeral bone loss. The Aequalis Flex Revive Shoulder System (Tornier, Minneapolis, MN) utilizes a plasma titanium-coated modular stem designed to achieve uncemented fixation into the humeral diaphysis. Bone is then able to on-grow to the humeral stem and provide long-term rotation stability, while simultaneously allowed for modular reconstruction proximally. Other designs have utilized a taper-fluted modular design for humeral fixation (Lima SMR, Arlington, TX). In the total hip arthroplasty literature, this type of design has shown lower rates of subsidence and loosening, particularly in patients with compromised bone proximally.[29] When applied in the shoulder, these stems offer robust humeral fixation into higher quality bone while achieving excellent rotational stability. These stems can be deployed distal to compromised bone and then built up with varying sized proximal bodies. However, it remains unclear if these stems will cause progressive proximal osteolysis. Furthermore, in our experience, these stems can be quite destructive to remove following osseous integration in the case of revision.

Alternatively, the Humeral Reconstruction Prosthesis (HRP, Exactech, Gainesville, FL) utilizes a press-fit collar over humeral resection bone. The prosthesis is cemented into place, while the collar is impacted over the remaining humeral diaphysis (see **FIGURE 45.6**). Initial rotational stability is maintained by the cement mantle and the tight humeral collar. Longer-term rotational stability is gained as the bone grows onto the humeral collar. With postoperative ingrowth at the implant-host junction, long-term rotational stability is theorized to be greater with this prosthetic design.

Reconstruction with metal (prosthetic components) has numerous distinct advantages. Definitive fixation is obtained at the time of surgery, and there is no requirement of the host bone to fuse to allograft bone, which is a common reason for reoperation after APC reconstruction.[18,21] In the hands of experienced surgeons, replacement with a modular prosthesis is also faster, not requiring the intricate carpentry skills necessary with an APC reconstruction. However, despite these advantages, it is expected that metallic modular reconstruction prostheses will be more expensive than using traditional components with an APC. Additionally, soft tissue healing to metal remains inadequate, and the long-term functionality of these repairs are unknown.

ACCOMPANIED TENDON TRANSFERS

In cases of proximal humeral bone loss, attachments for the rotator cuff, pectoralis major, latissimus major, teres major, and deltoid may be sacrificed. The loss of these muscles can lead to functional limitations of the shoulder following reconstruction, regardless of the technique utilized. In order to maximize function, transfer of local musculature may be added to humeral reconstruction procedures.

Transfer of the latissimus dorsi with or without transfer of the teres major has been described to restore active external rotation in combination with RTSA in patients with combined loss of active elevation and external rotation.[30-32] These patients typically present with an external rotation lag sign[33] preoperatively, which is associated with a deficient infraspinatus and teres minor. In case of substantial proximal humeral bone loss, the entire greater tuberosity (where both the infraspinatus and teres minor are inserted) can be missing, leading to a similar clinical presentation. In most cases, the remaining rotator cuff muscle can be reattached to the APC or modular proximal humeral reconstruction. However, in some cases, allografts without any tendinous attachments may be chosen or a surgeon may find there is no remaining rotator cuff available to attach. In these cases, tendon transfers may be an option to restore active axial rotation and to improve stability in this soft-tissue–deprived environment. Several tendon transfers have been described on a native shoulder to restore both active external and internal rotation,[34-39] and biomechanical studies have suggested that all of these could be beneficial in combination with an RTSA.[40] These include transfer of the latissimus dorsi (to the front to restore active internal rotation[35,37,38] or to the back to restore active external rotation[34,41]), transfer of the lower trapezius,[36,39] and transfer of the pectoralis major.[42,43]

Restoration of Active External Rotation

In cases of proximal humerus bone loss, where the posterior cuff is not reparable after RTSA with APC, patients can recover satisfactory active forward elevation and abduction but are often unable to recover active external rotation (**FIGURE 45.7**). This leads to an inability to position the arm in space that significantly impacts activities of daily living.[30] Two tendon transfers have been described to restore active external rotation: the latissimus dorsi ± teres major transferred to the lateral or anterolateral aspect of the humeral shaft[30-32,44] or the lower trapezius transferred posteriorly to the footprint of the infraspinatus.[36,39] The preferred option in combination with an RTSA is the modified L'Episcopo procedure as described by Boileau et al through an extended deltopectoral approach.[30] However, in cases of extensive proximal humeral bone loss, the tendon of the latissimus dorsi might no longer be available for tendon transfer. In this case, the only remaining option is the transfer of the lower trapezius lengthened by either a semitendinosus autograft or Achilles allograft.[36,39] This procedure can be performed in the beach chair position with the patient positioned laterally on the operative table in order to access the medial border of the scapula in the surgical

field. The first step is the harvest of the lower trapezius tendon from the scapular spine as has been described by Elhassan et al.[36] The lower trapezius is then released from both the underlying and subcutaneous tissues in order to obtain sufficient excursion and is placed in a wet gauze. The fascia of the infraspinatus is opened and partly excised to allow proper gliding of the graft.

The next step is the implantation of the RTSA with the APC. Before reduction of the joint, the graft is fixed to the allograft at the footprint of the infraspinatus. The graft can either be fixed using transosseous # 5 nonabsorbable braided sutures or directly sutured to the tendons attached to the proximal humerus allograft with # 2 nonabsorbable braided sutures. The space between the posterior deltoid and posterior cuff is developed using blunt scissors, and a long clamp is passed from the dorsal incision to retrieve the graft. The joint is then reduced, and the arm is placed in maximal external rotation. In this position, the medial free end of the allograft is sutured to the lower trapezius tendon in a Pulvertaft fashion with # 2 nonabsorbable braided sutures. The patient is then placed in a brace in 30° of abduction and 50° of external rotation for 6 weeks.

Restoration of Active Internal Rotation

Recently, Collin[45] has shown in an ultrasound study that active internal rotation was significantly higher in patients with a healed subscapularis tendon after RTSA than in patients with a ruptured tendon. Therefore, replacing an irreparable subscapularis with a tendon transfer in combination with an RTSA may be an option to restore active internal rotation in these patients. Severe proximal humeral bone loss can lead to a loss of the tendon insertions of some of the internal rotators: subscapularis, pectoralis major, latissimus dorsi, and teres major.[46] Loss of internal rotation can be extremely debilitating as it leads to the inability to place the arm behind the back, which is necessary for personal hygiene.[47,48] Therefore, replacement of an irreparable subscapularis in combination with an RTSA and APC could be an option to restore active internal rotation. Two main tendon transfers have been described to successfully restore active internal rotation in the native shoulder: transfer of the pectoralis major[42,43] to the lesser tuberosity or transfer of the latissimus dorsi anteriorly to the most anterior part of the footprint of the supraspinatus.[35,38] It has been shown in a biomechanical study that the moment arm of the latissimus dorsi transfer is greater than that of the pectoralis major transfer in a native shoulder. However, the semiconstrained design of the reverse shoulder arthroplasty (RSA) allows the transfer of the sternal head of the pectoralis major to become more efficient to restore internal rotation as all forces applied on the joint are transformed into rotational forces.[40] Consequently, in cases of severe proximal humerus bone loss in which

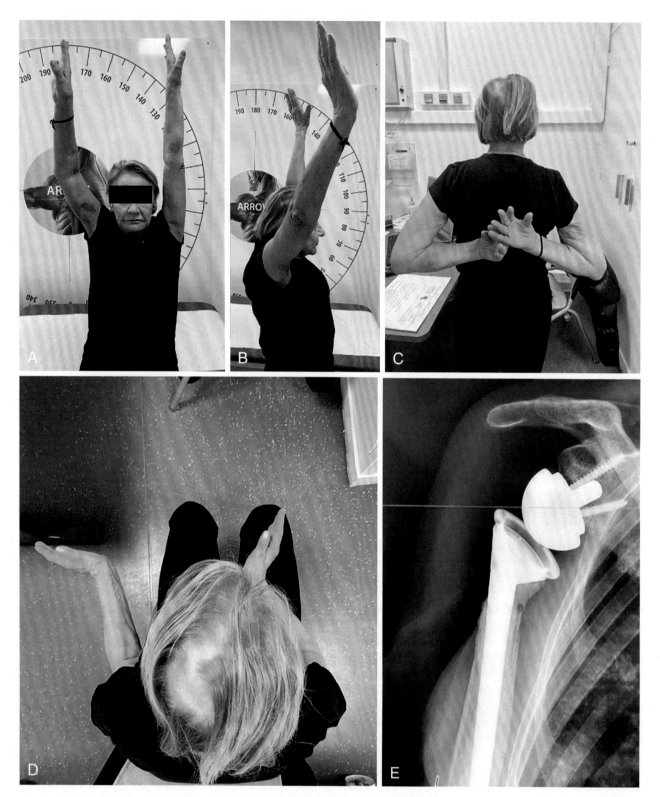

FIGURE 45.7 A 73-year-old woman after reverse shoulder arthroplasty (RSA) with proximal humeral bone loss, without any soft-tissue/tendon transfer reconstruction. She has clinically satisfactory active abduction (**A**), anterior flexion (**B**), and internal rotation (**C**) but no active external rotation with external rotation lag sign (**D**). The loss of the greater tuberosity and external rotators (**E**) results in this loss of function. Therefore, she is not able to position the arm in space leading to a severe limitation in activities of daily living despite good overall range of motion.

a deficit of active internal rotation can be expected, both tendon transfers can be proposed to restore internal rotation, although neither has been reported in combination with an APC to our knowledge.

Stabilization of the Articulation

Restoration of active axial rotation is of course important. However, reconstruction of the proximal humerus is often a salvage procedure with limited functional goals, and in these cases, the objective may be "only" to restore a pain-free stable shoulder. Indeed, the main complication in cases of severe proximal humeral bone loss is instability, which can occur for several reasons: (1) insufficient restoration of humeral length,[49] (2) loss of the stabilizing action of the anterior and posterior check-reins that are the anterior and posterior cuff,[5] and (3) loss of the contour of the greater tuberosity leading to a loss of the so-called wrapping angle[50] of the deltoid associated with a loss of compression from the deltoid. Both restoration of proper humeral length and of the contour of the greater tuberosity can be achieved with an APC or a modular humeral prosthesis. This allows for proper tensioning of the deltoid but to obtain optimal stabilization of the joint, attachment of the remaining rotator cuff to the tendon stumps of the proximal allograft is recommended. However, in some cases, the shoulder lacks anterior and posterior functional soft-tissue, and thus, it may be unstable despite adequate templating and bony reconstruction (**FIGURE 45.8**). In this situation, tendon transfers can be proposed in combination with proximal humeral reconstruction to replace the deficient rotator cuff in order to restore anterior and posterior compressive forces. The objective is, therefore, to restore a line of pull similar to that of the subscapularis anteriorly and the infraspinatus posteriorly. This can be achieved by transferring the latissimus dorsi anteriorly through a pectoralis major-sparing deltopectoral approach and the lower trapezius posteriorly.

AUTHORS' PREFERRED TECHNIQUES

Allograft Prosthetic Composite

In our practice, APC reconstruction is considered in cases of massive humeral bone loss in younger patients or those elderly patients lacking enough length of distal diaphyseal bone to accept a stemmed prosthesis. Careful preoperative planning is essential. Bilateral humeral x-rays with magnification markers are useful for measuring both the anticipated humeral defect and also for sizing the humeral allograft. Computed tomography (CT) scans, when available, are also helpful for sizing humeral allografts. Depending on the supplier, these grafts can be obtained with or without soft tissue attachments. Our strong preference is to order frozen allografts with preserved soft tissue attachments in the event native tissues can be repaired primarily to the allograft tendon. When

ordering the graft, it is important to obtain a graft that is similar in size to the native bone in order to appropriately fill the soft tissue envelope. Use of an oversized graft may lead to difficulties closing the deltopectoral interval secondary to increased bony volume.

At the time of surgery, a deltopectoral incision is utilized and extended distally as needed. Depending on the level of resection, the brachialis may be split midline or lifted from lateral to medial. Care should be taken to identify the radial nerve proximal to the lateral epicondyle as it courses form posterior to anterior when distal dissection is required.[51] Any remaining soft tissue attachments are tagged for later repair to the prosthesis, and any remaining nonusable proximal humeral bone is resected. The humerus is then osteotomized transversely. The proximal humeral defect is measured based off of the resected bone or preoperative template. At this point, the glenoid is prepared if a reverse shoulder configuration is to be used. In the setting of hemiarthroplasty, the rotator cuff tendons are mobilized and prepared with multiple #2 nonabsorbable braided sutures. Our strong preference is to utilize the RTSA when the glenoid bone stock is sufficient and the deltoid is functional.

On the back table, the humeral allograft is secured with vice grips and prepared. First, the humeral head is resected in its native retroversion, retaining all soft tissue attachments, which are amenable to repair. The humeral canal is then reamed and broached according to the implant surgical technique. We prefer to use cemented short-stem prostheses contained completely within the allograft so that at least two screws can be placed bicortically below the stem tip. Additional screws can then be angled around the stem. When a short-stem prosthesis cannot be completely contained within the allograft with sufficient space for screws, we utilize a long-stem component to bypass the osteotomy site by at least two cortical diameters.

Once the allograft is prepared, if a long-stem component is utilized, the distal humeral diaphysis is prepared using the implant-specific reamers. The allograft is then osteotomized to restore appropriate humeral length. Initially, we prefer the graft to be 1 to 2 cm long until it can be fully placed into the soft tissue defect to confirm the allograft has adequate length. Sometimes, it is difficult to place the allograft at the templated length due to soft tissue contractures, which have occurred following bone loss. In these cases, it is important to release the entire soft tissue envelope to adequately restore humeral height. Failure to do so may lead to soft tissue relaxation over time and late instability. Once the allograft length is confirmed, final adjustments to the graft length are made. The humeral stem broach is placed into the allograft, with or without extension into the native humeral diaphysis. At this point, varus/valgus alignment is assessed clinically and under fluoroscopy. Adjustments to the osteotomy can be made as required.

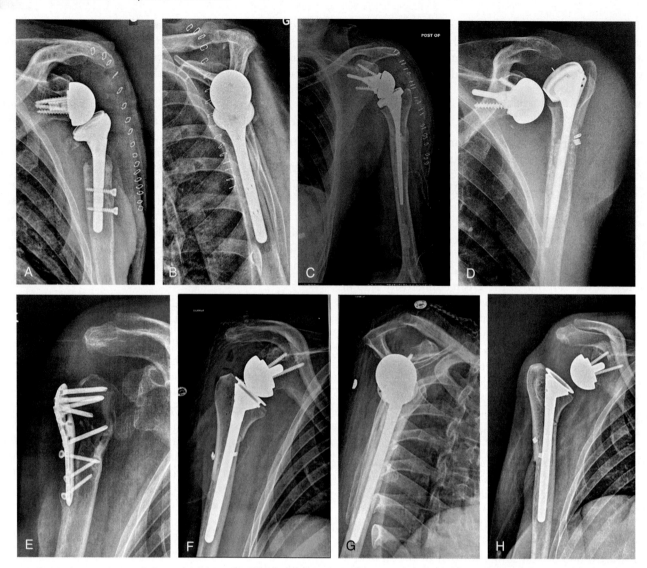

FIGURE 45.8 A and **B**, Anteroposterior (AP) and lateral standard radiographs of a reverse shoulder arthroplasty (RSA) implanted for a four-part fracture revised several times for instability. Severe proximal humerus bone loss. **C**, Revised to an allograft prosthetic composite (APC) (proximal humerus allograft) with a step-cut and radio-transparent cables with a lateralized implant (lateralized glenoid and humerus). **D**, 1 month postoperatively, instability despite proper restoration of humeral height possibly due to a lack of soft tissue reconstruction. **E**, Avascular necrosis (AVN) 3 years after open reduction and internal fixation (ORIF) for proximal humerus fracture. Nonunion and migration of the greater tuberosity visible behind the glenoid. **F,G**, Revised to an APC (proximal humerus allograft) with a step-cut and radio-transparent cables with a medialized implant (medialized glenoid and humerus). **H**, 1 month postoperatively, instability despite proper restoration of humeral height possibly due to a lack of soft tissue reconstruction.

Next, a 4.5-mm narrow-locking compression plate is sized and prebent for placement along the anterior face of the humerus. In very distal osteotomy sites, plating with locking distal humerus plates may need to be considered. A minimum of three screws on both sides of the graft-host junction is necessary. However, we strongly prefer four screws whenever possible. One positional screw is then placed on both sides of the osteotomy. Plate position is then confirmed. A second positional screw is placed distally. Finally, all proximal screws are prepared and placed with the understanding that the proximal most screws may need to be angled around the prosthesis. Cables and unicortical locking screws can also be

considered as needed. When all proximal screws have been placed, the distal screws are removed. The allograft is transferred to the back table. The trial components are removed, and the real humeral stem is cemented into place. Once the cement is hard, the APC is transferred back into the operative field. When using a long-stem prosthesis, the plate may need to be removed and the distal prosthesis cemented into the native humeral canal. Once the APC is in place, the two diaphyseal positioning screws are reinserted. A third screw is then prepared and placed in compression mode to compress the osteotomy site. When using distal cement, this must be done efficiently before the cement hardens.

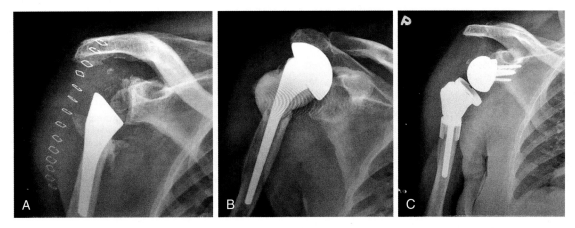

FIGURE 45.9 A, This 62-year-old woman was referred after a failed attempted to revise a hemiarthroplasty. **B,** Following resection of the stem, she has significant humeral bone loss to the deltoid tuberosity (Type 2B) and was treated with a temporary spacer while undergoing treatment for a C acnes infection. **C,** After clearing the infection, she was revised to a modular humeral reconstruction prosthesis.

Once the APC construct is secured, trial components are placed proximally, and the shoulder is reduced. Adjustments are made to gain appropriate soft tissue tension, and then the final components are placed. Any preserved native tendons are then secured to the allograft using #2 nonabsorbable sutures. In the setting of deficient soft tissues, local tendon transfers can be considered and affixed to the allograft tendon stumps.

Postoperatively, a deep drain is placed and removed the following morning. An arm sling with an abduction pillow is used until 6 weeks postoperatively when active-assisted range of motion is initiated. Strengthening is started at 12 weeks postoperatively, with gradual return to full activity (40 lb lifting restriction) at 6 months.

Modular Humeral Reconstruction

Proximal humeral reconstruction with modular metallic components is our preferred treatment for patients older than 60 years with bone loss graded as type 2B or 3 **(FIGURE 45.9).** We also prefer to treat most patients with oncologic conditions with this type of reconstruction, which is discussed in more detail in Chapter 48. Preoperative planning is performed in a similar manner as described for our APC technique. Patients are evaluated with a preoperative CT and bilateral humerus radiographs with magnification markers.

At the time of surgery, a utilitarian deltopectoral incision is utilized. In the setting of revision surgery, every attempt is made to preserve as much useable bone stock as possible. We prefer to use the HRP (Exactech, Gainesville FL) for these cases, as it is the only prosthesis with multiple proximal humerus bodies with varying diameters, designed to replicate the missing tuberosities and restore deltoid wrapping. Once the final bony deficits can be assessed, a resection level is chosen. Soft tissue is cleared circumferentially around the bone above and below the resection level to allow for the safe passage of a saw blade. A transverse osteotomy is performed, and the remaining proximal bone is resected. Any remaining soft tissue attachments are tagged for later repair to the prosthesis.

At this point, the glenoid is unobstructed. When performing an RTSA, we prefer to prepare and place the real glenoid baseplate and glenosphere. Attention is then turned to the humerus. Any remaining soft tissue within 2 to 3 cm of the osteotomy site is bluntly lifted off the humerus. The remaining humeral canal is reamed according to the technique guide. Rotational stability is, in part, obtained from the humeral collar, which fits around the remaining humeral diaphysis. When trialing this collar, the smallest/tightest collar should be chosen. However, we routinely downsize one size from the trial when implanting the real component in order to ensure rotational stability with the collar. Once the humeral diaphysis has been prepared, modular pieces can be added proximally to restore the missing humeral bone length based upon the preoperative plan. Small adjustments to the osteotomy site may be required based on the available length options of proximal bodies and middle segments needed to restore humeral length. Once the trial humeral components have been assembled, a trial RTSA tray is placed and the shoulder is reduced. Soft tissue tension is assessed by evaluating the conjoint tendon and deltoid tension whenever possible. Once again, it is important to perform appropriate soft tissue releases to restore the templated humeral length due to the risk of soft tissue relaxation over time. Once appropriate soft tissue tension has been obtained, the shoulder is dislocated and trial components are removed.

Following irrigation of the wound, the components for implantation are assembled on the back table. A cement restrictor is placed into the humeral canal and cement inserted using a standard pressurizing cement gun. We prefer to inject the cement when it is still slightly runny, as the humeral diaphysis is often smaller and prone to incomplete filling. The humeral component is then inserted in 20° of retroversion. This requires forceful malleting to engage the collar over the proximal humeral diaphysis. Once completely seated, a trial polyethylene is inserted and the shoulder is reduced. We do not wait for the cement to dry given the excellent rotational stability offered by the humeral collar. The shoulder is then taken through passive range of motion to assess for impingement and glenohumeral instability. Adjustments to the thickness of polyethylene can be made for fine-tuning of longitudinal tension. Once the final components have been selected, they are inserted. Any preserved native tendons are then secured to the metaphyseal part of the implant using #2 nonabsorbable stitches. In the setting of deficient soft tissues, local tendon transfers can be considered on the remaining native humeral bone. A deep drain is placed, and the wound is closed in layers in standard fashion.

The drain is usually removed the following morning. A sling with an abduction pillow is used for 6 weeks postoperatively and at that time active-assisted range of motion is initiated. Strengthening is started at 12 weeks postoperatively, with gradual return to full activity (40 lb lifting restriction) at 6 months.

CONCLUSION

Massive humeral bone loss is a challenging surgical problem in the setting of shoulder arthroplasty. When bone loss affects only the humeral metaphysis and/or tuberosities, standard implants can commonly be used. However, as bone loss progresses, surgeons must be prepared to employ more complex reconstruction techniques which can require exposure of named nerves and the transfer of local musculature. Reconstruction of massive bone loss which progressing into the humeral diaphysis has historically been performed using proximal humeral allografts. These APCs remain the choice of some surgeons and when performed with attached tendon stumps can be used to secure the remaining rotator cuff or transferred tendons. Furthermore, APCs have been shown to restore bone even in the setting of future re-revision. Newer modular humeral reconstruction prostheses now provide an alternative to APC reconstruction and allow for immediate stable fixation of the humerus. These prostheses have multiple options to reconstruct both length as well as humeral lateralization and can be performed without the fine carpentry skills required to successfully execute an APC reconstruction. When approaching shoulder arthroplasty in the setting of massive humeral bone loss, surgeons should be prepared with multiple implant options and be careful to completely restore humeral length and offset to minimize potential postoperative instability.

REFERENCES

1. Van Thiel GS, Halloran JP, Twigg S, Romeo AA, Nicholson GP. The vertical humeral osteotomy for stem removal in revision shoulder arthroplasty: results and technique. *J Shoulder Elbow Surg.* 2011;20(8):1248-1254. doi:10.1016/j.jse.2010.12.013

2. Malawer MM, Meller I, Dunham WK. A new surgical classification system for shoulder-girdle resections. Analysis of 38 patients. *Clin Orthop Relat Res.* 1991;(267):33-44.

3. Chalmers PN, Romeo AA, Nicholson GP, et al. Humeral bone loss in revision total shoulder arthroplasty: the proximal humeral arthroplasty revision osseous inSufficiency (PHAROS) classification system. *Clin Orthop Relat Res.* 2019;477(2):432-441. doi:10.1097/CORR.0000000000000590

4. Aibinder WR, Bartels DW, Sperling JW, Sanchez-Sotelo J. Midterm radiological results of a cementless short humeral component in anatomical and reverse shoulder arthroplasty. *Bone Joint J.* 2019;101-B(5):610-614. doi:10.1302/0301-620X.101B5.BJJ-2018-1374.R1

5. Ohl X, Bonnevialle N, Gallinet D, et al. How the greater tuberosity affects clinical outcomes after reverse shoulder arthroplasty for proximal humeral fractures. *J Shoulder Elbow Surg.* 2018;27(12):2139-2144. doi:10.1016/j.jse.2018.05.030

6. Roche CP, Diep P, Hamilton M, et al. Impact of inferior glenoid tilt, humeral retroversion, bone grafting, and design parameters on muscle length and deltoid wrapping in reverse shoulder arthroplasty. *Bull Hosp Jt Dis (2013).* 2013;71(4):284-293.

7. Werthel JD, Walch G, Vegehan E, Deransart P, Sanchez-Sotelo J, Valenti P. Lateralization in reverse shoulder arthroplasty: a descriptive analysis of different implants in current practice. *Int Orthop.* 2019;43(10):2349-2360. doi:10.1007/s00264-019-04365-3

8. Wagner ER, Statz JM, Houdek MT, Cofield RH, Sánchez-Sotelo J, Sperling JW. Use of a shorter humeral stem in revision reverse shoulder arthroplasty. *J Shoulder Elbow Surg.* 2017;26(8):1454-1461. doi:10.1016/j.jse.2017.01.016

9. Wagner ER, Houdek MT, Hernandez NM, Cofield RH, Sánchez-Sotelo J, Sperling JW. Cement-within-cement technique in revision reverse shoulder arthroplasty. *J Shoulder Elbow Surg.* 2017;26(8):1448-1453. doi:10.1016/j.jse.2017.01.013

10. Lucas RM, Hsu JE, Gee AO, Neradilek MB, Matsen FA. Impaction autografting: bone-preserving, secure fixation of a standard humeral component. *J Shoulder Elbow Surg.* 2016;25(11):1787-1794. doi:10.1016/j.jse.2016.03.008

11. Raiss P, Schnetzke M, Wittmann T, et al. Postoperative radiographic findings of an uncemented convertible short stem for anatomic and reverse shoulder arthroplasty. *J Shoulder Elbow Surg.* 2019;28(4):715-723. doi:10.1016/j.jse.2018.08.037

12. Stephens SP, Paisley KC, Giveans MR, Wirth MA. The effect of proximal humeral bone loss on revision reverse total shoulder arthroplasty. *J Shoulder Elbow Surg.* 2015;24(10):1519-1526. doi:10.1016/j.jse.2015.02.020

13. Owens CJ, Sperling JW, Cofield RH. Utility and complications of long-stem humeral components in revision shoulder arthroplasty. *J Shoulder Elbow Surg.* 2013;22(7):e7-e12. doi:10.1016/j.jse.2012.10.034

14. Werner BS, Abdelkawi AF, Boehm D, et al. Long-term analysis of revision reverse shoulder arthroplasty using cemented long stems. *J Shoulder Elbow Surg.* 2017;26(2):273-278. doi:10.1016/j.jse.2016.05.015

15. Cuff D, Levy JC, Gutiérrez S, Frankle MA. Torsional stability of modular and non-modular reverse shoulder humeral components in a proximal humeral bone loss model. *J Shoulder Elbow Surg.* 2011;20(4):646-651. doi:10.1016/j.jse.2010.10.026

16. Boileau P. Complications and revision of reverse total shoulder arthroplasty. *Orthop Traumatol Surg Res.* 2016;102(1 suppl):S33-S43. doi:10.1016/j.otsr.2015.06.031

17. McLendon PB, Cox JL, Frankle MA. Humeral bone loss in revision shoulder arthroplasty. *Am J Orthop (Belle Mead NJ).* 2018;47(2). doi:10.12788/ajo.2018.0012

18. Reif T, Schoch B, Spiguel A, et al. A retrospective review of revision proximal humeral allograft-prosthetic composite procedures: an analysis of proximal humeral bone stock restoration. *J Shoulder Elbow Surg.* 2020;29(7):1353-1358. doi:10.1016/j.jse.2019.10.029

19. El Beaino M, Liu J, Lewis VO, Lin PP. Do early results of proximal humeral allograft-prosthetic reconstructions persist at 5-year followup? *Clin Orthop Relat Res.* 2019;477(4):758-765. doi:10.1097/CORR.0000000000000354

20. Leung B, Horodyski M, Struk AM, Wright TW. Functional outcome of hemiarthroplasty compared with reverse total shoulder arthroplasty in the treatment of rotator cuff tear arthropathy. *J Shoulder Elbow Surg.* 2012;21(3):319-323. doi:10.1016/j.jse.2011.05.023

21. Abdeen A, Hoang BH, Athanasian EA, Morris CD, Boland PJ, Healey JH. Allograft-prosthesis composite reconstruction of the proximal part of the humerus: functional outcome and survivorship. *J. Bone Joint Surg Am.* 2009;91(10):2406-2415. doi:10.2106/JBJS.H.00815

22. King JJ, Nystrom LM, Reimer NB, Gibbs CP, Scarborough MT, Wright TW. Allograft-prosthetic composite reverse total shoulder arthroplasty for reconstruction of proximal humerus tumor resections. *J Shoulder Elbow Surg.* 2016;25(1):45-54. doi:10.1016/j.jse.2015.06.021

23. Wang Z, Guo Z, Li J, Li X, Sang H. Functional outcomes and complications of reconstruction of the proximal humerus after intra-articular tumor resection. *Orthop Surg.* 2010;2(1):19-26. doi:10.1111/j.1757-7861.2009.00058.x

24. Sanchez-Sotelo J, Wagner ER, Houdek MT. Allograft-prosthetic composite reconstruction for massive proximal humeral bone loss in reverse shoulder arthroplasty. *JBJS Essent Surg Tech.* 2018;8(1):e3. doi:10.2106/JBJS.ST.17.00051

25. Cox JL, McLendon PB, Christmas KN, Simon P, Mighell MA, Frankle MA. Clinical outcomes following reverse shoulder arthroplasty-allograft composite for revision of failed arthroplasty associated with proximal humeral bone deficiency: 2- to 15-year follow-up. *J Shoulder Elbow Surg.* 2019;28(5):900-907. doi:10.1016/j.jse.2018.10.023.

26. Wilke B, Cooper A, Gibbs CP, Spiguel A. Reverse-reamed intercalary allograft: a surgical technique. *J Am Acad Orthop Surg.* 2018;26(14):501-505. doi:10.5435/JAAOS-D-17-00052

27. Grosel TW, Plummer DR, Everhart JS, et al. Reverse total shoulder arthroplasty provides stability and better function than hemiarthroplasty following resection of proximal humerus tumors. *J Shoulder Elbow Surg.* 2019;28(11):2147-2152. doi:10.1016/j.jse.2019.02.032

28. Grosel TW, Plummer DR, Mayerson JL, Scharschmidt TJ, Barlow JD. Oncologic reconstruction of the proximal humerus with a reverse total shoulder arthroplasty megaprosthesis. *J Surg Oncol.* 2018;118(6):867-872. doi:10.1002/jso.25061

29. Abdel MP, Cottino U, Larson DR, Hanssen AD, Lewallen DG, Berry DJ. Modular fluted tapered stems in aseptic revision total hip arthroplasty. *J Bone Joint Surg Am.* 2017;99(10):873-881. doi:10.2106/JBJS.16.00423

30. Boileau P, Chuinard C, Roussanne Y, Neyton L, Trojani C. Modified latissimus dorsi and teres major transfer through a single deltopectoral approach for external rotation deficit of the shoulder: as an isolated procedure or with a reverse arthroplasty. *J Shoulder Elbow Surg.* 2007;16(6):671-682. doi:10.1016/j.jse.2007.02.127

31. Gerber C, Pennington SD, Lingenfelter EJ, Sukthankar A. Reverse Delta-III total shoulder replacement combined with latissimus dorsi transfer. A preliminary report. *J Bone Joint Surg Am.* 2007;89(5):940-947. doi:10.2106/JBJS.F.00955

32. Puskas GJ, Germann M, Catanzaro S, Gerber C. Secondary latissimus dorsi transfer after failed reverse total shoulder arthroplasty. *J Shoulder Elbow Surg.* 2015;24(12):e337-e344. doi:10.1016/j.jse.2015.05.033

33. Collin P, Treseder T, Denard PJ, Neyton L, Walch G, Lädermann A. What is the best clinical test for Assessment of the teres minor in massive rotator cuff tears? *Clin Orthop Relat Res.* 2015;473(9):2959-2966. doi:10.1007/s11999-015-4392-9

34. Boileau P, Baba M, McClelland WB, Thélu CÉ, Trojani C, Bronsard N. Isolated loss of active external rotation: a distinct entity and results of L'Episcopo tendon transfer. *J Shoulder Elbow Surg.* 2018;27(3):499-509. doi:10.1016/j.jse.2017.07.008

35. Elhassan BT. Feasibility of latissimus and teres major transfer to reconstruct irreparable subscapularis tendon tear: an anatomic

36. study. *J Shoulder Elbow Surg.* 2015;24(4):e102-e103. doi:10.1016/j.jse.2014.12.035

36. Elhassan BT, Wagner ER, Werthel JD. Outcome of lower trapezius transfer to reconstruct massive irreparable posterior-superior rotator cuff tear. *J Shoulder Elbow Surg.* 2016;25(8):1346-1353. doi:10.1016/j.jse.2015.12.006

37. Kany J, Guinand R, Croutzet P, Valenti P, Werthel JD, Grimberg J. Arthroscopic-assisted latissimus dorsi transfer for subscapularis deficiency. *Eur J Orthop Surg Traumatol.* 2016;26(3):329-334. doi:10.1007/s00590-016-1753-3

38. Mun SW, Kim JY, Yi SH, Baek CH. Latissimus dorsi transfer for irreparable subscapularis tendon tears. *J Shoulder Elbow Surg.* 2018;27(6):1057-1064. doi:10.1016/j.jse.2017.11.022

39. Valenti P, Werthel JD. Lower trapezius transfer with semitendinosus tendon augmentation: indication, technique, results. *Obere Extrem.* 2018;13(4):261-268. doi:10.1007/s11678-018-0495-8

40. Werthel J-D, Schoch BS, Hooke A, et al. Biomechanical effectiveness of tendon transfers to restore active internal rotation in shoulder with deficient subscapularis with and without reverse shoulder arthroplasty. *J Shoulder Elb Surg.* 2021;30(5):1196-1206. doi:10.1016/j.jse.2020.08.026.

41. Gerber C, Vinh TS, Hertel R, Hess CW. Latissimus dorsi transfer for the treatment of massive tears of the rotator cuff. A preliminary report. *Clin Orthop Relat Res.* 1988;(232):51-61.

42. Ernstbrunner L, Wieser K, Catanzaro S, et al. Long-term outcomes of pectoralis major transfer for the treatment of irreparable subscapularis tears: results after a mean follow-up of 20 years. *J Bone Joint Surg Am.* 2019;101(23):2091-2100. doi:10.2106/JBJS.19.00172

43. Moroder P, Schulz E, Mitterer M, Plachel F, Resch H, Lederer S. Long-term outcome after pectoralis major transfer for irreparable anterosuperior rotator cuff tears. *J Bone Joint Surg Am.* 2017;99(3):239-245. doi:10.2106/JBJS.16.00485

44. Favre P, Loeb MD, Helmy N, Gerber C. Latissimus dorsi transfer to restore external rotation with reverse shoulder arthroplasty: a biomechanical study. *J Shoulder Elbow Surg.* 2008;17(4):650-658. doi:10.1016/j.jse.2007.12.010

45. Hartzler RU, Barlow JD, An KN, Elhassan BT. Biomechanical effectiveness of different types of tendon transfers to the shoulder for external rotation. *J Shoulder Elbow Surg.* 2012;21(10):1370-1376. doi:10.1016/j.jse.2012.01.026

46. Ackland DC, Richardson M, Pandy MG. Axial rotation moment arms of the shoulder musculature after reverse total shoulder arthroplasty. *J Bone Joint Surg Am.* 2012;94(20):1886-1895. doi:10.2106/JBJS.J.01861

47. Kim MS, Jeong HY, Kim JD, Ro KH, Rhee SM, Rhee YG. Difficulty in performing activities of daily living associated with internal rotation after reverse total shoulder arthroplasty. *J Shoulder Elbow Surg.* 2020;29(1):86-94. doi:10.1016/j.jse.2019.05.031

48. Werthel J-D, Wagner ER, Elhassan BT. Long-term results of latissimus dorsi transfer for internal rotation contracture of the shoulder in patients with obstetric brachial plexus injury. *JSES Open Access.* 2018;2(3):159-164. doi:10.1016/j.jses.2018.05.002

49. Lädermann A, Williams MD, Melis B, Hoffmeyer P, Walch G. Objective evaluation of lengthening in reverse shoulder arthroplasty. *J Shoulder Elbow Surg.* 2009;18(4):588-595. doi:10.1016/j.jse.2009.03.012

50. Routman HD, Flurin P-H, Wright TW, Zuckerman JD, Hamilton MA, Roche CP. Reverse shoulder arthroplasty prosthesis design classification system. *Bull Hosp Jt Dis (2013).* 2015;73(suppl 1):S5-S14.

51. Simone JP, Streubel PN, Sánchez-Sotelo J, Steinmann SP, Adams JE. Fingerbreadths rule in determining the safe zone of the radial nerve and posterior interosseous nerve for a lateral elbow approach: an anatomic study. *J Am Acad Orthop Surg Glob Res Rev.* 2019;3(2):e005. doi:10.5435/JAAOSGlobal-D-19-00005

46 Arthroplasty for Chronic Glenohumeral Dislocations

Jason B. Smoak, MD and Matthew J. DiPaola, MD

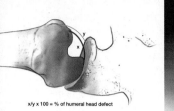

x/y x 100 = % of humeral head defect

EPIDEMIOLOGY AND BACKGROUND

A chronic glenohumeral dislocation (GHD) is generally defined as one whose recognition has been delayed by at least 3 weeks, although the exact definition is inconsistent in the current literature.[1,2] Some suggest that a chronic dislocation is best defined as any dislocation that was not identified at the time of the original injury.[2]

Chronic GHDs account for less than 2% of all shoulder dislocations.[3] Anterior GHDs are more frequent than posterior dislocations, but the incidence of chronic posterior GHDs is higher than chronic anterior GHDs.[2] Chronic posterior GHDs are often misdiagnosed by initial treating physicians, which may help to explain why nearly 80% of posterior dislocations may not be discovered until they have become chronic.[4]

Chronic GHDs often occur in elderly or mentally unstable patients.[5] Alcoholism, polytrauma, seizures, or electrical shock injuries are also well-known culprits for development of chronic GHD in young patients.[3-6] Delayed diagnosis is usually due to poor patient communication, negligence, inadequate examination, and incomplete or misinterpreted radiographs.[4]

Undiagnosed GHDs inevitably lead to loss of function in the affected shoulder. As the delay to diagnosis increases, humeral and glenoid bone defects are perpetuated by deterioration of articular cartilage, soft-tissue contractures, and rotator cuff tears. These patients frequently have poor bone quality and low rehabilitation potential, which makes treatment of these injuries even more challenging.[7]

A number of treatment options have been described for chronic GHD including closed or open reduction, tendon transfers, osteotomies, osteochondral grafting, and arthroplasty. Several factors including size of bone defects, presence of a torn rotator cuff, and chronicity of the dislocation must be considered when formulating a treatment approach. Although there are no large cohorts in the current literature, several case series have demonstrated successful treatment of chronic GHDs by shoulder arthroplasty including hemiarthroplasty, anatomic total shoulder replacement, and reverse total shoulder arthroplasty (RTSA).[3,5-12]

EVALUATION

History

In evaluating a patient for a suspected chronic GHD, the first step is a thorough history. The most common presenting complaint reported by a patient with a chronic GHD is loss of motion. Pain is almost always present initially; however, as more time passes and the chronic GHD becomes more "chronic," this becomes a less reliable finding. History of trauma is usually present although it may not be elicited due to the fact that seemingly trivial injury may cause dislocation in the elderly population, and some patients may be unable to communicate effectively. The clinician must have a high index of suspicion, especially in a patient whose history may be compromised such as one where alcohol or seizures may have played a role. The exact date of injury, age, prior activity level, and arm dominance are other important details to obtain. Patients should be explicitly questioned about a history of electric shock, seizures, and alcohol use as these are all potential contributing factors.

Physical Examination

Physical examination should always include detailed cervical spine and neurovascular examinations in addition to a complete shoulder evaluation. Neurological examination is particularly important in this population as there is a high risk for traction injury and neurological compromise. Comparison to the contralateral side is particularly useful when examination findings are subtle and may help to identify important asymmetries. Asymmetry typically worsens over time as atrophy accentuates the deformity. The clinician must be aware that patients with large body habitus may mask GHD more easily than patients with a smaller build.

In chronic anterior GHD, physical examination is often diagnostic and is characterized by fullness over the anterior glenohumeral joint in the subcoracoid region, which corresponds to the displaced humeral head.[5] This finding will be more evident in thinner patients. Flattening of the posterior and lateral contours of the shoulder along with prominence of the acromion posteriorly may be present **(FIGURE 46.1)**. The humeral head is frequently palpable in its anterior location. Range of motion (ROM) of the affected shoulder is highly variable depending on the chronicity of the dislocation. Initially, patients may lack significant internal rotation as well as forward flexion and abduction. This may be especially true when a humeral impression fracture is locked on the glenoid rim, which is commonly known as a locked GHD. With locked GHDs, repeated attempts to move the shoulder may enlarge humeral and glenoid bone defects, which allow for a much greater arc of motion. This can be a falsely reassuring sign. The clinician must guard against misinterpreting this finding as clinical improvement.

An axillary nerve palsy may present clinically with deltoid dysfunction and/or numbness over the lateral aspect of the shoulder. The axillary nerve is the most commonly injured nerve associated with anterior GHDs. Most axillary nerve deficits resolve over a period of months; however, persistent deficits may result in less predictable outcomes following operative treatment.[2,13,14] It is important to understand that a neurological examination may be unreliable in the setting of chronic GHD since it is often difficult to test deltoid function and sensation is not a reliable indicator of axillary nerve function.

The diagnosis of a chronic posterior GHD may be more challenging from physical examination perspective due to more subtle findings and its striking resemblance to other pathologies such as adhesive capsulitis. We have encountered patients treated for adhesive capsulitis whose posterior chronic GHD is only discovered when imaging studies are finally obtained. While the shoulder often lacks prominent deformity, some hallmark signs include a subtle posterior fullness with flattening of the anterior and lateral contours. Prominence of the acromion and coracoid

process anteriorly is also frequently present **(FIGURE 46.2)**. ROM is once again highly variable, yet in contrast to chronic anterior GHD, decreased external rotation is the classic finding and often presents as an internal rotation contracture. Loss of forward flexion and abduction are also often encountered in the early stages, yet enlargement of bone defects may ultimately allow for functional motion of the involved extremity. Neurovascular injury may be less common with chronic posterior GHD, but it remains critically important to examine for any deficits. Clinicians and therapists should be alert to a patient that presents with significant external rotation deficit and a firm endpoint. Overly aggressive therapy in the setting of a locked posterior GHD may result in massive erosion of the humeral head requiring a more aggressive surgical solution such as arthroplasty.

Radiographic Studies

Complete radiographic examination should be performed as part of any shoulder evaluation. A complete series of standard radiographs including a scapular anteroposterior (AP), scapular lateral (Y view), and axillary lateral or Velpeau axillary are essential in the initial evaluation of suspected chronic GHD. They should also be obtained prior to any shoulder manipulation to prevent any displacement of occult fractures. An axillary lateral or Velpeau radiograph is essential to avoid missed dislocations **(FIGURE 46.3)**.

A chronic anterior GHD will show an empty glenoid in AP shoulder radiographs as a result of anteroinferior dislocation of the humeral head. Scapular Y images may also demonstrate the anteroinferior location of the humeral head relative to the glenoid. An axillary lateral or Velpeau view is essential to confirm the diagnosis and may also help to elucidate the extent of any anterior glenoid and posterior humeral head bone defects **(FIGURE 46.4)**.

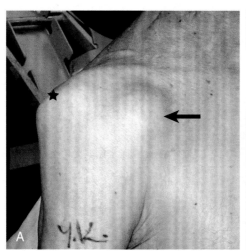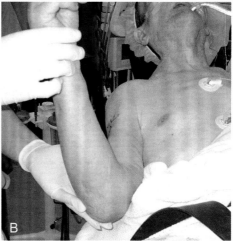

FIGURE 46.1 A, Deformity in a patient with a chronic anterior glenohumeral dislocation (GHD). Arrow pointing to anterior prominence and asterisk demonstrating flattening of posterior and lateral contours. **B**, Limited internal rotation in the same patient, a hallmark finding in chronic anterior GHD.

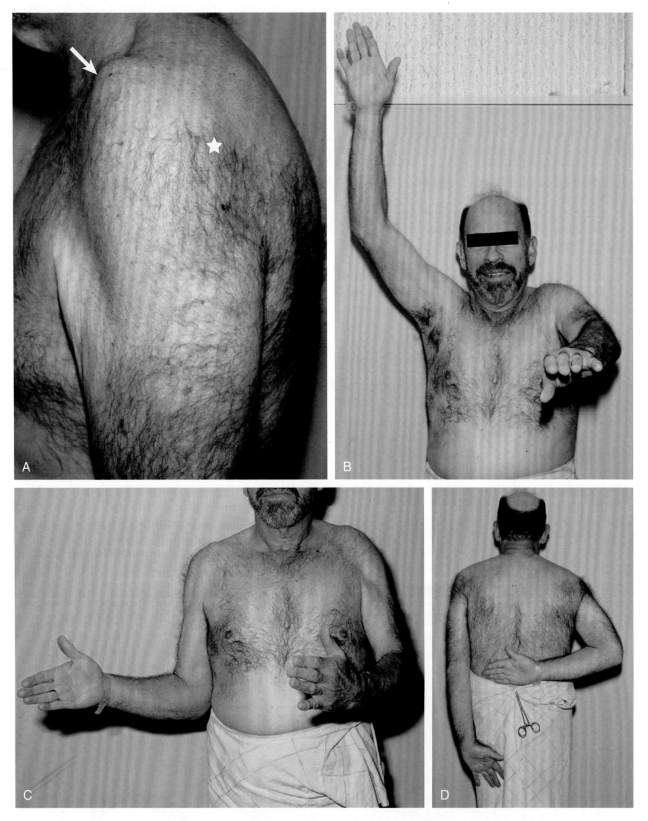

FIGURE 46.2 A, A patient with chronic posterior glenohumeral dislocation (GHD) with posterior fullness (asterisk) and flattening of the anterior and lateral contours (arrow). **B**, Limited forward elevation. **C**, Limited external rotation. **D**, Limited internal rotation.

Velpeau axillary radiograph technique

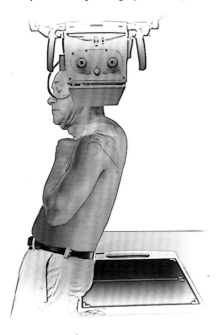

FIGURE 46.3 Illustration demonstrating the technique for obtaining a Velpeau axillary radiograph.

again, axillary lateral or Velpeau views are required to confirm the diagnosis. Concomitant posterior glenoid and anterior humeral head bone defects are also best represented on these radiographs.

Although diagnosis may be confirmed with standard radiographs, computed tomography (CT) is helpful to evaluate the extent of humeral and glenoid osteochondral injuries with greater accuracy. CT scan will allow for accurate and precise calculation of the percentage of articular surface defects. The arc of the humeral head defect divided by the total humeral articular surface arc is considered to be the percentage of humeral articular surface defect **(FIGURE 46.6)**. This value is used in most treatment algorithms for chronic GHD.

In cases of chronic anterior GHD, the surgeon may want to include a CT angiogram as part of preoperative planning to delineate the path and proximity of the vasculature to the dislocated humeral head. This can be included as part of a routine CT scan and help guide decision-making if a vascular complication were considered to be an intraoperative risk. While rare, vascular complications during open reduction have the potential to produce devastating complications. To this end, the authors routinely perform these procedures with a vascular surgeon and intraoperative angiography available in case of a potential bleeding complication.

CT scans are useful for defining the extent of bony injury, they do not provide sufficient detail regarding the soft tissues. Magnetic resonance imaging (MRI) is the study of choice to evaluate the extent of injury to soft tissues of which the status of the rotator cuff and condition of the articular cartilage is most important for decision-making. However, we do not recommend routine use of MRI in all patients with chronic GHD. Rather, we reserve its use for cases where the quality of the remaining soft tissues may significantly alter our treatment plan.

The AP radiographs of a chronic posterior GHD, similar to the physical examination, may only demonstrate subtle findings upon initial review. A crescent-type sign indicating the overlap of the humeral head and glenoid may be seen. A lightbulb sign, demonstrating loss of normal humeral head contour on AP radiographs such that it appears similar to a lightbulb, indicates that the humerus is in maximal internal rotation **(FIGURE 46.5)**. Although neither of these images are diagnostic, they should alert the provider to have a high level of suspicion for posterior GHD. Once

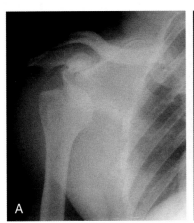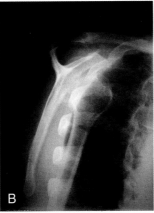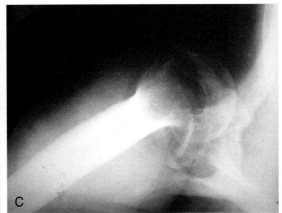

FIGURE 46.4 A, Scapular anteroposterior (AP) (Grashey). **B**, Scapular Y; and (**C**) axillary lateral radiographs show a chronic anterior glenohumeral dislocation.

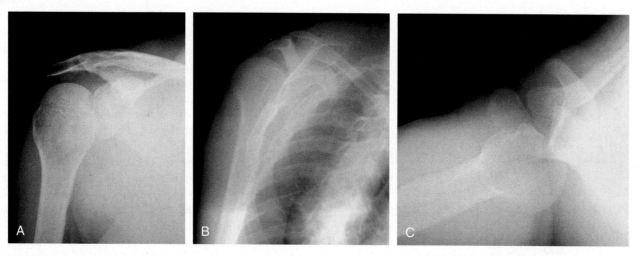

FIGURE 46.5 A, Lightbulb sign, the symmetric contour of the humeral head in a posteriorly dislocated shoulder on an anteroposterior (AP) shoulder radiograph. **B**, Scapular Y radiograph with chronic posterior glenohumeral dislocation (GHD) dislocation. **C**, Axillary lateral radiograph demonstrating posterior dislocation with anterior humeral impression fracture (reverse Hill-Sachs lesion). Note that the images correspond to the same patient in **FIGURE 46.2**.

TREATMENT OPTIONS AND DECISION-MAKING

Once the diagnosis of a chronic GHD has been made, a treatment strategy must be chosen. Several factors must be considered to formulate an effective treatment plan. Age, preinjury functional status, duration of dislocation, status of the rotator cuff, and extent of humeral and glenoid articular surface damage are some of the most important variables to consider.

Nonoperative treatment is generally divided into two categories: supervised neglect and closed reduction.

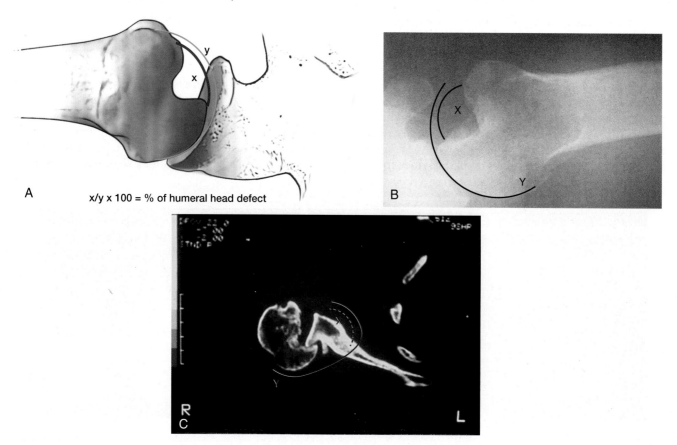

FIGURE 46.6 A, Illustration shows the method for calculation of the percentage of humeral head impression defect on an axillary image. Examples of this calculation are seen on the axial radiograph (**B**) and computed tomography (CT) scan (**C**) from patients with anterior humeral impression fractures.

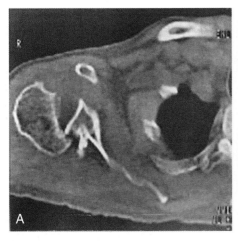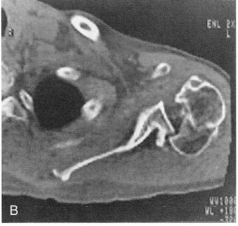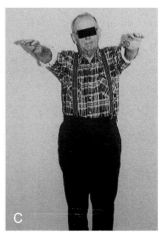

FIGURE 46.7 A and B, A 75-year-old male treated nonoperatively for bilateral posterior glenohumeral dislocations (GHDs) due to a seizure. Bilateral axial computed tomography (CT) scans reveal chronic posterior dislocations with >50% humeral articular surface defect. **C**, At 6 months follow-up, the patient had minimal pain and had recovered functional motion with forward elevation >90°.

Supervised neglect may be appropriate for patients that have significant medical comorbidities and pose an unacceptable surgical risk or patients with minimal pain and acceptable function **(FIGURE 46.7)**.

Closed reduction followed with a period of immobilization has been utilized in several case series with mixed results. Satisfactory outcomes were obtained in patients with small or nonexistent humeral head impression fractures and those that had been dislocated for less than 4 weeks.[15-19] Adequate anesthesia is required for any attempted closed reduction. In addition, it should be avoided if a locked dislocation is identified.

Operative treatment is usually required for GHDs older than 4 weeks or when a sizable humeral head articular surface defect is present resulting in a locked dislocation. Treatment may be further categorized by patient age and percentage of articular surface involvement.

Joint preservation operations consisting of open reduction and stabilization are typically reserved for younger patients, those with smaller bone defects, and well preserved articular cartilage. In the setting of a 20% to 40% humeral articular surface defect, a subscapularis or infraspinatus tendon transfer with or without the lesser or greater tuberosity is often required for stabilization of chronic posterior and anterior GHD, respectively. Younger patients with humeral defects ≥40% of the articular surface may be considered candidates for osteochondral allograft reconstruction. In contrast to humeral-sided bone loss, the glenoid is much less tolerant to bone loss. Defects larger than 20% to 25% are likely to fail an isolated soft-tissue reconstruction, and glenoid bone grafting is frequently necessary. Although meticulous preoperative workup may suggest that joint preservation is possible, it is wise to have arthroplasty components available in the event that intraoperative findings preclude such surgery.

Arthroplasty is generally indicated in older patients when humeral defects are greater than 40% to 50%, of the humeral articular surface arc, in the presence of large potentially irreparable rotator cuff tears, when significant glenoid erosion and bone loss is identified, and dislocations of greater than 6 months duration. Dislocations beyond 6 months typically have unsalvageable articular cartilage as well as marked osteopenia, which makes reconstruction both challenging and unpredictable. Prosthetic options generally fall into three categories: hemiarthroplasty, anatomic total shoulder arthroplasty (ATSA), and RTSA. Each of these options has advantages and disadvantages.

Hemiarthroplasty has the advantage of preserving glenoid articular cartilage and bone stock while allowing for conversion to total shoulder arthroplasty in the future. Disadvantages may be related to the unconstrained nature of the prosthesis and difficulty with obtaining a balanced, stable articulation. Significant soft-tissue releases, capsular plication, or tendon transfers may be required in order to obtain a stable construct. Indications include younger patients or patients with poor humeral bone quality not amenable to allograft reconstruction and those with intact glenoid articular cartilage **(FIGURE 46.8)**. It may also be used as a salvage operation for noncompliant patients or patients that lack enough glenoid bone stock for glenoid resurfacing.

The main advantage of ATSA over hemiarthroplasty is glenoid resurfacing. Disadvantages are similar to hemiarthroplasty with regards to the unconstrained nature of the prosthesis and difficulty with achieving stability. As previously mentioned, glenoid resurfacing requires sufficient glenoid bone stock; supplemental bone grafting in addition to custom or augmented glenoid prostheses may be required in the setting of significant glenoid erosion **(FIGURE 46.9)**. ATSA may be ideal for chronic GHD with an unsalvageable humeral head and irreversible articular cartilage changes on both the humeral head and the glenoid.

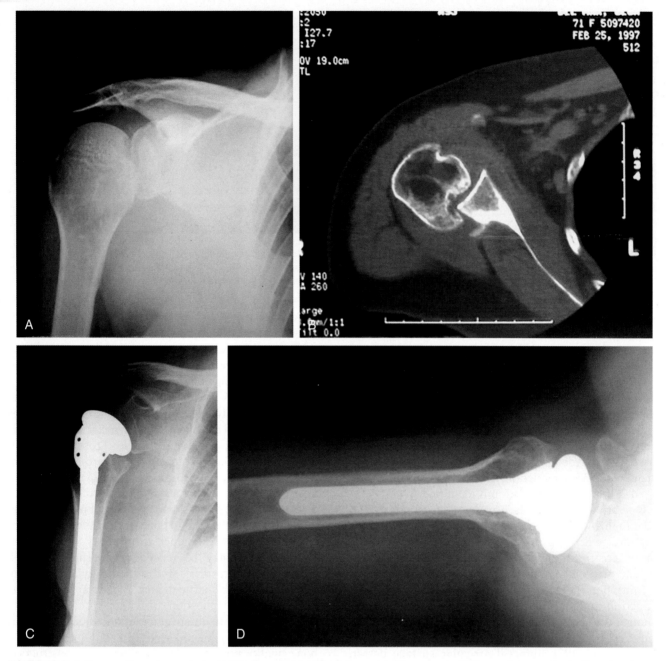

FIGURE 46.8 A, Preoperative anteroposterior (AP) radiograph and **(B)** axial computed tomography (CT) scan from a patient with a chronic posterior glenohumeral dislocation (GHD) with a large percentage of humeral head involvement. **C,** Postoperative AP and **(D)** axillary radiographs demonstrate the patient was successfully treated with hemiarthroplasty.

RTSA is an important option for the treatment of chronic GHD for several reasons. The main advantages of RTSA include the constrained nature of the prosthesis, as well as its reliable use in the setting of rotator cuff insufficiency. A significant disadvantage is the requirement of a functioning deltoid. In situations where there is significant uncertainty concerning the status of the axillary nerve preoperatively, the surgeon may consider obtaining a preoperative electromyogram (EMG) to assess the status of the axillary nerve. This may lend some reassurance regarding deltoid function. If an

axillary nerve deficit is present, it may be reasonable to delay RTSA until there is evidence of recovery at which time the procedure can be performed.

Our indications for use of RTSA in the setting of chronic GHD include elderly patients, patients in which there is significant humeral and glenoid bone loss, and those in which soft tissue balancing required for ATSA or hemiarthroplasty would prove to be challenging or lead to protracted recovery **(FIGURE 46.10).** As technique and implant designs continue to improve, the indications for RTSA can be expected to expand.

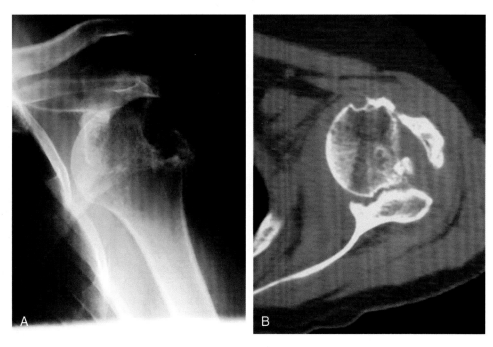

FIGURE 46.9 A, An anteroposterior (AP) radiograph and axial computed tomography (CT) (**B**) scan from a patient with a chronic anterior glenohumeral dislocation (GHD) with significant anterior glenoid bone loss.

OUTCOMES

Several studies have reported acceptable outcomes for the treatment of chronic GHD with arthroplasty. We identified 17 studies that reported outcomes of hemiarthroplasty, ATSA, or RTSA in the setting of a chronic GHD[1,3,5-12,17,20-24] **(TABLE 46.1)**.

Twelve studies reported on the results of 61 patients who underwent hemiarthroplasty for chronic anterior GHD[5,20,22,24] or chronic posterior GHD.[1,6,8-10,12,17,20,21] All studies showed improvements in both ROM and patient-reported outcomes scores. The majority of patients are reported to have at least a "satisfactory" outcome at final follow-up. Reoperations were infrequent and were primarily related to recurrent instability or glenoid articular cartilage wear.

Nine studies included 55 patients who underwent ATSA for treatment of chronic anterior[1,20,22,24] or chronic posterior GHD.[3,6,8,12,17,20] All studies showed improved ROM and patient-reported outcome scores. The majority of patients were rated to have a "satisfactory" outcome or better at final follow-up. Revision operations were infrequent and most commonly due to glenoid component loosening.

Four studies included 14 patients that underwent RTSA for chronic anterior[7,11,23] or chronic posterior[9] GHD. All studies demonstrated improved outcome scores at final follow-up. The relative paucity of RTSA literature compared to that of hemiarthroplasty and ATSA is likely because widespread use of RTSA had not occurred until this past decade. We anticipate that over the next decade the experience with RTSA for the treatment of chronic GHD will increase greatly.

TECHNICAL CONSIDERATIONS

Surgical Approach: Chronic Anterior GHD

A standard deltopectoral approach is utilized for chronic anterior GHDs. The humeral head is found to lie beneath the conjoint tendon. Depending on the duration of dislocation, the humeral head may become scarred in this anteroinferior position with significant adhesions and reactive tissue surrounding it. This may create a challenging exposure considering the close proximity to the brachial plexus and axillary vessels. Great care must be taken to avoid injury to these structures by avoiding excessive traction along with careful dissection. As noted, the assistance of a vascular surgeon should be considered for these difficult dissections. In particularly longstanding dislocations, especially when anterior glenoid erosion may result in greater medial displacement, a predrilled coracoid osteotomy or a conjoint tendon release may be beneficial to allow for adequate exposure and release of the humeral head.

The superior border of the pectoralis major insertion and the most anterior portion of the deltoid insertion into the humerus may also be released to enhance exposure and to provide additional soft tissue release. The bicipital groove and lesser tuberosity are important landmarks that can be identified by palpation. A subscapularis tenotomy or peel from the lesser tuberosity should be performed if the subscapularis is intact along with the underlying capsular insertion. The capsulotomy is extended proximally through the rotator interval to the anterior superior glenoid. The inferior capsule is released off the humeral neck in subperiosteal fashion

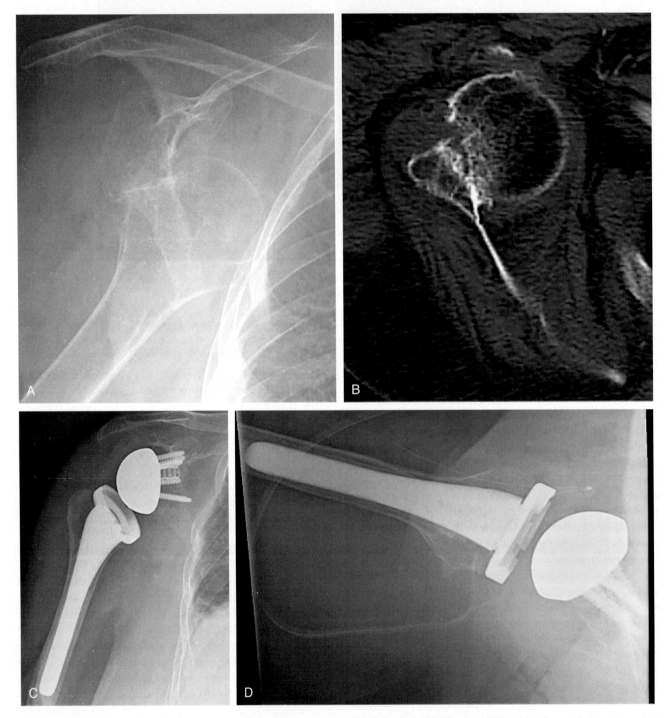

FIGURE 46.10 A, Preoperative anteroposterior (AP) and (**B**) axial computed tomography (CT) scan reveal a chronic anterior glenohumeral dislocation (GHD) with significant anterior glenoid erosion. **C,** Postoperative AP and (**D**) axillary radiographs demonstrate the patient was successfully treated with reverse total shoulder arthroplasty (RTSA).

to avoid injury to the axillary nerve. This will help in mobilizing the proximal humerus. The glenoid should be palpable through the rotator interval although it is frequently covered by fibrous tissue. This fibrous tissue should be excised, and the glenoid articular cartilage can then be inspected for signs of irreversible cartilage changes. If the long head biceps tendon remains intact, a tenodesis should be performed at the pectoralis insertion and the proximal portion of the tendon excised. A gentle reduction maneuver may now be performed while ensuring the humeral impression fracture is "unlocked" off of the anterior glenoid. The reduction can be facilitated by using a Cobb elevator interposed between the humeral head and the glenoid in a gentle "shoehorn" type maneuver (**FIGURE 46.11**). Release of the contracted posterior capsule off the glenoid margin is likely to be required to maintain reduction. Humeral head osteotomy may be performed prior to reduction to provide better exposure, facilitate mobilization of the proximal humerus, and expose the posterior capsule.

Several authors advocate increasing humeral component retroversion to avoid recurrent instability with a hemiarthroplasty or ATSA.[20,22] This is similar to our approach, although we believe treatment should be individualized to each patient's bony anatomy and quality of soft tissues.

When the glenoid shows signs of irreversible articular cartilage damage, then glenoid resurfacing is preferred. If glenoid bone loss will compromise base plate fixation, then supplemental bone grafting is required for reliable fixation and to support the glenoid component. Our preference is to use a portion of the resected humeral head fixed with two or three partially threaded cancellous screws. Rigid fixation with compression as well as adequate preparation of the donor and recipient surfaces are both critical to prevent nonunion and to obtain a stable construct for glenoid component fixation. Importantly, the compression screws must be sufficiently recessed to allow for adequate reaming of the glenoid. If humeral head bone quality is poor, then consider using allograft or iliac crest autograft. The surgeon should consider all of these alternatives during preoperative planning so all necessary options are available.

Small rotator cuff tears should be repaired at the time of surgery using suture anchors or transosseus technique. If a large or irreparable rotator cuff tear is present, then a pectoralis major or latissimus dorsi transfer should be considered in younger patients or RTSA in older patients. Meticulous repair of the anterior capsule and subscapularis may add considerable stability to a hemiarthroplasty or ATSA (**FIGURE 46.12**). Our threshold to perform an RTSA in low demand or elderly individuals is low given the more predictable and reproducible results that we can achieve (**FIGURE 46.13**).

Our postoperative rehabilitation protocol is individualized for each patient depending on the exact procedure performed, age, stability, and ROM at the end of the procedure. We prefer a shoulder immobilizer with an abduction pillow that is placed in the operative suite. Anatomic or hemiarthroplasty typically will start passive forward elevation the day after surgery. RTSA usually will not start shoulder ROM until 4 to 6 weeks after surgery. Our protocol is to begin active ROM at approximately 6 weeks postoperatively.

Surgical Approach: Chronic Posterior GHD

Similar to chronic anterior GHD, a deltopectoral approach is utilized for chronic posterior GHD. The coracoid, lesser tuberosity, and bicipital groove are identified, and a subscapularis tenotomy and capsulotomy are performed. Capsulotomy is extended through the rotator interval to the anterior superior glenoid. The capsule is released off the humeral calcar in subperiosteal fashion to avoid injury to the axillary nerve. The glenoid articular surface and anterior humeral impression defect should be palpable at this point. Excision of any fibrous tissue covering the glenoid is necessary both to inspect the articular cartilage and facilitate reduction of the humeral head. A gentle reduction maneuver may be performed after initially "unlocking" the humeral impression defect off of the posterior glenoid by internal rotation and a laterally directed force. An elevator or retractor may be used to facilitate reduction with a "shoehorn" type maneuver. Once the retractor or elevator is inserted between the humeral head and glenoid, the surgeon may externally rotate the humeral head along the surface of the instrument to guide the head back into the glenoid vault (**FIGURE 46.14; VIDEO 46.1**). Unlocking of the head is followed by anterior translation. It is important to minimize levering of the humeral head as it is often osteopenic, and these maneuvers have the potential to cause damage if not performed carefully and gently.

Some authors advocate for decreased retroversion of the humeral component for hemiarthroplasty and ATSA, whereas others recommend anatomic version.[8,12,17,20] Humeral retroversion in RSTA is often restored to an anatomic position.[7] We recommend an individualized approach be made based on the patient's anatomy and intraoperative trialing.

If irreversible glenoid articular cartilage damage is present, then glenoid resurfacing is preferred. When posterior glenoid wear would compromise glenoid component fixation, bone grafting may be necessary. We again prefer humeral head autograft stabilized with two or three partially threaded cancellous screws. If an RTSA is being performed, fixation of the graft may be obtained with the screws used to fix the baseplate.

TABLE 46.1 Study Characteristics and Results

	Rowe et al, 1982[1]	Hawkins et al, 1987[17]	Pritchett et al, 1987[20]	Flatow et al, 1993[22]
Level of evidence	IV	IV	IV	IV
DB score[a]	6	7	6	6
Study sample	Chronic posterior GHD (N = 2) Chronic anterior GHD (N = 1)	Chronic posterior GHD (N = 16 including 19 shoulders)	Chronic posterior GHD (N = 3) Chronic anterior GHD (N = 4)	Chronic anterior GHD (N = 9)
Age, years	Mean = 45.7 (range: 38-51)	Mean = 49.2 (range: 17-80)	Mean = 55 (range: 36-67)	Mean = 64 (range: 48-73)
Sex (male:female ratio)	1:2	32:8	5:2	6:11
Mechanism of injury	Fall (N = 1) Manipulation of shoulder (N = 1) Unknown (N = 1)	MVA, seizure, electroshock treatment, alcohol-related injury	Not reported	Fall, alcohol-related
Duration of dislocation before surgery	Mean = 12.7 y (range: 2-33)	Mean = 12 mo	Mean = 69 mo (range: 2-432 mo)	Mean = 46.8 mo (24-72)
Procedure	HA (N = 2) ATSA (N = 1)	HA (N = 9) ATSA (N = 10)	HA (N = 4) ATSA (N = 3)	HA (N = 1) ATSA (N = 8)
Associated procedure(s)	None	Posterior capsular plication (N = 6)	None	ATSA: Glenoid bone grafting (N = 3) Rotator cuff repair (N = 2)
Average follow-up	4.9 y (range: 2-10)	5.5 y	2.3 y	3.9 y (range: 2-6)
Percent humeral head defect	N/A	≥45%	≥30%	0% (N = 1) <40% (N = 4) ≥40% (N = 4)
Humeral component retroversion	N/A	HA: ≥ 6 mo dislocated—0° <6 mo dislocated—20° TSA: 0° (N = 6) 20° (N = 2) 30° (N = 2)	±30-50° altered from anatomic away from direction of dislocation	Increased as needed for stability
Range of motion	Not reported	**Preoperative**: Elevation: 105° (70°-160°) External rotation: −40° (−10 to −60) Internal rotation: T12 (L4-T8) **Postoperative**: *HA (N = 9)*: Elevation: 140° (range: 125-165) External rotation: 30° (range: 24-41) Internal rotation: L2 *TSA (N = 6)*: Elevation: 145° (range: 112-168) External rotation: 37° (range: 24-42) Internal rotation: L1-T12 *HA > ATSA (N = 3)*: Elevation: 106° (98-112) External rotation: 30° (22-34) Internal rotation: L2 (L1-L3)	Not reported	**Preoperative**: Elevation: 101° (range: 80-130) External rotation: 11° (0-25) Internal rotation: T10 **Postoperative**: Elevation: 147° (range: 110-180) External rotation: 69° (range 45-90)

Cheng et al, 1997[3]	Sperling et al, 2004[12]	Matsoukis et al, 2006[24]	Ivkovic et al, 2007[10]	Gavriilidis et al, 2010[8]
IV	IV	IV	IV	IV
8	8	7	N/A[b]	8
Chronic posterior GHD (N = 7)	Chronic posterior GHD (N = 12)	Chronic anterior GHD (N = 11)	Chronic bilateral posterior GHD (N = 1, including 2 shoulders)	Chronic posterior GHD (N = 11, including 12 shoulders)
Mean = 58 (range: 40-74)	Mean = 56 (range: 36-78)	Mean = 67.3 (range: 45-84)	Mean = 52 y	Mean = 49.8 ± 8.6
3:4	6:6	3:8	1:0	10:1
Idiopathic seizure (N = 5) Alcohol-related seizure (N = 2)	MVA (N = 4) Fall (N = 4) Seizure (N = 2) Unknown trauma (N = 2)	Traumatic (N = 11)	Grand mal seizure ×2	Traffic accident (N = 4) Epileptic seizure (N = 3) Electric shock (N = 1, bilateral) Skiing injury (N = 1) Unknown accidental fall (N = 2)
Mean = 23 mo (range: 1-86)	Mean = 26 mo (range: 4-88)	>3 wk	3 mo	14.5 mo ±23.3
ATSA (N = 7)	Uncemented HA (N = 5) Cemented HA (N = 1) Uncemented TSA (N = 4) Cemented TSA (N = 2)	Cemented HA (N = 7) Cemented TSA (N = 4)	HA (N = 1)	HA (N = 10) ATSA (N = 2)
None	None	Glenoid bone grafting (N = 4) Greater tuberosity fixation (N = 2)	Contralateral osteochondral autograft reconstruction (N = 1)	Latissimus dorsi transfer + HA (N = 2) Open rotator cuff repair + HA (N = 1) Pectoralis major transfer + HA (N = 1)
27 mo	9 y (range: 0.7-22 y)	47.7 mo (24-86)	3 y	37.4 ± 6.8 mo
Not reported	Not reported	Not reported	>50%	≥45%
Neutral or slight retroversion	22° (range: 5-30)	Anatomic	20°	Anatomic (20°-40°)
Preoperative: Elevation: 76.7° External rotation: −4° Internal rotation: S2 **Postoperative:** Elevation: 109° External rotation: 11.4° Internal rotation: T10	**Preoperative:** Abduction: 82° External rotation: −13° Internal rotation: sacrum **Postoperative:** Abduction: 96° External rotation: 28° Internal rotation: L4	**Preoperative:** Elevation: 48.6° External rotation: 13.2° **Postoperative:** Elevation: 90.0° External rotation: 25.5°	**Preoperative:** Flexion: 90° Abduction: 30° Internal rotation: sacrum External rotation: −20° **Postoperative:** Flexion: 140 Abduction: 90 Internal rotation: L5 External rotation: 45	**Preoperative:** Flexion: 84.2 ± 22.3° Abduction: 55.4 ± 21° External rotation: −6.7 ± 20.2° **Postoperative:** Flexion: 125 ± 47° Abduction: 95.8 ± 53.3° External rotation: 36.7 ± 19.7°

TABLE 46.1 Study Characteristics and Results (cont'd)

	Rowe et al, 1982[1]	Hawkins et al, 1987[17]		Pritchett et al, 1987[20]	Flatow et al, 1993[22]
Outcome scores	**Preoperative**: Not reported **Postoperative**: Average rating units (0-100): HA (mean = 67.5, range: 60-75) TSA (mean = 90)	Not reported		**Preoperative**: Rowe and Zarins score: 50/100 **Postoperative**: Rowe and Zarins score: 71/100 Patient satisfaction: Excellent: ≥90 ($N = 0$) Good: 89-70 ($N = 5$) Fair 69-50 ($N = 2$) Poor <50 ($N = 0$)	**Preoperative**: Not reported **Postoperative**: **ATSA**: Patient satisfaction: Excellent ($N = 4$) Satisfactory ($N = 4$) **HA**: Patient satisfaction: Missing, patient lost to follow-up ($N = 1$)
Reoperations	None	Conversion from HA to ATSA for glenoid wear ($N = 3$)		None	None
Postoperative complications	None	Dislocation after ATSA, not treated ($N = 1$)		Axillary nerve palsy, recovered ($N = 1$)	Anterior subluxation ($N = 1$) No superior migration, component breakage or loosening

	Macaulay et al, 2011[25]	Schliemann et al, 2011[9]	Torrens et al, 2012[21]	Venkatachalam et al, 2014[5]
Level of evidence	IV	IV	IV	IV
DB score[a]	N/A[b]	8	N/A[b]	N/A[b]
Study sample	Chronic anterior GHD ($N = 2$)	Chronic posterior GHD ($N = 2$)	Chronic bilateral posterior GHD ($N = 1$)	Chronic anterior GHD ($N = 1$)
Age, years	Mean = 77.5 (range: 73-82)	Mean = 53 (range: 30-86)	Mean = 45	Mean = 58
Sex (male:female ratio)	0:2	Not reported	1:0	1:0
Mechanism of injury	Fall ($N = 2$)	Not reported	Epileptic seizure ($N = 2$)	Fall ($N = 1$)
Duration of dislocation before surgery	Mean = 9 mo	Mean = 66 d (range: 0-365)	Mean = 3 mo	Mean = 6 mo

Cheng et al, 1997[3]	Sperling et al, 2004[12]	Matsoukis et al, 2006[24]	Ivkovic et al, 2007[10]	Gavriilidis et al, 2010[8]
Preoperative: VAS (pain): 7.7 VAS (function): 3.0 ASES: 20.1 **Postoperative**: VAS (pain): 3.5 VAS (function): 7.6 ASES: 55.6	**Preoperative**: **HA**: Pain score: 4.5/5 **ATSA**: Pain score: 4.6/5 **Postoperative**: **HA**: Pain score: 2.3/5 Satisfaction: Satisfactory (N = 4) Unsatisfactory (N = 2) **ATSA**: Pain score: 3/5 Satisfaction: Excellent (N = 1) Satisfactory (N = 2) Unsatisfactory (N = 3)	**Preoperative**: Constant score (age/gender adjusted): 28.2 **Postoperative**: Constant score (age/gender adjusted): 59.8 Satisfaction: Excellent (N = 2) Good (N = 6) Fair (N = 3)	**Preoperative**: Not reported **Postoperative**: Constant score: 55	**Preoperative:** Not reported **Postoperative**: Constant score overall: Mean = (59.5 ± 21.6) Overall adjusted for age and gender: Mean = (67.1 ± 24.1%) Constant pain subscore: 12.8 ± 3.9 Constant ADL subscore: 14.3 ± 6.1 Constant ROM subscore: 26 ± 9 Constant strength subscore: 9.3 ± 3.6 for strength More recent dislocations had better Constant scores and less pain
None	Revision for recurrent instability (N = 2 at 1.5 and 11 mo post-HA) Revision for component loosening (N = 1 at 14 y post-ATSA)	Glenoid component removal (N = 1) Bone graft screw removal (N = 1)	None	Removal of the metal-backed uncemented glenoid component for poly dissociation and implantation of a cemented all-polyethylene glenoid component at 36 wk postoperatively (N = 1)
Posterior subluxation treated with orthosis (N = 1)	Median neuropathy, resolved (N = 1)	Anterior subluxation (N = 1) Anterior dislocation (N = 3) Glenoid loosening (N = 3)	None	None

Werner et al, 2014[26]	Wooten et al, 2014[6]	Ji et al, 2016[11]	Van Tongel et al, 2016[7]	Olszewski et al, 2017[27]
IV	IV	IV	IV	IV
9	8	N/A[b]	7	N/A[b]
Chronic anterior GHD (N = 21)	Chronic posterior GHD (N = 32)	Chronic anterior GHD (N = 1)	Chronic anterior GHD (N = 6)	Chronic anterior GHD (N = 1)
Mean = 71 (range 50-85)	Mean = 54 (range: 25-79 y)	68	Mean = 73 (range: 65-86)	49
3:18	19:13	0:1	4:2	1:0
Fall (N = 21)	MVA (N = 13) Fall (N = 8) Seizure (N = 6) Unknown trauma (N = 5)	Fall (N = 1)	Not reported	Traumatic (N = 1)
Mean = 6 mo (range: 3-11)	Mean = 24 mo (range: 3-88)	Mean = 4 mo	Mean = 4.5 mo (range: 1-12)	>1 y

TABLE 46.1 Study Characteristics and Results (cont'd)

	Macaulay et al, 2011[25]	Schliemann et al, 2011[9]	Torrens et al, 2012[21]	Venkatachalam et al, 2014[5]
Procedure	RTSA (*N* = 2)	HA (*N* = 1) RTSA due to rotator cuff tear (*N* = 1)	HA (*N* = 1)	Cemented HA (*N* = 1)
Associated procedure(s)	Glenoid bone grafting (*N* = 2)	None	Contralateral osteochondal autograft reconstruction (*N* = 1)	Coracoid osteotomy/bone grafting (*N* = 1)
Average follow-up	1 y	55 mo (11-132)	2 y	24 mo
Percent humeral head defect	50%	>45%	50%	Not reported
Humeral component retroversion	20°	N/A	Anatomic	Not reported
Range of motion	**Preoperative**: Elevation: 30° External rotation: 0° Internal rotation: sacrum **Postoperative**: Elevation: 140°	Not reported	**Preoperative**: Flexion: 60° **Postoperative**: Flexion: 160° External rotation: 45° Internal rotation: L3	**Preoperative**: Flexion: 70° Abduction: 30° External rotation: 15° (fixed) **Postoperative**: Flexion: 160° Abduction: 155° External rotation: 10° Internal rotation: L3
Outcome scores	Not reported	**Preoperative**: Not reported **Postoperative**: Constant score (age/gender adjusted): 51 Rowe and Zarins score: 56/100	Not reported	**Preoperative**: Oxford shoulder score: 32 Oxford instability index: 20 WOSI: 18 **Postoperative**: Oxford shoulder score: 48 Oxford stability score: 46 WOSI: 25

Werner et al, 2014[26]	Wooten et al, 2014[6]	Ji et al, 2016[11]	Van Tongel et al, 2016[7]	Olszewski et al, 2017[27]
RTSA (N = 21)	HA (N = 18) ATSA (N = 14) Neer-II metal-backed glenoid component cemented (N = 3) Cofield all-polyethylene component cemented (N = 9) Cofield metal-backed ingrowth component (N = 2)	RTSA (N = 1)	RTSA (N = 6)	RTSA (N = 1)
Glenoid bone grafting (N = 21)	Repair of small-to-medium rotator cuff tear of the supraspinatus tendon (N = 3) Repair of large-to-massive tear (N = 1) Unrepairable tear (N = 1) Posterior capsule plication (N = 7)	Glenoid autograft (N = 1) Greater tuberosity osteotomy and fixation (N = 1)	Allograft bone grafting (N = 1)	None
4.9 y (2-10)	8.2 y (range: 0.7-31)	3 years	39 mo (range: 12-90)	24 mo
Not reported	≥45%	>30%	23.6%	30%
Not reported	5°-20° (N = 13) 21°-34° (N = 13)	Anatomic (20°)	10° (per manufacture guidelines)	20°
Preoperative: Elevation: 35° Abduction: 25° External rotation: 2.4° **Postoperative**: Elevation: 128° Abduction: 113° External rotation: 8.4°	**Preoperative**: External rotation: −15° (range −70-20) Abduction: 82° Internal rotation: sacrum **Postoperative**: External rotation: 50° (range: −60-90) Abduction: 90° Internal rotation: L4	**Preoperative**: Not reported **Postoperative**: Forward elevation: 30° Abduction: 40° External rotation: 10°	Not reported	**Preoperative**: Forward flexion: 50° Abduction: 35° External rotation:0° Internal rotation: to the side **Postoperative**: Forward flexion: 160° Abduction: 90° External rotation:30°
Preoperative: Constant score: 5.7 (range: 0-22) **Postoperative**: Constant score: 57.2 (range: 26-79) Outcome rated as: Excellent (N = 10)- Good (N = 8) Fair (N = 3)	**Preoperative**: Pain score: median = 4 (range: 3-5) **Postoperative**: Pain score: median = 3 (range: 1-5) 5°-20° humeral retroversion had postoperative pain score of 3, external rotation 40°, elevation 90° 21°-34° humeral retroversion had postoperative pain score of 2, external rotation 50°, elevation 90° Concomitant rotator cuff repair had postoperative pain score of 3, external rotation 15°, elevation 90° Concomitant posterior capsule plication had postoperative pain score of 3, external rotation 30°, elevation 110° *HA*: Patient satisfaction: Excellent (N = 4) Satisfactory (N = 8) Unsatisfactory (N = 6) *TSA*: Patient satisfaction: Satisfactory (N = 7) Unsatisfactory (N = 7)	**Preoperative**: ASES: 0 UCLA: 5 SST: 0 **Postoperative**: ASES: 60 UCLA: 26 SST: 7	**Preoperative**: Constant score: 33 (range: 17-47) **Postoperative**: Constant score: 76 (range: 55-90)	**Preoperative**: Subjective function: 90% **Postoperative**: Not reported

TABLE 46.1 Study Characteristics and Results (cont'd)				
	Macaulay et al, 2011[25]	**Schliemann et al, 2011**[9]	**Torrens et al, 2012**[21]	**Venkatachalam et al, 2014**[5]
Reoperations	None	None	None	None
Postoperative complications	None	None	None	None

	Raiss et al, 2017[28]
Level of evidence	IV
DB score[a]	9
Study sample	Chronic anterior GHD ($N = 18$) Chronic posterior GHD ($N = 4$)
Age, years	Mean = 71 (range: 51-91)
Sex (male:female ratio)	7:15
Mechanism of injury	Traumatic ($N = 15$) Not reported ($N = 7$)
Duration of dislocation before surgery	Mean = 23 mo (range: 1-148)
Procedure	RTSA ($N = 22$)
Associated procedure(s)	Glenoid bone grafting ($N = 4$ anterior; $N = 1$ posterior)
Average follow-up	Mean = 3.5 y (range: 2-9)
Percent humeral head defect	Not reported
Humeral component retroversion	0°-20°

Werner et al, 2014[26]	Wooten et al, 2014[6]	Ji et al, 2016[11]	Van Tongel et al, 2016[7]	Olszewski et al, 2017[27]
Conversion of RTSA to HA due to glenoid loosening (N = 1) Revision glenoid component for traumatic loosening (N = 1)	**HA**: Revision to TSA with posterior capsule plication, at 2 and 11 mo. postoperatively due to recurrent posterior subluxation or dislocation (N = 2) Resection because of instability in the setting of Parkinson disease and another for infection (N = 2) Revision to TSA due to pain from glenoid wear at 3/10 y (N = 2) **TSA**: Revision due to humeral fracture that went to nonunion (N = 1) Revision due to infection at 7 mo (N = 1) Revision to HA due to glenoid loosening after 14 y (N = 1)	None	None	None
Notching (N = 6) Heterotopic ossification (N = 5)	Median neuropathy, resolved (N = 1)	None	None	None

Statz et al, 2017[29]		Frias et al, 2018[23]	
IV		IV	
9		8	
Chronic anterior GHD (N = 19)		Chronic anterior GHD (N = 6)	
Mean = 62 (range: 34-80)		Mean = 69.5 (range: 64-80)	
3:16		1:5	
Not reported		Not reported	
Median = 32 wk		Mean = 1.6 mo (range: 1.2-2.3)	
HA (N = 3) ATSA (N = 7) RTSA (N = 9)		RTSA (N = 6)	
Glenoid bone grafting (N = 1 HA, N = 2 ATSA, N = 4 RTSA)		Glenoid bone grafting (N = 1)	
7.1 y (range: 2-30)		8 mo (range: 6-16)	
Not reported		Not reported	
Mean = 44° (range: 20°-75°)		20°	

TABLE 46.1 Study Characteristics and Results (cont'd)	
	Raiss et al, 2017[28]
Range of motion	**Preoperative**: Forward flexion: 37.7° Abduction: 35° External rotation: -0.5° **Postoperative**: Forward flexion: 103° Abduction: 35° External rotation:14.7° Internal rotation: Increased significantly ($P < 0.03$)
Outcome Scores	**Preoperative**: Constant score: 13.6 **Postoperative**: Constant score: 47.4 Patient satisfaction: Very good ($N = 8$) Good ($N = 5$) Satisfactory ($N = 5$) Unsatisfactory ($N = 4$)
Reoperations	Conversion to HA for glenoid failure in all four anterior bone grafted cases ($N = 4$ at 1 wk, 1 mo, 9 mo, 2 y) Revision humeral component for humeral fracture ($N = 1$) Resection arthroplasty for infection ($N = 1$)
Postoperative complications	Recurrent instability ($N = 1$)

ADL, activities of daily living, ASES, American Shoulder and Elbow Surgeons score, ATSA, anatomic total shoulder arthroplasty, DB, Downs and Black score, GHD, glenohumeral dislocation, HA, hemiarthroplasty, MVA, motor vehicle accident, N/A, not applicable, RTSA, reverse total shoulder arthroplasty, ROM, range of motion, SST, Simple Shoulder Test, TSH, total shoulder arthroplasty, UCLA, University of California at Los Angeles Shoulder score, VAS, visual analog scale, WOSI, Western Ontario Shoulder Instability Index.
[a]Scores from the Downs and Black Study Quality Assessment Tool. A maximum score of 9 indicates good quality and low risk of bias for case series.
[b]Scoring with the Downs and Black Study Quality Assessment Tool was not applicable for case series.

Statz et al, 2017[29]	Frias et al, 2018[23]
Preoperative: *HA/ATSA:* Elevation: 57° External rotation: 10° Internal rotation: Greater trochanter *RTSA:* Elevation:43° External rotation: −11° Internal rotation: Iliac crest **Postoperative**: *Hemi/ATSA:* Elevation: 81° External rotation: 21° Internal rotation: Sacroiliac joint *RTSA:* Elevation: 106° External rotation:46° Internal rotation: sacrum	**Preoperative**: Not reported **Postoperative**: Flexion: 105° (range: 55-170) External rotation: 18° (range: −0.5-26) Internal rotation: L3 (buttock-T12)
Preoperative: *Hemi/ATSA:* Pain score: 4.6/5 *RTSA:* Pain score: 4.8/5 **Postoperative**: *Hemi/ATSA:* Pain score: 2.6/5 ASES: 43 SST: 3.5/12 Subjective: 25/100 *RTSA:* Pain score: 1.8/5 ASES: 76 SST: 7.4/12 Subjective: 55/100	**Preoperative**: Not reported **Postoperative**: Constant score: 65 (range: 35-80)
Open reduction (*N* = 2 ATSA) Conversion to ATSA for glenoid wear (*N* = 1 HA)	None
Intraoperative humeral shaft fracture (*N* = 2 RTSA) Postoperative humeral shaft fracture (*N* = 1 RTSA) Moderate/severe subluxation or dislocation (*N* = 2 HA and *N* = 4 ATSA) Recurrent instability after revision open reduction (*N* = 1 ATSA)	None

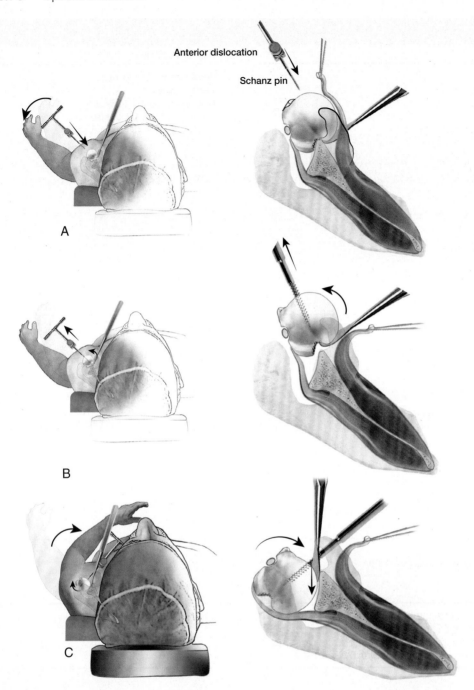

FIGURE 46.11 A, In difficult cases of chronic anterior dislocation the surgeon can insert a threaded Schanz pin on a T handle into the humeral head to aid in reduction. An elevator can be inserted through the rotator interval from a superior angle. However, it is usually necessary to release the subscapularis and capsule from the lesser tuberosity and humeral neck and insert the elevator from and anterior approach. **B**, The Schanz pin can aid in translating the humeral head for insertion of the elevator. Then elevator can then be used to disengage the humeral head from its position anterior to the glenoid. **C**, The humeral head can then be reduced into the glenoid.

Significant attenuation of the posterior capsule may be present in these patients. Posterior capsular plication may add considerable stability to an ATSA or hemi-arthroplasty if the posterior capsule is patulous. This can be performed using a side-to-side suture imbrication technique or a circular suture technique. It is also important to properly tension the subscapularis repair to avoid residual instability. RTSA is our preferred technique in most low-functioning or elderly patients. The predictable outcomes and constrained nature of the prosthesis may even suggest a lower threshold for its use in this population.

Patients are fitted with a shoulder orthosis in the operative suite immobilizing the arm in slight abduction and neutral external rotation. If capsular plications techniques are needed, we prefer immobilization in a

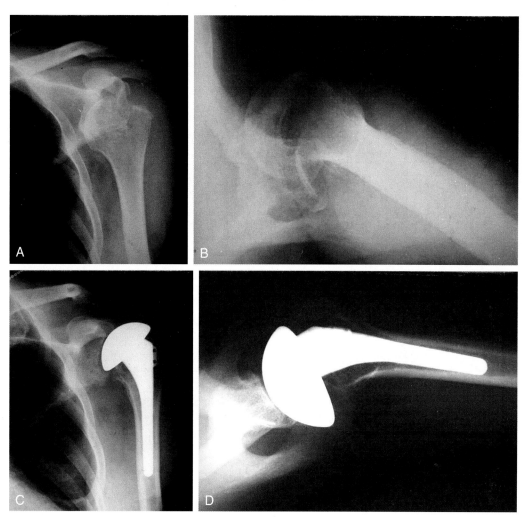

FIGURE 46.12 A, Preoperative anteroposterior (AP) and (**B**) axillary radiographs from a 77-year-old patient found to have a chronic anterior glenohumeral dislocation (GHD). **C and D,** 6-month follow-up radiographs reveal a concentrically reduced hemiarthroplasty. Fastidious repair of the anterior capsule and subscapularis is critical to obtain a stable prosthesis.

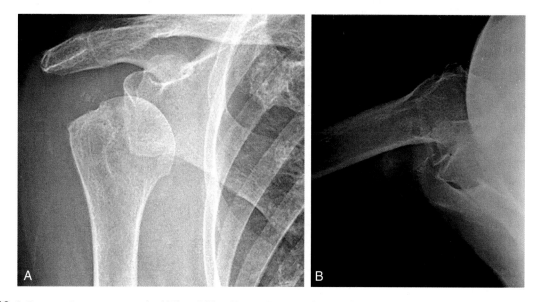

FIGURE 46.13 A, Preoperative anteroposterior (AP) and (**B**) axillary radiographs from a 73-year-old patient with a chronic anterior glenohumeral dislocation (GHD). **C,** Postoperative AP and (**D**) axillary radiographs at 6-month follow-up demonstrate the patient was successfully treated with reverse total shoulder arthroplasty (RTSA).

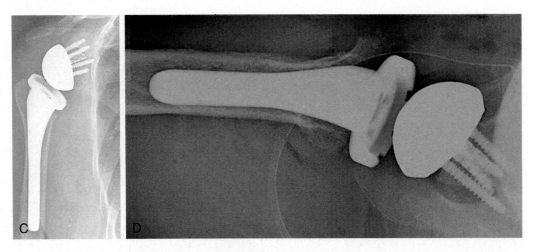

FIGURE 46.13 Cont'd

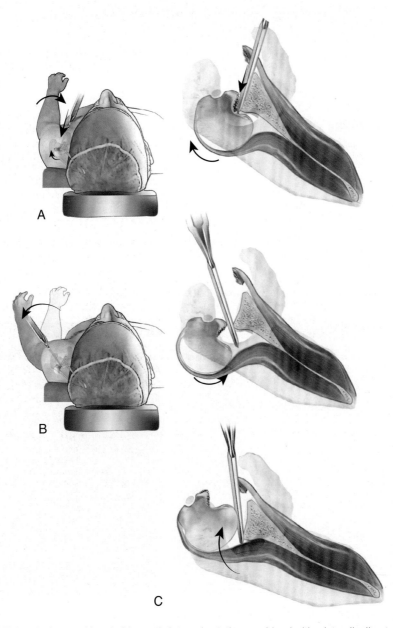

FIGURE 46.14 A, After mobilizing the humeral head with gentle internal rotation combined with a laterally directed force, the humerus is gently externally rotated so the elevator can be placed between the humeral head and the posterior glenoid rim. **B**, Once the elevator is between the humeral head and posterior glenoid rim, it can be used as a "shoehorn" combined with external rotation of the humerus to further "unlock" and mobilize the humeral head. **C**, Continued external rotation allows the humeral head to translate back into a reduced position on the glenoid.

"gunslinger"-type orthosis with 10° to 20° of external rotation. Our protocol is to begin shoulder motion at about 4 to 6 weeks postoperatively.

CONCLUSION

Chronic GHDs are complex injuries that present orthopedic surgeons with a unique set of challenges. Although the exact time period that defines a GHD as chronic is debated in the literature, most authors agree with the definition in which the diagnosis has been delayed by ≥3 weeks. Thorough evaluation including history, physical examination, and appropriate imaging studies are critical to fully understand the complex nature of these injuries and to develop a treatment plan. This chapter focused on patients with chronic GHD that may benefit from glenohumeral arthroplasty. The presence of humeral head defects ≥40% and dislocations >6 months duration are the most widely accepted indications. The use of hemiarthroplasty, ATSA, or RTSA depends on a combination of factors including age, quality of glenoid articular cartilage, and presence of associated rotator cuff injuries. Shoulder arthroplasty for the treatment of chronic GHD can provide successful outcomes when performed for the correct indications and with the necessary surgical skill.

REFERENCES

1. Rowe CR, Zarins B. Chronic unreduced dislocations of the shoulder. *J Bone Joint Surg Am.* 1982;64(4):494-505.
2. Sahajpal DT, Zuckerman JD. Chronic glenohumeral dislocation. *J Am Acad Orthop Surg.* 2008;16(7):385-398.
3. Cheng SL, Mackay MB, Richards RR. Treatment of locked posterior fracture-dislocations of the shoulder by total shoulder arthroplasty. *J Shoulder Elbow Surg.* 1997;6(1):11-17.
4. Aydin N, Kayaalp EM, Asansu M, Karaismailoglu B. Treatment options for locked posterior shoulder dislocations and clinical outcomes. *EFORT Open Rev.* 2019;4(5):194-200.
5. Venkatachalam S, Nicolas AP, Liow R. Treatment of chronic anterior locked glenohumeral dislocation with hemiarthroplasty. *Shoulder Elbow.* 2014;6(2):100-104.
6. Wooten C, Klika B, Schleck CD, Harmsen WS, Sperling JW, Cofield RH. Anatomic shoulder arthroplasty as treatment for locked posterior dislocation of the shoulder. *J Bone Joint Surg Am.* 2014;96(3):e19.
7. Van Tongel A, Claessens T, Verhofste B, De Wilde L. Reversed shoulder arthroplasty as treatment for late or ancient chronic glenohumeral dislocation. *Acta Orthop Belg.* 2016;82(3):637-642.
8. Gavriilidis I, Magosch P, Lichtenberg S, Habermeyer P, Kircher J. Chronic locked posterior shoulder dislocation with severe head involvement. *Int Orthop.* 2010;34(1):79-84.
9. Schliemann B, Muder D, Gessmann J, Schildhauer TA, Seybold D. Locked posterior shoulder dislocation: treatment options and clinical outcomes. *Arch Orthop Trauma Surg.* 2011;131(8):1127-1134.
10. Ivkovic A, Boric I, Cicak N. One-stage operation for locked bilateral posterior dislocation of the shoulder. *J Bone Joint Surg Br.* 2007;89(6):825-828.
11. Ji JH, Shafi M, Jeong JJ, Ha JY. Reverse total shoulder arthroplasty in the treatment of chronic anterior fracture dislocation complicated by a chronic full thickness retracted rotator cuff tear in an elderly patient. *J Orthop Sci.* 2016;21(2):237-240.
12. Sperling JW, Pring M, Antuna SA, Cofield RH. Shoulder arthroplasty for locked posterior dislocation of the shoulder. *J Shoulder Elbow Surg.* 2004;13(5):522-527.
13. de Laat EA, Visser CP, Coene LN, Pahlplatz PV, Tavy DL. Nerve lesions in primary shoulder dislocations and humeral neck fractures. A prospective clinical and EMG study. *J Bone Joint Surg Br.* 1994;76(3):381-383.
14. Fujihara Y, Doi K, Dodakundi C, Hattori Y, Sakamoto S, Takagi T. Simple clinical test to detect deltoid muscle dysfunction causing weakness of abduction – "akimbo" test. *J Reconstr Microsurg.* 2012;28(6):375-379.
15. Goga IE. Chronic shoulder dislocations. *J Shoulder Elbow Surg.* 2003;12(5):446-450.
16. Checchia SL, Santos PD, Miyazaki AN. Surgical treatment of acute and chronic posterior fracture-dislocation of the shoulder. *J Shoulder Elbow Surg.* 1998;7(1):53-65.
17. Hawkins RJ, Neer CS II, Pianta RM, Mendoza FX. Locked posterior dislocation of the shoulder. *J Bone Joint Surg Am.* 1987;69(1):9-18.
18. Schulz TJ, Jacobs B, Patterson RL Jr. Unrecognized dislocations of the shoulder. *J Trauma.* 1969;9(12):1009-1023.
19. Wilson JC, Mc KF. Traumatic posterior dislocation of the humerus. *J Bone Joint Surg Am.* 1949;31A(1):160-172.
20. Pritchett JW, Clark JM. Prosthetic replacement for chronic unreduced dislocations of the shoulder. *Clin Orthop Relat Res.* 1987;(216):89-93.
21. Torrens C, Santana F, Melendo E, Marlet V, Caceres E. Osteochondral autograft and hemiarthroplasty for bilateral locked posterior dislocation of the shoulder. *Am J Orthop (Belle Mead NJ).* 2012;41(8):362-364.
22. Flatow EL, Miller SR, Neer CS II. Chronic anterior dislocation of the shoulder. *J Shoulder Elbow Surg.* 1993;2(1):2-10.
23. Frias M, Sousa H, Torres TP, Lourenco P. Reversed shoulder arthroplasty on chronic glenohumeral dislocations: a small retrospective case series. *J Musculoskelet Disord Treat.* 2018;4(4):1-4.
24. Matsoukis J, Tabib W, Guiffault P, et al. Primary unconstrained shoulder arthroplasty in patients with a fixed anterior glenohumeral dislocation. *J Bone Joint Surg Am.* 2006;88(3):547-552.
25. Werner BS, Böhm D, Abdelkawi A, Gohlke F. Glenoid bone grafting in reverse shoulder arthroplasty for long-standing anterior houlder dislocation. *J Shoulder Elbow Surg.* 2014;23(11):1655-1661.
26. Olszewski N, Gustin M, Curry EJ, Li X. Management of complex anterior shoulder instability: A case-based approach. *Curr Rev Musculoskelet Med.* 2017;10(4):480-490.
27. Raiss P, Edwards TB, Bruckner T, Loew M, Zeifang F, Walch G. Reverse arthroplasty for patients with chronic locked dislocation of the shoulder (type 2 fracture sequela). *J Shoulder Elbow Surg.* 2017;26(2):279-287.
28. Statz JM, Schoch BS, Sanchez-Sotelo J, et al. Shoulder arthroplasty for locked anterior shoulder dislocation: a role for the reversed design. *Int Orthop.* 2017;41(6):1227-1234.

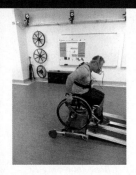

47 Arthroplasty in the Neurologically Impaired Shoulder

Alexander R. Graf, MD and Steven I. Grindel, MD

INTRODUCTION

A painless functional shoulder is contingent upon not only the integrity of the articular cartilage but also the strength of the rotator cuff and surrounding musculature that animate the shoulder girdle. Both central and peripheral nervous system disorders can compromise shoulder stability and function through secondary problems such as overload, weakness, spasticity, contracture, and aberrant movement patterns. These problems present unique challenges to shoulder arthroplasty and require a thorough understanding of how glenohumeral anatomy, kinematics, muscle tone, and postoperative demands differ from that of the "normal" shoulder to optimize outcomes **(TABLE 47.1)**. In addition, recognition of the unique psychosocial demands of this population cannot be overstated. While previous studies have shown increased complications following shoulder arthroplasty in patients with neurologically impaired shoulders, the tremendous improvements on quality of life that can result make treating this vulnerable patient population especially worthwhile.

Patient Evaluation

Understanding the patient's current level of functioning, independence, pain level, and their goals of surgery are all important elements in caring for this complex patient population. It is our experience that these patients often delay surgical intervention until the shoulder pathology is advanced. One reason is fear of further loss of independence during the recovery process from postoperative immobilization. Another is the likelihood of need for postoperative transfer to a skilled nursing facility which is a daunting place, especially for the younger patient.

The examination of the neurologically impaired shoulder should be concentrated on taking an inventory of what the patient has, what they need, and what they can spare. A multidisciplinary approach including surgeon, physical and occupational therapist, social worker, and physiatrist is ideal. Emphasize that arthroplasty can give back something but not always everything helps to set realistic expectations at first meeting and in our experience has been the best strategy.

THE WEIGHT-BEARING SHOULDER

Wheelchair-dependent patients pose several challenges to shoulder arthroplasty. Although they have relatively normal glenohumeral anatomy, the increased functional demand required of the shoulder to propel a wheelchair and for transfers leads to a high incidence of shoulder pathology over time. However, as medical care continues to improve the survival of patients who sustain cerebrovascular accidents (CVAs) or traumatic spinal cord injuries resulting in paraplegia, the prevalence of wheelchair-dependent patients will continue to increase.

Biomechanically, the push phase of wheelchair propulsion in which the arm is extended and internally rotated has been shown to increase vertical force across the shoulder over threefold and posterior force two-fold[1,2] **(FIGURE 47.1)**. This increased stress over time explains the greater incidence of rotator cuff lesions in wheelchair users as compared with ambulatory individuals (63% vs 15%).[3] Shoulder dysfunction in wheelchair users increases in direct correlation with age and duration of wheelchair use and not only limits independence but also can lead to depression over time.[4]

Previous studies have shown rotator cuff repair to be successful in wheelchair users in the short term but retears are common over time (as high as 40% in some series).[5-9] This pattern is echoed in the results of total shoulder arthroplasty (TSA) where rotator cuff failure is a near inevitability over time if the individual continues to bear weight through the shoulder.[10,11] This has led some to prefer primary reverse shoulder arthroplasty (RSA) in wheelchair-dependent patients. In the largest series to date, 83% of wheelchair ambulators were satisfied with their RSA; however, early complications (instability, glenoid baseplate loosening), late complications (periprosthetic fracture), and a notching rate of 42% make it far from ideal.[12]

Special Considerations

Preoperatively, patients are evaluated by a multidisciplinary team. Important elements of the patient's history include nature and laterality of pain, hand dominance, duration of wheelchair dependence, and previous treatment. Observation of wheelchair propulsion and patient

TABLE 47.1 Arthroplasty Challenges in the Neurologically Impaired Shoulder

Challenge	Common Examples
Overload	Wheelchair-dependent patients
	Crutch-dependent patients
Spasticity	Cerebral palsy
	Cerebrovascular accident
	Spinal cord injury
	Traumatic brain injury
Hyperkinetic	Basal ganglia disorder
	Epilepsy
Neuropathic	Congenital brachial plexus palsy
	Acquired brachial plexopathy
	Iatrogenic
	Postoncologic resection
	Syringomyelia
	Transverse myelitis
	Multiple sclerosis
	Neuromuscular disorders
	Neuropathic arthropathy

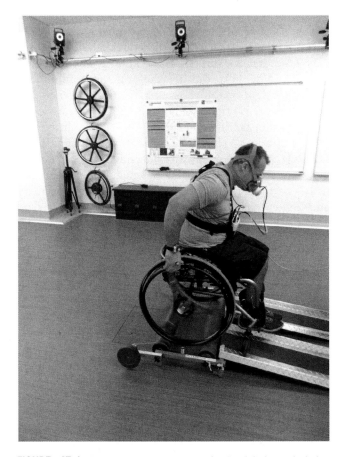

FIGURE 47.1 The propulsion phase of wheelchair ambulation demonstrated above in paraplegic patient secondary to traumatic spinal cord injury is associated with increased stress on the posterosuperior rotator cuff. (Photo courtesy of Brooke Slavens, PhD and Alyssa Schnorenberg, MS, The Mobility Lab at the University of Wisconsin-Milwaukee.)

transfers can provide information on opportunities for postural or wheelchair ergonomic changes that can help alleviate symptoms, especially if noticed early on. Nonsurgical treatment of shoulder pain in wheelchair-dependent patients has previously been well described **(TABLE 47.2)**.[8] However, often we have found this patient population to delay care due to fear of losing further independence which can lead to a problem that ultimately is harder to solve. Integrity of the rotator cuff, patient age, and level of demand help guide the shared patient-surgeon decision.

Recommendations

In the setting of glenohumeral arthritis with intact rotator cuff, TSA is an option for wheelchair ambulators but is not ideal if the patient is young and plans to continue to use a manual wheelchair. For higher demand patients with an intact rotator cuff, hemiarthroplasty (HA) with or without glenoid resurfacing via ream and run (Chapter 19) improves pain and function and leaves a good salvage option with preserved glenoid bone stock should the patient require revision to RSA **(FIGURE 47.2)**. Important technical considerations include adequate soft tissue release, maintenance of the labrum, avoiding overreaming of the glenoid to preserve subchondral bone, and not overstuffing the joint which can accelerate rotator cuff wear following anatomic TSA.

If the patient is a fall risk and has good bone stock, a stemless humeral component makes for an easier revision in the setting of periprosthetic fracture. An electric wheelchair can also preserve the rotator cuff after shoulder arthroplasty and should be discussed with the patient at the outset to maximize outcome. Magnetic resonance

TABLE 47.2 Strategies for Nonoperative Shoulder Pain Treatment

Social	Bring the patient to the shoulder-level environment
	Adapt the patient's home environment and car
	Avoid activities that irritate the shoulder
Physical	Treat associated elbow pathology
	Correct posture to minimize kyphosis
	Stretching and strengthening shoulder girdle
	Endurance training
	Weight loss, smoking cessation
Psychological	Treat associated mood disorders
	Foster supportive environment

Adapted from Fattal C, Coulet B, Gelis A, et al. Rotator cuff surgery in persons with spinal cord injury; relevance of a multidisciplinary approach. *J Shoulder Elbow Surg.* 2014;23:1263-1271.

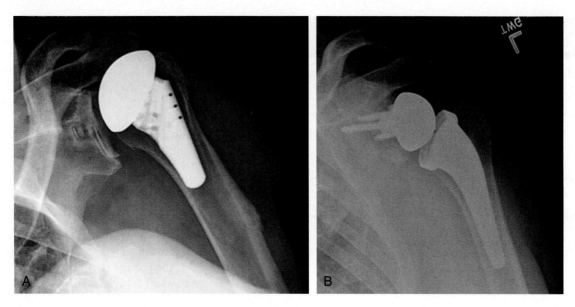

FIGURE 47.2 Rotator cuff failure after total shoulder arthroplasty (**A**) in wheelchair ambulator with cerebral palsy revised to reverse shoulder arthroplasty (**B**).

imaging (MRI) is essential preoperatively to determine the status of the rotator cuff. If there is any clinical or radiographic sign of rotator cuff pathology, RSA is the most reliable option for this population and is our preference for the majority of patients. During RSA, important technical considerations include lateralization to appropriately tension the deltoid, inferior glenosphere placement to avoid notching and impingement, and avoiding superior inclination of the glenosphere for stability.

THE SPASTIC SHOULDER

Spasticity results in increased muscle tone secondary to central neurologic dysfunction. Over time, this increased muscle tone can lead to painful contractures and eventual arthrosis. Although it is very uncommon for patients with spasticity to present for consideration of shoulder arthroplasty, patients with cerebral palsy (CP) as well as those who have survived a traumatic brain injury or CVA represent the majority of patients in this category. In individuals with CP, spasticity most often results in extension, adduction, and internal rotation contractures of the shoulder.[13] In addition, altered muscular activity can predispose to recurrent joint subluxation, abnormal joint morphology, and premature arthritis. Previous studies have shown physical therapy, occupational therapy, bracing, botulinum toxin injections, soft tissue releases, and musculotendinous lengthening of spastic muscle units to be effective in correcting the internal rotation deformity prior to the onset of arthritis.[14] In the setting of arthritis, both RSA and TSA have been performed with success, albeit in a few small case series with mixed functional results.[13,14] Overall, RSA has been associated with better function and fewer complications than TSA, but long-term data are lacking.[14]

Special Considerations

Preoperative evaluation includes understanding the patient's symptoms, individual functional goals, and the nature of their spasticity. As successful shoulder arthroplasty is as much a soft tissue operation as anything else, understanding how the aberrant muscle contractions can alter the normal force-couple relationships and soft tissue balance is critical in preventing postoperative glenohumeral instability and early component failure.[15]

In addition to physical examination, dynamic poly-EMG is recommended to understand which muscle units are spastic both at rest and under voluntary control. For contractures secondary to chronic spasticity and limited passive motion, capsular release as well as fractional lengthening of the contracted muscle units can be performed. For muscles that are spastic during active motion (dynamic spasticity), botulinum toxin can be used to block acetylcholine release and relax muscles in a dose-dependent manner for up to 6 months and can be repeated as necessary. Selective lidocaine blocks can also be used to simulate the effects of botulinum toxin prior to injection to target injections appropriately.

In the normal shoulder, the subscapularis and infraspinatus/teres minor serve as the anterior-posterior force couple. Superior escape is prevented during abduction by the supraspinatus, biceps tendon, and acromial arch. In CP, chronic shoulder extension, adduction, and internal rotation as well as elbow flexion lead to a tight anterior capsule and subscapularis and can lead to a relative lengthening of the posterior cuff elements. Intraoperatively, anterior capsule release with relative lengthening of the subscapularis muscle unit by lesser tubercle osteotomy with medialization as well as posterior capsulorrhaphy can help rebalance the shoulder during anatomic TSA. The biceps tendon can be tenotomized or tenodesed. Elbow flexion contractures should also be treated to minimize maladaptive shoulder patterns that can lead to instability and early prosthetic failure. However, even despite adequate soft tissue balancing, anatomic TSA remains fraught with complications. Therefore, in the majority of patients, RSA is our first-line option for reconstruction, particularly in patients with long-standing contracture or poorly controlled spasticity, as it has proven itself to be more reliable. Technically, it is important during RSA to not increase offset too much, as this increased tension on an already spastic deltoid can limit function significantly.

Recommendations

In the spastic shoulder with intact rotator cuff, soft tissue balancing with fractional lengthening and/or chemodenervation is a prerequisite to consideration of an anatomic TSA. However, even with reconstruction of a good soft tissue envelope and well-tensioned force couple, the subsequent risk of instability and early component failure over time make it a less desirable option. In a younger patient, HA and glenoid resurfacing via ream and run can be useful for pain control, modestly improve function, and be converted later to RSA if needed. In general, RSA with subscapularis release is our preferred technique as it allows for deltoid-driven motion of the shoulder and minimizes the variability in the other "moving parts" required for TSA. It is also important to appreciate the effect of long-standing spasticity on glenoid morphology. Augmented glenoid baseplates

with either metallic augmentation or Bio-RSA (Wright Medical, Memphis, TN) for B2 and type C glenoids are our first choice for these challenging glenoids. Osteotomy of the glenoid can be done in a staged manner for the younger patient, but the results can be less predictable. Templating software is helpful in planning the surgical procedure (**FIGURE 47.3**). In severe deformity, patient-specific guides or real-time computer-assisted positioning software can be used to aid in implant positioning.

THE HYPERKINETIC SHOULDER

Parkinson disease (PD) is a common neurologic disorder that affects 1% to 2% of the US population.[16] It is characterized by cell loss in the substantia nigra pars compacta portion of the basal ganglia and leads to cognitive (dementia), neuromuscular (tremors, increased muscle tone), and metabolic (osteoporosis fragility fractures) derangements that make shoulder arthroplasty particularly challenging. Because patients with PD have asynchronous motor function and lack complete volitional muscle control, they are prone to falls as well as shoulder instability.[17] In fact, previous studies have shown that PD is associated with increased rates of infection, dislocation, revision shoulder arthroplasty, fracture, component loosening, and systemic complications after conventional TSA, RSA, and HA.[16] This increased complication rate and poor functional result have also been shown to worsen with age (>65 years).[18] A 19% revision rate and a 47% incidence of unsatisfactory functional results after shoulder arthroplasty have been reported in the PD population. The goal in these patients should be

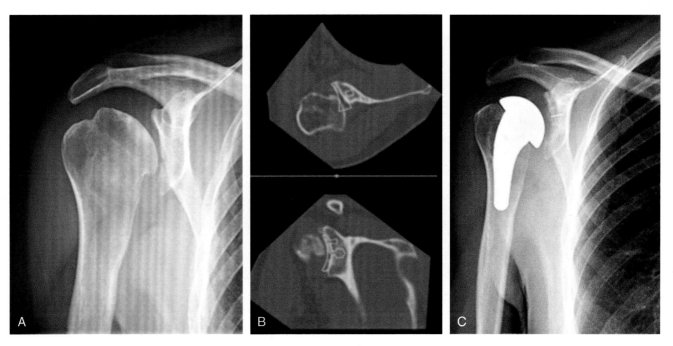

FIGURE 47.3 A 63-year-old male cane ambulator with type C glenoid presented with advanced glenohumeral arthritis (**A**). A custom glenoid and guide was templated from preoperative computed tomography scan (**B**) prior to successful anatomic total shoulder arthroplasty (**C**).

pain control, as functional gains are variable. This also emphasizes the importance of patient selection and optimization prior to surgery.[19-21]

Special Considerations

Regardless of the arthroplasty technique chosen, collaboration with neurology for optimization of the patient's disease, access to an extended care facility with increased supervision, a safe physical home environment, and an electric wheelchair to minimize falls and stress through implant are important perioperative considerations. In addition, preoperative assessment of bone mineral density and targeted therapy by an endocrinologist can help mitigate against periprosthetic fracture.

The preoperative X-ray can be used to assess humeral bone mineral density and may influence humeral component choice. Some authors advocate a stemless humeral prosthesis when humeral index (humeral diaphyseal cortical thickness:total diameter of humeral diaphysis ratio) is less than 0.23 as revision from a stemless to a stemmed implant is easier in osteoporotic bone than in a standard length stem which often necessitates osteotomy and fixation in poor quality bone.[22] However, this must be weighed against the fact that good metaphyseal bone is required for stemless humeral component fixation. In general, a shorter stem is better than a long stem in osteoporotic bone, as it achieves adequate fixation while also facilitating easier removal in the future should there be a need for revision.

In addition to a stemless or short-stemmed humeral component, an anterosuperior approach or a subscapularis sparing deltopectoral approach has also been advocated because of less postoperative instability and earlier return to active motion due to maintenance of the subscapularis insertion.[22] If utilizing a standard deltopectoral approach, incising the rotator cuff interval quite low along the upper border of the subscapularis tendon can lessen the possibility of later anterior-superior subluxation. Repair of the rotator interval is also important. Positioning the glenoid component in neutral and humeral component in 5° to 10° of anteversion if there is a slight tendency for posterior humeral subluxation has also been described to improve postoperative stability.[19]

Recommendations

In addition to clinical and radiographic indications for shoulder arthroplasty, the patient with PD must also have the cognitive function, social support, and optimized medical comorbid conditions prior to any surgical discussion. For tremors not controlled with oral agents, selective botulinum injection is an option, though it is relatively understudied for this application. In the rotator cuff intact patient younger than 60 years, we favor a stemless anatomic TSA in anticipation of the potential need for revision. In the younger patient that is high demand or unable to obtain electric wheelchair, ream and run glenoid resurfacing is preferred **(FIGURE 47.4)**. For the majority of patients we have treated with PD that are older with dysfunctional rotator cuffs, RSA is our option of choice **(FIGURE 47.5)**. For proximal humerus fractures not amenable to open reduction and internal fixation, we prefer an HA option in the younger high-demand patient, which can be converted to TSA down the road if the patient develops symptomatic glenohumeral arthrosis **(FIGURE 47.6)**. For most patients that are older than 60 years, or any previous evidence of cuff

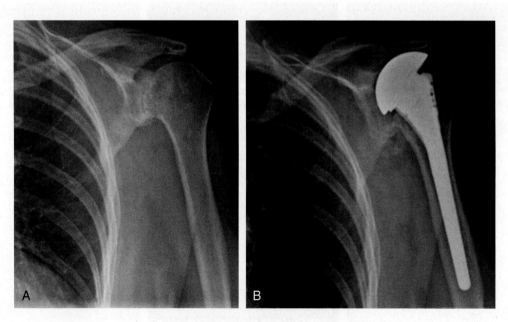

FIGURE 47.4 A 71-year-old woman with Parkinson disease and advanced glenohumeral arthritis **(A)** and intact rotator cuff underwent anatomic total shoulder arthroplasty with glenoid resurfacing with ream and run. Patient subsequently developed rotator cuff failure after fall with subsequent high-riding humeral head **(B)**.

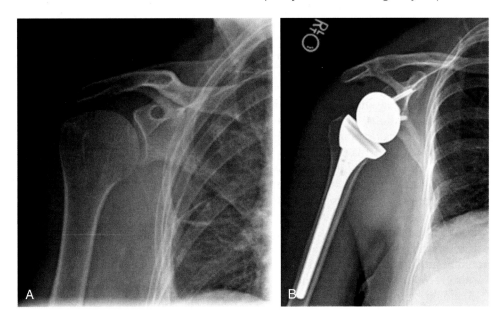

FIGURE 47.5 A 78-year-old woman with Parkinson disease and pseudoparalytic shoulder from rotator cuff tear (**A**) underwent reverse total shoulder arthroplasty (**B**).

pathology or arthritis, RSA is our primary method of reconstruction. Postoperatively, we caution against the prolonged use of slings in this population as it seems to make them more prone to losing their balance, resulting in falls and the potential for periprosthetic fractures.

THE NEUROPATHIC SHOULDER

Neuropathic Arthropathy

Neuropathic arthropathy (NA), or Charcot arthropathy, is a progressive receptor activator of nuclear factor kappa-B ligand (RANKL)–mediated joint destructive process secondary to loss of sensation, proprioception, or both. A syrinx is the most common underlying cause of NA affecting the shoulder (80%), though Arnold-Chiari malformations, posttraumatic syringomyelia, cervical spondylosis, infections such as tuberculosis or syphilis, and diabetes have also been reported.[23,24] Although the exact mechanism of joint destruction is not entirely clear, the predominant theories are that it is mediated either by an insult to the sensory neural pathways (neurotraumatic) or by increased joint perfusion (neurovascular).[24] Clinically, patients can present with typical shoulder arthritis symptoms; however, care

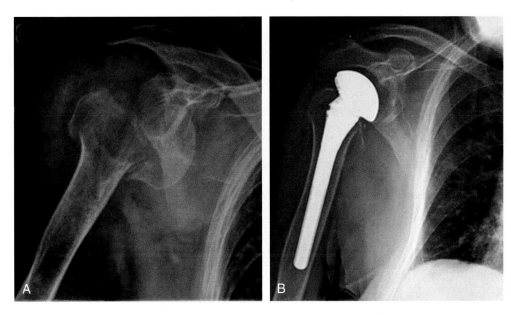

FIGURE 47.6 A 70-year-old man with Parkinson disease suffered a proximal humerus fracture dislocation after ground level fall (**A**) and was treated with hemiarthroplasty (**B**).

should be taken during the history (diabetes) as well as musculoskeletal and neurovascular examinations (decreased deep tendon reflexes or "cape"-like sensory abnormalities common in syringomyelia) to elicit findings that are different from the norm. NA of the shoulder has a diverse radiographic appearance, with atrophic and hypertrophic bony manifestations. Therefore, additional MR imaging is helpful in making diagnosis (effusion, soft tissue inflammation, and cartilage destruction) and assessing rotator cuff integrity for future surgical planning. Cervical spine X-ray with MRI or computed tomography (CT) myelogram is also recommended to evaluate for cervical spondylosis and syrinx, respectively. Nonoperative management consisting of anti-inflammatory medications, physical therapy, bracing, or joint injections should be attempted prior to any surgical consideration. It is also recommended that the underlying cause of the NA should be treated and stable for at least a year prior to surgery to optimize results.[24] Surgical options for treatment of NA of the shoulder range from synovectomy, HA, and RSA based on symptoms and the degree of bone and soft tissue compromise.[24] Outcomes are variable for shoulder reconstruction in this population and are limited to only a few case series with small samples sizes.[25-27] However, due to the known risk of early postoperative failure, shoulder arthroplasty should be considered very carefully. The use of RSA in carefully selected cases has shown some promise (**FIGURE 47.7**).

Brachial Plexus Deficits

While neurological compromise of the shoulder and upper extremity is the debilitating result of sensory and proprioceptive nerve dysfunction, atrophy is the end result of motor nerve injury and leads to a lack of functional muscle to animate the shoulder girdle. This most commonly occurs secondary to brachial plexus injury, such as in obstetric brachial plexus injury (OBPI), after tumor resection or trauma. If the nerve injury is identified promptly, nerve repair and/or transfers can restore nerve function and prevent abnormal glenohumeral loading, secondary contractures, and arthritis. However, once the window for nerve reconstruction has passed, tendon transfers are the workhorse for restoring lost function and providing stability to the shoulder girdle.

Obstetric Brachial Plexus Injury

Fortunately, OBPIs are rare (0.3-4 per 1000 live births in developed countries) and usually resolve within the first 2 years of life without need for surgical intervention.[28] However, for children with OBPI, the upper trunk (C5, C6) is most commonly affected, resulting in weakness in shoulder abduction and external rotation. If C7 is affected, triceps weakness will also be present. This leads to an imbalance in favor of the internal rotators: the subscapularis, pectoralis major, and latissimus dorsi. Long-term sequelae of this devastating injury can lead to internal rotation and adduction contractures of the shoulder, progressive posterior subluxation, and glenoid dysplasia.[28] Over time, this can lead to progressive glenohumeral arthritis, which in the setting of paralyzed shoulder girdle muscles and muscular imbalance complicates shoulder arthroplasty.

For advanced shoulder arthritis and pain in the setting of muscle weakness, imbalance, and glenoid deformity, previous studies have shown good pain relief but limited functional improvement following TSA, RSA, and HA in patients with OBPI.[28] These cases are technically challenging and considerably more costly when compared with shoulder fusion.[29] The discussion with the patient and family concerning shoulder reconstruction

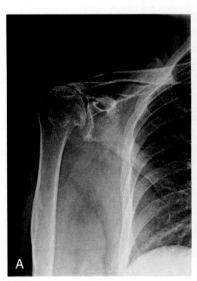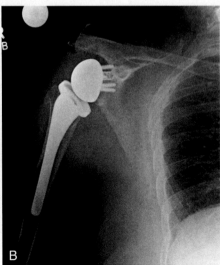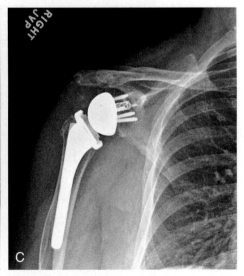

FIGURE 47.7 A 67-year-old woman with syringomyelia who underwent previous rotator cuff repair (RCR) presented with progressive shoulder dysfunction (**A**). She underwent reverse shoulder arthroplasty (**B**), and at 3-year follow-up, her shoulder was functioning well and implant was stable (**C**).

for patients with OBPI must take into account these historically poor functional results as well as alternatives. Shoulder fusion effectively treats the pain and residual motion is preserved through the scapulothoracic articulation. It is best when there is preserved elbow and hand motion and historically has been the gold standard for pediatric shoulder paralysis. If performed before skeletal maturity, limb shortening will result, as 80% of the humeral length is from proximal humerus physis growth and should be discussed with the family beforehand. The recommended position of fusion is controversial but ranges from 20° to 40° forward flexion, 20° to 30° internal rotation, and 20° to 45° abduction.[29]

Traumatic Brachial Plexopathy

Traumatic brachial plexopathy can occur after penetrating trauma but most frequently occurs in the setting of proximal humerus anterior fracture dislocations. Neurologic involvement after shoulder fracture dislocation is estimated to be 6.2%.[30] With anterior shoulder dislocations, axillary nerve injury is most common, with most being neurapraxia which typically recover over the period of a several weeks or a few months. An electromyography at 3 months after shoulder dislocation can help identify the degree of nerve injury and provide prognostic information. Long-term sequelae of chronic axillary nerve injury include lateral shoulder numbness as well as weakness in shoulder abduction (deltoid) and external rotation with the arm abducted (teres minor). Although RSA historically has been contraindicated in deltoid-deficient patients, recent reports suggest it can be effective for immediate treatment of anterior shoulder fracture dislocations with axillary nerve injury and stable even if axillary nerve does not recover.[31,32] In addition, in the setting of deltoid deficiency, it is emphasized that larger glenospheres, more constrained sockets, minimal humeral lengthening, and repaired subscapularis tendons maximize intrinsic shoulder stability and should be considered during RSA.[31]

Special Considerations

For patients with debilitating shoulder pain and advanced shoulder arthritis from long-standing sequelae of brachial plexus injuries, the constellation of muscle weakness, loss of proprioception and sensation, force-couple imbalance, chronic contractures, and glenoid deformity make it a rare but formidable challenge for shoulder surgeons. For these patients, it is important to set appropriate expectations and be sure that just because something *can* be done that it *should* (**FIGURE 47.8**). Emphasizing to the patient that shoulder reconstruction in this context more reliably improves pain than function can help prioritize treatment in the setting of bilateral shoulder dysfunction (**FIGURE 47.9**). Anatomic TSA can reliably treat pain but bony and soft tissue elements of the problem must be also addressed. In addition, persistent posterior subluxation despite soft tissue reconstruction is common and must be anticipated with future potential revision surgeries in mind.

Recommendations

Surgical reconstruction in the chronically contracted shoulder with force-couple imbalance and significant glenoid deformity often requires an extensile anterior shoulder approach with soft tissue releases, tendon transfers, and glenoid osteotomies to restore normal soft tissue tension and bony anatomy.[33] Anterior deltoid release from the clavicle origin helps prevent avulsion of the deltoid during exposure, as often the long-standing contractures make access to the glenohumeral joint particularly challenging.[33] A normal functioning elbow and hand are

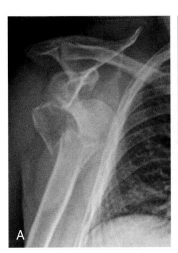 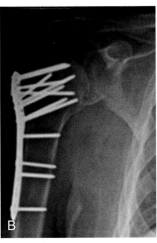 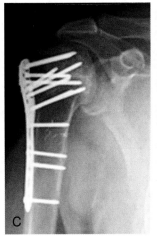 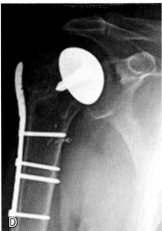

FIGURE 47.8 A 45-year-old man fell from ladder and sustained right proximal humerus fracture with anterior dislocation and axillary nerve injury (**A**). He underwent urgent open reduction and internal fixation (**B**). He subsequently presented to clinic 8 years after his injury with pain and progressive avascular necrosis with collapse of his humeral head (**C**) and no functional recovery of his deltoid. He underwent HemiCAP resurfacing (Arthrosurface, Franklin, MA) for treatment of his pain (**D**).

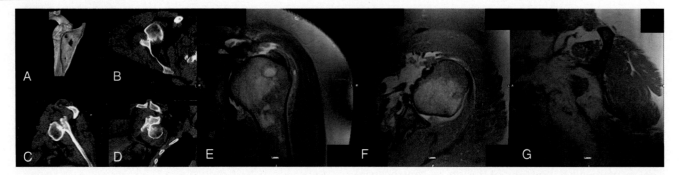

FIGURE 47.9 A 63-year-old woman with spastic quadriplegia secondary to C5-6 transverse myelitis presented to clinic with difficulty using her right arm after a fall 1 year prior while using walker and acute left shoulder pain. Computed tomography scan revealed chronic anterior shoulder dislocation with significant anterior-inferior glenoid bone loss (**A-D**) and a massive left rotator cuff tear with effusion and supraspinatus and subscapularis atrophy (**E-G**). The patient deferred surgical intervention on the right as her pain had resolved, and she had full function of her hand for activities of daily living. For the left shoulder, a reverse shoulder arthroplasty was planned to help alleviate pain and give back some motion through her intact deltoid.

a prerequisite to shoulder arthroplasty of any kind. In addition to a thorough physical examination, EMGs, CT, and MRI are helpful in quantifying the degree of muscle atrophy, glenoid dysplasia, and the viability of available tendons to transfer. During anatomic TSA, we prefer the latissimus dorsi over pectoralis major transfer for subscapularis deficiency. Lower trapezius or latissimus dorsi/teres major tendon transfers (L'Episcopo) are utilized for posterior cuff deficiency. Restoring the anterior-posterior force couple for stability and providing motor units to power the shoulder are important in anatomic TSA. Transferred tendons can be augmented with Achilles allograft if more length is needed. In RSA, we do not routinely perform tendon transfers, even in the setting of deficient deltoid function.

For glenoid dysplasia, reaming the "high side" to re-create neutral version is an option in the setting of good bone stock. Another option is using the humeral head as bone graft with reaming and possible staged glenoid resurfacing. Iliac crest bone grafting to the glenoid is also effective for advanced glenoid dysplasia with bone loss as it has been described in the revision RSA setting.[34] A sagittal split osteotomy with wedge graft that can be concentrically reamed to prevent excessive medialization has been described, but in the era of preoperative templating and custom glenoid augments is less ideal.[33] The humerus is usually cut in its native (abnormal) version of 10° anteversion to prevent disruption of the patient's native soft tissue balance. The subscapularis is released via osteotomy and medialized as needed in the setting of a chronic rigid internal rotation contracture or repaired to adjacent deltoid and pectoralis major to prevent anterior subluxation.

CONCLUSION

Shoulder arthroplasty in the neurologically impaired shoulder is rare and challenging. However, improved medical management is increasing the longevity of this diverse patient population and with it the incidence of degenerative shoulder pathology requiring shoulder surgeons that are up to meeting that challenge with compassion and resolve. Understanding the nuances of the various etiologies of neurologic impairment can help prevent complications and guide rehabilitation. In addition, a multidisciplinary approach is critical to optimize surgical candidates and help set appropriate expectations with patients perioperatively. With that in mind, results can be transformative for both surgeon and patient.

REFERENCES

1. Kulig K, Rau SS, Mulroy SJ, et al. Shoulder joint kinetics during the push phase of wheelchair propulsion. *Clin Orthop Relat Res.* 1998;354:132-143.
2. Collinger JL, Boninger ML, Koontz AM, et al. Shoulder biomechanics during the push phase of wheelchair propulsion: a multisite study of persons with paraplegia. *Arch Phys Med Rehabil.* 2008;89(4):667-676. doi:10.1016/j.apmr.2007.09.052
3. Akbar M, Balean G, Brunner M, et al. Prevalence of rotator cuff tear in paraplegic patients compared with controls. *J Bone Joint Surg Am.* 2010;92:23-30.
4. Wang JC, Chan RC, Tsai YA, et al. The influence of shoulder pain on functional limitation, perceived health and depressive mood in patients with traumatic paraplegia. *J Spinal Cord Med.* 2015;3:587-592.
5. Kerr J, Borbas P, Meyer DC, Gerber C, Tellez CB, Wieser K. Arthroscopic rotator cuff repair in the weight bearing shoulder. *J Shoulder Elbow Surg.* 2015;24:1894-1899.
6. Goldstein B, Young J, Escobedo EM. Rotator cuff repairs in individuals with paraplegia. *Am J Phys Med Rehabil.* 1997;76:316-322.
7. Jordan RW, Sloan R, Saithna A. Should we avoid shoulder surgery in wheelchair users? A systematic review of outcomes and complications. *Orthop Traumatol Surg Res.* 2018;104(6):839-846. doi:10.1016/j.otsr.2018.03.011
8. Fattal C, Coulet B, Gelis A, et al. Rotator cuff surgery in persons with spinal cord injury; relevance of a multidisciplinary approach. *J Shoulder Elbow Surg.* 2014;23:1263-1271.
9. Alentorn-Geli E, Wanderman NR, Assenmacher AT, Sánchez-Sotelo J, Cofield RH, Sperling JW. Reverse shoulder arthroplasty in weight-bearing shoulders of wheelchair-dependent patients: outcomes and complications at 2 to 5 years. *PM R.* 2018;10(6):607-615.
10. Hattrup SJ, Cofield RH. Shoulder arthroplasty in the paraplegic patient. *J Shoulder Elbow Surg.* 2010;19:434-438.

11. De Loubresse CG, Norton MR, Piriou P, Walch G. Replacement arthroplasty in the weight-bearing shoulder of paraplegic patients. *J Shoulder Elbow Surg*. 2004;13:369-372.

12. Kemp AL, King JJ, Farmer KW, Wright TW. Reverse total shoulder arthroplasty in wheelchair dependent patients. *J Shoulder Elbow Surg*. 2016;25:1138-1145.

13. Hattrup SJ, Cofield RH, Evidente VH, Sperling JW. Total shoulder arthroplasty for patients with cerebral palsy. *J Shoulder Elbow Surg*. 2007;16(5):e5-e9.

14. Marigi EM, Statz JM, Sperling JW, Sanchez-Sotelo J, Cofield RH, Morrey ME. Shoulder arthroplasty in patients with cerebral palsy: a matched cohort study to patients with osteoarthritis. *J Shoulder Elbow Surg*. 2020;29(3):483-490.

15. Abboud JA, Anakwenze OA, Hsu JE. Soft-tissue management in revision total shoulder arthroplasty. *J Am Acad Orthop Surg*. 2013;21(1):23-31.

16. Burrus MT, Werner BC, Cancienne JM, Gwathmey FW, Brockmeier SF. Shoulder arthroplasty in patients with Parkinson's disease is associated with increased complications. *J Shoulder Elbow Surg*. 2015;24(12):1881-1887. doi:10.1016/j.jse.2015.05.048

17. Skedros JG, Smith JS, Langston TD, Adondakis MG. Reverse total shoulder arthroplasty as treatment for rotator cuff-tear arthropathy and shoulder dislocations in an elderly male with Parkinson's disease. *Case Rep Orthop*. 2017;2017:5051987. doi:10.1155/2017/5051987

18. Koch LD, Cofield RH, Ahlskog JE. Total shoulder arthroplasty in patients with Parkinson's disease. *J Shoulder Elbow Surg*. 1997;6(1):24-28.

19. Kryzak TJ, Sperling JW, Schleck CD, Cofield RH. Total shoulder arthroplasty in patients with Parkinson's disease. *J Shoulder Elbow Surg*. 2009;18(1):96-99. doi:10.1016/j.jse.2008.07.010

20. Cusick MC, Otto RJ, Clark RE, Frankle MA. Outcome of reverse shoulder arthroplasty for patients with Parkinson's disease: a matched cohort study. *Orthopedics*. 2017;40(4):e675-e680. doi:10.3928/01477447-20170509-03

21. Jiang JJ, Toor AS, Shi LL, Koh JL. Analysis of perioperative complications in patients after total shoulder arthroplasty and reverse total shoulder arthroplasty. *J Shoulder Elbow Surg*. 2014;23(12):1852-1859.

22. Giannotti S, Bottai V, Dell'Osso G, Bugelli G, Guido G. Stemless humeral component in reverse shoulder prosthesis in patient with Parkinson's disease: a case report. *Clin Cases Miner Bone Metab*. 2015;12(1):56-59. doi:10.11138/ccmbm/2015.12.1.056

23. Alpert SK, Koval KJ, Zuckerman JD. Neuropathic arthropathy: review of current knowledge. *J Am Acad Orthop Surg*. 1996;4(2):100-108.

24. Santiesteban L, Mollon B, Zuckerman JD. Neuropathic arthropathy of the glenohumeral joint a review of the literature. *Bull Hosp Jt Dis (2013)*. 2018;76(2):88-99.

25. Crowther MA, Bell SN. Neuropathic shoulder in syringomyelia treated with resurfacing arthroplasty of humeral head and soft-tissue lining of glenoid: a case report. *J Shoulder Elbow Surg*. 2007;16(6):e38-e40.

26. Ueblacker P, Ansah P, Vogt S, et al. Bilateral reverse shoulder prosthesis in a patient with severe syringomyelia. *J Shoulder Elbow Surg*. 2007;16(6):e48-e51.

27. BSchoch, JDWerthel, JSperling, et al. Shoulder arthroplasty for Charcot arthropathy. Presented at: The Annual Meeting of the American Academy of Orthopaedic Surgeons, Las Vegas, Nevada, March 25-27, 2015.

28. Werthel JD, Schoch B, Frankle M, Cofield R, Elhassan BT. Shoulder arthroplasty for sequelae of obstetrical brachial plexus injury. *J Hand Surg Am*. 2018;43(9):871.e1-871.e7. doi:10.1016/j.jhsa.2018.02.006

29. González-Díaz R, Rodríguez-Merchán EC, Gilbert MS. The role of shoulder fusion in the era of arthroplasty. *Int Orthop*. 1997;21(3):204-209.

30. Stableforth PG. Four-part fractures of the neck of the humerus. *J Bone Joint Surg Br*. 1984;66(1):104-108.

31. Kurowicki J, Triplet JJ, Berglund DD, Zink T, Rosas S, Levy JC. Use of a reverse shoulder arthroplasty following a fracture-dislocation with a brachial plexus palsy: a case report. *JBJS Case Connect*. 2018;8(2):e36. doi:10.2106/JBJS.CC.17.00204

32. Gasbarro G, Crasto JA, Rocha J, Henry S, Kano D, Tarkin IS. Reverse total shoulder arthroplasty for geriatric proximal humerus fracture dislocation with concomitant nerve injury. *Geriatr Orthop Surg Rehabil*. 2019;10:2151459319855318. doi:10.1177/2151459319855318

33. Gosens T, Neumann L, Wallace WA. Shoulder replacement after Erb's palsy: a case report with ten years' follow-up. *J Shoulder Elbow Surg*. 2004;13(5):568-572.

34. Wagner E, Houdek MT, Elhassan BT, Sanchez-Sotelo J, Sperling JW, Cofield RH. Glenoid bone-grafting in revision to a reverse total shoulder arthroplasty: surgical technique. *JBJS Essent Surg Tech*. 2016;6(4):e35.

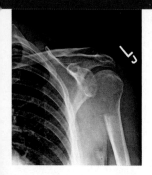

48 Arthroplasty for Shoulder Girdle Tumors

Cory G. Couch, MD, Thomas W. Wright, MD, and C. Parker Gibbs Jr, MD

INTRODUCTION

The treatment goal for malignant shoulder girdle tumors with subsequent reconstruction is complete extirpation of the malignancy and preservation of function. This is accomplished by ensuring adequate surgical margins, preserving vital structures, and subsequently reconstructing bone and soft tissue. Limb-salvage techniques in large shoulder tumors often result in narrow surgical margins due to the intimate relationship to neurovascular structures. Because of the involvement of adjacent soft tissue, proximal humerus resection often results in decreased shoulder function and stability provided by the rotator cuff and capsule, which may then result in dislocation. Despite these challenges, limb salvage can provide considerable functional advantages as well as local tumor control, in contrast to amputation. Restoring function after treating tumors of the shoulder girdle is critical because of the girdle's role in activities of daily living. When limb salvage is not feasible, amputation is an effective and valuable surgical option.

Although these tumors are infrequent, being knowledgeable of the approach to diagnose and treat them is important to optimizing patient outcomes. Advancements in surgical technique, radiotherapy, chemotherapy, and advanced imaging have led to an estimated 95% of patients being able to undergo limb-salvage surgery for bone or soft tissue sarcomas of the extremity.[1]

The proximal humerus is the most common site in the upper extremity for primary bone sarcomas and the third most common overall after the distal femur and proximal tibia. A recent Surveillance, Epidemiology, and End Results (SEER) database study by Howlander estimated yearly diagnosis of 3300 bone sarcomas in the United States, with the most common sarcomas being osteosarcoma, Ewing sarcoma, and chondrosarcoma.[2] Bone sarcomas of the shoulder girdle typically present with a large extraosseous mass and require resection of a margin of soft tissue covering the tumor to optimize local control.

Proximal humerus metastases, by comparison, are relatively common, with greater than 50% of upper extremity metastasis involving the humerus.[3] Treatment for patients with metastases to the shoulder girdle must be a collaborative decision-making effort. In addition to surgical care, radiation oncologists and medical oncologists are crucial parts of the overall treatment of the patient's disease. Specifically, the extent of surgery and recovery time must be balanced with end-of-life discussions. Each patient is an individual with differing clinical conditions and goals.

For optimal patient survival and functional outcomes, early recognition, accurate diagnosis, and appropriate initial management are the key factors.

HISTORICAL BACKGROUND

Prior to the early to mid-twentieth century, shoulder girdle malignant tumors were treated by forequarter amputation. Early in the twentieth century, a description of the Tikhoff-Linberg interscapulothoracic resection was published, which involved the removal of the head of the humerus, the distal one-third of the clavicle, the scapula, and soft tissue surrounding the sarcoma.[4-6] This surgical technique and its modifications remain in use today for resections of the shoulder girdle. Although the Tikhoff-Linberg resection was described for scapular resections, this technique is often reported for proximal humerus sarcoma resection. Advancements in imaging modalities, chemotherapy, and radiation have allowed surgeons to better plan and execute surgical resections and perform limb-preservation surgery, while optimizing local control. Advancements in reconstructive techniques and prostheses allow for both an improved variety of options for shoulder reconstruction as well as modest improvements in shoulder function after resection of shoulder girdle tumors.[7-9]

INDICATIONS AND CONTRAINDICATIONS FOR LIMB SALVAGE

Although limb salvage is the preferred treatment for shoulder girdle tumors, approximately 5% of proximal humerus sarcomas do not permit limb salvage. Relative contraindications for limb salvage include tumor encasement of the neurovascular bundle and chest wall invasion. Tumor involvement of the neurovascular bundle must be carefully evaluated when considering limb salvage, as many proximal humerus tumors have a large extraosseous component that will displace the neurovascular bundle without infiltrating the sheath. If the sheath is infiltrated, then limb salvage with an adequate margin is impossible without segmental resection and reconstruction of the neurovascular structures. If the neurovascular bundle is only displaced and not encased, the sheath around the bundle can be opened and used as a margin in sarcoma resection with preservation of the bundle and limb salvage. This is especially true in instances where effective chemo or radiation therapy is available and employed.

Historically a pathologic fracture through a sarcoma was considered a contraindication to limb-sparing surgery, but advancements in adjuvant therapies have made limb salvage possible in many of these cases. When adequate soft-tissue margins can be maintained around the pathologic fracture without spillage of tumor during resection of the tumor with preservation of a neurovascularly viable limb, salvage is recommended. This is most likely in cases where the fracture has gone on to heal prior to resection. A pathologic fracture in the setting of metastasis to the lung from sarcoma or to the bone from another primary tumor may also not be a contraindication for limb salvage. It is often better to preserve limb function in this patient population to optimize quality of remaining life as resection is not curative.

Most consider extensive invasion of the chest wall by a shoulder girdle tumor to be an absolute contraindication to limb salvage and tumor extension to the chest wall without extensive invasion as only a relative contraindication to limb salvage.[10] This recommendation is due to the soft tissue and almost certain neurovascular involvement in the axillary space in shoulder girdle tumors that extensively invade the chest wall and the potentially salvageable neurovascular bundle in tumors that extend to but do not invade the chest wall.

ANATOMIC CONSIDERATIONS

In addition to the need to preserve nerve and vascular function distally, preserving the axillary nerve as it travels just inferior to the glenohumeral joint is essential when planning a reverse total shoulder arthroplasty (RTSA) reconstruction. If the axillary nerve must be sacrificed, then a hemiarthroplasty should be used as a spacer to suspend the limb or a tendon transfer to reconstruct the deltoid moment arm is needed. Often, the axillary nerve cannot be preserved with an adequate margin in pathologic proximal humerus fractures through sarcoma, as the nerve intimately courses around the proximal humerus, innervating the deltoid. It is also vitally important to preserve the musculocutaneous nerve when possible for limb salvage as it courses just medially to the conjoined tendon. Not all branches must be preserved for maintenance of elbow function, and often, the proximal

branches must be sacrificed due to the large soft tissue mass expanding into the biceps brachii. Innervation to the brachialis alone can provide adequate elbow flexion strength for a functional elbow as this is the prime elbow flexor; however, supination strength will be diminished with the absence of a functioning biceps.

In metastatic disease to the shoulder girdle, a different approach is taken to margins, preserving function and reconstruction. In patients with diffuse metastatic disease, surgery itself for shoulder girdle tumors is not curative; therefore, a marginal or even intralesional margin is sometimes accepted to optimize both patient recovery speed and function preservation. Often a simpler reconstruction that allows for earlier function is better for patients with metastatic disease as a faster return of function is optimal due to potentially limited survival time of the patient. Although, in patients with oligometastatic disease, in particular, an isolated renal cell metastasis to the shoulder girdle, there is a proven survival benefit for a complete resection.[11] Regarding specific tumors, multiple myeloma bone lesions and renal cell carcinoma metastasis should be embolized ideally within 24 hours preoperatively to minimize blood loss in known hypervascular tumors, as preoperative embolization has been shown to reduce estimated blood loss.[12]

A proximal humerus sarcoma involving the intraarticular glenohumeral joint requires an extra-articular resection for an adequate surgical margin. Presumptive evidence of intra-articular extension includes visualization of the tumor in the glenohumeral joint or glenohumeral effusion on imaging. A study by Ozaki found that assessing the existence of a tumor inside the glenohumeral joint can be difficult in chondrosarcoma and osteosarcoma.[13] If the intra-articular glenohumeral joint is determined to have primary sarcoma involvement, an extra-articular resection should be performed. This is not the case for carcinoma metastatic to bone where wide margins are not required. To obtain a wide margin, the capsule and rotator cuff are left intact around the glenohumeral joint, and the glenoid is osteotomized medially to the capsular origin on the glenoid neck. Abdeen et al demonstrated inferior abduction and forward flexion outcomes in extra-articular resections of the humerus.[14]

In sarcomas arising from the scapula itself, a total or partial scapulectomy may be performed based on the anatomical involvement. If the scapular sarcoma violates the glenohumeral joint, an extra-articular resection of the proximal humerus must be performed en bloc with the scapulectomy, and a Tikhoff-Linberg approach is ideal.

RESECTION CLASSIFICATION

Malawer described an anatomic classification system (**FIGURE 48.1**) for shoulder girdle tumor resections that include the six categories listed below with subdivisions

Malawer Classification

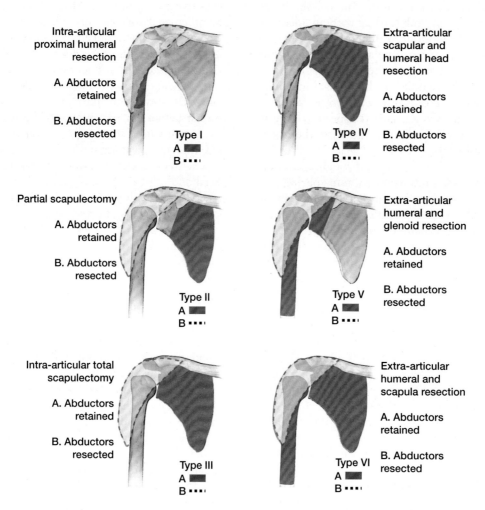

Intra-articular
proximal humeral
resection

A. Abductors
retained

B. Abductors
resected

Type I
A ▬▬
B ▪▪▪▪

Extra-articular
scapular and
humeral head
resection

A. Abductors
retained

Type IV
A ▬▬
B ▪▪▪▪

B. Abductors
resected

Partial scapulectomy

A. Abductors
retained

B. Abductors
resected

Type II
A ▬▬
B ▪▪▪▪

Extra-articular
humeral and
glenoid resection

A. Abductors
retained

B. Abductors
resected

Type V
A ▬▬
B ▪▪▪▪

Intra-articular total
scapulectomy

A. Abductors
retained

B. Abductors
resected

Type III
A ▬▬
B ▪▪▪▪

Extra-articular
humeral and
scapula resection

A. Abductors
retained

B. Abductors
resected

Type VI
A ▬▬
B ▪▪▪▪

FIGURE 48.1 Malawer anatomic classification system for shoulder girdle tumor resections.

of A (intact abductors) and B (abductors partially or completely resected):

Type I: Intra-articular proximal humeral resection
Type II: Partial scapular resection
Type III: Intra-articular total scapulectomy
Type IV: Extra-articular total scapulectomy and humeral head resection (classical Tikhoff-Linberg resection)
Type V: Extra-articular humeral and glenoid resection
Type VI: Extra-articular humeral and total scapular resection[10]

SHOULDER GIRDLE TUMOR WORK-UP

In patients who present with shoulder girdle tumors, a standardized evaluation approach will expedite diagnosis and aid in treatment planning. Orthogonal radiographs should be the first imaging modality to evaluate a shoulder mass, followed by advanced imaging of the mass with magnetic resonance image (MRI) with and without contrast to include the entire bone. If sarcoma is suspected, then a thin cut noncontrast computed tomography (CT) of the chest is recommended for evaluation of pulmonary metastasis. If metastatic carcinoma, myeloma, or lymphoma is suspected, then a CT of the chest, abdomen, and pelvis is recommended to evaluate for a potential primary source of carcinoma. A whole-body bone scan to evaluate for other sites of potential bone involvement is a recommended workup for all bone tumors. A standardized laboratory panel should also be ordered, including a complete blood count (CBC) with differential, comprehensive metabolic panel (CMP), serum protein electrophoresis (SPEP), and urine protein electrophoresis (UPEP). The next step in diagnosis is a biopsy performed with an appropriate technique either via core needle biopsy or a limited open biopsy.

BIOPSY PRINCIPLES

The recommended biopsy tract for proximal humerus tumors is through the anterior one-third of the deltoid muscle belly. It is not recommended to contaminate the pectoralis major with a biopsy through the deltopectoral interval due to the increased risk of hematoma formation and spread to neurovascular structures and the chest wall. The biopsy through the anterior one-third deltoid should be performed using a longitudinal incision of approximately 1 to 2 cm just lateral to the deltopectoral interval. The biopsy tract should be extra-articular, only involving the deltoid and the proximal humerus lateral to the bicipital groove, with the level of the biopsy based over the center portion of the tumor as long as the previously stated principles are not violated. Minimizing traumatic dissection and meticulous hemostasis during the biopsy is critical to minimize bleeding and thus contamination of surrounding soft tissues and the subacromial space.

INCISION/APPROACH OPTIONS

Tikhoff-Linberg Approach

In shoulder girdle tumors that involve the proximal humerus and for which resection with a margin involves resecting the deltoid, acromion, glenoid, and distal clavicle, a Tikhoff-Linberg approach provides extensile exposure. This approach is reserved for patients for whom a deltopectoral or deltoid splitting approach will not provide enough exposure for adequate margins in resection. With this approach, the recommended reconstructive option is an endoprosthesis anchored to the remaining scapula or a resection arthroplasty with the remaining humerus anchored to the scapula or clavicle. The goal is for the patient to maintain elbow and hand function; no shoulder function is expected apart from some scapulothoracic motion. It is possible to power a shoulder arthroplasty with the described tendon transfers when the deltoid is sacrificed, but this is beyond the scope of this chapter. The Tikhoff-Linberg approach and exposure is demonstrated in **FIGURE 48.2.**

Utilitarian Extensile Deltopectoral Approach

When the shoulder girdle tumor is amenable to resection with preservation of the deltoid and its innervation, a more functional glenohumeral joint can be reconstructed. A utilitarian or extensile deltopectoral approach allows for adequate visualization for resection of proximal humerus tumors and reconstruction. When deltoid function can be preserved, we prefer shoulder reconstruction using an RTSA. Because of prior biopsy placement in the anterior one-third of the deltoid muscle belly, the deltopectoral approach should excise the biopsy tract of the skin and portion of the deltoid previously contaminated during the sarcoma resection. The extensile deltopectoral approach **(VIDEO 48.1)** was used in the patient represented in **FIGURE 48.3.**

A posterior extension of this incision may also be useful. This utilitarian approach extends the anterior incision from the mid-clavicle, crossing over the trapezius, and across the mid-spine of the scapula and down its lateral border. This allows for elevation of a large fasciocutaneous flap and access to preserve neurovascular structures during resection; specifically, the axillary nerve and posterior humeral circumflex artery in the quadrangular space, as well as the radial nerve and profunda brachii artery in the triangular interval. This extension effectively converts the extensile deltopectoral approach into a modification of the Tikhoff-Linberg approach.

RECONSTRUCTIVE OPTIONS

Significant challenges exist for reconstruction of the shoulder girdle after tumor resection. One must consider the state of the host, adequacy of the remaining soft tissues, and whether radiation and/or chemotherapy were employed. It is critical to consider the remaining neurovascular and bony structures that determine the ultimate function of the eventual reconstruction. In frail hosts with extensive metastatic disease, a simple reconstruction may be the best solution. Many of these frail patients are not good candidates for staged or multiple procedures.

Once the shoulder girdle tumor has been resected with adequate margins, reconstruction can begin. Reconstructive alternatives include arthroplasty and nonarthroplasty options. These options should be extensively reviewed with the patient preoperatively and alternate plans made if the original plan is not viable after resection. Arthroplasty options include hemiarthroplasty and RTSA, both with allograft prosthetic composite (APC) reconstruction or an all-metal modular tumor prosthesis. The decision to perform an RTSA versus hemiarthroplasty is discussed in the next section. Nonarthroplasty options include resection arthroplasty, amputation, and arthrodesis and are briefly explored.

Arthroplasty Option

The decision to perform an RTSA versus hemiarthroplasty depends on the remaining viable deltoid and glenoid. With the advent of APC reconstruction and advances in tumor prostheses, major defects in the humerus can be accommodated but not so on the glenoid. For an RTSA to work, there must be adequate glenoid for stable baseplate fixation and at least two heads of the deltoid that are functional. Resection of the glenoid, axillary nerve, or entire deltoid eliminates the RTSA option. In cases with some scapular vault remaining, a custom baseplate RTSA can be used but is expensive. There are limited data to support the use of a pec major transfer to make up for a deficient deltoid.[15] The advantage of an RTSA over the hemiarthroplasty is enhanced stability and range of motion.[16] Grosel et al compared RTSA to hemiarthroplasty for proximal humeral reconstruction after tumor resection and found that RTSA had better elevation (85°) and a lower

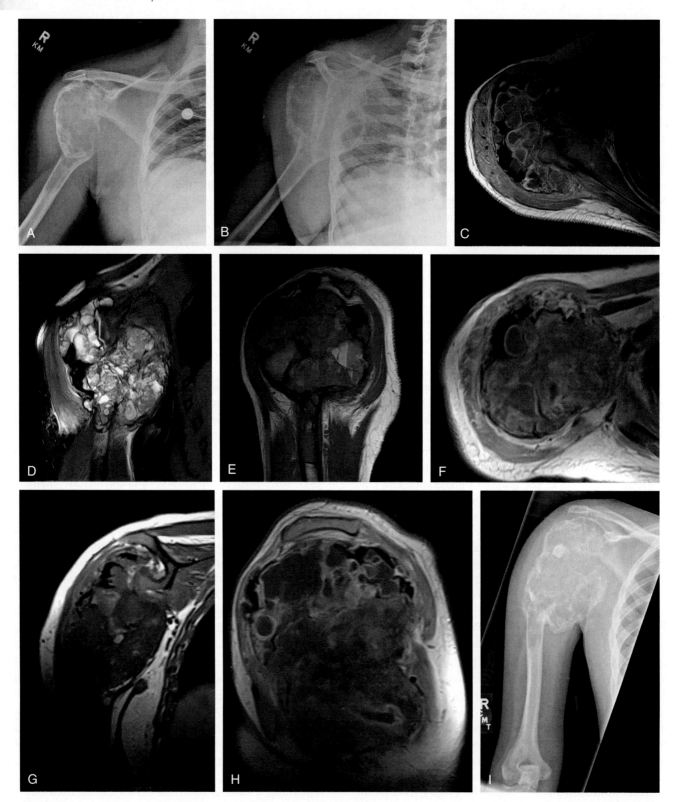

FIGURE 48.2 Hemiarthroplasty. **A**, Anteroposterior (AP) radiograph of the proximal humerus with osteosarcoma. **B**, Lateral radiograph of the proximal humerus with osteosarcoma. **C**, Axial magnetic resonance imaging (MRI) cut of the humerus demonstrating the extent of the osteosarcoma. **D**, Coronal MRI cut of the humerus demonstrating the extent of the osteosarcoma. **E**, Sagittal MRI cut of the humerus demonstrating the extent of the osteosarcoma. **F**, Axial MRI cut of the humerus demonstrating the extent of the osteosarcoma after chemotherapy. **G**, Coronal MRI cut of the humerus demonstrating the extent of the osteosarcoma after chemotherapy. **H**, Sagittal MRI cut of the humerus demonstrating the extent of the osteosarcoma after chemotherapy. **I**, AP radiograph of the proximal humerus with osteosarcoma after chemotherapy.

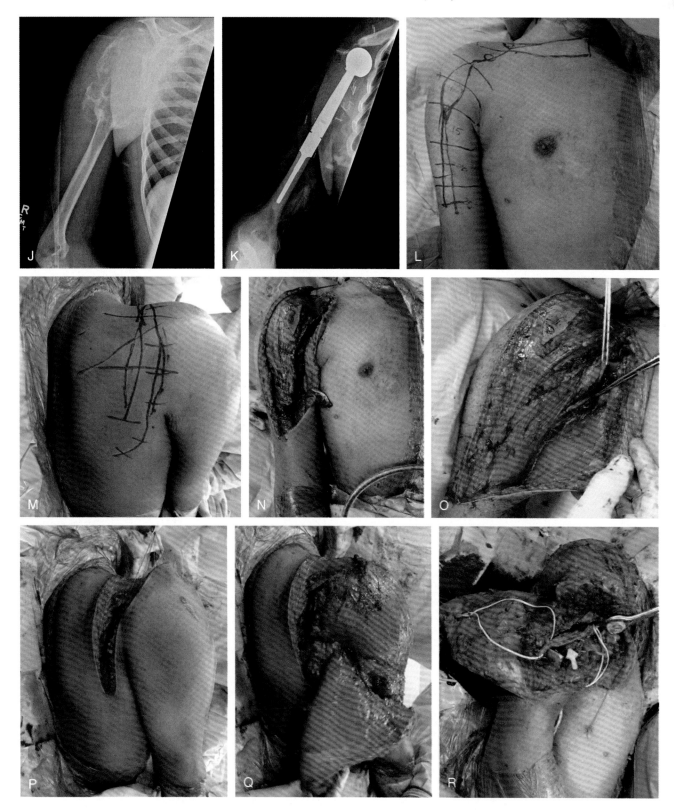

FIGURE 48.2 Cont'd **J**, Lateral radiograph of the proximal humerus with osteosarcoma after chemotherapy. **K**, AP radiograph of the proximal humerus 2 weeks after reverse total shoulder proximal humeral replacement prosthesis. **L**, Anterior view of the shoulder with potential incisions. **M**, Posterior view of the shoulder with potential incisions. **N**, Anterior superficial Tikhoff-Linberg approach to the shoulder. **O**, Anterior superficial Tikhoff-Linberg approach to shoulder with elevated fasciocutaneous flap. **P**, Posterior superficial Tikhoff-Linberg approach to the shoulder. **Q**, Posterior superficial Tikhoff-Linberg approach to the shoulder with elevated fasciocutaneous flap. **R**, Tikhoff-Linberg approach with cut end of the humerus elevated with the neurovascular bundle identified with an arrow.

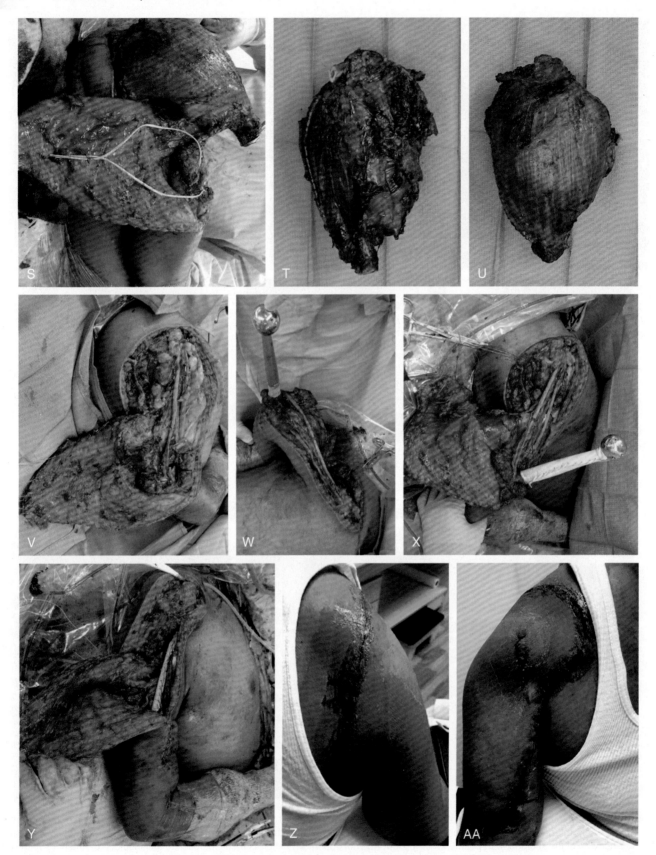

FIGURE 48.2 Cont'd **S**, Tikhoff-Linberg approach with cut end of the humerus elevated, posterior view. **T**, Medial view of the resected specimen. **U**, Lateral view of the resected specimen. **V**, Lateral view of the shoulder after the specimen is resected with skeletonized neurovascular structures. **W**, Hemiarthroplasty endoprosthesis cemented into the remaining humerus. **X**, Gore-Tex Dual Mesh sutured around endoprosthesis to minimize abrasion to neurovascular structures. **Y**, Hemiarthroplasty endoprosthesis reduced an sutured to remaining scapula and clavicle with Mersiline tape. **Z**, 2-week postoperative posterior view of the incision. **AA**, 2-week postoperative anterior view of the incision.

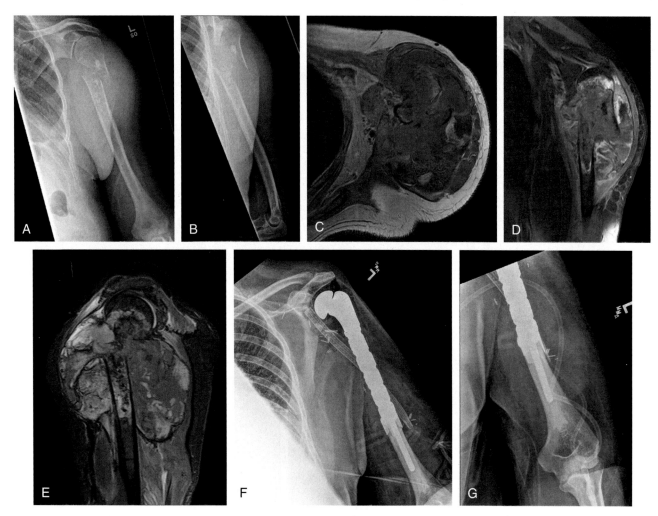

FIGURE 48.3 Hemiarthroplasty. **A**, Anteroposterior (AP) radiograph of the proximal humerus with dedifferentiated chondrosarcoma. **B**, Lateral radiograph of the proximal humerus with dedifferentiated chondrosarcoma. **C**, Axial magnetic resonance imaging (MRI) cut of the humerus demonstrating the extent of the dedifferentiated chondrosarcoma. **D**, Coronal MRI cut of the humerus demonstrating the extent of the dedifferentiated chondrosarcoma. **E**, Sagittal MRI cut of the humerus demonstrating the extent of the dedifferentiated chondrosarcoma. **F**, AP radiograph of the proximal humerus after dedifferentiated chondrosarcoma resection and proximal humeral endoprosthesis hemiarthroplasty. **G**, AP radiograph of the distal humerus after dedifferentiated chondrosarcoma resection and proximal humeral endoprosthesis hemiarthroplasty. See **VIDEO 48.1**.

complication rate (10%) compared to hemiarthroplasty (28° and 34%, respectively).[17]

If the deltoid, axillary nerve, or glenoid is resected, a hemiarthroplasty is the best arthroplasty option (see **FIGURE 48.2**). If the humeral resection is beyond the deltoid insertion, hemiarthroplasty that is modular and easily convertible to RTSA is a reasonable temporary or permanent solution. The biggest concern with hemiarthroplasty is provision of stability. Both Tan and Fujibuchi independently showed that the use of a synthetic mesh markedly improved stability with hemiarthroplasties and provided some additional motion over hemiarthroplasties stabilized with biologic tissue alone.[18,19] Appropriate tensioning of an RTSA when the deltoid insertion site has been resected is difficult, often resulting in dislocation of the RTSA. If dislocation occurs and there are no neurovascular consequences, then leaving the implant

dislocated for 4 to 6 months to allow deltoid healing is recommended before revising the modular arthroplasty to get the appropriate tension. It might be best with these large resections to plan a two-stage procedure either as a hemiarthroplasty with revision to an RTSA or an RTSA with a planned retensioning second procedure. However, it is very important to work with a modular implant that will allow for changes in length. If planned appropriately, the secondary procedure can be relatively minor.

Most reports on large proximal humeral resections have been on allograft composite reconstructions, usually hemiarthroplasties. Beaino et al evaluated APC reconstructions **(FIGURE 48.4)** at a minimum of 5-year follow-up and found a 10% revision rate.[8] However, today, a number of companies have developed a modular tumor implant for both hemiarthroplasty and RTSA reconstructions[20-22] **(FIGURES 48.5 and 48.6)**.

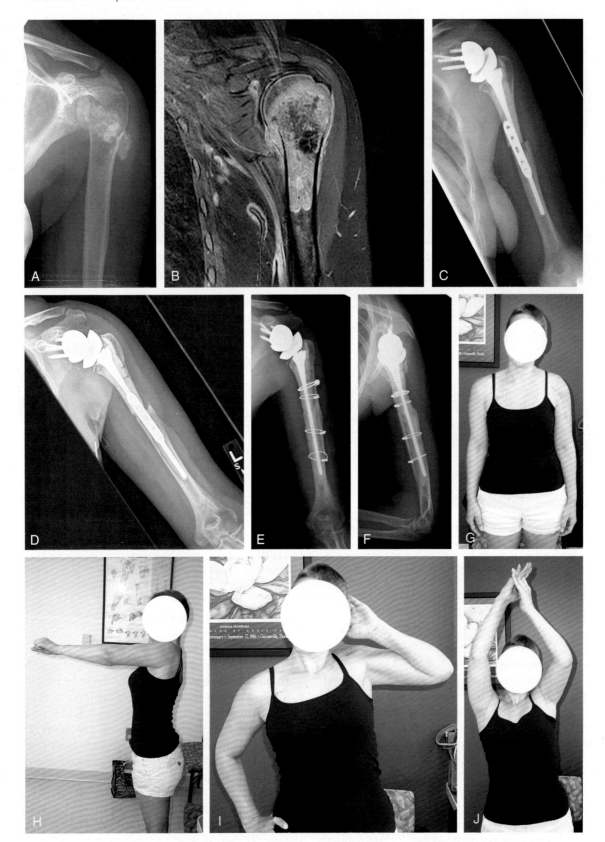

FIGURE 48.4 Allograft prosthesis composite. **A**, Radiograph of the proximal humerus with osteosarcoma. **B**, Magnetic resonance image (MRI) of the humerus demonstrating the extent of the osteosarcoma. **C**, Reverse allograft prosthetic composite (APC) reconstruction after resection of the osteosarcoma. **D**, 24 months after nonunion with loss of stability at the APC junction. **E**, Radiograph showing salvage with revision APC with the only allograft. **F**, Lateral radiograph showing the same reconstruction as E.**G**, Photograph of patient approximately 5 years postrevision. **H**, Patient performing active forward flexion. **I**, Patient actively touching the back of her head. **J**, Patient abducting her arm.

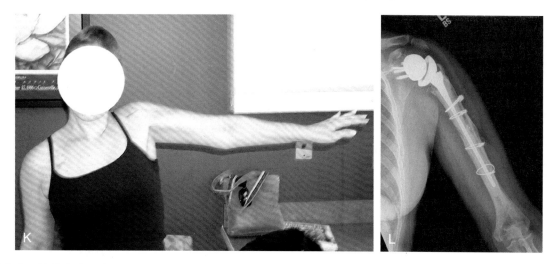

FIGURE 48.4 Cont'd **K**, Patient demonstrating active-assisted elevation. **L**, Anteroposterior (AP) radiograph 12 years s/p revision APC reverse.

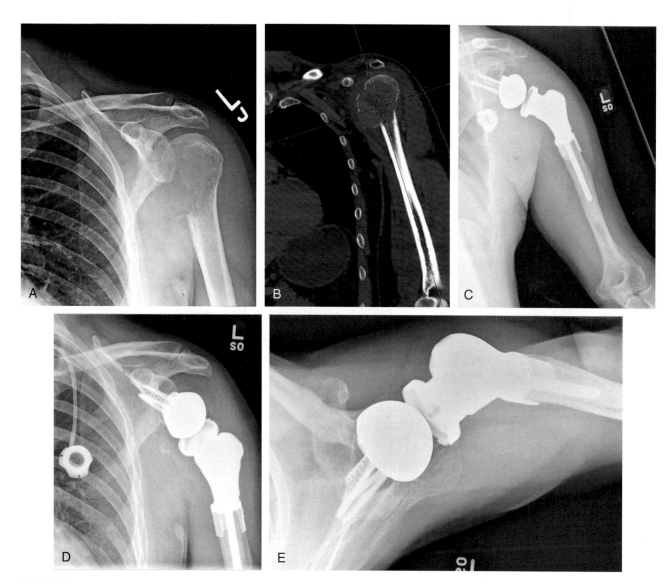

FIGURE 48.5 A, Grashey view of the proximal humerus lesion with impending pathologic fracture from renal cell metastasis. **B**, Computed tomography (CT) of the same lesion. **C**, Radiograph 2.5 years postresection and reconstruction with a humeral reconstruction prosthesis (HRP Exactech, Inc, Gainesville FL). Pt has no pain and 130° of active elevation, 10° active external rotation, and internal rotation to T10. **D**, Grashey closer view of the same reconstruction 2.5 years postop. **E**, Axillary lateral 2.5 years postreconstruction.

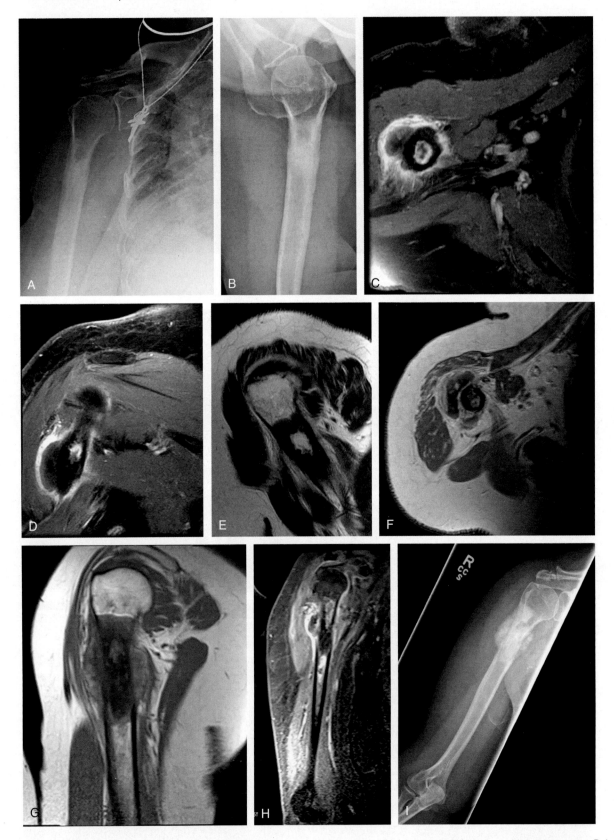

FIGURE 48.6 Humeral replacement prosthesis reverse. **A**, Anteroposterior (AP) radiograph of the proximal humerus with osteosarcoma. **B**, Lateral radiograph of the proximal humerus with osteosarcoma. **C**, Axial magnetic resonance imaging (MRI) cut of the humerus demonstrating the extent of the osteosarcoma. **D**, Coronal MRI cut of the humerus demonstrating the extent of the osteosarcoma. **E**, Sagittal MRI cut of the humerus demonstrating the extent of the osteosarcoma. **F**, Axial MRI cut of the humerus demonstrating the extent of the osteosarcoma after chemotherapy. **G**, Coronal MRI cut of the humerus demonstrating the extent of the osteosarcoma after chemotherapy. **H**, Sagittal MRI cut of the humerus demonstrating the extent of the osteosarcoma after chemotherapy. **I**, AP radiograph of the proximal humerus with osteosarcoma after chemotherapy.

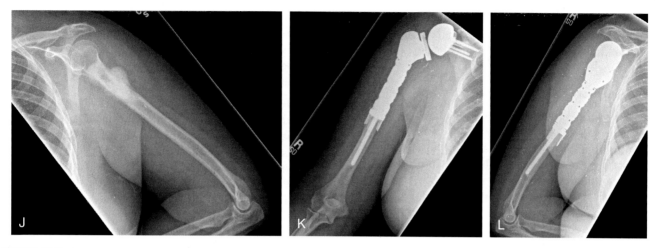

FIGURE 48.6 Cont'd **J**, Lateral radiograph of the proximal humerus with osteosarcoma after chemotherapy. **K**, AP radiograph of the proximal humerus 2 years after reverse total shoulder proximal humeral replacement prosthesis. **L**, Lateral radiograph of proximal humerus 2 years after reverse total shoulder proximal humeral replacement prosthesis.

Reconstruction of these large complex defects can be done with either a hemiarthroplasty or RTSA. RTSA is used increasingly more commonly due to its enhanced benefits of stability, pain relief, and function.[23,24] These implants have two major challenges: (1) long-term stability of the implant host humeral junction and (2) glenohumeral stability. The humeral stem must resist large rotational forces created by the long lever arm of the forearm. This presents a major problem as the forearm moment arm is pitted against the radius of the cemented humeral stem. Over the long-term, the cement mantle will fail. For long-term survivability, the implant must have the ability for bone on-growth. This can be done at the host junction by placing a collar over the stem on the outside of the humerus or via on-growth from compression at the implant host junction. With solid on-growth at the implant host junction, long-term survival can be anticipated. The second challenge of glenohumeral joint stability can be managed with repair of any remaining rotator cuff and maximizing the deltoid wrapping angle, which provides a compressive force to the RTSA, thereby maintaining glenohumeral stability. The wrapping angle can be maximized by using a larger proximal humeral modular body. Additionally, glenohumeral joint stability can be increased using a lateral center-of-rotation implant with a constrained liner.

Massive humeral bone loss distal to the deltoid insertion presents a major additional hurdle as the deltoid must be repaired and tensioned at the same time to maintain stability of an RTSA. In cases of revision surgery, it is less problematic as there is usually an extensive scar rind into which the deltoid can be tensioned. However, in cases of tumor resection, this rind does not exist. In the instance where an RTSA reconstruction dislocates following a take-down and repair at the deltoid insertion, our practice is to allow the shoulder to remain dislocated for 4 to 6 weeks to allow deltoid healing to the implant or APC. Revision surgery can then be performed with a healed deltoid that can be effectively tensioned.

The advantages of metallic reconstruction prosthesis for massive proximal bone loss compared to an allograft composite reconstruction include decreased OR time, less technical demand, ability to adjust tension in the future, no need for allograft host union, no allograft stress fractures, and a likely lower infection rate. The disadvantage may be soft tissue reconstruction and possibly cost, although shorter OR times may ameliorate this.

The results of proximal humeral reconstruction after tumor resection in a small series performed at our institution are promising from a pain standpoint and modest from a functional perspective. In a very preliminary analysis of proximal humeral reconstruction after tumor resection ($N = 12$), there were seven RTSA humeral reconstruction prostheses (HRP Exactech, Inc, Gainesville, FL), three APC RTSAs, and two others in the series. Average follow-up was 31 months with functional scores as follows: shoulder pain and disability index (SPADI), 35; simple shoulder test (SST), 18; American Shoulder and Elbow Surgeons (ASES) score, 71; University of California-Los Angeles, 24. Average active elevation was only 66° with active external rotation of 9°. Two patients (both APC RTSA) had instability issues. One of these two patients also had a fatigue failure of the allograft. An additional APC RTSA required another procedure to manage an APC host junction nonunion. There were no cases of the HRP loosening at the host bone-implant junction. We have noted that these patients functionally improve out to 2 years. The functional results are modest and continue to improve with follow-up, and the complication rate considering the complexity of the problem is reasonable, making an all-metal massive proximal humeral reconstruction implant a viable treatment option.

Nonarthroplasty Options

Patients with extensive involvement of the brachial plexus or vessels with a tumor may be best served with amputation, especially if they are frail hosts. In general, amputations about the shoulder tend to be poor prosthetic candidates. However, prosthesis technology is rapidly advancing, and this may change in the future.

Resection arthroplasty is a relatively simple option with a low complication rate. However, with large resections, the limb is very unstable and must be placed into space using the other limb. The hand, while it might be very functional, is trapped against the patient's side. Orthotics have not worked well with large bony resections about the shoulder. Active hosts are generally unhappy with resection arthroplasty, and this solution has been reserved for salvage or low-functioning poor hosts.

The final nonprosthetic option is a resection arthrodesis. Once union has been obtained, these patients have good pain relief and stability. Active motion is provided by the scapular motors. The biggest deficit is usually internal rotation, though this varies depending on the position of the fusion. Arthrodesis can be performed in the face of a nonfunctional deltoid and some glenoid deficiencies. A significant concern with shoulder arthrodesis after resection of a tumor is obtaining a solid fusion. The upper limb creates a very long moment arm that challenges any type of reconstruction. Resection arthroplasty fusions are performed with an allograft and internal fixation with or without a vascularized fibula.[25,26] Postoperative immobilization can be cumbersome and lengthy, and the complication rate is high.[25]

AUTHORS' PREFERRED APPROACH

We prefer, whenever possible to perform an RTSA with a tumor modular prosthesis. The introduction of these implants came with less surgical time, ease of implantation, modularity, and no need to be concerned about nonunion or fracture, so we rarely use an APC reconstruction. We believe that the infection rate will be less in these implants than in an APC. In resections of the humerus that are distal to the deltoid insertion, we have repaired the deltoid to the implant but expect the RTSA to either dislocate or require retensioning in the future. In other words, we plan on a second procedure in 6 to 8 months once the deltoid is fully healed. It is reasonable instead to place a modular tumor prosthesis hemiarthroplasty in these cases or in hosts with complex medical issues.

Our preferred technique for reconstruction with a functional deltoid and adequate glenoid is to place a reverse modular tumor prosthesis (HRP). After tumor resection with adequate margins, the operation is performed in the following steps.

1. Ream the distal humeral segment—we generally use the 80-mm stem as opposed to the 120-mm stem, as it is easier to revise in the future; however, if there is concern about distal metastatic disease, the longer stem might be indicated.
2. Plane the osteotomy.
3. Trial the ring collet on the minor outer diameter of the osteotomy and ensure that it fits snugly. This is vital for providing rotational stability. Note that the outer surface of the humerus is not round but slightly triangular.
4. Trial the collet and stem together and note the best fit by looking at the relationship of the stem, collet, and humerus. Note that both the stem and collet are eccentric to provide the best fit. As the stem is being cemented, we generally ream 2 mm greater than the implanted stem.
5. Place a cement restrictor at the appropriate depth.
6. Assemble the prosthetic stem and collar/collet on the back table, taking care to reproduce the orientation noted at trialing.
7. Inject and pressurize the antibiotic cement. Remove the upper 1 cm of cement. Place the stem and collet in the same orientation on the humerus as when it was trialed and then tapped into place. Remove excess cement.
8. Turn attention to the glenoid. This can be placed with or without intraoperative navigation (GPS). We recommend placing the baseplate flush or with a slight 1- to 2-mm overhang on the inferior glenoid. Ream and drill the glenoid. We recommend a minimum of three good screws. Use a lateralized glenosphere if the plan is to use a constrained liner, which we recommend with all major resections to enhance stability.
9. Modular trial segments on the stem allow distal proximal tensioning and testing, and multiple-sized bodies allow medial-lateral tensioning (maximize deltoid wrapping angle in order to improve implant stability).
10. Once satisfied with tensioning in both directions, remove the trial assembly, replace it with the actual appropriately sized prosthesis body, and place it on the cemented stem.
11. Repair any reasonable soft tissues to the implant (this will enhance stability).
12. If a hemiarthroplasty is planned, the technique is the same, but no glenoid component is placed, and a hemiarthroplasty is put on top of the stem rather than the cup for an RTSA.
13. Ensure meticulous closure of the deltoid to enhance stability.

14. Tranexamic acid is routinely used; therefore, do not place a drain.

In patients in whom the axillary nerve has been sacrificed or there is minimal functioning deltoid, we place a modular tumor prosthesis hemiarthroplasty and attempt to obtain stability using a Dacron graft. Invariably, these patients have some degree of instability.

We rarely perform arthrodesis anymore. Resection arthroplasties are reserved for the extremely frail host or for a multiple revision surgery patient as a salvage.

In an adequate host, with a functioning deltoid and some glenoid remaining, an RTSA with a modular tumor prosthesis can be a very gratifying reconstructive procedure that provides pain relief, modest function, and motion. With these newer implants, the question of durability still needs to be answered.

REFERENCES

1. Wong JC, Abraham JA. Upper extremity considerations for oncologic surgery. *Orthop Clin North Am.* 2014;45:541-564.
2. Howlader N, Noone A, Krapcho M, et al. *SEER Cancer Statistics Review, 1975-2010.* [Based on the November 2012 SEER data submission, posted to the SEER web site, April 2013]. National Cancer Institute; 2013:9.
3. Surgical management of upper extremity bone metastases: a treatment algorithm. In: Biermann JS, ed. *Orthopaedic Knowledge Update: Musculoskeletal Tumors.* 3rd ed. Wolters Kluwer; 2018:472.
4. Baumann P. Resection of the upper extremity in the region of the shoulder joint. *Khirurgh Arkh Velyaminova.* 1914;30:145.
5. Linberg BE. Interscapulo-thoracic resection for malignant tumors of the shoulder joint region. *J Bone Joint Surg.* 1928;10:344-349.
6. Samilson RL, Morris JM, Thompson RW. Tumors of the scapula. A review of the literature and an analysis of 31 cases. *Clin Orthop.* 1968;58:105-115.
7. Öztürk R, Arıkan ŞM, Toğral G, Güngör BŞ. Malignant tumors of the shoulder girdle: surgical and functional outcomes. *J Orthop Surg.* 2019;27:2309499019838355.
8. El Beaino M, Liu J, Lewis VO, Lin PP. Do early results of proximal humeral allograft-prosthetic composite reconstructions persist at 5-year followup? *Clin Orthop Relat Res.* 2019;477:758-765.
9. Sirveaux F. Reconstruction techniques after proximal humerus tumour resection. *J Orthop Traumatol Sur Res.* 2019;105:S153-S164.
10. Malawer MM, Sugarbaker PH. *Musculoskeletal Cancer Surgery: Treatment of Sarcomas and Allied Diseases.* Springer Science & Business Media; 2001.
11. Kavolius J, Mastorakos D, Pavlovich C, Russo P, Burt M, Brady MS. Resection of metastatic renal cell carcinoma. *J Clin Oncol.* 1998;16:2261-2266.
12. Pazionis TJ, Papanastassiou ID, Maybody M, Healey JH. Embolization of hypervascular bone metastases reduces intraoperative blood loss: a case-control study. *Clin Orthop Relat Res.* 2014;472:3179-3187.
13. Ozaki T, Putzke M, Rödl R, Winkelmann W, Lindner N. Incidence and mechanisms of infiltration of sarcomas in the shoulder. *Clin Orthop Relat Res.* 2002;395:209-215.
14. Abdeen A, Hoang BH, Athanasian EA, Morris CD, Boland PJ, Healey JH. Allograft-prosthesis composite reconstruction of the proximal part of the humerus: functional outcome and survivorship. *J Bone Joint Surg.* 2009;91:2406-2415.
15. Elhassan BT, Wagner ER, Werthel JD, Lehanneur M, Lee J. Outcome of reverse shoulder arthroplasty with pedicled pectoralis transfer in patients with deltoid paralysis. *J Shoulder Elbow Surg.* 2018;27:96-103.
16. Dubina A, Shiu B, Gilotra M, Hasan SA, Lerman D, Ng VY. What is the optimal reconstruction option after the resection of proximal humeral tumors? A systematic review. *Open Orthop J.* 2017;11:203.
17. Grosel TW, Plummer DR, Everhart JS, et al. Reverse total shoulder arthroplasty provides stability and better function than hemiarthroplasty following resection of proximal humerus tumors. *J Shoulder Elbow Surg.* 2019;28:2147-2152.
18. Tang X, Guo W, Yang R, Tang S, Ji T. Synthetic mesh improves shoulder function after intraarticular resection and prosthetic replacement of proximal humerus. *Clin Orthop Relat Res.* 2015;473:1464-1471.
19. Fujibuchi T, Matsumoto S, Shimoji T, et al. New endoprosthesis suspension method with polypropylene monofilament knitted mesh after resection of bone tumors in proximal humerus. *J Shoulder Elbow Surg.* 2015;24:882-888.
20. Trovarelli G, Cappellari A, Angelini A, Pala E, Ruggieri P. What is the survival and function of modular reverse total shoulder prostheses in patients undergoing tumor resections in whom an innervated deltoid muscle can be preserved? *Clin Orthop Relat Res.* 2019;477:2495-2507.
21. Grosel TW, Plummer DR, Mayerson JL, Scharschmidt TJ, Barlow JD. Oncologic reconstruction of the proximal humerus with a reverse total shoulder arthroplasty megaprosthesis. *J Surg Oncol.* 2018;118:867-872.
22. Streitbuerger A, Henrichs M, Gosheger G, et al. Improvement of the shoulder function after large segment resection of the proximal humerus with the use of an inverse tumour prosthesis. *Int Orthop.* 2015;39:355-361.
23. Bonnevialle N, Mansat P, Lebon J, Laffosse J-M, Bonnevialle P. Reverse shoulder arthroplasty for malignant tumors of proximal humerus. *J Shoulder Elbow Surg.* 2015;24:36-44.
24. Kaa A, Jørgensen P, Søjbjerg J, Johannsen H. Reverse shoulder replacement after resection of the proximal humerus for bone tumours. *Bone Joint J.* 2013;95:1551-1555.
25. Bilgin SS. Reconstruction of proximal humeral defects with shoulder arthrodesis using free vascularized fibular graft. *J Bone Joint Surg.* 2012;94:e94.
26. Mimata Y, Nishida J, Sato K, Suzuki Y, Doita M. Glenohumeral arthrodesis for malignant tumor of the shoulder girdle. *J Shoulder Elbow Surg.* 2015;24:174-178.

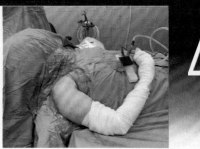

49 Prevention of Infection

Yoav Rosenthal, MD

INTRODUCTION

Although relatively uncommon, periprosthetic joint infection (PJI) is a serious complication of shoulder arthroplasty resulting in revision surgery, an extended hospital stay, prolonged use of antibiotics, and a negative impact on patients' outcome and satisfaction.[1-3] In recent years, the prevalence of shoulder arthroplasty has been steadily growing in the United States (from 13,837 shoulder arthroplasties in 1993 to 79,105 in 2014[4,5]) and is expected to continue to grow.[6] Therefore, despite the relatively consistent incidence of PJI at approximately 1% (ranging from 0.7%-1.8%) for primary cases and between 4% and 15% in revision cases,[7] the total prevalence of PJI of the shoulder is expected to increase as well.[7] This concerning increase in the prevalence of PJI of the shoulder has significant financial implications with rising healthcare expenditures. In North America, the most common management strategy for PJI of the shoulder involves a two-stage protocol.[8,9] Between 2003 and 2012, the mean hospital cost of these staged procedures was $35,825, compared with $16,068 for primary shoulder arthroplasty.[8,9] The potentially devastating effect on the patient's quality of life along with the increased financial burden on the healthcare system compels the surgeon performing shoulder arthroplasty to take all the necessary measures to prevent infection in patients undergoing shoulder arthroplasty. Recognizing the organisms that cause infection in shoulder arthroplasty is essential to select the appropriate prophylactic regimen and to have the most significant preventive impact.

Common Pathogens in Shoulder Arthroplasty

Approximately 85% of PJIs involve a single bacterium.[10] The most common pathogens are *Cutibacterium acnes* (formerly known as *Propionibacterium acnes*), *Staphylococcus epidermidis*, and *Staphylococcus aureus*. Other bacteria identified are coagulase-negative staphylococci, *Corynebacterium*, *Pseudomonas* spp., *Peptostreptococcus* spp., *Finegoldia magna*, *Bacillus* species, *Enterobacter cloacae*, *Proteus mirabilis*, *Staphylococcus albus*, diphtheroid, and *Enterococcus*.[3,9-12]

The remaining 15% of PJIs are polymicrobial, are not well understood, and may involve other types of bacteria.[10] Staphylococci species are very commonly found in *shoulder PJI* (between 27% and 52%[3,11,12]); however, they are not unique to shoulder infection. Nonetheless, most of the prophylactic measures utilized—that is, antibiotics and skin solutions—target staphylococci species. *C. acnes* involves, as a single agent, 27% to 59% of primary PJIs of the shoulder and is more common in revision arthroplasty infections, where it involves up to 70% of isolated bacteria.[3,11-15] Recently, *C. acnes* has been the focus of multiple studies designed to comprehend its role in shoulder infection and prevention.

Cutibacterium acnes

C. acnes is a slow-growing, non–spore-forming, gram-positive anaerobic bacillus. Unlike most of the aforementioned bacteria, which are considered part of the normal superficial skin flora, *C. acnes* colonizes within the acidic, anoxic environment of sebum-rich hair follicles but is also found among the other normal skin flora bacteria. Hair follicles and sebaceous glands are common around the head, neck, groin, back, and shoulder, especially the axilla. Therefore, *C. acnes* infection has been identified primarily about the spine and shoulder.[13,14,16,17] *C. acnes* has also been cultured frequently from glenohumeral joint fluid and tissue specimens taken from patients undergoing primary shoulder arthroplasty. This has raised the possibility that *C. acnes* may play a role in the etiology of glenohumeral osteoarthritis.[18] Several other studies yielded at least one positive *C. acnes* culture from specimen drawn in 20% to 33% of index primary shoulder arthroplasties.[19,20] Maccioni and colleagues demonstrated a low rate of positive *C. acnes* culture by utilizing strict specimen collection techniques. Out of 32 arthroplasty cases, only 3 patients (9.3%) had positive cultures for *C. acnes* in only a third of the total specimens obtained from these patients. Overall, this low rate of infection (3.125% of the specimens), compared to the rates presented in the aforementioned studies, may reflect high rates of *C. acnes* contamination, rather than infection.[21]

C. acnes may gain access to the glenohumeral joint and arthroplasty implants by several routes. First, it may colonize the deep tissues to begin with, prior to any surgery, or can be introduced by prior surgery (as arthroscopy), injection, or by hematogenous spread. Second, it may enter the joint through surgeon's manipulation of the subdermal layer during the surgical approach. Third, although *C. acnes* may be naturally present in deep tissue, it could also penetrate as a simple foreign contamination, originating from a contaminated surgical environment or a member of the surgical team.[14,19]

Multiple studies examined the efficacy of several measures taken throughout the phases of patient care, from preoperative preparations through peri- and intraoperative regimens and the postoperative course. Due to lack of high-quality evidence of some of these strategies, we will extrapolate some data from hip and knee arthroplasties, as well as nonarthroplasty shoulder surgery. In addition, sections of the recently published updated guidelines for the prevention of periprosthetic hip and knee joint infection by the American Academy of Orthopaedic Surgeons (AAOS)[22] and the proceedings of the 2018 International Consensus Meeting on the Prevention of Periprosthetic Shoulder Infections will be presented.[23]

PREOPERATIVE RISK FACTORS AND PROPHYLACTIC MEASURES

General Patient Characteristics

Matsen and colleagues retrospectively reviewed 342 shoulder revision arthroplasties for deep infections. By analyzing 101 cases of positive *C. acnes* cultures, several significant patient risk factors were identified: younger age, male sex, primary osteoarthritis as an indication for surgery, and a relatively lower American Society of Anesthesiologists score.[24]

Obesity

Several studies examined obesity as a risk factor for shoulder PJI. Jiang and colleagues examined 4796 patients who underwent shoulder arthroplasty and found no significant difference in the short-term incidence of superficial or deep wound infection, wound dehiscence, or total wound complications among four different body mass index (BMI) groups of patients (18.5-25 kg/m², 25-30 kg/m², 30-35 kg/m², and 35 kg/m² and above). In fact, no significant difference was found for all complications examined in this study.[25] Similarly, a meta-analysis performed by Klein and colleagues found no significant difference in the infection incidence in patients with BMI below and above 30 kg/m².[26]

This may differ, however, for morbidly obese patients (BMI >40 kg/m²). Theodoulou and colleagues analyzed 10 shoulder arthroplasty studies and found a small increased odds ratio (OR = 1.94) for infection in morbidly obese patients, compared with nonobese patients.[27]

Statz and colleagues examined the outcome of primary reverse total shoulder arthroplasty (RTSA) in 41 morbidly obese patients and reported two cases of infection that requires revision surgery.[28]

Diabetes Mellitus

Diabetes mellitus (DM) is a highly prevalent disease with over 380 million affected worldwide in 2013. The increased postoperative risk of infection has already been established in other surgical fields;[29] however, literature regarding the risk in shoulder arthroplasty is scarce. Richards and colleagues retrospectively investigated 1186 patients with DM who had undergone primary shoulder arthroplasty. The incidence of PJI among these patients was not significantly increased, compared to 3342 patients without DM (1.1% vs 1.0%, respectively) in this cohort.[12]

Cancienne and colleagues, however, queried a much larger national database, including 18,729 primary shoulder arthroplasty patients, of which 43% were previously diagnosed with DM (*n* = 8068). The corrected incidence of superficial wound complication among diabetic patients was 1.4%, compared with 0.9% among nondiabetic patients (OR = 1.22). The corrected incidence of deep infection requiring additional surgery among diabetic patients was 0.7%, compared with 0.4% among nondiabetic patients (OR = 1.47). Furthermore, they found that patients with a threshold HBA1c level greater than 8.0 mg/dL had a significantly higher risk of both wound complications and deep infection requiring surgical intervention.[30] These findings emphasize the importance of examining the preoperative levels of HBA1c in patients with DM and support measures to optimize glycemic control preoperatively.

Smoking

Smoking appears to be a significant risk factor for infection following shoulder arthroplasty. In a cohort including 1834 shoulder arthroplasties (814 smokers and 1020 nonsmokers), Hatta and colleagues identified an increased risk for PJI in smokers.[31] Althoff and colleagues reviewed a database of 14,465 patients, which included 1513 smokers. Smokers had a significantly increased risk for wound complications, as well as superficial and deep surgical site infection.[32] On the other hand, Morris and colleagues did not find an increased incidence of PJI among smokers undergoing RTSA.[33] However, the latter study examined 301 patients, which included only 15 smokers.

Smoking may be a modifiable risk factor as it appears to be an independent risk factor for postoperative infection.[31] Therefore, smoking cessation intervention should be considered in patients undergoing shoulder arthroplasty.

Immunosuppressant Therapy

Organ transplant patients with ongoing immunosuppressive therapy have an increased risk of PJI following both hip and knee arthroplasty.[34] Data regarding the risk of shoulder PJI are limited. In a retrospective cohort of 30 primary shoulder arthroplasties in 25 solid organ transplant patients, compared with a nontransplant cohort of 120 patients, Hatta and colleagues did not identify a significantly increased risk of infection.[35] Notably, Malcolm and colleagues examined perioperative complications of shoulder arthroplasty in organ transplant patients and noticed only a fivefold higher risk of genitourinary infection.[36]

Human Immunodeficiency Virus

According to the 2019 Joint United Nations Programme on HIV/AIDS data sheet, approximately 2.2 million people are living with human immunodeficiency virus (HIV) in North America and Western and Central Europe.[37] Bala and colleagues investigated complications following total shoulder arthroplasty in patients with HIV infection. Retrospectively reviewing a database of 51 million patient records, they identified 2528 patients with HIV infection who underwent shoulder arthroplasty. The authors identified a significant increased risk of shoulder PJI both within 90 days postoperatively and within 2-year postoperatively.[38]

Asymptomatic Bacteriuria

Asymptomatic bacteriuria refers to the presence of true bacteriuria without any signs and symptoms of urinary tract infection. In a large meta-analysis, including 2043 patients in 11 studies undergoing hip and knee arthroplasty with preoperative asymptomatic bacteriuria, Gomez-Ochoa and colleagues found an increased proportion (twofold) of surgical site infection in patients with asymptomatic bacteriuria, compared with the comparison group. However, the same microorganism was identified in the both sites in only 12.7% of the patients with surgical site infection. As expected, the most common bacteria cultured in urine was *Escherichia coli*, whereas the most common bacteria causing surgical site infection was gram-positive cocci.[39] This makes the causal relationship between asymptomatic bacteriuria and surgical site infection questionable. Therefore, routine urinary screening prior to elective total joint arthroplasty is not recommended, as antibiotic treatment of asymptomatic bacteriuria has not been shown to reduce the risk of PJI.[40]

Preoperative Intra-Articular Corticosteroid Injection

Garrigues and colleagues at the 2018 International Consensus Meeting on Orthopedic Infections identified four studies that directly investigated the effect of corticosteroids injections to the shoulder prior to shoulder arthroplasty. They found a significant increase in the risk of postoperative PJI following shoulder arthroplasty if performed within 3 months of an injection, compared with noninjection. No significant difference was observed for arthroplasties performed 3 to 12 months after an injection.[23] These findings strongly suggest that shoulder arthroplasty should not be performed within 3 months following a corticosteroid injection to the shoulder.

In a recent large, retrospective cohort, Forsythe and colleagues investigated 12,060 patients who received a corticosteroid injection prior to arthroscopic rotator cuff repair. Patients receiving an injection within 1 month prior to surgery had a significantly increased risk of infection following surgery, whereas patients receiving an injection 1 to 3 months, 4 to 6 months, or 7 to 12 months prior to surgery were not at an increased risk of infection postoperatively.[41] Although this study focused on arthroscopic rotator cuff repairs, the results provide further support for avoiding corticosteroid injections prior to planned shoulder arthroplasty.

The issue of the frequency of intra-articular corticosteroid injections preoperatively and the risk of PJI has not been reported for shoulder arthroplasty. However, Chambers and colleagues demonstrated and increased risk of PJI (in patients receiving multiple injections within the 12 months preceding hip replacement).[42]

History of Axillary Lymph Node Dissection

Padegimas and colleagues reviewed 32 shoulder arthroplasty cases in female patients with a history of cancer, who had previously undergone axillary lymph node dissection (ALND). In this retrospective cohort, two patients developed incisional cellulitis and were treated successfully with oral antibiotics. There were no cases of PJI documented. Based on these data, the authors' conclusion was that previously performed ALND is not a contraindication for shoulder arthroplasty performed through a deltopectoral incision.[43]

Properly addressing preoperative patient risk factor may play an important role in the reduction of the risk of PJI following shoulder arthroplasty. Published studies suggest that smoking cessation, optimization of glycemic control (>8.0 mg/dL), and perhaps weight reduction (to BMI <40 kg/m^2) may diminish the risk of infection. Furthermore, avoiding arthroplasty within 3 months of an intra-articular steroid injection is recommended. Asymptomatic bacteriuria and a history of ALND do not appear to be a risk factor for infection following shoulder arthroplasty.

PERIOPERATIVE AND INTRAOPERATIVE PROPHYLACTIC MEASURES

Preoperative Home Chlorhexidine Wash

Since a substantial percentage of PJIs is caused by normal skin flora, the important question to answer is what are the most effective prophylactic measures that can be used preoperatively and intraoperatively? Murray and colleagues investigated the effect of preoperative home application of chlorhexidine versus standard soap-and-water shower before shoulder surgery (mostly shoulder arthroscopy). The overall positive culture rate from the posterior shoulder and axilla was significantly reduced for the chlorhexidine group. This reduction was most prominent in coagulase-negative *Staphylococcus* and *Corynebacterium*, but not in *C. acnes*.[44] The *latter* finding was confirmed by Matsen and colleagues, as chlorhexidine was found efficient in reducing coagulase-negative *Staphylococcus* and several other bacteria but unsuccessful in reducing *C. acnes*.[45]

The complete home chlorhexidine protocol consists of showering with soap and water the evening before surgery, followed by wiping the axilla, shoulder, and ipsilateral chest and back, with a 2% chlorhexidine gluconate–impregnated cloth 1 hour after showering. In the morning of surgery, the patient is instructed to apply the 2% chlorhexidine gluconate–impregnated cloth again in the manner performed the previous night and within 2 hours of departing for the hospital. The authors concluded that it may be valuable to apply home chlorhexidine cloths, especially considering that they are inexpensive and safe.[44]

Nasal Decolonization

Between 17% and 28% of patients undergoing elective total joint arthroplasty have a positive preoperative nasal screening for *S. aureus*.[46-49] The identified risk factors for nasal *S. aureus* colonization are DM, immunosuppression, and renal insufficiency.[48] Preoperative *Staphylococcus aureus* nasal screening and decolonization programs have been proven to lower postoperative surgical site infection rates in cardiac surgery, as well as hip and knee replacement surgery.[47,50,51] A single preoperative application of 10% povidone-iodine should be effective and sufficient for short-term suppression (up to 4-6 hours) of *S. aureus* during the perioperative period.[46,52] Furthermore, a cost analysis performed by Stambough and colleagues revealed a significant economic gain for the health system with the use of a nasal screening and decolonization protocol as a result of reduced hospital costs.[53]

Preoperative Prophylactic Antibiotics

The evidence to support a specific prophylactic perioperative antibiotic regimen is of limited strength. Both AAOS guidelines and the proceedings from the 2018 International Consensus Meeting recommend cefazolin (2 g intravenous [IV] or 3 g if patient weight exceeds 120 kg) 30 to 60 minutes prior to incision as the first line of perioperative prophylaxis.[22,23] For patients with history of methicillin-resistant *S. aureus* (MRSA) infection or colonization, vancomycin (15 mg/kg) within 2 hours

prior to incision is recommended, and for patients with proven serious β-lactam allergy, clindamycin (15 mg/kg) within 2 hours prior to incision is the treatment of choice. Redosing should be given every 4 hours for the cefazolin regimen.[23]

Since the aforementioned regimens provide partial coverage of the most common organisms causing shoulder PJI, doxycycline was examined as an additional prophylactic option. In a randomized controlled study, Rao and colleagues did not observe a significant reduction of *C. acnes* cultures in the skin, dermis, or glenohumeral joint of shoulder arthroplasty patients receiving a combination of doxycycline and cefazolin, compared to cefazolin only.[54]

The routine addition of vancomycin to the standard prophylactic regimen is still a matter of debate.[55] In addition, patients receiving prophylactic treatment with both cefazolin and vancomycin, have a markedly increased risk of developing acute kidney injury, compared with patients receiving cefazolin alone.[56] Therefore, the addition of vancomycin should be reserved only for patients with a high risk of MRSA infection.

Axillary Hair Removal

Preoperative removal of axillary hair has been proposed as a method to decrease the rate of infection in shoulder surgery, especially due to the colonization of *C. acnes* in hair follicles. However, there is no consensus among surgeons regarding this regimen.[57] Saltzman and colleagues examined the efficacy of different skin solutions in 150 patients. They noticed that 25% of the patients had voluntarily shaved their axillary hair as preparation for surgery. No statistically significant difference in the rate of positive cultures was detected between those who had shaved their axilla and those who had not.[58]

Marecek and colleagues also compared shaving and no shaving regimens and found no significant difference in the burden of *C. acnes* between shaved and unshaved axillae. Surprisingly, there was a significantly greater total bacterial burden in the shaved group.[59]

Both studies support the conclusion that preoperative shaving of the axilla has no beneficial effect on decreasing the risk of infection.

Surgical Skin Preparation

Skin cleansing at the operation site with antiseptic solutions is routinely performed in the operating room before draping and skin incision. This skin preparation aims to reduce the microorganism load present on the skin. Multiple studies have evaluated the efficacy of various skin solutions in reducing bacterial load before and after the incision. However, evidence demonstrating statistically significant differences in surgical site infection when comparing different routines is either limited or low.[60]

Chlorhexidine

It is important to use an effective skin preparation solution to eliminate as much skin flora as possible and prevent seeding of the surgical incision. Saltzman and colleagues studied the native skin flora about the shoulder and the efficacy of different skin solutions. Based on their study, the most isolated bacteria on the skin of the shoulder, prior to preparation, was coagulase-negative staphylococci, C. acnes, and Corynebacterium. This level 1 study compared a solution composed of 2% chlorhexidine gluconate and 70% isopropyl alcohol, a solution containing 0.7% iodophor and 74% isopropyl alcohol, and povidone-iodine scrub and paint (0.75% iodine scrub and 1% iodine paint). The 2% chlorhexidine gluconate and 70% isopropyl alcohol solution was found most effective in eliminating the overall surface bacteria, as manifested by the rate of positive cultures obtained after skin preparation. The 2% chlorhexidine gluconate and 70% isopropyl alcohol solution was as effective as the 0.7% iodophor and 74% isopropyl alcohol solution in eliminating coagulase-negative staphylococci, and both were more effective than the povidone-iodine solution. None of the preparation solutions showed superiority in eliminating C. acnes, since the total number of positive C. acnes cultures obtained after preparation was too small to allow clinical significance.[58] Two additional studies failed to show effective eradication of C. acnes with chlorhexidine skin preparations.[61,62]

Benzoyl Peroxide

Benzoyl peroxide was found effective for the treatment of acne, due to its ability to penetrate the follicles of sebaceous glands in the dermis.[63] Therefore, several studies were conducted to test its efficacy in eradicating C. acnes around the shoulder.

A double-blind randomized controlled study performed recently by Van Diek and colleagues examined 30 patients who were screened and tested positive for the presence of C. acnes on the skin of their shoulder. Then they applied benzoyl peroxide gel five times, and skin swabs were cultured. Applying benzoyl peroxide gel was found to effectively reduce the presence of C. acnes by 51.4%, compared with the control group.[64]

An earlier study performed by Duvall and colleagues, which examined 34 volunteers, demonstrated significant reduction in C. acnes burden on the shoulder after application of benzoyl peroxide 5%.[65]

Sabetta and colleagues treated patients with a benzoyl peroxide 5% gel to the entire shoulder and axillary region, starting two mornings before scheduled shoulder arthroscopy. They demonstrated a significant reduction in the rate of positive C. acnes cultures from the skin of the anterior deltoid and axilla of the benzoyl peroxide–treated shoulder compared with the nontreated group.[66]

Last, a study designed to reduce the C. acnes load combined benzoyl peroxide and chlorhexidine. The authors did not identify any benefit of combining the two agents; rather, chlorhexidine alone was more effective than the combination for the eradication of C. acnes.[67]

Hydrogen Peroxide

Benzoyl peroxide rapidly decomposes to benzoic acid and hydrogen peroxide. The former is a skin irritant, whereas the latter is the active ingredient. Two studies investigated the efficacy of the addition of 3% hydrogen peroxide. Chalmers and colleagues cultured samples from the skin, dermis, and glenohumeral joint after applying the addition of hydrogen peroxide to a 2% chlorhexidine gluconate and 70% isopropyl alcohol solution in 30 patients undergoing shoulder arthroplasty, compared with 35 patients in the control group. In male patients only, compared with the control group, the hydrogen peroxide treatment group showed a significant reduction in the rate of positive cultures (especially C. acnes) from the skin, dermis, and the glenohumeral joint.[68] Stull and colleagues examined the efficacy of the addition of 3% hydrogen peroxide to chlorhexidine gluconate and povidone-iodine in shoulder arthroscopy. The patients treated with hydrogen peroxide had a reduced rate of positive C. acnes cultures from biopsies taken from the posterior arthroscopic portal, compared with controls (17.1% vs 34.2%, respectively, $P = 0.033$).[69]

Both authors concluded that hydrogen peroxide was both safe and inexpensive and could be added to skin preparation protocols before shoulder surgery.

Skin Barrier Draping

Plastic Adhesive Draping

Plastic adhesive draping has been widely adopted by orthopedic surgeons as a strategy to protect the surgical wound during surgery from organisms that may be present on the surrounding skin by creating a physical sterile barrier.

Yet, studies examining the role of adhesive drapes in reducing surgical site infection and bacterial colonization in surgery have presented conflicting results with little evidence supporting its use.

Bacterial colonization of the skin, while using plastic adhesive drapes in simulated cardiothoracic surgery, was examined by Falk-Brynhildsen and colleagues. They cultured samples taken from prepared skin of 10 healthy volunteers on eight different occasions during a 6-hour simulated surgery and compared bacterial recolonization with or without adhesive plastic draping. They found a significantly increased number of positive cultures drawn from the plastic adhesive drape samples compared with the no drape samples. They concluded that the use of adhesive plastic drapes may accelerate recolonization of the skin during surgery.[70]

Iodine-Impregnated Adhesive Draping

Milandt and colleagues studied the efficacy of *iodine-impregnated adhesive drapes* in bacterial recolonization prevention in 20 patients undergoing a simulated total knee arthroplasty. The skin of both knees was prepared, but only one knee was covered with an iodine-impregnated adhesive drape. Three sets of culture samples taken from both the iodine-impregnated adhesive draped limb and no drape limb showed similar bacteria growth.[71] However, since these studies were simulations, and no incision was performed, the effect of blood and other fluids in the surgical field could not be evaluated.

Rezapoor and colleagues did study the intraoperative effect of iodine-impregnated adhesive drapes and demonstrated a significant reduction in the rate of contamination of the surgical field, compared to no drapes (12% contamination vs 27.5%, respectively). However, separation between the adhesive drape and the skin edges did increase the rate of bacterial contamination.[72]

A Cochrane systematic review conducted by Webster and Alghamdi reviewed seven studies comparing the use of iodine-impregnated adhesive drapes with no drapes in over 3000 patients and found no evidence that adhesive draping reduces surgical site infection rates. They did find, in contrast, some evidence suggesting the adhesive drapes may increase the risk of infection.[73] Clearly, the data concerning use of adhesive drapes with or without iodine impregnation is conflicting. Nonetheless, it seems to have become a standard procedure in orthopedic surgery **(FIGURE 49.1)**.

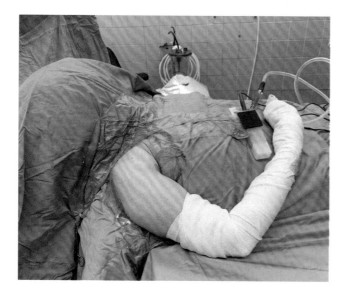

FIGURE 49.1 An iodine-impregnated adhesive drape is utilized to cover the axilla and seal as a barrier between the surrounding skin and the sterile drapes edges.

Replacement of Scalpels and Electrocautery Tips

In effort to avoid introducing skin and subcutaneous contaminants into the deeper tissues, more than half of the orthopedic surgeons replace scalpel blades after the primary skin incision.[74] The theory behind this practice is to prevent contamination of deeper tissues through the continued use of a scalpel, which has been in contact with skin and sebaceous gland flora. Two studies, by Ritter in 1975 and by Grabe in 1985, examined this theory by culturing skin and deep-tissue blades. Both found that most cultures grew staphylococci species. However, in both studies, there was no significant difference in the rate of positive cultures between skin and deep cultures.[75,76]

Recently, Ottesen and colleagues investigated the rate of contamination of skin and deep blades in 277 patients, by using modern skin preparation techniques. Only eight patients (2.8%) had a positive skin blade culture and only five patients (1.8%) had a positive deep-tissue blade culture, which were equal to the positive cultures in the control blade. Both the skin and deep-tissue blades cultured the same bacteria in only one patient. In a different study, Schindler and colleagues found a higher rate of positive cultures from skin (15.3%) and deep-tissue blades (10.8%), but also from the control blade (6.4%). They also reported a higher rate of growth of the same organism on both skin and deep-tissue blades (9.7%). Since the cost involved in the practice of replacing blades is low, they recommended replacing the blades.[77]

Some authors may advocate for the use of electrocautery immediately after the skin incision. In a retrospective study, Shashi and colleagues cultured the electrocautery tip that was collected at the conclusion of hip arthroplasty procedures. Although none of the patients developed an infection within 90 days, 6% of the specimens had positive cultures.[78] In light of these findings, perhaps attention should be given to the electrocautery device with an emphasis on returning it to its holder when not at use and replacing the tip during the procedure.

Wound Protector Sleeve

Since *C. acnes* is believed to emerge from the subdermal layer, it was postulated that a wound protector sleeve, covering the subdermal layer, may reduce the transport of *C. acnes* to the deeper layers. The wound protector sleeve is composed of two thermoplastic rings connected by a polyester film. One ring is laid on the skin and the other is placed deep to the deltoid and pectoralis major. Thus, a "tunnel" is formed, covering the subdermal layer and protecting it from trauma caused by surgical instruments and retractors used in the deeper layers. In shoulder arthroplasty, there is some limited evidence that supports the utilization of a wound protector sleeve. It has been shown to have the potential to isolate the superficial tissue layer from the surgeon's gloves, instruments, and retractors, resulting in a decrease in the rate of *C. acnes* transmission to the deeper tissues.[79]

Antibiotic-Impregnated Cement

Nowinski and colleagues retrospectively collected 501 consecutive primary reverse total shoulder arthroplasties performed by four surgeons. Antibiotic-loaded cement (containing tobramycin, gentamycin, or vancomycin/tobramycin) was used in 236 cases. At an average follow-up of 37 months, no deep wound infections occurred among the patients who had antibiotic-impregnated cement. However, among the 265 cases with non–antibiotic-loaded cement group, eight patients (3.0%) developed a deep wound infection. This difference was clearly significant. Antibiotic regimens in this study were 1 g of tobramycin per 40 g of bone cement, 1 g of vancomycin per 40 g of bone cement, or mixed 1 g of vancomycin and 1.2 g of tobramycin powder.[80] Nonetheless, the AAOS clinical practice guidelines for arthroplasty warns about the possible harm of indiscriminate use of antibiotic-loaded cement because of the potential for microbial resistance, increased risk of loosening by altering the mechanical properties of the cement, and increased costs.[22] At present, the use of antibiotic-loaded cement in primary shoulder arthroplasty cases is not the standard of care. However, its use in revision shoulder arthroplasty and patients at increased risk for infection can be justified.

Subscapularis Tagging Suture Disposal

Roach and colleagues investigated the subscapularis tenotomy tagging sutures as a potential source of infection. In this experiment, prior to subscapularis repair, the authors removed the tagging sutures for culture for comparison with a control group of sutures placed in a sterile container next to the surgical technician. Twenty-four percent of the experiment group cultures were positive, with *Staphylococcus* species and *C. acnes* being the most dominant. Interestingly, 32% of the control group sutures were contaminated as well, but with a wider variety of organisms. Based on the results of this study, the authors recommended replacing the tagging sutures, prior to repairing the subscapularis tendon. Since the 32% of the control sutures were also contaminated, the authors also suggested opening the sutures immediately prior to their use.[81]

Wound Irrigation

Surgical wound irrigation has been traditionally used in surgery with the goal of reducing the bacterial load in a surgical wound by a combination of water pressure, dilution, or the application of antimicrobial agents. Usually irrigation takes place at the end of the surgical procedure, prior to closure, but is also used in arthroplasty prior to implantation. In the Cochrane review of wound irrigation for prevention of surgical site infection, Atkinson and colleagues reviewed 20 studies with over 7000 participants and found that wound irrigation may reduce the rate of infection by 1.3%, whereas the use of antibacterial irrigation (36 studies, 6163 patients) may reduce the incidence of infection by 6%.[82]

Povidone-Iodine

A large retrospective study performed by Brown and colleagues in 2012 evaluated the efficacy of dilute povidone-iodine (Betadine) lavage in hip and knee arthroplasties. According to the described protocol, after implantation of the prosthetic implants, just prior to wound closure, the wound was soaked with 500 mL of 0.35% diluted povidone-iodine solution for 3 minutes and then irrigated with 1 L of saline. The application of povidone-iodine resulted in a sixfold reduction in the incidence of PJI, compared with the pre–povidone-iodine group (0.15% vs 0.97%, respectively). Given the low cost and safety of povidone-iodine, the authors concluded that it is a reasonable measure of infection prophylaxis.[83]

A recent basic science study was conducted by Cichos and colleagues to determine and compare the efficacy of povidone-iodine, vancomycin powder, and chlorhexidine gluconate against seven bacteria species including MRSA and *S. epidermidis*. *C. acnes* was not included in the study. Bacteria time to death for all seven species was immediate upon contact with 1% povidone-iodine and was significantly faster than chlorhexidine gluconate and vancomycin. These results may suggest that exposure of entire joint to povidone-iodine is more important than the duration of exposure. It may be more beneficial to soak the entire surgical field with povidone-iodine solution, rather than waiting for 3 minutes before irrigation of the povidone-iodine solution.[84]

Syringe Versus Pulse Lavage

In the aforementioned Cochrane review, Atkinson and colleagues reviewed two studies investigating the efficacy of pulse lavage and deduced that it may reduce the risk of infection by 11%, compared with no lavage.[82] Of these two studies, only the study by Hargrove and colleagues involved orthopedic surgery. In this prospective randomized multicenter study, patients undergoing hip hemiarthroplasty were divided to a 2-L pulse lavage group (*n* = 164) and a 2-L syringe irrigation group (*n* = 192), both of which utilized normal saline solution. The pulse lavage group had a significantly lower rate of overall infection (5.6% vs 15.6%, respectively) and deep infection (1.8% vs 5.2%, respectively, *P* = 0.009).[85] Although not performed in shoulder arthroplasty patients, these results support the use of pulsatile lavage.

Vancomycin Powder

The intraoperative application of vancomycin powder is commonly used in orthopedic surgery, and its efficacy in reducing surgical site infections has been established in spine surgery.[86] However, a retrospective small-scaled study performed in total hip arthroplasty demonstrated a nonsignificant reduction in the rate of infection in the vancomycin group, compared with the nonvancomycin group (0.3% vs 1.6%, $P = 0.4$). The calculated number needed to treat with topical vancomycin administration was 102 patients in order to prevent one infection.[87]

A retrospective analysis of 272 patients undergoing elbow contracture release, performed by Yan and colleagues, demonstrated a significant reduction of infection in the vancomycin group (0/179), compared with the control group (6/93).[88]

Finally, an economic break-even analysis performed by Hatch and colleagues aimed to assess the cost effectiveness of topical administration of vancomycin powder in shoulder arthroplasty. The authors determined 1 g of vancomycin to be cost effective in preventing PJIs, given an absolute risk reduction of 0.01% to 0.19%.[89]

Administration of topical vancomycin produces a low serum vancomycin level,[90] and the overall adverse event rate in topical vancomycin-treated patients is low (0.3%). Documented adverse events include nephrotoxicity, ototoxicity, and seroma formation.[91]

Based on current literature, there is no evidence to support the administration of topical vancomycin powder specifically in shoulder arthroplasty; however, based on data extrapolated from other orthopedic specialties, there may be a role for its administration in high-risk patients for PJI.[23]

Use of Drain

Multiple studies published between 1997 and 2019, assessing the potential benefit of the use of drains in shoulder surgery, did not support their routine use.

Gartsman and colleagues prospectively investigated the use of drains in 300 consecutive patients undergoing open rotator cuff repair, open anterior shoulder instability repair, and shoulder arthroplasty. There was no statistically significant difference in all measured parameters including infection between the 150 patients who received a drain and the 150 who did not. The authors recommended use of a drain only in cases of excessive bleeding, that is, as fracture cases, revisions, and lysis of adhesions.[92]

Trofa and colleagues conducted a prospective randomized controlled study to determine the benefit of drain use in shoulder arthroplasty. In this study, no significant differences were identified between the drain group ($n = 50$) and the control group ($n = 50$) in all measured outcomes: surgical duration, estimated blood loss, duration of hospital stay, or immediate complications.[93]

Frye and colleagues retrospectively investigated 378 shoulder arthroplasty patients, in which a drain was used in 111 patients. They did not identify a significant relationship between drain use and postoperative complications, including infections, and as such did not support the routine use of drains in shoulder arthroplasty.[94]

Chan and colleagues studied data from a nationwide database and noticed a decreased trend in the use of drains from 25% during 2006 to 16% during 2016. The authors identified no difference in the OR for early postoperative infection between patients with and without drains.[95]

Skin Closure Technique

The objective of a good wound closure is to promote rapid skin healing and an acceptable cosmetic result, while minimizing the risk of complications such as dehiscence and infection.[96]

Staples Versus Sutures

Controversy exists regarding the superior method of wound closure, especially between staples and sutures.

A large meta-analysis by Smith and colleagues investigated six databases during and identified six studies examining this issue in orthopedic surgery. The procedures included hip and knee arthroplasty, hip fracture surgery, and upper and lower extremity open reduction and internal fixations. Overall, 683 wounds were studies, and of those, 332 wounds underwent suture closure and 351 wounds underwent staple closure. Skin sutures included either subcuticular polypropylene or nylon sutures. The authors found that the risk of developing superficial wound infection following staple closure was three times greater than suture closure (17/350 vs 3/333, respectively, $P = 0.01$).[96] Of the six studies presented in this meta-analysis, only one study included the upper limb, and these results were not presented independently from the lower extremity cases.

A later, more updated, meta-analysis, conducted by Krishnan and colleagues, investigated 13 studies (6 of these studies were analyzed in the previous study by Smith and colleagues). All of the included studies provided data on the rate of infection and found no significant difference between suture closure (17/563) and staples (21/692).[97]

Antibiotic-Coated Sutures

The efficacy of antibiotic-coated sutures on the incidence of surgical site infections was investigated in abdominal surgery. Elsolh and colleagues conducted a meta-analysis and identified five eligible studies. Patients with antibiotic-coated sutures had a slightly lower risk of infection, compared with standard sutures (10.4% vs 13%, respectively); however, this difference was not statistically significant ($P = 0.15$). It is unclear whether these results can be extrapolated to shoulder surgery and specifically shoulder arthroplasty.

Wound Dressing

The surgical wound is not hermetically sealed immediately after skin closure, theoretically allowing for penetration of bacteria into the wound. Therefore, wound dressing protocols vary from surgeon to surgeon from simple gauze pads covered by adhesive tape to silver-impregnated dressings. Silver ion's antimicrobial properties have been known for years.

A case-control study of primary hip and knee arthroplasties, performed by Tisosky and colleagues, compared the incidence of superficial and deep wound infections in patients who received a standard dressing, consisting of nonadherent layer and dry gauze (*n* = 525) with patients receiving silver nylon dressings (*n* = 309). Within 12 months of follow-up, the overall infection rate was 8.4% in the standard dressing group, compared with 3.9% in the silver-impregnated dressing group (*P* = 0.012).[98]

To date, no studies have been conducted to investigate the effect of silver-impregnated dressings in shoulder surgery patients. However, these dressing have been shown to possess a killing effect against *C. acnes* in an in vitro model.[99]

Space Suits

Introduced by Sir John Charnley in the 1960s, the body exhaust suit ("space suit"), which later evolved into a sterile surgical helmet system covered by a sterile disposable hood, was designed to create a negative pressure environment within the surgeon's suit in order to decrease airborne bacterial colony–forming units and intraoperative contamination in total joint arthroplasties.[16,100,101] However, studies raising doubts of potential contamination utilizing these systems followed. Moore and colleagues identified an increased bacterial colony count in the background of the operating room that could potentially contaminate the gowns and gloves, when the system's fan was switched on, before wearing the hood and gown. Therefore, the authors recommended switching the fan on only after wearing the hood and gown.[102] More concerning data were published by Kearns and colleagues, demonstrating high rates of intraoperative hood contamination with potential PJI pathogens. The authors of this study recommended replacing surgical gloves if the hood is touched or adjusted during surgery.[100]

Moreover, Hooper and colleagues retrospectively analyzed over 88,000 patients in the New Zealand Joint Registry who had undergone either total hip or knee arthroplasty. In total hip arthroplasty, the authors found a significantly increased rate of revision surgery for deep infection in cases where space suits were used. Total knee arthroplasty performed wearing space suits significantly increased both the rate of revision surgery for deep infection and the incidence of infection, compared

with not wearing a space suit. The authors concluded that there is no benefit in the use of space suits in hip and knee arthroplasty.[103] Similar findings were published in a systematic review performed by Young and colleagues, concluding that surgical helmet systems have not been shown to reduce contamination or deep infection during arthroplasty.[104] Once again, the absence of shoulder arthroplasty specific studies makes it difficult to determine the role of space suits in preventing infection.

Glove Replacement

Within the operating room, surgical gloves play a role in reducing the risks of transmission of bacteria by providing a protective barrier that prevents gross contamination of the surgical field. Moreover, wearing two sets of gloves significantly reduces the number of perforations to the inner glove, compared to the number of perforations occurring when only one glove is worn.[105] It seems, however, that surgical gloves do not retain their sterility throughout the procedure. Davis and colleagues demonstrated that 28.7% of gloves used for surgical preparation before hip or knee arthroplasty were contaminated. The authors recommended that overgloves should be used and replaced before the application of an adhesive covering.[106] Beldame and colleagues investigated different stages of glove contamination in total hip replacements, and despite identifying multiple glove contaminations at different stages, at 1-year follow-up, no surgical infections occurred. The authors recommended, based on isolated bacteria results, to replace gloves at specific stages of the procedure: after draping, bone preparation, joint reduction (which was the phase of most frequent contaminations), and after cementing.[107] Kim and colleagues conducted a systematic review of the glove changes in arthroplasty and added a recommendation to replace gloves at least once an hour, before implantation of the prosthesis, and if a visible perforation was noticed.[108] It is unclear if these recommendations have gained traction in hip and knee arthroplasty, and thus far, glove change protocols have not been used in shoulder arthroplasty procedures.

Operative Time

Longer operative times have been associated with an increased risk of complications in hip, knee, and shoulder arthroplasty.

Wang and colleagues retrospectively reviewed over 17,000 primary total hip and knee arthroplasties with a minimum follow-up of 1 year. The mean operative time for patients with infection occurring within 1 year was significantly longer than those without infection (74.3 and 68.0 minutes, respectively).[109]

Swindell and colleagues investigated the association of operative time and rate of infection following shoulder arthroplasty using a large multicenter registry with prospectively collected data. Over 14,000 patients were divided into three cohorts: procedures lasting less than 90 minutes; procedures lasting 90 to 120 minutes; and those lasting more than 120 minutes. The authors found a significant increase in the risk of complications as operative time increased. Despite finding a correlation between the risk of surgical site infection and operative time, the results were not statistically significant.[110] Despite this limited statistical significance, efforts to reduce the operative time without compromising the quality of patient surgical care would probably be beneficial.[109]

Laminar Airflow

Laminar flow is described as an entire body of air moving with a constant velocity in a single direction along parallel flow lines.[111] The use of operating room ventilation systems leading to ultraclean air environment was introduced by Sir John Charnley in the 1960s, and combined with other strict aseptic regimens, was shown to reduce the rate of PJIs from 8.9%, using a "primitive" operating room ventilation system, to 1.3% utilizing air cleansing systems.[112] However, studies published in the past 10 years focused on lower extremity joint arthroplasty, and fracture fixation repeatedly demonstrated no significant reduction of surgical infections with the use of laminar flow systems, compared with standard ventilation systems.[111,113,114] Recently, in an investigation of over 88,000 hip and knee arthroplasty cases, Hooper and colleagues showed a statistically increased risk of deep infection necessitating revision surgery with the use of laminar flow ventilation, in both total hip and knee arthroplasties, compared with nonlaminar flow ventilation.[103]

Furthermore, the implementation of laminar flow is associated with a substantial cost, as the mean installation cost alone in North America is $140,000. Considering the latest evidence advocating against the efficacy of laminar flow in the reduction PJIs, this cost may not be justified.[115]

No studies have been conducted to investigate the importance of laminar flow in shoulder arthroplasty. However, since laminar flow was designed to reduce wound contamination with contaminated air, and the fact the *C. acnes* plays a substantial role in shoulder PJI originates within the subdermal tissue, and not from the operating room environment, the utilization of laminar flow in shoulder arthroplasty can be even less justified.[115]

Operative Room Traffic

Frequent door openings may correlate with the number of colony-forming units found inside the operating room during surgery and may subsequently increase the rate of PJI.[116] The average number of door openings during primary joint arthroplasty is 60 to 71.1 per case.[117,118] In contrast to previously published studies reporting diminished pressure with single door opening,[119] Weiser

and colleagues demonstrated that single door opening did not depressurize the operating room's positive pressure. However, simultaneous opening of two doors (outer door and inner door) would potentially allow the entrance of contaminated air into the operating room. Therefore, the authors recommended operating room personnel education to avoid opening both doors simultaneously.[120] In attempt to solve frequent door opening, Eskildsen and colleagues installed audible alarms on the door, which activated with door opening. At first, the number of door openings was significantly reduced, but over time, door openings gradually increased, implying that staff adapted to the activated alarm. Eventually, the final door opening rates remained lower, compared with the rates before the experiment had started.[121]

Blood Transfusion

The incidence of blood transfusion following primary shoulder arthroplasty is 2.3% to 11.3% but may be as high as 43%.[122-126] Blood transfusions are associated with an increased complication rate and an extended length of hospitalization.[127] Furthermore, evidence exists that allogenic blood transfusions have known negative immunomodulatory effects, thereby lowering the threshold for PJI.[128,129] Grier and colleagues retrospectively reviewed 7794 patients who received blood transfusions following shoulder arthroplasty and found a significant increased risk of PJI both at 90 days and 2 years.[128] Similarly, Everhart and colleagues found a dose-dependent relationship between blood transfusions and surgical site infection following primary and revision shoulder arthroplasty.[130]

POSTOPERATIVE PROPHYLACTIC MEASURES

IV Antibiotic Treatment—Single Versus Multiple Doses

In a retrospective study, investigating over 20,000 patients, Tan and colleagues found no significant difference in overall PJI between a single dose of antibiotics and multiple doses, but did notice a trend toward a lower PJI in the single-dose group. The benefit of a single antibiotic dose over multiple doses is obvious, as it reduces cost and the potential for antimicrobial resistance.[131]

However, Inabathula and colleagues found that high-risk patients benefit from extended antibiotic prophylaxis following hip and knee arthroplasty.[132] In their study, patients with morbid obesity and DM showed significant reduction in the incidence of 90-day infection rate with a 7-day oral treatment of cefadroxil for standard patients, sulfamethoxazole and trimethoprim for patients who tested positive for MRSA, or clindamycin for allergic patients.

Length of Hospital Stay

Duchman and colleagues investigated 4619 cases for 30-day morbidity following short-stay shoulder arthroplasty (defined as discharge on postoperative day 0 or 1), compared with inpatient shoulder arthroplasty (defined as discharge on postoperative day 2 or greater). A significant difference between the incidences of superficial or deep wound infection was not identified.[133]

Dental Prophylaxis

Hematogenously seeded PJIs may develop following dental procedures, independently of the time of implantation of the prosthetic component. However, treating patients who have had orthopedic implants undergoing dental procedures with prophylactic antibiotics is still controversial. A recent systematic review conducted regarding the role of antibiotic prophylaxis concluded that based on the available evidence, prophylactic treatment is not indicated prior to dental procedures in patients with orthopedic implants.[134]

An AAOS voting panel, based on five criteria, has proposed case-dependent appropriate recommendations regarding prophylactic antibiotic treatment.[135,136] The criteria are type of dental procedure, specifically whether it involves manipulation of gingival or periapical tissues or perforation of the oral mucosa; immunocompromised status; history of DM and the quality of diabetic control based on the HbA$_{1C}$ levels; timing of the orthopedic procedure; and history of PJI that required surgery (**FIGURE 49.2**). If found appropriate, the antimicrobial drug of choice is amoxicillin (2 g, 30-60 minutes prior to dental procedure). If the patient is unable to consume oral medication, ampicillin (2 g intramuscular [IM] or IV, 30-60 minutes prior to dental procedure) or ceftriaxone (1 g IM or IV, 30-60 minutes prior to dental procedure) are recommended. In case of β-lactam anaphylaxis, oral azithromycin (2 g, 30-60 minutes prior to dental procedure) or clarithromycin (500 mg, 30-60 minutes prior to dental procedure) can be prescribed instead of cephalosporins.[136] A useful AAOS online application may be found at https://aaos.webauthor.com/go/auc/auc.cfm?auc_id=224965. Clearly, high-powered evidence is necessary to determine the true efficacy of these regimens. Until then, the AAOS appropriate use criteria may be most useful.

CONCLUSION

Understanding the risk factors and the appropriate measures to minimize PJIs is imperative. This chapter presented many studies that investigated various surgical risk factors, with variable levels of evidence.

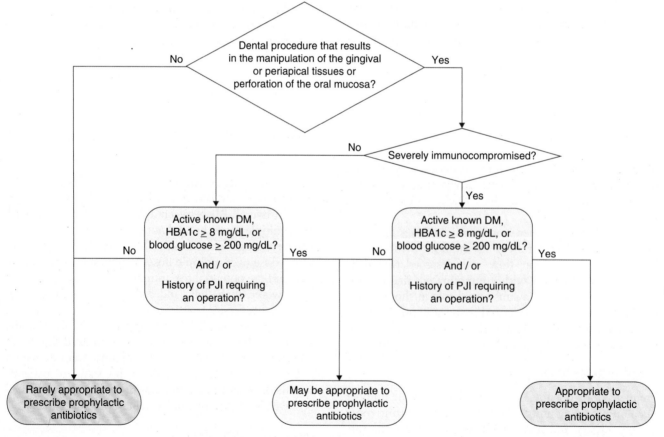

FIGURE 49.2 Management of Patients with Orthopaedic Implants Undergoing Dental Procedures: A simplified flowchart depicting the American Academy of Orthopaedic Surgeons Appropriate Used Criteria guidelines for antibiotic prophylaxis prior to dental procedures in patients with an implanted joint prosthesis.[135] DM, diabetes mellitus; PJI, periprosthetic joint infection. (Reproduced with permission from Quinn RH, Murray JN, Pezold R, Sevarino KS, Members of the Writing, Voting Panels of the AUC for the Management of Patients With Orthopaedic Implants Undergoing Dental Procedures. The American Academy of Orthopaedic Surgeons appropriate use criteria for the management of patients with orthopaedic implants undergoing dental procedures. *J Bone Joint Surg Am.* 2017;99:161-163.)

Shoulder PJI has a low baseline incidence, and statistically, most prophylactic measures may have little impact on the overall rate of infection. It is nearly impossible to enroll an adequate number of patients to conduct a study which will provide the desired power and clinical significance. Since surgical infection is undoubtedly a multifactorial phenomenon, a single measure can only have limited statistical influence on the prevalence of postoperative infections. Thus, the combination of multiple measures may have a more significant effect on the prevention of infection in shoulder arthroplasty. The efficacy of a combination of multiple measures cannot be analyzed with conventional investigational and statistical methods. Yet, as surgeons, we are still obliged to take all steps, within reasonable constraints of both time and cost, to prevent PJIs, even occasionally without adequate evidence to support our decisions.

Author's Recommendations

1. Patient selection—Patients with increased risk of infection should be carefully indicated for shoulder arthroplasty and should be well-informed regarding the potential for and the implications of PJI. Delaying surgery in favor of improving glycemic control and smoking cessation may be valuable since these are modifiable risk factors.

2. Preoperative home skin preparation with 2% chlorhexidine gluconate cloths should be utilized the night before and morning of surgery.

3. Nasal *S. aureus* screening and decolonization with 10% povidone-iodine before surgery.

4. IV antibiotic prophylaxis: cefazolin (2 g IV, 3 g if patient weight exceeds 120 kg) 30 to 60 minutes prior to skin incision; history of MRSA: vancomycin (15 mg/kg) within 2 hours prior to incision; β-lactam allergy: clindamycin (15 mg/kg) within 2 hours prior to incision.

5. Skin preparation with 2% chlorhexidine gluconate and 70% isopropyl alcohol. The addition of benzoyl peroxide or hydrogen peroxide may be considered.

6. Seal the drape edges and cover the axilla with iodine-impregnated adhesive drapes (**FIGURE 49.1**). Change gloves before application of adhesive tapes.

7. Replace scalpel blades after initial skin incision and keep the electrocautery device in its holder when not in use.

8. If cement is used, consider antibiotic-impregnated cement: 1 g of tobramycin per 40 g of bone cement or 1 g of vancomycin per 40 g of bone cement.

9. Routine irrigation with normal saline before implantation and closure.

10. After prosthesis implantation, soak the surgical wound with 500 mL of 0.35% diluted povidone-iodine solution for 1 to 3 minutes, followed by normal saline irrigation.

11. Dispose of subscapularis tagging sutures before repair.

12. Operating room traffic should be limited and door opening should be minimized.

13. Maintain a strict blood transfusion regimen to minimize utilization.

14. Hospital length of stay should be minimized.

REFERENCES

1. Hackett DJ Jr, Crosby LA. Infection prevention in shoulder surgery. *Bull Hosp Jt Dis (2013)*. 2015;73 suppl 1:S140-S144.
2. Alp E, Cevahir F, Ersoy S, Guney A. Incidence and economic burden of prosthetic joint infections in a university hospital: a report from a middle-income country. *J Infect Public Health*. 2016;9:494-498.
3. Kwon YW, Kalainov DM, Rose HA, Bisson LJ, Weiland AJ. Management of early deep infection after rotator cuff repair surgery. *J Shoulder Elbow Surg*. 2005;14:1-5.
4. Kim SH, Wise BL, Zhang Y, Szabo RM. Increasing incidence of shoulder arthroplasty in the United States. *J Bone Joint Surg Am*. 2011;93:2249-2254.
5. Palsis JA, Simpson KN, Matthews JH, Traven S, Eichinger JK, Friedman RJ. Current trends in the use of shoulder arthroplasty in the United States. *Orthopedics*. 2018;41:e416-e423.
6. Farley KX, Wilson JM, Daly CA, Gottschalk MB, Wagner ER. The incidence of shoulder arthroplasty: rise and future projections compared to hip and knee arthroplasty. *JSES Open Access*. 2019;3:244.
7. Padegimas EM, Maltenfort M, Ramsey ML, Williams GR, Parvizi J, Namdari S. Periprosthetic shoulder infection in the United States: incidence and economic burden. *J Shoulder Elbow Surg*. 2015;24:741-746.
8. Baghdadi YMK, Maradit-Kremers H, Dennison T, et al. The hospital cost of two-stage reimplantation for deep infection after shoulder arthroplasty. *JSES Open Access*. 2017;1:15-18.
9. Paxton ES, Green A, Krueger VS. Periprosthetic infections of the shoulder: diagnosis and management. *J Am Acad Orthop Surg*. 2019;27:e935-e944.
10. Flurin L, Greenwood-Quaintance KE, Patel R. Microbiology of polymicrobial prosthetic joint infection. *Diagn Microbiol Infect Dis*. 2019;94:255-259.
11. Coste JS, Reig S, Trojani C, Berg M, Walch G, Boileau P. The management of infection in arthroplasty of the shoulder. *J Bone Joint Surg Br*. 2004;86-B:65-69.
12. Richards J, Inacio MC, Beckett M, et al. Patient and procedure-specific risk factors for deep infection after primary shoulder arthroplasty. *Clin Orthop Relat Res*. 2014;472:2809-2815.
13. Horneff JG, Hsu JE, Huffman GR. *Propionibacterium acnes* infections in shoulder surgery. *Orthop Clin N Am*. 2014;45:515-521.
14. Hsu JE, Bumgarner RE, Matsen FA III. Propionibacterium in shoulder arthroplasty: what we think we know today. *J Bone Joint Surg Am*. 2016;98:597-606.
15. Jacquot A, Sirveaux F, Roche O, Favard L, Clavert P, Mole D. Surgical management of the infected reversed shoulder arthroplasty: a French multicenter study of reoperation in 32 patients. *J Shoulder Elbow Surg*. 2015;24:1713-1722.
16. Clark JJC, Abildgaard JT, Backes J, Hawkins RJ. Preventing infection in shoulder surgery. *J Shoulder Elbow Surg*. 2018;27:1333-1341.
17. Kadler BK, Mehta SS, Funk L. *Propionibacterium acnes* infection after shoulder surgery. *Int J Shoulder Surg*. 2015;9:139-144.
18. Levy O, Iyer S, Atoun E, et al. Propionibacterium acnes: an underestimated etiology in the pathogenesis of osteoarthritis? *J Shoulder Elbow Surg*. 2013;22:505-511.
19. Falconer TM, Baba M, Kruse LM, et al. Contamination of the surgical field with *Propionibacterium acnes* in primary shoulder arthroplasty. *J Bone Joint Surg Am*. 2016;98:1722-1728.
20. Mook WR, Klement MR, Green CL, Hazen KC, Garrigues GE. The incidence of Propionibacterium acnes in open shoulder surgery: a controlled diagnostic study. *J Bone Joint Surg Am*. 2015;97:957-963.

21. Maccioni CB, Woodbridge AB, Balestro JC, et al. Low rate of *Propionibacterium acnes* in arthritic shoulders undergoing primary total shoulder replacement surgery using a strict specimen collection technique. *J Shoulder Elbow Surg.* 2015;24:1206-1211.

22. American Academy of Orthopaedic Surgeons. *Diagnosis and Prevention of Periprosthetic Joint Infections Clinical Practice Guideline.* Accessed September 16, 2019. https://wwwaaosorg/pjiguideline

23. Garrigues GE, Zmistowski B, Cooper AM, Green A; ICM Shoulder Group. Proceedings from the 2018 International Consensus Meeting on Orthopedic Infections: prevention of periprosthetic shoulder infection. *J Shoulder Elbow Surg.* 2019;28:S13-S31.

24. Matsen FA III, Whitson A, Neradilek MB, Pottinger PS, Bertelsen A, Hsu JE. Factors predictive of Cutibacterium periprosthetic shoulder infections: a retrospective study of 342 prosthetic revisions. *J Shoulder Elbow Surg.* 2019;29:1177-1187.

25. Jiang JJ, Somogyi JR, Patel PB, Koh JL, Dirschl DR, Shi LL. Obesity is not associated with increased short-term complications after primary total shoulder arthroplasty. *Clin Orthop Relat Res.* 2016;474:787-795.

26. Klein A, Jauregui JJ, Raff E, Henn RF, Hasan SA, Gilotra M. Early outcomes and complications of obese patients undergoing shoulder arthroplasty: a meta-analysis. *J Clin Orthop Trauma.* 2020;11:S260-S264.

27. Theodoulou A, Krishnan J, Aromataris E. Risk of complications in patients who are obese following upper limb arthroplasty: a systematic review and meta-analysis. *Obes Res Clin Pract.* 2020;14:9-26.

28. Statz JM, Wagner ER, Houdek MT, et al. Outcomes of primary reverse shoulder arthroplasty in patients with morbid obesity. *J Shoulder Elbow Surg.* 2016;25:e191-e198.

29. Lopez LF, Reaven PD, Harman SM. Review: the relationship of hemoglobin A1c to postoperative surgical risk with an emphasis on joint replacement surgery. *J Diabetes Complications.* 2017;31:1710-1718.

30. Cancienne JM, Brockmeier SF, Werner BC. Association of perioperative glycemic control with deep postoperative infection after shoulder arthroplasty in patients with diabetes. *J Am Acad Orthop Surg.* 2018;26:e238-e245.

31. Hatta T, Werthel JD, Wagner ER, et al. Effect of smoking on complications following primary shoulder arthroplasty. *J Shoulder Elbow Surg.* 2017;26:1-6.

32. Althoff AD, Reeves RA, Traven SA, Wilson JM, Woolf SK, Slone HS. Smoking is associated with increased surgical complications following total shoulder arthroplasty: an analysis of 14,465 patients. *J Shoulder Elbow Surg.* 2020;29:491-496.

33. Morris BJ, O'Connor DP, Torres D, Elkousy HA, Gartsman GM, Edwards TB. Risk factors for periprosthetic infection after reverse shoulder arthroplasty. *J Shoulder Elbow Surg.* 2015;24:161-166.

34. Ledford CK, Watters TS, Wellman SS, Attarian DE, Bolognesi MP. Risk versus reward: total joint arthroplasty outcomes after various solid organ transplantations. *J Arthroplasty.* 2014;29:1548-1552.

35. Hatta T, Statz JM, Itoi E, Cofield RH, Sperling JW, Morrey ME. Shoulder arthroplasty in patients with immunosuppression following solid organ transplantation. *J Shoulder Elbow Surg.* 2020;29:44-49.

36. Malcolm TL, Chatha K, Breceda AP, et al. The impact of solid organ transplant history on inpatient complications, mortality, length of stay, and cost for primary total shoulder arthroplasty admissions in the United States. *J Shoulder Elbow Surg.* 2018;27:1429-1436.

37. UNAIDS. *UNAIDS Data 2019.* Accessed November 23, 2020. https://www.unaids.org/en/resources/documents/2019/2019-UNAIDS-data

38. Bala A, Penrose CT, Visgauss JD, et al. Total shoulder arthroplasty in patients with HIV infection: complications, comorbidities, and trends. *J Shoulder Elbow Surg.* 2016;25:1971-1979.

39. Gomez-Ochoa SA, Espin-Chico BB, Garcia-Rueda NA, Vega-Vera A, Osma-Rueda JL. Risk of surgical site infection in patients with asymptomatic bacteriuria or abnormal urinalysis before joint arthroplasty: systematic review and meta-analysis. *Surg Infect (Larchmt).* 2019;20:159-166.

40. Sousa RJG, Abreu MA, Wouthuyzen-Bakker M, Soriano AV. Is routine urinary screening indicated prior to elective total joint arthroplasty? A systematic review and meta-analysis. *J Arthroplasty.* 2019;34:1523-1530.

41. Forsythe B, Agarwalla A, Puzzitiello RN, Sumner S, Romeo AA, Mascarenhas R. The timing of injections prior to arthroscopic rotator cuff repair impacts the risk of surgical site infection. *J Bone Joint Surg Am.* 2019;101:682-687.

42. Chambers AW, Lacy KW, Liow MHL, Manalo JPM, Freiberg AA, Kwon YM. Multiple hip intra-articular steroid injections increase risk of periprosthetic joint infection compared with single injections. *J Arthroplasty.* 2017;32:1980-1983.

43. Padegimas EM, Merkow D, Nicholson TA, et al. Outcomes of shoulder arthroplasty following axillary lymph node dissection. *Shoulder Elbow.* 2019;11:344-352.

44. Murray MR, Saltzman MD, Gryzlo SM, Terry MA, Woodward CC, Nuber GW. Efficacy of preoperative home use of 2% chlorhexidine gluconate cloth before shoulder surgery. *J Shoulder Elbow Surg.* 2011;20:928-933.

45. Matsen FA, Whitson AJ, Hsu JE. While home chlorhexidine washes prior to shoulder surgery lower skin loads of most bacteria, they are not effective against *Cutibacterium (Propionibacterium). Int Orthop.* 2020;44:531-534.

46. Rezapoor M, Nicholson T, Tabatabaee RM, Chen AF, Maltenfort MG, Parvizi J. Povidone-iodine-based solutions for decolonization of nasal Staphylococcus aureus: a randomized, prospective, placebo-controlled study. *J Arthroplasty.* 2017;32:2815-2819.

47. Sporer SM, Rogers T, Abella L. Methicillin-resistant and methicillin-sensitive *Staphylococcus aureus* screening and decolonization to reduce surgical site infection in elective total joint arthroplasty. *J Arthroplasty.* 2016;31:144-147.

48. Walsh AL, Fields AC, Dieterich JD, Chen DD, Bronson MJ, Moucha CS. Risk factors for *Staphylococcus aureus* nasal colonization in joint arthroplasty patients. *J Arthroplasty.* 2018;33:1530-1533.

49. Chen AF, Heyl AE, Xu PZ, Rao N, Klatt BA. Preoperative decolonization effective at reducing staphylococcal colonization in total joint arthroplasty patients. *J Arthroplasty.* 2013;28:18-20.

50. Nicholson MR, Huesman LA. Controlling the usage of intranasal mupirocin does impact the rate of *Staphylococcus aureus* deep sternal wound infections in cardiac surgery patients. *Am J Infect Control.* 2006;34:44-48.

51. Hacek DM, Robb WJ, Paule SM, Kudrna JC, Stamos VP, Peterson LR. *Staphylococcus aureus* nasal decolonization in joint replacement surgery reduces infection. *Clin Orthop Relat Res.* 2008;466:1349-1355.

52. Ghaddara HA, Kumar JA, Cadnum JL, Ng-Wong YK, Donskey CJ. Efficacy of a povidone iodine preparation in reducing nasal methicillin-resistant *Staphylococcus aureus* in colonized patients. *Am J Infect Control.* 2020;48:456-459.

53. Stambough JB, Nam D, Warren DK, et al. Decreased hospital costs and surgical site infection incidence with a universal decolonization protocol in primary total joint arthroplasty. *J Arthroplasty.* 2017;32:728-734 e1.

54. Rao AJ, Chalmers PN, Cvetanovich GL, et al. Preoperative doxycycline does not reduce *Propionibacterium acnes* in shoulder arthroplasty. *J Bone Joint Surg Am.* 2018;100:958-964.

55. Sewick A, Makani A, Wu C, O'Donnell J, Baldwin KD, Lee GC. Does dual antibiotic prophylaxis better prevent surgical site infections in total joint arthroplasty? *Clin Orthop Relat Res.* 2012;470:2702-2707.

56. Courtney PM, Melnic CM, Zimmer Z, Anari J, Lee GC. Addition of vancomycin to cefazolin prophylaxis is associated with acute kidney injury after primary joint arthroplasty. *Clin Orthop Relat Res.* 2015;473:2197-2203.

57. Herrera MF, Bauer G, Reynolds F, Wilk RM, Bigliani LU, Levine WN. Infection after mini-open rotator cuff repair. *J Shoulder Elbow Surg.* 2002;11:605-608.

58. Saltzman MD, Nuber GW, Gryzlo SM, Marecek GS, Koh JL. Efficacy of surgical preparation solutions in shoulder surgery. *J Bone Joint Surg Am.* 2009;91:1949-1953.

59. Marecek GS, Weatherford BM, Fuller EB, Saltzman MD. The effect of axillary hair on surgical antisepsis around the shoulder. *J Shoulder Elbow Surg.* 2015;24:804-808.

60. Dumville JC, McFarlane E, Edwards P, Lipp A, Holmes A. Preoperative skin antiseptics for preventing surgical wound infections after clean surgery. *Cochrane Database Syst Rev*. 2013;(3):CD003949.

61. MacLean SBM, Phadnis J, Ling CM, Bain GI. Application of dermal chlorhexidine antisepsis is ineffective at reducing *Proprionibacterium acnes* colonization in shoulder surgery. *Shoulder Elbow*. 2019;11:98-105.

62. Phadnis J, Gordon D, Krishnan J, Bain GI. Frequent isolation of *Propionibacterium acnes* from the shoulder dermis despite skin preparation and prophylactic antibiotics. *J Shoulder Elbow Surg*. 2016;25:304-310.

63. Bikowski J. A review of the safety and efficacy of benzoyl peroxide (5.3%) emollient foam in the management of truncal acne vulgaris. *J Clin Aesthet Dermatol*. 2010;3:26-29.

64. van Diek FM, Pruijn N, Spijkers KM, Mulder B, Kosse NM, Dorrestijn O. The presence of Cutibacterium acnes on the skin of the shoulder after the use of benzoyl peroxide: a placebo-controlled, double-blinded, randomized trial. *J Shoulder Elbow Surg*. 2020;29:768-774.

65. Duvall G, Kaveeshwar S, Sood A, et al. Benzoyl peroxide use transiently decreases *Cutibacterium acnes* load on the shoulder. *J Shoulder Elbow Surg*. 2020;29:794-798.

66. Sabetta JR, Rana VP, Vadasdi KB, et al. Efficacy of topical benzoyl peroxide on the reduction of *Propionibacterium acnes* during shoulder surgery. *J Shoulder Elbow Surg*. 2015;24:995-1004.

67. Hancock DS, Rupasinghe SL, Elkinson I, Bloomfield MG, Larsen PD. Benzoyl peroxide + chlorhexidine versus chlorhexidine alone skin preparation to reduce Propionibacterium acnes: a randomized controlled trial. *ANZ J Surg*. 2018;88:1182-1186.

68. Chalmers PN, Beck L, Stertz I, Tashjian RZ. Hydrogen peroxide skin preparation reduces Cutibacterium acnes in shoulder arthroplasty: a prospective, blinded, controlled trial. *J Shoulder Elbow Surg*. 2019;28:1554-1561.

69. Stull JD, Nicholson TA, Davis DE, Namdari S. Addition of 3% hydrogen peroxide to standard skin preparation reduces Cutibacterium acnes-positive culture rate in shoulder surgery: a prospective randomized controlled trial. *J Shoulder Elbow Surg*. 2020;29:212-216.

70. Falk-Brynhildsen K, Friberg O, Soderquist B, Nilsson UG. Bacterial colonization of the skin following aseptic preoperative preparation and impact of the use of plastic adhesive drapes. *Biol Res Nurs*. 2013;15:242-248.

71. Milandt N, Nymark T, Jorn Kolmos H, Emmeluth C, Overgaard S. Iodine-impregnated incision drape and bacterial recolonization in simulated total knee arthroplasty. *Acta Orthop*. 2016;87:380-385.

72. Rezapoor M, Tan TL, Maltenfort MG, Parvizi J. Incise draping reduces the rate of contamination of the surgical site during hip surgery: a prospective, randomized trial. *J Arthroplasty*. 2018;33:1891-1895.

73. Webster J, Alghamdi A. Use of plastic adhesive drapes during surgery for preventing surgical site infection. *Cochrane Database Syst Rev*. 2015;(4):CD006353.

74. Tejwani NC, Immerman I. Myths and legends in orthopaedic practice: are we all guilty? *Clin Orthop Relat Res*. 2008;466:2861-2872.

75. Grabe N, Falstie-Jensen S, Fredberg U, Schröder H, Sørensen I. The contaminated skin-knife – Fact or fiction? *J Hosp Infect*. 1985;6:252-256.

76. Ritter MA, French ML, Eitzen HE. Bacterial contamination of the surgical knife. *Clin Orthop Relat Res*. 1975;(108):158-160.

77. Schindler OS, Spencer RF, Smith MD. Should we use a separate knife for the skin? *J Bone Joint Surg Br*. 2006;88:382-385.

78. Shahi A, Chen AF, McKenna PB, et al. Bacterial contamination in tips of electrocautery devices during total hip arthroplasty. *J Arthroplasty*. 2015;30:1410-1413.

79. Smith ML, Gotmaker R, Hoy GA, et al. Minimizing Propionibacterium acnes contamination in shoulder arthroplasty: use of a wound protector. *ANZ J Surg*. 2018;88:1178-1181.

80. Nowinski RJ, Gillespie RJ, Shishani Y, Cohen B, Walch G, Gobezie R. Antibiotic-loaded bone cement reduces deep infection rates for primary reverse total shoulder arthroplasty: a retrospective, cohort study of 501 shoulders. *J Shoulder Elbow Surg*. 2012;21:324-328.

81. Roach R, Yu S, Pham H, Pham V, Virk M, Zuckerman JD. Microbial colonization of subscapularis tagging sutures in shoulder arthroplasty: a prospective, controlled study. *J Shoulder Elbow Surg*. 2019;28:1848-1853.

82. Norman G, Atkinson RA, Smith TA, et al. Intracavity lavage and wound irrigation for prevention of surgical site infection. *Cochrane Database Syst Rev*. 2017;10:CD012234.

83. Brown NM, Cipriano CA, Moric M, Sporer SM, Della Valle CJ. Dilute betadine lavage before closure for the prevention of acute postoperative deep periprosthetic joint infection. *J Arthroplasty*. 2012;27:27-30.

84. Cichos KH, Andrews RM, Wolschendorf F, Narmore W, Mabry SE, Ghanem ES. Efficacy of intraoperative antiseptic techniques in the prevention of periprosthetic joint infection: superiority of betadine. *J Arthroplasty*. 2019;34:S312-S318.

85. Hargrove R, Ridgeway S, Russell R, Norris M, Packham I, Levy B. Does pulse lavage reduce hip hemiarthroplasty infection rates? *J Hosp Infect*. 2006;62:446-449.

86. Hey HW, Thiam DW, Koh ZS, et al. Is intraoperative local vancomycin powder the answer to surgical site infections in spine surgery? *Spine (Phila Pa 1976)*. 2017;42:267-274.

87. Cohen EM, Marcaccio S, Goodman AD, Lemme NJ, Limbird R. Efficacy and cost-effectiveness of topical vancomycin powder in primary cementless total hip arthroplasty. *Orthopedics*. 2019;42:e430-e436.

88. Yan H, He J, Chen S, Yu S, Fan C. Intrawound application of vancomycin reduces wound infection after open release of post-traumatic stiff elbows: a retrospective comparative study. *J Shoulder Elbow Surg*. 2014;23:686-692.

89. Hatch MD, Daniels SD, Glerum KM, Higgins LD. The cost effectiveness of vancomycin for preventing infections after shoulder arthroplasty: a break-even analysis. *J Shoulder Elbow Surg*. 2017;26:472-477.

90. Johnson JD, Nessler JM, Horazdovsky RD, Vang S, Thomas AJ, Marston SB. Serum and wound vancomycin levels after intrawound administration in primary total joint arthroplasty. *J Arthroplasty*. 2017;32:924-928.

91. Ghobrial GM, Cadotte DW, Williams K Jr, Fehlings MG, Harrop JS. Complications from the use of intrawound vancomycin in lumbar spinal surgery: a systematic review. *Neurosurg Focus*. 2015;39:E11.

92. Gartsman GM, Milne JC, Russell JA. Closed wound drainage in shoulder surgery. *J Shoulder Elbow Surg*. 1997;6:288-290.

93. Trofa DP, Paulino FE, Munoz J, et al. Short-term outcomes associated with drain use in shoulder arthroplasties: a prospective, randomized controlled trial. *J Shoulder Elbow Surg*. 2019;28:205-211.

94. Frye BD, Hannon P, Santoni BG, Nydick JA. Drains are not beneficial in primary shoulder arthroplasty. *Orthopedics*. 2019;42:e29-e31.

95. Chan JJ, Cirino CM, Huang HH, et al. Drain use is associated with increased odds of blood transfusion in total shoulder arthroplasty: a population-based study. *Clin Orthop Relat Res*. 2019;477:1700-1711.

96. Smith TO, Sexton D, Mann C, Donell S. Sutures versus staples for skin closure in orthopaedic surgery: meta-analysis. *Br Med J*. 2010;340:c1199.

97. Krishnan R, MacNeil SD, Malvankar-Mehta MS. Comparing sutures versus staples for skin closure after orthopaedic surgery: systematic review and meta-analysis. *BMJ Open*. 2016;6:e009257.

98. Tisosky AJ, Iyoha-Bello O, Demosthenes N, Quimbayo G, Coreanu T, Abdeen A. Use of a silver nylon dressing following total hip and knee arthroplasty decreases the postoperative infection rate. *J Am Acad Orthop Surg Glob Res Rev*. 2017;1:e034.

99. Bowler PG, Welsby S, Hogarth A, Towers V. Topical antimicrobial protection of postoperative surgical sites at risk of infection with Propionibacterium acnes: an in-vitro study. *J Hosp Infect*. 2013;83:232-237.

100. Kearns KA, Witmer D, Makda J, Parvizi J, Jungkind D. Sterility of the personal protection system in total joint arthroplasty. *Clin Orthop Relat Res*. 2011;469:3065-3069.

101. McGovern PD, Albrecht M, Khan SK, Muller SD, Reed MR. The influence of surgical hoods and togas on airborne particle concentration at the surgical site: an experimental study. *J Orthop Sci*. 2013;18:1027-1030.

102. Moores TS, Khan SA, Chatterton BD, Harvey G, Lewthwaite SC. A microbiological assessment of sterile surgical helmet systems using particle counts and culture plates: recommendations for safe use whilst scrubbing. *J Hosp Infect.* 2019;101:354-360.

103. Hooper GJ, Rothwell AG, Frampton C, Wyatt MC. Does the use of laminar flow and space suits reduce early deep infection after total hip and knee replacement?: the ten-year results of the New Zealand Joint Registry. *J Bone Joint Surg Br.* 2011;93:85-90.

104. Young SW, Zhu M, Shirley OC, Wu Q, Spangehl MJ. Do 'surgical helmet systems' or 'body exhaust suits' affect contamination and deep infection rates in arthroplasty? A systematic review. *J Arthroplasty.* 2016;31:225-233.

105. Phillips S. The comparison of double gloving to single gloving in the theatre environment. *J Perioper Pract.* 2011;21:10-15.

106. Davis N, Curry A, Gambhir AK, et al. Intraoperative bacterial contamination in operations for joint replacement. *J Bone Joint Surg Br.* 1999;81:886-889.

107. Beldame J, Lagrave B, Lievain L, Lefebvre B, Frebourg N, Dujardin F. Surgical glove bacterial contamination and perforation during total hip arthroplasty implantation: when gloves should be changed. *Orthop Traumatol Surg Res.* 2012;98:432-440.

108. Kim K, Zhu M, Munro JT, Young SW. Glove change to reduce the risk of surgical site infection or prosthetic joint infection in arthroplasty surgeries: a systematic review. *ANZ J Surg.* 2019;89:1009-1015.

109. Wang Q, Goswami K, Shohat N, Aalirezaie A, Manrique J, Parvizi J. Longer operative time results in a higher rate of subsequent periprosthetic joint infection in patients undergoing primary joint arthroplasty. *J Arthroplasty.* 2019;34:947-953.

110. Swindell HW, Alrabaa RG, Boddapati V, Trofa DP, Jobin CM, Levine WN. Is surgical duration associated with postoperative complications in primary shoulder arthroplasty? *J Shoulder Elbow Surg.* 2020;29:807-813.

111. James M, Khan WS, Nannaparaju MR, Bhamra JS, Morgan-Jones R. Current evidence for the use of laminar flow in reducing infection rates in total joint arthroplasty. *Open Orthop J.* 2015;9:495-498.

112. Charnley J, Eftekhar N. Postoperative infection in total prosthetic replacement arthroplasty of the hip-joint. With special reference to the bacterial content of the air of the operating room. *Br J Surg.* 1969;56:641-649.

113. Singh S, Reddy S, Shrivastava R. Does laminar airflow make a difference to the infection rates for lower limb arthroplasty: a study using the National Joint Registry and local surgical site infection data for two hospitals with and without laminar airflow. *Eur J Orthop Surg Traumatol.* 2017;27:261-265.

114. Pinder EM, Bottle A, Aylin P, Loeffler MD. Does laminar flow ventilation reduce the rate of infection? an observational study of trauma in England. *Bone Joint J.* 2016;98-B:1262-1269.

115. Davis DE, Zmistowski B, Abboud JA, Namdari S. Cost effectiveness of laminar flow systems for total shoulder arthroplasty: filtering money from the OR? *Arch Bone Jt Surg.* 2020;8:38-43.

116. Smith EB, Raphael IJ, Maltenfort MG, Honsawek S, Dolan K, Younkins EA. The effect of laminar air flow and door openings on operating room contamination. *J Arthroplasty.* 2013;28:1482-1485.

117. Bedard M, Pelletier-Roy R, Angers-Goulet M, Leblanc PA, Pelet S. Traffic in the operating room during joint replacement is a multidisciplinary problem. *Can J Surg.* 2015;58:232-236.

118. Panahi P, Stroh M, Casper DS, Parvizi J, Austin MS. Operating room traffic is a major concern during total joint arthroplasty. *Clin Orthop Relat Res.* 2012;470:2690-2694.

119. Mears SC, Blanding R, Belkoff SM. Door opening affects operating room pressure during joint arthroplasty. *Orthopedics.* 2015;38:e991-e994.

120. Weiser MC, Shemesh S, Chen DD, Bronson MJ, Moucha CS. The effect of door opening on positive pressure and airflow in operating rooms. *J Am Acad Orthop Surg.* 2018;26:e105-e113.

121. Eskildsen SM, Moskal PT, Laux J, Del Gaizo DJ. The effect of a door alarm on operating room traffic during total joint arthroplasty. *Orthopedics.* 2017;40:e1081-e1085.

122. Ryan DJ, Yoshihara H, Yoneoka D, Zuckerman JD. Blood transfusion in primary total shoulder arthroplasty: incidence, trends, and risk factors in the United States from 2000 to 2009. *J Shoulder Elbow Surg.* 2015;24:760-765.

123. Dacombe PJ, Kendall JV, McCann P, et al. Blood transfusion rates following shoulder arthroplasty in a high volume UK centre and analysis of risk factors associated with transfusion. *Shoulder Elbow.* 2019;11:67-72.

124. Burns KA, Robbins LM, LeMarr AR, Childress AL, Morton DJ, Wilson ML. Estimated blood loss and anemia predict transfusion after total shoulder arthroplasty: a retrospective cohort study. *JSES Open Access.* 2019;3:311-315.

125. Ahmadi S, Lawrence TM, Sahota S, et al. The incidence and risk factors for blood transfusion in revision shoulder arthroplasty: our institution's experience and review of the literature. *J Shoulder Elbow Surg.* 2014;23:43-48.

126. Gruson KI, Accousti KJ, Parsons BO, Pillai G, Flatow EL. Transfusion after shoulder arthroplasty: an analysis of rates and risk factors. *J Shoulder Elbow Surg.* 2009;18:225-230.

127. King JJ, Patrick MR, Struk AM, et al. Perioperative factors affecting the length of hospitalization after shoulder arthroplasty. *J Am Acad Orthop Surg Glob Res Rev.* 2017;1:e026.

128. Grier AJ, Bala A, Penrose CT, Seyler TM, Bolognesi MP, Garrigues GE. Analysis of complication rates following perioperative transfusion in shoulder arthroplasty. *J Shoulder Elbow Surg.* 2017;26:1203-1209.

129. Rohde JM, Dimcheff DE, Blumberg N, et al. Health care-associated infection after red blood cell transfusion: a systematic review and meta-analysis. *J Am Med Assoc.* 2014;311:1317-1326.

130. Everhart JS, Bishop JY, Barlow JD. Medical comorbidities and perioperative allogeneic red blood cell transfusion are risk factors for surgical site infection after shoulder arthroplasty. *J Shoulder Elbow Surg.* 2017;26:1922-1930.

131. Tan TL, Shohat N, Rondon AJ, et al. Perioperative antibiotic prophylaxis in total joint arthroplasty: a single dose is as effective as multiple doses. *J Bone Joint Surg Am.* 2019;101:429-437.

132. Inabathula A, Dilley JE, Ziemba-Davis M, et al. Extended oral antibiotic prophylaxis in high-risk patients substantially reduces primary total hip and knee arthroplasty 90-day infection rate. *J Bone Joint Surg Am.* 2018;100:2103-2109.

133. Duchman KR, Anthony CA, Westermann RW, Pugely AJ, Gao Y, Hettrich CM. Total shoulder arthroplasty: is less time in the hospital better? *Iowa Orthop J.* 2017;37:109-116.

134. Slullitel PA, Onativia JI, Piuzzi NS, Higuera-Rueda C, Parvizi J, Buttaro MA. Is there a role for antibiotic prophylaxis prior to dental procedures in patients with total joint arthroplasty? A systematic review of the literature. *J Bone Jt Infect.* 2020;5:7-15.

135. Quinn RH, Murray JN, Pezold R, Sevarino KS, Members of the Writing, Voting Panels of the AUC for the Management of Patients With Orthopaedic Implants Undergoing Dental Procedures. The American Academy of Orthopaedic Surgeons appropriate use criteria for the management of patients with orthopaedic implants undergoing dental procedures. *J Bone Joint Surg Am.* 2017;99:161-163.

136. American Academy of Orthopaedic Surgeons. *Appropriate Use Criteria For the Management of Patients with Orthopaedic Implants Undergoing Dental Procedures.* 2016. Accessed November 23, 2020. https://www5.aaos.org/uploadedFiles/PreProduction/Quality/AUCs_and_Performance_Measures/appropriate_use/auc-patients-with-orthopaedic-implants-dental-procedures.pdf

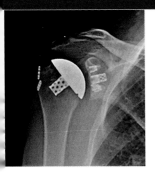

50 Outpatient Shoulder Arthroplasty

Jessica Welter, DO and Thomas (Quin) Throckmorton, MD

INTRODUCTION

The number of shoulder arthroplasties performed each year is increasing at a comparable or even higher rate than that of lower extremity arthroplasty, with more than 150,000 being performed each year. Traditionally, total joint arthroplasty (TJA) has remained an inpatient procedure because of concerns over pain control, blood loss, and potential postoperative complications. However, with a growing awareness of health care costs and an emphasis on savings without sacrificing quality, attention has turned to ambulatory joint replacement.

DRIVING FACTORS

The recent history of total shoulder arthroplasty (TSA) has shown that primary and revision shoulder arthroplasty has increased at annual rates of 6% to 13% from 1993 to 2007.[1] During the same time, charges also have increased at annual rates of $900 to $1700. This rising number of arthroplasties combined with the increased cost has the potential to place a financial strain on the health care system.[2] At the same time, the mean length of stay (LOS) following TJA is declining.[3] In a study of over 2000 patients undergoing TSA from 2005 to 2011, the LOS was 2.2 days.[3] In a survey of American Shoulder and Elbow Surgeons members, 69.8% of shoulder surgeons responded that their patients had an average LOS of less than 1.5 days (unpublished data, Brolin 2017). More recently, Brolin et al[4] in a comparative outpatient to inpatient study found an average LOS of 1.1 days in their group of 30 hospitalized patients.

With growing awareness of health care expenditures, there has been much emphasis on providing quality care in the most efficient and cost-effective manner possible. The United States has the world's highest per capita health care cost—about double that of other wealthy nations.[5] According to a paper published in 2016, tax-funded health expenditures totaled $1.877 trillion in 2013 and were projected to increase to $3.642 trillion by 2024.[5] However, the United States has already exceeded this projection with expenditures of $3.6 trillion in 2018. Furthermore, the National Health Expenditure is now projected to grow 5.5% per year and to reach nearly $6.0 trillion by 2027.[6] Public demands for improved cost control of physician services are increasing, while insurance companies seek to measure quality of care metrics. As a result, physicians are now required to provide cost-effective care cost-effective care without compromising quality. One such method of efficiency and cost savings is transitioning traditionally inpatient procedures, such as TJA, to outpatient procedures.

PATIENT SELECTION

Proper medical evaluation preoperatively is imperative to identify factors that place patients at an increased risk of a complication or readmission after shoulder arthroplasty. Anthony and colleagues found increased complications following TSA with chronic steroid use, a preoperative hematocrit of less than 38%, American Society of Anesthesiologists class 4, and an operative time longer than 2 hours.[7] Congestive heart failure also was associated with an increased mortality rate. Waterman and colleagues evaluated 30-day morbidity and mortality following elective shoulder arthroplasty and found preexisting cardiac disease to be a significant risk factor.[8] Both cardiac disease and increased age were associated with a higher risk of mortality, and both peripheral vascular disease (PVD) and operative time of more than 174 minutes were associated with increased complications. Courtney et al[9] found in their national database study that patients who were aged more than 70 years, those with malnutrition, cardiac history, smoking history, or diabetes mellitus are at higher risk for both readmission and complications after total hip arthroplasty (THA) and total knee arthroplasty (TKA).

Using published risk factors and consulting with our ambulatory surgery center (ASC) anesthesiology team, our center proposed an algorithm for selecting outpatient TSA candidates (**FIGURE 50.1**)[10] and then validated it with a cohort of patients. Use of this algorithm produced a low rate of perioperative complications and no hospital admissions. The first two decision points in this algorithm are age and preoperative anemia. Patients older than 70 years are considered contraindicated for an outpatient TSA, and a preoperative hematocrit <30 warrants anemia workup and reevaluation. The second branch of decision-making involves

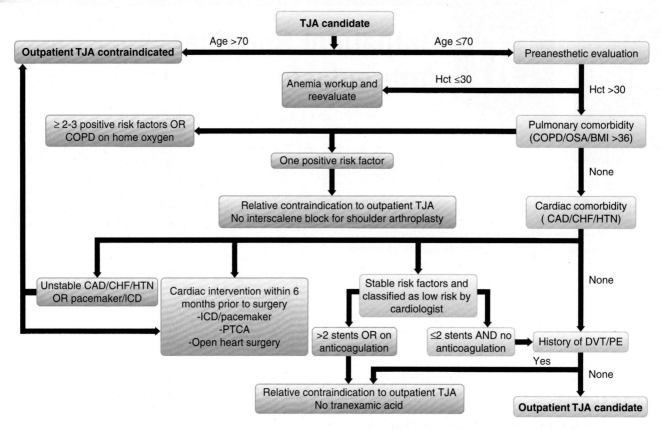

FIGURE 50.1 Algorithm for patient selection for outpatient total joint arthroplasty (TJA). BMI, body mass index; CAD, coronary artery disease; CHF, congestive heart failure; COPD, chronic obstructive pulmonary disease; DVT, deep vein thrombosis; HTN, hypertension; ICD, implantable cardioverter defibrillator; PE, pulmonary embolism; PTCA, percutaneous transluminal coronary angioplasty; OSA, obstructive sleep apnea. (From Fournier MN, Brolin TJ, Azar FM, et al. Identifying appropriate candidates for ambulatory outpatient shoulder arthroplasty: validation of a patient selection algorithm. *J Shoulder Elbow Surg.* 2019;28:65-70.)

pulmonary and cardiac conditions. Lastly, a history of thromboembolic disease and the use of anticoagulation are evaluated. In this algorithm, a patient can still be a candidate for outpatient TSA even with a single pulmonary comorbidity and/or stable cardiovascular risk factors. To validate the algorithm, 61 outpatient shoulder arthroplasty patients were identified and followed up for the 90-day episode of care; all complications were noted. The average patient age was 58 years (range 37-69 years); 49 had anatomic TSAs; and 12 had reverse TSAs. All patients were able to be discharged home on the day of surgery. None required 23-hour stays, and no patient was subsequently admitted to the hospital. There were seven complications (11.5%), one requiring reoperation within 90 days (hematoma evacuation). Nonsurgical complications included one patient with postoperative bradycardia that resolved and one patient who became acutely hypotensive with induction of anesthesia. This surgery was then aborted and the patient had successful, uncomplicated shoulder arthroplasty in a hospital environment 1 month later. Four additional complications occurred in the 90-day episode-of-care period: two patients developed arthrofibrosis requiring additional therapy, one patient

sustained a fall and traumatic rupture of subscapularis repair but declined further intervention, and one patient had mild anterior subluxation on postoperative radiographs.

Other authors have also published patient selection criteria. Biron et al[11] used a machine learning model to successfully predict which patients would be considered "short stay" candidates following TSA, and Meneghin et al[12] developed an outpatient arthroplasty risk assessment score that classified patients as a "low-moderate" and "not appropriate" for early discharge. Regardless of the algorithm chosen, a reliable and safe method to determine which patients are eligible for outpatient shoulder arthroplasty and those better suited to the hospital setting is critical for developing an outpatient shoulder program.

PAIN MANAGEMENT PROTOCOL

Significant advances in pain management protocols have facilitated the transition to outpatient TJA. Preoperative analgesia, multimodal pain regimens, nerve blocks, periarticular injections of long-acting local anesthetics, and patient education all help to decrease postoperative pain and subsequently the consumption of opioids.

Minimizing opioid use not only increases patient satisfaction but also decreases opioid-related adverse effects and facilitates rehabilitation. Assessment of patient expectations is vital to preoperative evaluation. Specifically, patients who have a history of anxiety or depression, a history of preoperative opioid use, or multiple medical comorbidities are at increased risk for less effective pain control.[13] It is, therefore, important to identify these patients before scheduling surgery and to educate and psychologically prepare them for the planned protocol in order to effectively manage their postoperative pain. Experience and expertise of the anesthesia team can strongly influence the development of pain management protocols.

Multimodal Pain Regimens

Preemptive analgesia has been shown to reduce postoperative pain and opioid consumption postoperatively. This includes acetaminophen, nonsteroidal anti-inflammatory drugs, and gabapentinoid medications given to patients in the immediate perioperative period.[13] Ongoing research is directed at optimizing the timing and dosage of these medications.

Periarticular Injections and Nerve Blocks

There is an emerging body of evidence comparing the use of periarticular injections to regional nerve blockade for treatment of postoperative pain following shoulder arthroplasty.[14-19] While most studies show general equivalence in overall pain metrics, which of these is chosen is likely dependent on a combination of surgeon, institutional, and anesthesia preferences.

Weller et al[19] compared 156 patients who received interscalene catheters with 58 patients who received a liposomal bupivacaine (LB) periarticular injection at the time of TSA. No differences in visual analog scale scores were found at 24 hours, 2 weeks, 6 weeks, or 12 weeks, but the interscalene group had more major complications, which were typically pulmonary in nature. Sabesan et al,[18] in a randomized controlled trial of 70 patients who received either continuous interscalene nerve blocks (ISBs) or LB injection, found that the groups had equivalent narcotic use, pain scores, and time to first narcotic use within the first 24 hours, but the continuous ISB group had more complications and increased cost. The LB group had higher ASES and Penn Shoulder scores at final follow-up. Hannan et al[15] performed a retrospective cohort analysis of 37 patients who received LB injections following inpatient TSA compared with 21 patients who received ISBs. They found that LB was associated with less pain, less opioid consumption, and shorter hospital stays. Namdari et al[16] reported a randomized trial comparing ISB with LB injection; the patients undergoing nerve blocks had less pain immediately after surgery but were more likely to experience rebound pain at 24 hours. In a randomized

controlled trial, Okoroha et al[17] compared local LB injection and ISB and found an increase in pain in the LB group between 0 and 8 hours postoperatively, but a significant increase in intravenous morphine equivalents in the ISB group between 13 and 16 hours. At the conclusion of the day of surgery, there were no significant differences in any variables. The authors suggested that LB provides similar overall pain relief with no increase in complications or LOS.

At our institution, we do not perform nerve blocks for inpatient or outpatient shoulder arthroplasty. Preoperative medications given in the holding area consist of acetaminophen 1g PO, gabapentin 300 mg PO, celecoxib 200 mg PO (meloxicam 15 mg if sulfa allergy), and long-acting oxycodone 10 mg PO. Prior to wound closure, we inject the scapular notch, deltoid, pectoralis major, and soft tissues with a mixture of 20 mL LB, 40 mL 0.25% bupivacaine, and 30 mg of ketorolac. Discharge prescriptions consist of acetaminophen, gabapentin, celecoxib (or meloxicam if sulfa allergy), carisoprodol, oxycodone, and aspirin. Supplemental medications to mitigate pharmacologic side effects include a stool softener, proton pump inhibitor, and antinausea medication. Patients are encouraged to use cryotherapy at frequent intervals to assist with pain and decrease swelling. This multimodal program has significantly reduced postoperative opioid consumption and is allowing us to transition toward opioid-sparing protocols.

SAFETY

TJA has traditionally remained an inpatient procedure because of concerns over pain control, blood loss, and potential postoperative complications. Courtney et al[9] compared the complications of outpatient TJA with inpatient TJA and found that bleeding requiring transfusion was the most common complication in both study groups. Incidences of all other complications were low. There was no difference in the rate of wound complications or infection, deep venous thrombosis (DVT), pulmonary embolism, cardiac arrest, or re-intubation. When controlling for confounding variables, outpatient TJA was not a significant risk factor for readmission.

TSA is known to have a lower complication rate than THA or TKA,[7,8,14,20,21] which would suggest that TSA can be safely performed as an outpatient procedure. Published data[4] from our institution show no significant difference when comparing complication rates between ASC patients and hospital patients undergoing TSA. Using matched cohorts, Brolin et al[4] found that the complication rates among ambulatory outpatient and inpatient TSA were 13% versus 10%, respectively, which were not significantly different. Minor complications reported in the outpatient group included arthrofibrosis in two patients and mild asymptomatic anterior subluxation in one patient. Another patient in the outpatient cohort fell 11 weeks after surgery and disrupted the subscapularis repair. This was considered a major complication. Minor complications in the inpatient group included superficial DVT, blood transfusion, and mild asymptomatic anterior subluxation. There were no hospital admissions from the ASC cohort and no readmissions from the hospital cohort.

Further comparisons of inpatient and outpatient TSA in recent years have all demonstrated low complication rates in the outpatient setting. Leroux et al[22] compared 7024 inpatients with 173 outpatients who had TSA, with outpatient TSA defined as having an LOS <23 hours. Overall, four patients (2.3%) had adverse events, two (1.9%) readmissions, and no deaths. They found no difference in hospital readmissions between outpatients and inpatients. Kramer et al[23] found no difference between inpatient and outpatient TSA in terms of 90-day readmissions, 90-day emergency room visits, and 1-year mortality. Basques et al[24] used a Medicare data set to compare outcomes and found that after controlling for age, gender, and medical comorbidities, patients who had TSA as outpatients had lower rates of 30- and 60-day readmissions and lower complication rates than inpatients.

Cancienne et al[25] found the 90-day complication rate for outpatient TSA to be 15.9% compared with 17.7% for inpatients. They found that the chance of receiving a blood transfusion or having a urinary tract infection was increased in the inpatient group. Another study looked specifically at blood transfusion and found that a preoperative hematocrit of less than 39.6% resulted in 11% chance of receiving a blood transfusion compared with 0.7% with a level greater than that threshold.[26] It is for this reason that a low preoperative hematocrit is one of the first branches in our patient selection algorithm.

Another concern of surgeons transitioning to outpatient TSA is the risk for postoperative infection and postoperative antibiotic protocols. When patients remain in the hospital for inpatient TSA, they frequently are given 23 hours of postoperative IV antibiotics for prophylaxis; however, if the surgery is performed in a true ambulatory surgery setting, postoperative antibiotics must be given orally or not at all. We do not routinely prescribe postoperative oral antibiotics, which is supported by the Centers of Disease Control and Prevention guideline for the prevention of surgical site infection.[27] Unpublished data from our institution (Throckmorton and Fryberger) show no increased rate of infection based on an institutional database review of 896 inpatient and 126 outpatient TSAs. The inpatients received 24 hours of prophylaxis, while the outpatients received only one dose of preoperative IV antibiotics and no postoperative prophylaxis. We found no significant difference in overall infection rates (1.45% and 1.59%) between the two groups.

Despite a relatively low complication profile associated with outpatient TSA, it is imperative to reemphasize the importance of patient selection to minimize potential catastrophic complications as well as readmission rates. The 90-day readmission rates after TSA range from 2.5% to 6.6%.[28-31] Age, increased comorbidities, and obesity have been shown to be factors associated with readmission. Cancienne et al[25] found that medically related readmissions represented 81.8% of all readmissions in the ambulatory group, with the primary risk factors being obesity, diabetes, PVD, congestive heart failure, depression, chronic anemia, and chronic lung disease. Selecting the ideal candidate for outpatient shoulder arthroplasty requires a multidisciplinary approach, with collaborative efforts involving the patient, anesthesia team, preoperative clearance clinic, and the surgeon.

OUTCOMES

Overall, patient satisfaction for inpatient TSA is quite high, and the same can be said about satisfaction with outpatient TSA. Our institution surveyed patients who had TSA at both ambulatory and inpatient surgical settings. Patients were very satisfied with the arthroplasty itself, as well as the environment of the surgery. If given a choice, however, the ASC group preferred having their surgery in the ASC setting, while a high percentage of patients in the inpatient group would have preferred to change to an ASC setting. Similarly, Leroux et al[32] evaluated 41 anatomic and reverse shoulder arthroplasties performed at an outpatient surgery center and reported patient-reported outcomes obtained using a phone questionnaire. They found that 97% of patients were satisfied with their outpatient procedure. More recently, Nagda et al[33] reported 2-year outcomes at their institution following their first 29 outpatient TSAs; all patients reported that they were still satisfied with their outcome and surgery.

In addition to providing a safe environment and high patient satisfaction, the cost analysis of outpatient shoulder arthroplasty is quite promising, particularly with the development of bundled payment models. A recent study by Walters et al[34] performed a cost-minimization analysis of 76 patients who had anatomic TSA at an ASC. They found that primary anatomic TSA using a bundled care program in an outpatient setting coincides with markedly lower charges, with the average total implant charges being significantly less for the bundled group ($24,822 vs $28,405). Other studies have reinforced this concept. Cancienne et al[25] reported a significant reduction in both procedural and hospital-related reimbursements for shoulder arthroplasty, which resulted in a mean cost reduction of $3615 per patient in diagnosis-related group reimbursements. Gregory et al[35] compared patient-level costs of primary elective TSA between inpatient and outpatient settings. Their study evaluated 21,331 inpatient and 1542 outpatient TSAs that were performed between 2010 and 2015. Inpatient costs ($76,109) were significantly higher than outpatient costs ($22,907). Even after exclusion of inpatient-specific charges, inpatient TSA remained 41.1% more expensive than the outpatient setting.

It also should be noted that patient insurance and payer status are important factors in this process. Outpatient TSA is not currently an approved procedure for patients insured by government payers, although outpatient TKA was recently granted approval. In contrast, patients with commercial insurance are not restricted from outpatient TSA, and physicians interested in this practice may find it beneficial to negotiate bundled payments or insurance carve-outs to facilitate program implantation.[35]

CONCLUSION

In conclusion, the dynamics of the current health care environment dictates a need for safe, value-based care. As part of the response to this environment, outpatient shoulder arthroplasty has emerged as a safe and cost-effective procedure. Complication rates are comparable to those with surgeries performed as an inpatient and patient satisfaction is high. There are several key points to the success of an outpatient shoulder arthroplasty program, specifically proper patient selection and perioperative education. Also, a collaborative approach to the development of multimodal pain control regimens has significantly improved postoperative pain management, allowing for same-day discharge following shoulder replacement.

REFERENCES

1. Kim SH, Wise BL, Zhang Y. Increasing incidence of shoulder arthroplasty in the United States. *J Bone Joint Surg Am.* 2011;93(24):2249-2254.
2. Day JS, Lau E, Ong KL, et al. Prevalence and projections of total shoulder and elbow arthroplasty in the United States to 2015. *J Shoulder Elbow Surg.* 2010;19:1115-1120.
3. Dunn JC, Lanzi J, Kusnezov N, et al. Predictors of length of stay after elective total shoulder arthroplasty in the United States. *J Shoulder Elbow Surg.* 2015;24:754-759.
4. Brolin TJ, Mulligan RP, Azar FM, Throckmorton TW. Neer award 2016: outpatient total shoulder arthroplasty in an ambulatory surgery center is a safe alternative to inpatient total shoulder arthroplasty in a hospital. A matched cohort study. *J Shoulder Elbow Surg.* 2016;26:204-208.
5. Himmelstein DU, Woolhandler S. The current and projected taxpayer shares of US health costs. *Am J Public Health.* 2016;106:449-452.
6. Centers for Medicare & Medicaid Services. National Health Expenditure Data. Accessed January 22, 2020. https://www.cms.gov/research-statistics-data-and-systems/statistics-trends-and-reports/nationalhealthexpenddata/nhe-fact-sheet/
7. Anthony CA, Westermann RW, Gao Y, et al. What are risk factors for 30-day morbidity and transfusion in total shoulder arthroplasty? A review of 1922 cases. *Clin Orthop Relat Res.* 2015;473:2099-2105.
8. Waterman BR, Dunn JC, Bader J, et al. Thirty-day morbidity and mortality after elective total shoulder arthroplasty: patient-based and surgical risk factors. *J Shoulder Elbow Surg.* 2015;24:24-30.
9. Courtney M, Boniello AJ, Berger RA. Complications following outpatient total joint arthroplasty: an analysis of a national database. *J Arthroplasty.* 2017;32:1426-1430.
10. Fournier MN, Brolin TJ, Azar FM, et al. Identifying appropriate candidates for ambulatory outpatient shoulder arthroplasty:validation of a patient selection algorithm. *J Shoulder Elbow Surg.* 2019;28:65-70.
11. Biron DR, Sinha I, Kleiner JE. A novel machine learning model developed to assist in patient selection for outpatient total shoulder arthroplasty. *J Am Acad Orthop Surg.* 2020;28:e580-e585.
12. Meneghini RM, Ziemba-Davis M, Ishmael MK, et al. Safe selection of outpatient joint arthroplasty patients with medical risk stratification: the "outpatient arthroplasty risk assessment score". *J Arthroplasty.* 2017;32(8):2325-2331.
13. Codding JL, Getz CL. Pain management strategies in shoulder arthroplasty. *Orthop Clin North Am.* 2018;49:81-91.
14. Farmer KW, Hammond JW, Queale WS, et al. Shoulder arthroplasty versus hip and knee arthroplasties: a comparison of outcomes. *Clin Orthop Relat Res.* 2007;455:183-189.
15. Hannan CV, Albrecht MJ, Petersen SA, et al. Liposomal bupivacaine vs interscalene nerve block for pain control after shoulder arthroplasty: a retrospective cohort analysis. *Am J Orthop (Belle Mead NJ).* 2016;45:424-430.
16. Namdari S, Nicholson T, Abboud J, et al. Randomized controlled trial of interscalene block compared with injectable liposomal bupivacaine in shoulder arthroplasty. *J Bone Joint Surg Am.* 2017;99:550-556.
17. Okoroha KR, Lynch JR, Keller RA, et al. Liposomal bupivacaine versus interscalene nerve block for pain control after shoulder arthroplasty: a prospective randomized trial. *J Shoulder Elbow Surg.* 2016;25:1742-1748.
18. Sabesan VJ, Sharhriar R, Petersen-Fitts GR, et al. A prospective randomized controlled trial to identify the optimal postoperative pain management in shoulder arthroplasty: liposomal bupivacaine versus continuous interscalene catheter. *J Shoulder Elbow Surg.* 2017;26:1810-1817.
19. Weller WJ, Azzam MG, Smith RA, et al. Liposomal bupivacaine mixture has similar pain relief and significantly fewer complications at less cost compared to indwelling interscalene catheter in total shoulder arthroplasty. *J Arthroplasty.* 2017;32:3557-3562.
20. Chalmers PN, Gupta AK, Rahman Z, et al. Predictors of early complications of total shoulder arthroplasty. *J Arthroplasty.* 2014;29:856-860.
21. Fehringer EV, Mikuls TR, Michaud KD, et al. Shoulder arthroplasties have fewer complications than hip or knee arthroplasties in US veterans. *Clin Orthop Relat Res.* 2010;468:717-722.
22. Leroux TS, Basques BA, Frank RM. Outpatient shoulder arthroplasty: a population based study comparing adverse event and readmission rates to inpatient total shoulder arthroplasty. *J Shoulder Elbow Surg.* 2016;25:1780-1786.
23. Kramer JD, Chan PH, Prentice HA, et al. Same-day discharge is not inferior to longer length of in-hospital stay for 90-day readmissions following shoulder arthroplasty. *J Shoulder Elbow Surg.* 2020;29:898-905.
24. Basques BA, Erickson BJ, Leroux T, et al. Comparative outcomes of outpatient and inpatient total shoulder arthroplasty. *Bone Joint J.* 2017;99-B:934-938.
25. Cancienne JM, Brockmeier SF, Gulotta LV, et al. Ambulatory total shoulder arthroplasty: a comprehensive analysis of current trends, complications, readmissions, and costs. *J Bone Joint Surg Am.* 2017;99:629-637.
26. Padegimas EM, Clyde CT, Zmistowski BM, et al. Risk factors for blood transfusion after shoulder arthroplasty. *Bone Joint J.* 2016;98-B:224-228.
27. Berrios-Torres SI, Umschield CA. Centers for Disease Control and Prevention guideline for the prevention of surgical site infection. *J Am Med Assoc.* 2017;152:784-791.
28. Anakwenze O, Fokin A, Chocas M, et al. Complications in total shoulder and reverse total shoulder arthroplasty by body mass index. *J Shoulder Elbow Surg.* 2017;26:1230-1237.
29. Mahoney A, Bosco JA, Zuckerman JD. Readmission after shoulder arthroplasty. *J Shoulder Elbow Surg.* 2014;23:377-381.
30. Matsen FA, Li N, Gao H, et al. Factors affecting length of stay, readmission, and revision after shoulder arthroplasty: a population-based study. *J Bone Joint Surg Am.* 2015;97:1255-1263.
31. Westermann RW, Anthony CA, Duchman KR, et al. Incidence, causes and predictors of 30-day readmission after shoulder arthroplasty. *Iowa Orthop J.* 2016;36:70-74.

32. Leroux TS, Zuke WA, Saltzman BM. Safety and patient satisfaction of outpatient shoulder arthroplasty. *JSES Open Access*. 2018;2:13-17.

33. Nagda S, Patel S. Patient satisfaction in outpatient total shoulder arthroplasty. *Ambul Surg*. 2020;26:10-14.

34. Walters JD, Walsh RN, Smith RA, et al. Bundled payment plans are associated with notable cost savings for ambulatory outpatient total shoulder arthroplasty. *J Am Acad Orthop Surg*. 2020;28:795-801.

35. Gregory JM, Wetzig AM, Wayne CD. Quantification of patient-level costs in outpatient total shoulder arthroplasty. *J Shoulder Elbow Surg*. 2019;28:1066-1073.

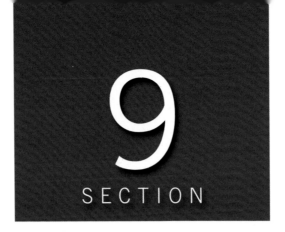

Looking Ahead

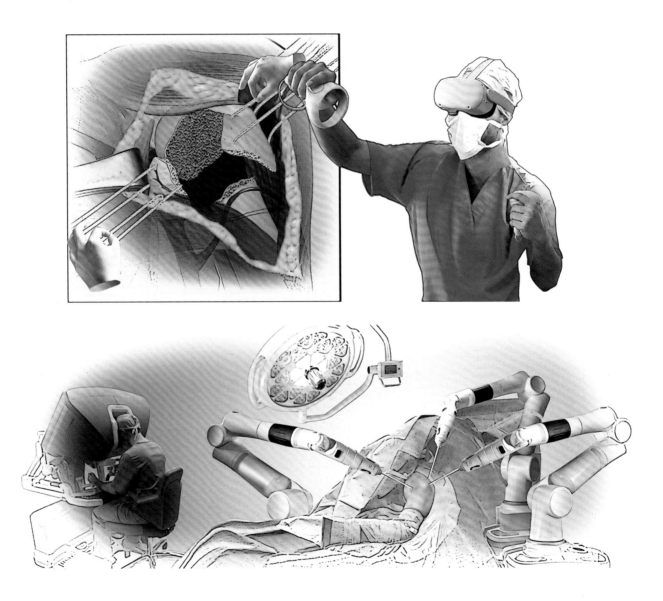

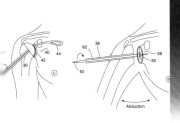

51 Total Shoulder Arthroplasty in 10 Years:
Implant Design and Surgical Techniques

Thomas Vanasse, MS, Josie Elwell, PhD, and Joseph D. Zuckerman, MD

INTRODUCTION

Incredible progress has been made in the realm of shoulder arthroplasty, from the first modern era designs to the multitude of devices for hemi-, resurfacing, anatomic, reverse, fracture, and revision shoulder arthroplasty available today. It is expected that these advancements will continue to accelerate over the next 10 years through improved implant designs, advanced materials and coatings, and new surgical approaches. The continued incorporation of computers and technology—from navigation to robotics to machine learning—will contribute greatly to new advances in shoulder arthroplasty. These advancements will build upon our current knowledge and experience to enhance our understanding of joint mechanics and improve implant longevity so that shoulder arthroplasty can ultimately benefit even greater numbers of patients. In this chapter, we will try to "predict" what the next 10 years will bring, and to do so, we will rely on designs that have already received patent protection. It is possible that some of these designs will be the products we use in 10 years.

IMPLANT TYPES

Solutions for the Glenoid

As anatomic glenoids have progressed from keeled to all-polyethylene pegged to poly/metal hybrid implants, the desire for a truly uncemented anatomic total shoulder arthroplasty (ATSA) glenoid has only increased. Several designs currently available including the Zimmer Biomet Modular Hybrid and Trabecular Metal Glenoids and the Exactech Cage Glenoid minimize the amount of cement necessary for fixation by utilizing porous material or cage features to allow for bony in-growth or through-growth. The short- to midterm results have generally been promising, with good clinical outcomes and comparable, or even reduced, incidence of radiolucent lines compared to all-poly glenoids.[1,2] It is likely that the next generation of glenoids will be designed to include enhanced features and porous coatings/structures to provide initial press-fit and long-term fixation, eliminating the need for cement and screws to obtain initial fixation.

The prevalence of platform humeral stems has increased because of the benefits of performing revision arthroplasty without the need to remove a well-fixed and well-positioned humeral component. In an ideal scenario, the glenoid component would offer the same level of convertibility. Unfortunately, metal-backed glenoids have historically performed poorly, and even modern designs have shown higher revision rates than traditional cemented glenoids.[3] This is likely due to backside polyethylene wear and overstuffing from the combined thickness of the metal and polyethylene composite. Despite this track record, these devices are still being pursued because of the theoretical benefits in revision cases, with newer options available from Zimmer Biomet, LimaCorporate, and Arthrex. The long-term performance of this generation of implants remains to be documented, although regardless of the level of success, it is unlikely that others will be deterred from conceptualizing and developing new convertible glenoid designs[4-7] in the years to come (**FIGURE 51.1A** and **B**). These future devices would ideally incorporate enhanced locking mechanisms to minimize motion between the polyethylene component and baseplate and use advanced bearing materials to reduce wear and decrease construct thickness to avoid overstuffing.

Solutions for the Humerus

Since the enthusiasm for smaller humeral components shows no signs of abating, it is anticipated that the number of stemless implants on the market will rise over the next decade and the indications for their use will continue to expand. As stemless implant usage in ATSA has grown, so has the interest in a platform stemless device that could be converted to a reverse total shoulder arthroplasty (RTSA) or could potentially be used as a primary RTSA in patients with adequate bone quality and quantity. The LimaCorporate SMR Stemless is one such convertible stemless implant currently being used. The early clinical results will determine whether it has the potential for mid- and long-term success. In general, to be successful as an RTSA, these devices will need to incorporate features, such as fins, threads, or bone cages, as well as porous

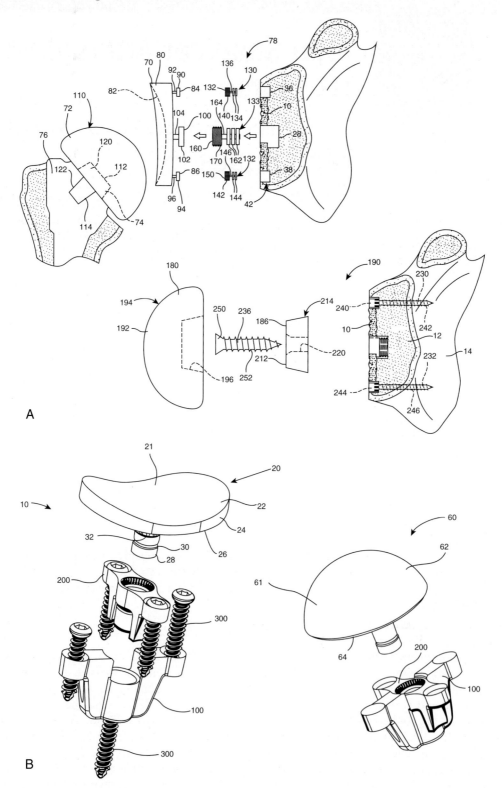

FIGURE 51.1 Anatomic and reverse configurations of convertible glenoid designs described in (**A**) US patent 8,632,598[4] and (**B**) US patent 8,920,508 B2.[5]

regions, which ensure strong initial and long-term fixation. Additionally, they will likely need to have a partially or fully inset center of rotation to withstand the forces imparted as a result of the relatively constrained nature of RTSA configurations. There are certainly numerous recent inventions that have been disclosed in this space,[8-10] including designs with thread-like features (**FIGURE 51.2A**) and through-holes/slots (**FIGURE 51.2B**)

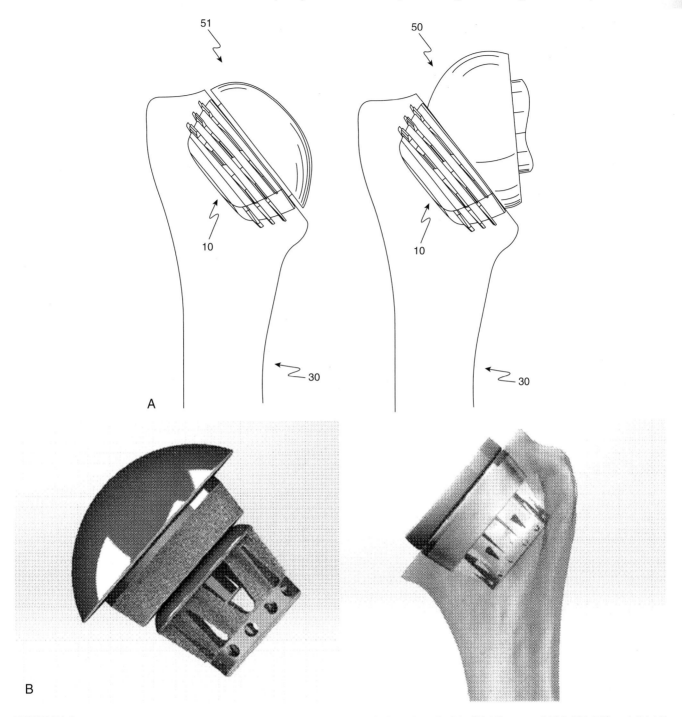

FIGURE 51.2 Anatomic and reverse configurations of convertible stemless designs described in (**A**) US patent 8,512,410 B2[8] and (**B**) US patent 9,956,083 B2.[10]

to enhance fixation. Time will tell whether these proposed and patented designs make it through the rigorous process of product development.

Revision Options

The rapidly increasing number of shoulder arthroplasties performed worldwide each year also implies that there will be an increasing revision burden. With that rise comes the need for a wider variety of revision implants to provide surgeons and their patients with options to address these challenging cases especially when excessive bone loss is present. On the glenoid side, surgeons can currently utilize augmented glenoid components, bone grafts in conjunction with a baseplate, or custom solutions for more extreme cases, such as the Vault Reconstruction System from Zimmer Biomet, ProMade from LimaCorporate, or Glenius from Materialise.

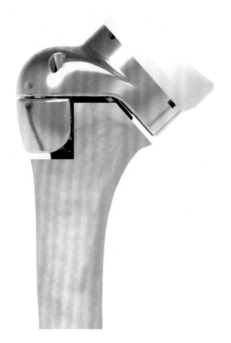

FIGURE 51.3 Humeral Augmented Tray for humeral bone loss. (Used with permission from © Exactech, Inc.)

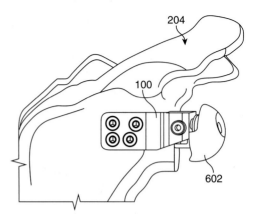

FIGURE 51.4 Glenoid prosthesis with flanges for scapular-deficient patient as described in US patent application 2020/0046510 A1.[15]

Several systems are currently available on the humeral side, including the Humeral Reconstruction Prosthesis from Exactech and the Segmental Revision System from Zimmer Biomet. These systems can be used to rebuild a humerus with massive bone loss or, if needed, be used to replace an entire humerus.

In cases of proximal humeral bone loss following fracture treatment or revision arthroplasty, it is well recognized that when the greater tuberosity fails to heal or is absent, range of motion and stability are negatively affected.[11-13] Implants that can address greater tuberosity and proximal bone deficiency should provide an option for these patients to fill this bone void, increase deltoid wrap, and improve stability without replacing more of the humerus than is necessary. The Equinoxe Humeral Augmented Tray **(FIGURE 51.3)** provides this option, and there is little doubt that more of these types of systems will be designed and developed over the next 10 years to provide solutions to complex situations for which options are currently limited. On the glenoid side, these may include implants with additional points of fixation along the scapula[14-16] **(FIGURE 51.4)** or better methods/tools for the creation of patient-specific bone graft[17,18] **(FIGURE 51.5)**. Some of these concepts, along with others yet to be contemplated, may become additions to the armamentarium of the shoulder arthroplasty surgeon.

New to World Concepts

New technologies that may result in completely new types of shoulder arthroplasty beyond the very familiar hemiarthroplasty, resurfacing, ATSA, and RTSA are advancing. For example, pyrocarbon interposition shoulder arthroplasty is being evaluated as a treatment option for young patients, in which a pyrocarbon sphere articulates against both the prepared humerus and glenoid. Although short-term clinical data have shown results comparable to hemiarthroplasty,[19] midterm data have shown progressive glenoid and greater tuberosity erosion and only 90% implant survival rate at 4 years.[20] Pyrocarbon may not be the material of choice, but advances in biomaterials will likely identify new options to consider in shoulder implants.

There is interest in the creation of a mobile-bearing or multiarticulating shoulder[21-23] **(FIGURE 51.6A and B)**, which certainly has been used successfully in other joint replacements. The goal of these designs would be to achieve increased range of motion. Bipolar shoulder prostheses are within this category and have been used sparingly with limited success and are considered for salvage-type procedures. Future mobile-bearing devices

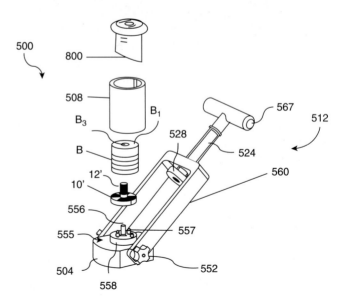

FIGURE 51.5 Bone press for the creation of patient-specific bone graft as described in US patent application 2017/0273795.[18]

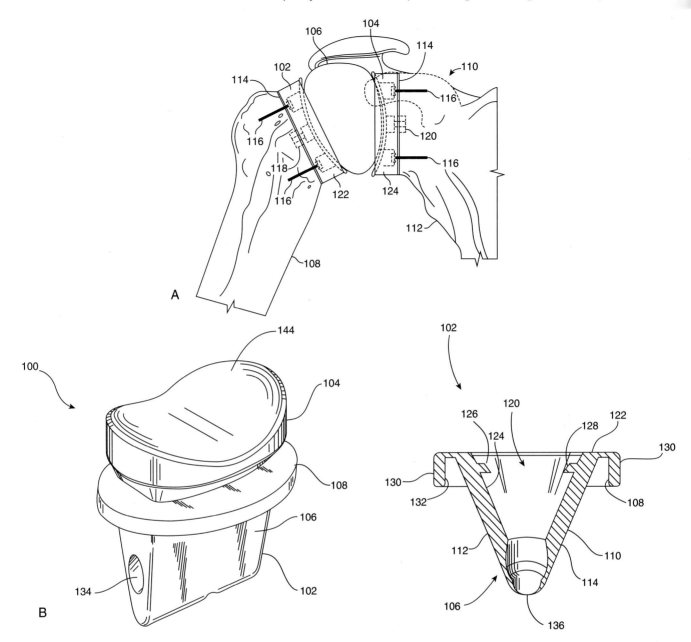

FIGURE 51.6 A, Stemless shoulder with an additional articulation component as described in US patent application 2017/0105843 A1[22]; (**B**) mobile-bearing glenoid component as described in US patent 9,439,769 B2.[23]

would certainly require improved design and materials and assessment in carefully designed clinical trials to determine indications and efficacy. It is likely that "revolutionary" designs like these will not achieve the clinical outcomes for wide utilization, but the same was probably said about devices and implants that currently enjoy widespread use today. Time will determine whether these "outside-the-box" implants achieve success.

IMPLANT MATERIALS

Advances and innovation in overall implant design in the next decade will likely be accompanied by improvements in material science. Bearing materials in joint

replacements are of particular importance in determining the longevity of the implant. Decreasing bearing wear plays a role in (1) reducing the generation of particles that could induce unfavorable inflammatory reactions and (2) preserving the articular geometry to maintain joint kinematics over time. Advancements in wear resistance could improve the long-term survival of shoulder arthroplasties, which is *particularly* important in younger patients.

Polyethylene

Currently, the most commonly used bearing materials are cobalt-chrome (CoCr) and polyethylene, the latter of which is more susceptible to wear. Polyethylene wear is a concern because wear particles can induce osteolysis which, in turn, can compromise implant fixation that can lead to aseptic loosening in both ATSA and RTSA.[24] Both the normal and abnormal biomechanics of either type of shoulder replacement can result in polyethylene wear. In ATSA, excessive translation of the humeral head and repeated edge loading of the glenoid component, resulting from implant malposition or a rotator cuff deficiency, can exacerbate polyethylene wear beyond what would be expected in the presence of normal joint mechanics. The cyclic edge loading may induce the rocking horse phenomenon. Glenoid component loosening in ATSA is multifactorial but remains one of the most common complications.[25] In RTSA, repeated impingement of the humeral liner on the lateral border of the scapula can generate osteolysis-inducing wear particles that affect fixation of the baseplate. Even as our knowledge and understanding of optimal biomechanics via implant design and surgical techniques expand, advances in bearing materials to improve longevity will be also be valuable.

Ultra-high–molecular-weight polyethylene (UHMWPE) has been adopted for use as a bearing material in total joint replacement for decades. More recently, cross-linked UHMWPE has dominated the total joint arthroplasty landscape. Cross-linking UHMWPE, most commonly achieved via irradiation, offers superior wear characteristics. However, this may come at the cost of compromising mechanical properties.[26]

Irradiation can be used to both sterilize UHMWPE and induce cross-linking. Inducing cross-linking requires higher levels of radiation than is used for sterilization. Irradiation, either for the purpose of sterilization or cross-linking, can result in generation of free radicals that react with oxygen, a process known as oxidation. Oxidation contributes to the degradation of mechanical properties as oxygen diffuses into UHMWPE, both during storage and in vivo. It should be noted that sterilization can be achieved via radiation-free methods, but these methods do not induce cross-linking and therefore do not improve wear resistance.

Removing free radicals responsible for oxidation after cross-linking involves postirradiation thermal treatments in which the polyethylene is remelted or annealed. However, thermal treatments can have immediate negative effects on mechanical properties, particularly fatigue strength, by disrupting the crystalline structure.[27] A potential avenue to avoid the trade-off between improving oxidation resistance and negatively affecting mechanical properties is impregnation of cross-linked UHMWPE with vitamin E. Vitamin E, an antioxidant, reacts with free radicals that would otherwise cause oxidation. The addition of vitamin E, combined with cross-linking, potentially offers the best of both worlds by improving both wear and oxidation resistance, while maintaining mechanical properties by eliminating the need for thermal treatments.[28]

Within the field of orthopedics, vitamin E polyethylene was first utilized in tibial trays and acetabular liners for knee and hip arthroplasties. Following this trend, anatomic glenoid components and reverse humeral liners are now manufactured with vitamin E polyethylene. For example, DJO Global offers several types of vitamin E cross-linked polyethylene based upon the mechanics of the system. Moderately cross-linked vitamin E polyethylene glenoid components are offered as part of the Turon Shoulder and AltiVate Anatomic Systems based upon the sliding and gliding kinematics of the systems. Highly cross-linked vitamin E polyethylene humeral liners are incorporated into the RSP and AltiVate Reverse Shoulder systems based upon the rotational kinematics of a ball-and-socket joint. The rationale for use of vitamin E polyethylene is the superior wear and oxidation characteristics, which theoretically could result in improved implant longevity. If this is documented, then we can expect cross-linked vitamin E polyethylene to become the polyethylene of choice in shoulder arthroplasty systems.

Ceramics

Improvements in the wear and oxidation resistance of UHMWPE may be accompanied by adoption of alternatives to the metallic components in shoulder arthroplasty over the next decade. One such alternative is the use of ceramics, namely alumina and zirconia. Ceramics have been in use in hip replacements for quite some time. Several bearing combinations exist for hip arthroplasty, including ceramic-on-polyethylene (ceramic femoral head and polyethylene acetabular liner) and ceramic-on-ceramic bearings.[29] Ceramics are attractive options for several reasons, most notably that they are bioinert, have low coefficients of friction, and are scratch resistant.

When used in combination with polyethylene bearings, ceramics have the potential to reduce polyethylene wear, thereby reducing the likelihood of osteolysis and subsequent implant loosening.[30] However, concerns exist regarding fracture of ceramic components. Ceramics have high compressive strengths, but tensile strengths are much lower, causing them to be brittle. In hip arthroplasty, the incidence of ceramic component fracture is relatively low,[31] and although concerns still exist, they have been largely alleviated by improved manufacturing techniques that reduce impurities, which can be responsible for crack initiation and subsequent propagation. Improved formulations, specifically alumina-zirconia composites, have the potential to improve mechanical properties (ie, fracture toughness) of ceramic joint replacement components.

In shoulder arthroplasty, several systems utilized primarily in Europe offer ceramic components. For anatomic replacement, Mathys offers a ceramic humeral head as part of the Affinis Short, which is a stemless system **(FIGURE 51.7A)**. CeramTec currently has a humeral head under development to be made of BIOLOX delta, a fourth-generation alumina-zirconia composite ceramic.[34] At present, ceramic humeral heads articulate on polyethylene glenoid components. Its use on the glenoid side is more challenging because of the need to keep the glenoid component as thin as possible to avoid overstuffing. Thus, over the next decade, it is not out of the realm of possibility that anatomic glenoids *could* be made of ceramics, but it is much more likely that the humeral head will receive most of the emphasis.

For RTSA, ceramic components are more readily available and are used for both glenospheres and humeral liners. For example, LimaCorporate includes UHMWPE glenospheres and ceramic humeral liners in the SMR Reverse System. Wear resulting from "normal" use theoretically may be alleviated by incorporation of UHMWPE on the glenoid side, rather than the humeral side, by reducing generation of wear particles resulting from repeated impingement of the humeral liner with the axillary scapular border. Merolla et al. reported on 36 patients who received UHMWPE glenospheres at a mean follow-up of 36 months, concluding that clinical outcomes were good, but also noted a 17.5% rate of scapular notching.[35] Thus, while UHMWPE glenospheres may not *prevent* scapular notching, the benefits may be in the reduced osteolysis if the notching does not result from the generation of polyethylene wear debris. Mid- and long-term studies will be needed to confirm the efficacy of UHMWPE glenospheres used in combination with a range of humeral liner materials including metal and ceramic.

The UNIC Reverse system offers ceramic glenospheres and humeral liners allowing for a ceramic-on-ceramic coupling. The potential benefits of ceramic-on-ceramic systems are in the elimination of polyethylene particles altogether. At present, ceramic-on-ceramic is a concept more widely accepted in hip arthroplasty from which we can learn important information. Studies have shown high survivorship most likely as a result of decreased wear.[36] A concern, in addition to fracture, is audible squeaking of the joint during use, which could potentially be more noticeable in the shoulder.

Pyrocarbon

A newer concept within the realm of hemiarthroplasty relates to the use of pyrolytic carbon (pyrocarbon) to resurface or replace the humeral head. Although this material is also being utilized for new implant types, such as the previously mentioned interposition shoulder arthroplasty, it may also have application for use in hemiarthroplasty in patients with primarily humeral-sided disease. The use of metallic components to replace the humeral head often results in progressive glenoid erosion. Pyrocarbon has been proposed as an alternative due to its low coefficient of friction and mechanical properties that resemble cortical bone, which may mitigate damage to the glenoid.[37] Wright Medical currently offers a pyrocarbon humeral head as part of the Aequalis Ascend Flex system **(FIGURE 51.7B)**. A recent study by Garret et al.[38] showed favorable clinical outcomes of pyrocarbon hemiarthroplasty at 2-year follow-up in patients with an average age of 57.9 years at the time of surgery. As mid- and long-term data become available, it is possible that more shoulder arthroplasty systems will introduce this material as an option for younger patients with humeral-sided disease including osteonecrosis.

A potential benefit of alternative bearing surfaces, in addition to decreased wear, is the ability to use these components in patients with metal allergies and, specifically, nickel sensitivity. Ceramic-on-ceramic or ceramic-on-polyethylene bearings, in combination with nickel-free titanium components, would offer a solution

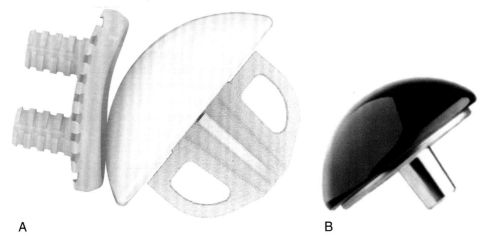

A   B

FIGURE 51.7 A ceramic humeral head and glenoid component offered within the Mathys Affinis Short system[32] for anatomic total shoulder arthroplasty (**A**) and the pyrocarbon humeral head featured in the Aequalis Ascend Flex system[33] for hemiarthroplasty (**B**). (A, Image reprinted with permission from Mathys Medical. © 2021 Mathys AG Bettlach. B, Image reprinted with permission from Stryker Corporation. © 2021 Stryker Corporation. All rights reserved.)

to this very uncommon but important finding. As mid- and long-term clinical data becomes available for shoulder systems that currently offer bearing materials other than the traditional UHMWPE on cobalt-chrome articulations, the clinical benefit of these materials will be evaluated, and it is probable an increased number of shoulder arthroplasty systems will include these alternatives in the future.

SURFACE FINISHES/COATINGS

Longevity of shoulder implants may be improved by advances in bearing materials, but various other strategies in the realm of implant coatings, particularly on the components that interface directly with the bone, are currently being explored to improve fixation and decrease revision rates. Preventing two main reasons for revision, specifically implant loosening and infection, will certainly be an area of focus over the next 10 years. Implant loosening may occur, even in the absence of osteolysis, when bony on-growth (osseointegration) is insufficient to maintain fixation over time. Infection, in which bacterial growth interferes with the implant-bone interface, results in loosening and the need for revision. Current options for infection prevention include the addition of antibiotics to bone cement. However, release of the antibiotics in vivo is usually short-lived and somewhat unpredictable. As shoulder arthroplasty moves toward metallic, press-fit components to improve fixation via increased osseointegration, alternative methods to reduce infection rates have also been sought. Recently, there has been a push to develop coatings that could offer multi-faceted benefits in terms of secure long-term fixation and infection prevention to reduce revision rates. However, adhesion of bacteria to an implant surface and subsequent development of biofilms that increase the difficulty of eradicating infection is, unfortunately, promoted by many of the same surface characteristics that promote osseointegration. As we move forward, the development of new surfaces for osseointegration will need to be able to balance these competing goals.

Coatings for Osseointegration

Both the chemical structure and surface topology of implants and coatings can play a role in promoting osseointegration. Several classes of coatings currently exist. Coatings such as plasma spray rely solely on microscale topology to increase surface area and surface energy of a metallic implant, which eventually allows for a strong implant-bone interface as the bone remodels into pores and/or channels within the coating. Other types of coatings are known as bioactive coatings, which promote increased fixation by bonding directly to newly remodeled bone. The most commonly used bioactive coating is hydroxyapatite, a bioceramic which has had a role in joint replacements for many years. Other bioactive coatings including metal ions, extracellular matrices, and titanium nanotubes have been, and will continue to be, investigated as options to improve osseointegration of many types of orthopedic implants.[39] In addition to coating material, topology characteristics, such as pore size, will continue to be investigated and optimized to enhance implant fixation.[40]

Antimicrobial Coatings

Researchers have also focused on coatings that would impede the growth of bacterial colonies and biofilms on metallic implant surfaces as a mechanism to prevent infection. Perhaps the most widely recognized infection prevention technique involves the use of silver nanoparticles. Silver nanoparticles have the ability to disrupt key processes necessary for the survival and replication of bacterial cells. Other agents, such as chitosan and titanium oxide, are also being investigated for use in antimicrobial coatings.[41] The advantages of these types of coatings lie in their ability to target several strains of bacteria.

Additionally, there is great potential for future coatings to deliver antibiotics or antiseptics via bioresorbable polymers or nanotubes that can provide controlled drug release over time. For example, titanium nanotubes can be loaded with antibiotics and the size of the nanotubes may be controlled, such that surface texture/topology also promotes osseointegration.[42] Coatings such as these, as well as composites that offer the best of both worlds, will continue to be a focus of biomaterials research over the next decade.

Bearing Surface Coatings

In addition to advancements to the bone-implant interface coatings, there is also potential for continued development of coatings for metallic articular components. The goals of coating metallic articular components are related to the ability to utilize a traditional bearing material (ie, CoCr) while improving wear performance and reducing the potential for release of metal ions, which poses a risk for patients with metal (most often nickel) sensitivities. Current metallic bearing options for nickel-sensitive patients include titanium humeral heads and glenospheres for ATSA and RTSA, which generally perform poorly in comparison to CoCr in terms of wear. Potential coatings may include titanium nitride (TiN), diamond-like carbon, and nanostructured diamond.[43] Articular surface coatings would ideally have low coefficients of friction, high wear resistance, and increased biocompatibility (much the same as the advantages of ceramic components), while preserving the high fracture strength of the underlying metal.

Although many variations of implant coatings are currently being researched, few are currently available for clinical use. The development of coatings that will eventually be used in implants presents a uniquely challenging scenario. Coatings must be treated as implants when being evaluated for safety because delamination of the coating from the implant surface is a risk. As such, efforts to develop coatings are generally lengthy and costly. Nevertheless, it is likely that the next generation of implant coatings will eventually enter the arthroplasty market in an effort to reduce revision rates and improve the efficacy of not just shoulder arthroplasty but many types of joint replacements.

ROLE OF ADDITIVE MANUFACTURING

Just as the materials used in shoulder arthroplasty will continue to advance by leaps and bounds, so too will the methods by which these devices are made. Most of this progress will likely be in the realm of additive manufacturing, which is also known as three-dimensional (3D) printing. This advanced form of manufacturing already plays a role in shoulder arthroplasty today. Patient-specific guides are additively manufactured, usually from nylon, so that they can be custom made to match the glenoid anatomy of a particular patient. These often include a printed model of the patient's scapula for preoperative review. In addition, several implants are 3D printed from titanium powder including the LimaCorporate SMR Stemless **(FIGURE 51.8A)**, Exactech Equinoxe Stemless **(FIGURE 51.8B)**, and the Materialise Glenius custom glenoid. These implants include regions with a porous structure that consist of a repeated pattern or more randomized, trabecular-like design. Ideally, these structures have been created with an optimized pore size and percent porosity to encourage long-term bony in-growth, similar in concept to optimizing coating topography for osseointegration.

The frequency of use of custom-made shoulder implants will rise dramatically in the next decade due to both an increased revision burden and an increased availability of these devices. Additive manufacturing will help to meet this demand and allow for the treatment of even the most complex bone loss, providing surgeons with devices that perfectly match their patient's anatomy, which will likely also simplify these difficult procedures. The speed at which these custom devices are created and delivered will no doubt improve as additive manufacturing technology progresses and as new manufacturing and distribution models are developed, including on-site production at healthcare facilities.[27] There will certainly be regulatory challenges to this type of arrangement, and additively manufactured parts still require post processing (machining, cleaning, passivation, inspection) after they are printed. However, these are hurdles worth overcoming if patients in need of personalized shoulder arthroplasty implants can obtain them sooner and more cost-effectively.

Additive manufacturing will allow for more advanced designs that could not be made through traditional subtractive machining. Complex shapes can be 3D printed to create implants that better match patient anatomy and instruments that are more ergonomic. Material can also be selectively removed from a device to reduce weight without sacrificing strength or functionality. Porous structures can be applied to any location on the implant to enhance or even customize fixation. As with implant coatings, the usage and fine-tuning of these porous structures will certainly increase over the next decade of shoulder arthroplasty. However, it will require long-term clinical studies to confirm their effectiveness.

Additive manufacturing will most likely be an integral part of the future of shoulder arthroplasty. Rapid

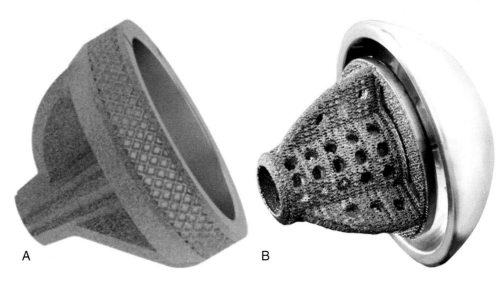

FIGURE 51.8 Additively manufactured shoulder implants: **(A)** LimaCorporate SMR Stemless Shoulder[44] and **(B)** Exactech Equinoxe Stemless Shoulder.[45] (A, Image of the product used under license of Limacorporate S.p.A. – Italy. B, Used with permission from © Exactech, Inc.)

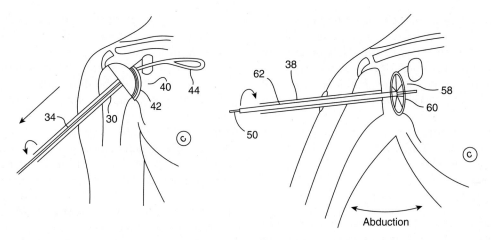

FIGURE 51.9 Shoulder joint preparation using the transhumeral approach described in US patent 9,445,910 B2.[47]

prototyping will increase the pace of innovation as designs can be iterated and refined in short periods of time through plastic and metal 3D printing. As these printers get smaller and less costly, they will be more easily accessible to those brainstorming shoulder implant and instrument designs, from those in academics to the entrepreneurs working from home, thereby broadening the base from which the next revolutionary concepts will be generated.

SURGICAL TECHNIQUES

A decade from now, will most orthopedic surgeons be performing shoulder arthroplasty through a standard deltopectoral approach, or will another method become popular or even the standard? As described in Chapter 20, several subscapularis-sparing techniques have been developed to allow for all or a portion of the subscapularis to remain attached while performing an ATSA. Specialized instrumentation has also been created to assist in these approaches, although they have not become widely adopted primarily because they can be more technically challenging.[46] The surgical approach utilized for shoulder arthroplasty will most likely evolve over the next decade in ways that are difficult to predict. There are already new approaches being developed that require discussion.

Transhumeral Approaches

One method being investigated is the transhumeral approach. Chudik describes a method and instrumentation for replacing the glenohumeral joint through a portal in the proximal humerus, all without the need to dislocate the joint.[47] This passage allows for perpendicular access to both the humerus and glenoid **(FIGURE 51.9)**, while a small anterosuperior incision is used for joint exposure, head resection, and insertion of modular instruments as well as definitive implant components. Instruments used to support this approach

are low profile and can be passed through both the transhumeral and anterosuperior portals and assembled in situ. Fitzpatrick has also described a transhumeral approach that includes a jig connected to the anatomical neck of the humerus to accurately drill along a perpendicular axis through the humeral head **(FIGURE 51.10)**.[48] Additionally, Paterson et al. have described a method and the associated instrumentation using both a deltopectoral incision and transdeltoid access that allows for glenoid preparation without the need for full glenoid cavity exposure.[49]

Posterior Approach

Greiwe has described a humeral implant system inserted through a posterior incision between the middle and posterior portions of the deltoid.[50] With the patient placed in a lateral position and the arm adducted across the body,

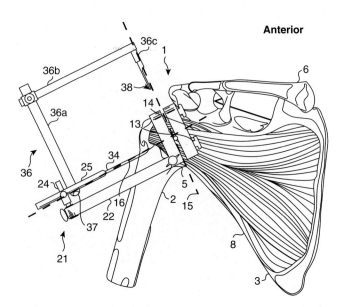

FIGURE 51.10 Specialized jig for transhumeral approach as described in US patent 9,730,708 B2.[48]

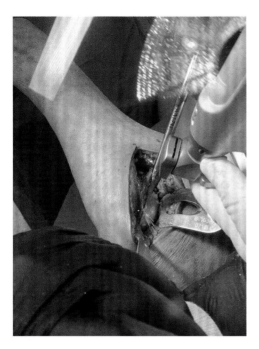

FIGURE 51.11 View of the shoulder joint using the posterior approach with specialized retractors. (Image courtesy of Dr. Michael Greiwe.)

approach-specific retractors are utilized to expose the joint and protect surrounding tissue (**FIGURE 51.11**). The joint is then prepared for the proposed stemless implant that consists of three components: a head, a base, and an insert that is placed between the head and base. The base component is inserted into the prepared humerus and provides fixation. Rather than connecting the head directly to the base, the head is first coupled to the insert. The insert has a rail feature that allows the head/insert assembly to slide into a slot in the base, thereby permitting attachment, even if space or exposure of the joint is limited. Six-month results

using this approach at one site have shown encouraging results,[51] but larger multicenter studies with longer follow-up will be needed to support broader usage.

Arthroscopic Approaches

Others are exploring methods and systems for arthroscopic shoulder arthroplasty. Both Termanini and Burt have disclosed approaches and instrumentation to prepare for and insert shoulder implants using multiple small incisions. The methods of Termanini[52] include an external osteotomy guide with a centralizing device for humeral head resection (**FIGURE 51.12A**); **FIGURE 51.12B** shows arthroscopic preparation of the glenoid articular surface over a guide wire after humeral head resection and removal, with the humerus pulled downward to increase space in the joint. Burt has described humeral head resurfacing components and glenoid templates that can be folded into low-profile configurations for insertion through small arthroscopic portals and then deployed to full size once in the joint space.[53]

How broadly these new approaches are adopted within shoulder arthroplasty will be related to how steep the learning curve is and how well the associated instrumentation and implants can be refined over the years to come. Some of these may prove too difficult to utilize consistently, while others may find some niche success in the hands of high-volume shoulder specialists. With the expansion of preoperative planning and navigation and the advent of robotic assisted surgery in the shoulder, it is likely that novel surgical approaches to shoulder arthroplasty can be developed, which utilize this advanced technology to improve visualization, increase accuracy, spare surrounding soft tissues, and potentially improve patient outcomes.

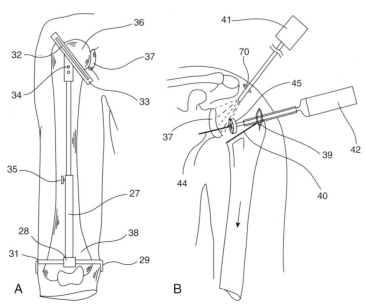

FIGURE 51.12 A, Osteotomy guide with centralizing device for arthroscopic approach as described in patent 10,595,866 B2.[52] **B**, Arthroscopic glenoid preparation over a guide wire as described in patent 10,595,866 B2.[52]

CONCLUSION

Implant designs, materials, and surgical approaches on the current forefront of technology and research are likely indicative of the future landscape of shoulder arthroplasty. At present, shoulder arthroplasty is generally a successful procedure in terms of relieving pain and restoring range of motion for a wide range of patients and indications. The goals of advancements in the field will be rooted in further improving the efficacy of the procedure, whether on a broad scale or for specific (eg, younger) patient populations and providing alternative solutions for complex scenarios. Improved implant fixation mechanisms and bearing materials, bone-preserving and modular designs for ease of convertibility, solutions for bone loss, and reduction of complication rates via implant coatings are likely to remain a focus. Additionally, increased utilization of additive manufacturing will likely allow for broader use of patient-specific implants. Coupled with the possibility of developing less invasive, soft tissue–sparing surgical techniques, there are a multitude of areas in which concepts currently being explored may come to fruition. The future holds the key to advancements in not only implant designs and options but also tools and technology that aid in preoperative planning and accuracy of in situ placement of these devices, the combination of which offers the potential to further improve patient outcomes.

REFERENCES

1. Nelson CG, Brolin TJ, Ford MC, et al. Five-year minimum clinical and radiographic outcomes of total shoulder arthroplasty using a hybrid glenoid component with a central porous titanium post. *J Shoulder Elbow Surg.* 2018;27:1462-1467. doi:10.1016/j.jse.2018.01.012

2. Friedman RJ, Cheung E, Grey SG, et al. Clinical and radiographic comparison of a hybrid cage glenoid to a cemented polyethylene glenoid in anatomic total shoulder arthroplasty. *J Shoulder Elbow Surg.* 2019;28:2308-2316. doi:10.1016/j.jse.2019.04.049

3. Page RS, Pai V, Eng K, et al. Cementless versus cemented glenoid components in conventional total shoulder joint arthroplasty: analysis from the Australian Orthopaedic Association National Joint Replacement Registry. *J Shoulder Elbow Surg.* 2018;27:1859-1865. doi:10.1016/j.jse.2018.03.017

4. McDaniel J, Hellman B. *Convertible Glenoid Implant.* US patent 8,632,598. January 21, 2014.

5. Iannotti J, Williams G, Koka D, et al. *Glenoid Vault Fixation.* US patent 8,920,508 B2. December 30, 2014.

6. Hopkins AR. *Convertible Glenoid.* US patent 10,342,669 B2. July 09, 2019.

7. Hodorek BC, Gargac SM. *Convertible Glenoid Implant.* US patent application 2016/0324649 A1. November 10, 2016.

8. Metcalfe NJT, Michel G. *Stemless Shoulder Implant.* US patent 8,512,410 B2. August 20, 2013.

9. Knox KP, Gargac SM, Mutchler AW, et al. *Stemless Prosthesis Anchor Components, Methods, and Kits.* US patent application 2019/0175354 A1. June 13, 2019.

10. Humphrey CS. *Instruments and Techniques for Orienting Prosthesis Components for Joint Prostheses.* US patent 9,956,083 B2. May 01, 2018.

11. Simovitch RW, Roche CP, Jones RB, et al. Effect of tuberosity healing on clinical outcomes in elderly patients treated with a reverse shoulder arthroplasty for 3- and 4-part proximal humerus fractures. *J Orthop Trauma.* 2019;33:e39-e45. doi:10.1097/BOT.0000000000001348

12. Sabesan VJ, Lima DJL, Yang Y, et al. The role of greater tuberosity healing in reverse shoulder arthroplasty: a finite element analysis. *J Shoulder Elbow Surg.* 2020;29:347-354. doi:10.1016/j.jse.2019.07.022

13. Raiss P, Edwards TB, da Silva MR, et al. Reverse shoulder arthroplasty for the treatment of nonunions of the surgical neck of the proximal part of the humerus (type-3 fracture sequelae). *J Bone Joint Surg Am.* 2014;96:2070-2076. doi:10.2106/JBJS.N.00405

14. Roche CP, Hamilton M, Diep P, et al. *Platform RTSA Glenoid Prosthesis With Modular Attachments Capable of Improving Initial Fixation, Fracture Reconstructions, and Joint Biomechanics.* US patent application 2019/0159907 A1. May 30, 2019.

15. Maale GE. *Glenoid Fossa Prosthesis.* US patent application 2020/0046510 A1. February 13, 2020.

16. Frankle MA, Gutierrez S, Williams G. *Glenosphere With Flange for Augmented Fixation and Related Methods.* US patent 9,782,263 B1. October 10, 2017.

17. Couture P. *Patient-specific Surgical Guide for Intra-operative Production of Patient-specific Augment.* US patent 9,173,665 B2. November 03, 2015.

18. Neichel N, Vennin MJM, Leon C, et al. *Bone Graft Shaper & Patient Specific Bone Graft.* US patent application 2017/0273795 A1. September 28, 2017.

19. Garret J, Godeneche A, Boileau P, et al. Pyrocarbon interposition shoulder arthroplasty: preliminary results from a prospective multicenter study at 2 years of follow-up. *J Shoulder Elbow Surg.* 2017;26:1143-1151. doi:10.1016/j.jse.2017.01.002

20. Barret H, Gauci M-O, Langlais T, et al. Pyrocarbon interposition shoulder arthroplasty in young arthritic patients: a prospective observational study. *J Shoulder Elbow Surg.* 2020;29:e1-e10. doi:10.1016/j.jse.2019.05.044

21. Hopkins A, Hardy P. *Shoulder Prosthesis and Components Thereof.* US patent 9,763,797 B2. September 19, 2017.

22. Britton O, Nolan DA, Hopkins A, et al. *Stemless Shoulder Implant.* US patent application 2017/0105843 A1. April 20, 2017.

23. Wirth MA, Iannotti JP, Williams GW Jr, et al. *Mobile Bearing Glenoid Prosthesis.* US patent 9,439,769 B2. September 13, 2016.

24. Amstutz HC, Campbell P, Kossovsky N, et al. Mechanism and clinical significance of wear debris-induced osteolysis. *Clin Orthop.* 1992;(276):7-18.

25. Bohsali KI, Bois AJ, Wirth MA. Complications of shoulder arthroplasty. *J Bone Joint Surg Am.* 2017;99:256-269. doi:10.2106/JBJS.16.00935

26. Bracco P, Bellare A, Bistolfi A, et al. Ultra-high molecular weight polyethylene: influence of the chemical, physical and mechanical properties on the wear behavior. A review. *Materials Basel.* 2017;10:791. doi:10.3390/ma10070791

27. Hussain M, Naqvi RA, Abbas N, et al. Ultra-high-molecular-weight-polyethylene (UHMWPE) as a promising polymer material for biomedical applications: a concise review. *Polymers.* 2020;12:323. doi:10.3390/polym12020323

28. Gigante A, Bottegoni C, Ragone V, et al. Effectiveness of vitamin-E-doped polyethylene in joint replacement: a literature review. *J Funct Biomater.* 2015;6:889-900. doi:10.3390/jfb6030889

29. Kumar N, Arora GNC, Datta B. Bearing surfaces in hip replacement – Evolution and likely future. *Med J Armed Forces India.* 2014;70:371-376. doi:10.1016/j.mjafi.2014.04.015

30. Mueller U, Braun S, Schroeder S, et al. Influence of humeral head material on wear performance in anatomic shoulder joint arthroplasty. *J Shoulder Elbow Surg.* 2017;26:1756-1764. doi:10.1016/j.jse.2017.05.008

31. Traina F, De Fine M, Di Martino A, et al. Fracture of ceramic bearing surfaces following total hip replacement: a systematic review. *BioMed Res Int.* 2013;2013:157247. doi:10.1155/2013/157247

32. Mathys Medical Ltd. Affinis short [photograph]. Accessed June 22, 2020. https://www.mathysmedical.com/en/products/shoulder

33. Wright Medical Technologies, Inc. Pyrocarbon humeral head [photograph]. Tornier Aequalis Ascend Flex Convertible Shoulder System Surgical Technique. http://osimplantes.com.br/. Accessed 22 June 2020.

34. CeramTec. Accessed May 2, 2020. https://www.ceramtec-medical.com/en/biolox

35. Merolla G, Tartarone A, Sperling JW, et al. Early clinical and radiological outcomes of reverse shoulder arthroplasty with an eccentric all-polyethylene glenosphere to treat failed hemiarthroplasty and the sequelae of proximal humeral fractures. *Int Orthop.* 2017;41:141-148. doi:10.1007/s00264-016-3188-1

36. Molloy D, Jack C, Esposito C, et al. A mid-term analysis suggests ceramic on ceramic hip arthroplasty is durable with minimal wear and low risk of squeak. *HSS J.* 2012;8:291-294. doi:10.1007/s11420-012-9291-y

37. Carpenter SR, Urits I, Murthi AM. Porous metals and alternate bearing surfaces in shoulder arthroplasty. *Curr Rev Musculoskelet Med.* 2016;9:59-66. doi:10.1007/s12178-016-9319-x

38. Garret J, Harly E, Le Huec J-C, et al. Pyrolytic carbon humeral head in hemi-shoulder arthroplasty: preliminary results at 2-year follow-up. *JSES Open Access.* 2019;3:37-42. doi:10.1016/j.jses.2018.09.002

39. Zhang BGX, Myers DE, Wallace GG, et al. Bioactive coatings for orthopaedic implants – Recent trends in development of implant coatings. *Int J Mol Sci.* 2014;15:11878-11921. doi:10.3390/ijms150711878

40. Otsuki B, Takemoto M, Fujibayashi S, et al. Pore throat size and connectivity determine bone and tissue ingrowth into porous implants: three-dimensional micro-CT based structural analyses of porous bioactive titanium implants. *Biomaterials.* 2006;27:5892-5900. doi:10.1016/j.biomaterials.2006.08.013

41. Kazemzadeh-Narbat M, Lai BFL, Ding C, et al. Multilayered coating on titanium for controlled release of antimicrobial peptides for the prevention of implant-associated infections. *Biomaterials.* 2013;34:5969-5977. doi:10.1016/j.biomaterials.2013.04.036

42. Gulati K, Ramakrishnan S, Aw MS, et al. Biocompatible polymer coating of titania nanotube arrays for improved drug elution and osteoblast adhesion. *Acta Biomater.* 2012;8:449-456. doi:10.1016/j.actbio.2011.09.004

43. Catledge SA, Thomas V, Vohra YK. Nanostructured diamond coatings for orthopaedic applications. *Woodhead Publ Ser Biomater.* 2013;2013:105-150. doi:10.1533/9780857093516.2.105

44. LimaCorporate. SMR stemless [photograph]. 2018. Accessed April 28, 2020. https://limacorporate.com/medical/77/smr-stemless.html

45. Exactech, Inc. Equinoxe stemless shoulder [photograph]. 2018. Accessed April 25, 2020. https://www.exac.com/extremities/equinoxe-stemless-shoulder/

46. Ding DY, Mahure SA, Akuoko JA, et al. Total shoulder arthroplasty using a subscapularis-sparing approach: a radiographic analysis. *J Shoulder Elbow Surg.* 2015;24:831-837. doi:10.1016/j.jse.2015.03.009

47. Chudik SC. *Method of Minimally Invasive Shoulder Replacement Surgery.* US patent 9,445,910 B2. September 20, 2016.

48. Fitzpatrick MJ. *Method of Humeral Head Resurfacing And/or Replacement and System for Accomplishing the Method.* US patent 9/730,708 B2. August 15, 2017.

49. Paterson P, Pressacco M, Fattori A, et al. *Method for Surgical Application of a Glenoid Prosthesis Component of a Shoulder Joint Prosthesis and Relating Surgical Instruments.* US patent application 2019/0216615 A1. July 18, 2019.

50. Greiwe RM. *Humeral Head Implant System.* US patent 10,368,999 B2. August 06, 2019.

51. Greiwe RM, Hill MA, Boyle MS, et al. Posterior approach total shoulder arthroplasty: a retrospective analysis of short-term results. *Orthopedics.* 2020;43:e15-e20. doi:10.3928/01477447-20191122-03

52. Termanini Z. *Arthroscopic Shoulder Arthroplasty and Method Thereof.* US patent 10,595,886 B2. March 24, 2020.

53. Burt DM. *Arthroscopic Total Shoulder Arthroplasty.* US patent 10,039,556 B2. August 07, 2018.

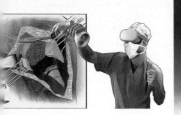

52 Total Shoulder Arthroplasty in 10 Years: Advanced Technology

Alexander T. Greene, BS and Joseph D. Zuckerman, MD

INTRODUCTION

Before the advent of contemporary computers and advanced diagnostic imaging, surgeons had to rely on tactile hand skills and inherent medical knowledge and instinct to assess, diagnose, and treat patients. Arguably, the largest improvements in surgical intervention since the adoption of germ theory and general anesthesia have come about as the result of embracing advanced technologies, which give surgeons the ability to see, assess, and operate to a level of precision and accuracy beyond what is achievable without them.

The first of these advancements came from modern imaging techniques such as computed tomography (CT) and magnetic resonance imaging (MRI) that the rise of the integrated circuit and advanced computational power made possible. At their introduction, these techniques allowed for two-dimensional (2D) visualization of image slices throughout the body at a resolution and regional focus previously not available with standard radiographic imaging. The advent of computer modeling and digital rendering further advanced these imaging modalities, allowing for reconstruction and visualization of three-dimensional (3D) structures from the 2D images. In the present day, these imaging advancements fueled the development of powerful preoperative and intraoperative software to aid surgeons in planning, guidance, and decision-making in patient care.

The goal of using advanced technologies in total shoulder arthroplasty (TSA) is to leverage the additional data derived from these applications to improve implant durability, longevity, and ultimately clinical outcomes. When evaluating the future impact of advanced technologies on the field of shoulder arthroplasty over the next 10 years, the effects can be considered in the context of the different stages of patient care: preoperative, intraoperative, and postoperative.

PREOPERATIVE

Preoperative Planning

Arguably the largest impact on TSA preoperative patient care as the result of advanced technology is the development of 3D preoperative planning software. Recent literature shows that the mere exercise of going through the thought process of preoperative planning in 3D leads to better accuracy in surgical placement of the final glenoid implant.[1-5] Such software has evolved rapidly in recent years and continues to be a major area of focus for development. This type of software is now widely available from most orthopedic implant manufacturers, which allows the surgeon to virtually perform a TSA procedure and place the glenoid and humeral implants in 3D space with millimeter and degree precision (**FIGURE 52.1**). All current systems allow for planning and adjustment of glenoid component positioning in the scapula, and some systems allow for templating the humeral component as well as manipulation of the bones in 3D space which can provide a basic biomechanical assessment of the effect of the type and position of the implants chosen.

At the time of writing, all commercially available software is CT-based and is constructed solely on the bony anatomy of a patient. Future advancements in imaging modalities will include visualization of the soft tissues around the shoulder, allowing for further evaluation and assessment by the surgeon beyond the bony structures. This could be accomplished through improvements in any of three currently available imaging modalities. The first improvement can be through advancements in CT scan imaging, where dual-energy CT or image postprocessing can enhance the visual acuity of soft tissue structures.[6,7] The second can be through improvements in MRI, which traditionally is an imaging modality more suited for soft tissue visualization. Advancements and availability of high-resolution MRI with a small image slice thickness will need to be made more readily available to replace the current standard of care for shoulder arthroplasty imaging, which is a CT scan.[8] A combination of imaging modalities may also be used, but due to the cost and logistic challenges of patients having more than one preoperative scan (both CT and MRI), one imaging modality will need to rise above the other as the better solution to visualize both bony and soft tissue anatomy. Although high-resolution CT is currently more readily available, MRI has the advantage of no radiation exposure for the patient as

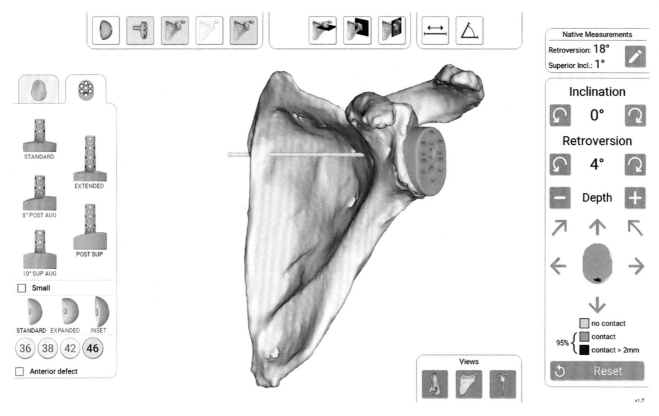

FIGURE 52.1 Contemporary preoperative planning software. (Used with permission from © Exactech, Inc.)

well as higher resolution of soft tissue anatomy due to the different weighting abilities of the scanner detectors. The third imaging modality improvement could be with ultrasound, which technically has the highest spatial resolution of these three imaging modalities. However, challenges in beam penetration through the entirety of the shoulder, a lower signal-to-noise ratio, and variations in operator technique all present technical challenges that will need to be overcome before ultrasound can be adopted to produce a high-resolution 3D model of the shoulder.[9]

When a patient with metal implants in the shoulder is scanned with any of these imaging modalities, metal artifact is generated, distorting the image and limiting the efficacy of these scans in this clinical situation. Metal artifact reduction (MAR) techniques will continue to improve over time, especially as 3D imaging becomes more prevalent in orthopedics[10,11] **(FIGURE 52.2)**. Although 2D biplanar x-ray imaging is a fourth imaging modality that has shown some promise in other total joint applications, this imaging technique does not have the local accuracy that CT imaging does for the shoulder, especially with regards to the local accuracy needed for accurate resolution of the glenoid and glenoid vault.

Once the soft tissue structures are incorporated into preoperative planning software, full assessment and

optimization of the biomechanics of the joint can be performed. For an anatomic total shoulder arthroplasty (ATSA), it is well established in the literature that reproducing the anatomy is correlated with positive clinical outcomes.[12,13] This includes reproduction of the native humeral head and restoration of the joint line, reconstruction of the glenoid anatomy with a properly positioned glenoid component, and proper tensioning of the rotator cuff.[14-17] All of these parameters can currently be preoperatively planned, but limited information is provided to the user on what the optimal targets are and how to quantify them. Regarding glenoid component positioning, current literature shows there has yet to be a consensus on the proper way to plan for an individual patient. Not only is there high variability in planning the same patient among different surgeons but also high variability in planning the same patient at different times by the same surgeons.[18,19] This lack of consensus will ultimately be settled by controlling for individual variables with long-term clinical outcome studies. Additionally, as computing power, imaging inputs, and shoulder-specific knowledge all increase, preoperative planning software will evolve to include a more patient-specific biomechanical analysis, which a process that is currently time-consuming and traditionally only available with statistical shape models (SSM)

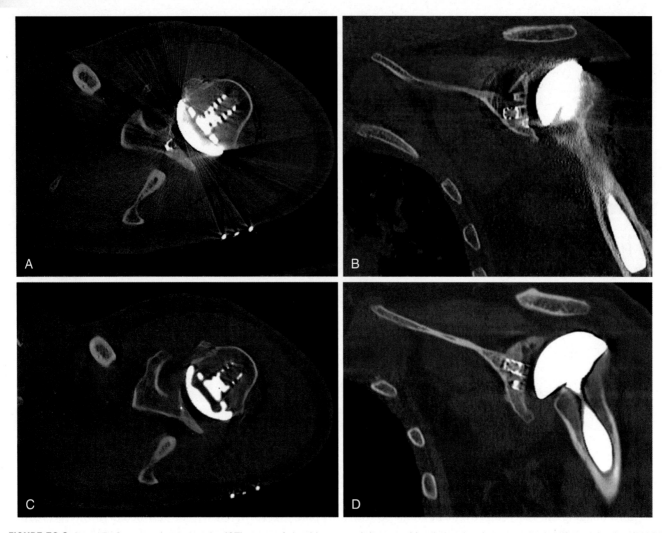

FIGURE 52.2 A and **B**, Computed tomography (CT) scans of shoulders containing metal implants showing non-metal artifact reduction (MAR) images and (**C** and **D**) MAR images.

in a research setting.[20,21] The customization and specificity provided by looking at the patient's native joint offsets, muscle tensioning, comorbidities, and other patient-specific parameters will empower surgeons to optimize implant type and position based on not only established means but also on what is best for a particular patient.

The greatest area for improvement in optimizing soft tissue tensioning in TSA resides in reverse total shoulder arthroplasty (RTSA), as tensioning parameters are not only patient-specific but are also more greatly influenced by implant parameters due to the non-anatomic reproduction of the joint in RTSA. Different implant systems and manufacturers use a variety of parameters to adjust the medialization and lateralization of the glenoid and humeral components, amount of distalization of the humeral components, and overall tension of the joint.[22-26] A certain amount of glenoid/humeral lateralization for one patient may not be ideal for another, and

vice versa. For example, a lateralized glenosphere may tension the deltoid more but could cause complications in an osteoporotic patient with a thinner acromion.[27,28] However, determining the optimal tension of a RTSA will not only be influenced by offsets that create the most efficient moment arms but also by the efficiency, tensioning, and function of the individual muscles involved.[22,29-31] Future preoperative planning software that incorporates soft tissue data will be able to factor in the influence of these parameters and determine what may be optimal for a particular patient.

Another area of improvement involving soft tissues is quantifying the amount of fatty infiltration and volume of the muscle bodies.[32] Specifically, being able to quantify the percentage of fatty infiltration of the rotator cuff and deltoid muscles will help surgeons discern if and how functional the muscles are before surgery, potentially aiding in the decision-making process to determine if a RTSA is preferred in a patient with an intact but potentially nonfunctioning rotator cuff.[33,34] This will benefit both ATSA and RTSA, as it will help surgeons determine the condition of specific muscles, their strength potential, how well they are functioning, and how their role will affect the greater biomechanics of the shoulder complex once other parameters are modified.

Lastly, there will be advancements in how the preoperative planning software user interface is delivered to and used by the surgeon. Traditional systems use software on a 2D computer screen or tablet, but future systems will evolve toward a mixed reality, augmented reality (AR), or immersive virtual reality environment.[35] These systems give the surgeon the ability to virtually perform the surgery in a digital environment that mimics the operating room (OR), often giving tactile, haptic feedback on surgical movements and providing valuable information on not only the optimal plan for the case but how to perform the procedure in a stepwise fashion **(FIGURE 52.3)**. This may influence a surgeon's preoperative plan in TSA; for example, in a scenario where a significantly retroverted glenoid implant is planned and then changed as a result of realizing challenging glenoid exposure with such retroversion during the virtual case. Such applications also have potential to aid in medical training by providing a safe, low-cost environment for physicians to practice in a virtual environment, where specific movements and procedures could be repeated until mastery is achieved.

INTRAOPERATIVE

Due to the tangible nature of orthopedic surgery, the intraoperative domain may be most poised for a positive impact from advanced technology than any other. The assistance and precision from advanced instrumentation provide a tremendous advantage by increasing a surgeon's ability to both execute small tactile movements and to accurately follow a preoperative plan.

3D Printing

As advancements in 3D printing continue to decrease cost and logistical challenges associated with traditional manufacturing techniques, the ability to machine implants and instruments on-demand and potentially even in a hospital or an OR environment will develop. Patient-specific instrumentation has been a popular application of 3D printing in TSA, but recent literature has shown mixed results with currently available techniques.[4,36] In addition, ordering imaging and custom instrumentation in advance of a procedure sometimes presents issues with lead times and available resources. With the ability to customize instrumentation on-site for a procedure, exact drill/saw guides and jigs can be created after surgical exposure of the bony landmarks, accommodating for variance in surgical approach and any change in the patient's anatomy since the time of imaging. This will also enable a surgeon to pivot to a different treatment if needed by adjusting the custom instrumentation accordingly in real-time.

3D printing patient-specific implants and instruments on-demand will also greatly reduce the inventory needed for a TSA, as many manufacturer-specific instruments will no longer be needed to successfully perform the case. The large inventory of different sizes and types of implants required to be available for a specific case will no longer be necessary as only one implant will be produced for each case. This has the potential to reduce both OR time and the total cost of the procedure while also increasing surgeon confidence in the preoperatively planned and selected implant.

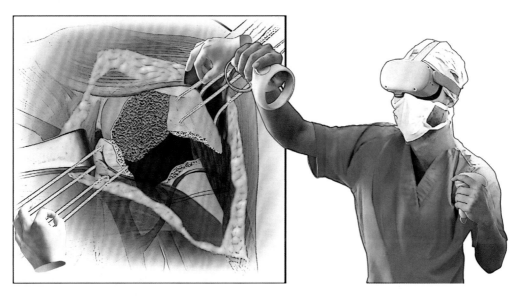

FIGURE 52.3 Preoperative planning and surgical simulation in virtual reality.

In addition to instrumentation, on-site 3D printing will allow surgeons to address complex anatomy at the time of surgery. Custom implants are traditionally reserved for severe deformities when a standard off-the-shelf product will not suffice. Improvements in 3D printing and reductions in manufacturing costs will bring mass customization to all patients. A risk with current 3D printed custom implants is having the implant not fit the patient at the time of surgery either due to further degeneration of the patient's anatomy since the time of preoperative imaging or because of inaccurate implant construction from the imaging. On-site 3D printing could allow a more precise implant to be created to fit the patient's anatomy after exposure and could more easily accommodate for intraoperative variables that are difficult to predict such as change in bony geometry due to fracture or tumor removal. It will also improve the patient experience in the healthcare system and potentially reduce the overall length of the treatment regimen. The patient could be scanned, have implants and instruments printed, and the case performed all within the same institution **(FIGURE 52.4)**.

Smart Instruments

Another application of advanced technology in the intraoperative domain is through smart instruments. A smart instrument can be defined as any tool that is traditionally purely mechanical in nature but is augmented by electronic components to provide additional information or guidance to the user. One such instrument is a device to define the soft tissue tension in the shoulder. This would be clinically beneficial in both ATSA and RTSA but may have more utility in RTSA as proper tension is usually a technique that is "experience based". Thus far, targets for optimal tensioning have yet to be quantified, but the effects of improper tension are well documented.[37-40] An electromechanical humeral liner trial for RTSA that provides surgeons with the tension of the reduced RTSA construct in pounds and the point of contact of the load has recently been developed and is currently in early stages of clinical use **(FIGURE 52.5)**. This has the potential to allow surgeons to define the optimal tension for a particular patient and vary the implant type and offsets accordingly. Research shows that RTSA tension is indeed patient-specific and does have a direct impact on range of motion (ROM).[41] It will be important to evaluate the stability and tension of the joint throughout a dynamic ROM assessment and not just a static load assessment in one position **(FIGURE 52.6)**. The effect of procedural differences such as subscapularis repair will also likely change the joint tension and biomechanics throughout the various ranges of motion. This type of tension measuring device will also be useful in ATSA and could help surgeons determine when to upsize or downsize the humeral head or when additional capsular releases or imbrication procedures are needed. Due to size constraints, the humeral head trials are the more likely location for the load sensors instead of the smaller glenoid components. A future application of such tensioning devices may be an automatically detecting and self-expanding trial implant or tensioning instrument to simplify the trialing process and more efficiently establish the proper tension for the ROM assessment portion of the procedure. Combined with recommendations from clinical outcomes, a patient's unique biomechanics may be assessed real-time in the OR, providing the surgeon the opportunity to adjust implant type and position based on direct assessment rather than only preoperative imaging. Other smart instrument applications could be sensors used on the muscles themselves to determine individual muscle tension, strain, activation, and efficiency.

In addition, a common challenge in ATSA is determining if humeral bone has sufficient density and structure to support the use of a variety of press-fit implants that all load the bone in different ways (standard stem, short stem, stemless, or resurfacing humeral implant).[42-44] Assessments of the humeral bone are traditionally qualitative and rely on surgeon feel and judgment intraoperatively. An instrument with sensors could apply a local load to an area of the bone and provide feedback to the surgeon on thresholds for bone quality and what the anticipated fixation of different types of implants would be to assist in optimal humeral implant selection.

Navigation

Intraoperative navigation provides additional patient and instrument positional information to the surgeon in real-time to help guide more precise and accurate placement of the instruments and implants during the procedure.[45,46] This can be a tremendous benefit in TSA, where incisions are limited, and exposure of the glenohumeral joint can be challenging.[47] On the scapular side, the smaller bony anatomy of the glenoid provides a relatively small target for the glenoid implants, which can be difficult to orient properly even for experienced surgeons.[48] The detrimental impact of glenoid implant malposition is well documented in ATSA, potentially leading to early loosening.[49-54] In RTSA, implant malposition can not only cause early loosening but can adversely affect stability and ROM and result in complications such as scapular notching and dislocation.[22,31,37,38,55-60]

Conventional navigation employs the use of a camera tracking system and registration algorithm to orient the patient's physical anatomic structures to a virtual model from either preoperative imaging in image-based navigation or an SSM representing the anatomic structure in imageless navigation. Such systems provide feedback to the surgeon by overlaying the surgical tools on the patient imaging displayed on a screen as is common

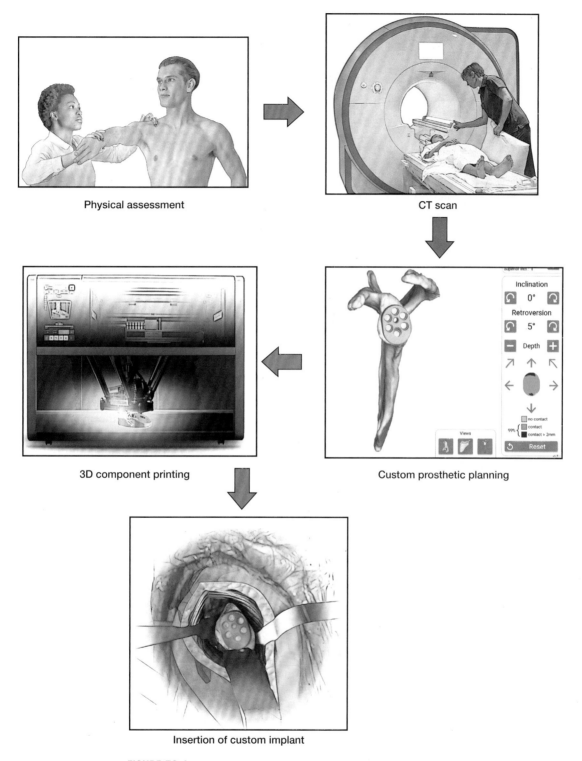

Physical assessment

CT scan

3D component printing

Custom prosthetic planning

Inclination

0°

Retroversion

5°

Depth

no contact
contact
contact > 2mm

Views

Reset

Insertion of custom implant

FIGURE 52.4 Three-dimensional (3D) printing process in the hospital.

in stereotaxic neurosurgery procedures or on a digital 3D rendering of the patient's anatomic structure represented by an SSM. These systems require the creation of a local coordinate system to orient the patient to the imaging or SSM. This typically requires a surgeon to attach either an active (usually infrared light-emitting diode) or passive (infrared reflective) tracker to the patient's bone and then perform a registration algorithm to orient the imaging to the patient's body. This is typically performed manually via a handheld probe by touching specific structures on the patient as prompted by the navigation interface. However, this technique

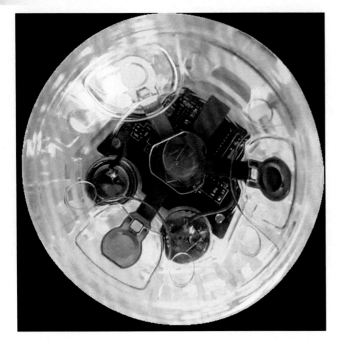

FIGURE 52.5 Electromechanical load sensing trial for reverse total shoulder arthroplasty (RTSA). (Used with permission from © Exactech, Inc.)

can be prone to user error if the precise instructions are not followed or if the patient's physical structures do not match the imaging. Additional trackers are then placed onto calibrated surgical instruments to orient the system.[61] This entire procedure can be time consuming,

often requires troubleshooting, and can be frustrating to the surgeon.

For the scapular side of TSA, intraoperative navigation provides the surgeon with precise entry points in the glenoid, as well as depths and angles for reaming, drilling, screw placement, and ultimately final implant positioning **(FIGURE 52.7)**. Jones et al reported surgeons can achieve accuracy of RTSA glenoid component positioning within 1.9° ± 1.9° for version and 2.4° ± 2.4° for inclination in relation to a preoperative plan.[46] Regarding tracker fixation, there are not many bony structures available in a standard deltopectoral incision for tracker fixation. The only currently available commercial application for glenoid-sided navigation uses the coracoid process as a reference point. Although it is in close proximity to the operating area, the coracoid can often be compromised preoperatively or intraoperatively in ATSA and RTSA. In addition, osteoporosis can also compromise fixation.[61-64] Future developments in glenoid-sided navigation may include real-time local density calculations to allow surgeons to assess ideal placement of implant components and screw trajectory for best fixation and minimize chance of fracture from screw malpositioning.[62,63]

Humeral-sided navigation has yet to be developed and is an area of future advancement. Consequences of humeral implant malposition are also well documented and can result in stress shielding and potential implant loosening.[44,64-67] In addition, as bone-preserving ATSA implants such as stemless humeral components become

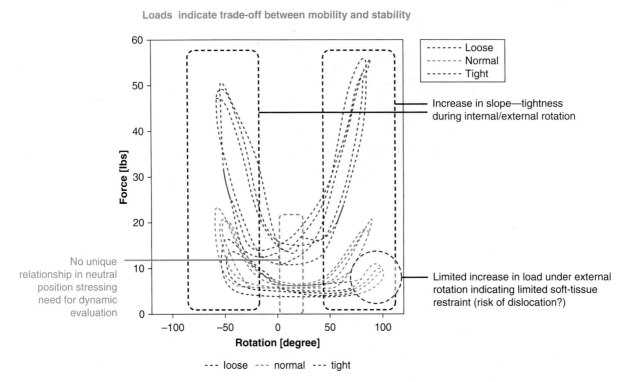

FIGURE 52.6 Loose versus normal versus tight condition shoulder.

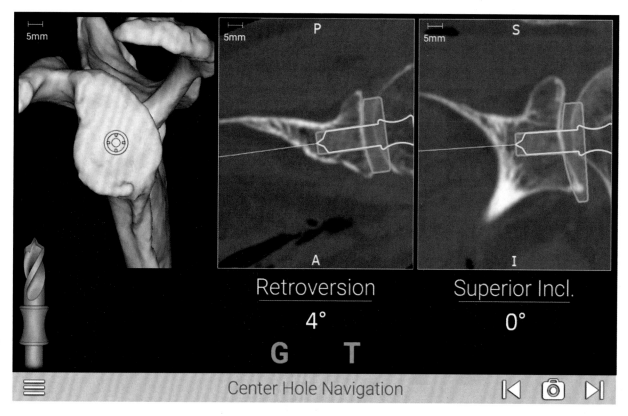

FIGURE 52.7 Modern navigation interface. (Used with permission from © Exactech, Inc.)

more popular, the implants no longer reference the humeral canal upon preparation and insertion and are thus more sensitive to malalignment.[68,69] A humeral navigation system could help the surgeon execute the humeral cut at the proper height and angle, prepare the internal cavity of the humerus in the proper shape and location, and aid in insertion of the implant in the proper depth and orientation. The main technical challenge to overcome in humeral navigation is where and how to rigidly fixate a tracker to the humeral bone that does not compromise the bone's integrity and also maintains visibility throughout the wide ROM in a TSA. Another opportunity once both sides of the joint are navigated and have trackers referencing the scapula and humerus is the ability to perform intraoperative biomechanical assessments, with feedback on where and how much the bones are moving throughout the ROM. This could be especially helpful in a trialing scenario in which a surgeon has the opportunity to adjust implant-specific parameters and offsets, optimizing for ROM and function.

The largest area for future improvement in a navigation system for TSA resides in the tracking systems and registration process. Tracker placement and fixation remains a challenge in any surgical navigation procedure, not just in orthopedics. Most systems require direct line of sight between the trackers and the system's camera, which can often become obstructed during

the procedure. To improve this, there is potential to develop tracker-less navigation in the future. This may be achieved using either inertial measurement units (IMUs), an electromagnetic field generator, or ultrawideband positioning, all of which do not require direct line of sight.[70-74] The most promising technique may be a hybrid system of cameras and detectors, using a combination of either visible or infrared light detection such as laser light detection and ranging (also known as LIDAR) or forward-looking infrared (also known as FLIR), ultrasound or sound navigation and ranging (also known as SONAR), and radio detection and ranging (also known as RADAR) to scan the incision and patient's anatomy and then automatically perform the registration without trackers or user input **(FIGURE 52.8)**. Such a system could be paired with intraoperative O-arm CT to obtain the required imaging in the OR with the patient on the operating table, eliminating the need for preoperative imaging and speeding up the registration process.[75] For such an automatic registration system to work, the system must also be able to adjust for both patient and surgeon movement after the registration, so a continuous update of both the registration and the display of information will be required. Ultimately, the image resolution and processing power of such systems will need to be dramatically improved before the accuracy and precision desired in TSA will make this a feasible option. However, this

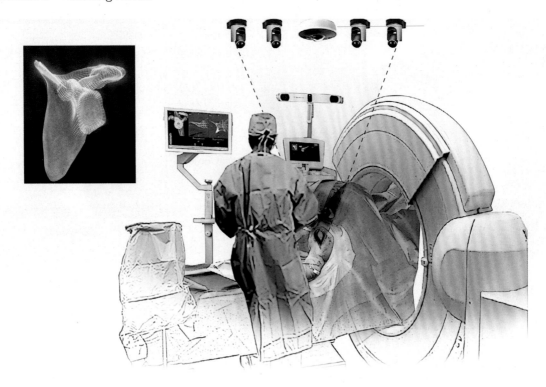

FIGURE 52.8 Tracker-less navigation registration.

advancement has the potential to make navigation the standard of care, by eliminating the steps of registration and tracker fixation from the procedure.

The next most meaningful advancement in intraoperative navigation for TSA will overlay the navigation interface directly onto the incision site itself, enabling the surgeon to perceive both the patient and the navigation interface in the same field of view. This may be achieved using an AR interface to display both reality and digital information in the same line of sight and depth of field. Such an application has the potential to reduce the incision size and enable more minimally invasive TSAs, potentially even in an arthroscopic approach as the surgeon will be able to "see" directly through tissues and into the joint without exposing in a traditional fashion **(FIGURE 52.9)**. These AR environments could be created by having the surgeon use a wearable display such as the Microsoft Hololens.[76] However, before this can become a feasible AR delivery mechanism for orthopedic procedures, the processing power and image resolution of such systems will need to be improved to provide the accuracy and precision required in surgery.[77-83] In developing AR, the goal is to have an accurate digital image appear realistic and not be distracting to the user when it is overlaid on a real image. In addition, with the precise accuracy required in a surgical procedure, the digital image must be aligned properly with the target (in this case the patient) and must correct in real-time for surgeon head movement,

surgeon eye movement, and patient movement, which all contribute to the perceived digital image moving on the AR display. At the time of writing, there is no system available that accommodates for these aspects of movement during the procedure, which contribute to a jittery AR image that is not only inaccurate but also potentially distracting in an OR environment. In addition, the ergonomics of using a wearable display in the OR have yet to be optimized for all orthopedic procedures, as long-term comfort and compatibility with total joint hoods and headlamps will need to be considered.[84]

Another potential delivery mechanism of an AR environment could be an external screen or digital see-through plane placed between the surgeon and the patient, similar to the cockpits of modern military aircraft. Such a screen could be used for portions of the procedure where navigation assistance is needed and moved out of the surgical field when not needed. The advantage of this type display over a wearable setup is less fatigue on the user from having to wear a digital display or head-based mount for the entire procedure. As well, this display eliminates surgeon head movement and reduces the effect of surgeon eye movement since the focal length from the image to the surgeon's eyes is increased. Both of these measures decrease the jitter of the overlaid digital image.

The last and most advanced AR development will be projection of the visual navigation information directly onto the patient. This technique requires much more

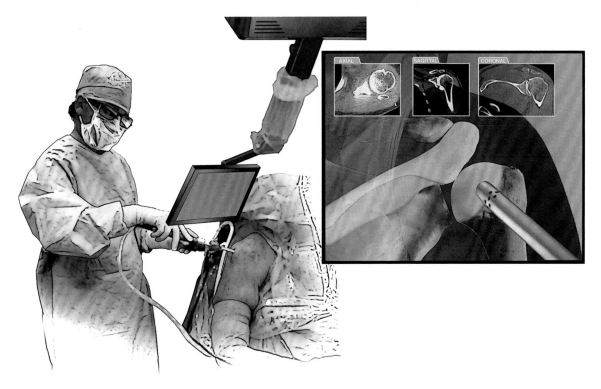

FIGURE 52.9 Minimally invasive total shoulder arthroplasty (TSA) through an arthroscopic incision using an augmented reality interface.

powerful cameras and computational processing for proper orientation of the image onto the patient and projectors powerful enough to transmit an image that can be seen in an OR lighting environment. This approach has the potential to look the most natural and be the least invasive to OR workflow compared to using an external screen or wearable display. Due to technical challenges, it is most likely that a tracker-based AR system will be developed first, followed by a tracker-less system as the camera accuracy and registration algorithms improve to the point that the trackers can be eliminated altogether.

Robotics

Robotics are similar to navigation with respect to the imaging, registration, and trackers required for the procedure. Similarly, robotics will also benefit from the tracking, alignment, and user interface advancements discussed for navigation. Robotics build on the advantages provided by navigation systems by adding a more precise level of control of the surgical instruments, as the actuators in a robotic platform can operate on a level of precision unachievable by the human hand.[85] The application of haptics and tactile feedback in a robotic platform can help the user know when instruments are in a proper position or conversely, in a potentially dangerous one. Just like navigation, however, robotic systems are only as accurate as the reliability of their registration and tracking techniques. Robotics have gained expanded utilization and market share in hip and knee arthroplasty and spine procedures, despite substantial capital expenses and clinical studies showing mixed results in improvement of clinical outcomes.[86-91] Nevertheless, robotics add a level of customization and improved accuracy and shoulder arthroplasty will undoubtedly see similar benefits once an application is developed.[92] As 3D printed custom implants become more commonplace, custom bone preparation enabled by robotics may be required for their proper use and fixation. Typically, the type of tool used in a robotic arm is modified from traditional hand tools, such as small high-speed burrs for finely detailed machining of the bone. These types of instruments can also be paired with sensors to potentially provide local bone density measurements of the contacted bone, providing real-time updates to the surgeon as the bone is being prepared.

In addition to more accurate and precise movements, robotics provide the opportunity to reduce incision size. The use of cameras and smaller surgical instruments on robotic arms that do not have to be manipulated by the human hand can be inserted into smaller incisions. Much of the incision size in TSA is dictated by the surgeon's requirement for adequate exposure of the anatomic structures and to have space to use the instruments that are designed for manipulation by the human hand. A smaller incision also has the potential to minimize soft tissue trauma and facilitate recovery. A TSA that preserves all of the rotator cuff during the approach has the potential to improve clinical outcomes, but lower-profile incisions have typically made the procedure more difficult as a result of reduced visualization.[93-95]

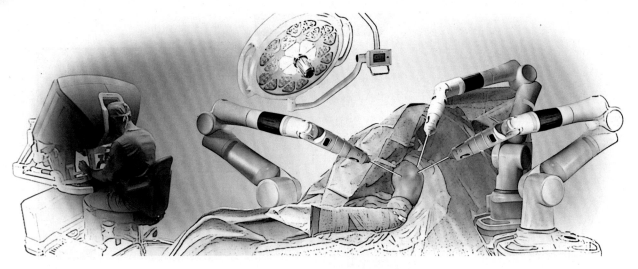

FIGURE 52.10 Robotic application in total shoulder arthroplasty (TSA).

With low-profile robotic arms and cameras to visualize the anatomic structures, this requirement becomes less critical. Robotic arms will also likely make it easier to perform the registration process in anatomic areas that are usually less accessible. ATSA and RTSA may eventually become arthroscopic-assisted or completely arthroscopic, as has been the trend for other operative procedures around the shoulder (**FIGURE 52.10**). This will progress until the incision size approaches a limit where the implants will need to be designed for low profile/arthroscopic insertion, as many humeral and glenoid implants are a certain minimum size to begin with and require an axis of insertion that may not be available in an arthroscopic or low-profile approach. As incision size starts to limit the insertion of standard-sized implants, it may accelerate the development of lower profile, more bone-preserving implants that can be inserted using these approaches. We recognize that there are many steps needed to advance to this level, but orthopedic surgeons and engineers certainly have a track record of ingenuity and creativity, and this may be the next horizon.

Smart Implants

A mostly untapped area of development resides in the development of smart implants, or implants containing electronic components to provide real-time data to the surgeon and patient once implanted. Smart implants are commonplace in the cardiovascular and neurostimulator spaces but have yet to be commercially available in orthopedics.[96,97] Specific to TSA, Westerhoff et al. placed strain gauges and wireless data transmitters inside the humeral component of an ATSA implant to measure the joint reaction forces during different movements.[98,99] Although successful, these implants were investigational devices and were only available in a research setting. Even though only a small number of these devices were implanted, the data and insights gleaned from the research have been invaluable to our understanding of

the mechanics of TSA. From an industry perspective, many regulatory hurdles exist in creating widely available implants containing sensors, which will likely need to be approved through the Food and Drug Administration's Premarket Approval process. This process can take many years and requires a significant financial investment to complete clinical trials. The most basic sensors that could be built into commercially available implants are radio frequency identification (also known as RFID) microchips, which can provide information such as serial number, device type, and patient information to the user. In more advanced applications, strain gauges, load sensors, and IMUs and could be built into the humeral and glenoid components for both ATSA and RTSA to provide not only joint reaction forces but also real-time orientation of the components throughout active dynamic motion and activities of daily living (**FIGURE 52.11**). The greatest advantage of a dynamic movement assessment using wireless smart implants is being able to observe joint loads under active muscle tension. In addition to using sensor data for biomechanical research and development of the next-generation prostheses and techniques, this data could also be used in the early detection of component loosening and infection. Early wireless detection of these complications could provide tremendous benefit for patients by enabling earlier intervention and the potential to minimize the adverse effects that are inevitable with delayed diagnosis. Implantable temperature and pH sensors could also provide early detection for infection and loosening by detecting changes in the homeostatic environment.

In addition to providing feedback to surgeons, sensors could also provide immediate feedback to the patient. For example, if a patient performed a motion that imposed a load or position exceeding a clinically relevant threshold on the joint and implant, the implant could either emit a sound, vibration, or signal to a wireless communicating device to alert the patient that this

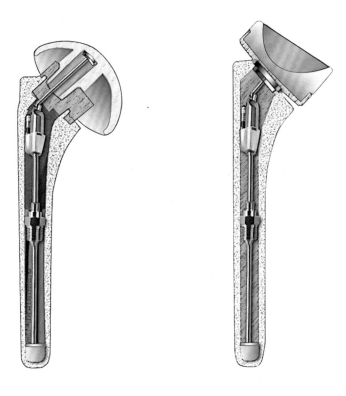

FIGURE 52.11 Smart implants with sensors.

motion is discouraged. Additionally, these sensors could be used postoperatively in a physical therapy or exercise program to provide feedback to the patient on how his/her rehabilitation program is progressing over time and where improvements can be made.

POSTOPERATIVE

The postoperative domain has seen the least amount of application of advanced technologies and for this reason may be poised to experience the largest growth. Wireless connectivity and continuous data monitoring will provide insights to surgeons and patients alike beyond the brief snapshot that is typically gleaned in physical therapy and postoperative follow-up visits.

Wearables

Similar to the application of sensors in implants, wearables use various sensors to collect and communicate data to the surgeon and patient. As their name suggests, these devices are "worn" by the patient in a sleeve, sticker, or similar attachment mechanism to collect data on the patient. At the most basic level, wearable IMU sensors on the patient's shoulder and wrist can provide active ROM and position data, assisting with postoperative physical therapy in a manner similar to implants containing sensors **(FIGURE 52.12)**. The large advantages

wearables have over implantable sensors are reduced complexity, no need for implantation, and the nonpermanent aspect that allows the patient to remove the device when desired. In addition, if a sensor breaks, malfunctions need to be recharged, or if a newer version is introduced, the sensor can simply be replaced and does not require revision surgery. In a postoperative setting, wearables can help patients progress through physical therapy in a home setting by using the feedback from the wearable combined with guidance from a patient-focused application. Although these techniques have gained traction in other joint arthroplasties, they have yet to be integrated into TSA. When this does occur, they will have a substantial impact on postoperative care.[100-102] As wearable data becomes more accessible to patients, the benefit will also extend into the preoperative domain. Prehabilitation exercises to condition a patient for surgery have been shown to increase postoperative clinical outcomes in other joint replacements.[103,104] The use of wearable devices will make the prehabilitation process easier and more accessible to the patient with the potential to increase compliance. Lastly, wearables have the potential to streamline the clinical data collection process. Traditional clinical data collection methods often involve in-person follow-up visits for patients, which are resource-intensive. In addition, follow-up visits are often missed, which undermines the value of data collection.

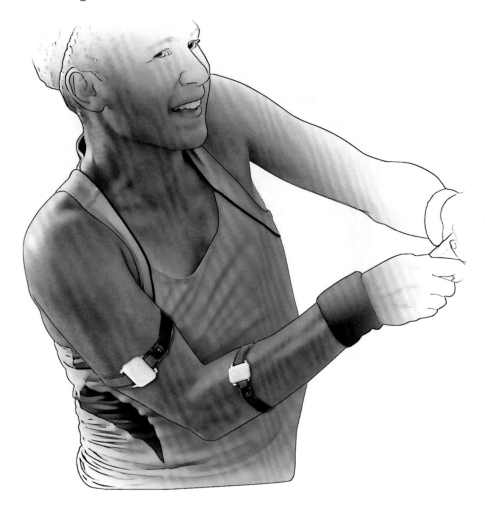

FIGURE 52.12 Wearables deployed on humerus and forearm.

The automated collection of ROM, patient-reported metrics, and other useful outcome measures from wearables will lower the barrier for data collection and enhance the quality of data being collected. Technology that simplifies the data collection and analysis process will have a synergistic benefit across all of healthcare.

Machine Learning

The advanced technology that will have the greatest impact across the entire continuum of care for arthroplasty patients will be the application of machine learning. Machine learning has created the opportunity to observe patterns and correlations in immensely large datasets in a fraction of the time compared to traditional methods, where such correlations would be otherwise undetectable. With the large magnitude of variables that affect patient outcomes in ATSA and RTSA, the features that most heavily influence an optimal outcome will be identified much more quickly by the use of machine learning algorithms.[100,105,106] Once these algorithms are validated by clinical outcomes, future software will allow the surgeon to input general

health and demographic information for an individual patient, which combined with imaging data could generate not only predicted outcomes for the patient for different arthroplasty procedures but also a recommendation for optimal implant type and position. Intraoperative data on implant type and final position could also be features considered by the algorithm. Postoperatively, once the data flow from the patient's outcome measures is fed back to the inputs of the machine-learning algorithm, the process becomes self-sustaining and improves over time **(FIGURE 52.13)**. This will have implications across the entire continuum of patient care. Preoperatively, machine-learning algorithms will help surgeons determine if a patient is a good candidate for elective surgery based upon predefined improvement thresholds of minimally clinically important difference and substantial clinical benefit for various outcome metrics. If the patient is projected to be a surgical candidate, the algorithm can aid in the decision-making process of ATSA versus RTSA as recently described by Kumar et al.[106-111] Intraoperatively, machine learning could help a surgeon

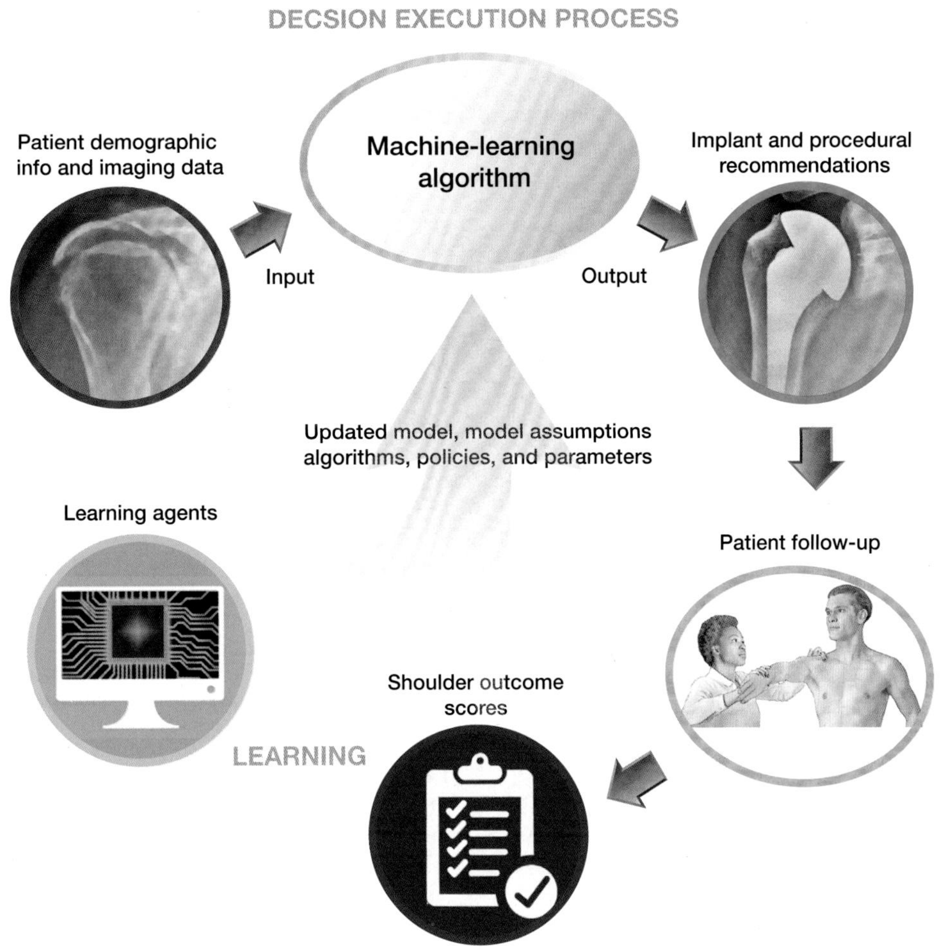

DECSION EXECUTION PROCESS

FIGURE 52.13 Machine-learning process.

pivot in approach if the procedure does not go as planned and aid in the initial registration process of an AR display to decrease operative time and increase surgical accuracy.[80] Postoperatively, the machine learning process could help create a tailored physical therapy program for a specific patient based on parameters that demonstrated success in other patients.

COST-BENEFIT ANALYSIS OF ADVANCED TECHNOLOGIES

As pressures increase to control the cost of healthcare, what is considered absolutely necessary for a surgical procedure will be scrutinized to the fullest extent. Advanced technologies may make a surgeon more accurate and informed but in most cases will also add to the cost of treatment. Manufacturers will be pressured to provide technology solutions to practitioners that add sufficient clinical value to justify the additional expense of the technology. In addition, the trend to perform TSA in an outpatient setting or ambulatory surgery center will impose space and cost restrictions more stringent than those currently in place when these procedures are performed in the inpatient setting, further pressuring

technology to be affordable, footprint conscious, and clinically beneficial. As TSA moves toward a bundled payment reimbursement structure as many hip and knee arthroplasty procedures have, capping the price on reimbursement for the implants, instruments, and added technology will present additional challenges. This will emphasize the importance of clinical data collection to be able to justify the capital expense of these technologies. For example, a large robotic platform requiring a significant up-front capital purchase may have less of a value proposition in TSA than a streamlined, low-profile system provided at no capital cost, especially in lower-volume settings.[112]

CONCLUSION

Throughout the continuum of care, the impact of advanced technology in the next 10 years on ATSA and RTSA will change not only how the procedures are performed but also the thought process in how the patient is treated. The treatment regimen will continue to evolve toward a more holistic, customized approach, harnessing the power of data and clinical outcomes to improve patient satisfaction. Advanced technologies will help surgeons treat patients better, faster, and more accurately and will engage both the surgeon and the patient on a more personal level. Efforts will be made to provide advanced technologies in a cost-efficient matter, with data-driven value propositions based on clinical outcomes.

REFERENCES

1. Berhouet J, Gulotta LV, Dines DM, et al. Preoperative planning for accurate glenoid component positioning in reverse shoulder arthroplasty. *Orthop Traumatol Surg Res.* 2017;103:407-413. doi:10.1016/j.otsr.2016.12.019

2. Iannotti J, Baker J, Rodriguez E, et al. Three-dimensional preoperative planning software and a novel information transfer technology improve glenoid component positioning. *J Bone Joint Surg Am.* 2014;96:e71. doi:10.2106/JBJS.L.01346

3. Iannotti JP, Walker K, Rodriguez E, et al. Three-dimensional preoperative planning and patients specific instrumentation improve glenoid component positioning. *J Shoulder Elbow Surg.* 2017;26:e321-e323. doi:10.1016/j.jse.2017.06.011

4. Iannotti JP, Walker K, Rodriguez E, et al. Accuracy of 3-dimensional planning, implant templating, and patient-specific instrumentation in anatomic total shoulder arthroplasty. *J Bone Joint Surg.* 2019;101:446-457. doi:10.2106/JBJS.17.01614

5. Iannotti JP, Weiner S, Rodriguez E, et al. Three-dimensional imaging and templating improve glenoid implant positioning. *J Bone Joint Surg Am.* 2015;97:651-658. doi:10.2106/JBJS.N.00493

6. Nicolaou S, Liang T, Murphy DT, et al. Dual-energy CT: a promising new technique for assessment of the musculoskeletal system. *Am J Roentgenol.* 2012;199:S78-S86. doi:10.2214/AJR.12.9117

7. Mallinson PI, Coupal TM, McLaughlin PD, et al. Dual-energy CT for the musculoskeletal system. *Radiology.* 2016;281:690-707. doi:10.1148/radiol.2016151109

8. Bishop JY, Jones GL, Rerko MA, et al. 3-D CT is the most reliable imaging modality when quantifying glenoid bone loss. *Clin Orthop Relat Res.* 2013;471:1251-1256. doi:10.1007/s11999-012-2607-x

9. Hacihaliloglu I. Ultrasound imaging and segmentation of bone surfaces: a review. *Technology (Singap World Sci).* 2017;05:74-80. doi:10.1142/S2339547817300049

10. Zhang Y, Yu H. Convolutional neural network based metal artifact reduction in X-ray computed tomography. *IEEE Trans Med Imag.* 2018;37:1370-1381. doi:10.1109/TMI.2018.2823083

11. Higaki T, Nakamura Y, Tatsugami F, et al. Improvement of image quality at CT and MRI using deep learning. *Jpn J Radiol.* 2019;37:73-80. doi:10.1007/s11604-018-0796-2

12. Flurin PH, Roche CP, Wright TW, et al. Correlation between clinical outcomes and anatomic reconstruction with anatomic total shoulder arthroplasty. *Bull Hosp Jt Dis (2013).* 2015;73(suppl 1):S92-S98.

13. Neer II CS, Watson KC, Stanton FJ. Recent experience in total shoulder replacement. *J Bone Joint Surg Am.* 1982;64:319-337.

14. Roche CP, Flurin PH. Biomechanical impact of posterior glenoid wear on anatomic total shoulder arthroplasty. *Bull Hosp Jt Dis (2013).* 2013;71(suppl 2):S5-S11.

15. Krishnan SG, Bennion PW, Reineck JR, et al. Hemiarthroplasty for proximal humeral fracture: restoration of the Gothic arch. *Orthop Clin North Am.* 2008;39:441-450. doi:10.1016/j.ocl.2008.05.004

16. Ganapathi A, McCarron JA, Chen X, et al. Predicting normal glenoid version from the pathologic scapula: a comparison of 4 methods in 2- and 3-dimensional models. *J Shoulder Elbow Surg.* 2011;20:234-244. doi:10.1016/j.jse.2010.05.024

17. Scalise JJ, Codsi MJ, Bryan J, et al. The three-dimensional glenoid vault model can estimate normal glenoid version in osteoarthritis. *J Shoulder Elbow Surg.* 2008;17:487-491. doi:10.1016/j.jse.2007.09.006

18. Parsons M, Greene A, Polakovic S, et al. Intersurgeon and intrasurgeon variability in preoperative planning of anatomic total shoulder arthroplasty: a quantitative comparison of 49 cases planned by 9 surgeons. *J Shoulder Elbow Surg.* 2020;29(12):2610-2618.

19. Parsons M, Greene A, Polakovic S, et al. Assessment of surgeon variability in preoperative planning of reverse total shoulder arthroplasty A quantitative comparison of 49 cases planned by 9 surgeons. *J Shoulder Elbow Surg.* 2020;29(10):2080-2088.

20. Walker DR, Struk AM, Matsuki K, et al. How do deltoid muscle moment arms change after reverse total shoulder arthroplasty? *J Shoulder Elbow Surg.* 2016;25:581-588. doi:10.1016/j.jse.2015.09.015

21. Glenday J, Kontaxis A, Roche S, et al. Effect of humeral tray placement on impingement-free range of motion and muscle moment arms in reverse shoulder arthroplasty. *Clin Biomech.* 2019;62:136-143. doi:10.1016/j.clinbiomech.2019.02.002

22. Roche CP, Diep P, Hamilton M, et al. Impact of inferior glenoid tilt, humeral retroversion, bone grafting, and design parameters on muscle length and deltoid wrapping in reverse shoulder arthroplasty. *Bull Hosp Jt Dis (2013).* 2013;71:284-293.

23. Routman HD, Flurin P-H, Wright T, et al. Reverse shoulder arthroplasty prosthesis design classification system. *Bull Hosp Jt Dis (2013).* 2015;73:S5-S14.

24. Hansen ML, Routman H. The biomechanics of current reverse shoulder replacement options. *Ann Jt.* 2019;4:17. doi:10.21037/aoj.2019.01.06

25. Langohr GDG, Giles JW, Athwal GS, et al. The effect of glenosphere diameter in reverse shoulder arthroplasty on muscle force, joint load, and range of motion. *J Shoulder Elbow Surg.* 2015;24:972-979. doi:10.1016/j.jse.2014.10.018

26. Giles JW, Langohr GDG, Johnson JA, et al. Implant design variations in reverse total shoulder arthroplasty influence the required deltoid force and resultant joint load. *Clin Orthop Relat Res.* 2015;473:3615-3626. doi:10.1007/s11999-015-4526-0

27. Werthel JD, Schoch BS, van Veen SC, et al. Acromial fractures in reverse shoulder arthroplasty: a clinical and radiographic analysis. *J Shoulder Elbow Arthroplasty.* 2018;2. doi:10.1177/2471549218777628

28. King JJ, Dalton SS, Gulotta LV, et al. How common are acromial and scapular spine fractures after reverse shoulder arthroplasty? a systematic review. *Bone Joint J.* 2019;101-B:627-634. doi:10.1302/0301-620X.101B6.BJJ-2018-1187.R1

29. Hamilton MA, Diep P, Roche C, et al. Effect of reverse shoulder design philosophy on muscle moment arms. *J Orthop Res.* 2015;33(4):605-613. doi:10.1002/jor.22803

30. Roche CP, Wright W. Optimizing deltoid efficiency with reverse shoulder arthroplasty using a novel inset center of rotation glenosphere design. *Bull Hosp Jt Dis (2013).* 2015;73(suppl 1):S37-S41.

31. Roche CP, Diep P, Hamilton MA, et al. Impact of posterior wear on muscle length with reverse shoulder arthroplasty. *Bull Hosp Jt Dis (2013).* 2013;73(suppl 1):S63-S67.

32. Simovitch RW, Helmy N, Zumstein MA, et al. Impact of fatty infiltration of the teres minor muscle on the outcome of reverse total shoulder arthroplasty. *J Bone Joint Surg Am.* 2007;89:934-939. doi:10.2106/JBJS.F.01075

33. Goutallier D, Postel JM, Bernageau J, et al. Fatty muscle degeneration in cuff ruptures. Pre- and postoperative evaluation by CT scan. *Clin Orthop Relat Res.* 1994;(304):78-83.

34. Wiater BP, Koueiter DM, Maerz T, et al. Preoperative deltoid size and fatty infiltration of the deltoid and rotator cuff correlate to outcomes after reverse total shoulder arthroplasty. *Clin Orthop Relat Res.* 2015;473:663-673. doi:10.1007/s11999-014-4047-2

35. Lohre R, Warner JJP, Athwal GS, et al. The evolution of virtual reality in shoulder and elbow surgery. *JSES Int.* 2020;4:215-223. doi:10.1016/j.jseint.2020.02.005

36. Lau SC, Keith PPA. Patient-specific instrumentation for total shoulder arthroplasty: not as accurate as it would seem. *J Shoulder Elbow Surg.* 2018;27:90-95. doi:10.1016/j.jse.2017.07.004

37. Cheung EV, Sarikissian EJ, Sox-Harris A, et al. Instability after reverse total shoulder arthroplasty. *J Shoulder Elbow Surg.* 2018;27:1946-1952. doi:10.1016/j.jse.2018.04.015

38. Levy JC, Otto R, Virani N, et al. Acromial fractures after reverse shoulder arthroplasty: evaluation of clinical and radiographic risk factors. *J Shoulder Elbow Surg.* 2013;22:e38-e39. doi:10.1016/j.jse.2012.12.043

39. Henninger HB, Barg A, Anderson AE, et al. Effect of deltoid tension and humeral version in reverse total shoulder arthroplasty: a biomechanical study. *J Shoulder Elbow Surg.* 2012;21:483-490. doi:10.1016/j.jse.2011.01.040

40. Kohan EM, Chalmers PN, Salazar D, et al. Dislocation following reverse total shoulder arthroplasty. *J Shoulder Elbow Surg.* 2017;26:1238-1245. doi:10.1016/j.jse.2016.12.073

41. Verstraete MA, Conditt MA, Parsons IM, et al. Assessment of intraoperative joint loads and mobility in reverse total shoulder arthroplasty through a humeral trial sensor. *Semin Arthroplasty JSES.* 2020;30(1):2-12. doi:10.1053/j.sart.2020.03.001

42. Razfar N, Reeves JM, Langohr DG, et al. Comparison of proximal humeral bone stresses between stemless, short stem, and standard stem length: a finite element analysis. *J Shoulder Elbow Surg.* 2016;25:1076-1083. doi:10.1016/j.jse.2015.11.011

43. Denard PJ, Raiss P, Gobezie R, et al. Stress shielding of the humerus in press-fit anatomic shoulder arthroplasty: review and recommendations for evaluation. *J Shoulder Elbow Surg.* 2018;27:1139-1147. doi:10.1016/j.jse.2017.12.020

44. Langohr GDG, Reeves J, Roche CP, et al. The effect of short-stem humeral component sizing on humeral bone stress. *J Shoulder Elbow Surg.* 2020;29:761-767. doi:10.1016/j.jse.2019.08.018

45. Sadoghi P, Vavken J, Leithner A, et al. Benefit of intraoperative navigation on glenoid component positioning during total shoulder arthroplasty. *Arch Orthop Trauma Surg.* 2015;135:41-47. doi:10.1007/s00402-014-2126-1

46. Jones R, Greene A, Polakovic S, et al. Accuracy and precision of placement of the glenoid baseplate in reverse total shoulder arthroplasty using a novel computer assisted navigation system combined with pre-operative planning: a controlled cadaveric study. *Semin Arthroplasty JSES.* 2020;30(1):73-82.

47. Strauss EJ, Roche C, Flurin PH, et al. The glenoid in shoulder arthroplasty. *J Shoulder Elbow Surg.* 2009;18:819-833. doi:10.1016/j.jse.2009.05.008

48. Schoch B, Haupt E, Leonor T, et al. Computer navigation leads to more accurate glenoid targeting during total shoulder arthroplasty compared with 3-dimensional preoperative planning alone. *J Shoulder Elbow Surg.* 2020;29(11):2257-2263.

49. Allred JJ, Flores-Hernandez C, Hoenecke HR, et al. Posterior augmented glenoid implants require less bone removal and generate lower stresses: a finite element analysis. *J Shoulder Elbow Surg.* 2016;25:823-830. doi:10.1016/j.jse.2015.10.003

50. Farron A, Terrier A, Büchler P. Risks of loosening of a prosthetic glenoid implanted in retroversion. *J Shoulder Elbow Surg.* 2006;15:521-526. doi:10.1016/j.jse.2005.10.003

51. Hermida JC, Flores-Hernandez C, Hoenecke HR, et al. Augmented wedge-shaped glenoid component for the correction of glenoid retroversion: a finite element analysis. *J Shoulder Elbow Surg.* 2014;23:347-354. doi:10.1016/j.jse.2013.06.008

52. Kersten AD, Flores-Hernandez C, Hoenecke HR, et al. Posterior augmented glenoid designs preserve more bone in biconcave glenoids. *J Shoulder Elbow Surg.* 2015;24:1135-1141. doi:10.1016/j.jse.2014.12.007

53. Rahme H, Mattsson P, Wikblad L, et al. Stability of cemented in-line pegged glenoid compared with keeled glenoid components in total shoulder arthroplasty. *J Bone Joint Surg Am.* 2009;91:1965-1972. doi:10.2106/JBJS.H.00938

54. Shapiro TA, McGarry MH, Gupta R, et al. Biomechanical effects of glenoid retroversion in total shoulder arthroplasty. *J Shoulder Elbow Surg.* 2007;16:S90-S95. doi:10.1016/j.jse.2006.07.010

55. Friedman RJ, Stroud N, Glattke K, et al. The impact of posterior wear on reverse shoulder glenoid fixation. *Bull Hosp Jt Dis (2013).* 2015;73(suppl 1):S15-S20.

56. Mollon B, Mahure SA, Roche CP, et al. Impact of scapular notching on clinical outcomes after reverse total shoulder arthroplasty: an analysis of 476 shoulders. *J Shoulder Elbow Surg.* 2017;26:1253-1261. doi:10.1016/j.jse.2016.11.043

57. Nyffeler RW, Werner CML, Gerber C. Biomechanical relevance of glenoid component positioning in the reverse Delta III total shoulder prosthesis. *J Shoulder Elbow Surg.* 2005;14:524-528. doi:10.1016/j.jse.2004.09.010

58. Roche CP, Flurin PH, Wright TW, et al. An evaluation of the relationships between reverse shoulder design parameters and range of motion, impingement, and stability. *J Shoulder Elbow Surg.* 2009;18:734-741. doi:10.1016/j.jse.2008.12.008

59. Roche CP, Marczuk Y, Wright TW, et al. Scapular notching and osteophyte formation after reverse shoulder replacement: radiological analysis of implant position in male and female patients. *Bone Joint J.* 2013;95-B:530-535. doi:10.1302/0301-620X.95B4.30442

60. Simovitch RW, Zumstein MA, Lohri E, et al. Predictors of scapular notching in patients managed with the Delta III reverse total shoulder replacement. *J Bone Joint Surg Am.* 2007;89:588-600. doi:10.2106/JBJS.F.00226

61. Edwards TB, Gartsman GM, O'Connor DP, et al. Safety and utility of computer-aided shoulder arthroplasty. *J Shoulder Elbow Surg.* 2008;17:503-508. doi:10.1016/j.jse.2007.10.005

62. Kennon JC, Lu C, McGee-Lawrence ME, et al. Scapula fracture incidence in reverse total shoulder arthroplasty using screws above or below metaglene central cage: clinical and biomechanical outcomes. *J Shoulder Elbow Surg.* 2017;26:1023-1030. doi:10.1016/j.jse.2016.10.018

63. Crosby LA, Hamilton A, Twiss T. Scapula fractures after reverse total shoulder arthroplasty: classification and treatment. *Clin Orthop Relat Res.* 2011;469:2544. doi:10.1007/s11999-011-1881-3

64. Casagrande DJ, Parks DL, Torngren T, et al. Radiographic evaluation of short-stem press-fit total shoulder arthroplasty: short-term follow-up. *J Shoulder Elbow Surg.* 2016;25:1163-1169. doi:10.1016/j.jse.2015.11.067

65. Denard PJ, Noyes MP, Walker JB, et al. Radiographic changes differ between two different short press-fit humeral stem designs in total shoulder arthroplasty. *J Shoulder Elbow Surg.* 2018;27:217-223. doi:10.1016/j.jse.2017.08.010

66. Schnetzke M, Coda S, Raiss P, et al. Radiologic bone adaptations on a cementless short-stem shoulder prosthesis. *J Shoulder Elbow Surg.* 2016;25:650-657. doi:10.1016/j.jse.2015.08.044

67. Raiss P, Schnetzke M, Wittmann T, et al. Postoperative radiographic findings of an uncemented convertible short stem for anatomic and reverse shoulder arthroplasty. *J Shoulder Elbow Surg.* 2019;28:715-723. doi:10.1016/j.jse.2018.08.037

68. Brolin TJ, Cox RM, Abboud JA, et al. Stemless shoulder arthroplasty: review of early clinical and radiographic results. *JBJS Rev.* 2017;5:e3. doi:10.2106/JBJS.RVW.16.00096

69. Kadum B, Hassany H, Wadsten M, et al. Geometrical analysis of stemless shoulder arthroplasty: a radiological study of seventy TESS total shoulder prostheses. *Int Orthop.* 2016;40:751-758. doi:10.1007/s00264-015-2935-z

70. Nguyen D, Ferreira LM, Brownhill JR, et al. Improved accuracy of computer assisted glenoid implantation in total shoulder arthroplasty: an in-vitro randomized controlled trial. *J Shoulder Elbow Surg.* 2009;18:907-914. doi:10.1016/j.jse.2009.02.022

71. Zhang C, Kuhn MJ, Merkl BC, et al. Real-time noncoherent UWB positioning radar with millimeter range accuracy: theory and experiment. *IEEE Trans Microw Theor Tech.* 2010;58:9-20. doi:10.1109/TMTT.2009.2035945

72. Mahfouz MR, Kuhn MJ, To G, et al. Integration of UWB and wireless pressure mapping in surgical navigation. *IEEE Trans Microw Theor Tech.* 2009;57:2550-2564. doi:10.1109/TMTT.2009.2029721

73. Ren H, Kazanzides P. Investigation of attitude tracking using an integrated inertial and magnetic navigation system for hand-held surgical instruments. *IEEE ASME Trans Mechatron.* 2012;17:210-217. doi:10.1109/TMECH.2010.2095504

74. Pflugi S, Liu L, Ecker TM, et al. A cost-effective surgical navigation solution for periacetabular osteotomy (PAO) surgery. *Int J Comput Assist Radiol Surg.* 2016;11:271-280. doi:10.1007/s11548-015-1267-1

75. Oertel MF, Hobart J, Stein M, et al. Clinical and methodological precision of spinal navigation assisted by 3D intraoperative O-arm radiographic imaging: technical note. *J Neurosurg Spine.* 2011;14:532-536. doi:10.3171/2010.10.SPINE091032

76. Wang L, Sun Z, Zhang X, et al. A HoloLens based augmented reality navigation system for minimally invasive total knee arthroplasty. In: Yu H, Liu J, Liu L, et al, eds. *Intelligent Robotics and Applications.* Springer International Publishing; 2019. p. 519-530. (Lecture Notes in Computer Science). doi:10.1007/978-3-030-27529-7_44

77. Ogawa H, Hasegawa S, Tsukada S, et al. A pilot study of augmented reality technology applied to the acetabular cup placement during total hip arthroplasty. *J Arthroplasty.* 2018;33:1833-1837. doi:10.1016/j.arth.2018.01.067

78. Logishetty K, Western L, Morgan R, et al. Can an augmented reality headset improve accuracy of acetabular cup orientation in simulated THA? A randomized trial. *Clin Orthop Relat Res.* 2019;477:1190-1199. doi:10.1097/CORR.0000000000000542

79. Alexander C, Loeb AE, Fotouhi J, et al. Augmented reality for acetabular component placement in direct anterior total hip arthroplasty. *J Arthroplasty.* 2020;35(6):1636-1641.e3. doi:10.1016/j.arth.2020.01.025

80. Liu H, Auvinet E, Giles J, et al. Augmented reality based navigation for computer assisted hip resurfacing: a proof of concept study. *Ann Biomed Eng.* 2018;46:1595-1605. doi:10.1007/s10439-018-2055-1

81. Verhey JT, Haglin JM, Verhey EM, et al. Virtual, augmented, and mixed reality applications in orthopedic surgery. *Int J Med Robot.* 2020;16:e2067. doi:10.1002/rcs.2067

82. Laverdière C, Corban J, Khoury J, et al. Augmented reality in orthopaedics. *Bone Joint J.* 2019;101-B:1479-1488. doi:10.1302/0301-620X.101B12.BJJ-2019-0315.R1

83. Berhouet J, Slimane M, Facomprez M, et al. Views on a new surgical assistance method for implanting the glenoid component during total shoulder arthroplasty. Part 2. From three-dimensional reconstruction to augmented reality: feasibility study. *Orthop Traumatol Surg Res.* 2019;105:211-218. doi:10.1016/j.otsr.2018.08.021

84. Yoon JW, Chen RE, Kim EJ, et al. Augmented reality for the surgeon: systematic review. *Int J Med Robot.* 2018;14:e1914. doi:10.1002/rcs.1914

85. Kwartowitz DM, Herrell SD, Galloway RL. Toward image-guided robotic surgery: determining intrinsic accuracy of the da Vinci robot. *Int J Comput Assist Radiol Surg.* 2006;1:157-165. doi:10.1007/s11548-006-0047-3

86. Hansen DC, Kusuma SK, Palmer RM, et al. Robotic guidance does not improve component position or short-term outcome in medial unicompartmental knee arthroplasty. *J Arthroplasty.* 2014;29:1784-1789. doi:10.1016/j.arth.2014.04.012

87. Gilmour A, MacLean AD, Rowe PJ, et al. Robotic-arm–assisted vs conventional unicompartmental knee arthroplasty. The 2-year clinical outcomes of a randomized controlled trial. *J Arthroplasty.* 2018;33:S109-S115. doi:10.1016/j.arth.2018.02.050

88. Liow MHL, Xia Z, Wong MK, et al. Robot-assisted total knee arthroplasty accurately restores the joint line and mechanical axis. A prospective randomised study. *J Arthroplasty.* 2014;29:2373-2377. doi:10.1016/j.arth.2013.12.010

89. Blyth MJG, Anthony I, Rowe P, et al. Robotic arm-assisted versus conventional unicompartmental knee arthroplasty: exploratory secondary analysis of a randomised controlled trial. *Bone Joint Res.* 2017;6:631-639. doi:10.1302/2046-3758.611.BJR-2017-0060.R1

90. Pearle AD, van der List JP, Lee L, et al. Survivorship and patient satisfaction of robotic-assisted medial unicompartmental knee arthroplasty at a minimum two-year follow-up. *Knee.* 2017;24:419-428. doi:10.1016/j.knee.2016.12.001

91. Kim HJ, Jung WI, Chang BS, et al. A prospective, randomized, controlled trial of robot-assisted vs freehand pedicle screw fixation in spine surgery. *Int J Med Robot.* 2017;13:e1779. doi:10.1002/rcs.1779

92. Chen AF, Kazarian GS, Jessop GW, et al. Robotic technology in orthopaedic surgery. *J Bone Joint Surg Am.* 2018;100:1984-1992. doi:10.2106/JBJS.17.01397

93. Ding DY, Mahure SA, Akuoko JA, et al. Total shoulder arthroplasty using a subscapularis-sparing approach: a radiographic analysis. *J Shoulder Elbow Surg.* 2015;24:831-837. doi:10.1016/j.jse.2015.03.009

94. Lädermann A, Denard PJ, Tirefort J, et al. Subscapularis- and deltoid-sparing vs traditional deltopectoral approach in reverse shoulder arthroplasty: a prospective case-control study. *J Orthop Surg Res.* 2017;12:112. doi:10.1186/s13018-017-0617-9

95. Simovitch R, Fullick R, Zuckerman JD. Use of the subscapularis preserving technique in anatomic total shoulder arthroplasty. *Bull Hosp Jt Dis (2013).* 2013;71(suppl 2):94-100.

96. Károly K, Ellenbogen KA. Device sensing: sensors and algorithms for pacemakers and implantable cardioverter defibrillators. *Circulation.* 2010;122:1328-1340. doi:10.1161/CIRCULATIONAHA.109.919704

97. Morrell MJ; RNS System in Epilepsy Study Group. Responsive cortical stimulation for the treatment of medically intractable partial epilepsy. *Neurology.* 2011;77:1295-1304. doi:10.1212/WNL.0b013e3182302056

98. Bergmann G, Graichen F, Bender A, et al. In vivo glenohumeral contact forces – measurements in the first patient 7 months postoperatively. *J Biomech.* 2007;40:2139-2149. doi:10.1016/j.jbiomech.2006.10.037

99. Westerhoff P, Graichen F, Bender A, et al. In vivo measurement of shoulder joint loads during activities of daily living. *J Biomech.* 2009;42:1840-1849. doi:10.1016/j.jbiomech.2009.05.035

100. Bini SA, Shah RF, Bendich I, et al. Machine learning algorithms can use wearable sensor data to accurately predict six-week patient-reported outcome scores following joint replacement in a prospective trial. *J Arthroplasty.* 2019;34:2242-2247. doi:10.1016/j.arth.2019.07.024

101. Shah RF, Zaid MB, Bendich I, et al. Optimal sampling frequency for wearable sensor data in arthroplasty outcomes research. A prospective observational cohort trial. *J Arthroplasty.* 2019;34:2248-2252. doi:10.1016/j.arth.2019.08.001

102. Ramkumar PN, Haeberle HS, Ramanathan D, et al. Remote patient monitoring using mobile health for total knee arthroplasty: validation of a wearable and machine learning–based surveillance platform. *J Arthroplasty.* 2019;34:2253-2259. doi:10.1016/j.arth.2019.05.021

103. Jahic D, Omerovic D, Tanovic AT, et al. The effect of prehabilitation on postoperative outcome in patients following primary total knee arthroplasty. *Med Arch.* 2018;72:439-443. doi:10.5455/medarh.2018.72.439-443

104. Clode NJ, Perry MA, Wulff L. Does physiotherapy prehabilitation improve pre-surgical outcomes and influence patient expectations prior to knee and hip joint arthroplasty? *Int J Orthop Trauma Nurs.* 2018;30:14-19. doi:10.1016/j.ijotn.2018.05.004

105. Fontana MA, Lyman S, Sarker GK, et al. Can machine learning algorithms predict which patients will achieve minimally clinically important differences from total joint arthroplasty? *Clin Orthop Relat Res.* 2019;477:1267-1279. doi:10.1097/CORR.0000000000000687

106. Kumar V, Roche C, Overman S, et al. What is the accuracy of three different machine learning techniques to predict clinical outcomes after shoulder arthroplasty? *Clin Orthop Relat Res.* 2020;478(10):2351-2363. doi:10.1097/CORR.0000000000001263

107. Kumar V, Roche C, Overman S, et al. Using machine learning to predict clinical outcomes after shoulder arthroplasty with a minimal feature set. *J Shoulder Elbow Surg.* 2020;S1058274620306467. doi:10.1016/j.jse.2020.07.042

108. Kumar V, Roche C, Overman S, et al. Use of machine learning to assess the predictive value of 3 commonly used clinical measures to quantify outcomes after total shoulder arthroplasty. *Semin Arthroplasty JSES.* 2021;S1045452721000067. doi:10.1053/j.sart.2020.12.003.

109. Roche C, Kumar V, Overman S, et al. Validation of a machine learning derived clinical metric to quantify outcomes after TSA. *J Shoulder Elbow Surg.* 2021;S1058274621001014. doi:10.1016/j.jse.2021.01.021.

110. Simovitch R, Flurin PH, Wright T, et al. Quantifying success after total shoulder arthroplasty: the substantial clinical benefit. *J Shoulder Elbow Surg.* 2018;27:903-911. doi:10.1016/j.jse.2017.12.014

111. Simovitch R, Flurin PH, Wright T, et al. Quantifying success after total shoulder arthroplasty: the minimal clinically important difference. *J Shoulder Elbow Surg.* 2018;27:298-305. doi:10.1016/j.jse.2017.09.013

112. Moschetti WE, Konopka JF, Rubash HE, et al. Can robot-assisted unicompartmental knee arthroplasty Be cost-effective? A markov decision analysis. *J Arthroplasty.* 2016;31:759-765. doi:10.1016/j.arth.2015.10.018

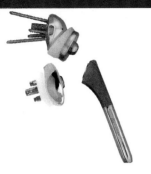

53 Shoulder Arthroplasty and the Economics of Healthcare

Jeffrey S. Chen, MD and Joseph A. Bosco III, MD, FAAOS

INTRODUCTION

Healthcare Economics

Healthcare economics is the branch of economics focused on the efficient allocation of available resources to maximize health benefits to a society. Broadly speaking, the field encompasses the performance of healthcare systems in their entirety as determined by the efficiency, efficacy, value, and behavior in the production and consumption of healthcare within that system. The core definitions of markets, including the economic models of supply and demand, apply but are complicated by several additional factors that make healthcare unique.[1] First, the healthcare sector is confounded by the presence of third parties such as insurers, governments, and medical technology companies, each with their own, often competing, interests. Second, there exists an asymmetry of information such that consumers (patients) usually do not know what they need and cannot evaluate the value of the treatment they receive. Finally, providers are not paid directly by consumers but rather by third parties. As such, market rules are established by third parties rather than market prices. For these reasons among others, resources are frequently misallocated resulting in the scenario in which all parties act in their own self-interest to the detriment of the whole, while healthcare markets become increasingly inefficient.

United States Federal Healthcare Spending

Healthcare spending within the United States continues to rise without any sign of cessation. According to the most recent data from the Organisation for Economic Co-operation and Development (OECD), the United States spent 17.1% of gross domestic product (GDP) on healthcare in 2017 compared with 4.2% to 12.3% of GDP for all remaining member countries.[2] The reasons for the continued increase in spending are many. Rather than being cost saving, recent advances in medical technology, including new devices and implants, have increased spending. With increasing life expectancy, the percentage of older patients within the population continues to increase and place higher demand on the healthcare system. Nine percent of the US population was

greater than 65 years old in 1960 versus 15% in 2015 and that number continues to increase.[1] Additionally, healthcare and life itself are inelastic goods, such that demand is relatively static even when prices change. As society becomes richer, the marginal value of years of life declines slower than other goods, thus people spend a higher fraction of income on healthcare. Finally, recent analysis has determined that the rise in healthcare expenditures is mostly due to increased expense of procedures rather than increased utilization of services.[3]

Value in Healthcare

In an effort to decrease the cost of US healthcare, there has been a recent shift from a volume-based fee-for-service (FFS) system to a system focused on value-based care. In a traditional FFS system, healthcare providers charge for each service or procedure delivered and patients and/or payors pay for each healthcare service upon receipt. This leads to conflicting interests for all involved parties and increasing amounts of system inefficiency. In a value-based system, the focus is on patient-centered outcomes, which is measured by quality rather than volume of services rendered.

$$Value = \frac{Outcomes}{Cost}$$

Economist Michael Porter defined value in healthcare as health outcomes achieved per dollar spent.[4] Value is centered on the patient, which should then determine the rewards for all other parties (payors, providers, suppliers). Outcomes are multidimensional and vary based on the condition treated. Costs encompass total costs for the full cycle of care for treatment of the condition, not just the cost of individual services. For example, in evaluation of shoulder arthroplasty for treatment of glenohumeral osteoarthritis, possible outcome measures include but are not limited to 30- and 90-day readmissions, 30- and 90-day surgical site infections, length of stay, and patient-reported outcomes such as pain and functional scores. Costs include not only the prosthesis and operating room (OR) time but also the hospitalization, postoperative care including nursing facilities, rehabilitation, and management of any postoperative complications. In this model, benefits of any individual service ultimately depend on the effectiveness of all other interventions throughout the care cycle.

In the past, value in healthcare has been challenging to both measure and deliver. Commonly utilized metrics did not adequately portray value. For example, measures for a single department are too narrow to be pertinent to the individual patient, whereas measures for an entire hospital are too broad. Shifting focus from billing to patient outcomes tailored for a specific disease process and intervention simultaneously improves healthcare efficiency and coordination of care among providers. Thus, the ability to measure, report, and compare outcomes is the most important step to improve value.[5]

Decreasing Costs and Increasing Access

In other industries, decreasing cost to improve value can be achieved by decreasing outcomes within a tolerable range. This is not ethically acceptable in healthcare as there exists a standard of care that must be met. Value cannot be created by decreasing outcomes to save money. Alternative strategies to decrease healthcare costs include limiting access to care, stratifying procedures, and rationing care, although these are not ethically sound provided there is enough healthcare to distribute. Increasing access to care especially at an earlier stage can also potentially decrease costs by way of preventative care.

In an effort to control federal healthcare spending, the US Center for Medicare & Medicaid Services Innovation (CMMI) was established by the 2010 Affordable Care Act. CMMI's stated purpose was to develop and test "innovative payment and service delivery models to reduce expenditures ... while preserving and enhancing the quality of care" for recipients of Medicare, Medicaid, and Children's Health Insurance Program. Specifically, they have supervised the creation and trialing of several Alternative Payment Models (APMs), forms of healthcare payment reform that incorporate value into reimbursements. This national effort to improve value by decreasing costs,

improving outcomes, and increasing access was the catalyst that set in motion the shift toward value-based care in the United States.

ALTERNATIVE PAYMENT MODELS

Bundled Payments

Perhaps the most relevant APM for shoulder arthroplasty is the bundled payment model. A bundled payment is a combined payment for the physician, hospital, and all other healthcare provider services for a single episode of care. An episode of care is defined as all services provided to a patient in the treatment of a defined condition or as part of a procedure for an agreed-upon period. The payment is calculated based on expected costs of all items and services furnished to a beneficiary during an episode of care. The purpose of a bundled payment is to create incentive for providers to coordinate and deliver care more efficiently. In this form of agreement, the providers assume risk that their costs exceed their payment, but they also have the potential to profit when costs are below the fixed payment, thus providing incentive to increase the value of their care not only with the intervention provided but also throughout the entire episode of care. Gainsharing, or an incentivized financial agreement between a hospital or group and an individual physician, allows this reward to be realized by the individual practitioner so long as appropriate ethical safeguards exist.[6]

Joint replacement has been a special area of interest for bundled payments given the relatively homogeneous nature of the procedures, increasing volume, and the rising cost burden for Medicare and Medicaid programs. Thus, the CMMI has made continued efforts to implement bundled payments for arthroplasty **(FIGURE 53.1)**. The Bundled Payments for Care Improvement (BPCI) initiative was initiated in 2013 in an attempt to improve fragmented care for multiple medical conditions with minimal coordination across providers and healthcare settings. Specifically, it was a voluntary program in which providers could opt in to one of four payment and delivery models with target prices derived solely from

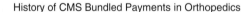

History of CMS Bundled Payments in Orthopedics

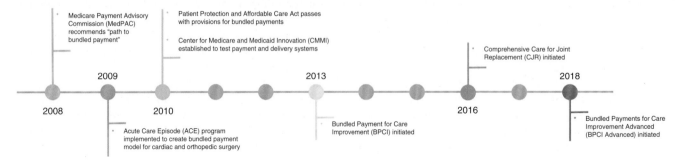

FIGURE 53.1 History of Centers for Medicare & Medicaid Services (CMS) bundled payments in orthopedics.

an individual institution's historical pricing. Based on expanding participation and initial success with BPCI, the Comprehensive Care for Joint Replacement (CJR) was initiated in 2016. In contrast to BPCI, this was a mandatory program, designed for hospitals, focused solely on joint replacement, requiring the participation of nearly 800 hospitals in 67 urban areas. Target prices were also derived from an institution's historical pricing, but were integrated with regional historical pricing with a progressive shift toward prices solely derived from regional prices. The initiative also implemented a pay-for-performance system incorporating the use of quality scores. After 2 years, the program was modified and now only mandates participation in 34 of the original 67 metropolitan statistical areas.

The aforementioned bundled care initiatives have mobilized hospitals and physicians and set changes into motion which are still evolving today.[7] Studies have demonstrated appropriate response by hospitals to these changes, including altering post–acute care (PAC) settings, decreasing hospitalization times, and decreasing utilization of skilled nursing facilities (SNFs) and inpatient rehabilitation facilities (IRFs).[8,9] They describe overall reductions in Medicare episode payments versus comparison groups in areas of both historically high and low payments, in both elective and fracture settings, all without affecting quality of care. However, closer scrutiny of participating institutions shows differences that are not initially apparent.

Analysis of both models has shown that BPCI hospitals tend to be larger and more teaching intensive (vs safety-net hospital status as seen in many CJR hospitals), with a larger annual Medicare volume and higher cost attributable to institutional PAC. Both groups had a similar risk exposure and baseline episode quality and cost.[10] These differences have implications on the generalizability of results seen between both models and begin to broach the idea that mandatory participation may have detrimental effects on access to care. A study at a high-volume, single-specialty orthopedic hospital in 2019 compared the economic implications of the institution's participation with BPCI with CJR and showed a substantially reduced margin for savings for CJR versus BPCI, with a projected annual savings decrease of 83.3%.[11] As CJR drives down price targets for all hospitals in a given area, proposed savings are threatened as methods to cut costs are rapidly exhausted. This may ultimately jeopardize access to care for patients at low-volume hospitals who may find joint replacement unaffordable to perform given the rapidly decreasing reimbursements. It remains to be seen how policymakers will interpret and utilize the results of these two initiatives in the future.

Other Models

Several other APMs have been proposed and implemented, although their effect on shoulder arthroplasty is less profound than that of bundled payments. An accountable care organization is a network of doctors, hospitals, and other healthcare providers that share responsibility for coordinating care and meeting quality and cost metrics for a defined patient population. A patient-centered medical home facilitates coordination of care through a patient's primary care physician. Private payors were slow to adopt, but now several commercial models also exist that share frameworks with the aforementioned APMs but with less rigidly defined parameters. All APMs are united by the common goal of increasing quality of patient care while decreasing per capita costs—increasing value—with reimbursements tied to quality metrics and incentives to coordinate care.

Unintended Consequences

As hospitals make changes to adapt to and survive in new systems, there may be unanticipated adverse consequences along the way. One such consequence is the stifling of new innovation. Maximizing value by focusing on outcomes such as 30- or 90-day outcomes may falsely shift treatment toward short-term solutions. For example, when comparing open reduction and internal fixation (ORIF) to reverse total shoulder arthroplasty (RTSA) for treatment of proximal humerus fractures, RTSA may be thought to provide inferior value due to increased short-term cost but may be of greater value in the long term. This is further complicated by a perverse financial incentive in which insurance companies are unlikely to be insuring the same patients for several years in the future; thus, they are willing to pay for a less expensive, more "valuable" solution in the short-term despite worse long-term outcomes. The reason being that the potential long-term savings will not be realized by the current insurance company, as the patient is unlikely to be insured by that company when the savings are manifested. The capacity to explore and research innovation in the form of new prostheses and new technologies such as robotics may be suppressed with similar reasoning.

As previously mentioned, another area of concern is an increase in healthcare disparities specifically with respect to access to care. With attention fixated on outcome and quality measures, there is a decreased incentive to operate on patients with unfavorable social determinants of health, such as those with complicated medical comorbidities or lower socioeconomic status. When attempting to maximize quality metrics, improve outcomes, and limit complications, patient selection and risk stratification unfortunately become a large focus. This brings an ethical dilemma into the conversation as care may be delayed for those who need it the most.[12]

These implications on access to care certainly extend to the growing field of shoulder arthroplasty. Waldrop et al showed that Medicaid and Medicare patients younger than 65 years who underwent primary total shoulder arthroplasty (TSA) demonstrated poorer preoperative function and postoperative patient-reported outcomes than similar patients with private insurance despite similar functional improvements from baseline.[13] In models incorporating quality measures such as CJR, these findings may influence surgeon and hospital decisions to proceed with surgery. Sheth et al demonstrated that more disadvantaged patients (lower socioeconomic status determined by Area Deprivation Index) had a higher body mass index, higher preoperative opioid use, higher rates of diabetes, more preoperative pain, and lower preoperative functional scores when undergoing TSA for glenohumeral osteoarthritis.[14] Certainly, providers and payors both need to be cognizant of the potential impact of socioeconomic factors and preexisting conditions when determining fair bundle payments and reimbursements going forward.

Centers of Excellence and High-Volume Providers

A center of excellence (COE) is a program within a healthcare institution that is assembled to supply an exceptionally high concentration of expertise and related resources centered on a specific area of medicine, delivering associated care in a comprehensive, interdisciplinary fashion to afford the best patient outcome possible.[15] As an increasing proportion of care becomes reimbursed by APMs, there is an incentive for healthcare systems to integrate both horizontally (providers of the same service) and vertically (providers of different points of a supply chain) in an attempt to maximize efficiency and value, forming highly specialized COEs. Formation of these centers requires coordination and a tremendous amount of resources, but ideally, they maximize value by increasing quality of care while minimizing costs with mutual benefits for both providers and patients. In a study of hospital volume and outcomes specifically for RTSA, an inverse relationship was demonstrated between hospital volume and all-cause 90-day readmission rates, cost, and overall resource utilization.[16]

A similar discussion can be had regarding high-volume providers. Extensive research has shown a volume-value relationship in hip and knee arthroplasty with improved outcomes associated with increased surgeon volume.[17] Similar studies have also been conducted for shoulder arthroplasty, although the interpretation of their results has been conflicting.[18-20] Meta-analyses of these studies have shown that low volume (definition ranging from less than one to five procedures per year) was associated with increased length of stay, OR time, in-hospital complications, and cost, although not all of these differences were statistically significant.[21,22] In addition, there are very little data on readmission rates, and perhaps most important, no patient-reported or functional outcomes were collected. Thus, although not conclusive, the literature appears to point toward increased value with increased surgeon volume in shoulder arthroplasty. The

formation of COEs and concentration of high-volume providers, however, are not free from unintended consequences. As they form, a high level of care becomes concentrated at one geographic focus. This may decrease access to care for those with already limited access by increasing travel distance, transportation costs, time off from work, etc. Patients may be diverted from hospitals that traditionally serve patients of a lower socioeconomic background. If combined with mandatory participation in bundled payment models based on regional pricing such as CJR, these safety-net hospitals may be priced out from certain procedures and low-volume surgeons may be excluded from performing procedures altogether, even further decreasing access to care.

EFFECTS ON SHOULDER ARTHROPLASTY

Current Trends

The number of TSAs performed in the United States continues to increase.[23-25] FDA approval of RTSA in 2004 along with expanding indications for both TSA and RTSA and continued development of dedicated shoulder and elbow fellowship training all play a role in the continued growth of TSA.[26,27] Zmistowski et al used Medicare databases and hospital referral regions (HRRs) to study trends and variability in TSA use from 2012 to 2014. They showed that although overall access to TSA is expanding, including access to surgeons with high-volume TSA caseload (defined as more than 20 Medicare TSA cases per year), there continues to be notable geographic variations with socioeconomic underpinnings. Specifically, HRRs with a lower proportion of white patients and a higher percentage of poor patients (defined by eligibility for Medicaid) reported decreased use of TSA despite the presence of a sufficient Medicare population to support an arthroplasty surgeon. In addition, they found that more than 44% of Medicare patients at their institution traveled outside of their local HRR for their procedure.[28] These findings echo the previously stated concern of limiting access to care with the concentration of high-volume providers in COEs. As the field of TSA continues to grow, the changing face of the healthcare system will undoubtedly have implications.

Currently, the episode of care for shoulder arthroplasty is Medicare Severity-Diagnosis Related Groups (DRG) code 483 (major joint replacement or reattachment of upper extremity with or without major complications or comorbidities). This does not account for the type of procedure (anatomic TSA vs RTSA) or the indication for procedure (glenohumeral osteoarthritis, rotator cuff arthropathy, fracture, etc.). In addition, the Current Procedural Terminology code is the same for both TSA and RTSA (23,472). This method of coding grossly generalizes all shoulder arthroplasty procedures and indications without adjusting for increased risks that may accompany different patient populations. For example, a retrospective database study has shown that patients who underwent TSA for proximal humerus fracture were significantly more likely to have a longer hospital stay, 30-day surgical and medical complications, need for revision surgery within 30 days, postoperative transfusions, nonhome discharge, and 30-day readmissions than patients undergoing TSA for osteoarthritis.[29] Thus, there is a clear difference in resource utilization when TSA is performed for different indications. In this example, the fracture group comprises a different patient population than the arthritis group, with physiologic and functional differences as well as need for a more time-sensitive procedure with less time for optimization. This is analogous to what transpired with hip arthroplasty bundles. Initially, hip arthroplasty for arthritis was treated the same as hip arthroplasty for fractures. After several studies demonstrated that costs and outcomes for these two procedures are different, all fracture patients were assigned to a higher intensity DRG.[30-32] With the shift toward bundled payment models, similar changes will have to occur for shoulder arthroplasty to appropriately code procedures and assign their true expected value.

Despite this, initial trials of bundled payments with shoulder arthroplasty have shown early success. Odum et al compared 132 FFS patients and 333 BPCI patients who underwent TSA in their practice and found that BPCI patients had lower rates of SNF admissions, IRF admissions, home health aide (HHA) utilization, and readmissions, with a 4% decrease in expenditures overall after controlling for postacute events.[33] Walters et al compared bundled and unbundled groups receiving TSA specifically in the outpatient setting and found significant cost savings in the bundled group versus the unbundled group both in total surgical day charges as well as total 90-day global period charges. Implant pricing, negotiated as part of the bundle, was the primary driver of cost reduction.[34] Outcomes were not included as part of this particular study.

Controlling Cost in Shoulder Arthroplasty

In order to control costs, one must first understand the breakdown of the total costs associated with a full episode of care. For shoulder arthroplasty in particular, costs include operative costs (OR time, surgical supplies and equipment, implants, cement, anesthesia, perioperative staffing, radiography), hospitalization costs (hospital fees, medications, laboratory studies, supplies, radiography, inpatient therapy, nursing), and follow-up costs (posthospitalization therapy, skilled nursing requirements, follow-up visits, complications, readmissions, and reoperations). A retrospective study of 361 patients undergoing shoulder arthroplasty procedures over a 5-year period showed that of total cost, 70% was operative costs, 24% was inpatient costs, and

6% was 90-day follow-up costs.[35] Factors associated with an increased total cost include younger age and an indication for surgery of "other" (proximal humerus fractures and their sequelae, inflammatory arthropathy, osteonecrosis). Use of RTSA versus anatomic TSA was associated with increased operative cost, likely due to differences in implant pricing. Implant pricing has consistently been shown to be the primary cost contributor in arthroplasty, comprising at least 40% of overall cost across all areas of arthroplasty and as high as 60% for RTSA.[36]

Efforts to reduce costs in shoulder arthroplasty should be multifaceted and target all areas of the total cost breakdown. As implant pricing contributes such a significant cost, it is logical to address that first. Several strategies exist to decrease implant cost in arthroplasty, all of which have been implemented with success.[37] A physician awareness program simply provides surgeons with vendor pricing lists and overall hospital economic impact with the selection of a particular vendor's implant without limiting their choice of vendors.[38] A preferred vendor discount program is a legal agreement between a hospital and an implant company usually consisting of a volume guarantee for a hospital-wide preferred status to purchase implants at a discounted price.[39] Reference pricing, also known as a price cap or price ceiling, is a maximum price per implant imposed unilaterally by the hospital purchasing department, leaving the decision up to vendors whether to continue to provide implants to that hospital.[40] Implant standardization and demand matching programs stratify patients into groups based on age, health, and functional status and assign an implant based on that specific analysis.[41]

Efforts also have been made to address cost containment for other contributors of cost in shoulder arthroplasty. The transition of TSA from an inpatient to an outpatient setting is one such effort to reduce hospitalization costs. Several studies have shown that in well-indicated patients, outpatient TSA is a safe alternative to inpatient TSA without significant differences in complications or readmissions.[42-44] A database study compared 706 patients who underwent ambulatory TSA with a matched group of 4459 patients who underwent inpatient TSA between 2010 and 2014.[45] The authors found that ambulatory TSA was associated with significantly lower costs ($14,722 vs $18,336) with similar rates of complications and readmissions.

A similar study showed analogous results with respect to decreased costs of ambulatory surgery, with significant differences persisting even with elimination of inpatient-specific costs (ie, nursing, medications, accommodations).[46] This may be due to differences in productivity between inpatient and outpatient centers, including surgeon-staff familiarity with procedures being performed and efficient use of surgical equipment, disposables, and other resources. The authors also showed a significant cost savings when inpatient TSA was performed at high-volume centers versus low-volume centers ($68,508 vs $80,803), stemming mostly from nursing- and procedure-related charges. This reinforces the cost-saving nature of COEs and high-volume providers previously mentioned. Other methods of reducing operative cost in TSA stem from OR optimization and include increasing availability of sterilized trays, hiring dedicated arthroplasty OR staff, minimizing turnover times, and limiting waste of implants and disposables. Hospitalization and follow-up costs can be reduced with the development of integrated clinical pathways to standardize patient optimization, pain protocols, postoperative radiographs, laboratory testing, antibiotics, and discharge planning in an effort to limit unnecessary testing and reduce length of stay.[47-51]

Measuring and Enhancing Value in Shoulder Arthroplasty

With the shift toward APMs, value has to be continually measured to gage success. But how is value measured in shoulder arthroplasty? We understand the Porter definition of value in healthcare as outcomes achieved over cost incurred. But as outcomes and cost are not one-time measurements, but rather accumulated over the course of years, advanced methods and models must be utilized to compare value to that of existing options.

The quality-adjusted life year (QALY) is a generalized measure of the value of health outcomes. It incorporates length of life and quality of life into a single weighted measure. QALYs are usually estimated by various scales and questionnaires completed by either patients or examiners. Ideally, one QALY equates to 1 year of perfect health, whereas a QALY of zero equals death. The incremental cost-effectiveness ratio (ICER) compares two different interventions in terms of "cost of gained effectiveness." Simply put, it is a measure of how much it would cost to gain one more QALY with a given intervention, usually measured in dollars per QALY ($/QALY). Although its origin and applicability have been debated, a threshold of $50,000/QALY has frequently been used as a benchmark for cost-effectiveness analysis such that if the ICER of a given intervention exceeds this, that intervention is considered cost-effective.[52,53] This is complicated by the concept that the willingness to pay (WTP) for a QALY is likely not a constant value and may be dependent on amount, duration, or type of health gain. Recent literature has also critiqued failure to adjust for inflation and economic variation between nations and has suggested increasing this threshold from $50,000/QALY to $100,000/QALY or higher or changing to a ranged or tiered system spanning $50,000/QALY to $150,000/QALY to account for different WTP of government, society, and health systems.[54]

Value of Shoulder Arthroplasty for Arthritis

The literature is surprisingly sparse regarding cost-effectiveness of TSA for the treatment of arthritis. Mather et al used a Markov model to analyze a cohort of 64-year-old patients undergoing TSA versus hemiarthroplasty (HA) for glenohumeral osteoarthritis.[55] The authors found that while both TSA and HA are cost-effective options leading to increased quality of life with acceptable costs, TSA dominated HA (ie, TSA was simultaneously more effective and less costly) with an ICER well below the WTP cutoff of $50,000/QALY as the most cost-effective treatment from both a payor and a patient perspective. The authors acknowledge a limitation of the study in the assignment of utility values from literature lacking strong level I outcome data and even by deriving values from hip and knee arthroplasty literature. Unfortunately, this is a limitation of many Markov model studies given the variety of parameters they require as previously discussed.

Bhat et al used a Markov model to compare TSA versus HA in a cohort of young, 30- to 50-year-old patients with severe end-stage glenohumeral arthritis and found that TSA is the more cost-effective treatment with greater cost savings, less revision procedures, and a greater QALY gain than HA.[56] At this time, no studies have been performed comparing value of RTSA with TSA for glenohumeral arthritis even as indications continue to expand. Several studies have compared outcomes of RTSA versus TSA for glenohumeral arthritis with an intact cuff and found slight improvements in complication rates, reoperation rates, patient-reported outcomes, or function between the two treatments although few statistically significant.[57] One study did find additional rates of radiographic loosening in the TSA group versus the RTSA group at a mean follow-up time of 49 months, which may or may not have implications on future need for revision.[58] Thus, the determination of value between the two options boils down to whether the marginal improvement in outcomes is worth the additional cost of RTSA.

Value of Shoulder Arthroplasty for Rotator Cuff Pathology

The literature regarding cost-effectiveness of RTSA for rotator cuff pathology is much more robust, likely a result of its higher costs in the setting of expanding indications. Despite improvements in function and pain seen with RTSA for various indications, its use is associated with a higher complication rate and significantly increased cost.[59] Thus, many authors have sought to answer whether RTSA provides better value than existing options.

The first area of focus is in the treatment of rotator cuff pathology. Coe et al used a Markov model to compare RTSA and HA for treatment of rotator cuff arthropathy in an average cohort of 70-year-old patients with a WTP cutoff of $100,000/QALY and found that RTSA may be a cost-effective option.[60] Sensitivity analysis demonstrated that the model was highly sensitive to complication rate and implant price. A change in RTSA complication rate from over 9.6% to less than 8.4% swung RTSA from a dominated option to a cost-effective one. A change in HA complication rate from 4.6% to 5.3% had the same effect on RTSA outcome. Reducing RTSA implant cost from over $13,000/implant to less than $7000/implant brings the ICER below a WTP cutoff of $50,000/QALY. These sensitivities show that the model is volatile and highly influenced by the literature from which complication rates and utilities were obtained.

Renfree et al conducted a prospective study of 27 patients undergoing RTSA for rotator cuff arthropathy and found that at 2 years, RTSA resulted in a significant improvement in QALY and was cost-effective using a cutoff of $50,000/QALY and either Short Form-36 Healthy Survey ($26,920/QALY) or EuroQol ($16,747/QALY) for calculation of self-reported patient utility.[61] In contrast to Coe's study, Renfree's calculations used real costs and outcomes rather than modeled costs and averaged outcomes. However, the short follow-up period of 2 years may fail to incorporate future complications and need for revision surgery, which were included in Coe's analysis. The study was also limited by a small sample size.

Kang et al performed a Markov decision model to compare physical therapy (PT), arthroscopic débridement and biceps tenotomy (AD-BT), HA, and RTSA for treatment of massive irreparable rotator cuff tear in a cohort of 70-year-old patients with a WTP threshold of $50,000/QALY and found that RTSA is a cost-effective option with an ICER of $25,522/QALY.[62] PT initially appears to be the most cost-effective option with sensitivity analysis; however, when considered in clinical context, RTSA is the preferred and most cost-effective option. Additionally, the authors concluded that AD-BT can be considered as a cheap alternative for low-function patients seeking pain relief without functional improvements.

The aforementioned studies focus on end-stage rotator cuff pathology including arthropathy and irreparable tears, but how about large or massive tears where repair may be possible? Makhni et al conducted an expected-value decision analysis (an alternative model to the Markov model) to compare arthroscopic rotator cuff repair (ARCR) with RTSA in the treatment of 65-year-old patients with large and massive rotator cuff tears without arthropathy and found that ARCR may be more cost-effective than primary RTSA (ICER of $15,500/QALY vs $37,400/QALY).[63] When accounting for worse outcomes with salvage RTSA performed for retear progressing to rotator cuff arthropathy after ARCR, primary RTSA only becomes more cost-effective with both a high rate of retear and a high rate of progression to arthropathy after

retear (eg, 68.5% retear rate and 89% progression rate) in the ARCR group. Dornan et al came to a similar conclusion with a Markov decision model comparing ARCR and RTSA in the treatment of 60-year-old patients with massive rotator cuff tears and pseudoparalysis without osteoarthritis, concluding that ARCR with conversion to RTSA on potential failure was the most cost-effective strategy with an ICER of $3959.55/QALY.[64] Sensitivity analysis showed that RTSA becomes most cost-effective when the utility of RTSA was at least 0.04 QALYs/year greater than the utility of ARCR, which may be applicable in cases of significant fatty atrophy or shoulder instability. Thus, it appears that RTSA is likely cost-effective for rotator cuff arthropathy and irreparable massive rotator cuff tears and is likely not cost-effective for large and massive rotator cuff tears amenable to rotator cuff repair as a first line of treatment.

Value of Shoulder Arthroplasty for Fractures

Utility of arthroplasty in the treatment of proximal humerus fractures has also been studied. Traditionally, fractures not amenable to ORIF have been managed with HA, although results are variable and highly dependent on tuberosity healing.[65] RTSA provides a salvage option in these cases as results are independent of tuberosity healing. When comparing RTSA to ORIF for treatment of proximal humerus fractures, it is important to consider the complications of both procedures as well as the need for conversion to RTSA after failed ORIF or HA.

A 2019 retrospective database study compared 1624 patients who underwent primary arthroplasty (both HA and RTSA) with 98 patients who underwent secondary arthroplasty for failed ORIF for treatment of proximal humerus fractures.[66] The authors found a significantly higher all-cause 2-year reoperation rate in the salvage arthroplasty group (19.4%) versus the primary arthroplasty group (4.4%). The study is limited by the 2-year cutoff when searching for reoperation as the primary arthroplasty group may have been subject to additional reoperations in mid- to long-term follow-up. Another retrospective study in 2016 compared 26 patients who underwent primary RTSA (acute fracture, malunion, or nonunion) for proximal humerus fracture with 23 patients who underwent secondary RTSA (failed HA or failed ORIF) and found that the primary RTSA group outperformed the secondary group in four different outcome scores as well as active external rotation range of motion and strength.[67] Although they are not cost-effectiveness analyses, these studies demonstrate that when determining value of RTSA versus ORIF for proximal humerus fractures, one must consider the detrimental results both in cost and functional outcome with failure of ORIF. Survivorship of the implant and life expectancy of the patient are other considerations. However, if successful, the value of ORIF is likely higher given its lower costs compared to RTSA.

When comparing RTSA and HA for proximal humerus fractures, the improved functional outcomes of RTSA due to independence from tuberosity healing must be balanced against increased overall costs as well as the limited life expectancy of patients typically presenting with this injury. Similar to failed ORIF, failed HA and subsequent conversion to RTSA is also associated with a high complication rate and functional impairments.[68] Solomon et al compared 16 patients treated by RTSA and 8 patients treated by HA for proximal humerus fracture and showed that RTSA was significantly more expensive than HA in terms of implant cost, OR cost, and total cost of hospitalization with similar function but significantly better pain and outcome scores than HA at a mean follow-up time of 43 months.[69] However, the sample size was small and rehabilitation costs, skilled nursing needs, and need for revision surgery were not taken into account and no cost analysis was performed; thus, no conclusions can be made about the comparative value between the two options with this study.

Nwachukwu et al used a Markov model to compare RTSA and HA in the treatment of complex proximal humerus fractures in a cohort of 70-year-old patients using a WTP threshold of $100,000/QALY.[70] The authors performed a multiperspective analysis and showed that while both options improved QALY, RTSA is cost-effective from both the payor and the hospital perspective, whereas HA is only cost-effective from the hospital perspective and does not maximize QALY for the patient. Thus, HA may be pursued by hospitals seeking a less expensive alternative to provide high but perhaps not maximal QALY gains. Interestingly, when performing sensitivity analysis, the authors found that from the hospital perspective, HA was preferred after 87 years of age and nonoperative management was preferred after 93 years of age, likely due to the trade-off of life expectancy with the costs associated with RTSA.

Osterhoff et al obtained similar results using a Markov model of the Canadian system to compare RTSA and HA in treatment of complex proximal humerus fractures with a WTP threshold of Can$50,000/QALY.[71] They found that RTSA was cost-effective with an ICER of Can$13,679/QALY with 92.6% of sensitivity analysis model simulations favoring RTSA. Given that the study model was populated using Canadian system values, interpretation of the results in the context of another healthcare system is limited. A threshold of Can$50,000/QALY is even lower than the commonly used threshold of $50,000/QALY, but a system with large healthcare costs such as the United States is likely to result in larger ICERs. However, the trend toward the cost-effectiveness of RTSA can still be appreciated.

Thus, it appears that RTSA may be a cost-effective option for the treatment of proximal humerus fractures although the evidence is weaker than for rotator cuff arthropathy. To our knowledge, no cost-effectiveness analysis has compared RTSA to ORIF, and of the two analyses comparing RTSA to HA, one uses a high WTP threshold of $100,000/QALY and the other is based on the Canadian healthcare system. Regardless, it is clear that when analyzing RTSA value for proximal humerus fractures, it is important to consider the increased costs and decreased outcomes of salvage RTSA, the durability of implants, and the life expectancy and functional status of the patient. A summary of all cost-effectiveness analyses can be seen in **TABLE 53.1**.

CONCLUSION

The future of shoulder arthroplasty and healthcare in general is rapidly evolving. The number of patients insured under government-sponsored programs continues to increase and may reach 50% in the upcoming years. As the paradigm shifts toward a system centered on value-based care, the field of shoulder arthroplasty will undoubtedly feel the effects. The growth and adaptation of various APMs show that this change is already here. Future implementation of these values may exist in ways not previously encountered. For example, consider the concept of longitudinal disease management in which a fee is collected per patient per month for management of a specific condition regardless of the treatment they receive. Operative procedures would shift from an income generator to a cost center. The effects on the decision to offer and perform surgery are obvious. These types of APMs will force us to examine the value of any treatment we prescribe to our patients.

The rise of new entities may also shape the face of the health industry. There is a trend toward consolidation throughout the healthcare industry, including hospitals, physicians, insurance companies, pharmaceutical industry, and medical device companies. Major shifts such as the acquisition of Aetna by CVS in 2018 will lead to the formation of large new healthcare entities. Formation of these entities, especially by way of vertical integration, will undoubtedly affect patient steerage. Patients will be directed toward "high-value providers" by these entities that may have implications on access to care. Understanding how "value" is determined and how quality is measured will be essential for surgeons. The costs of our surgical procedures must be supported by improved patient-reported outcomes if we expect payers to continue to pay for these procedures.

Shoulder arthroplasty utilization continues to rise with an increasing focus on the value of reverse prosthesis designs and their higher costs yet expanding indications. As efforts continue to lower costs and improve outcomes, it is important to be mindful of unintended consequences such as limiting access of care to the socioeconomically disadvantaged and stifling advances in technology and innovation. Active understanding of the healthcare system and continued efforts to monitor and research value will help surgeons maintain the high standard of care that exists in orthopedics today.

TABLE 53.1 Summary of Shoulder Arthroplasty Cost-Effectiveness Analyses

Study	Comparison	Cohort	ICER Threshold	Result
Arthritis				
Mather et al,[55] 2010	TSA vs HA	OA	$50,000/QALY	TSA dominates HA in cost-effectiveness
Bhat et al,[56] 2016	TSA vs HA	OA in young patients	$50,000/QALY	TSA dominates HA in cost-effectiveness
Rotator Cuff				
Coe et al,[60] 2012	RTSA vs HA	RCA	$100,000/QALY	RTSA may be cost-effective
Renfree et al,[61] 2013	RTSA	RCA	$50,000/QALY	RTSA is cost-effective
Kang et al,[62] 2017	RTSA vs HA vs AD-BT vs PT	Massive irreparable RCT	$50,000/QALY	RTSA is cost-effective
Makhni et al,[63] 2016	RTSA vs ARCR	Large/massive RCT without RCA	$50,000/QALY	ARCR is more cost-effective than RTSA
Dornan et al,[64] 2017	RTSA vs ARCR	Massive RCT with PP without OA	$50,000/QALY	ARCR with RTSA conversion upon failure is most cost-effective
Fracture				
Nwachukwu et al,[70] 2016	RTSA vs HA	PHF	$100,000/QALY	RTSA is cost-effective for payor and hospital; HA is cost-effective for hospital only
Osterhoff et al,[71] 2017	RTSA vs HA	PHF	Can$50,000/QALY	RTSA is cost-effective

AD-BT, arthroscopic débridement and biceps tenotomy; ARCR, arthroscopic rotator cuff repair; HA, hemiarthroplasty; ICER, incremental cost-effectiveness ratio; OA, osteoarthritis; PHF, proximal humerus fracture; PP, pseudoparalysis; PT, physical therapy; QALY, quality-adjusted life year; RCT, randomized controlled trial; RTSA, reverse total shoulder arthroplasty; TSA, total shoulder arthroplasty.

REFERENCES

1. Mankiw NG. *The Economics of Healthcare.* 2017. Accessed March 30, 2020. https://scholar.harvard.edu/files/mankiw/files/economics_of_healthcare.pdf
2. Health Expenditure. *Organisation for Economic Co-operation and Development (OECD) website.* Accessed March 30, 2020. https://www.oecd.org/els/health-systems/health-expenditure.htm
3. Papanicolas I, Woskie LR, Jha AK. Health care spending in the United States and other high-income countries. *J Am Med Assoc.* 2018;319(10):1024-1039.
4. Porter ME. What is value in health care? *N Engl J Med.* 2010;363(26):2477-2481.
5. Bosco JA III, Sachdev R, Shapiro LA, Stein SM, Zuckerman JD. Measuring quality in orthopaedic surgery: the use of metrics in quality management. *Instr Course Lect.* 2014;63:473-485.
6. Mercuri JJ, Iorio R, Zuckerman JD, Bosco JA. Ethics of total joint arthroplasty gainsharing. *J Bone Joint Surg Am.* 2017;99(5):e22.
7. Bosco JA, Harty JH, Iorio R. Bundled payment arrangements: keys to success. *J Am Acad Orthop Surg.* 2018;26(23):817-822.
8. Iorio R, Bosco J, Slover J, Sayeed Y, Zuckerman JD. Single institution early experience with the bundled payments for care improvement initiative. *J Bone Joint Surg Am.* 2017;99(1):e2.
9. The Lewin Group. *CMS Comprehensive Care for Joint Replacement Model: Performance Year 1 Evaluation Report.* 2018. Accessed March 30, 2020. https://innovation.cms.gov/files/reports/cjr-firstannrpt.pdf
10. Navathe AS, Liao JM, Polsky D, et al. Comparison of hospitals participating in medicare's voluntary and mandatory orthopedic bundle programs. *Health Aff (Millwood).* 2018;37(6):854-863.
11. Padilla JA, Gabor JA, Kalkut GE, et al. Comparison of payment margins between the bundled payments for care improvement initiative

and the comprehensive care for joint replacement model shows a marked reduction for a successful program. *J Bone Joint Surg Am.* 2019;101(21):1948-1954.
12. Bronson WH, Fewer M, Godlewski K, et al. The ethics of patient risk modification prior to elective joint replacement surgery. *J Bone Joint Surg Am.* 2014;96(13):e113.
13. Waldrop LD II, King JJ III, Mayfield J, et al. The effect of lower socioeconomic status insurance on outcomes after primary shoulder arthroplasty. *J Shoulder Elbow Surg.* 2018;27(6 suppl):S35-S42.
14. Sheth MM, Morris BJ, Laughlin MS, Elkousy HA, Edwards TB. Lower socioeconomic status is associated with worse preoperative function, pain, and increased opioid use in patients with primary glenohumeral osteoarthritis. *J Am Acad Orthop Surg.* 2020;28(7):287-292.
15. Elrod JK, Fortenberry JL Jr. Centers of excellence in healthcare institutions: what they are and how to assemble them. *BMC Health Serv Res.* 2017;17(suppl 1):425.
16. Farley KX, Schwartz AM, Boden SH, Daly CA, Gottschalk MB, Wagner ER. Defining the volume-outcome relationship in reverse shoulder arthroplasty: a nationwide analysis. *J Bone Joint Surg Am.* 2020;102(5):388-396.
17. Bozic KJ, Maselli J, Pekow PS, Lindenauer PK, Vail TP, Auerbach AD. The influence of procedure volumes and standardization of care on quality and efficiency in total joint replacement surgery. *J Bone Joint Surg Am.* 2010;92(16):2643-2652.
18. Hammond JW, Queale WS, Kim TK, McFarland EG. Surgeon experience and clinical and economic outcomes for shoulder arthroplasty. *J Bone Joint Surg Am.* 2003;85(12):2318-2324.
19. Jain N, Pietrobon R, Hocker S, Guller U, Shankar A, Higgins LD. The relationship between surgeon and hospital volume and outcomes for shoulder arthroplasty. *J Bone Joint Surg Am.* 2004;86(3):496-505.

20. Ramkumar PN, Navarro SM, Haeberle HS, Ricchetti ET, Iannotti JP. Evidence-based thresholds for the volume-value relationship in shoulder arthroplasty: outcomes and economies of scale. *J Shoulder Elbow Surg.* 2017;26(8):1399-1406.

21. Kooistra BW, Flipsen M, van den Bekerom MPJ, van Raay J, Gosens T, van Deurzen DFP. Shoulder arthroplasty volume standards: the more the better? *Arch Orthop Trauma Surg.* 2019;139(1):15-23.

22. Weinheimer KT, Smuin DM, Dhawan A. Patient outcomes as a function of shoulder surgeon volume: a systematic review. *Arthroscopy.* 2017;33(7):1273-1281.

23. Day JS, Lau E, Ong KL, Williams GR, Ramsey ML, Kurtz SM. Prevalence and projections of total shoulder and elbow arthroplasty in the United States to 2015. *J Shoulder Elbow Surg.* 2010;19(8):1115-1120.

24. Padegimas EM, Maltenfort M, Lazarus MD, Ramsey ML, Williams GR, Namdari S. Future patient demand for shoulder arthroplasty by younger patients: national projections. *Clin Orthop Relat Res.* 2015;473(6):1860-1867.

25. Schairer WW, Nwachukwu BU, Lyman S, Craig EV, Gulotta LV. National utilization of reverse total shoulder arthroplasty in the United States. *J Shoulder Elbow Surg.* 2015;24(1):91-97.

26. Iannotti JP. Shoulder and elbow fellowships. *Clin Orthop Relat Res.* 2006;449:241-243.

27. Jain NB, Yamaguchi K. The contribution of reverse shoulder arthroplasty to utilization of primary shoulder arthroplasty. *J Shoulder Elbow Surg.* 2014;23(12):1905-1912.

28. Zmistowski B, Padegimas EM, Howley M, Abboud J, Williams G Jr, Namdari S. Trends and variability in the use of total shoulder arthroplasty for Medicare patients. *J Am Acad Orthop Surg.* 2018;26(4):133-141.

29. Malik AT, Bishop JY, Neviaser AS, Beals CT, Jain N, Khan SN. Shoulder arthroplasty for a fracture is not the same as shoulder arthroplasty for osteoarthritis: implications for a bundled payment model. *J Am Acad Orthop Surg.* 2019;27(24):927-932.

30. Grace TR, Patterson JT, Tangtiphaiboontana J, Krogue JD, Vail TP, Ward DT. Hip fractures and the bundle: a cost analysis of patients undergoing hip arthroplasty for femoral neck fracture vs degenerative joint disease. *J Arthroplasty.* 2018;33(6):1681-1685.

31. Schroer WC, Diesfeld PJ, LeMarr AR, Morton DJ, Reedy ME. Hip fracture does not belong in the elective arthroplasty bundle: presentation, outcomes, and service utilization differ in fracture arthroplasty care. *J Arthroplasty.* 2018;33(7 suppl):S56-S60.

32. Yoon RS, Mahure SA, Hutzler LH, Iorio R, Bosco JA. Hip arthroplasty for fracture vs elective care: one bundle does not fit all. *J Arthroplasty.* 2017;32(8):2353-2358.

33. Odum SM, Hamid N, Van Doren BA, Spector LR. Is there value in retrospective 90-day bundle payment models for shoulder arthroplasty procedures? *J Shoulder Elbow Surg.* 2018;27(5):e149-e154.

34. Walters JD, Walsh RN, Smith RA, Brolin TJ, Azar FM, Throckmorton TW. Bundled payment plans are associated with notable cost savings for ambulatory outpatient total shoulder arthroplasty. *J Am Acad Orthop Surg.* 2020;28(9):795-801.

35. Chalmers PN, Kahn T, Broschinsky K, et al. An analysis of costs associated with shoulder arthroplasty. *J Shoulder Elbow Surg.* 2019;28(7):1334-1340.

36. Carducci MP, Gasbarro G, Menendez ME, et al. Variation in the cost of care for different types of joint arthroplasty. *J Bone Joint Surg Am.* 2020;102(5):404-409.

37. Alvarado CM, Bosco J. Understanding and controlling cost in total joint arthroplasty. *Bull Hosp Jt Dis (2013).* 2015;73(2):70-77.

38. Healy WL, Iorio R. Implant selection and cost for total joint arthroplasty: conflict between surgeons and hospitals. *Clin Orthop Relat Res.* 2007;457:57-63.

39. Boylan MR, Chadda A, Slover JD, Zuckerman JD, Iorio R, Bosco JA. Preferred single-vendor program for total joint arthroplasty implants: surgeon adoption, outcomes, and cost savings. *J Bone Joint Surg Am.* 2019;101(15):1381-1387.

40. Bosco JA, Alvarado CM, Slover JD, Iorio R, Hutzler LH. Decreasing total joint implant costs and physician specific cost variation through negotiation. *J Arthroplasty.* 2014;29(4):678-680.

41. Healy WL, Iorio R, Ko J, Appleby D, Lemos DW. Impact of cost reduction programs on short-term patient outcome and hospital cost of total knee arthroplasty. *J Bone Joint Surg Am.* 2002;84(3):348-353.

42. Basques BA, Erickson BJ, Leroux T, et al. Comparative outcomes of outpatient and inpatient total shoulder arthroplasty: an analysis of the Medicare dataset. *Bone Joint J.* 2017;99-B(7):934-938.

43. Brolin TJ, Mulligan RP, Azar FM, Throckmorton TW. Neer Award 2016: outpatient total shoulder arthroplasty in an ambulatory surgery center is a safe alternative to inpatient total shoulder arthroplasty in a hospital. A matched cohort study. *J Shoulder Elbow Surg.* 2017;26(2):204-208.

44. Leroux TS, Basques BA, Frank RM, et al. Outpatient total shoulder arthroplasty: a population-based study comparing adverse event and readmission rates to inpatient total shoulder arthroplasty. *J Shoulder Elbow Surg.* 2016;25(11):1780-1786.

45. Cancienne JM, Brockmeier SF, Gulotta LV, Dines DM, Werner BC. Ambulatory total shoulder arthroplasty: a comprehensive analysis of current trends, complications, readmissions, and costs. *J Bone Joint Surg Am.* 2017;99(8):629-637.

46. Gregory JM, Wetzig AM, Wayne CD, Bailey L, Warth RJ. Quantification of patient-level costs in outpatient total shoulder arthroplasty. *J Shoulder Elbow Surg.* 2019;28(6):1066-1073.

47. Behery OA, Kouk S, Chen KK, et al. Skilled nursing facility partnerships may decrease 90-day costs in a total joint arthroplasty episode under the bundled payments for care improvement initiative. *J Arthroplasty.* 2018;33(3):639-642.

48. Bookman JS, Romanelli F, Hutzler L, Bosco JA, Lajam C. The utility and cost effectiveness of immediate postoperative laboratory studies in hip and knee arthroplasty. *Bull Hosp Jt Dis (2013).* 2019;77(2):132-135.

49. Chen KK, Harty JH, Bosco JA. It is a brave new world. Alternative payment models and value creation in total joint arthroplasty: creating value for TJR, quality and cost-effectiveness programs. *J Arthroplasty.* 2017;32(6):1717-1719.

50. Payne A, Slover J, Inneh I, Hutzler L, Iorio R, Bosco JA III. Orthopedic implant waste: analysis and quantification. *Am J Orthop (Belle Mead NJ).* 2015;44(12):554-560.

51. Boylan MR, Bosco JA III, Slover JD. Cost-effectiveness of preoperative smoking cessation interventions in total joint arthroplasty. *J Arthroplasty.* 2019;34(2):215-220.

52. Brauer CA, Rosen AB, Olchanski NV, Neumann PJ. Cost-utility analyses in orthopaedic surgery. *J Bone Joint Surg Am.* 2005;87(6):1253-1259.

53. Grosse SD. Assessing cost-effectiveness in healthcare: history of the $50,000 per QALY threshold. *Expert Rev Pharmacoecon Outcomes Res.* 2008;8(2):165-178.

54. Nwachukwu BU, Bozic KJ. Updating cost effectiveness analyses in orthopedic surgery: resilience of the $50,000 per QALY threshold. *J Arthroplasty.* 2015;30(7):1118-1120.

55. Mather RC III, Watters TS, Orlando LA, Bolognesi MP, Moorman CT III. Cost effectiveness analysis of hemiarthroplasty and total shoulder arthroplasty. *J Shoulder Elbow Surg.* 2010;19(3):325-334.

56. Bhat SB, Lazarus M, Getz C, Williams GR Jr, Namdari S. Economic decision model suggests total shoulder arthroplasty is superior to hemiarthroplasty in young patients with end-stage shoulder arthritis. *Clin Orthop Relat Res.* 2016;474(11):2482-2492.

57. Wright MA, Keener JD, Chamberlain AM. Comparison of clinical outcomes after anatomic total shoulder arthroplasty and reverse shoulder arthroplasty in patients 70 years and older with glenohumeral osteoarthritis and an intact rotator cuff. *J Am Acad Orthop Surg.* 2020;28(5):e222-e229.

58. Steen BM, Cabezas AF, Santoni BG, et al. Outcome and value of reverse shoulder arthroplasty for treatment of glenohumeral osteoarthritis: a matched cohort. *J Shoulder Elbow Surg.* 2015;24(9):1433-1441.

59. Ponce BA, Oladeji LO, Rogers ME, Menendez ME. Comparative analysis of anatomic and reverse total shoulder arthroplasty: in-hospital outcomes and costs. *J Shoulder Elbow Surg.* 2015;24(3):460-467.

60. Coe MP, Greiwe RM, Joshi R, et al. The cost-effectiveness of reverse total shoulder arthroplasty compared with hemiarthroplasty for rotator cuff tear arthropathy. *J Shoulder Elbow Surg.* 2012;21(10):1278-1288.

61. Renfree KJ, Hattrup SJ, Chang YH. Cost utility analysis of reverse total shoulder arthroplasty. *J Shoulder Elbow Surg.* 2013;22(12):1656-1661.

62. Kang JR, Sin AT, Cheung EV. Treatment of massive irreparable rotator cuff tears: a cost-effectiveness analysis. *Orthopedics.* 2017;40(1):e65-e76.

63. Makhni EC, Swart E, Steinhaus ME, et al. Cost-effectiveness of reverse total shoulder arthroplasty versus arthroscopic rotator cuff repair for symptomatic large and massive rotator cuff tears. *Arthroscopy.* 2016;32(9):1771-1780.

64. Dornan GJ, Katthagen JC, Tahal DS, et al. Cost-effectiveness of arthroscopic rotator cuff repair versus reverse total shoulder arthroplasty for the treatment of massive rotator cuff tears in patients with pseudoparalysis and nonarthritic shoulders. *Arthroscopy.* 2017;33(4):716-725.

65. Boileau P, Krishnan SG, Tinsi L, Walch G, Coste JS, Mole D. Tuberosity malposition and migration: reasons for poor outcomes after hemiarthroplasty for displaced fractures of the proximal humerus. *J Shoulder Elbow Surg.* 2002;11(5):401-412.

66. Nowak LL, Hall J, McKee MD, Schemitsch EH. A higher reoperation rate following arthroplasty for failed fixation versus primary arthroplasty for the treatment of proximal humeral fractures: a retrospective population-based study. *Bone Joint J.* 2019;101-B(10):1272-1279.

67. Dezfuli B, King JJ, Farmer KW, Struk AM, Wright TW. Outcomes of reverse total shoulder arthroplasty as primary versus revision procedure for proximal humerus fractures. *J Shoulder Elbow Surg.* 2016;25(7):1133-1137.

68. Ernstbrunner L, Rahm S, Suter A, et al. Salvage reverse total shoulder arthroplasty for failed operative treatment of proximal humeral fractures in patients younger than 60 years: long-term results. *J Shoulder Elbow Surg.* 2020;29(3):561-570.

69. Solomon JA, Joseph SM, Shishani Y, et al. Cost analysis of hemiarthroplasty versus reverse shoulder arthroplasty for fractures. *Orthopedics.* 2016;39(4):230-234.

70. Nwachukwu BU, Schairer WW, McCormick F, Dines DM, Craig EV, Gulotta LV. Arthroplasty for the surgical management of complex proximal humerus fractures in the elderly: a cost-utility analysis. *J Shoulder Elbow Surg.* 2016;25(5):704-713.

71. Osterhoff G, O'Hara NN, D'Cruz J, et al. A cost-effectiveness analysis of reverse total shoulder arthroplasty versus hemiarthroplasty for the management of complex proximal humeral fractures in the elderly. *Value Health.* 2017;20(3):404-411.

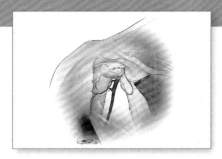

Index

Note: Page numbers followed by "*f*" indicate figures and "*t*" indicate tables.